SPORTS MEDICINE
Just the Facts

EDITORS

Francis G. O'Connor, MD, FACSM

Director, Sports Medicine Fellowship Program
Associate Professor of Family Medicine
Department of Family Medicine
Uniformed Services University of the Health Sciences
Bethesda, Maryland

Robert E. Sallis, MD, FAAFP, FACSM

Co-Director, Sports Medicine Fellowship
Kaiser Permanente Medical Center
Fontana, California

Robert P. Wilder, MD, FACSM

Associate Professor Physical Medicine and Rehabilitation
Medical Director the Runner's Clinic at UVA
Team Physician, UVA Athletics, The University of Virginia
Charlottesville, Virginia

Patrick St. Pierre, MD

Assistant Professor of Orthopedic Surgery
Uniformed Series University of the Health Sciences
Bethesda, Maryland
Associate Director Nirschl Orthopedic
Sports Medicine Fellowship
Arlington, Virginia

SPORTS MEDICINE
Just the Facts

Francis G. O'Connor

Robert E. Sallis
Robert P. Wilder
Patrick St. Pierre

McGraw-Hill
Medical Publishing Division

*New York   Chicago   San Francisco   Lisbon   London   Madrid
Mexico City   Milan   New Delhi   San Juan   Seoul
Singapore   Sydney   Toronto*

JAN 0 3 2005

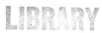
The *McGraw·Hill* Companies

SPORTS MEDICINE
Just the Facts

1 2 3 4 5 6 7 8 9 0   QPD/QPD   0 9 8 7 6 5 4

ISBN 0-07-142151-3

This book was set in Times New Roman by International Typesetting and Composition.
The editors were James Shanahan and Michelle Watt.
The production supervisor was Sherri Souffrance.
Project management was provided by International Typesetting and Composition.
The indexer was Jerry Ralya.
The text and cover designer was Joan O'Connor.
This book was printed and bound by Quebecor/Dubuque

This book is printed on acid-free paper.

NOTICE

Medicine is an ever-changing science. As new research and clinical experience broaden
our knowledge, changes in treatment and drug therapy are required. The authors and the
publisher of this work have checked with sources believed to be reliable in their efforts
to provide information that is complete and generally in accord with the standards
accepted at the time of publication. However, in view of the possibility of human error
or changes in medical sciences, neither the authors nor the publisher nor any other party
who has been involved in the preparation or publication of this work warrants that the
information contained herein is in every respect accurate or complete, and they disclaim
all responsibility for any errors or omissions or for the results obtained from use of the
information contained in this work. Readers are encouraged to confirm the information
contained herein with other sources. For example and in particular, readers are advised
to check the product information sheet included in the package of each drug they plan to
administer to be certain that the information contained in this work is accurate and that
changes have not been made in the recommended dose or in the contraindications for
administration. This recommendation is of particular importance in connection with new
or infrequently used drugs.

Library of Congress Cataloging-in-Publication Data

Sports medicine : just the facts / edited by Francis G. O'Connor … [et al.].
    p. ; cm.
  Includes bibliographical references and index.
  ISBN 0-07-142151-3
  1. Sports medicine—Handbooks, manuals, etc.   I. O'Connor, Francis G.
  [DNLM: 1. Sports Medicine—Handbooks, 2. Athletic Injuries—Handbooks.
  QT 29 S7639 2005]
  RC1211.S665 2005
  617.1'027—dc22

                                                                    2004044838

CONTENTS

v

CONTRIBUTORS

Brian E. Abell, Orthopedic Resident, Dwight D. Eisenhower Army Medical Center, Augusta, Georgia

Jeffrey S. Abrams, MD, Director, Princeton Orthopedic and Rehabilitative Associates, Attending Orthopedic Surgeon, University Medical Center at Princeton, Princeton, New Jersey

W. Bruce Adams, MD, Senior Medical Officer, Director of Sports Medicine, Officer Candidate School, Quantico, Virginia

Terry A. Adirim, MD, MPH, Associate Professor, Pediatrics and Emergency Medicine, George Washington University School of Medicine and Health Sciences Washington, DC

Venu Akuthota, MD, Associate Professor, Department of Rehabilitation Medicine, University of Colorado Health Sciences Center, Aurora, Colorado

Keith S. Albertson, MD, Chief, Orthopedic Service, Dewitt Army Community Hospital, Fort Belvior, Virginia

Alan P Alfano, MD, Associate Professor of Clinical Physical Medicine and Rehabilitation, Department of Physical Medicine and Rehabilitation, Medical Director, UVA-HEALTHSOUTH Rehabilitation Hospital, University of Virginia Health System, Charlottesville, Virginia

Robert A. Arciero, MD, Professor, Orthopedic Surgery, Orthopedic Consultant, University of Connecticut, Department of Orthopedics, University of Connecticut Health Center, Farmington, Connecticut

Edward S. Ashman, Sports Medicine Fellow, Nirschl Orthopedic Center for Sports Medicine and Joint Reconstruction, Arlington, Virginia

Chad A. Asplund, MD, Chief Resident, Family Practice Residency Program, DeWitt Army Community Hospital, Fort Belvoir, Virginia

Geoffrey S. Baer, MD, PhD, Resident in Orthopedic Surgery, University of Virginia Health System, Charlottesville, Virginia

Thad Barkdull, MD, Clinic Director, US Army Health Clinic, Dugway Proving Grounds, Utah

Carl J. Basamania, Chief, Adult Reconstructive Shoulder Surgery, Division of Orthopedic Surgery, Duke University Medical Center, Durham, North Carolina

Todd C. Battaglia, Resident in Orthopedic Surgery, University of Virginia Health System, Charlottesville, Virginia

Kenneth B. Batts, DO, Chairman, Department of Family Practice and Emergency Medical Services, Tripler Army Medical Center, Honolulu, Hawaii

Anthony J. Beutler, MD, Director, Sports Medicine, Family Practice Department, Malcolm Grow Medical Center, Assistant Professor of Family Medicine, Uniformed Services University of the Health Sciences

Andrew M. Blecher, Primary Care Sports Medicine Resident, Department of Orthopedic Surgery, Cleveland Clinic Foundation, Cleveland, Ohio

Barry P. Boden, MD, The Orthopedic Center, Rockville, Maryland, Adjunct Associate Professor, Uniformed Services University of the Health Sciences, Bethesda, Maryland

Jay E. Bowen, DO, Attending Physician, Kessler Institute for Rehabilitation, Assistant Professor, Department of Physical Medicine & Rehabilitation, UMDNJ-New Jersey Medical School, West Orange, New Jersey

Michael G. Bowers, DO, Chief Resident, Department of Family Medicine, Dewitt Army Community Hospital

Mark D. Bracker, MD, Founding Director, Primary Care Sports Medicine Fellowship, Clinical Professor, Department of Family and Preventive Medicine, University of California, San Diego, La Jolla, California

Fred H. Brennan, Jr., DO, FAOASM, Director, Primary Care Sports Medicine, Dewitt Army Community Hospital, Ft. Belvoir, Virginia, Assistant Team Physician, George Mason University, Fairfax, Virginia

Kevin J. Broderick, DO, Family Medicine Associates, Middletown, Massachusetts

David L. Brown, MD, Director, Sports Medicine, Madigan Army Medical Center, Fort Lewis, Washington

Linda L. Brown, MD, Director, Allergy and Immunology Clinic, Madigan Army Medical Center, Fort Lewis, Washington

Jennifer Burke, MD, Clinical Assistant Professor, Department of Community and Family Medicine, Team Physician, St. Louis University, Director of Sports Medicine, Forest Park Hospital, St. Louis, Missouri

Brian D. Busconi, MD, Associate Professor of Orthopedic Surgery, University of Massachusetts Medical School, Chief of Sports Medicine, UMass Memorial Medical Center, Worcester, Massachusetts

Janus D. Butcher, MD, FACSM, Assistant Professor of Family Medicine, University of Minnesota, Duluth, Team Physician, US Cross Country Skiing, Staff Physician, Duluth Clinic, Duluth, Minnesota

Robert C. Cantu, MA, MD, FACS, FACSM, Chief, Neurosurgery Service, Director, Services of Sports Medicine, Emerson Hospital, Concord, Massachusetts, Co-Director, Neurologic Sports Injury Center, Brigham and Women's Hospital Boston, Massachusetts, Medical Director National Center for Catastrophic Sports Injury Research, Adjunct Professor Department of Exercise and Sport Science, University of North Carolina at Chapel Hill, Chapel Hill, North Carolina, Neurosurgery Consultant, Boston College Football and Boston Cannons

Dennis A. Cardone, DO, Associate Professor, Director, Sports Medicine Fellowship and Sports Medicine Center, Department of Family Medicine, UMDNJ-Robert Wood Johnson Medical School, New Brunswick, New Jersey

Julie Casper, MD, Clinical Instructor and Sports Medicine Fellow, Department of Family Medicine, David Geffen School of Medicine at UCLA, Los Angeles, California

A. Bobby Chhabra, MD, Assistant Professor of Orthopedic Surgery, Division of Hand, Microvascular, and Upper Extremity Surgery, Virginia Hand Center, University of Virginia Health System, Charlottesville, Virginia

Scott Chirichetti, DO, Chief Resident, Physical Medicine & Rehabilitation, University of Virginia, Charlottesville, Virginia

Steven B. Cohen, MD, Resident Physician, Department of Orthopedic Surgery, University of Virginia Health Sciences Center, Charlottesville, Virginia

Brian J. Cole, MD, MBA, Associate Professor, Departments of Orthopedics & Anatomy and Cell Biology, Director, Rush Cartilage Restoration Center, Rush University Medical Center, Chicago, Illinois

Ugo Della Croce, PhD, Associate Professor, Physical Medicine & Rehabilitation, Systems Engineer, Motion Analysis Lab, University of Virginia, Charlottesville, Virginia

Loren A. Crown, MD, Emergency Medicine Fellowship Director, University of Tennessee College of Health Sciences, Covington, Tennessee

Diane Dahm, MD, Assistant Professor, Orthopedic Surgery, Mayo Clinic, Rochester, Minnesota

Gregory G. Dammann, MD, Director, Sports Medicine, Department of Family Medicine, Tripler Army Medical Center, Honolulu, Hawaii

Thomas M. DeBerardino, MD, Chief, Orthopedic Surgery Service, Keller Army Community Hospital; Team Physician, United States Military Academy, West Point, New York

Patricia A. Deuster, PhD, MPH, Department of Military and Emergency Medicine, Uniformed Services University of the Health Sciences, Bethesda, Maryland

William W. Dexter, MD, FACSM, Director, Sports Medicine Program, Assistant Director, Family Practice Residency Program, Maine Medical Center, Portland, Maine

Margarete DiBenedetto, MD, Professor and Former Chair (retired), Department of Physical Medicine and Rehabilitation, University of Virginia, Charlottesville, Virginia

Jay Dicharry, MPT, CSCS, Staff Physical Therapist, University of Virginia/Healthsouth, Charlottesville, Virginia

David R. Diduch, MD, Associate Professor of Orthopedic Surgery, Co-Director, Division of Sports Medicine, Director, Sports Medicine Fellowship, University of Virginia Health System, Charlottesville, Virginia

John P. DiFiori, MD, Associate Professor and Chief, Division of Sports Medicine, Department of Family Medicine, David Geffen School of Medicine at UCLA, Los Angeles, California

Nancy M. DiMarco, PhD, RD, LD, Professor, Department of Nutrition and Food Sciences, Nutrition Coordinator, The Institute for Women's Health, Coordinator, Masters Program in Exercise and Sports Nutrition, Texas Women's University, Denton, Texas

Robert J. Dimeff, MD, Assistant Clinical Professor of Family Medicine, Case Western Reserve University; Associate Professor of Family Medicine, The Ohio State University; Medical Director, Section of Sports Medicine, Vice-Chairman, Department of Family Practice, Cleveland Clinic Foundation, Cleveland, Ohio

Kevin J. Elder, MD, Bayfront Medical Center Sports Medicine Program, FP Residency, St. Petersburg, Florida

Kayvan A. Ellini, MD, Department of Internal Medicine, University of New Mexico Health Sciences Center, Albuquerque, New Mexico

Jay Erickson, MD, Assistant Professor of Family Medicine, Uniformed Services University School of Medicine, Director, Primary Care Clinics, Robert E. Bush Naval Hospital, Twentynine Palms, California

Eve V. Essery, Doctoral Candidate, Department of Nutrition and Food Sciences, Texas Women's University, Denton, Texas

Karl B. Fields, MD, Director, Family Medicine, Residency and Sports Medicine Fellowship, Moses Cone Health System, Greensboro, North Carolina

Catherine M. Fieseler, MD, Head Team Physician, Cleveland Rockers, Division of Sports Medicine, Cleveland Clinic Foundation, Cleveland, Ohio

Scott B. Flinn, MD, Consultant to the Surgeon General, Navy Sports Medicine, Naval Special Warfare Group ONE Logistics Support, Medical Department, San Diego, California

Nicole L. Frazer, PhD, Director of Clinical Psychology, Assistant Professor of Family Medicine, Uniformed Services University of the Health Sciences, Bethesda, Maryland

Michael Fredericson, MD, Associate Professor, Physical Medicine & Rehabilitation, Team Physician, Stanford University, Palo Alto, California

Michael C. Gaertner, DO, Instructor, Emergency Medicine Fellow, University of Tennessee, Tipton Family Practice, Covington, Tennessee

Robert Giering, MD, Fellow, Pain Management, Department of Anesthesiology, University of Virginia, Charlottesville, Virginia

John E. Glorioso, MD, Brigade Surgeon, SBCT Brigade, Second Infantry Division, Fort Lewis, Washington

John P. Goldblatt, MD, Assistant Professor, University of Rochester, Division of Sports Medicine, Rochester, New York

Tom Grossman, ATC, Department of Athletics, University of Virginia, Charlottesville, Virginia

Carlos A. Guanche, MD, Clinical Associate Professor, University of Minnesota, The Orthopedic Center, Eden Prairie, Minnesota

David D. Haight, MD, Department of Family Medicine, Madigan Army Medical Center, Tacoma, Washington

Kimberly Harmon, MD, FACSM, Clinical Assistant Professor, Department of Family Medicine, Clinical Assistant Professor Department of Orthopaedics and Sports Medicine, Team Physician, University of Washington, Seattle, Washington

Joseph M. Hart, MS, ATC, Athletic Trainer, University of Virginia, Sports Medicine/Athletic Training, Charlottesville, Virginia

R. Todd Hockenbury, MD, Assistant Clinical Professor of Orthopedic Surgery, University of Louisville, Blugrass Orthopedic Surgeons, PSC, Louisville, Kentucky

Halli Hose, Internist, San Diego VA Healthcare System, Assistant Clinical Professor, University of California, San Diego

Thomas M. Howard, MD, Chief, Department of Family Medicine, Associate Director, Sports Medicine Fellowship, Dewitt Army Community Hospital, Fort Belvoir, Virginia

Garrett S. Hyman, MD, MPH, Sports, Spine, and Musculoskeletal Fellow, Kessler Institute for Rehabilitation, Department of Physical Medicine & Rehabilitation, UMDNJ-New Jersey Medical School, West Orange, New Jersey

Christopher D. Ingersoll, PhD, ATC, FACSM, Director, Graduate Programs in Sports Medicine/Athletic Training, University of Virginia, Charlottesville, Virginia

Carrie A. Jaworski, MD, Family Practice and Sports Medicine, Associate Director, Resurrection Family Practice Residency, Team Physician and Medical Director, Athletic Training Program, North Park University, Chicago, Illinois

Jeffrey G. Jenkins, MD, Assistant Professor of Clinical Physical Medicine and Rehabilitation, University of Virginia School of Medicine, Charlottesville, Virginia

Michael W. Johnson, MD, Primary Care Sports Medicine and Family Practice, Private Practice, Tacoma, Washington

Wayne B. Jonas, MD, Director, Samueli Institute, Associate Professor Family Medicine, USUHS, Bethesda, Maryland

Shawn F. Kane, MD, Primary Care Sports Medicine Fellow, USUHS, Bethesda, Maryland

Amanda Weiss Kelly, MD, Assistant Professor of Pediatrics, Case Western Reserve University, Rainbow Babies and Children's Hospital

D. Casey Kerrigan, MD, Professor and Chair, Department of Physical Medicine & Rehabilitation, University of Virginia, Charlottesville, Virginia

David O. Keyser, LCDR, MSC, USN, Department of Military and Emergency Medicine, Uniformed Services University of the Health Sciences, Bethesda, Maryland

John J. Klimkiewicz, Associate Professor of Orthopedic Surgery, Director, Sports Medicine, Georgetown University, Washington, DC

Alex J. Kline, Medical Student, UVA Health System, Department of Orthopedic Surgery, Charlottesville, Virginia

Roger J. Kruse, MD, Head Team Physician, University of Toledo, Program Director, Sports Care, Sports Medicine Fellowship at the Toledo Hospital, Vice Chair, Sports Medicine and Sports Science of the U.S. Figure Skating Association, Toledo, Ohio

John P. Kugler, MD, MPH, Director of Primary Care and Community Medicine, Dewitt Army Health Care System, Fort Belvoir, Virginia

Stephen J. Lee, Fourth year medical student, Northwestern University Feinberg School of Medicine, Rush-Presbyterian-St. Luke's Medical Center, Chicago, Illinois

Jeffrey A. Levy, DO, Sports Medicine Fellow, Uniformed Services University of the Health Sciences, Bethesda, Maryland

John M. MacKnight, MD, Associate Professor, Clinical Internal Medicine and Orthopaedic Surgery, Medical Director, Sports Medicine, Primary Care Team Physician, University of Virginia, Charlottesville, Virginia

Scott A. Magnes, MD, FACSM, Staff Orthopedic Surgeon, Naval Hospital, Great Lakes, Illinois

Gerard A. Malanga, MD, Director of Sports, Spine, and Orthopedic Rehabilitation, Kessler Institute for Rehabilitation, Associate Professor, Physical Medicine & Rehabilitation, UMDNJ-New Jersey Medical School, West Orange, New Jersey

Eric M. Mangrum, PT, OCS, FAAOMPT, Staff Physical Therapist, University of Virginia/Healthsouth, Charlottesville, Virginia

Ronica A. Martinez, MD, Family and Sports Medicine, Kaiser Permanente Fontana, Fontana, California

Augustus D. Mazzocca, MD, Assistant Professor, Department of Orthopedics, University of Connecticut Health Center, John Dempsey Hospital, Farmington, Connecticut

Douglas B. McKeag, MD, MS, AUL Professor and Chair, Department of Family Medicine, Director, IU Center for Sports Medicine, Indiana University School of Medicine

John P. Metz, MD, Assistant Director, JFK Family Practice Residency, Edison, New Jersey

C. Michele Miller, DO, Chief Resident, Department of Physical Medicine & Rehabilitation, UMDNJ-New Jersey Medical School, Newark, New Jersey

Mark D. Miller, MD, Associate Professor of Orthopedic Surgery, UVA Health System, Charlottesville, Virginia

Danny Mistry, MD, Assistant Professor, Physical Medicine & Rehabilitation, Co-Medical Director, University of Virginia Athletics, Charlottesville, Virginia

Kambiz Motamedi, MD, Assistant Professor, Musculoskeletal Imaging, David Geffen School of Medicine at UCLA, Los Angeles, California

James R. Morales, MD, Silver Bay Medical Center, Toms River, New Jersey

Scott F. Nadler, DO, Professor, Physical Medicine & Rehabilitation, UMDNJ-New Jersey Medical School, Newark, New Jersey

Bradley J. Nelson, MD, Chief, Department of Surgery, Keller Army Community Hospital, West Point, New York

Robert J. Nicoletta, MD, Orthopaedic Associates of Rochester, Sports Medicine/Arthroscopy, Rochester, New York

Robert P. Nirschl, MD, MS, Associate Clinical Professor of Orthopedic Surgery, Georgetown University, Founder and Director, Nirschl Orthopedic Sports Medicine Clinic, Medical Director, Virginia Sports Medicine Institute, Arlington, Virginia

Rochelle Nolte, MD, Sports Medicine Fellow, Uniformed Services University of the Health Sciences, US Coast Guard Training Center, Health Services Division, Cape May, New Jersey

Derek H. Ochiai, Sports Medicine Fellow, Nirschl Orthopedic Center for Sports Medicine and Joint Reconstruction, Arlington, Virginia

Elizabeth M. O'Connor, DDS, Clinical Associate, Department of Dentistry, St. Joseph's Hospital Health Center, Syracuse, New York

Ralph P. Oriscello, MD, FACC, FACP, Director, Division of Cardiology, Veteran's Administration Medical Center, East Orange, New Jersey

Brett D. Owens, MD, Resident in Orthopedic Surgery, University of Massachusetts Medical School, Worcester, Massachusetts

Michael E. Pannunzio, MD, Assistant Professor, Department of Orthopedic Surgery, University of Virginia Health Sciences System, Charlottesville, Virginia

Chris G. Pappas, MD, Department of Family Medicine, Madigan Army Medical Center, Tacoma, Washington

Andrew D. Perron, MD, FACEP, FACSM, Residency Program Director, Maine Medical Center, Portland, Maine

Paul F. Pasquina, MD, Director, Physical Medicine and Rehabilitation Residency Program, Walter Reed Army Medical Center, Washington, DC

Nicholas A. Piantanida, MD, Director, Primary Care Sports Medicine, DeWitt Army Hospital, Ft. Belvoir, Virginia

Mark D. Porter, Orthopaedic Service, William Beaumont Army Medical Center, Texas Tech UHS, El Paso, Texas

Joel Press, MD, FACSM, Medical Director, Center for Spine, Sports, and Occupational Rehabilitation, Rehabilitation Institute of Chicago, Chicago, Illinois

David E. Price, MD, Sports Medicine Fellow, Bayfront Medical Center, St. Petersburg, Florida

Christopher M. Prior, DO, Director, Sports Medicine, Department of Family Medicine, Darnall Army Community Hospital, Fort Hood, Texas

Scott W. Pyne, MD, Team Physician & Director of Sports Medicine, US Naval Academy, Annapolis, Maryland

Christopher B. Ranney, MD, Department of Family Practice, Offut Air Force Base, Nebraska

Brian V. Reamy, MD, Associate Professor and Chair, Department of Family Medicine, Uniformed Services University of Health Sciences, Bethesda, Maryland

John P. Reasoner, MD, Member, USA Boxing Sports Medicine Committee, Clinic Director, Emergicare Medical Clinic, Colorado Springs, Colorado

Jennifer L. Reed, MD, Assistant Professor, PM&R, Eastern Virginia Medical School, Norfolk, Virginia

John C. Richmond, MD, Professor, Orthopedic Surgery, Tufts University School of Medicine, Chairman, Department of Orthopedic Surgery, New England Baptist Hospital

Nancy E. Rolnik, Sports Medicine Fellow, Kaiser Permanente, Fontana, California

Aaron Rubin, MD, Staff Physician and Partner, Southern California Permanente Medical Group, Program Director, Kaiser Permanente Sports Medicine Fellowship Program, Kaiser Permanente Department of Family Medicine, Fontana, California

Anthony A. Schepsis, MD, Associate Professor of Orthopedic Surgery, Director of Sports Medicine, Boston University Medical Center, Boston, Massachusetts

Leanne L. Seeger, MD, FACR, Professor and Chief, Musculoskeletal Imaging, Medical Director, Outpatient Radiology, David Geffen School of Medicine at UCLA, Los Angeles, California

Peter H. Seidenberg, MD, Director of Sports Medicine, St. Louis University Family Practice Residency Program, 375th Medical Group, Scott Air Force Base, Illinois

Kate Serenelli, MS, ATC, CSCS, Staff Athletic Trainer, Department of Athletics, University of Virginia, Charlottesville, Virginia

Craig K. Seto, MD, Assistant Professor, Family Medicine, University of Virginia Health System, Charlottesville, Virginia

Michael Shea, MD, Sports Medicine Fellowship Program, Moses Cone Health System, Greensboro, North Carolina

Jay Smith, MD, Associate Professor, Physical Medicine & Rehabilitation, Mayo College of Medicine, Rochester, Minnesota

Carolyn M. Sofka, MD, Assistant Professor of Radiology, Weill Medical College of Cornell University, Assistant Attending Radiologist, Hospital for Special Surgery, New York, New York

Rebecca Spaulding, MD, Sports Medicine Fellowship Program, Moses Cone Health System, Greensboro, North Carolina

Mark B. Stephens, MD, MS, Staff Family Physician, Medical Director, Flight Line Clinic, Naval Hospital, Sigonella, Italy, Associate Professor of Family Medicine, Uniformed Services University of the Health Sciences, Bethesda, Maryland

David Stewart, MD, Sports Medicine Fellow, Muses Cone Health System, Greensboro, North Carolina

Dean C. Taylor, MD, Director, US Army Joint and Soft Tissue Trauma Center Fellowship, Head Team Physician, United States Military Academy, West Point, New York

John Tobey, MD, Spine and Sports Fellow, Department of Rehabilitation Medicine, University of Colorado Health Science Center, Aurora, Colorado

John Turner, MD, CAQSM, Assistant Professor, Department of Family Medicine, Indiana University, Indianapolis, Indiana

Winston J. Warme, MD, Chief, Orthopedic/Rehabilitation Service, Program Director, Orthopedic Surgery Residency, William Beaumont Army Medical Center, Texas Tech UHSC, El Paso, Texas

Charles W. Webb, DO, Director of Sports Medicine, Department of Family Practice, Martin Army Community Hospital, Ft. Benning, Georgia

Brian Whirrett, MD, Sports Medicine Fellow, University of Washington, Seattle, Washington DC

Russell D. White, MD, Clinical Associate Professor, Department of Family Medicine, University of South Florida College of Medicine, Florida Institute of Family Medicine, P.C., Assistant Team Physician, Tampa Bay Devil Rays, St. Petersburg, Florida

John H. Wilckens, MD, Assistant Clinical Professor of Orthopedics, Johns Hopkins Bayview Medical Center, Baltimore, Maryland

Cynthia M. Williams, DO, MEd, Assistant Professor of Family Medicine, Uniformed Services University of the Health Sciences, Bethesda, Maryland

Pamela M. Williams, Assistant Professor of Family Medicine, Uniformed Services University of the Health Sciences, Bethesda, Maryland

Tory Woodard, MD, Chief Resident, Department of Family Medicine, Malcolm Grow Air Force Medical Center, Andrews Air Force Base, Maryland

David C. Young, MD, Sports Medicine, The Permanente Medical Group, Department of Orthopedics, South San Francisco, California

Joseph J. Zuback, Orthopaedic Service, William Beaumont Army Medical Center, Texas Tech UHS, El Paso, Texas

PREFACE

In the spring of 1993, primary care sports physicians across the country were scrambling to identify good resources to prepare for the first examination for a Certificate of Added Qualification in Sports Medicine. This examination was co-sponsored by the American Boards of Family Practice, Internal Medicine, Pediatrics, and Emergency Medicine. At review courses a common theme was that at that time, there was no identifiable source that reliably identified the discipline of sports medicine, let alone a good review book or study guide. Since that time, of course, there have been a number of excellent books published in the field of primary care sports medicine.

At the Annual Meeting of the American College of Sports Medicine in 2002, Darlene Cook of McGraw-Hill approached me about a new line of textbooks that their company was developing called *Just the Facts*. Darlene, who had mentored Robert Wilder and myself through our first book, *Running Medicine*, stated that McGraw-Hill's market research had identified a need by clinicians for sources of essential information in an outline format that provided quick reference. Darlene also felt these books would provide excellent sources of study for clinicians facing initial certification examinations or recertification exams. As I was beginning to prepare for my ten-year recertification in sports medicine since my initial examination in 1993, I thought it would be an interesting endeavor.

The first task was to assemble a team of quality editors and authors. My first call was to Dr. Robert Wilder, a physical medicine and rehabilitation physician and my colleague on a number of academic pursuits. We decided to include a second sports medicine physician, as this would be an ambitious project, as well as an orthopedic surgeon to hopefully recruit the most expertise in operative orthopedics. We were very fortunate to have Dr. Robert Sallis, an authority in primary care sports medicine and fellowship program director, accept our invitation. Dr. Patrick St. Pierre, a sports trained orthopedic surgeon and educator, graciously agreed to coordinate our orthopedic chapters. As a multidisciplinary group, our goal became to develop a text that would have value among a variety of clinicians involved with sports medicine including medical doctors, surgeons, allied healthcare professionals and athletic trainers. Our vision was a well-referenced, evidenced-based source of material that would provide a resource for both study and practice.

A quick look at the author list identifies for the reader a number of "who's who" leaders in the field of sports medicine. Interspersed among the "giants" in the field are recently graduated fellows and junior clinicians hungry to establish their own reputations in their communities. A common theme among all our selected authors was that all were striving for excellence, and all are "practicing" clinicians. A second look at the list also reveals the multidisciplinary nature of our team with family physicians, internists, cardiologists, radiologists, orthopedic surgeons, neurosurgeons, nutritionists, psychologists, physiologists, physiatrists, allergists, therapists, and athletic trainers, among others all contributing.

Despite the charge of creating a concise book that included only "just the facts," we were overwhelmed by the quality, and faced the unenviable position of editing a considerable amount of material. We tried to replace volume and detail with concisely written tables and algorithms where applicable. A review of any of the chapters will quickly bring the reader to the conclusion that this text is much more than "just the facts." We couldn't be prouder of the final product and certainly hope it meets the initial objectives we discussed for the reader. We believe it does, as this book will be an excellent reference for review and for clinical reference in patient care settings.

When we talked about dedicating the book we were all in agreement that this text should be for those members of our family who have supported us throughout the years; through the long days, the evening training rooms, the volunteer community events, and the Friday nights and Saturday afternoons at local sporting events. We especially want to thank our wives, Janet, Susan, Kathy, and Linda and all our children, Ryan, Sean, Brendan, Lauren, Stephen, Ryan, Caroline, Samantha, Matt, Shannon, Patrick, Matthew, and Danielle. We would additionally like to thank Darlene Cook for her vision and support, and Michelle Watt, our developmental editor at McGraw-Hill for keeping us on task.

SPORTS MEDICINE
Just the Facts

GENERAL CONSIDERATIONS IN SPORTS MEDICINE

1 THE TEAM PHYSICIAN

Christopher Ranney, MD
Anthony I Beutler, MD
John H Wilckens, MD

WHAT IS A TEAM PHYSICIAN?

- Very little has been published about the duties and responsibilities of a team physician and no formal studies exist as to the qualifications and skills necessary to be effective in these duties.
- The following consensus statement from the American College of Sports Medicine (ACSM) defines the unique role of a team physician:

> The Team Physician must have unrestricted medical license and be an MD or DO who is responsible for treating and coordinating the medical care of the athletic team members. The principal responsibility of the team physician is to provide for the well-being of individual athletes—enabling each to realize his or her full potential. The team physician should possess special proficiency in the care of musculoskeletal injuries and medical conditions encountered in sports. The team physician also must actively integrate medical expertise with other healthcare providers, including medical specialists, athletic trainers, and allied health professionals. The team physician must ultimately assume responsibility within the team structure for making medical decisions that affect the athlete's safe participation. (Herring et al, 2000*b*)

- Doctors from many specialties serve in the role of team physician with primary care physicians comprising the majority. The most common fields of medicine with the percentage of the total in parentheses is family practice (25.5%), orthopedic surgery (16.2%), osteopathic medicine (10.9%), internal medicine (10.1%), general practice (6.3%), pediatrics (5.4%), emergency medicine (4.9%), general urgery (4.5%), obstetrics/gynecology (2.8%), cardiology (2.0%), and all others (11.5%) (Melion, Walsh, Shelton, 1997).
- The team physician is part of a team of professionals that cares for the athletes and contributes to their success by maximizing training and competition preparation. He or she also assists by accurately diagnosing ailments and promptly, yet completely, rehabilitating injuries to get athletes back to competition as quickly and safely as possible. In addition to expertise in the common medical conditions encountered in athletes, other necessary qualities include: flexibility and availability, good communication skills, a desire to educate, and an understanding of injury prevention principles (Herring et al, 2000*b*).

TIME REQUIREMENTS OF A TEAM PHYSICIAN

- A team physician must have an office schedule that can accommodate athletes with urgent and time sensitive medical needs.
- Most team physicians have designated training room time each week, at least one to two evenings, where they can evaluate new and follow-up existing injuries of team members. This is an especially important setting in which to communicate with the trainer on the rehabilitation progress of athletes' injuries (Herring et al, 2001). An athlete's behavior and responses can vary widely depending on the familiarity of the environment; hence, training rooms should ideally be held in the athlete's "native environment," at a location convenient to athletes and close to practice or training facilities.

- Team physicians often neglect team practices. While it is not necessary that all practices be attended, occasional, brief appearances during practice will allow the physician to gain insight into the environment and conditions in which the athletes train, the team's training regimen, and interactions between coaches and players. A better appreciation of all these factors can prove invaluable in the physician's medical decision making. Additionally, brief appearances at practice help the physician build collegial relationships with coaches and players, establishing his or her role as a part of the team and distinguishing the physician from other officials, support staff, and media representatives who only participate in game-day activities.
- Amount of time spent at the actual competition depends on the team physician's role and availability, as well as state laws and regulations of the governing athletic association. Some laws mandate that a physician be in attendance for every game. Other laws allow nonphysician medical personnel, such as an athletic trainer, to cover an event with on-call physician backup (Herring et al, 2000*a*).
- A doctor who is the team physician for an entire institution must decide whether to attend all the games for a few teams, or to attend a few games for every team. We recommend that team physicians attend at least part of one practice and at least one game for each team they supervise. Providing good *team medicine* is very difficult without observing the interactions and conditions of play and practice.

CORE KNOWLEDGE OF THE TEAM PHYSICIAN

- To perform his or her duties effectively, a team physician needs an understanding of the medical conditions common to the athlete. This knowledge should encompass many areas of medicine, including but not limited to—orthopedics, cardiopulmonary medicine, neurology, dermatology, and sound principles of rehabilitation (Herring et al, 2000*b*).
- The team physician also needs expertise in pharmacology. Practical pharmacology for the team physician includes not only knowing how to treat illnesses, but also an understanding of performance enhancing drugs and herbal medicines. Team physicians must be familiar with the substances that are banned by the governing athletic association so that an athlete does not inadvertently lose eligibility to compete (Melion et al, 1997).
- A team physician must have a general knowledge of behavioral medicine and psychology. Mood disturbances and mental illnesses (like depression) affect athletes and can be very common in injured athletes.

- A team physician's knowledge of exercise science and nutrition can help prevent injuries, as well as maximize an athlete's performance. Disordered eating and overtraining can prove devastating if not recognized early and treated effectively (Herring et al, 2000*b*).

MEDICAL RESPONSIBILITIES OF THE TEAM PHYSICIAN

- The first responsibility of a team physician is to determining whether an athlete is fit to participate. This evaluation most commonly occurs during the preparticipation physical. This examination may or may not be preformed by the team physician, but the team physician should review the documentation of this examination so that he or she will know of any condition that may limit competition or predispose the athlete or other participants to injury. This preparticipation physical must be done prior to athletic training or participation—preferably 6–8 weeks beforehand so that all potentially disqualifying conditions can be fully evaluated without missing jeopardizing scheduled participation (Herring et al, 2000*a*).
- Sideline and event coverage is the most obvious responsibility of the team physician. A physician should cover all collision and high-risk sports. Other athletic events can be covered by any allied health professional who is trained in recognition and initial treatment of athletic injuries (Herring et al, 2000*a*). A team physician must continually remind himself or herself that he or she is more than a spectator. The physician should be a "dispassionate observer," meaning that the emotions of competition must not affect medical decision making. Attention should be directed to the safety of the participants, not the immediate passions of the game.
- The team physician should focus attention on aspects of play and individuals who are more prone to injury. In other words, the seasoned team physician will carefully follow the game, but not always follow the ball. For instance, in American football relatively little injury information can be gained by watching the flight of the ball on punts, kickoffs, and passes. Rather, injuries occur and attention should be focused on linemen, quarterbacks after releasing the ball, and wide-receivers after catching the ball. In every sport, special attention should be given to situations and players at high risk for injury.
- The team physician must be prepared to handle nonparticipant emergencies for it is not uncommon for the team physician to be called on to treat an ill-fallen coach, referee, or spectator.
- The team physician insures accurate diagnosis through use of additional studies and specialty consults, communicates information clearly and confidentially

regarding the player's condition to those who need to know, coordinates the rehabilitation process, and determines when the athlete is able to compete again. This essential process involves *active* communication with athletes, parents, athletic trainers, physical therapists, coaches, administrators, and other medical specialists as necessary (Rice, 2002).

- Pursuing active follow-up with medical specialists is a critical duty. Team physicians may refer athletes to subspecialty providers to assist in treatment or with clearance for athletic participation; however, information from these visits does not naturally flow back to the team physician. Assuming that the specialty provider will call with any important information, or that all pertinent information will flow back through the health care system, will result in confusion for the team physician and danger for the athletes. Shadow files, tickler lists, and other reminder systems can help team doctors actively and personally follow up on referrals, thus preventing the always embarrassing and often dangerous situations that result from incomplete medical communication between subspecialists and the team physician.
- Documentation of medical care is often mistakenly neglected in the team setting. The team physician needs to keep formal and confidential medical records that detail communication with consultants, give treatment and follow-up instructions, and provide details for insurance and reimbursement purposes (Rice, 2002).
- The team physician should have final say of when an athlete is initially cleared to begin competition and when a previously injured athlete may return to play (Herring et al, 2000a).

ADMINISTRATIVE RESPONSIBILITIES OF THE TEAM PHYSICIAN

- The team physician's primary concern is the coordination of medical supervision. This organization includes: making sure qualified medical personnel are attending practices and competitions as needed, designing a plan for sideline evaluation, and having necessary medical equipment readily available. The team physician encourages defined roles and responsibilities for all involved in the medical care of the team, along with establishing a medical chain of command. The team physician may not make all the daily decisions but should have full authority concerning medical policy-making.
- The team physician needs to lead the planning for and practicing of medical emergencies and urgencies. In addition to having an emergency treatment and transport

plan, the team physician also must know the medical capabilities of surrounding hospitals—particularly around away competitions sites—so that injured athletes are brought to medical facilities that are best equipped to handle their specific medical problem (Herring et al, 2000a).

- The team physician should implement protocols that facilitate timely and quality medical care for situations when he or she is not immediately available. Preestablished guidelines for return to play are very helpful, especially when injuries to impact athletes result in high pressure for returning to competition before appropriate healing has occurred (Herring et al, 2000b). The ACSM consensus statement on return-to-play issues more fully details the responsibilities of the team physician when returning athletes to competition (Herring et al, 2002).
- The team physician oversees the playing environment. He or she should evaluate both practice and game facilities for safety. A safe playing environment also involves appropriate and properly fitting protective equipment, available hydration, and an activity level appropriate for the climate.

COMMUNICATION RESPONSIBILITIES OF THE TEAM PHYSICIAN

- For a team to receive optimal medical care, the team physician and trainer must communicate openly and clearly. Even before the season, they need to discuss medical treatment protocols, which preferably are documented in writing (Rice, 2002). When an injury occurs there can be no confusion over who will go on the field for initial evaluation and who will communicate to the coach the extent of an athlete's injury and playing status.
- A team physician needs to develop good rapport with the coach. Offering injury prevention suggestions and player health education may demonstrate to the coach a shared desire to assist the team attaining their goals. Most importantly, a team physician must keep the coach informed of an injured player's ability to continue to compete safely. Without breaching player confidentially, the team physician should provide the coach a timeframe for further evaluation or the player's return. In general, this should be communicated in terms of a sport-specific timeline, such as: the player is out for a play, out for a series, reassessment will be done at half-time or game's end, or the player is likely lost for the remaining part of the season.
- A team physician may also be required to discuss a player's medical condition with the school officials. Administrators often need to know specifics regarding

physician recommendations: how long will the player miss class or be in the hospital. They seldom need to know medical or personal details of the athlete's situation. Remember that the athlete's confidentiality is the first concern. Members of the media rarely, if ever, need information from the team physician.

- Well-defined criteria for dealing with the media should be established. If a team physician is encouraged to participate in an interview, insist that written questions be submitted before-hand so that appropriate remarks can be constructed for the record. These planned responses can be reviewed with team coaches, trainers, and administrators to ensure their consistency, accuracy, and regard for the athlete's privacy.
- A team physician may need to discuss an athlete's medical condition with his parents, especially if working with minors. It may be beneficial to send a letter to parents prior to the season, describing the role of the team physician and the continued importance of their personal primary care physician to the athlete's overall health.
- As mentioned above, the team physician coordinates specialty care as medically indicated. In doing so, he or she should provide the pertinent information necessary to the respective medical consultant's care and receive written documentation of recommendations from medical specialists.

OTHER CONSIDERATIONS FOR THE TEAM PHYSICIAN

- Sports medicine abounds with opportunities for research. Simply keeping accurate epidemiologic and injury data has the potential to impact training regimens, competition rules, or mandates for protective equipment (Rice, 2000).
- Every would-be team physician must research the medical liability risk and insurance coverage associated with the position. A written contract or memorandum of understanding with the institution or team that defines responsibilities and level of coverage expected is essential—even if no compensation is to be received (Rice, 2002). Good Samaritan laws exist in many states but the exact law varies widely between different jurisdictions. Most Good Samaritan laws apply only if the physician is receiving no compensation for his or her services. Compensation may be defined by a specific dollar amount, or as little as receiving a team shirt to wear at games!
- Compensation as a team physician is variable. Almost all work with teams competing at less than collegiate level is voluntary. Deferring offers for nominal remuneration in favor of paying a trainer's salary can be a beneficial and time saving option (Rice, 2002). Most

team physicians work with athletic teams solely for professional and personal satisfaction owing to their interest in sports and athletes.

REFERENCES

Each of these consensus statements is published by multiple organizations. They may be downloaded or viewed free at www.acsm.org/publications/consensusstatements.htm

Herring SA, Bergfeld JA, Boyd J, et al: *Sideline Preparedness for the Team Physician: A Consensus Statement.* American Academy of Family Physicians, American Academy of Orthopedic Surgeons, American College of Sports Medicine, American Osteopathic Academy of Sports Medicine, 2000*a*.

Herring SA, Bergfeld JA, Boyd J, et al: *Team Physician Consensus Statement.* American Academy of Family Physicians, American Academy of Orthopedic Surgeons, American College of Sports Medicine, American Osteopathic Academy of Sports Medicine, 2000*b*.

Herring SA, Bergfeld JA, Boyd J, et al: *The Team Physician and Conditioning of Athletes for Sports: A Consensus Statement.* American Academy of Family Physicians, American Academy of Orthopedic Surgeons, American College of Sports Medicine, American Osteopathic Academy of Sports Medicine, 2001.

Herring SA, Bergfield JA, Boyd J, et Al: The team physician and return-to-play issues: A consensus statement. *Med Sci Sports Exer* 34:1212–1214, 2002.

Melion MB, Walsh WM, Shelton GL: *The Team Physician's Handbook,* 2nd ed. Philadelphia, PA, Hanley & Belfus, 1997, pp 1–7.

Rice SG: The high school athlete: Setting up a high school sports medicine program, in Mellion MB, EWalsh WM, Madden C, et al (eds.): *The Team Physician's Handbook,* 3rd ed. Philadelphia, PA, Hanley & Belfus, 2002, pp 67–77.

Rice SG: Development of an injury surveillance system: Results from a longitudinal study of high school athletes, in Ashare AB (ed.): *Safety in Ice Hockey* vol. 3, ASTM STP 1341. West Conshohocken, PA, American Society for Testing and Materials, 2000, pp 3–18.

2 ETHICAL CONSIDERATIONS IN SPORTS MEDICINE

Ralph G Oriscello, MD FACC, FACP

INTRODUCTION

- Ethics in general is the conforming to accepted standards of conduct. No one achieves ethical perfection but sports physicians are good by nature and guided by high ethical standards. Sports themselves are considered to reflect values generally considered to be important to society: character building, health promotion, and the pursuit of competitive excellence and enjoyment.

- Ethical considerations in the area of sports medicine are similar to those in medicine in general, including the basic principles and rules.
- Beneficence, the principle of performing acts or making recommendations only potentially beneficial to an athlete, is the trump principle.
- Nonmaleficence, the principle of prohibiting recommendations or actions detrimental to an athlete's short- and long-term health, is considered with every action taken in the trainer's room when tending to an injured athlete.
- Confidentiality informed consent and truthfulness are absolutely essential for the ethical management of any sports related medical decision.

THE SPORTS PHYSICIAN'S RESPONSIBILITIES

- An athlete's autonomy, his or her interests and desires, and the third principle of medical ethics must always be taken into consideration in any decision made by a sports physician. Such decisions should always be made in the athlete's best interest.
- Whether the decision involves a diagnostic test or the athlete's eligibility, its end result is the maintenance of good health with the least risk to the athlete.
- Conflict between physician and athlete should always be minimal or absent.
- While autonomy is respected, most athletes can and should rely on their sports physician to lead them in the decision making process.
- It is quickly recognized by the sports physician that one solution rarely fits all with the same problem. The same set of circumstances can lead to a different suggested solution by the same sports physician.
- Exactness and infallibility, while desirable, are not traits of even the finest sports physicians (Maron, 1994).
- The sports physician's primary duty is to make the best effort to maintain or restore health and functional ability (Howe, 1988).
- The athlete's welfare must guide all efforts.
- To be a good sports physician, he or she must have a genuine appreciation for the importance of athletics in his or her client's life. The precepts of Dr. O'Donoghue for sports physicians are timeless: accept athletics, avoid expediency, adopt the best methods, act promptly, and try to achieve perfection (O'Donoghue, 1984).
- The injured athlete must know the diagnosis, understand its implications, and participate in all therapeutic decisions.

- Despite the athlete's wishes, the sports physician cannot do less than seek the best possible outcome.
- All sports medicine physicians gain knowledge and better judgment with experience, soon recognizing many recommendations or forms of therapy have risks as well as benefits.
- Harm can come to the athlete-patient from unnecessary or excessive restriction as well as from failure to restrict activity when appropriate.
- The sports physician does not operate in a vacuum. To make sports oriented medical decisions, one must be well versed in current recommendations for eligibility and continued participation and not depend on his or her own limited personal experience or unscientific reasoning (Mitten, 1999).
- Recognizing the wide range of opinions and individual fallibility, athlete-patients can assert their right to another opinion.
- Continuing education of the sports physician aids in the development of a suitable level of skill and knowledge and their maintenance (26th Bethesda Conference, 1994).
- While sports physicians will be able to treat most referrals, they must be aware of their own level of competence. They must know when and where to refer for specialized consultation or therapy. It is essential to know their colleague's ability, personality, and empathy for athletes in order to make competent referrals (Rizve and Thompson, 2002).
- The referred patient should not be abandoned. The consultant may gain insight from the referring physician. This affords the athlete continuing support from his or her primary sports physician.
- There is no obligation to accept without question the recommendations of consultants, especially if incongruent with the referring physician's knowledge of the patient.
- All the above lead to trust established between athlete and physician, allowing for more comfortable resolution of the decision making process.

POTENTIAL FOR DIVIDED LOYALTIES

- While rare in high school and uncommon in college sports, there is major distrust between professional athletes and team physicians (George, 2002).
- Athletes may feel that there are too many instances when the quality of their treatment is often secondary to the doctor's obligation to team owners and coaches.
- A salaried position can interfere with the traditional doctor–patient relationship.
- To many the role of the salaried physician leads to a conflict of interest. Such a conflict exists when the

employed sports physician's objective professional duties are compromised by personal interests, e.g., the financial reward of his or her association with a professional team as well as the publicity and high visibility one gets from such a position.

- It is an ethical breach for anything but the athlete's health interest to be considered, again, recognizing judgment errors in too conservative or too liberal therapy can occur.
- The ultimate welfare of the athlete may seem in conflict with the wishes of parents or spouse, coaches or team management. The fact that an organization or someone other than the athlete pays the physician is immaterial. The loyalty of the sports physician is to the continued healthy physician–patient relationship.
- Decisions must be made solely based on sound medical judgment. A reasonable third party, e.g. a university or professional team, will understand this. If it does not, the physician should remove his or her services from that party.
- Occasionally, wishes of the athlete-patient conflict with what the physician believes are in the athlete's best interest. If after negotiation and additional consultation the sports physician feels uncomfortable with another's recommendation, continued care of the athlete-patient could be difficult or impossible. The athlete should be reassigned to another physician.
- For the professional athlete, the unfavorable mix of high salaries and short careers can make for risky decision making by both the athlete and the physician. Coaches often encourage physicians to rush players back on to the field to win games. Players themselves often desire to rush back too quickly.
- Teammates should not be allowed to pressure injured athletes by suggesting they are malingering while collecting a substantial income. Under these circumstances many physicians play by the rules of the coaching staff.
- An untimely death or worsening injury sets the stage for lack of trust in the team physician.
- By actions alone, the team physician demonstrates that his or her utmost responsibility is to protect the players. If a player should not be on the playing field, that players will not be there.

DRUG USE

- It is common knowledge that there is illicit drug use by athletes at all levels: recreational drugs, anabolic steroids, pain controlling agents, ergogenics, and alcohol.

- Therapeutic medications are an integral part of sports medicine. Used appropriately, they control pain and inflammation, speed recovery, and hasten return to function.
- It is the obligation of the sports physician to know each drug thoroughly, especially its potential effect(s) on the safety or effectiveness of the athlete's performance. Appropriately prescribed drugs must not expose the athlete to potential disqualification, e.g., as in the prevention of exercise-induced asthma, when an effective legal medication can be found.
- Nowadays, available testing makes it impossible to catch all participants who use banned substances. That is rapidly changing.
- There are those who would remove all bans on enhancing agents, hormones for instance, allowing for a "free-for-all" with unrestricted use.
- There are two major arguments against such an attitude: one should not condone cheating; and the essence of sport itself.

CONFIDENTIALITY

- There is *no* grade to confidentiality: more for a high profile athlete; less for one with a lesser public persona.
- Confidentiality must be inviolate, despite the fact that athletes are very public persons.
- Society wants to know the most intimate details of athletes' lives, including medical evaluations and treatments.
- No athletes forfeit their right to medical privacy.
- All inquiries made of sports physicians by the press or other interested parties should go unanswered unless specifically permitted by the athlete.
- Even with permission, the sports physician must be extraordinarily sensitive about details revealed.
- Despite claims regarding the public's "right to know," the right to privacy remains with the athlete–patient.
- The press is very resourceful in gaining information—inaccurate on more than a few occasions. If inaccurate information is printed, the physician may, with the athlete's permission, attempt to correct it.
- On occasion, the sports physician will advise the athlete–patient about the amount of information to release to coaches. This is important when restriction from practice or competition is necessary. The athlete usually grants such permission. Here we refer to the athlete's private sports physician, not one employed by a school or professional team.
- No greater breach of confidentiality can occur than if any health information is released to anyone remotely related to the athlete's career without forewarning the individual.

- When a sports physician is employed by a school, team, or similar entity, the expectations of both athlete–patient and sports physician are agreed on at the outset. That sports physician must always maintain his or her position as an advocate for the athlete–patient's welfare.
- An employed sports physician must still respect the athlete–patient's autonomy in medical decision making, while advising against any decision that could compromise the patient's future health and athletic career.

RELATIONSHIP WITH COLLEAGUES

- Among the problems that can arise for a team physician are those involving other physicians participating in the care of the athlete–patient. There must be sensitivity demonstrated to the relationship of all medical professionals involved.
- The sports physician must never criticize the actions of another physician to the athlete–patient. Private discussions with the primary care physician regarding recommended therapy should be undertaken.
- The sports physician is in a position to positively influence his or her colleague's care of athletes in the future by such positive input.
- If playing restrictions have been imposed on an athlete by a primary care physician, while not countermanding them, the sports physician must always insist on an individual assessment of the athlete's return to play status.
- Consultation between the sports physician and the athlete's primary care physician usually solves the problem and provides an opportunity for education.
- Sports medicine is a team effort involving physicians and many paramedical disciplines. The sport's physician recognizes that these can be helpful while coordinating the athlete's care. The sports physician must insist that such assistants adhere to the same high ethical standards he or she practices.
- The sports medicine physician has an obligation to expose quackery and unproved practices employed in the guise of improving performance, thus protecting athletes and their careers.

FEAR OF LEGAL ENTANGLEMENT

- There is always a question as to what the sports medicine physician should do in the presence of a life-threatening situation or a potentially disabling condition. Under these circumstances, the physician must be cautious and recommend against participation.
- When operating at the highest ethical level with support from the medical literature and the medical community, such an event should never alter a physician's role in the future evaluation of other athletes.
- A sports physician not afraid to make the difficult call should be sought out by other physicians and athletes.

SUMMARY

- Sports medicine offers awesome responsibilities and a magnitude of potential problems exceeding many other specialties.
- Familiarity with many disease states that can affect an athlete's ability to participate is required.
- Athletes can only be allowed to participate if they do not endanger themselves or others.
- The physician must be familiar with unethical means to enhance performance.
- The physician must be aware of resources available to aid him or her in rendering an authoritative opinion.
- The physician must be devoted to the rules of confidentiality, informed consent, and truthfulness.
- The physician must be aware that occasional decisions may require legal enforcement.
- The physician must be aware that there is no table of contents to refer to for every decision. A backbone, on occasion, is more important than an ethics primer.

REFERENCES

26th Bethesda Conference: Recommendations for determining eligibility for competition in athletes with cardiovascular abnormalities. *J Am Coll Cardiol* 24:845, 1994.

George T.: Care by team doctors raises conflict issue. *N Y Times (print)* Sect.8 (col 5), Jul 28, 2002.

Howe WB.: Primary care sports medicine: a partimer's perspective. *Phys Sports med* 16:103, 1988.

Maron B.: Surviving competitive athletics with hypertrophic cardiomyopathy. *Am J Cardiol* 73:1098, 1994.

Mitten MJ.: Medicolegal issues, in Williams RA (ed.): *The Athlete and Heart Disease: Diagnosis, Evaluation & Management.* Philadelphia, PA, Lippincott Williams & Wilkins, 1999, p 307.

O'Donoghue DH.: Treatment of Injuries to Athletes, 4th ed. Phildelphia, W.B. Saunders, 1984, p 7.

Rizve AA, Thompson PD.: Hypertrophic cardiomyopathy: Who plays and who sits. *Cur Sports Med Rep* 93, 2002.

3 LEGAL ISSUES

Aaron Rubin, MD, FAAFP, FACSM

INTRODUCTION

- The advice of an attorney should be considered before making any legal decisions.
- Sports is a microcosm of society.
- There are rules of sports and society that must be created, interpreted and, at times, argued.
- Medical practice in sports is held to the same standards as any other medical practice.
- Legal issues in the area include—but are not limited to—malpractice, contracts, licensure, insurance, Good Samaritan laws, and confidentiality issues.
- These issues may be complicated by the practice of sports medicine in the public arena and the traditions of team and game coverage.
- This chapter is by no means meant to substitute for the advice of an attorney, but is presented to draw attention to potential legal issues that may arise in the practice of sports medicine.

DEFINITIONS

- **Law:** A body of rules or standards of action or conduct ordained or established by some authority. The law of a state is found in statutory and constitutional enactments as interpreted by its courts and contemplates both statutory and case law.
- **Lawful:** Legal, permitted by the law. Not forbidden by law, not illegal.
- **Contract:** An agreement between two or more parties which creates legally binding obligations to do or not to do a particular thing. A valid contract must involve competent parties, proper subject matter, consideration, and mutuality of agreement and of obligation.
- **Expressed:** An express contract is openly expressed in writing or orally stated in distinct and explicit language.
- **Implied:** An implied contract is one inferred by the conduct of the parties to exist.
- **Bilateral:** A bilateral contract is one involving mutual promises between parties.
- **Unilateral:** A unilateral contract is a one-sided promise where one party undertakes an obligation without receiving in return any express engagement or promise of performance from the other.

- **Civil law:** Body of law that a nation or state has established for itself. Law determining private rights and liabilities as distinguished from criminal or natural law. Laws concerned with civil or private rights and remedies as contrasted with criminal laws.
- **Criminal law:** The branch of law which defines what public wrongs are considered crimes and assigns punishment for those wrongs. It declares what conduct is criminal, and prescribes the punishment to be imposed for such conduct.
- **Natural law:** The moral or ethical law, formulated in accordance with reason, natural justice, and the original state of nature.
- **Case law:** Law based on judicial precedent rather than legislative enactment. The body of law founded in adjudicated cases as distinguished from statute, common law. It includes the aggregate of reported cases that interpret statutes, regulations, and constitutional provisions.
- **Tort:** A wrongful injury, a private or civil wrong. A tort is some action or conduct by someone (defendant) which causes injury or damage to another (plaintiff). Torts may be *intentional* (when the defendant intends to violate a legal duty) or *negligent* (when the defendant fails to exercise the proper degree of care established by law). A legal wrong committed on the person or property independent of contract. It may be either (1) a direct invasion of some legal right of the individual; (2) the infraction of some public duty by which special damage accrues to the individual; or (3) the violation of some private obligation by which like damage occurs to the individual.
- **Negligence:** The inadvertent or unintentional failure to exercise that care which a reasonable, prudent, and careful person would exercise; conduct which violates certain legal standards of due care. Negligence constitutes grounds for recovery in a tort action, if it causes injury to the plaintiff.
- **Liability:** Any type of obligation or debt owed to another party. An obligation or mandate to do or refrain from doing something. An obligation one is bound in law or justice to perform.
- **Plaintiff**: Person who brings a lawsuit; the complainant; the prosecution in a criminal case. The party who complains or sues in a civil action and is so named on the record.
- **Defendant:** The person accused in a criminal case or sued in a civil action. The person defending or denying wrongdoing.
- **Captain of the ship doctrine:** This doctrine imposes liability on the surgeon in charge of an operation for negligence of his or her assistants when those assistants are under the surgeon's control, even though the

assistants are also employees of the hospital (Nolan and Nolan-Haley, 1990).

DUTIES, ROLE, AND RESPONSIBILITIES OF THE TEAM PHYSICIAN

- The duties of the team physician to a team may be outlined in a letter of agreement or contract between the organization and physician.
- The duties to the individual athlete should be considered as with any other patient–physician relationship.
- Balancing this duty to team and athlete must be considered in every situation.
- A consensus statement on the duties of the team physician has been created by several organizations and available in its entirety from these groups:
  a. American Academy of Family Physicians (AAFP)
  b. American Academy of Orthopedic Surgeons (AAOS)
  c. American College of Sports Medicine (ACSM)
  d. American Medical Society for Sports Medicine (AMSSM)
  e. American Orthopedic Society for Sports Medicine (AOSSM)
  f. American Osteopathic Academy of Sports Medicine (AOASM)
- Qualifications from this consensus statement include the following:
  a. Medical or osteopathic degree with unrestricted license to practice medicine
  b. Fundamental knowledge of emergency care regarding sporting events
  c. Trained in CPR
  d. Working knowledge of trauma, musculoskeletal injuries and medical conditions affecting the athlete
- Medical duties from this statement stated that the team physician has ultimate responsibility to include coordination of the preparticipation screening; management of on-field injuries; medical management of injury and illness; coordination of rehabilitation and return to participation; coordination of medical care, education, and documentation; and record keeping.
- Administrative duties include establishing relationships, education, development of a chain of command, plan and train for emergencies, address equipment and supply issues (as needed to provide adequate medical coverage), provide for event coverage, and assess environments concerns and playing conditions.
- Standard definitions of negligence generally apply. The physician is held to what the reasonable, prudent man would do. As guidelines become more

established, these may become the basis for duties and responsibilities of the team physician.

DUTIES, ROLE, AND RESPONSIBILITIES OF THE TEAM AND ATHLETES

- The responsibilities of the team (organization, ownership, administration) should also be outlined in a contract.
- The team should provide a safe venue (including adequate security), appropriate safety equipment, supplies needed to treat injured or ill athletes (unless otherwise specified in the agreement) and appropriate response for an emergency situation.
- The team (including coaching staff) should not interfere with care of the athlete including return to play issues.
- The athlete should be prepared for participation and participate safely and according to the rules of the sport. If not, they may share in responsibility for injury.
- The athlete or team has a duty to report conditions to the team physician and not conceal illnesses, injury, or symptoms that may occur.

CONTRACTS

- Traditionally, many team physicians work with as little as a handshake or loose agreement.
- One should consider "putting it in writing."
- This contract should outline duties, responsibilities for providing supplies, compensation, travel expectations, provision of coverage in your absence, length of contract, responsibilities for providing preparticipation examinations, liability coverage, and game decision processes (such as who has the final word on return to play issues).
- An attorney can be extremely helpful in creating such a document.

LIABILITY

MALPRACTICE COVERAGE

- Malpractice is defined as unreasonable lack of skill or professional misconduct.
- Failure to render professional services under circumstances in the community by the "average, prudent reputable member of the profession" with resultant injury or damage to the recipient of those services.

- Negligence is the predominant theory of liability in medical malpractice suits. It requires the following to occur:
  a. Physician's duty to the plaintiff
  b. Violation or breach of applicable standard of care
  c. Connection (causation) between the violation of care and harm
  d. Injury (damages) that can be compensated
- Physicians should have adequate coverage to defend any case brought against them and to compensate any judgments decided against them.
- Coverage may not be in effect if a physician is practicing beyond the scope of his or her expertise or in an unlicensed area.
- Physicians traveling out of state or country with teams should be aware of this possibility and check with their malpractice carrier.
- Malpractice insurance should include an adequate *tail* to cover physicians when they change jobs

FALLACY OF THE GOOD SAMARITAN

- Good Samaritan doctrine: One who sees a person in imminent and serious peril through negligence of another cannot be charged with contributory negligence as a matter of law, in risking his own life or serious injury in attempting to affect a rescue, provided the attempt is not recklessly or rashly made. Under this doctrine, negligence of a volunteer must worsen the position of person in distress before liability will be imposed. This protection from liability is provided by statute in most states (Nolan and Nolan-Haley, 1990).
- These laws and protection vary from state to state.
- These are a defense in a lawsuit and must be presented by your attorney as such.
- A person expected to act, such as a team physician at a game, may not be covered by the Good Samaritan doctrine, whether compensated or not.
- The Good Samaritan doctrine should not be a substitute for adequate malpractice coverage.
- The doctrine should be adequate in most states to cover a physician who renders aid when an unexpected medical situation arises, such as at an auto accident or if as a spectator at an event where another spectator has a cardiac arrest.
- Some jurisdictions may require a physician to provide care under these circumstances.

PATIENT (ATHLETE)—PHYSICIAN RELATIONSHIP

- The patient (athlete)–physician relationship should be one of mutual trust and teamwork.

- The athlete (or parents or guardian if a minor) has rights to autonomy, self determination, privacy, and appropriate medical care.
- Even if a minor, an athlete has certain rights to seek medical care in most jurisdictions for treatment related to pregnancy, drugs, and sexually transmitted disease. Check with local laws.
- Privacy is a difficult issue owing to the public nature of athletic events—evaluation is done on the field or courtside. All attempts must be made to maintain privacy.
- Professional and college organizations may consider waivers to allow certain information regarding athletic injuries or illnesses to be discussed with press representatives. Some organizations require reporting of injuries and illness (such as professional sports and some college sports). Care must be taken to avoid disclosing information.
- It is probably best to have an administrative person, such as a sports information director or public information officer, deal with the press to prevent the physician from inadvertently releasing private issues. If the physician is to talk with the press he or she should speak with caution and only with the athlete's permission.

DRUGS AND THE ATHLETE

MEDICATIONS: PRESCRIBING; DISPENSING

- Legal medications are generally divided into two groups, prescription and over-the-counter (OTC). Prescription medications are further divided into controlled substances (narcotics, sedatives, and the like) that have a higher potential for abuse and misuse and standard prescription drugs (such as antibiotics, anti-inflammatory medication, and medication for blood pressure and diabetes).
- In some states, a special prescription is needed for dispensing of the highest level of controlled substances.
- Medication prescribing and dispensing falls under many laws including state medical laws, pharmacy laws, and consumer safety laws.
- In general a physician may prescribe medication or provide medications under the state laws which usually include examination of the patient.
- A licensed pharmacist may provide medication as prescribed by a licensed physician.
- There are generally strict labeling requirements often including the name of the patient, name and strength of the medication, directions for use, date dispensed, quantity dispensed, and warnings of common side effects. In addition, many states require the pharmacist to counsel the patient on the medication.

• Dispensing medications by individuals not licensed to do so, even if OTC, may not be allowed and could open those doing so to prosecution under appropriate laws. This may also open the individuals to liability for negligence if an untoward effect occurs.

DRUG TESTING (SEE CHAPTER 20)

• The team physician may be asked to participate in drug testing program for teams.
• Careful consideration regarding the physician's role as an enforcer of rules versus a counselor for medical care must be undertaken.
• Proper protection of rights and "due process" of the athlete must be maintained.
• Testing may include recreational as well as performance enhancing drugs.
• Testing may be voluntary or mandated by certain organizations, such as the National College Athletic Administration (NCAA) or International Olympic Committee (IOC).

CAPTAIN OF THE SHIP

• Though the doctrine relates to surgeons and assistants, the philosophy could be expanded to team physicians and those they work with.
• Choose your partners in sports medical care wisely to avoid being drawn into bad situations.

RISK MANAGEMENT

• Manage risk by being prepared, documenting care, working with likeminded professionals, anticipating problems, and communicating with athletes and, where appropriate, their families.
• Advice of legal counsel should be sought in planning team coverage, writing contracts, and if any events occur.
• Bad outcomes often lead to legal actions (lawsuits).

REFERENCES

Nolan JR, Nolan-Haley JM: *Black's Law Dictionary*, 6th ed. St Paul, MN, West Publishing, 1990.

BIBLIOGRAPHY

Birnie B: Legal issues for the team physician, in Rubin AL (ed.): *Sports Injuries and Emergencies, a Quick-Response Manual.* New York, NY, McGraw-Hill, 2003.

Davis T, Mathewson AD, Shropshire KL: *Sports and the Law: A Modern Anthology.* Durham, NC, Carolina Academic Press, 1999.

Gallup EM: *Law and the Team Physician.* Champaign, IL, Human Kinetics, 1995.

Gilbert Law Summaries: Law Dictionary. Chicago, IL, Harcourt Brace 1994.

Herring SA, Bergfeld J, Boyd J, et al: *Team Physicians Consensus Statement.* www.acsm.org/pdf/teamphys.pdf 2001.

4 FIELD-SIDE EMERGENCIES

Michael C Gaertner, DO
Loren A Crown, MD

INTRODUCTION

• While most sports injuries are nonemergent and musculoskeletal in nature, there are certain life- and limb-threatening injuries that the *field-side physician* (FP) must be prepared to handle immediately. The most important step in the management of field-side emergencies is preparation, and depending on the setting of the event and the level of competition, resources may be limited. The FP must at a minimum have ready access to appropriate health care personnel to assist in an emergency, appropriate medical supplies and emergency equipment, immediate access to a telephone, and the ability to transport an athlete to a medical facility. It would also be advisable to be certified in *basic life support* (BLS), *advanced cardiac life support* (ACLS), and *advanced trauma life support* (ATLS) and to have a working knowledge of the common and uncommon injuries specific to the event being covered.

GENERAL APPROACH TO THE FALLEN ATHLETE

• When approaching the fallen athlete, the field-side evaluation should be both rapid and focused. The "primary survey" should follow the "ABCDE" approach taught by ATLS (Committee on Trauma, 1997) and should occur where the athlete is found. They should initially be left in that position unless they are prone and unconscious or there is a problem performing the "ABCs" (Luke and Micheli, 1999; Blue and Pecci, 2002), in which case they should be logrolled to a supine position.

- The logroll should ideally be a four person technique in which the team leader is at the victim's head maintaining in-line immobilization of the head and neck, while the other three members of the team are controlling the torso, hips, and legs. The athlete should be turned in the direction of the three assistants according to the count of the leader and then onto a spine board placed under the athlete.

- If an athlete is wearing an appropriately fitted helmet, neither the helmet nor its chin strap should be removed. Padding or sandbags should be placed around the helmet and the shoulders; hips and legs immobilized. The face-guard can easily be removed by prying or cutting it off for access to the airway. The helmet and shoulder pads should be considered a single unit—the removal of either one necessitates the removal of the other, as leaving only one of them in place forces the neck out of a neutral position (Haight and Shiple, 2001; Gastel et al, 1998). If the athlete is not wearing a helmet, a rigid cervical collar should be applied with in-line immobilization of the spine.

- After the primary survey is complete and the patient stabilized, a more detailed secondary survey should be performed either on the field or on the sideline, depending on the status of the athlete and the environmental conditions.

- The factors to be considered while evaluating the fallen athlete include whether or not the injury was witnessed/unwitnessed and/or traumatic/atraumatic. The age, general conditioning, and specific medical conditions of the athlete should be considered, as well as the general characteristics of the sport, such as the amount of contact (i.e., collision, limited contact, and noncontact), the degree of speed involved, and the duration of the event. Finally, the environmental conditions must be considered as both a potential causative and/or exacerbating factor in the injury.

- After the initial examination of the patient is completed, the FP should identify any problem areas and categorize them as being of either an immediate or potential life threatening/disabling nature and treat accordingly. Frequent reevaluation of the injured athlete is a must.

IMMEDIATE LIFE THREATENING INJURIES

RESPIRATORY COMPROMISE

UPPER AIRWAY OBSTRUCTION

- Although rare in organized sports, respiratory arrest can result from *upper airway obstruction* (UAO). Signs include respiratory distress with little or no air movement, significant accessory muscle use, and stridorous, wheezing, or snoring breath sounds. If the athlete is unconscious, the airway should be opened with a jaw-thrust maneuver to keep the tongue from occluding the airway and an oral/nasal airway inserted as necessary. In-line repositioning of the head/neck may be necessary to establish airway patency if the neck is significantly contorted. The oropharynx should be inspected for foreign bodies and removed if visualized; however, blind finger sweeps are not recommended in either children or adults. Significant facial/mandibular trauma with resultant loss of support of the tongue or with blood, secretions, and loose teeth in the pharynx can produce UAO, particularly in the unconscious athlete who has lost protective airway reflexes. Other causes of UAO, such as airway edema from anaphylaxis, inhalation burn injuries, or an expanding neck or retropharyngeal hematoma from neck trauma should be considered, with early intubation a priority. Surgical airway capability is a necessity as well.

LARYNGEAL FRACTURE

- This rare injury occurs after direct trauma to the anterior neck. Signs include stridor, hoarseness, subcutaneous emphysema, and perhaps bony crepitus and a palpable fracture. Although airway obstruction may not be immediate, it can rapidly progress to this stage because of resultant edema and as with other causes of obstruction, early intubation is a priority; surgical airway capability is again a necessity.

PNEUMOTHORAX

- A simple pneumothorax may be spontaneous (i.e., rupture of a bleb) or traumatic, with spontaneous pneumothoraces occurring more often in sports that involve changes in intrathoracic pressure (i.e., scuba diving and weightlifting) (Partridge et al, 1997) and traumatic pneumothoraces occurring secondary to rib fractures. Symptoms may include unilateral chest pain, dyspnea, and cough. Immediate treatment is rarely needed unless the patient is severely dyspneic or the pnuemothorax is open or under tension. Those with a stable simple pneumothorax should be given oxygen and transported to a medical facility for further evaluation and management.

OPEN PNEUMOTHORAX

- This is defined as a pneumothorax accompanied by an open wound to the chest (sucking chest wound). Treatment consists of placing an occlusive dressing over the open wound and taping it down on three sides to create a one-way valve that allows air to exit without reentering till a definitive thoracostomy tube can be placed.

TENSION PNEUMOTHORAX

- This occurs when a pneumothorax is accompanied by progressive accumulation of air in the pleural space with the resultant increase in intrathoracic pressure causing a shift of mediastinal structures away from the pneumothorax as well as a decrease in venous return and cardiac output. In addition to the previously listed symptoms, these athletes may have tracheal deviation away from the affected side with jugular venous distention and hypotension. This is a true medical emergency that requires immediate treatment by needle decompression of the chest with a large (14–16 gauge) needle or catheter inserted in the anterior chest wall in the second intercostal space at the midclavicular line, followed by placement of a thoracostomy tube.

CARDIAC ARREST

- Although devastating when it occurs in a young athlete, a traumatic sudden death is extremely rare with incidence varying depending on the age of the athlete and the sporting event (O'Connor et al, 1998). The most common cause of sudden cardiac death in young athletes is congenital cardiovascular structural abnormalities with hypertrophic cardiomyopathy leading the list, followed by coronary artery anomalies and myocarditis (McCaffrey et al, 1991). The most common cause in older athletes (age > 30–35) is atherosclerotic heart disease causing acute ischemic events.
- The field-side treatment of any cause of cardiac arrest should follow *advanced cardiac life support* (ACLS) guidelines with attention to early *cardiopulmonary resuscitation* (CPR) and defibrillation as indicated. An equally important task for the FP is to identify those athletes who are having warning signs of cardiac disease and dysrhythmias, such as sudden unexplained syncope or collapse, exertional syncope, early fatigue, or anginal chest pain during or immediately following exertion (O'Connor et al, 1998). Strong consideration

should be given to withholding these athletes from further competition until a thorough evaluation is performed.

ANAPHYLAXIS

- Anaphylactic reactions are acute systemic hypersensitivity reactions that can be idiopathic, exercise-induced, or allergen-induced, and although rare, they can progress very rapidly and prove fatal if unrecognized. Insect stings (esp. hymenoptera) may be a cause of sports related anaphylaxis.
- The symptoms of anaphylaxis may include urticaria/angioedema, upper airway edema, dyspnea, wheezing, flushing of skin, dizziness/hypotension/syncope, gastrointestinal symptoms, rhinitis, and headache (Winbery and Lieberman, 1995). Symptom onset is typically rapid (within 5–30 min of exposure), and in its most severe form can progress to severe bronchospasm, airway edema, and fatal cardiovascular collapse.
- Treatment consists of prompt attention to the ABCs, followed by treatment with 100% oxygen, epinephrine (1:1000) 0.3–0.5 mL in adults or 0.01 mg/kg in children given subcutaneously or intramuscularly and repeated every 10–15 minutes as needed, IV (intravenous) fluids if hypotensive, beta-agonists by nebulizer if bronchospasm is present, antihistamines (H1 and H2 blockers), and glucocorticoids if available. The athlete must be rapidly transported to a medical facility as continued observation will be required.

SEVERE HEMORRHAGE

- Hemorrhage in the athlete may be the result of lacerations, fractures, vascular disruptions, or visceral organ or muscle disruptions. It can manifest as either massive external bleeding or insidious and occult internal bleeding. Control of external bleeding should follow the basic principles of hemostasis, which include steady direct pressure over the bleeding site and over larger arteries proximal to the site of injury, as well as elevation of the affected body part. Blind clamping of bleeding vessels and tourniquet application (with the possible exception of a traumatic amputation) are not recommended.
- Scalp lacerations can cause significant hemorrhage and often go unnoticed if the athlete is lying on his back or is strapped to a spine board.
- Occult bleeding may produce delayed signs and symptoms, and what may at first appear to be an atraumatic

incident may actually have been caused by recent unnoticed or unwitnessed trauma (Blue and Pecci, 2002).

- Potential injuries, which may be major sources of occult blood loss, include hemorrhage into the thoracic and abdominal cavities, the soft tissues surrounding major long bone fractures, the retroperitoneal space secondary to a pelvic fracture, and as a result of penetrating torso injury (Committee on Trauma, 1997).
- Signs and symptoms of hypovolemic shock include altered sensorium, pale and cool extremities with a decreased capillary refill, weak, thready, and rapid pulses, hypotension, tachycardia, and tachypnea.
- Treatment should follow ATLS protocol and at a minimum two large bore peripheral IVs should be started and oxygen administered. Consideration should be given to starting crystalloid fluids, although there is some debate as to whether or not aggressive fluid resuscitation may actually be more detrimental to patients with certain types of injuries, and one should consider the concept of permissive hypotension when managing hypovolemic shock in the alert patient (Fowler and Pepe, 2002).

POTENTIAL LIFE THREATENING/ DISABLING INJURIES

HEAD INJURY

- Head injuries in sports are quite common and often provoke anxiety and uncertainty. Fortunately, the most common head injury in sports is a concussion and 90% or more of concussions do not involve a *loss of consciousness* (LOC) (McAlindon, 2002; Harmon, 1999). The FP must learn not only how to recognize them (which is not always easy) and become familiar with a system to grade them, but must also search for clues to more serious underlying injury, and finally determine if and when an athlete may return to play.
- When approaching the fallen athlete with a suspected head injury, the FP should rapidly assess the ABCs and determine the level of consciousness as well as note any spontaneous movement and speech. Assessment for potential spine injury should be done, and once on the sidelines, a full neurologic examination performed, including a full sensory, motor, and cranial nerve examination as well as cognitive functioning and memory testing.
- Obvious signs of skull fracture or intracerebral bleeding such as pupillary asymmetry, postauricular or periorbital ecchymosis, clear otorrhea, rhinorrhea, or hemotympanum, and any depression in the skull should be searched for. It must be emphasized that

even if the initial examination is completely normal, frequent reassessment is mandatory as victims of head injury will often rapidly deteriorate and many of the above listed findings may not appear until later.

- A concussion is by far the most common head injury in sports and is defined by the American Academy of Neurology (AAN) as "a trauma induced alteration in mental status that may or may not involve loss of consciousness" (Quality Standards Subcommittee, 1997). Several grading systems for concussions exist (Quality Standards Subcommittee, 1997; Cantu, 1986; Colorado Medical Society School and Sports Medicine Committee, 1990) and cannot be adequately discussed in this chapter alone, but broadly speaking, the three most commonly used systems assess severity based on the presence or absence of an LOC and/or posttraumatic amnesia, as well as the duration of *postconcussive symptoms* (PCS).
- Despite the multiple differences amongst the recognized guidelines, most authorities would agree with the following statements:
  1. No athlete should return to play while *any* symptoms are still present either at rest or with exertion.
  2. No athlete should return to play on the same day if the concussion involved an LOC (even if brief) or if postconcussive symptoms are still present 15–20 min after the injury.
  3. An athlete with a mild concussion (Grade 1) with no LOC and resolution of PCS within 15–20 min both at rest and with provocative exertional maneuvers may safely return to play that same day, provided this was the first concussion.
  4. Regardless of whether an athlete returns to play or is disqualified from play for that day, frequent reevaluation and serial examinations are *absolutely mandatory*.
- Two specific head injuries deserve mention because of the rapidity with which they present and their associated morbidity and mortality:

EPIDURAL HEMATOMA
- This most commonly results from a tear of the middle meningeal artery after high-velocity impact to the temporoparietal region and is associated with a skull fracture 80% of the time. Athletes will often experience a brief LOC followed by a lucid interval which may last up to several hours, and then progress to rapid neurologic deterioration and eventually coma and brainstem herniation. Treatment is surgical and immediate transfer to a medical facility is required.

SECOND IMPACT SYNDROME
- This is defined as a second head injury occurring before the symptoms of a first head injury have resolved.

A controversial topic, it is a catastrophic injury that may occur because of a loss of cerebral autoregulation caused by the initial injury (Harmon, 1999; Crump, 2001; Graber, 2001). When the second injury occurs, and it is often a very mild injury, cerebral edema rapidly develops with subsequent brainstem herniation within a matter of seconds to minutes. Treatment consists of immediate intubation and hyperventilation, administration of an osmotic diuretic (i.e., mannitol), and transport to a medical facility. Despite aggressive treatment, mortality and morbidity are around 50% and 100% respectively (Cantu, 1998; 1992).

NECK INJURY

- Neck injuries, although relatively uncommon and usually self-limited (McAlindon, 2002), represent one of the most feared and potentially catastrophic injuries in sports. The FP must promptly recognize the potential for spine injury, adhere strictly to spinal precautions (discussed previously in this chapter), and finally determine whether an athlete requires immobilization and transfer to a medical facility, can return to play, or simply requires further sideline observation.
- Indications for spinal immobilization include a post-traumatic LOC, subjective neck pain or bony tenderness on examination, significant neck/upper back trauma, significant head injury, mental status changes, neurologic abnormalities, or significant mechanism of injury (Luke and Micheli, 1999; McAlindon, 2002).
- One of the more daunting tasks as an FP is distinguishing the minor from the more serious spinal injuries thus determining which athletes may safely return to play after a neck injury. Usually minor, "burners" or "stingers" are nerve injuries resulting from trauma to the neck and/or shoulder that causes either a compressive or a traction injury to the 5th or 6th cervical nerve roots or the brachial plexus itself (Haight and Shiple, 2001; McAlindon, 2002; Kuhlman and McKeag, 1999). It consists of an immediate onset of burning pain radiating down the arm and is usually unilateral in distribution and often associated with other symptoms such as numbness, paresthesias, and muscle weakness or paresis. It is typically self-limiting with most cases resolving in a matter of minutes, although some symptoms may persist for weeks to months.
- A "burner" should *not* be considered as an initial diagnosis if an athlete has any of the following:
  a. Bilateral upper extremity involvement
  b. Any lower extremity involvement
  c. Neck pain or tenderness

- Although there are no definitive guidelines as to which athletes with neck injuries are safe to return to play, it is generally agreed on that only those players with absolutely no neck pain or neurologic symptoms and with completely normal examinations may return to play safely, with repeated evaluation being absolutely necessary (Haight and Shiple, 2001; McAlindon, 2002).

OPHTHALMOLOGIC INJURY

- Any injury to the eye warrants an immediate and thorough ocular examination, as seemingly minor injuries can be potentially vision-threatening. Examination of the eyes should include an assessment of visual acuity, visual fields, the eyelids and periorbital bony structures, the surface of the globe (conjunctiva, sclera, cornea), the pupils (size, shape, reactivity), extraocular movements, and fundoscopic examination and possibly intraocular pressure measurement as indicated (Cuculino and DiMarco, 2002).
- Potential injuries to the eye and/or ocular structures include (Cuculino and DiMarco, 2002) the following:

EYELID LACERATIONS
- Any lacerations involving the lid margin or lacrimal system or those with significant tissue loss should be repaired by an ophthalmologist.

CORNEAL ABRASION
- A superficial defect in the cornea presenting with pain, photophobia, tearing, and a foreign body sensation. Diagnosis is by fluoroscein examination and treatment consists of topical antibiotics, analgesia, and tetanus prophylaxis.

CORNEAL FOREIGN BODY
- The presentation is similar to corneal abrasion, and corneal perforation must be ruled out if there is a history of high-velocity objects involved. Removal can usually be accomplished with slit-lamp assistance under topical anesthesia.

CORNEAL LACERATION
- Many of these are self-sealing and difficult to visualize, thereby requiring a high index of suspicion. Examination may show a teardrop pupil, hyphema, or flat anterior chamber. The eye should be covered with a hard shield and the athlete told not to move the eye. Intraocular pressures should *not* be measured and immediate ophthalmology consult is required.

HYPHEMA

- Blood within the anterior chamber, usually owing to trauma, although atraumatic hyphemas may occur in the presence of coagulopathies. Presenting symptoms include decreased vision, pain, and a history of trauma. The size of the hyphema should be noted, the eye shielded, and immediate ophthalmology consult obtained.

INTRAOCULAR FOREIGN BODY

- Presenting symptoms include pain, irritation, and injection, and suspicion should be based on a history of any high-velocity projectile or metal striking metal. Fluoroscein staining may reveal a positive Seidel sign, a washing away and streaking of fluoroscein as aqueous humor leaks out of the globe. The eye should be shielded, intraocular pressure measurements avoided, and ophthalmology consultation obtained.

GLOBE RUPTURE

- Usually occurs from direct blunt trauma to the eye because of a sudden increase in intraocular pressure. Examination may reveal a total subconjunctival hemorrhage, enophthalmos, teardrop pupil, or a flat anterior chamber. Treatment is the same as that of an intraocular foreign body or corneal laceration.

RETROBULBAR HEMORRHAGE

- Usually occurs after trauma and presents with acute proptosis, pain, swelling, and limitation of *extraocular muscle* (EOM) movement. It is essentially an "orbital compartment syndrome" and irreversible vision loss can occur within 1 h. Immediate referral to an ophthalmologist is required.

ORBITAL RIM FRACTURE

- Usually a result of blunt trauma with examination revealing periorbital bony tenderness, crepitus, or paresthesias in the distribution of the infraorbital nerve, as well as limitation of EOM movement if there is entrapment. Athletes should be sent for radiographic evaluation, with treatment depending on the extent of injury.

NASAL INJURY

- The field-side care of problematic nasal injuries generally involves identification of nasal fractures, control of epistaxis, or treatment of septal hematomas.
- Isolated nasal fractures are usually not corrected acutely unless associated with significant deformity or other soft tissue injury. Treatment includes ice, analgesics, nasal decongestants, and avoidance of further injury.

- Given that 95% of nosebleeds are anterior in origin, most can be controlled with either direct pressure and, if necessary, cauterization of an identified bleeding site or packing with a nasal tampon.
- A potential complication of nasal injuries that must be carefully looked for is a septal hematoma, which is a red-blue, bulging mass on the nasal septum. These should be drained promptly by incision or aspiration followed by packing to prevent reaccumulation, as avascular necrosis and/or an abscess of the nasal septum may develop within a few days if left untreated.

EAR INJURY

- An auricular hematoma is a subperichondral accumulation of blood following blunt trauma. If large enough and left untreated it can cause avascular necrosis as well as asymmetrical regrowth of new cartilage with a resultant cosmetic deformity of the ear known as a *cauliflower ear.* Treatment involves drainage of the hematoma followed by a pressure dressing to prevent reaccumulation.
- Tympanic membrane perforation, although not an acute emergency, must be recognized so that proper follow up care is obtained to ensure proper healing and avoidance of hearing loss. Most will be caused by either blunt or noise induced trauma and greater than 90% will heal spontaneously. Antibiotics (either systemic or topical) are typically not necessary for uncomplicated perforations. Those that are caused by penetrating trauma should be promptly referred to an otolaryngologist.

ABDOMINAL/PELVIC INJURY

- Although potentially serious and even life-threatening, most abdominal injuries can be managed nonoperatively with close observation. These injuries generally result from either rapid deceleration, direct blunt trauma to the abdomen, or indirect trauma from a displaced lower rib fracture (Amaral, 1997).
- Injuries to the abdominal wall include simple contusions and rectus sheath hematomas, both of which are benign and usually managed conservatively, although the latter can occasionally require surgical intervention. The importance of these injuries to the FP lies in excluding associated intra-abdominal injuries, with mechanism of injury being perhaps the most important clue since a single field-side abdominal examination, even if benign, is often misleading and inadequate in excluding significant intra-abdominal injury (Amaral, 1997).

SPLENIC/HEPATIC INJURY

- The spleen and liver comprise the two most common organs injured in blunt abdominal trauma. There may be left or right upper quadrant and/or shoulder pain respectively, as well as signs of hypotension if bleeding is significant. All athletes with significant pain and/or appropriate mechanism of injury should be sent for *computed tomography imaging* (CT scan) and/or observation.

GENITOURINARY INJURY

- Injuries to the renal system seldom require immediate intervention and suspicion should be based on the mechanism of injury as well as the presence and degree of hematuria (Amaral, 1997). One must keep in mind that injury to the kidney may be present without hematuria and that hematuria does not always signify significant renal injury. In terms of evaluating hematuria, usually only those athletes with gross hematuria or with persistent microscopic hematuria accompanied by hypotension or associated nonrenal injuries require radiographic evaluation of the genitourinary system (Amaral, 1997).

URETHRAL/GENITAL INJURY

- Gross blood at the urethral meatus, a scrotal or perineal hematoma, and an absent or high-riding prostate on rectal examination are all signs of urethral trauma and require consideration of a pelvic CT with contrast to look for bladder or urethral extravasation or hematomas followed by a retrograde urethrogram. Blunt trauma to the scrotal area may result in displacement of the testicle into the perineum or inguinal canal or may rupture the testicular capsule, both of which may require surgical intervention. Examination is often difficult because of pain and swelling; however, severe scrotal or testicular swelling or a nonpalpable testicle warrants further evaluation. In the absence of direct trauma, testicular torsion must be ruled out in the athlete presenting with acute onset of testicular pain. In either case, color flow doppler ultrasound studies may define the nature or extent of the problem.

MUSCULOSKELETAL INJURY

- Musculoskeletal injuries are the most commonly encountered injuries in sports. Most are minor and self-limited and it is certainly beyond the scope of this chapter to discuss various specific fractures; however, a few general statements about fracture care can be made and a handful of limb-threatening injuries discussed.

- In terms of fracture care, the FP must always ascertain the mechanism of injury and never assume that the obvious deformity is the only injury. Always check the neurovascular status of the affected body part distal to the fracture site. If there is vascular compromise, reduction of dislocations and/or fractures should be attempted in the field with gentle traction. Otherwise, fractures should be splinted in the position in which they are found, unless some degree of reduction is required because of neurovascular compromise. Finally, no athlete should return to play if there is a question of a fracture, no matter how minor the injury may seem, as this may transform a nondisplaced or a closed fracture into a displaced or open one.
- The following injuries represent a potential threat to a limb:

OPEN FRACTURE

- Previously known as a compound fracture, this is a fracture associated with overlying soft tissue injury with communication between the fracture site and the skin. These are at high risk for subsequent infection and osteomyelitis and require washout in the operating room. On the field, the open wound should be covered with moist sterile gauze and the extremity splinted with no attempts made to push extruding bone or soft tissue back into the wound or reduce the fracture, unless neurovascular compromise is present.

TRAUMATIC AMPUTATIONS

- This is a very rare and dramatic injury which is easy to recognize. The proximal stump should be irrigated with a sterile solution and a sterile pressure dressing applied, with a tourniquet used only for severe, uncontrolled bleeding. The amputated portion should be irrigated, wrapped in a sterile fashion, placed in a bag, and put on ice with rapid transport to an appropriate medical facility.

COMPARTMENT SYNDROME

- This is a state of increased pressure within a closed tissue compartment that compromises blood flow through nutrient capillaries supplying muscles and nerves within that compartment. The potential causes of compartment syndrome are numerous, although in terms of athletes, this is typically an injury with the most common site being the anterior compartment of the leg. Presentation typically occurs within a few hours after injury and will consist of severe and constant pain over the involved compartment, with an increase in pain with both active contraction and passive stretching of the involved muscles. There may also be significant dysesthesias as well as an absent or diminished pulse, pallor, and/or paralysis of the affected neuromuscular group, although these are considered to be late findings which indicate that significant myoneural ischemia has already occurred. Treatment is an emergent fasciotomy and requires rapid transport of the athlete to a medical facility.

KNEE DISLOCATION

- Although extremely rare and usually associated with a high-velocity/high-energy mechanism of injury, this is a very serious injury which may require a high index of suspicion as many dislocations will have spontaneously reduced prior to evaluation. The knee will typically be very swollen and painful and will often demonstrate severe instability in multiple directions on examination. The seriousness of the injury lies in the high rate of associated complications, specifically popliteal artery injury and peroneal nerve injury (which may occur despite spontaneous reduction and normal pulses). Early reduction of a visible dislocation is important. Rapid transport of the patient with a known or suspected dislocation to a medical facility for orthopedic and/or vascular consultation is essential.

HIP DISLOCATION

- Like the knee, this dislocation is rare in sports and usually involves a high-velocity/high-energy mechanism of injury. Posterior dislocations are by far the most common type, and the seriousness of this injury lies in the risk for *avascular necrosis* (AVN) of the femoral head as circulation is disrupted. This occurs in a matter of hours with 6 h being the danger zone—as approximately 60% of reductions beyond 6 h develop AVN, while only 5% of reductions occurring under 6 h develop this complication (Scopp and Moorman, 2002).

ENVIRONMENTAL INJURY

HYPOTHERMIA

- Defined as core body temperature <95°F, this usually occurs as a result of prolonged exposure to cold environmental conditions. When approaching the hypothermic athlete, the FP must keep the following points in mind:
  1. Treatment should routinely start with passive external rewarming (i.e., moving the athlete from a cold to a warm environment, removing all wet clothing, and covering with dry blankets). Active external rewarming and core rewarming should usually be deferred until the hospital environment because patients with moderate to severe hypothermia are at high risk of having significant electrolyte, acid-base, and cardiovascular changes associated with rewarming.
  2. Significantly hypothermic patients are at very high risk of fatal cardiac arrhythmias and should be moved and handled very gently to avoid triggering ventricular fibrillation (Jacobsen et al, 1997).
  3. Pulses are often difficult to detect in significantly hypothermic patients, so CPR should not be started prematurely as it may actually trigger a cardiac dysrhythmia. And if CPR is started, it should continue until warming has been completed; "they're not dead until they're warm and dead."

HYPERTHERMIA

- Heat related illnesses represent a spectrum of disease ranging from heat cramps and edema all the way to heat stroke and death. Heat stroke is a true medical emergency with high mortality rates if unrecognized. It typically presents in warm, humid conditions with elements of overexertion and dehydration on the part of the athlete. Signs of dehydration (tachycardia, hypotension, and oliguria) are often present, as well as a temperature >105°F and prominent *central nervous system* (CNS) and autoregulatory changes. The FP must keep the following in mind when approaching the hyperthermic athlete:
  a. Active and passive cooling measures (i.e., removing from the heat, removing clothing, placing ice packs around the groin, neck, and axillae) should be instituted immediately with the goal of therapy being to lower the core temperature to ≤102°F as quickly as possible (Jacobsen et al, 1997).
  b. Intravenous fluids should be started early; however, caution must be used as overaggressive rehydration may put the victim at an increased risk of pulmonary edema and *adult respiratory distress syndrome* (ARDS). All victims of heatstroke should be transported to a medical facility for further care.

LIGHTNING INJURY

- Although rare, lightning injury is one of the more frequent injuries by a natural phenomenon with the largest number of sports injuries occurring in water sports and most injuries occurring during the months of June–September (Jacobsen et al, 1997). Although it is by definition an *electrical injury*, it differs significantly from high-voltage electrical injuries in both the pattern and severity of injuries as well as the immediate treatment. Although the voltage of lightning is extraordinarily high, it is usually an instantaneous contact that tends to flash over the outside of a victim's body, often creating superficial burns, but sparing extensive damage to internal organs and structures. Lightning may injure a person by striking either the person directly or something they are holding, or by splashing over from a nearby person or object that has been struck. It may also strike the ground and spread circumferentially, often creating multiple victims. Although it can potentially affect any organ system, injuries to the cardiovascular and neurologic systems tend to be the most common, with the immediate cause of death most commonly being cardiopulmonary arrest (Jacobsen et al, 1997). Minor injuries include dysesthesias, minor burns, temporary LOC, confusion, amnesia, tympanic membrane perforation, and ocular injury. More serious injuries usually result from sequelae of the blunt trauma of the electrical blast and from cardiac arrest. The FP should keep the following points in mind when approaching a victim of lightning injury:

1. Standard ACLS protocols should be followed.
2. Victims do not "retain charge" and are not dangerous to touch, so CPR should not be delayed for this reason.
3. Contrary to popular belief, lightning can and often does strike the same place twice, so personal safety must be taken into consideration.
4. Hypotension in a lightning victim should prompt a search for occult hemorrhage or fractures as a result of blunt trauma. Spinal precautions are required.
5. Pupils may become "fixed and dilated" because of the nature of lightning injuries and this should not preclude resuscitation attempts as these changes do not necessarily indicate brain death in lightning victims.
6. In lightning victims with cardiopulmonary arrest, cardiac automaticity and contractions will often resume spontaneously and in a short period of time, while respiratory arrest from paralysis of the medullary respiratory center may be prolonged. Therefore, unless the victim is ventilated quickly they will progress to a secondary hypoxic cardiac arrest despite normal cardiac activity. If promptly resuscitated and supported, full recovery may ensue.
7. In consideration of the previous two points, in a multicasualty situation from a lightning strike, the FP should always resuscitate the dead first, a reversal of the standard rule of triage where the obvious moribund are left to the last.

SUMMARY

• In conclusion, though most sports related injuries are minor, for the few urgent/emergent events the FP will encounter, planning is paramount. Medical equipment appropriate for the event and knowledge of life support techniques is essential. A study of the topics presented here should be helpful in preparing for field-side emergencies.

REFERENCES

Amaral JF: Thoracoabdominal injuries in the athlete. *Clin Sports Med* 16(4):739–753, 1997.

Blue JG, Pecci MA: The collapsed athlete. *Orthop Clin North Am* 33(3):471–478, 2002.

Cantu RC: Guidelines for return to contact sports after a cerebral concussion. *Phys Sportsmed* 14(10):75, 76, 79, 83, 1986.

Cantu RC: Second-impact syndrome. *Clin Sports Med* 1: 37–44, 1998.

Cantu RC: Second impact syndrome: Immediate management. *Phys Sportsmed* 20(9):55–66, 1992.

Colorado Medical Society School and Sports Medicine Committee: Guidelines for the management of concussion in sports. *Colo Med*, 87:4, 1990.

Committee on Trauma: *Advanced Trauma Life Support for Doctors: Student Course Manual.* American College of Surgeons, 1997.

Crump WJ: Managing adolescent sports head injuries: A case-based report. *Fam Prac Recert* 23(4):27–32, 2001.

Cuculino GP, DiMarco CJ: Common ophthalmologic emergencies: A systematic approach to evaluation and management. *Em Med Rep* 23(13):163–178, 2002.

Fowler R, Pepe PE: Prehospital care of the patient with major trauma. *Emerg Med Clin North Am* 20(4):953–974, 2002.

Gastel JA, Palumbo MA, Hulstyn MJ, et al: Emergency removal of football equipment: a cadaveric cervical spine injury model. *Ann Emerg Med* 32(4):411–417, 1998.

Graber M: Minor head trauma in children and athletes. *Emerg Med* 14, 17, 18, 20, Oct. 2001.

Haight RR, Shiple BJ: Sideline evaluation of neck pain. *Phys Sportsmed* 29(3):45–62, 2001.

Harmon KG: Assessment and management of concussion in sports. *Am Fam Physician* 60(3):887–892, 1999.

Jacobsen TD, Krenzelok EP, Shicker L, et al: Environmental injuries. *Dis Mon* 814–912, 1997.

Kuhlman GS, McKeag DB: The "burner": A common nerve injury in contact sports. *Am Fam Physician* 60(7):2035–2040, 1999.

Luke A, Micheli L: Sports injuries: Emergency assessment and field-side care. *Pediatr Rev* 20(9):291–302, 1999.

McAlindon RJ: On field evaluation and management of head and neck injured athletes. *Clin Sports Med* 21(1):1–14, 2002.

McCaffrey FM, Braden DS, Strong WB. Sudden cardiac death in young athletes. *Am J Dis Child* 145:177–83, 1991.

O'Connor FG, Kugler JP, Oriscello RG: Sudden death in young athletes: Screening for the needle in a haystack. *Am Fam Physician* 57(11):2763–2770, 1998.

Partridge RA, Coley A, Bowie R, et al: Sports-related pneumothorax. *Ann Emerg Med* 30(4):539–541, 1997.

Quality Standards Subcommittee: Practice parameter: The management of concussion in sports (summary statement). *Neurology* 48:581–585, 1997.

Scopp JM, Moorman CT: Acute athletic trauma to the hip and pelvis. *Orthop Clin North Am* 33(3):555–563, 2002.

Winbery SL, Lieberman PL: Anaphylaxis. *Immunol Allergy Clin North Am* 15(3):447–475, 1995.

5 MASS PARTICIPATION EVENTS
Scott W Pyne, MD, FAAFP

GOALS

- Mass participation events are those sporting events in which many people participate and are generally spread out over several miles and variable terrain.
- Advanced planning and preparation are critical to successfully accommodate the medical needs of the event participants.
- The medical director has numerous responsibilities of planner, communication, and organizer in addition to the care of injured athletes.

MEDICAL COVERAGE

- The needs of the athletes competing must be considered well prior to the event.
- Specific considerations of the type of event, number of participants, course peculiarities, and environmental predictions are all very important in determining the medical coverage required.

SAFE ENVIRONMENT

- As a key advisor to the Event Director, the medical director must ensure that the event is conducted with the safety of the competitors being of utmost importance. Often this is furthest from the minds of race organizers especially with competing priorities of sponsor, financial and community concerns.
- In extreme conditions the race may need to be cancelled or rescheduled. It is best that these possibilities and contingency plans be discussed and prepared prior to the race day.
- It is often necessary to review the course for any potential trouble-spots and hazards that could cause injury. The start and finish are common sites of medical concern. The start area should be on a large level surface devoid of obstacles, thereby allowing the athletes to more easily accommodate the surge that invariably occurs. The finish area should also be large enough to prevent the athletes from bunching up and being forced to stand in one place. It should also have necessary facilities and resources to allow the athletes to properly cool down and recover after the event and easy access to medical treatment areas.
- Biking, swimming, and skiing events carry additional risk elements (Mayers and Noakes, 2000), such as water safety and trauma potential associated with high speeds. Water temperature, sea conditions, road conditions, transition, acceleration and deceleration areas, and protective equipment must be carefully scrutinized.

EPIDEMIOLOGY

INJURY RATE

- Running (42 km) 1–20%, running (<21 km) 1–5%, triathlon (225 km) 15–30%, nordic skiing (55 km) 5%, triathlon (51 km) 2–5%, cycling (variable) 5% (Roberts, 1989).
- Injury rate increases with increased distance and environmental temperature. (Holtzhausen and Noakes, 1997; Hiller et al, 1987)

PREDICTING INJURY RATE

- Previous years' experience is very helpful in planning for subsequent years. This also stresses the importance of a reliable injury data tracking system.
- Similar events in similar elements can be used in the initial planning and preparation stages.
- Fortunately the risk for exertional death in marathons is quite small. (Maron et al, 1996)

MEDICAL PHILOSOPHY

LEVEL OF CARE

- The level of medical care that will be available on the course must be defined and agreed on between the medical director and the event director early in the planning stage.

- This may differ among the aid stations throughout the course with the most robust resources usually being provided at the finish area.
- The usage and type of intravenous fluids, availability of oxygen, medications, and advanced cardiac and trauma life support equipment are all areas requiring discussion.
- Coordination with the local *emergency medical system* (EMS) and emergency rooms and hospitals is absolutely required.
- Mobile medical assets in the form of bike, canoe/ kayak teams or EMS units provide an excellent means to access injured competitors throughout the course (Laird, 1989).

MEDICATION PLAN

- A decision must be made as to the provision of medication on the race course and in the medical aid stations. It is recommended that these medications be tightly controlled and kept to a minimum if dispensed at all.
- In longer events it is not uncommon for athletes to carry and take their own medication during the event. This must be anticipated to best treat the competitor and prevent overprescribing.
- The availability of urgent or emergency medication, such as aspirin, epinephrine auto-injector, albuterol meter dose inhaler, glucose, and *advanced cardiac life support* (ACLS) medications should be considered.

LABORATORY PLAN

- Medical aid stations may or may not have basic laboratory capability. The ability to assess an athletes' blood glucose and sodium levels will assist with their rapid evaluation and allow for the appropriate treatment of a collapsed athlete (Davis, et al, 2001).
- Hand held glucose and electrolyte monitors are readily available and have become part of the standard medical kit for many endurance events (Speedy et al, 2003).

COMMUNICATION PLAN

- It is vital that medical support assets have the ability to communicate with each other, EMS assets, local hospitals, and the event director before, during, and after the competition.
- Various communication networks have been used to include cellular phones, computer networks, ham radio, and hand-held radios. These systems should be tested well before the event and a backup plan should be established in the case of failure of the primary means of communication.
- A communication plan outlining how EMS will be requested and dispatched, where injured athletes will be taken and when to contact the medical director will increase the efficiency of the medical care provided.

MEDICAL CHAIN OF COMMAND

- An individual must be identified to serve as the medical director. His or her responsibilities include advanced planning, event day medical decision making, and medical troubleshooting. The medical support staff, event director, and media—all benefit from having one identified contact, rather than a committee, to answer all medical issues.
- It is also recommended that each aid station have an assigned medical leader well versed in the event medical philosophy. This medical leader can organize the support staff and coordinate medical care provided locally.

MEDICAL TRAINING

MEDICAL STAFF

- It is common that the medical support for mass participation events is gathered from a diverse background and experience level. Most are better versed in medical care within a clinical or hospital facility than in the field environment.
- The medical plan, chain of command and level of care provided must be reviewed with the medical staff. It is helpful although not always practical to provide an education session prior to race day.
- Triage and treatment guidelines specific for the event provided in writing are useful as well as administration information to include the course map, parking, proximity to water, food and facility stations, communication, and transportation plans.

COMPETITORS

- Participants should also be given medical information prior to the event. This is most easily provided with the race information and can be coordinated through the event director. Additions to event websites, handouts to accompany the race packet pick-up and information posters displayed in common areas are several examples.

- Common medical conditions and their prevention, location of medical aid stations on the course and available services at these areas assist the participants in their planning and preparation for a safe event.
- Medical presentations to the athletes and interest groups are often well received.
- Race-day information regarding weather conditions and health warnings has been used with success at numerous events (Cianca et al, 2001).

STAFFING

MEDICAL AND NONMEDICAL SUPPORT

- The appropriate staffing of medical treatment areas with both medical and nonmedical staff is important in the safe conduct of the medical aid station. The composition and number of this staff will vary depending on the location and nature of the event.
- The number of staff can be best derived from previous experience or through comparison with similar events in similar conditions. A helpful guide from the American College of Sports Medicine (Armstrong et al, 1996) is to provide the following medical personnel per 1000 runners: 1 or 2 physicians, 4–6 podiatrists, 1–4 emergency medical technicians, 2–4 nurses, 3–6 physical therapists, 3–6 athletic trainers, and 1–3 assistants. Approximately 75% of these personnel should be stationed at the finish area.
- Nonmedical staff can assist with the transport of injured athletes, documentation, medical tracking, and provide information within the medical aid station and to event staff.

STAFF FEEDBACK

- After the event it is most important to elicit feedback from both medical and nonmedical staff. This often identifies areas that had not been considered in the initial planning and execution phases of the event.
- The follow-up of these comments in a written after-action report is highly recommended as it allows the documentation of areas of concern, develops solutions, and prepares for subsequent events.

TRIAGE AND TREATMENT GUIDELINES

- The majority of the medical conditions presenting at a given event can be predicted well in advance. Preparing, training, and practicing for these conditions

are important in the evaluation, treatment, and disposition of injured participants.

SEVERE VS. NONSEVERE

- The initial evaluation of an athlete in the medical aid station should focus on the severity of their injury (Holtzhausen and Noakes, 1997). Fortunately most complaints are nonsevere in nature and can be quickly treated and released.
- Severe medical conditions include cardiac events, hypothermia, hyperthermia, hyponatremia, near-drowning, and head and neck trauma. These can be quickly differentiated from nonsevere conditions by the evaluation of mental status, rectal temperature (Roberts, 2000), blood pressure, and pulse. Serum glucose and sodium levels may also aid in the diagnosis.
- Depending on the medical care plan of the event, some of these severe conditions may be treated at the medical aid station or transported via EMS to the most appropriate medical treatment facility.

MEDICAL VS. MUSCULOSKELETAL

- Medical conditions, such as exercise associated collapse, heat stroke, chest pain and hyponatremia can be triaged from muscle cramps, blisters, and extremity pain in the treatment areas.
- This separation of care allows the assignment and preparation of support staff in the area of care for which they are most experienced. This also allows those with more severe conditions to be treated in the same area where they can be more closely monitored.
- The establishment of a medical holding area has proven successful (O'Connor et al, 2003). This area is reserved for athletes who are waiting for transportation for nonsevere conditions or who are not prepared to leave the medical area, but do not require further care. This group is continuously observed and encouraged to make their way back to the after event areas.

EVALUATION OF EXERCISE ASSOCIATED COLLAPSE

- The majority of cases of exercise associated collapse are the result of predictable physiologic events associated with exertion and respond rapidly to positioning with the head down and legs and pelvis elevated position (Holtzhausen and Noakes, 1997). These athletes generally have normal mental status.

- Individuals with altered mental status should be rapidly evaluated with a rectal temperature for hyperthermia or hypothermia. Persistent altered mental status with relatively normal rectal temperatures should be treated as suspected hyponatremia until proven otherwise (Holtzhausen and Noakes, 1997).
- Hyperthermic individuals should be rapidly cooled on site, preferably with ice water immersion (Mayers and Noakes, 2000; Holtzhausen and Noakes, 1997).

FINANCE AND LOGISTICS

FINANCIAL PLANNING

- The conduct of mass participation events both requires and has the potential to generate money. Medical directors must ensure that the safety of the participants and the support staff is not compromised by decisions to increase revenue for the event. The medical director must be involved in any plans affecting the event that may have medical implications.
- Planning for the costs of medical supplies, transportation, and personnel compensation must be made and agreed on early in the event planning process.

MEDICAL AID STATION LOCATION

- The spacing of medical aid stations throughout the course is determined by many variables. The course must be previewed and the location of medical aid stations established based on anticipated need, appropriate location, and course specific considerations (Cianca et al, 2001).
- Medical aid stations must be easily identifiable to competitors and EMS units.
- Medical evacuation routes must be established to avoid conflict with the event in progress and ensure the most efficient transport requirements.

TRANSPORTATION PLAN

- It is not unusual for participants to decide that a medical treatment area is a good place to end their participation in the event. If this decision is realized in the middle of the course, a plan for the removal of these athletes must be used.
- Many races have a "sweep" vehicle that follows the last competitor and can transport these participants to the finish area. Other transport arrangements may be available depending on the nature of the event, but must be anticipated prior to the event.

MEDICAL-LEGAL

- An additional responsibility of the medical director is the assurance of medical staff liability coverage.
- General event insurance packages usually exclude medical coverage (Dooley, 1999).
- Options for medical liability coverage should be discussed with legal representation in advance of the event and include individual or group policies—Good Samaritan laws.

CONCLUDING COMMON SENSE PRINCIPLES

- Medical planning and preparation are absolute requirements for the successful conduct of mass participation events.
- Following established medical plans, treatment guidelines, and remembering limitations with a focus on competitor and staff safety invariably results in a fulfilling experience for everyone involved.

REFERENCES

Armstrong LE, Epstein Y, Greenleaf JE, et al: America College of Sports Medicine: Position statement on heat and cold illnesses during distance running. *Med Sci Sports Exerc* 28:i–vii, 1996.

Cianca JC, Roberts WO, Horn D: Distance running: Organization of the medical team, in O'Connor FG, Wilder RP (eds.): *Textbook of Running Medicine*, New York, NY, McGraw-Hill, 2001, pp 489–503.

Davis DP, Videen JS, Marino A, et al: Exercise associated hyponatremia in marathon runners: A two-year experience. *J Emerg Med* 21(1):47–57, 2001.

Dooley JW: Professional liability coverage (medical malpractice). *Road Race Manage* Oct, 3, 1999.

Hiller WD, O'Toole ML, Fortess EE, et al: Medical and physiologic considerations in triathlons. *Am J Sports Med* 15(2):164–168, 1987.

Holtzhausen LM, Noakes TD: Collapsed ultraendurance athlete: Proposed mechanisms and an approach to management. *Clin J Sports Med* 7(4):292–301, 1997.

Laird RH: Medical care at ultraendurance triathlons. *Med Sci Sports Exerc* 21(5):S222–S225, 1989.

Maron BJ, Poliac LC, Roberts WO: Risk for sudden cardiac death associated with marathon running. *J Am Coll Cardiol* 28:428–431, 1996.

Mayers LB, Noakes TD: A guideline to treating ironman triathletes at the finish line. *Physician Sports Med* 28(8):33–50, 2000.

O'Connor FG, Pyne SW, Brennan FH: Exercise-associated collapse: An algorithmic approach to race day management part I of II. *Am J Med Sports* 5:221–217, 229, 2003.

Roberts WO: Assessing core temperature in collapsed athletes: what's the best method? *Physician Sports Med* 28(9):71–76, 2000.

Roberts WO: Exercise-associated collapse in endurance events. A classification system. *Physician Sports Med* 17:49–57, 1989.

Speedy DB, Noakes TD, Holtzhausen LM: Exercise-associated collapse. *Physician Sports Med* 31(3), 2003.

6 CATASTROPHIC SPORTS INJURIES

Barry P Boden, MD

INTRODUCTION

- In the United States approximately 10% of all brain injuries and 7% of all new cases of paraplegia and quadriplegia are related to athletic activities (Mueller, 1996).
- Information on catastrophic injuries in athletes is collected by the National Center for Catastrophic Sports Injury Research (NCCSIR), the US Consumer Product Safety Commission (CPSC), and the professional league data registries.
- The NCCSIR defines catastrophic sports injury as "any severe spinal, spinal cord, or cerebral injury incurred during participation in a school- or college-sponsored sport." Concussions are not considered to be catastrophic injuries.
- The NCCSIR classifies injuries as direct, resulting from participating in the skills of a sport (i.e., trauma from a collision), or indirect, resulting from systemic failure owing to exertion while participating in a sport.
- The NCCSIR subdivides catastrophic injuries into three categories: fatal, nonfatal, and serious. A nonfatal injury is any injury where the athlete suffered a permanent, severe, functional disability. A serious injury is a severe injury with no permanent functional disability, e.g., a fractured cervical vertebra without paralysis (Mueller, 1996).
- The CPSC operates a statistically valid injury and review system known as the *national electronic injury surveillance system* (NEISS) (www.cpsc.gov). The NEISS estimates are calculated using data from a sample of hospitals that are representative of emergency departments in the United States. The CPSC does not provide data on injury specifics nor does it include information on injuries that initially presented to physician offices.
- The National Collegiate Athletic Association (NCAA) and the National Federation of State High School Associations (NFSH) review injury epidemiology annually and publish a rules book for each sport with the intent of promoting safe play (www.ncaa.org; www.nfhs.org).

EPIDEMIOLOGY

- For all sports followed by the NCCSIR, the total direct and indirect incidence of catastrophic injuries is 1 per 100,000 high school athletes and 4 per 100,000 college athletes (Mueller and Cantu, 2000).
- The combined fatality rate for direct and indirect injuries in high school is 0.40 for every 100,000 high school athletes and 1.42 for every 100,000 college participants (Mueller and Cantu, 2000).
- Football is associated with the greatest number of catastrophic injuries for all major team sports.
- Pole vault, gymnastics, ice hockey, and football have the highest incidence of injury per 100,000 male participants (Mueller and Cantu, 2000).
- Cheerleading is associated with the highest number of direct catastrophic injuries for all female sports (Mueller and Cantu, 2000).

INDIRECT INJURIES

- Indirect or nontraumatic deaths in athletes have been identified to be predominantly caused by cardiovascular conditions such as *hypertrophic cardiomyopathy* (HCM), cardiac artery anomalies, myocarditis, aortic stenosis, and dysrhythmias. The most common etiology of sudden cardiac death is HCM for those under age 35, and coronary artery disease for those over age 35. Noncardiac conditions that cause fatalities are heat illness and miscellaneous diagnoses such as rhabdomyolysis, status asthmaticus, and electrocution caused by lightning.

CARDIAC CONDITIONS

- Most young athletes who die suddenly have HCM. These athletes typically have prodromal symptoms such as presyncope or syncope with or without exercise prior to the fatal event. A systolic murmur is often appreciated only in the standing position or with a Valsalva maneuver.

- Congenital coronary artery anomalies are a frequent cause of sudden cardiac death. These athletes may or may not have symptoms of syncope or chest pain with exercise making diagnosis difficult.
- Athletes with aortic stenosis and mitral valve prolapse have abnormal auscultatory findings that should lead to the suspected diagnosis.
- The preparticipation physical is critical for detecting cardiac conditions that may be life threatening.

HEAT ILLNESS

EPIDEMIOLOGY
- Heat illness is the third most common cause of death in athletes.
- Risk factors for heat illness include obesity, fever, recent respiratory or *gastrointestinal* (GI) viral illness, sickle cell trait, stimulants, supplements such as ephedrine, illicit drugs, alcohol, sleep deprivation, sunburn, and underconditioned athletes (Coyle, 2000).
- Heat illness usually occurs during unseasonable hot conditions at times of extreme exertion. A typical scenario is an obese football lineman wearing a football uniform and playing two a day practices during late summer tryouts in the Southeast United States.

CLINICAL FEATURES
- Heat cramps is a misnomer and should be termed exercise cramps. Muscle cramping is triggered by fatigue and can occur at any temperature.
- Heat syncope is associated with an abrupt loss of consciousness in a heat-exposed athlete whose core temperature is normal or mildly elevated. The condition often occurs toward the completion of exercise owing to reduced cardiac return and postural hypotension. Heat syncope usually occurs during the first few days of heat exposure before the body has been allowed to acclimatize.
- Heat exhaustion is defined as the inability to continue to exercise in the heat since the *cardiovascular* (CV) system fails to respond to workload. The condition occurs at core or rectal temperatures between 100.4 and 104°F. Symptoms of heat exhaustion can include muscle cramping, mild confusion, headache, dizziness, chills, nausea, and often collapse.
- Heatstroke is exercise-associated collapse with thermoregulatory failure and *central nervous system* (CNS) dysfunction. Heatstroke and mental status changes begin at temperatures in excess of 104°F. The athlete may or may not be sweating. The condition

may result in a variety of life-threatening problems, such as rhabdomyolysis, renal failure, *disseminated intravascular coagulopathy* (DIC), liver failure, and brain injury.
- The athlete with repeated heat illness requires a workup for a muscle enzyme deficiency.

DIAGNOSIS AND TREATMENT
- A correct diagnosis is based on the history, physical examination, core body temperature, and differential including hyponatremia and cardiac conditions.
- Treatment involves rapid cooling, moving to a cooler environment, removing clothing, tepid water spray, fans, and ice to the neck, groin, and axilla. Hydration should include both oral intake and *intravenous* (IV) fluids. Rehydration with sports drinks containing electrolyes is preferred over water. Athletes with core temperatures greater than 104°F should be considered for cold water immersion. *Emergency medical services* (EMS) should be contacted for athletes with heat exhaustion and heat stroke.

PREVENTION
- The incidence of heat illness can be significantly reduced by frequent hydration, acclimatization, identifying at-risk athletes, and monitoring daily weights, medication use, and status of recent illnesses.

DIRECT INJURIES

FOOTBALL

EPIDEMIOLOGY
- Football has the highest number of catastrophic head and neck injuries per year for all high school and college sports (Mueller and Cantu, 2000).

MECHANISMS
- Spearing or tackling a player with the top of the head has been identified as a major cause of permanent cervical quadriplegia. When the neck is flexed 30° the cervical spine becomes straight and the forces are transmitted directly to the spinal structures. In 1976, spearing was banned and the rate of catastrophic cervical injuries dramatically dropped (Torg et al, 2002; Torg and Gennarelli, 1994).
- *Cervical cord neurapraxia* (CCN) is an acute, transient neurologic episode associated with sensory changes with or without motor weakness or complete paralysis in the arms, legs, or both (Torg et al, 2002). Complete recovery usually occurs within 10 to 15 min but may take up to 2 days. The *pincer* mechanism

involves cord compression either through hyperflexion or hyperextension of the neck. An episode of CCN is not an absolute contraindication to return to football. It is unlikely that athletes who experience CCN are at risk for permanent neurologic sequelae with return to play. The overall risk of a recurrent CCN episode with return to football is approximately 50% and is correlated with the canal diameter size. The smaller the canal diameter the greater the risk of recurrence.

PREVENTION

• Banning spearing-tackling and teaching players to play "heads up" ball with no contact on the top of the helmet has dramatically reduced the incidence of permanent cervical quadriplegia.
• The development of a safety standard for the football helmet by the National Operating Committee on Standards for Athletic Equipment (NOCSAE) has also been a significant factor in reducing head and neck injuries.
• Training medical personnel to understand on-field management of athletic head and neck injuries and guidelines for return to contact or collision sport after an injury.

POLE VAULTING

EPIDEMIOLOGY

• Pole vaulting is a unique sport in that athletes often land from heights ranging from 10 to 20 ft. Pole vaulting has one of the highest rates of direct, catastrophic injuries per 100,000 participants for all sports monitored by the NCCSIR (Boden et al, 2001).
• The vast majority of catastrophic pole vaulting injuries are head injuries in male athletes. The overall incidence of catastrophic pole vault injuries is two per year, while the incidence of fatalities is one per year. Most injuries occurred at the high school level (Boden et al, 2001).

MECHANISMS OF INJURY

• Three common mechanisms of injury have been described (Boden et al, 2001). The most common mechanism occurs when a pole vaulter lands with his body on the edge of the landing pad and his head whips off the pad, striking the surrounding hard surface (in most cases either concrete or asphalt). The second most common mechanism occurs when the vaulter releases the pole prematurely or does not have enough momentum and lands in the vault or planting box. The third most common mechanism occurs when the vaulter completely misses the pad and lands directly on the surrounding hard surface.

PREVENTION

• As of Jan 2003, both the NCAA and NFHS decided to increase the minimum pole vault landing pad size from 16′ × 12′ to 19′8″ × 16′5″. Because the majority of injuries are a result of athlete's either completely or partially missing the landing pad, this rule change has the potential to significantly reduce the number of catastrophic injuries.
• Any hard or unyielding surfaces such as concrete, metal, wood, or asphalt around the landing pad must be padded or cushioned.
• A new rule has been adopted placing the crossbar farther back over the landing pad. This should reduce the chance of an athlete landing in the vault or planting box.
• A coach's box or painted square in the middle of the landing pad is being promoted. This zone would help train athletes to instinctively land near the center of the landing pad. Other safety measures include marking the runway distances so athletes can better gage their takeoff, and prohibiting the practice of tapping or assisting the vaulter at takeoff.
• Pole vaulting is a complicated sport requiring extensive training. Certification by coaches is encouraged.
• The value of helmets in reducing head injuries in high school pole vaulters is controversial. Without conclusive data as to their protective effect, the use of helmets is optional for athletes at this time (www. skyjumpers.com).

SOCCER

EPIDEMIOLOGY

• Injuries to the head, neck, and face in soccer account for between 5 and 15% of all injuries. Most head and neck injuries occur when two players collide, especially when jumping to head the ball.
• Fatalities in soccer are usually associated with either movable goalposts falling on a victim or player impact with the goal post (Janda et al, 1995). The CPSC identified at least 21 deaths over a 16-year period associated with movable goalposts (www. cpsc.gov).
• The incidence of concussions in high level soccer athletes is approximately one per team per season (Boden et al, 1998). There is a 50% chance for a professional athlete to sustain a concussion over a 10-year span. Most concussions occur as a result of contact with an opposing player, not with the soccer ball.

- There is no evidence that an isolated episode of heading a soccer ball can cause any head injury; however, there is controversy over whether repetitive soccer heading over a prolonged career can lead to neuropsychologic deficits.

PREVENTION

- Children should never be allowed to climb on the net or goal framework. Soccer goalposts should be secured at all times. During the off-season, goals should either be disassembled or placed in a safe storage area. Goals should be moved only by trained personnel, and should be used only on flat fields (www.cpsc.gov). The use of padded goalposts may also reduce the incidence of impact injuries with the goalposts (Janda et al, 1995).
- Children should use smaller soccer balls to reduce the risks of repetitive heading. Leather or water-soaked soccer balls should never be used. Proper heading techniques should be employed: contact on the forehead with the neck muscles contracted. Soccer players should be trained to hit the ball, not to be hit by the ball. A long-term prospective study on the cumulative effects of heading a soccer ball is currently underway.

WRESTLING

EPIDEMIOLOGY

- Indirect catastrophic wrestling injuries are often the result of rapid weight loss which causes dehydration and potential cardiovascular compromise (Kiningham and Gorenflo, 2001; Oppliger et al, 1996).
- There are approximately 2.11 direct catastrophic wrestling injuries per year at the high school and college levels (Boden et al, 2002). The direct catastrophic injury rate in high school and college wrestlers is approximately 1 per 100,000 participants. The majority of injuries occur in match competitions, where intense, competitive situations place wrestlers at a higher risk (Boden et al, 2002; Jarrett et al, 1998; Pasque and Hewett, 2000).
- There is a trend toward more direct injuries in the low- and middle-weight classes.
- Cervical fractures or major cervical ligament injuries constitute the majority of direct catastrophic wrestling injuries (Boden et al, 2002).

MECHANISM

- The position most frequently associated with injury is the defensive posture during the takedown maneuver, followed by the down position (kneeling), and the lying position (Boden et al, 2002). There is no clear predominance of any one type of takedown hold that contributes to wrestling injuries.
- The athlete is typically injured by one of three scenarios: (1) The wrestler's arms are in a hold such that he or she is unable to keep from landing on his or her head when thrown to the mat. (2) The wrestler attempts a roll but is landed on by the full weight of his opponent, causing a twisting, usually hyperflexion, neck injury. (3) The wrestler lands on the top of his head, sustaining an axial compression force to the cervical spine.

PREVENTION

- A minimum body fat for high school and college wrestlers has been established to reduce weight loss injuries. The NFHS also instituted a rule that competitors cannot lose more than 1.5% body weight per week. Both the NCAA and NFHS have banned the use of laxatives, diuretics, and other rapid weight loss techniques such as rubber suits.
- Referees should strictly enforce penalties for slams and gain more awareness of dangerous holds (Boden et al, 2002). There is particular vulnerability for the defensive wrestler who may be off balance, have one or both arms held, and then have his opponent land on top of him. Stringent penalties for intentional slams or throws are encouraged. The referee should have a low threshold of tolerance to stop the match during potentially dangerous situations.
- Coaches can prevent serious injuries by emphasizing safe, legal wrestling techniques (Boden et al, 2002). Coaches should teach wrestlers to keep their head up during any takedown maneuver to prevent axial compression injuries to the cervical spine. Proper rolling techniques, with avoidance of landing on the head, need to be emphasized in practice sessions.

CHEERLEADING

EPIDEMIOLOGY

- Over the past 20 years cheerleading has evolved into an activity demanding high levels of skill, athleticism, and complex gymnastics maneuvers (www.aacca.org).
- In 2002 cheerleading was one of the four most popular organized sports activities for women in high school.
- Cheerleaders in college and high school account for more than half of the catastrophic injuries that occur in female athletes (Mueller and Cantu, 2000).
- There are approximately 1.95 direct catastrophic cheerleading injuries per year. The catastrophic injury rate is 0.4 per 100,000 in high school cheerleaders,

- 2 per 100,000 college participants, or an overall rate of 0.6 per 100,000 cheerleaders (Boden et al, in press).
- In 2000 the CPSC estimated a total of 1258 head injuries in cheerleaders of which 604 were recorded as concussions and 6 as skull fractures. In the same year there were 1814 neck injuries with 76 fractures in cheerleaders that initially presented to an emergency department in the United States (www.cpsc.gov).
- Compared with other sports, cheerleading has a low overall incidence of injuries, but a high risk of catastrophic injuries.
- The majority of injuries occur in female athletes because there are more female than male cheerleaders and the women are usually at the top of the pyramid or being thrown into the air during basket tosses. The majority of injuries occur during the winter months, because cheerleaders perform on indoor hard surfaces.
- College athletes are five times more likely to sustain a catastrophic injury than their high school counterparts (Boden et al, in press). This finding is likely owing to the increased complexity of stunts at the college level.
- Catastrophic head injuries are twice as common as cervical injuries.

MECHANISMS

- The most common stunts resulting in catastrophic injury are the pyramid or the basket toss. The cheerleader at the top of the pyramid is most frequently injured. A basket toss is a stunt where a cheerleader is thrown into the air, often between 6 and 20 ft, by either three or four tossers. Poor judgment or inadequate training of the spotter is often the main problem leading to injury.
- Less common mechanisms include advanced floor tumbling routines, participating on a wet surface, or performing a mount. The majority of injuries occur when an athlete lands on an indoor hard gym surface (Boden et al, in press).

PREVENTION

- Height restrictions on pyramids are limited to two levels in high school and 2.5 body lengths in college (www.ncaa.org; www.nfhs.org). The top cheerleaders are required to be supported by one or more individuals (base) who are in direct weight-bearing contact with the performing surface. The base cheerleaders must remain stationary and maintain constant contact with the suspended or top athlete. Spotters must be present for each person extended above shoulder level. The suspended person is not allowed to be inverted (head below horizontal) or to rotate on the dismount. Limiting the total number of cheerleaders in a pyramid as well as the quick transitions between pyramids and other complex stunts may also help reduce injuries.

- Basket toss rules limit the stunt to four tossers, starting the toss from the ground level (no flips) and having one of the tossers behind the top person during the toss (www.ncaa.org; www.nfhs.org). The top person (flyer) is trained to be directed vertically and not allow the head to drop backward out of alignment with the torso or below a horizontal plane with the body. Other safety measures that may reduce the incidence of basket toss injuries include evaluating the height thrown, using mandatory landing mats for complex stunts, and improving the skills of the spotters.
- All stunts should be restricted when wet conditions are present.
- Injuries from floor tumbling routines can be prevented by proper supervision, progression to complex tumbling only when simple maneuvers are mastered, and using spotters as necessary.
- Minitrampolines, springboards, or any apparatus used to propel a participant have been prohibited since the late 1980s.
- A landing mat should be employed during all complex stunts.
- Cheerleading coaches need to place equal time and attention on the technique and attentiveness of spotters in practice compared with the athletes' performing the stunts.
- Coaches are encouraged to complete a safety certification, especially for any teams that perform pyramids, basket tosses, and/or tumbling.
- Pyramids and basket tosses should be limited to experienced cheerleaders who have mastered all other skills and should not be performed without qualified spotters or landing mats.

BASEBALL

EPIDEMIOLOGY

- Baseball has a low rate of noncatastrophic injuries, but a high incidence of catastrophic injuries.
- Head injuries constitute the majority of catastrophic injuries.
- There are approximately two direct catastrophic injuries reported to the NCCSIR per year or 0.6 injuries per 100,000 participants (Mueller and Cantu, 2000). The total incidence of catastrophic injuries and fatalities is 5 and 13 times higher, respectively, at the college level than at the high school level (Boden et al, unpublished).

MECHANISMS

- The most common mechanism is a pitcher hit by a batted ball, followed by a collision of two fielders, and a collision of a runner and a fielder (Boden et al, unpublished). An area of controversy in baseball is the safety of aluminum or enhanced bats. Nonwood bats are typically lighter than woods bats and can be swung faster with greater ball velocity off the bat.

- Commotio cordis is arrhythmia or sudden death from low-impact blunt trauma to the chest in subjects with no preexisting cardiac disease (Maron et al, 1995; Janda et al, 1998). The proposed mechanism is impact just prior to the peak of the T wave on an EKG which induces ventricular fibrillation. The pediatric population may be more susceptible because of a thinner layer of soft tissue to the chest wall, increased compliance of the immature rib cage, and slower protective reflexes.

PREVENTION

- Protecting pitchers from a batted ball may be accomplished by requiring pitchers to wear helmets at all times, using protective screens during batting practice, and regulating the bat and ball (Boden et al, unpublished).
- In 2003, the NCAA and NFHS placed new regulations on bats. All bats must be certified as having a ball exit speed that cannot exceed 97 miles per hour as measured by the Baum hitting machine. In addition, certified bats may not weigh more than 3 oz less than the length of the bat (i.e., a 34-in. long bat cannot weigh less than 31 oz) (www.nfhs.org).
- Decreasing the ball's hardness and weight may significantly reduce injury severity. The coefficient of restitution or the measure of rebound that a ball has off a hard surface cannot exceed 0.555 at the high school and college levels.
- Preventive strategies for commotio cordis include teaching youth baseball players to turn their chest away from a batted ball. The use of chest protectors is controversial. Automatic external defibrillators hold promise for preventing fatalities but require further research (Maron et al, 1995; Janda et al, 1998).

ICE HOCKEY

EPIDEMIOLOGY

- Although the number of catastrophic injuries in ice hockey is low compared with other sports, the incidence per 100,000 participants is high (Mueller and Cantu, 2000).
- The majority of catastrophic injuries occur to the cervical spine.

MECHANISMS

- Most injuries occur when an athlete is struck from behind by an opponent and contacts another object, especially the boards, with the crown of the head (Reid and Saboe, 1989; Tator et al, 1991).

- Head and facial injuries are common from collisions or being hit by the puck or stick.
- Catastrophic accidents from collisions with goalposts were common before the advent of displaceable goalposts.

PREVENTION

- Enforcing current rules against pushing or checking from behind.
- Encouraging the use of helmets and face masks.
- Padding the boards and developing a potential space between the boards and the plexiglass extension may reduce the frequency and severity of head and neck injuries.
- Ensuring that the goals can slide out of position to protect athletes from colliding against an immovable object.
- Discouraging aggression and fighting in hockey.

SWIMMING

MECHANISMS

- Most catastrophic swimming injuries are related to the racing dive into the shallow end of pools (Mueller and Cantu, 2000).
- Hyperventilating just prior to swimming can rid the body of carbon dioxide. This fools the brain into thinking it doesn't need to breathe, even when its oxygen stores are dangerously low, which may lead to loss of consciousness and drowning.

PREVENTION

- At the high school level, swimmers must start the race in the water if the water depth at the starting end is less than 3.5 ft. If the water depth is 3.5 ft to less than 4 ft at the starting end, the swimmer may start from the deck or in the water. If the water depth at the starting end is 4 ft or more the swimmer may start from a platform up to 30 in. above the water surface (www.nfhs.org).
- The NCAA is in the process of requiring water depth at the starting end to be a minimum of 5 ft when starting platforms are in use (www.ncaa.org).
- The NFHS mandates that swimmers break the surface of water to breathe at or before 15 m to prevent shallow water blackout.

GYMNASTICS

- There is a paucity of information on catastrophic gymnastics injuries.

• Most injuries are associated with a missed vault, a fall from the parallel bars or horizontal bar, or a faulty dismount (Mueller and Cantu, 2000).

GENERAL PREVENTION TIPS
• Preparticipation physicals
• Qualified coaches
• Proper strength and conditioning programs
• Supervision of athletes at all times
• EMS protocols in place at all times
• Continued research concerning catastrophic injuries and methods to prevent these injuries

REFERENCES

Boden BP, Kirkendall DT, Garrett WE: Concussion incidence in elite college soccer players. *Am J Sports Med* 26:238, 1998.

Boden BP, Lin W, Young M, et al: Catastrophic injuries in wrestlers. *Am J Sports Med* 30:791, 2002.

Boden BP, Pasquine P, Johnson J, et al: Catastrophic injuries in pole-vaulters. *Am J Sports Med* 29:50–54, 2001.

Boden BP, Tacchetti R, Mueller FO: Catastrophic injuries in baseball. *Am J Sports Med* 32, 2004. (in press)

Boden BP, Tacchetti R, Mueller FO: Catastrophic injuries in cheerleaders. *Am J Sports Med*. 31:881–888, 2003.

Coyle, JF: Thermoregulation, in Sullivan JA, Anderson SJ (eds.): *Care of the Young Athlete*. American Academy of Pediatrics and American Academy of Orthopedic Surgeons, 2000, pp 65–80.

Janda DH, Bir C, Wild B, et al: Goal post injuries in soccer: A laboratory and field testing analysis of a preventive intervention. *Am J Sports Med* 23:340, 1995.

Janda DH, Bir CA, Viano DC, et al: Blunt chest impacts: Assessing the relative risk of fatal cardiac injury from various baseballs. *J Trauma* 44:298–303, 1998.

Jarrett GJ, Orwin JF, Dick RW: Injuries in collegiate wrestling. *Am J Sports Med* 26:674–680, 1998.

Kiningham RB, Gorenflo DW: Weight loss methods of high school wrestlers. *Med Sci Sports Exerc* 33:810–813, 2001.

Maron BJ, Poliac LC, Kaplan JA, et al: Blunt impact to the chest leading to sudden death from cardiac arrest during sports activities. *N Engl J Med* 333:337–342, 1995.

Mueller FO: Introduction, in Mueller FO, Cantu RC, VanCamp SP (eds.): *Catastrophic Injuries in High School and College Sports*. Champaign, IL, HK Sport Science Monograph Series, 1996.

Mueller FO, Cantu RC: NCCSIR nineteenth annual report. *National Center for Catastrophic Sports Injury Research: fall 1982–spring 2000*. Chapel Hill, NC, National Center for Sports Injury Research, 2000.

Oppliger RA, Case HS, Horswill CA, et al: American College of Sports Medicine position statement: Weight-loss in wrestlers. *Med Sci Sports Exerc* 28:ix–xii, 1996.

Pasque CB, Hewett TE: A prospective study of high school wrestling injuries. *Am J Sports Med* 28:509–515, 2000.

Reid DC, Saboe L: Spine fractures in winter sports. *Sports Med* 7:393–399, 1989.

Tator CH, Edmonds VE, Lapczak L, et al: Spinal injuries in ice hockey players, 1966–1987. *Can J Surg* 34(1):63–69, 1991.

Torg JS, Gennarelli TA: Head and cervical spine injuries, in DeLee JC, Drez Jr D (eds.): *Orthopaedic Sports Medicine: Principles and Practice*. Philadelphia, WB, Saunders, 1994, pp 417–462.

Torg JS, Guille JT, Jaffe S: Current concepts review: Injuries to the cervical spine in American football players. *J Bone Joint Surg* 84-A:112, 2002.

www.aacca.org; American Association of Cheerleading Coaches and Advisors.

www.cpsc.gov; United States consumer product safety commission summary reports. *National Electronic Injury Surveillance System*. Washington, DC, US Consumer Product Safety Commission.

www.ncaa.org

www.nfhs.org

www.skyjumpers.com.

---

7 ORTHOPEDIC SPORTS MEDICINE TERMINOLOGY

Scott A Magnes, MD

One of the challenges facing orthopedic surgeons is the communication barrier that exists when interacting with others outside our specialty. Orthopedic surgery has a vocabulary that is unique, and few health care workers outside of the field speak this language fluently. This is also true in our subspecialty of orthopedic sports medicine. The purpose of this chapter is to attempt to make readers more fluent in our language in order to enhance meaningful communication.

GENERAL TERMINOLOGY

• **Accessory or supernumerary bone:** Develops from separate center of ossification from parent bone; may or may not obtain bony union with parent bone.
• **Active motion:** *Range of motion* (ROM) of a joint that a patient is able to achieve on his own.
• **Active-assisted motion:** ROM of a joint that a patient is able to achieve with the assistance of the examiner.
• **Allograft:** Cadaver graft.
• **Anatomic Axis (of lower extremity):** Angle formed by intersection of lines through the femoral and tibial shafts with patient standing. The difference between the mechanical and anatomic axis is usually $5 \pm 2°$.

- **Apophysis:** Secondary growth center forming bony outgrowth that remains a part of the native bone, e.g., process, tubercle, and tuberosity.
- **Aphophysitis:** Inflammation of an apophysis
- **Arthritis:** Joint inflammation
- **Arthrosis:** Joint degeneration
- **Atrophy:** Muscle wasting, loss of muscle mass
- **Autograft:** Graft from one's own body
- **Avascular necrosis, aseptic necrosis, osteonecrosis (AVN):** Blood supply to the affected bone is insufficient, resulting in bony necrosis, etiologies include idiopathic, traumatic, steroids, heavy alcohol usage, dysbaric illness (Caisson disease), blood dyscrasias (e.g., sickle cell disease), high doses of radiation therapy, and Gaucher's disease. Untreated, the natural disease progression is to DJD.
- **Avulsion fracture:** Injury to tendinous insertion site where a small piece of bone is fractured in continuity with the tendon, rather than rupture at the tendon-bone interface.
- **Bone bruise:** Microfractures seen on MRI. This is common with ACL injuries where the lesions are located on the lateral femoral condyle and the posterior portion of the lateral tibial plateau.
- **Bursitis:** Inflammation of a bursa
- **Chondromalacia:** Softening or damage to the articular cartilage of the patella—diagnosis made under direct visualization at the time of surgery. This term is often used to describe similar lesions in other bones.
- **Chondrosis:** Chondral degeneration
- **Diaphysis:** Midshaft, tubular portion of long bone
- **Dislocation:** Complete loss of apposition of articulating bones that normally comprise a joint.
- **Effusion:** Fluid within a joint
- **Epiphysis:** Center of ossification, longitudinal growth center
- **Extension lag:** Lack of normal active extension of a joint with normal passive extension, usually measured in degrees
- **Flexion contracture:** Lack of normal active and passive extension of a joint usually measured in degrees
- **Incidence:** The number of new cases of a disease or injury and the like that occur during a specified period of time in a defined population.
- **Instability:** Functional term referring to joint *laxity*—may be unidirectional or multidirectional, with the etiology being post-traumatic or congenital.
- **Laxity:** Degree of looseness, usually referring to a ligament. Symptomatic laxity is termed *instability*.
- **Long bone:** Length > width, found in limbs
- **Mechanical axis (of lower extremity):** Angle formed by intersection of lines drawn from center of femoral head to center of knee joint, and center of knee joint to center of ankle with patient standing

- **Metaphysis:** Area adjacent to physis, consists of cancellous bone.
- **Osteochondritis dissecans (OCD):** A fragment of subchondral bone and its overlying chondral cartilage are separated from the underlying bone. The etiology is unclear, but most likely traumatic. Most often it occurs in the knee and the most common location is the lateral aspect of the medial femoral condyle.
- **Osteotomy:** Transection of a bone, often refers to the tibia or femur to correct for varus or valgus deformities. The surgeon alters the mechanical axis of the limb in an attempt to alleviate malalignment, arthrosis, and pain.
- **Passive motion:** ROM of a joint performed by the examiner
- **Physis:** Growth plate
- **Prevalence:** The number of cases of a disease or injury and the like present in a defined population during a particular point in time
- **Proprioception:** Reflex mechanism whereby position sense receptors are able to detect the position of a joint in space and therefore provide a coordinated muscular response to aid in stabilization of a joint. This important skill is often ignored or underrehabilitated following injury.
- **Recurvatum:** Hyperextension of a joint
- **Sesamoid bone:** Bones located within tendons
- **Short bone:** More cuboidal in shape, found in carpus and tarsals
- **Sprain:** Injury to a ligament owing to excessive stress
- **Strain:** Injury to a muscle or tendon owing to excessive stress
- **Stress views:** Radiographs used to assess ligamentous integrity by stressing the involved ligaments and assessing for increased laxity, often comparing to the normal contralateral side
- **Subluxation:** Partial dislocation of a joint
- **Tendonitis (tendinitis):** Inflammation of a tendon
- **Tendonopathy (tendinopathy):** Diseased tendon
- **Tendonosis (tendinosis):** Tendon degeneration (usually focal)
- **Tenosynovitis:** Tendon sheath inflammation
- **Tensile strength:** Maximum stress that a structure can sustain before failure

TERMINOLOGY REFERRING TO FRACTURES

- **Alignment:** Relationship of the longitudinal axis of one fracture fragment to another
- **Angulation:** Position of distal fracture fragment in relation to the proximal fragment or direction of the apex of the angle formed by the fracture fragments

- **Apposition:** Contact of the ends of the fracture fragments
- **Avulsion:** Bony fragment is pulled away from its native bone by muscle contraction (e.g., mallet finger) or a passive opposing force to a ligament (e.g., tibial avulsion fracture of ACL).
- **Butterfly fragment:** Wedge-shaped fracture fragment that is separated from the main fracture fragment in a comminuted fracture
- **Closed:** Intact skin
- **Comminuted:** More than two fracture fragments
- **Compression:** Usually refers to vertebral fracture where impaction occurs
- **Delayed union:** Failure of union in the duration of time that healing usually takes place for that bone.
- **Depression:** An impaction-type fracture where the hard surface of one bone is driven into a second softer surface of bone (e.g., tibial plateau fracture).
- **Diastasis:** Abnormal separation of two bones, e.g., symphysis pubis diastasis secondary to ruptured ligaments, widened ankle mortise secondary to syndesmosis disruption
- **Displacement:** Degree of loss of anatomic position
- **Distraction:** Opposing ends of fracture fragments are not in contact, e.g., secondary to musculotendinous forces, interposed soft tissue, and the like suboptimal for fracture healing.
- **Extra-articular:** Does not penetrate the joint
- **Fibrous union:** Healing with fibrous tissue rather than bony callus
- **Fracture (fx or #):** Complete or incomplete discontinuity (break) of bone or cartilage
- **Impaction:** One fracture fragment is forcibly driven (telescoped) into another adjacent fragment, e.g., Colles fracture.
- **Incomplete fractures:** Only one cortex of the bone has been broken and the other remains intact.
- **Intra-articular:** Involves articular surface of a joint
- **Malunion:** Healing of the fracture in an unacceptable position
- **Nonunion:** Failure of bony union with cessation of healing process
- **Pseudoarthrosis:** Nonunion of a fx resulting in a *false joint*
- **Oblique:** Fracture line is oblique to the long axis of the bone.
- **Open:** Fracture site communicates with ambient environment (old term was *compound*).
- **Pathologic:** Fractures occurring in bones that have been weakened by disease.
- **Remodeling:** Occurs in skeletally immature patients with healed fractures such that future bony growth will serve to correct bony deformity, if it is not rotational in nature. Potential for remodeling is greatest in

younger children, fractures occurring in close proximity to the physis and if the bony displacement is in the plane of motion of the affected joint.
- **Segmental:** Comminuted fracture where a long bone is separated into at least three segments
- **Spiral:** Caused by a torsional force and is akin to an oblique fracture that encircles the long bone.
- **Transverse:** Fracture is perpendicular to the long axis of the bone.
- **Union:** Healing of fracture

FRACTURE EPONYMS

- **Aviator's astralgus:** General term referring to fracture or fracture-dislocation involving the talus
- **Barton's fracture:** Dorsal articular margin fracture of the distal radius
- **Bennett's fracture:** Triangular-shaped intra-articular fracture involving the radial portion of the base of the thumb metacarpal with proximal dislocation of the metacarpal shaft
- **Boxer's fracture:** Fracture of the neck of the small metacarpal. This term is often incorrectly used to describe a similar fracture in other metacarpal bones.
- **Chance fracture:** This is usually caused by a flexion injury to the spine resulting in a sagitally oriented fracture through the posterior spinous process and neural arch exiting the superior articular surface of the involved vertebral body just anterior to the neural foramina (spinal canal).
- **Chauffeur's fracture:** Triangular-shaped oblique articular fracture involving the radial portion of the distal radius
- **Chopart's fracture and dislocation:** Injury involving the midtarsal joints (talonavicular and calcaneocuboid) of the foot
- **Clay-shoveler's fracture:** Fracture of the posterior spinous process(es) of the lower cervical and/or upper thoracic vertebrae
- **Colles fracture:** Comminuted fracture of the distal radius occurring in osteopenic bone as a result of a fall on an outstretched hand resulting in dorsal angulation of the fracture fragments
- **Dashboard fracture:** Posterior wall acetabular fracture
- **Essex-Lopresti fracture:** Comminuted radial head fracture with associated dislocation of the distal radioulnar joint
- **Galeazzi's fracture:** Radius fracture at the junction of the middle and distal thirds with concomitant subluxation of the distal ulna
- **Greenstick fracture:** Incomplete, angulated fracture that occurs in skeletally immature patients that results

in bowing of the affected bone, with the affected cortex always occurring on the convex surface
- **Jones fracture:** Fracture of the base of the small metatarsal occurring at the metaphyseal–diaphyseal junction. The significance is that this is a vascular watershed area resulting in an increased propensity to nonunion requiring a short leg cast and nonweight bearing.
- **Lis-Franc's fracture/dislocation:** Occurring at the tarsometatarsal joint of the foot. There are two types: Homolateral (all rays dislocate laterally) and divergent (lesser rays are dislocated laterally).
- **Maissoneuve fracture:** Fracture of the proximal one-third of the fibula associated with rupture of the tibia–fibula syndesmosis and fracture of the medial malleolus or rupture of the deltoid ligament
- **Mallet finger (baseball finger):** Flexion deformity of the distal phalanx resulting from a separation of the common extensor tendon at its insertion at the dorsal base of the distal phalanx with or without an avulsion fracture
- **March fracture:** Stress or fatigue fracture usually referring to the metatarsals
- **Monteggia's fracture:** Fracture of the proximal third of the ulna with anterior dislocation of the radial head.
- **Nightstick fracture:** Fracture of the ulnar shaft
- **Piedmont fracture:** Isolated, closed fracture of the radius at the junction of the middle or distal-thirds
- **Rolando's fracture:** Y-shaped intra-articular fracture at the base of the thumb metacarpal
- **Segond's fracture (lateral capsular sign):** Avulsion fracture of the lateral capsule off the lateral tibial plateau associated with an ACL injury.
- **Torus fracture ("buckle" fracture):** Incomplete fracture with buckling of one cortex predominantly in skeletally immature patients. It usually occurs with a fall on an outstretched hand and is a stable fracture.

CLASSIFICATION SYSTEMS

ACROMIOCLAVICULAR JOINT INJURIES

- **Type 1:** *Acromioclavicular* (AC) ligament sprain
- **Type 2:** Partial tear of the AC ligament; sprain of *coracoclavicular* (CC) ligaments
- **Type 3:** AC and CC ligaments disrupted with superior displacement of the clavicle <100% of the width of the clavicle
- **Type 4:** AC and CC ligaments disrupted with clavicle displaced into or through trapezius
- **Type 5:** As in type 3 except that clavicle is displaced superiorly 100–300%.

- **Type 6:** AC and CC ligaments disrupted with clavicle displaced inferiorly

ACROMION MORPHOLOGY

- Bigliani described the morphology of the acromion. It is felt that increasing curvature is associated with higher risk for rotator cuff pathology and impingement. The classification system is based on morphology of the acromion as seen on the *supraspinatus outlet* (SSO) view radiograph. The increased curvature is most often associated with arthrosis of the acromion.
- **Type 1:** Flat acromion
- **Type 2:** Curved acromion
- **Type 3:** Hooked acromion

ARTICULAR CARTILAGE LESIONS

- Outerbridge published his classification system for chondromalacia patellae. Today it is used to classify chondrosis thoughout the knee and other joints, as well. This classification is often used incorrectly, and a new classification system is needed. Until then, the author recommends the lesions be described on the basis of anatomic location, dimension of lesions, and depth of penetration in order to avoid any misunderstandings in communication.

MODIFIED OUTERBRIDGE CLASSIFICATION

- **Grade I:** Cartilage softening and swelling
- **Grade II:** Fragmentation and fissuring <1 cm in diameter
- **Grade III:** Fragmentation and fissuring >1cm in diameter
- **Grade IV:** Erosion of cartilage to bone (i.e., full thickness damage)

AMERICAN MEDICAL ASSOCIATION LIGAMENT INJURY CLASSIFICATION

- **Grade I:** Minor tearing without increase in translation of affected joint (with laxity testing on PE)
- **Grade II:** Partial tear with mild-moderate increased translation
- **Grade III:** Complete tear with marked increase in translation

LAXITY

Looseness, usually referring to a ligament compared with the normal contralateral side
- **Grade I:** (1+): up to 5 mm
- **Grade II:** (2+): from 6 to 10 mm
- **Grade III:** (3+): >10 mm

NERVE INJURIES (SEDDON CLASSIFICATION)

- **Neurapraxia:** No structural damage to nerve with complete recovery expected
- **Axonotomesis:** Disruption of the axon and myelin sheath with resulting degeneration of the axon distal to the site of injury; recovery expected
- **Neurotmesis:** Partial or complete tear of nerve with disruption of axon, myelin sheath, and connective tissue elements; recovery not expected

NERVE INJURIES (SUNDERLAND CLASSIFICATION)

- **Type 1:** Neurapraxia
- **Type 2:** Axonotomesis
- **Type 3:** Neurotmesis—loss of nerve fiber continuity with perineurium and epineurium intact
- **Type 4:** Neurotmesis—loss of nerve fiber continuity with only epineurium intact
- **Type 5:** Neurotmesis—complete transection of nerve

STRAIN (CLASSIFICATION):

- **1st Degree:** Minimal damage to the muscle, tendon, or musculotendinous unit
- **2nd Degree:** Partial tear to the muscle, tendon, or musculotendinous unit
- **3rd Degree:** Complete disruption to the muscle, tendon, or musculotendinous unit

BIBLIOGRAPHY

Beaty, Kasser (eds.): *Rockwood & Green's Fractures in Children*, 5th ed. Baltimore, MD, Lippincott, Williams & Wilkins, 2001.

Bigliani LU, Morrison D, April EW: The morphology of the acromion and its relationship to rotator cuff tears. *Orthop Trans* (10):228, 1986.

Bucholz, Heckman (ed.): *Rockwood & Green's Fractures in Adults*, 5th ed. Baltimore, MD, Lippincott, Williams & Wilkins, 2001.

DeLee, Drez (eds.): *Orthopaedic Sports Medicine: Principles and Practices*, 2nd ed. Philadelphia, Elsevier Science, 2003.

Fairbank TJ: Knee joint changes after meniscectomy. *JBJS(B)* 30(4):664–670, 1948.

Helms CL: *Fundamentals of Skeletal Radiology*, 2nd ed. Mosby, Churchill, W. B. Saunders, 1995.

Newman Dorland WA, (Ed.): *Dorland's Illustrated Medical Dictionary*, 29th edn., Mosby, Churchill, W. B. Saunders, 2000.

Outerbridge RE: The etiology of chondromalacia of the patellae. *JBJS(B)* (43):752–755, 1961.

Seddon JH: Three types of nerve injury. *Brain* 66(4):237–288, 1943.

Sunderland S: A classification of peripheral nerve injuries producing loss of function. *Brain* 74:491–516, 1951.

Tria AJ, Klein KS: *An Illustrated Guide to the Knee.* New York: Churchill Livingstone, 1992.

8 BASICS IN EXERCISE PHYSIOLOGY

Patricia A Deuster, PhD, MPH
David O Keyser, PhD

SKELETAL MUSCLE PHYSIOLOGY

THE SKELETAL MUSCLE FIBER

BASIC UNITS
- The primary components of skeletal muscle include the sarcomere, the myofilaments, the myofibril (basic unit of contraction), the muscle fiber (cell), fascicles (bundles of about 150 muscle fibers each), and a muscle (Fig. 8-1). The sarcomere, an area from Z-disk to Z-disk and the functional contraction unit of a myofibril, contains two types of myofilaments: thick (myosin) and thin (actin) myofilaments, which are repeated throughout the muscle myofibril.
- Other important structures within a sarcomere are I-bands, A-bands, H-zones (absence of actin), and M-bands (sarcomere's center). Transverse tubules (T-tubules: see Excitation-Contraction Coupling), found at the A–I junction of the sarcomere, and the *sarcoplasmic reticulum* (SR) are the primary regulators of calcium influx into muscle units. The muscle cell membrane is the sarcolemma.

MUSCLE PROTEINS
- Key skeletal muscle proteins include actin, myosin, troponin, and tropomyosin. Actin and myosin make up the myofilaments within the myofibril, with myosin being the site of ATP binding. A troponin complex on the actin molecule acts as a calcium binding site to initiate contraction, and tropomyosin is found in the thin filaments of muscle fibers, where it inhibits contraction until modified by troponin.

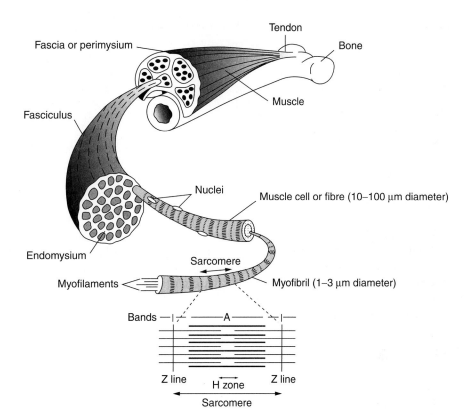

FIG. 8-1 Basic anatomy and structure of skeletal muscle. (Reprinted with permission from www.medicdirect.com and www.medicdirect.co.uk.)

MUSCULAR CONTRACTION

MOTOR NEURONS

- Two specific motor neurons for initiating and regulating muscle contraction are the alpha and gamma neurons. Alpha motor neurons are responsible for initiating contractions in the contractile (extrafusal) fibers of the muscles, whereas the gamma neurons innervate muscle spindle (intrafusal) fibers of the muscle (see below).

MOTOR UNIT

- The motor unit, the basic functional unit of movement, comprises an alpha motor neuron, a synaptic junction (motor endplate), and the muscle fibers it innervates.
- One motor neuron can innervate 10 to several thousand muscle fibers. Release of acetylcholine by the neurons initiates contraction and degradation of acetylcholine by cholinesterase terminates the action potential.

EXCITATION-CONTRACTION COUPLING (EC COUPLING)

- Muscle contraction is triggered by an electrical impulse involving acetylcholine release, arrival at the sarcolemma (muscle cell membrane) after crossing the synaptic junction, and the subsequent entry of calcium into the myofibril. The electrical impulse travels quickly into the interior of the muscle cell, down the T-tubules with release of calcium from the SR to the myofibril.
- Once calcium stores are released from the SR, a non-stoppable contraction is initiated: calcium entry activates crossbridge linkages and contraction of the sarcomere.
- **Sliding filament theory:** The sliding filament theory states that muscle contraction occurs when the two major myofilaments (actin and myosin) slide past one another through a series of crossbridge linkages. Myosin crossbridge linkages combine, detach, and recombine in an oscillatory pattern such that at any point in time about 50% of the myosin heads are attached to actin binding sites. None of the myofilaments actually change length.
- **All or none law:** If a motor neuron initiates an action potential and releases acetylcholine at the neuromuscular junction, then all muscle fibers innervated by that motor neuron will contract simultaneously. Muscle fibers achieve gradation of contraction strength by recruiting fewer or more motor neurons to initiate contraction and/or by changing the frequency of action potentials to sustain contractions.

TABLE 8-1   Characteristics of Major Skeletal Muscle Fiber Types*

FIBER CHARACTERISTICS	SLOW TWITCH	FAST TWITCH	
Other terminology	Type I	Type IIa	Type IId(x)
	Slow Oxidative (SO)	Fast/Oxidative/Glycolytic (FOG)	Fast/Oxidative/Glycolytic (FOG)
Aerobic capacity	HIGH	MED/HIGH	MED
Myoglobin content	HIGH	MED	LOW
Color	RED	RED	PINK/WHITE
Fatigue resistance	HIGH	MED/HIGH	MED
Glycolytic capacity	LOW	MED	MED/HIGH
Glycogen content	LOW	MED	HIGH
Triglyceride content	HIGH	MED	MED/LOW
Time to peak tension	SLOW	MED	MED/HIGH
Myosin ATPase activity	LOW	MED	MED
Myosin heavy chain (MHC)	MHCIβ	MHCIIa	MHCIId(x)
Tension cost[†]	LOW	MED	MED
ATP/ADP	LOW	MED	MED

*This chart represents current nomenclature for human skeletal muscle fiber types. Former Type IIb human muscle fibers are currently referred to as Type IId(x) because of MHC types found in human muscle. Type IIb muscle fibers and Type IIb MHC are found in rodents and other species (Pette and Staron, 2001; Staron, 1997; Zhen-He et al, 2000).

[†]Tension cost = ATPase activity to isometric tension ratio.

SENSORY RECEPTORS

- **Muscle spindles:** These specialized intrafusal muscle fibers are located between and among extrafusal fibers deep within the interior of the muscle. As proprioceptors, they sense and relay the length or velocity of a muscle's movement (e.g., patellar reflex).
- **Golgi tendon organs:** These sensory organs detect differences in tension and muscle length. Although quiescent during periods of slow to moderate muscle activity, they increase discharge when muscle load is excessive. *Golgi tendon organs* (GTO) act to protect against injury due to overloading.

SKELETAL MUSCLE FIBER TYPES

- Skeletal muscle is extremely dynamic, with various fiber types characterized by differences in morphology, histochemistry, enzyme activity, surface characteristics, and functional capacity (Pette and Staron, 2001; Staron, 1997). Table 8-1 presents selected characteristics of muscle fiber types as currently designated in human skeletal muscle.
- Within the normal population, the distribution of specific fiber types depends on a variety of factors, and shows extraordinary adaptive potential in response to innervation/neuronal activity, hormones, neural signalling, training/functional demands, and aging (Pette and Staron, 2001). Muscle fiber type appears to change in response to these effectors in a sequential manner from either slow to fast or fast to slow (Demirel et al, 1999; Pette and Staron, 2001; Zhen-He et al, 2000).

- Recent advances in fiber typing have brought about a change in nomenclature for human muscle fiber types: Type IIb is now referred to as Type IId(x) due to the expression of the *myosin heavy chain* (MHC) form IId(x). MHC IIb is expressed in rodents and other species, but does not appear as a distinct fiber type in humans (Pette and Staron, 2001; Staron, 1997; Zhen-He et al, 2000).

ENERGY METABOLISM

ENERGY SYSTEMS

- Energy for muscular activity can be derived from three specific systems (Table 8-2, Fig. 8-2). The *immediate, or phosphagen, system* consists of *adenosine triphosphate* (ATP) and *creatine phosphate* (PC or phosphocreatine); it allows for very short bursts of maximal power.
- The *short term, or glycogen-lactic acid, system* consists of glucose entering the glycolytic pathway and the subsequent oxidation of pyruvic acid to lactic acid. The short term system is often classified as anaerobic because it can occur in the absence (or presence) of oxygen (O_2). The energy formed allows for only 1–1.6 min of maximal muscle activity at a reduced power output as compared to the phosphagen system.
- The *aerobic, or long term, system* involves glucose entering the glycolytic pathway through to pyruvic acid and its subsequent oxidation to acetyl *coenzyme A* (CoA) for entry into the *tricarboxylic acid* (TCA)

TABLE 8-2 Comparison of the Maximal Rates of Power and Length of Time Power Can be Maintained for the Immediate-, Short-Term, and Long-Term Energy Systems

ENERGY SYSTEMS	MOLE OF ATP/MIN	TIME TO FATIGUE
Immediate: Phosphagen (Phosphocreatine and ATP)	4	5 to 10 s
Short-term: Glycogen-lactic acid (Glycolytic)	2.5	1.0 to 1.6 min
Long-term: Aerobic	1	Unlimited time

cycle. Other organic compounds can also enter the TCA cycle. *Free fatty acids* (FFA) from triglycerides are broken down into two-carbon acetyl fragments and joined with CoA to form acetyl CoA. This process,

known as â-oxidation, can only occur under aerobic conditions.

• Amino acids can also enter the TCA cycle after deamination/transamination and conversion into forms such as acetyl CoA and/or acetoacetate. The reduced coenzymes, NADH and $FADH_2$, formed during glycolysis and the TCA cycle, are shuttled to the electron transport chain within the mitochondria. There they are oxidized to NAD and FAD, respectively, and ATP is regenerated from ADP with 2.5 ATP/NADH and 1.5 ATP /$FADH_2$. The O_2 used is tightly linked to aerobic ATP production.

• One molecule of glucose going through the glycolytic pathway to lactate yields 2 ATP, whereas one molecule of glucose going through the aerobic pathway yields 30 ATP.

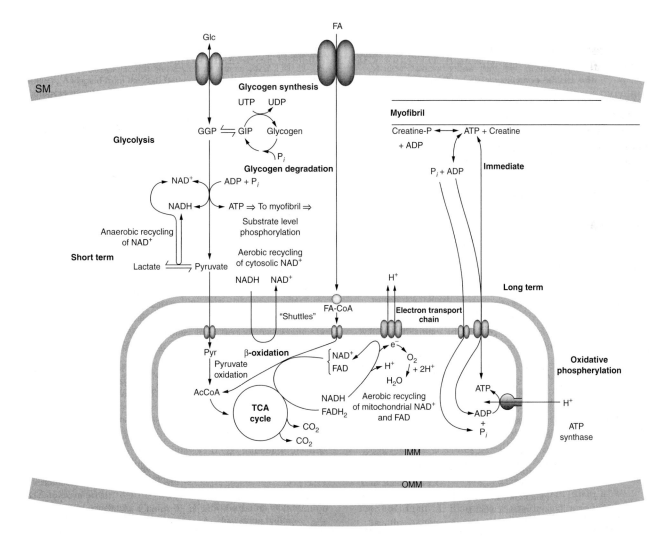

FIG. 8-2 A schematic of the energy systems in skeletal muscle: immediate, short term and long term. SM: Sarcolemma, Glc: Glucose; FA: Free Fatty Acid; OMM: Outer mitochondrial membrane; IMM: Inner Mitochondrial Membrane. (Designed by Mark Roseman, PhD.)

TABLE 8-3 Energy Stores for a 60-Kg Person with 15% Body Fat

ENERGY SOURCE	ENERGY (GRAMS)	ENERGY (KCAL)
Liver and muscle glycogen	400–750	500–1000
Glucose in body fluids	15–20	60–80
Total carbohydrate stores	**415–770**	**560–1080**
Subcutaneous adipose triglycerides	9000	81,000
Intramuscular triglycerides	150	1350
Total triglyceride stores	**9150**	**82,350**
Total energy stores	**9435–9920**	**82,970–83,430**

ENERGY STORES AND SOURCES

- ATP, glucose, and free fatty acids are stored in various amounts, with ATP storage being sufficient for only 5 to 7 s of activity. Glycogen, the storage form of carbohydrate and a polymer of glucose, is found in both liver and muscle tissue.
- Triglycerides, the storage form of lipids, consist of three fatty acids and a glycerol backbone. Amount and energy yields for glycogen (4 kcal/g) in liver and skeletal muscle and triglycerides (9.4 kcal/g) in skeletal muscle and adipose tissues are shown in Table 8-3.
- Storing 1 g of glycogen requires at least 2 g of water, thus the energy yield is less than half of what would be expected from the weight: if there were 120 g of glycogen, then 80 g would be water and the energy yield would be 160 rather than 480 kcal.

- Type 2 fibers store more glycogen but less triglyceride than Type 1 fibers. Proteins are not a storage form of energy, and require catabolism of tissue for energy.
- The breakdown of glycogen to form glucose for energy is called *glycogenolysis* and the process of converting amino acids or lactate into glucose is called *gluconeogenesis*.

BASIC DEFINITIONS IN EXERCISE PHYSIOLOGY

PULMONARY VENTILATION

- The total volume of air moved into and out of the lungs each minute, commonly called *minute ventilation* (VE), is a function of *tidal volume* (VT) and *respiratory rate* (fB). At rest, VE is between 5 and 7 L/min, whereas during exercise it increases to between 60 and 180 L/min, depending on the health of the person (Fig. 8-3). VT increases by expanding both inspiratory and expiratory volumes: these *extra* volumes are called *inspiratory* and *expiratory reserve volumes* (IRV and ERV), respectively. The increase in VT allows VE to increases five-to tenfold during exercise. An increase in fB further augments VE.

MAXIMAL VOLUNTARY VENTILATION

- *Maximal voluntary ventilation* (MVV), a measure of maximum breathing capacity, is the volume of air exchanged during repeated maximal respirations in a specified time period (10 to 15 s). It is expressed as

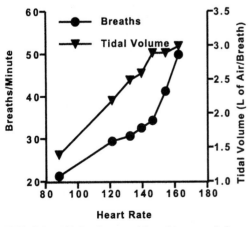
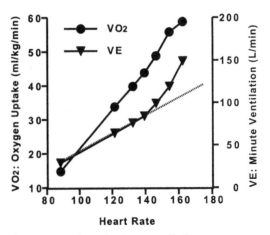

FIG. 8-3 Tidal volume and breathing rate (left panel) and oxygen uptake and minute ventilation (right panel) in response to progressive maximal treadmill exercise. Dotted line through VE in right panel indicates departure from linearity.

L/min and represents a limit for comparison with maximal VE during exercise (VE_{max}).

BREATHING RESERVE

• The difference between MVV and VE_{max}: *breathing reserve* (BR) is sometimes expressed as VE_{max}/MVV. Theoretically, BR is the additional VE available during maximal exercise. If a person achieves maximal work capacity prior to attaining MVV, the person has a normal BR, whereas if MVV = VE, the person may have compromised pulmonary function. A typical BR is 11 L/min, with normal VE_{max}/MVV ranging between 0.6 and 0.75 (60 to 75%).

OXYGEN UPTAKE (VO₂)

• Oxygen uptake (VO_2) is based on the Fick equation and can be expressed as: $VO_2 = CO \times (a\text{-}VO_2) = HR \times SV \times (a\text{-}VO_2)$, where CO = cardiac output, $a\text{-}VO_2$ is the arteriovenous O_2 content difference, SV is stroke volume, and HR is heart rate. For an average size adult (70 kg), CO at rest would be about 5 L/min and during strenuous exercise, 20 to 30 L/min.
• VO_2, determined during exercise by measuring respiratory gases, is related to the fractional percent of O_2 in inspired and expired air and VE. Inspired air contains 20.93% O_2 and expired air around 17.0%.
• VO_2 is usually expressed in absolute units (L/min) or relative to body weight (mL/kg/min). Resting VO_2 usually ranges between 0.25 and 0.4 L/min and maximal exercise VO_2 values can exceed 5 L/min (15–70 mL/kg/min) (Fig. 8-3). Higher values indicate higher aerobic fitness.

CARBON DIOXIDE PRODUCTION (VCO₂)

• Carbon dioxide (CO_2) is produced metabolically in the tissues, transported in blood by venous return to the lung, and eliminated from the lung by breathing (VE). Inspired air contains 0.03% CO_2 and expired air about 5% CO_2. Like VO_2, VCO_2 is usually expressed as L/min or mL/kg/min. Resting and strenuous exercise values depend on metabolism and pulmonary function, but resting values are less than VO_2.

LACTIC ACID

• Lactate, a product of glycolysis, is formed from pyruvate in the recycling of NAD (Fig. 8-2), or when insufficient O_2 is available for pyruvate to enter the TCA cycle. The extent of lactate formation depends on the availability of both pyruvate and NADH. Blood lactate at rest is about 0.8 to 1.5 mM, but during intense exercise can be in excess of 18 mM.
• During exercise, muscle cells dispose of lactate by releasing it into the circulation where it becomes an important fuel for the heart and nonexercising muscles. Lactate released from the muscle can also be converted to glucose in the liver by the Cori cycle.

OXYGEN PULSE

• The ratio of VO_2 (mL/min) to HR (bpm), when both measures are obtained simultaneously, is O_2 pulse (mL/beat). It is an important measure since it reflects the product of stroke volume and $a\text{-}VO_2$ difference (see equation under VO_2).
• O_2 pulse increases with increasing work effort (range 4 to 30 mL/beat) and is affected by a variety of factors, including anemia and heart disease. A low value during exercise indicates HR is too high for VO_2 and can be an indication of heart disease.

RESPIRATORY QUOTIENT/RESPIRATORY EXCHANGE RATIO

• The *respiratory quotient* (RQ) is the ratio of CO_2 produced by cellular metabolism to O_2 used by tissues. This metabolic marker is used to quantify the relative amounts of carbohydrate and fatty acids being oxidized for energy. The RQ cannot exceed 1.0: an RQ of 0.7 implies dependence on free fatty acids and a value of 1.0 dependence on carbohydrate.
• The *respiratory exchange ratio* (RER) reflects pulmonary exchange of CO_2 and O_2 at rest and during exercise. The RER also ranges between 0.7 and 1.0 during steady state exercise and can reflect substrate preference; however, it exceeds 1.0 during strenuous exercise because of increasing metabolic activity not matched by VO_2 and additional CO_2 derived from bicarbonate buffering of lactic acid. The terms RQ and RER are often used interchangeably, but their distinction is important.

VENTILATORY EQUIVALENTS

• Ventilatory equivalents (VE/VO_2 and VE/VCO_2) are unitless numbers derived from the ratio of VE to VO_2 and VCO_2. VE/VO_2 indicates the volume (L) of air required to use 1 L of O_2 and VE/VCO_2 indicates the appropriateness of ventilation (L of air required to remove L of CO_2).

- During maximal exercise testing below the anaerobic threshold, VE is linearly related to VO_2 and VCO_2, after which VE/VO_2 increases followed by an increase in VE/VCO_2. The increase in VE/VCO_2 reflects respiratory compensation for rise in blood lactate.

MAXIMAL HEART RATE

- The highest HR achieved during a standardized maximal exercise testing is the maximal HR. If an exercise test is not possible, then age-predicted heart-rate formulas can be used. Two formulas used are: Maximal HR = 220 – age *or* 208 – 0.7 × age.
- The first formula has been used for many years and the second was only recently developed. This new formula may be more accurate for older persons and is independent of gender and habitual physical activity (Tanaka, Monahan, and Seals, 2001). It is important to note that an estimated maximal HR may be 5 to 10% (10 to 20 bpm) higher or lower than the actual value.
- Maximal HR differs for various activities, since it is influenced by body position and amount of muscle mass involved.

HEART RATE RESERVE

- The difference between maximal HR during maximal exercise testing and resting HR is the *heart rate reserve* (HRR). If maximal HR is 205 bpm and resting HR is 55 bpm, then HRR would be 205 – 55 = 150 bpm. The smaller the difference, the lower the reserve and the narrower the range for exercising.

TARGET TRAINING HEART RATE

- A training program requires calculating a target heart range. To calculate the lower and upper target heart rates, 60–90% of maximal heart rate or 50–85% of heart rate reserve can be used. For the first, 60 and 90% of maximal HR will be determined as: 0.60 × Maximal HR (bpm) and 0.90 × Maximal HR (bpm).
- For the second method or Karvonen formula, which may be a more appropriate and valid approach, 50 and 85% of HRR is used: 0.50 × HRR + resting HR and 0.85 × HRR + resting HR.

MUSCULAR CONTRACTIONS

ISOMETRIC/STATIC CONTRACTIONS
- Isometric contractions refer to muscle fiber recruitment wherein no change in fiber length takes place: no joint or limb motion occurs. Examples of isometric

contractions are a person holding a weight in a particular position and postural stability.

ISOTONIC/DYNAMIC CONTRACTIONS
- Isotonic contractions are when muscle fibers change length and no movement at joints occurs. Specific types of dynamic contractions include *concentric, eccentric,* and *isokinetic*.
- *Concentric* contractions are movements where the muscle fibers shorten as the muscle contracts, such as when a weight is being lifted. This is also known as positive work.
- When the direction is reversed and the weight is lowered, the contraction becomes an *eccentric* contraction (negative work), where muscle fibers lengthen as the muscle contracts. More fast-twitch motor units are activated during eccentric contractions.

ISOKINETIC CONTRACTIONS
- Isokinetic machines make these contractions possible: the muscular movement is performed at constant speed against a variable resistance. The applied resistance during the contraction is increased or lowered at various points across the full range of motion so a constant speed of movement can be maintained. Diagnostic strength equipment use isokinetic tension, so more accurate measures of strength can be made at varying joint angles.

BORG SCALE OR RATING OF PERCEIVED EXERTION

- A Borg scale or *rating of perceived exertion* (RPE) scale is for an individual to rate his or her own "degree of physical strain" (Table 8-4). The original Borg scale ranges from 6 to 20, with each number anchored

TABLE 8-4   The Original and New Borg Scales for Rating of Perceived Exertion

ORIGINAL SCALE		NEW SCALE	
6	No exertion at all	0	Nothing at all
7	Extremely light	0.5	Very, very weak
8		1	Very weak
9	Very light	2	Weak
10		3	Moderate
11	Light	4	Somewhat strong
12		5	Strong
13	Somewhat hard	6	
14		7	Very strong
15	Hard (heavy)	8	
16		9	
17	Very hard	10	Very, very strong
18		*	Maximal
19	Extremely hard		
20	Maximal exertion		

by a simple verbal expression: a person exercising at 130 bpm should report a RPE of 13. A variant scale using 0 to 10 as the numeric ratio has been proposed.

MEASUREMENTS OF ENERGY, WORK, AND POWER

DEFINITIONS OF ENERGY, WORK, AND POWER

- Physical exercise involves both mechanical and chemical work by the muscles, with the degree of muscular effort dependent on duration, frequency, and intensity. Together these define energy, work, and power.
- **Energy:** The capacity to do work, with energy measured in Joules: 4.186 J = 1 kcal and 1 J = 2.3889 × 10^{-4} kcal.
- **Work:** When a force acts against resistance to produce motion: Force × Distance. Work is often expressed in kilogram-meters or kgm, where 1 kcal = 426.85 kgm = 4.18 kJ Power—Rate at which work is performed or the rate of energy transfer—Work/Time. Power is usually expressed as Watts (W), where 1W = 1 J/s; 6.12 kpm/min; and 0.01433 kcal/min.

ENERGY EXPENDITURE

- *Energy expenditure* (EE) is usually determined in one of two ways: direct and indirect calorimetry. For direct calorimetry, both external work and heat output are measured, and heat production is used as an estimate of metabolic rate. For indirect calorimetry, either open or closed circuit spirometry can be used.
- With open circuit spirometry, VO_2 and VCO_2 are measured and the RER is calculated. Simplistically RER can be added to 4 and then multiplied by L of O_2/min to derive kcal/min.
- Example: If VO_2 and RER determined from gas analysis were 0.3 L of O_2/min and 0.75 and 2.5 L/min and 0.95, at rest and during exercise, respectively, then EE at rest would be 4.75 (4.0 + 0.75) × 0.3 = 1.4 kcal/min and during exercise, 4.95 × 2.5 = 12.4 kcal/min. Net EE would be 12.4 – 1.4 or 11.0 kcal/min.
- EE can also be estimated from VO_2 by assuming 1 L of O_2 is ~5 kcal. If resting VO_2 was 0.3 L/min, energy costs would be (0.3 × 5) 1.5 kcal/min.

CALCULATING WORK AND POWER

- Work and power are calculated based on the particular activity.

- For example, work for cycle ergometry is measured as: resistance (kg) × rev/min × flywheel distance (m) × time. If a 80-kg male cycled at 100 rpm against a 3-kg load for 20 min (flywheel distance of 6 m), then: Work = 3 kg × 100 rpm × 6 m/rev × 20 min = 36,000 kgm Power = 36,000/20 min = 1,800 kgm/min = 1800/6.12 = 294 W (4.2 kcal/min).
- If a 70-kg man stepped up and down a 0.5-m bench 30 times/min for 10 min then: Work = 70 kg × 0.5m × 30 steps × 10 min = 10,500 kgm Power = 10,500/10 min = 1,050 kpm/min = 1,050/6.12 = 171.6 W (2.5 kcal/min).

WORK EFFICIENCY

- Gross work efficiency is the ratio of mechanical work output to energy expended; it typically ranges between 15 and 30%.
- Net work efficiency is the ratio of mechanical work output to total energy expended minus resting EE.
- Example: A woman with a resting VO_2 of 0.3 L/min rides a cycle ergometer for 30 min at 150 W (1 W = 0.01433 kcal) and uses 2 L O_2/min. Gross efficiency = Mechanical work output: 150 W (250 × 0.01433) ~ 2.2 kcal/min; Total energy expended: 2 L/min ~10 kcal/min or 2.2 × 100/10 = 22%. Net efficiency = 2.0 – 0.3 = 1.7 L/min ~8.5 kcal/min or 2.2 × 100/8.5 = 25.9%.
- Factors influencing exercise efficiency include work rate, speed of movement, and muscle fiber composition, and a variety of biomechanical factors, such as equipment and clothing.

EXERCISE ECONOMY

- Economy of movement is defined in terms of VO_2 (energy required) for a specific power output or velocity (mL/min/W or mL/kg/min to km/min or mile/min). Selected factors affecting economy include shoes, stride length, and frequency for running; and body mass, velocity, and aerodynamic positioning for cycling. Values may range from 200 to 350 mL/kg/km for running and 10 to 15 mL/W for cycling.

METABOLIC ENERGY EQUIVALENT

- *Metabolic energy equivalent* (MET) is the energy cost of activities in terms of multiples of resting metabolic rate. If 1 MET (resting metabolic rate) is taken as 3.5 mL of O_2/kg/min), then 3 MET would be 10.5 mL/kg/min and 6 MET would be 21 mL/kg/min.

These units are used by the Center for Disease Control to recommend exercise intensity.

- Energy expenditure for activities such as eating, dressing, and walking around the house range from 1 to 4 MET, whereas the cost of climbing a flight of stairs, walking on level ground, scrubbing floors, or playing a game of golf ranges from 4 to 10 MET. Strenuous sports, such as swimming, singles tennis, and football often exceed 10 MET.

BASIC CONCEPTS IN AEROBIC AND ANAEROBIC EXERCISE

MAXIMAL AEROBIC POWER

- Maximal aerobic power, or VO_{2max}, is the greatest amount of O_2 a person can consume during physical exercise. It is a useful measure for characterizing the functional capacity of the cardiovascular, pulmonary, and O_2 transport systems, and is considered "power" because it is a rate: L of O_2/min.
- If two individuals had absolute VO_{2max} values of 4.2 and 3.2 L/min and both weighed 70 kg, then normalizing for body weight would yield values of 60 and 45.7 mL/kg/min respectively. If person one weighed 70 kg and person two 53 kg, then normalized VO_{2max} values would be 60 mL/kg/min for both persons. VO_{2max} values above 50 mL/kg/min are considered high.

TESTING FOR MAXIMAL AEROBIC POWER
- The best tests for measuring VO_{2max} are incremental tests. A number of issues and concepts are important for VO_{2max} testing.
- **Requirements for maximal testing:** Minimal requirements for a valid maximal exercise test are that the exercise must involve large muscle groups and the rate of work must be measurable and reproducible. In addition, the test conditions should be standardized and the test should be tolerated by most people. Motivation should not be a major factor, and little to no skill should be required. The primary ways to assess aerobic power are by treadmill walking/running, cycle or arm ergometry, and step tests. The test protocol should be incremental or progressively increasing work so a true VO_{2max} is achieved. Different values will be obtained when the mode of exercise changes, and the absolute value will reflect the muscle mass involved. Combining upper and lower body work will yield higher values than treadmill, cycle, and arm work alone.
- **Concept of plateau:** During a progressive exercise test, when a step increase in work does not result in a further (or minimal) increase in VO_2, then VO_2 has begun to level off. The leveling off or plateauing effect is considered the single best criteria for attaining a true VO_{2max}. For many treadmill protocols, an increase in VO_2 <0.150 L/min is indicative of a plateau.

- **Criteria for achieving VO_{2max}:** If a leveling off or plateauing of VO_2 cannot be seen, then other criteria are used to document a true VO_{2max}. At least two of the following criteria should be met for a true VO_{2max} test: blood lactate levels above 7 or 8 mM; HR equal to or within 15 beats of the age-estimated maximal HR; RER $\geq$ 1.15; and/or RPE $\geq$ 17.
- **VO_{2peak}:** When an exercise tests is terminated and the criteria described are not met, the higher VO_2 achieved is referred to as VO_{2peak}.
- **Ventilatory threshold:** Ventilatory threshold is the point where VE begins to increase disproportionately to VO_2 during incremental exercise testing. It is a measure of "excess" ventilation and has been termed anaerobic threshold.
- **Estimating VO_{2max}:** VO_{2max} can be estimated using the known linear relation between HR and VO_2. HR at submaximal work rates can be plotted against VO_2 and then the estimated maximal HR can be used to extrapolate to VO_{2max}. Cycle tests are most appropriate because there are expected VO_2 values as a function of Watts (see Table 8-5). Walking tests, step tests, endurance runs, and nonexercise data can also be used to estimate VO_{2max}. Potential errors exist for all these estimates and care needs taken in interpreting these data.

DETERMINANTS OF AND FACTORS AFFECTING VO_{2MAX}
- **Intrinsic and extrinsic factors:** Intrinsic factors affecting VO_{2max} include genetics, gender, body composition/muscle mass, age, and existing pathologies. Extrinsic factors include training/activity levels, dietary intake (alcohol, caffeine), nutritional and hydration status, and environmental conditions.
- **Determinants:** All systems serving a role in the delivery of O_2 can affect VO_{2max}. Central factors include cardiac output, pulmonary ventilation, arterial pressure, *hemoglobin* (Hb) content, O_2 diffusion into and through the lungs, the alveolar ventilation: perfusion ratio, and

TABLE 8-5   Expected VO_2 Values at Designated Power Outputs Between 1 and 3 Min with Cycle Ergometry

POWER (W)	OXYGEN UPTAKE (L/MIN)
50	0.9
100	1.5
150	2.1
200	2.8
250	3.5
300	4.2
350	5.0
400	5.7

Hb-O_2 affinity. Peripheral determinants include muscle blood flow, capillary density, O_2 diffusion to and extraction by muscle cells, Hb-O_2 affinity, and skeletal muscle fiber profiles.

AEROBIC AND ANAEROBIC EXERCISE

EXERCISE DOMAINS

• Three specific exercise domains were reported by Gaesser and Poole (1996). Graphical presentations of the domains (moderate, heavy, and severe) are presented in Fig. 8-4 for an incremental exercise test and for constant load tests at three workloads. In panel one, the *lactate threshold* (T_{Lac}) represents the boundary between the moderate and heavy domain, and critical power (Wa) represents the boundary for the severe domain. These concepts are described below.

• **Lactate threshold:** As shown in Fig. 8-4, T_{Lac} represents the lowest exercise intensity that can be maintained where blood lactate appearance exceeds its removal and there is a sustained increase of about 1 mM lactates above preexercise levels.

• **Maximal lactate at steady state:** *Maximal lactate at steady state* (MLSS) is the highest blood lactate concentration that can be sustained without progressive accumulation: a new steady state is achieved (between 3 and 8 mM). The upper boundary of the heavy domain may demarcate MLSS.

• **Critical power:** As the lower boundary of the severe domain, Wa is the maximum power output that can be sustained without a continued and progressive anaerobic contribution. Exercise above Wa will elicit VO_{2max}.

• **Onset of blood lactate accumulation:** At specific exercise intensity, muscle lactate production exceeds utilization and blood lactate begins to accumulate because appearance exceeds removal. Wa, MLSS, and *onset of blood lactate accumulation* (OBLA) may all demarcate the transition between the heavy and severe exercise domains.

• **Steady state exercise:** When rate of lactate production is balanced by the rate of oxidative removal and VO_2 is stabilized within 3 to 6 min. As such, cardiac output, HR, and pulmonary gas exchange are in a steady state and exercise can continue for an extended period of time.

• **Slow component of oxygen uptake:** A continued rise in VO_2 beyond the 3rd min is observed when exercise is above the lactate threshold. The rise in VO_2 (Fig. 8-4) usually stabilizes within 20 min when exercise is within the heavy domain, or gradually increases to VO_{2max} when exercise is within the severe domain. The cause of the slow component of oxygen uptake has not been clearly defined, but may reflect that the working limbs are a key to initiation of this rise in VO_2.

OXYGEN KINETICS

• **Oxygen deficit:** When an individual begins to exercise, a certain VO_2 is required but the aerobic energy system cannot meet the demands aerobically. VO_2 gradually increases until it reaches a steady state. The difference in VO_2 between steady state O_2 and O_2 required but not used prior to steady state conditions is termed the O_2 deficit.

• **Oxygen debt:** On termination of exercise, VO_2 remains elevated to restore energy systems to their

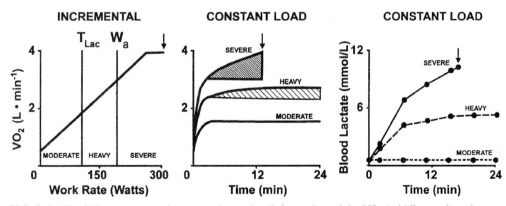

FIG. 8-4   The VO_2 responses to incremental exercise (left panel), and the VO_2 (middle panel) and blood lactate (right panel) responses to constant load exercise as a function of exercise intensity domains. T_{Lac} represents the lactate threshold and Wa represents critical power or work rate where maximal lactate at steady state occurs. (Reprinted with permission, DA Poole [Poole and Richardson, 1997; Gaesser and Poole, 1996]).

preexercise states, after having borrowed ATP at the beginning of exercise. This term, O_2 debt, was coined by AV Hill in the early 1900s, but is transitioning to excess postexercise oxygen consumption (see below).

- **Excess postexercise oxygen consumption:** *Excess postexercise oxygen consumption* (EPOC), the integral of VO_2 during recovery after the termination of exercise, consists of a fast and slow component. It is highly correlated with exercise intensity, and the fast portion may reflect resynthesis of stored PC and restoration of muscle and blood O_2 stores. The slow component may reflect elevated body temperature, catecholamines, accelerated metabolism (conversion of lactic acid to glucose/gluconeogenesis) and other hormonal/metabolic processes.

RESISTANCE EXERCISE

- Resistance exercise is used to improve muscular fitness, which is a combination of strength, endurance, and power. Strength is the greatest force a muscle can exert in one effort; endurance is the muscle's ability to make repeated efforts; and power is a measure of how quickly muscular strength can be applied.

WEIGHT TRAINING PARAMETERS
- When training with weights, the magnitudes of increase in muscle strength and endurance depend on the specific training parameters: repetitions, sets, volume, and intensity.
- **Repetition maximum:** The amount of force a subject can lift a given number of repetitions defines *repetition maximum* (RM). For example, 1RM is the maximal force a subject can lift with one repetition and 5RM would be the maximal force someone could lift five times. Resistance training with weights represents isotonic strength.
- **Repetitions:** Repetitions reflect the number of consecutive times a particular weight is lifted without a rest period. For examples, repetitions could be 5, 10, 12, 25, or 50.
- **Sets:** The number of sets delineates how many times the repetitions are repeated after a rest period. For example, a training session could consist of three sets of 12 repetitions.
- **Volume:** Volume equates to the total number of times a weight was lifted (Sets × Reps). For example, if the session was three sets of 12 repetitions, the volume would be 3 × 12 or 36 repetitions. Volume indicates how much work was done: the greater the volume, the greater the total work.

- **Intensity:** Intensity reflects the actual resistance lifted, and is expressed as a percent of the maximum weight (1RM). If the 1RM for a particular exercise is 80 kg, then a weight of 40 kg would be a 50% and 60 kg a 75% intensity.

RESISTANCE TRAINING CONCEPTS
- **SAID or Specific adaptation to imposed demand:** The specificity principle states that physiological, neurological, and psychological adaptations to training are specific to the "imposed demand." For example, to develop speed, power, and specific metabolic pathways, the imposed demand must target those specific areas.
- **Strength-endurance continuum:** A weight training concept based on the premise that muscle strength and muscle endurance exist on a continuum, with muscle strength being 1RM and muscle endurance representing the ability to exert a lower force repeatedly over time. Low numbers of repetitions (6–10 RM) are associated with increases in strength and high numbers (20–100 RM) are associated with increases in endurance. As repetitions increase, there is a transition from strength to endurance.
- **Muscle hypertrophy:** Compensatory growth in skeletal muscle in response to a specifically imposed load. The primary components to muscle hypertrophy include a neural response, followed by an upregulation of second messenger systems to activate the family of immediate early genes that dictate the responses of contractile protein genes, and message passing down to alter protein expression.
- Muscle hypertrophy may take 2 months to begin. The new contractile proteins appear to be incorporated into existing myofibrils and there may be a limit to how large a myofibril can become: they may split at some point. Hypertrophy results primarily from growth of each muscle cell, rather than an increase in the number of cells.
- Muscle hypertrophy is observed in all three major fiber types (Types I, IIa, and IId(x/b) when low, but not high, numbers of repetitions are performed. Physiologic adaptations and performance are linked to both the volume and intensity of resistance training.

BIOMECHANICAL FACTORS IN MUSCLE STRENGTH
- Neural control, muscle cross-sectional area, arrangement of muscle fibers, muscle length, joint angle, velocity of muscle contraction, joint angular velocity, strength-to-mass ratio, body size, joint motion (joint mobility, dexterity, flexibility, limberness, and range of motion), point of tendon insertion, and the interactions of these factors influence muscle strength.

DELAYED-ONSET MUSCLE SORENESS

- *Delayed-onset muscle soreness* (DOMS) is a term used to describe temporary soreness that results primarily from eccentric exercise and resistance training. It is usually noted the day after the exercise and may last 3 to 4 days.
- Factors that may elicit DOMS inflammation, osmotic changes within muscle tissue, microtrauma to the tissue, and/or alterations in calcium metabolism.

PLYOMETRICS

- Plyometrics is a specific method of training for power or explosiveness. Most plyometric exercises involve jumping, bounding, and hopping. The force generated by a lengthening contraction (eccentric) can be markedly increased if it is followed by a shortening contraction (concentric).
- Plyometric training is a process that specifically focuses on rapid pairing of eccentric and concentric contractions, or stretch/shortening cycles, to produce increases in power.

EXERCISE TRAINING

PRINCIPLES OF TRAINING

- **FITT:** This is an acronym to describe a physical training variable that can be altered to achieve various fitness goals. FITT stands for *frequency, intensity, time* (duration), and *type* of exercise.
- **Overload:** The overload principle states that gains in strength/endurance come about only when progressively greater demands are placed on the cardiopulmonary and musculoskeletal systems.
- **Periodization:** This is a technique that involves altering training variables (repetitions/set, exercises performed, volume, and rest interval between sets) to achieve well-defined gains in muscular strength, endurance, and overall performance for a specific event. The specific phases include activation (getting the body ready for a new activity–about 4 weeks), followed by strength development (4 to 7 weeks) and then muscular endurance (8 to 12 weeks).
- **Quantifying exercise intensity:** Exercise intensity can be estimated from METs, a percentage of maximal HR, a percentage of VO_{2max}, or as a function of RPE.
- **Absolute and relative intensity:** If two individuals (Tom and Mark) have VO_{2max} values of 4.2 and 3.2 L/min respectively, and both work at 2.5 L/min, then they would be working at the same absolute power output, but at different relative intensities because they have

different VO_{2max} values. Tom would be working at 2.5/4.2 or 60% and Mark at 2.5/3.2 or 78% of VO_{2max}.

ADAPTATIONS TO TRAINING

ENDURANCE TRAINING

- Adaptations to endurance exercise include improvements in neuromuscular and cardiovascular function and in respiratory muscle efficiency and cost of breathing; decreases in body mass/body fat; improvements in heat tolerance; increases in self-esteem; lower blood lactate accumulation at higher power outputs, and increased insulin sensitivity.

RESISTANCE TRAINING

- Resistance training induces a variety of adaptations, with clear increases in strength. Neural adaptations include increases in strength with/without hypertrophy, greater synchronicity in activating motor units, and increased presynaptic and postsynaptic neurotransmitter receptors. Contractile adaptations include muscle hypertrophy within the whole muscle and myofibers through increased synthesis and accretion of intracellular myofibrilar proteins and activation of local satellite cells to add new nuclei to existing myofibers.
- Fiber type specific adaptations induced by resistance training depend on volume and intensity, but a common change is an increase in the percentage of Type IIa fibers, at the expense of the Type IId(x/b) fibers. Resistance training is not usually associated with increases in VO_{2max}, but may enhance overall cardiovascular function by improving strength that lessens the load of daily activities.

ESTIMATING STRENGTH AND ENDURANCE

AEROBIC AND ANAEROBIC POWER

- Simple in-office and field tests can be used to estimate VO_{2max}. These include the 2-mi run, 12-min run, and the 3-min step test. Other tests include submaximal cycle ergometry. Tests for anaerobic power include vertical jumps, the Wingate anaerobic cycle test, a running-based anaerobic sprint test (400 m), and the 300-yd shuttle run.

MUSCULAR STRENGTH AND ENDURANCE

- Tests to assess muscular strength include free weights (1 RM: back squats/bench presses), hand grip

dynamometry (maximal strength), and isokinetic equipment (60 to 120°/s).
• Muscular endurance can be measured by maximal number of push-ups, pull-ups, and/or sit-ups, as well as hand grip dynamometry (sustained submaximal endurance), and isokinetic equipment (180 to 300°/s).

REFERENCES

Demirel HA, Powers SK, Naito H, et al: Exercise-induced alerations in skeletal muscle myosin heavy chain phenotype: Dose-response relationship. *J Appl Physiol* 86(3):1002–1008, 1999.

Gaesser GA, Poole DC: The slow component of oxygen uptake kinetics in humans, in Holloszy JO (ed.): *Exercise and Sport Science Reviews,* vol. 24. Baltimore, MD, Williams & Wilkins, 1996, p. 35.

Pette D, Staron RS: Transitions of muscle fiber phenotypic profiles. *Histochem Cell Biol* 115:359–372, 2001.

Poole DC, Richardson RS: Determinants of oxygen uptake: Implications for exercise testing. *Sports Med* 24:308–320, 1997.

Staron RS: Human skeletal muscle fiber types: Delineation, development, and distribution. *Can J Appl Physiol* 22:307–327, 1997.

Tanaka H, Monahan KD, Seals DR: Age-predicted maximal heart rate revisited. *J Am Coll Cardiol* 37:153–156, 2001.

Zhen-He H, Bottinelli R, Pelligrino MA, et al: ATP consumption and efficiency of human single muscle fibers with different myosin isoform composition. *Biophys J* 79:945–961, 2000.

BIBLIOGRAPHY

American College of Sports Medicine: *Guidelines for Exercise Testing and Prescription*, 6th ed. Baltimore, MD, Lippincott William & Wilkins, 2000.

Astrand P-O, Rodahl K, Dahl HA, Stromme SB: *Textbook of Work Physiology: Physiological Bases of Exercise*, 4th ed. Champaign IL, Human Kinetics, 2003.

ATS/ACCP: Statement on cardiopulmonary exercise testing. *Am J Respir Crit Care Med* 167:211–277, 2003.

Billat LV: Use of blood lactate measurements for prediction of exercise performance and for control of training. *Sports Med* 22:157–175, 1996.

Campos GE, Luecke TJ, Wendeln HK, et al: Muscular adaptations in response to three different resistance training regimens: Specificity of repetition maximum training zones. *Eur J Appl Physiol* 88:50–60, 2002.

McArdle WD, Katch FI, Katch VL: *Exercise Physiology: Energy, Nutrition, and Human Performance,* 5th ed. Baltimore, MD, Lippincott, Williams & Wilkins, 2001.

McHugh MP, Tyler TF, Greenberg SC, et al: Differences in activation patterns between eccentric and concentric quadriceps contractions. *J Sports Sci* 20:83–91, 2002.

Rodriguez LP, Lopez-Rego J, Calbet JA, et al: Effects of training status on fibers of the musculus vastus lateralis in professional road cyclists. *Am J Phys Med Rehabil* 81:651–660, 2002.

Wasserman K, Hansen JE, Sue DY, et al: *Principles of Exercise Testing and Interpretation: Including Pathophysiology and Clinical Applications*, 3rd ed. Baltimore, MD, Lippincott, Williams & Wilkins, 1999.

9 ARTICULAR CARTILAGE INJURY

Stephen J Lee, BA
Brian J Cole, MD, MBA

INTRODUCTION

• Articular cartilage lines the articulating surfaces of diarthrodial joints and serves several important functions: (1) provision of a smooth, low-friction surface, (2) joint lubrication, and (3) stress distribution with load bearing.
• Articular cartilage injury most commonly occurs in the knee and thus has been most extensively studied in this area. Cartilage injuries of the knee affect approximately 900,000 Americans annually, resulting in more than 200,000 surgical procedures each year to treat high-grade lesions (grade III or IV) (Cole et al, 1999).
• In a restrospective study of 31,516 knee arthroscopies, Curl and associates (1997) identified articular cartilage damage in 63% of the patients. Among those affected, 41% had grade III and 19% grade IV lesions. More recently, Hjelle and colleagues (2002) prospectively evaluated 1000 knee arthroscopies and found chondral or osteochondral defects in 61% of the patients with 55% of the defects classified as grade III and 5% grade IV. The weight-bearing zone of the medial femoral condyle was found to be the most commonly affected area (58% of all articular cartilage lesions). Other commonly affected areas include the weight-bearing zone of the lateral femoral condyle and patellofemoral joint (Hjelle et al, 2002; Brittberg, 2000).

COMPOSITION AND ORGANIZATION

• Articular cartilage consists primarily of a large *extracellular matrix* (ECM) and a sparse population of chondrocytes.

TABLE 9-1   Organization of Articular Cartilage

ZONE	CHONDROCYTE	COLLAGEN	PROTEOGLYCAN	WATER	PROPERTIES
Middle	Random, oblique	Larger diameter, less organized	—	—	Less stiff than superficial zone
Superficial	Flat, parallel to surface	Thin, parallel to surface	Lowest conc.	Highest conc.	Low fluid permeability Resistance to shear forces
Deep	Spherical, in columns	Perpendicular to surface, extending into calcified zone	Highest	Lowest	Anchors cartilage to subchondral bone
Tidemark	Separates deep zone from calcified zone, number increases with age				
Calcified	Small cells in cartilaginous matrix with apatitic salts				

1. Chondrocytes (5% of total wet weight) are derived from mesenchymal stem cells which differentiate during skeletal morphogenesis and are responsible for producing matrix components that regulate cartilage homeostasis. The chondrocytes respond to a variety of factors, including matrix composition, mechanical load, and soluble mediators such as growth factors and cytokines.

2. The primary components of the ECM are water (65–80% of the total wet weight), *proteoglycans* (PG) (aggrecan, 4–7% of the total wet weight), and collagens (primarily type II, 10–20% of the total wet weight), with other proteins and glycoproteins in lesser amounts. The collagens provide form and tensile strength. The proteoglycans bind water and help distribute stresses as water flows through the porous-permeable ECM under compressive loads.

• The ultrastructure of articular cartilage can be divided into four distinct zones: superficial, middle, deep, and calcified. Each has a characteristic composition that imparts unique mechanical properties (Table 9-1).

INJURY AND REPAIR

• Mechanical injuries to articular cartilage occur when abnormal blunt traumatic and shear forces result in high compressive stress throughout the tissue and high shear stress at the cartilage–subchondral bone junction (Finerman and Noyes, 1992). This results in an isolated cartilage injury known as a focal chondral defect, which is different from chondromalacia and osteoarthritis. Chondromalacia describes the macroscopic appearance of a gradation of cartilage damage including softening and fissuring to variable degrees of cartilage depth. Most often it is asymptomatic and does not require treatment. Primary osteoarthritis is a progressive degenerative condition that increases in prevalence nonlinearly after the age of 50 years. Macroscopically, focal chondral lesions appear as an isolated defect whereas osteoarthritis appears as diffuse fraying, fibrillation, and thinning of the articular cartilage.

• The lack of vascular, neural, and lymphatic access to articular cartilage creates a limited environment for spontaneous repair. Injuries that do not penetrate the subchondral bone show little sign of spontaneous repair, whereas those that extend into the depth of subchondral bone initiate a vascular proliferative response that produces a mix of normal hyaline cartilage (primarily type II collagen) and a structurally and biomechanically inferior "scar cartilage," or fibrocartilage (primarily type I collagen).

• Articular cartilage injury can be separated into three distinct types: (1) *cartilage matrix and cell injuries*— microdamage to the cells and matrix without visible disruption of the articular surface, (2) *chondral injuries*—visible mechanical disruption limited to articular cartilage, and (3) *osteochondral injuries*— visible mechanical disruption of articular cartilage and subchondral bone.

1. Cartilage matrix and cell injuries

    a. Decreased PG concentration, increased hydration, and possibly disorganization of the collagen network. The decreased PG concentration and increased hydration are strongly correlated with a decrease in cartilage stiffness and an increase in its hydraulic permeability. As a result, greater loads are transmitted to the collagen-PG matrix, increasing the vulnerability of the ECM to further damage.

    b. It is not known at what point the accumulated microdamage is irreversible. Presumably, the chondrocytes can restore the matrix as long as the loss of matrix PG does not exceed the rate of synthesis, the collagen network remains intact, and sufficient chondrocytes remain viable (Martin and Buckwalter, 2000).

2. Chondral injuries
   a. May result in chondral fissures, flaps, fractures, and chondrocyte damage
   b. Lack of vascular access and migration of mesenchymal cells limits the repair response (Buckwalter and Mow, 1992; Buckwalter, Rosenberg, and Hunziker, 1990). The surrounding chondrocytes respond by proliferating and increasing the synthesis of matrix components; however, the proliferating cells and newly synthesized matrix do not fill the tissue defect, and soon after injury the increased proliferative and synthetic activity ceases. The adjacent normal cartilage may then be overloaded and also degenerate over time.

3. Osteochondral injuries
   a. Acute injuries may fracture deep into subchondral bone
   b. Hemorrhage and fibrin clot formation trigger an inflammatory response, altering the synovial fluid and joint environment. The fibrin clot extends into the cartilage defect and releases vasoactive mediators and growth factors, including *transforming growth factor beta* (TGF-β) and *platelet derived growth factor* (PDGF). These factors may stimulate repair of osteochondral defects.
   c. However, the chondral repair tissue is intermediate between normal hyaline cartilage and fibrocartilage, resulting in a structure less stiff and more permeable than normal articular cartilage (Buckwalter et al, 1988; Buckwalter and Mankin, 1997a; 1997b; Buckwalter, Rosenberg, and Hunziker, 1988). The repair tissue rarely persists and most often begins to show evidence of depletion of PGs, increased hydration, fragmentation and fibrillation, increasing collagen content, and loss of chondrocyte-like cells within a year (Buckwalterl, 2002).

PATIENT EVALUATION

• Cartilage injuries can occur in isolation or in association with other intra-articular pathology, thus it is important for the evaluating physician to maintain a high index of suspicion especially in the presence of concomitant pathology such as varus or valgus alignment, patellofemoral malalignment, ligamentous instability, and meniscal deficiency.

• The most common clinical presentation following an acute full-thickness chondral or osteochondral injury is a loose body. When chronic, symptoms may be subtle but often include localized pain, swelling, and mechanical symptoms (locking, catching).

• A thorough history should elicit the onset of symptoms (traumatic or insidious), mechanism of injury, previous injuries, and symptom-provoking activities.

• A thorough physical examination (Table 9-2) is essential to evaluate for concomitant pathology that would alter the treatment plan. Antalgic postures or gaits may be present due to painful weightbearing in the involved knee, or adaptive gait patterns such as in-toeing or out-toeing or a flexed-knee gait may develop as the patient shifts weight away from the affected area. Range of motion testing is usually normal in patients with isolated focal chondral defects. Crepitus, catching, locking, or grinding can occur with focal irregularities in the articular surface.

• Most often, the history, physical examination, and plain radiographs are all that are required to make the appropriate diagnosis. Ideal plain films include 45°

TABLE 9-2   Components of a Comprehensive Musculoskeletal Examination

Habitus
Alignment
　Varus
　Valgus
Gait
　Antalgic
　Flexed-knee
　Recurvatum (hyperextension)
　Compensatory
　Thrust
　Varus (lateral)/Valgus (medial)
Swelling
　Soft tissue
　Effusion
Ligamentous laxity
　Anteroposterior (ACL/PCL)
　Medial-Lateral (MCL/LCL)
Range of motion
Strength, muscle atrophy
Specific compartments
　Tibiofemoral
　Patellofemoral
Meniscus
　Joint line tenderness
Provocative maneuvers
Related joints
　Spine
　Hips
　Feet
Neurovascular

ABBREVIATION: ACL = anterior cruciate ligament; PCL = posterior cruciate ligament; MCL = medial collateral ligament; LCL = lateral collateral ligament.

TABLE 9-3   Modified International Cartilage Repair Society Classification System for Chondral Injury

GRADE OF INJURY	MODIFIED ICRS
Grade 0	Normal cartilage
Grade I	Superficial fissuring
Grade II	<1/2 cartilage depth
Grade III	>1/2 cartilage depth up to subchondral plate
Grade IV	Through subchondral plate, exposing subchondral bone

TABLE 9-4   Nonsurgical Management of Chondral Lesions

Oral medications	Non-steroidal anti-inflammatory drugs (NSAIDS)
	Acetaminophen
	Glucosamine-sulfate—believed to stimulate chondrocyte and synoviocyte metabolism
	Chondroitin-sulfate—believed to inhibit degradative enzymes and prevent fibrin thrombi formation in periarticular tissues
Physical modalities	Activity modification—avoidance of high-impact exercises
	Physical therapy—quadriceps strengthening hamstring flexibility
Bracing	Knee sleeve for improved proprioception
	Unloader brace to protect damaged knee compartment
Injections	Corticosteroids
	High-molecular weight hyaluronans

flexion weight bearing *posteroanterior* (PA), patellofemoral, and non-weight-bearing lateral projections (Mandelbaum, Romanelli, and Knapp, 2000). These views allow assessment of joint space narrowing, subchondral sclerosis, osteophytes, and cysts. Special studies such as long-cassette mechanical axis view may be necessary to evaluate overall alignment. If significant joint space narrowing is present on the 45° flexion PA radiograph, MRI is not indicated. An MRI is valuable in assessing the status of the knee ligaments and menisci, but generally tends to underestimate the degree of cartilage abnormalities seen at the time of arthroscopy (Khanna et al, 2001). The role of the bone scan remains controversial: isolated articular surface defects that do not penetrate subchondral bone may not be identified by bone scan. Arthroscopy continues to remain the gold standard for the diagnosis of articular cartilage injuries.

- The Outerbridge classification system (Outerbridge, 1961) was initially developed for macroscopic grading of chondromalacia patellae and has since been modified on numerous occasions. A recent modification by the International Cartilage Repair Society (ICRS) (Brittberg, 2000; Brittberg and Peterson, 1998) classifies chondral injuries into five distinct grades (Table 9-3).

NONSURGICAL MANAGEMENT

- Nonsurgical management (Table 9-4) is largely ineffective in symptomatic patients and should be reserved for relatively low-demand patients, patients wishing to avoid or delay surgery, and patients with advanced degenerative osteoarthritis which is a contraindication for articular cartilage restoration procedures.
- Traditional methods for treatment of chondral lesions include the judicious use of nonsteroidal anti-inflammatory drugs combined with activity modification. Oral chondroprotective agents such as glucosamine

and chondroitin sulfate potentially offer some relief in subjective symptoms. Glucosamine is thought to stimulate chondrocyte and synoviocyte activity, and chondroitin is thought to inhibit degradative enzymes and prevent fibrin thrombi formation in periarticular tissues (Gosh, 1992; Bucci, 1994; Muller-Fassbender et al, 1994). Recent studies indicate that pain, joint line tenderness, range of motion, and walking speed may be improved with these medications (Barclay, Tsourounis, and McGart, 1998; DaCamara and Dowless, 1998). However, there are no clinical data showing that these oral agents affect the formation of cartilage (Tomford, 2000). Viscosupplementation with high-molecular weight hyaluronans remains an option despite the lack of well-controlled studies demonstrating efficacy.

- Prolonged nonsurgical management of symptomatic chondral lesions may lead to additional joint deterioration, making surgical intervention more difficult or less successful. Suggested indications for referral to an orthopedic surgeon with expertise in cartilage restoration techniques are presented in Table 9-5.

TABLE 9-5   Indications for Referral to an Orthopedic Surgeon

High-energy injury with direct trauma to the knee
Acute motion loss
Gross deformity
Acute neurovascular deficit
Mechanical symptoms (catching, locking, sensation of a loose body)
Failed nonsurgical management greater than 3 months in duration
Repeated giving way or complaints of instability

SURGICAL MANAGEMENT

- Various surgical modalities exist for the treatment of chondral lesions and can be grouped into three categories: (1) palliative, (2) reparative, and (3) restorative (Table 9-6). The goals are to reduce symptoms, improve joint congruence by restoring the articular surface with the most normal tissue (i.e., hyaline cartilage) possible, and to prevent further cartilage degeneration. Concomitant management of associated pathology such as malalignment, ligament insufficiency, and/or meniscal injury is essential for a successful outcome.

PALLIATIVE

- Arthroscopic debridement and lavage is used to remove degenerative debris, cytokines, and proteases that may contribute to cartilage breakdown. It is ideally indicated in the patient with defect area less than 2 cm^2 and who has exhausted all nonoperative treatments. Postoperative rehabilitation involves weight-bearing as tolerated and early strengthening exercises. In the absence of meniscal pathology, the results following arthroscopic debridement are at best guarded.
- Thermal chondroplasty (laser, radiofrequency energy) of superficial chondral defects allows more precise contouring of the articular surface when used in conjunction with debridement. However, there is concern regarding the depth of chondrocyte death and cellular necrosis in the treated area and thus remains investigational.

REPARATIVE

- *Marrow stimulating techniques* (MST—microfracture, abrasion arthroplasty, and subchondral drilling) involve surgical penetration of subchondral bone to allow the migration of mesenchymal cells and fibrin clot formation in the area of the chondral defect. The resulting quality and volume of repair tissue (fibrocartilage) is variable. These procedures are used in low demand patients with larger lesions (>2 cm^2) or in higher demand patients with smaller lesions (<2 cm^2). Microfracture is preferred over subchondral drilling and abrasion arthroplasty for several reasons: (1) it is less destructive to the subchondral bone because it creates less thermal injury than drilling, (2) it allows better access to difficult areas of the articular surface, (3) it provides a controlled method of depth penetration, and (4) selection of the correctly angled awl permits the microfracture holes to be made perpendicular to the subchondral plate (Steadman, Rodkey, and Rodrigo, 2001; Steadman, 1997). Postoperative rehabilitation consists of nonweight bearing for 6 to 8 weeks and may include *continuous passive motion* (CPM) to improve the extent and quality of the repair tissue. As MSTs are low-cost and relatively low-morbidity procedures, they remain the mainstay for the initial management of small chondral lesions.

RESTORATIVE

- *Autologous chondrocyte implantation* (ACI) is a two-stage procedure involving biopsy of normal articular cartilage, culture of chondrocytes in vitro, and transplantation into the chondral defect beneath a periosteal patch. This restorative procedure results in hyaline-like cartilage which is believed to be superior to fibrocartilage (Grande, 1997). Postoperative rehabilitation entails aggressive CPM and nonweight bearing for 6 weeks with a gradual increase to full-weight bearing from 6 to 12 weeks. ACI is a costly procedure with a relatively lengthy recovery period and is most often used as a secondary procedure for the treatment of medium to larger focal chondral defects (>2 cm^2).
- Osteochondral grafts restore articular congruity by transplanting a cylindrical plug of subchondral bone and articular cartilage which can be obtained from the

TABLE 9-6   **Surgical Management of Chondral Lesions**

PROCEDURE	INDICATIONS	OUTCOME
Arthroscopic debridement and lavage	Minimal symptoms, short-term relief	Palliative
Thermal chondroplasty (laser, radiofrequency energy)	Partial thickness defects, investigational	Palliative
Marrow stimulating techniques	Smaller lesions, persistent pain	Reparative
Autologous chondrocyte implantation	Small and large lesions with or without subchondral bone loss	Restorative
Osteochondral autograft	Smaller lesions, persistent pain	Restorative
Osteochondral allograft	Larger lesions with subchondral bone loss	Restorative

TABLE 9-7 Results of Arthroscopic Debridement and Lavage

AUTHOR	N	MEAN FOLLOW-UP	RESULTS
Owens et al, 2002	19 patients	24 months	Fulkerson score 12 mos – 80.9, 24 mos – 77.5
Hubbard, 1996	76 knees	4.5 years	>50% improved
Timoney et al, 1990	109 patients	48 months	63% good 37% fair/poor
Baumgartner et al, 1990	49 patients	33 months	52% good 48% fair/poor
Jackson, 1989	137 patients	3.5 years (2 to 9)	68% remained improved
Sprague, 1981	78 patients	14 months	74% good 26% fair/poor

patient (i.e., autograft) or from a cadaveric source (i.e., allograft). The two-dimensional surface area can be covered, but the challenge lies in accurately restoring the three-dimensional surface contour.

a. Osteochondral autografts offer the advantage of using the patient's own tissue; however, the limited amount of donor tissue confines this technique to smaller lesions (<2 cm^2). The risk of donor-site morbidity increases as more tissue is harvested. Postoperative rehabilitation includes early range of motion and nonweight bearing for 2 weeks with an increase to full-weight bearing from 2 to 6 weeks. It is most commonly indicated for the primary treatment of smaller lesions considered symptomatic and for similarly sized lesions for which an MST or ACI procedure has failed.

b. Osteochondral allograft can be used to treat larger lesions (>2 cm^2) that are difficult to treat with other methods. Tissue matching and immunologic suppression are unnecessary as the allograft tissue is avascular and alymphatic. Postoperative rehabilitation consists of immediate CPM and nonweight bearing for 6 to 12 weeks. This procedure is most often used as a secondary treatment option for failed ACI in larger defects.

• Tables 9-7 through 9-12 provide a summary of outcomes studies for arthroscopic debridement and lavage, microfracture, ACI, and osteochondral autografts and allografts.

TABLE 9-8 Results of Microfracture

AUTHOR	N	MEAN FOLLOW-UP	RESULTS
Steadman et al, 2003	71 knees Age $\leq$ 45 years	11 years (7 to 17 years)	80% improved Lysholm 59 → 89 Tegner 6 → 9 Majority of improvement 1st year Maximal improvement 2 to 3 years Younger patients did better
Steadman, Rodkey, and Rodrigo, 2001	75 patients	11.3 years	Lysholm 58.8 → 88.9 Tegner 3.1 → 5.8 Work 4.9 → 7.6 Sports 4.2 → 7.1
Blevins et al, 1998	140 recreational athletes Mean age 38 years Mean defect size 2.8 cm^2 38 high-level athletes Mean age 26 years Mean defect size 2.2 cm^2	4 years 3.7 years	54 2nd look arthroscopy: 35% with surface unchanged Older, less active did worse 77% returned to sports @ 9.3 months
Gill et al, 1998; Gill and MacGillivray, 2001	103 patients	6 years (2 to 12 years)	86% rated knee as normal/nearly normal Acute (treated within 12 weeks) did better
Steadman et al, 1997	203 patients	3 years (2 to 12 years)	75% improved, 19% unchanged, 6% worse 60% improved sports Poor prognosis—joint space narrowing, age >30 years, no postoperative CPM

TABLE 9-9   Results of Autologous Chondrocyte Implantation

AUTHOR	N	LOCATION	MEAN FOLLOW-UP	RESULTS
Peterson et al, 2002	18	F	>5 years	89% good/excellent
	14	OCD	>5 years	86% good/excellent
	17	P	>5 years	65% good/excellent
	11	F/ACL	>5 years	91% good/excellent
Minas, 2001	169	F, Tr, P, T	>1 year	85% significant improvement
				13% failure
Micheli et al, 2001	50	F, Tr, P	>3 years	84% significant improvement
				2% unchanged
				13% declined
Peterson et al, 2000	25	F	>2 years	92% good/excellent
	19	P	>2 years	62% good/excellent
				Improved to 85% with distal realignment
	16	F/ACL	>2 years	75% good/excellent
	16	Multiple	>2 years	67% good/excellent
Gillogly, Voight, and Blackburn, 1998	25	F, P, T	>1 year	88% good/excellent
Brittberg et al, 1994	16	F	39 months	88% good/excellent
				12% poor
	7	P without distal realignment	36 months	29% good/excellent
				42% fair
				29% poor

ABBREVIATIONS: F = femur; Tr = trochlea; P = patella; T = tibia; ACL = anterior cruciate ligament; OCD = osteochondritis dissecans.

TABLE 9-10   Results of Osteochondral Autografts

AUTHOR	N	LOCATION	MEAN FOLLOW-UP	RESULTS
Hangody et al, 2001	461	F	>1 year	92% good/excellent
	93	P/Tr	>1 year	81% good/excellent
	24	T	>1 year	80% good/excellent
Kish, Modis, and Hangody, 1999	52	F in competitive athletes	>1 year	100% good/excellent
				63% returned to full sports
				31% returned to sports at lower level
				90% <30 years returned to full sports
				23% >30 years returned to full sports
Bradley, 1999	145		18 months	43% good/excellent
				43% fair
				12% poor
Hangody et al, 1998	57	F, P	48 months	91% good/excellent

ABBREVIATIONS: F = femur; Tr = trochlea; P = patella; T = tibia.

TABLE 9-11   Results of Osteochondral Allografts

AUTHOR	N	LOCATION	MEAN FOLLOW-UP	RESULTS
Aubin et al, 2001	60 Mean age 27 years	F	10 years	84% good/excellent
				20% failure
Bugbee, 2000	122 Mean age 34 years	F	5 years	91% success rate at 5 years
				75% success rate at 10 years
				5% failure
Chu et al, 1999	55 Mean age 35 years	F, T, P	75 months	76% good/excellent
				16% failure
Gross, 1997	123 Mean age 35 years	F, T, P	7.5 years	85% success rate
Garrett, 1994	17 Mean age 20 years	F	3.5 years	94% success rate
Meyers, Akeson, and Convery F, 1989	39 Mean age 38 years	F, T, P	3.6 years	78% success rate
				22% failures

ABBREVIATIONS: F = femur; P = patella; T = tibia.

TABLE 9-12   Survivorship Analysis of Osteochondral Allografts

AUTHOR	N	LOCATION	5/7.5 YEARS	10 YEARS	14/15 YEARS	20 YEARS
Gross et al, 2002	60 Mean age 27 years	F	85%	85%	74%	
Ghazavi et al, 1997	123 Mean age 35 years	F, T, P	95%	71%		66%
Beaver et al, 1992	92 Mean age 50 years	F, T	75%	64%	63%	

ABBREVIATIONS: F = femur; P = patella; T = tibia.

DECISION MAKING

• The choice of surgical intervention is complex and involves the consideration of many factors, including defect size, depth, location, chronicity, response to previous treatments, concomitant pathology, patient age, physical demand level, and expectations. Multiple options often exist for similar lesions and there is not necessarily a consensus regarding the optimal treatment. Thus, the treatment algorithm presented in Fig. 9-1 should be regarded as an overview of the surgical-decision tree currently available to treat symptomatic chondral lesions. It is important to note that even though treatment options are not currently amenable to a menu-driven decision making process, there are several lesion- and patient-specific factors that are critical to the decision making process. These include: location and size of the injury or extent of disease progression, primary versus secondary treatment and patient activity demand. This algorithm is currently evolving and will undoubtedly change as we acquire new information from animal studies and clinical trials.

REFERENCES

Aubin PP, Cheah HK, Davis AM, et al: Long-term follow-up of fresh femoral osteochondral allografts for posttraumatic knee defects. *Clin Orthop* 391:S318–S327, 2001.

Barclay TS, Tsourounis C, McGart GM: Glucosamine. *Ann Pharmacother* 32:574–579, 1998.

Baumgaertner MR, Cannon WDJ, Vittori JM, et al: Arthroscopic debridement of the arthritic knee. *Clin Orthop* 253:197–202, 1990.

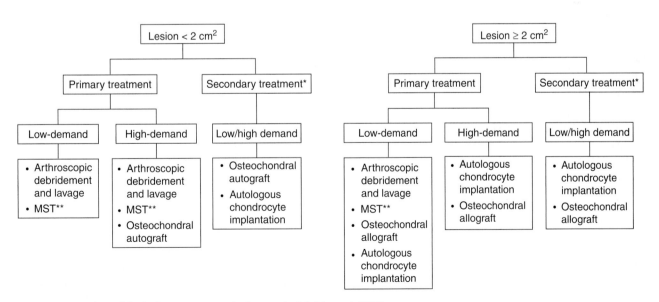

*In patients who have failed primary treatment (arthroscopic debridement, MST)
**Marrow stimulating techniques (i.e., microfracture, abrasion, drilling)

FIG. 9-1   Surgical management algorithm for the treatment of symptomatic focal chondral lesions.

Beaver RJ, Mahomed M, Backstein D, et al: Fresh osteochondral allografts for post-traumatic defects in the knee. A survivorship analysis. *J Bone Joint Surg* 74B:105–110, 1992.

Blevins FT, Steadman JR, Rodrigo JJ, et al: Treatment of articular cartilage defects in athletes: An analysis of functional outcome and lesion appearance. *Orthopedics* 21:761–7, 1998.

Bradley JP (ed.): Osteochondral autograft transplantation clinical outcome study, in *Metcalf Memorial Meeting.* Sun Valley, ID, 1999.

Brittberg M: Evaluation of cartilage injuries and cartilage repair. *Osteologie* 9:17–25, 2000.

Brittberg M, Peterson L: Introduction to an articular cartilage classification. *CRS Newsl* 1:8, 1998.

Brittberg M, Lindahl A, Nilsson A, et al: Treatment of deep cartilage defects in the knee with autologous chondrocyte transplantation. *N Engl J Med* 331:889–895, 1994.

Bucci L. Chondroprotective agents: Glucosamine salts and chondroitin sulfates. *Townsend Lett Doct* 1:52–54, 1994.

Buckwalter, JA: Articular cartilage injuries. *Clin Orthop* 402:21–37, 2002.

Buckwalter JA, Mankin HJ: Articular cartilage I: Tissue design and chondrocyte-matrix interactions. *J Bone Joint Surg* 79A:600–611, 1997*a*.

Buckwalter JA, Mankin HJ: Articular cartilage II: Degeneration and osteoarthrosis, repair, regeneration, and transplantation. *J Bone Joint Surg* 79A:612–632, 1997*b*.

Buckwalter JA, Mow VC: Cartilage repair in osteoarthritis, in Moskowitz RW, Howell DS, Goldberg VM, Mankin HJ (eds.): *Osteoarthritis: Diagnosis and Management,* 2nd ed. Philadelphia, Saunders 1992, pp 71–107.

Buckwalter JA, Rosenberg LA, Hunziker EB: Articular cartilage: Injury and repair, in Woo SL, Buckwalter JA (eds.): *Injury and Repair of the Musculoskeletal Soft Tissues.* Park Ridge, IL, American Academy of Orthopaedic Surgeons 1988, pp 465–482.

Buckwalter JA, Rosenberg LA, Hunziker EB: Articular cartilage: Composition, structure, response to injury, and methods of facilitation repair, in Ewing JW (ed.): *Articular Cartilage and Knee Joint Function: Basic Science and Arthroscopy.* New York, NY, Raven Press 1990, pp 19–56.

Buckwalter JA, Hunziker EB, Rosenberg LC, et al: Articular cartilage: Composition and structure, in Woo SL, Buckwalter JA (eds.): *Injury and Repair of the Musculoskeletal Soft Tissues.* Park Ridge, IL, American Academy of Orthopaedic Surgeons 1988, pp 405–425.

Bugbee WD: Fresh osteochondral allografting. *Oper Tech Sports Med* 8:158–162, 2000.

Chu CR, Convery FR, Akeson WH, et al: Articular cartilage transplantation. Clinical results in the knee. *Clin Orthop* 360:159–368, 1999.

Cole BJ, Frederick R, Levy A, et al: Management of a 37 year old man with recurrent knee pain. *J Clin Outcomes Manag* 6:46–57, 1999.

Curl W, Krome J, Gordon E, et al: Cartilage injuries: A review of 31,516 knee arthroscopies. Arthroscopy 13:456–460, 1997.

DaCamara CC, Dowless GV: Glucosamine sulfate for osteoarthritis. *Ann Pharmacother* 32:580–587, 1998.

Finerman GAM, Noyes FR (eds.): *Biology and Biomechanics of the Traumatized Synovial Joint: The Knee as a Model.* Rosemont, IL, American Academy of Orthopaedic Surgeons 597, 1992.

Garrett JC: Fresh osteochondral allografts for treatment of articular defects in osteochondritis dissecans of the lateral femoral condyle in adults. *Clin Orthop* 303:33–37, 1994.

Ghazavi MT, Pritzker KP, Davis AM, et al: Fresh osteochondral allografts for post-traumatic osteochondral defects of the knee. *J Bone Joint Surg* 79B:1008–1013, 1997.

Gill TJ, MacGillivray JD: The technique of microfracture for the treatment of articular cartilage defects in the knee. *Oper Tech Sports Med* 11:105–107, 2001.

Gill TJ, Steadman JR, Rodrigo JJ, et al: Indications and long-term clinical results of microfracture. *2nd Symp Int Cartilage Repair Soc,* Boston, MA, November, 1998.

Gillogly SD, Voight M, Blackburn T: Treatment of articular cartilage defects of the knee with autologous chondrocyte implantation. *J Orthop Sports Phys Ther* 28:241–251, 1998.

Gosh P: Second-line agents in osteoarthritis, in Dixon JS and Furst DE (eds.). Second Line Agents in the Treatment of Rheumatic Diseases. New York, NY, Marcel Dekker 1992, pp 363–427.

Grande D, Pitman M, Peterson L, et al: The repair of experimentally produced defects in rabbit articular cartilage by autologous chondrocyte implantation. *J Orthop Res* 7:208–218, 1997.

Gross AE: Fresh osteochondral allgorafts for post-traumatic knee defects: Surgical technique. *Oper Tech Orthop* 7:334, 1997.

Gross AE, Aubin P, Cheah HK, et al: A fresh osteochondral allograft alternative. *J Arthroplasty 17, Suppl* 1:50–53, 2002.

Hangody L, Feczki P, Bartha L, et al: Mosaicplasty for the treatment of articular defects of the knee and ankle. *Clin Orthop 391 Suppl* S328–S336, 2001.

Hangody L, Kish G, Karpati Z, et al: Mosaicplasty for the treatment of articular cartilage defects: application in clinical practice. *Orthopedics* 21:751–756, 1998.

Hjelle K, Solheim E, Strand T, et al: Articular cartilage defects in 1,000 knee arthroscopies. *Arthroscopy* 18:730–734, 2002.

Hubbard MJ: Articular debridement versus washout for degeneration of the medial femoral condyle. A five-year study. *J Bone Joint Surg* 78B:217–219, 1996.

Jackson RW: Meniscal and articular cartilage injury in sport. *J R Coll Surg Edinb* 34:S15–S17, 1989.

Khanna BAJ, Cosgarea AJ, Mont MA, et al: Magnetic resonance imaging of the knee. Current techniques and spectrum of disease. *J Bone Joint Surg 83A, Suppl 2 Pt* 2:128–141, 2001.

Kish G, Modis L, Hangody L: Osteochondral mosaicplasty for the treatment of focal chondral and osteochondral lesions of the knee and talus in the athlete. Rationale, indications, techniques, and results. *Clin Sports Med* 18:45–66, 1999.

Mandelbaum BR, Romanelli DA, Knapp TP: Articular cartilage repair: Assessment and classification. *Op Tech Sports Med* 8:90–97, 2000.

Martin JA, Buckwalter JA: The role of chondrocyte-matrix interactions in maintaining and repairing articular cartilage. *Biorheology* 37:129–140, 2000.

Meyers MH, Akeson W, Convery F. Resurfacing of the knee with fresh osteochondral allograft. *J Bone Joint Surg* 71A:704–713, 1989.

Micheli LJ, Browne JE, Erggelet C, et al: Autologous chondrocyte implantation of the knee: Multicenter experience and minimum 3-year follow-up. *Clin J Sports Med* 11:223–228, 2001.

Minas T: Autologous chondrocyte implantation for focal chondral defects of the knee. *Clin Orthop* 391:S349–S361, 2001.

Muller-Fassbender H, Bach GL, Hasse W, et al: Glucosamine sulfate compared to ibuprofen in osteoarthritis of the knee. *Osteoarthritis Cartilage* 2:61–69, 1994.

Outerbridge RE: The etiology of chondromalacia patellae. *J Bone Joint Surg* 43B:752–757, 1961.

Owens BD, Stickles BJ, Balikian P, et al. Prospective analysis of radiofrequency versus mechanical debridement of isolated patellar chondral lesions. *Arthroscopy* 18:151–155, 2002.

Peterson L, Brittberg M, Kiviranta I, et al: Autologous chondrocyte transplantation. Biomechanics and long-term durability. *Am J Sports Med* 30:2–12, 2002.

Peterson L, Minas T, Brittberg M, et al: Two- to 9-year outcome after autologous chondrocyte transplantation of the knee. *Clin Orthop* 374:212–234, 2000.

Sprague NF, 3rd: Arthroscopic debridement for degenerative knee joint disease. *Clin Orthop* 160:118–123, 1981.

Steadman JR, Briggs KK, Rodrigo JJ, et al: Outcomes of microfracture for traumatic chondral defects of the knee: Average 11-year follow-up. *Arthroscopy* 19:477–484, 2003.

Steadman JR, Rodkey WG, Rodrigo JJ. Microfracture: Surgical technique and rehabilitation to treat chondral defects. *Clin Orthop* 391:S362–S369, 2001.

Steadman JR, Rodkey WG, Singleton SB, et al: Microfracture technique for full-thickness chondral defects: technique and clinical results. *Operative Tech Orthop* 7:300–304, 1997.

Timoney JM, Kneisl JS, Barrack RL, et al: Arthroscopy update #6. Arthroscopy in the osteoarthritic knee. Long-term follow-up. *Orthop Rev* 4:371–3, 376–9, 1990.

Tomford WW: Chondroprotective agents in the treatment of articular cartilage degeneration. *Oper Tech Sports Med* 8:120–121, 2000.

10 MUSCLE AND TENDON INJURY AND REPAIR

Bradley J Nelson, MD
Dean C Taylor, MD

INTRODUCTION

- Muscle and tendon injuries occur frequently in the athletic population. Most injuries are self-limiting and a full recovery is to be expected; however, these injuries can dramatically affect an athlete's performance and their ubiquitous nature makes these injuries an important part of the athlete's care.

- This chapter will review injury and repair of muscle and tendon tissue. Emphasis will be placed on the basic science of these injuries.

SKELETAL MUSCLE INJURY AND REPAIR

- Muscle injury is the most common musculoskeletal complaint in the athlete. Common muscle injuries include muscle strains, delayed muscle soreness, contusions, and cramps.
- This section on muscle injury will provide a brief review of anatomy and physiology, a description of the reparative process, and then a discussion of the types of muscle injuries common in athletes.

ANATOMY AND PHYSIOLOGY

- Skeletal muscle is composed primarily of contractile proteins (myosin, actin, tropomyosin, and troponin) and a connective tissue matrix (Best, 1997).
- The muscle fiber is the basic structural element of skeletal muscle. The fiber is a syncytium of fused muscle cells with multiple nuclei (Garrett and Best, 2000). Within the fibers are myofibrils which are composed of repeating units of light and dark bands called sarcomeres. The bands are made up of thick (myosin) and thin (actin) filaments.
- The muscle fiber originates from bone or tendon, traverses one or more joints, and inserts into a tendon that connects to bone. Fiber arrangement can be parallel or oblique (pennate, bipennate, and the like) in orientation. Fibers can be classified as type I (slow-twitch oxidative) and type II (fast-twitch). Type II fibers are further classified into type IIa (fast-twitch oxidative glycolytic) and IIb (fast-twitch glycolytic).
- Satellite cells are separate cells along the periphery of the muscle fiber that regenerate into muscle cells in response to injury.
- The musculotendinous junction is a specialized region of highly folded membranes that increase the surface area for force transmission (Best, 1997). Most muscle strain injuries occur in this region.
- The sarcoplasmic reticulum is a specialized cellular organelle that is responsible for calcium movement across the cell membrane and electric transmission within the cell.
- A motor unit is a single nerve axon and all the muscle fibers it innervates. The nerve contacts the muscle fiber at the motor end plate.
- A muscle contraction begins when an electric impulse travels down a nerve axon to its motor end plates.

A chemical transmission occurs across the synapses that generate electric potentials in the muscle membranes. These electric potentials cause the sarcoplasmic reticulum to release calcium. The calcium binds to troponin, which results in a conformational change in tropomyosin that allows the interaction between the myosin (thick) and actin (thin) filaments. These filaments slide past each other to shorten or resist lengthening. This process is powered by the hydrolysis of ATP (Garrett and Best, 2000).

REPARATIVE PROCESS

- The pathophysiology of healing muscle is similar regardless of the type of injury. The reparative process involves both inflammatory cells (neutrophils, macrophages) and myogenic (satellite) cells.
- Inflammatory cell invasion of the damaged muscle tissue begins shortly after injury.
  1. Neutrophils initially infiltrate the injury site via cellular chemotaxis. The cellular mechanism responsible for attracting the neutrophils is not completely known but probably involves a complex signaling process. Mediators such as *basic fibroblast growth factor* (bFGF), *platelet-derived growth factor* (PDGF), and *interleukin-1* (IL-1) stimulate macrophages and fibroblasts within the muscle tissue, which in turn, attract and activate inflammatory cells (Tidball, 1995).
  2. Macrophages are the most prevalent inflammatory cells present in injured muscle. Distinct subclasses of macrophages have been identified and play specific roles in the healing process. One subclass of macrophages is involved in the phagocytosis of damaged tissue and further stimulation of the inflammatory response. A second subclass of macrophages helps modulate the reparative process (Tidball, 1995).
- Satellite cells are myogenic mononuclear cells responsible for muscle fiber regeneration. Muscle injury stimulates these cells to differentiate into myoblasts, which fuse together and develop into multinucleated muscle fibers (Lehto and Jarvinen, 1991).
- Fibroblast proliferation and collagen matrix synthesis occur along with the inflammatory response and muscle regeneration. This connective tissue scar formation may inhibit the complete repair of injured muscle (Lehto and Jarvinen, 1991).

MUSCLE STRAIN INJURY

- Muscle strain is the most common injury sustained in sports. This type of muscle injury can range from delayed muscle soreness (discussed below), to partial muscle strain, to complete muscle disruption.
- These injuries occur most commonly during eccentric contraction in muscles that cross two joints (rectus femoris, biceps femoris, gastrocnemius). These muscles have a high proportion of type II (fast-twitch) fibers and these injuries occur most frequently during sprinting (Noonan and Garrett, Jr, 1999).

MECHANISM OF INJURY
- High forces are generated in relatively few muscle fibers during eccentric muscular contraction; however, muscle contraction alone is insufficient to create muscle strain injury. Passive stretch of the muscle past its resting length is required to injure the muscle (Garrett et al, 1988). This increased strain disrupts the muscle fibers near the muscle-tendon junction.
- Cellular disruption results in the hydrolysis of structural proteins and inflammation that further damages the muscle tissue (Nikolaou et al, 1987).
- Animal studies reveal that muscle tissue sustaining a nondisruptive strain injury demonstrates decreased load to failure when subjected to stress (Obremsky et al, 1994; Taylor et al, 1993). In addition, these partially injured muscles generate significantly less contractile force. This may explain the clinical observation that significant muscle strain injuries are frequently preceded by a minor injury. These studies also underscore the importance of rest and complete recovery prior to the resumption of athletic activities.

REPARATIVE RESPONSE
- Similar to the general reparative response of muscle described above.
- The presence of inelastic fibrotic tissue (scar) may make the muscle more susceptible to additional injury.

TREATMENT AND PREVENTION
- As mentioned above, reduced activity is key in the treatment of muscle strain injuries. This helps control inflammation and prevents further tissue damage.
- Immobilization can diminish pain, reduce inflammation, and allow torn muscle ends to reapproximate. Prolonged muscle immobilization (greater than 7–14 days) results in muscle that demonstrates lower loads to failure and should be avoided (Noonan and Garrett, Jr, 1999).

NONSTEROIDAL ANTI-INFLAMMATORY DRUGS
- Animal studies demonstrate that *nonsteroidal anti-inflammatory drugs* (NSAIDs) reduce the inflammatory response associated with muscle strain injury but

may delay complete healing of the muscle tissue (Nikolaou et al, 1987; Obremsky et al, 1994). The indication for the use of these drugs in muscle strain injury is unclear.
- Cryotherapy provides an analgesic effect but its effect on inflammation is unclear (Noonan and Garrett, Jr, 1999).

MUSCLE STRENGTHENING
- Muscle strengthening is an important factor in the recovery of injured muscle and the prevention of reinjury.
- Basic science research has demonstrated that fatigued muscle has decreased load to failure and energy absorption than control muscle tissue (Mair et al, 1996). These data would support the belief that the athlete with a muscle strain injury should not return to competition until complete muscle strength and conditioning have returned.

MUSCLE STRETCHING AND WARM-UP
- Muscle is viscoelastic material, and passive stretching can reduce stress for a given muscle length (Taylor et al, 1990). In addition, preconditioned muscle and muscle that is warm fails at higher loads than control muscle (Safran et al, 1988). These studies suggest the importance of stretching and warm-up in the prevention of muscle strain injury.
- A recent review of clinical and basic science literature questions the above conclusions and states that stretching prior to exercise does not prevent injury and may make the muscle more susceptible to injury (Shrier, 1999). Additional studies are needed before definitive conclusions can be made.

DELAYED MUSCLE SORENESS

- Delayed muscle soreness is defined as skeletal muscle pain 24–72 h after unaccustomed physical activity. The pain lasts approximately 5–7 days and can range from mild soreness to severe discomfort (Armstrong, 1984). Loss of muscle strength, loss of joint range of motion, tenderness, and elevated muscle enzymes are also present.
- Strength loss can be explained by both the presence of pain and a decrease in the inherent force-producing capacity of the muscle fibers (Armstrong, 1984).
- No permanent muscle injury occurs and complete muscle recovery is seen within 14 days.
- Delayed muscle soreness occurs most commonly in muscles performing eccentric activity and is related to both the intensity and duration of activity.

PATHOPHYSIOLOGY
- High tension over a small cross-sectional area (seen in eccentric muscular contraction) results in cytoskeletal disruption.
- Sarcolemma (cell membrane) disruption results in an influx of intracellular Ca^{2+} that induces proteolytic enzyme mediated myoprotein degradation (Armstrong, 1984).
- Cellular damage results in the activation of inflammatory processes. This stimulates nociceptors within the muscle resulting in the production of pain (Armstrong, 1984).

TREATMENT AND PREVENTION
- Further exercise appears to be the most effective method of diminishing the symptoms of delayed muscle soreness. This is most likely owing to exercise-induced production of endorphins or other alterations in neural pathways (Armstrong, 1984).
- Delayed muscle soreness diminishes with repetition of exercise. The reasons for this are unclear. There is still continued muscle tissue damage with repetitive exercise but to a progressively lesser extent. The discomfort associated with this tissue damage, however, is greatly diminished.
- Nonsteroidal anti-inflammatory drugs demonstrate similar effects in an exercise-induced muscle injury model as they do in other muscle injury models. There is early benefit to the muscle by limiting inflammation but the later negative effects on maximum muscle function mitigate this (Mishra et al, 1995).

MUSCLE CONTUSION INJURY

- Muscle contusions are common injuries in collision and contact sports. These injuries most frequently involve the lower extremity muscle groups, such as the quadriceps, gastrocnemius, or anterior muscles of the lower leg (Best, 1997).
- The initial clinical presentation includes pain, swelling, loss of joint range of motion, and the possibility of a palpable muscle defect. This can be followed by persistent swelling and warmth, a firm mass, and continued loss of motion.
- Animal studies of muscle contusion injury demonstrate muscle fiber rupture resulting in hematoma formation, edema, and inflammation (Walton and Rothwell, 1983).

REPARATIVE RESPONSE
- Similar to the general process of muscle healing described above; however, there appears to be less scar formation with a muscle contusion injury than with a muscle strain injury.

TREATMENT

Immobilization Versus Mobilization of Contused Muscle

a. Brief immobilization (less than 5 days) leads to faster healing without further tissue damage while prolonged immobilization results in muscle atrophy and delayed muscle activity in a rat model (Jarvinen, 1975; Lehto, Duance, and Restall, 1985). In addition, early mobilization results in increased tensile stiffness of contused muscle and more rapid resolution of the contusion injury (Jarvinen, 1976).

b. Clinical studies from the U. S. Military Academy demonstrate that a brief period of immobilization (24–48 h) with the involved muscle in a lengthened position followed by mobilization results in earlier recovery than prolonged muscle immobilization (Jackson and Feagin, 1973; Ryan et al, 1991).

PHARMACOLOGIC TREATMENT

• Animal studies have demonstrated that both corticosteroids and nonsteroidal anti-inflammatory drugs cause a decrease in the early inflammatory response (Beiner et al, 1999); however, there is delayed muscle regeneration and a decrease in the later tensile properties of the healed muscle. Recent animal studies also show that anabolic steroids and growth factors can produce a beneficial effect in the healing of contused muscle (Beiner and Jokl, 2001). The clinical use of these substances has not been approved, however.

• Myositis ossificans is a concerning complication of muscle contusion injury. The etiology of this abnormal bone formation is unclear but is related to the degree of muscle injury, the region injured (quadriceps and brachialis), and the number of times the muscle is subjected to trauma (Beiner and Jokl, 2001). Clinically there is usually tenderness, swelling, loss of motion, persistent warmth, and a firm mass in the area of the bone formation. The abnormal bone is radiographically evident by 4 weeks and resembles mature bone by 6 months (Best, 1997). The bone frequently resolves spontaneously. Surgical resection, if necessary, should be delayed until the osteoblastic activity has ceased (6 months to 1 year).

MUSCLE CRAMPS

• Muscle cramps commonly affect both athletes and nonathletes. The gastrocnemius muscle and hamstrings are most commonly involved but cramping can involve nearly any muscle group. Cramps begin with the muscle in a shortened position.

• The cramp begins as a fasciculation from a single focus within the muscle and then spreads throughout the muscle. Electric evidence suggests that the source of the abnormal activity is coming from the nerve within the muscle (Best, 1997).

• The etiology of muscle cramping is unclear but dehydration and hyponatremia are frequently present. Hypokalemia and hypocalcemia have also been implicated (Best, 1997).

• Treatment includes passive stretching of the muscle along with fluid and sodium replacement.

• Athletes with repeated episodes of cramping should undergo evaluation for electrolyte or endocrine disorders.

TENDON INJURY AND REPAIR

• Tendon injuries are secondary to direct trauma (lacerations) or tensile overload.

• Tensile overload injuries are very common athletic injuries and can occur acutely or as a result of chronic overload.

• Acute tendon overload usually results in injury to the musculotendinous junction or a bony avulsion since tendons can withstand high tensile loads. Rarely does a normal tendon rupture midsubstance.

• Chronic tendon overload injuries are common overuse injuries and will be the focus of this section.

ANATOMY AND PHYSIOLOGY

• Tendons consist primarily of type I collagen fibrils, a proteoglycan matrix, and relatively few fibroblasts.

a. Type I collagen consists of two alpha-I polypeptide chains and one alpha-2 chain. These three chains are organized into a triple helix stabilized by hydrogen and covalent bonds (Wood et al, 2000).

b. The collagen triple helix molecules are aligned in a quarter-staggered arrangement to make up the collagen microfibril. This results in alignment of oppositely charged amino acids and contributes to the tendon's strength.

a. The microfibrils are then arranged in a parallel, well ordered, and densely packed fashion. This organization also contributes to the tendon's tensile strength. The microfibrils are combined with a proteoglycan and water matrix to form collagen fascicles. The tendon consists of groupings of these fascicles surrounded by connective tissue that contains blood vessels, nerves, and lymphatics (Wood et al, 2000).

- The insertion of tendons onto bone is usually via four zones: tendon, fibrocartilage, mineralized fibrocartilage, and bone.
- Tendons that bend at acute angles (flexor tendons in the hand) are enclosed in a distinct sheath that acts as a pulley (Wood et al, 2000). Synovial fluid within the sheath assists in tendon gliding. Tendons that are not enclosed in a sheath (Achilles tendon) are covered by a paratenon.
- Mechanical forces affect the characteristics of tendon. Tendons subjected to tensile loads have smaller densely packed collagen fibrils, increased collagen synthesis, smaller proteoglycans (Decorin), and a higher collagen to proteoglycan ratio. Tendons sustaining compressive loads exhibit increased proteoglycan levels, larger proteoglycan molecules, and larger less dense collagen fibrils (Hyman and Rodeo, 2000).
- Aging also affects the material characteristics of tendon with decreased collagen synthesis, increased collagen fibril diameter, decreased proteoglycan content, decreased water content, and decreased vascularity. This results in a stiffer, weaker tendon (Hyman and Rodeo, 2000).

CHRONIC TENSILE OVERLOAD INJURIES

TERMINOLOGY
- There is significant confusion regarding the terminology of chronic tendon injuries. Tendinitis, tendonitis, and tendinosis are frequently used terms to describe the clinical picture of pain, swelling, and stiffness in a tendon.
- Terminology based on pathology has been proposed (Jarvinen et al, 1997):
  a. Paratenonitis: Inflammation of the paratenon or tendon sheath. Peritendinitis and tenosynovitis are included in this category.
  b. Paratenonitis with tendinosis: Tendon degeneration with concomitant paratenon inflammation
  c. Tendinosis: Tendon degeneration without inflammation
  d. Tendinitis: Inflammation within the tendon
- *Tendinopathy* has been proposed as a generic term describing the clinical picture of pain, swelling, and impaired performance (Maffulli, Kahn, and Puddu, 1998).

ETIOLOGY
- The etiology of chronic tendon injuries is multifactorial and involves a combination of intrinsic and extrinsic factors.
- Important intrinsic factors include *anatomic abnormalities* (malalignment, muscle weakness/imbalance,

decreased flexibility, and joint laxity), age, gender, weight, and predisposing diseases (Almekinders, 1998; Kannus, 1997).
- Important extrinsic factors include excessive mechanical load (frequency, duration, and intensity), training errors (over training, rapid progression, fatigue, running surface, and poor technique), and equipment problems (footwear, racquets, and seat height) (Almekinders, 1998; Kannus, 1997).
- There are very few well-controlled studies that examine the etiologic factors involved in chronic tendon injuries.

PATHOPHYSIOLOGY
- Repetitive load on a tendon that results in 4–8% strain causes microscopic tendon fiber damage. Continued load on the tendon at this level overwhelms the tendon's ability for repair. Damage occurs to the collagen fibrils, the noncollagenous matrix, and microvasculature (Hyman and Rodeo, 2000).
- Cellular damage results in inflammation of the surrounding paratenon (paratenonitis). Tissue edema, fibrin exudate, and capillary occlusion result in local tissue hypoxia. Audible crepitation may be noted on examination (Kannus, 1997).
- The paratenon becomes thickened as fibroblast proliferation and fibrotic adhesions develop. This results in decreased tendon gliding and triggering.
- Intrinsic tendon damage (tendinosis) may occur with continued tendon overload. Tendon degeneration may appear as a number of histologic entities (hypoxic degeneration, mucoid degeneration, fiber calcification, and the like) (Kannus, 1997).
- The causal link between initial inflammation (paratenonitis) and tendon degeneration (tendinosis) is unclear. Researchers have demonstrated that chronic paratenonitis can result in tendon degeneration in an animal model (Backman et al, 1990); however, a large clinical study showed no previous evidence of paratenonitis in over 60% of patients who sustained an Achilles tendon rupture (Kannus and Jozsa, 1991). The initial paratenonitis may be causative factor for tendon degeneration or may coexist independently.
- The exact cellular mechanism of tendon degeneration has not been completely defined. Important factors include tissue hypoxia, free radical induced tendon damage, and tissue hyperthermia (Kannus, 1997).

DIAGNOSIS
- The history often reveals repetitive mechanical overload. The athlete will usually be involved in either an endurance sport (running, cycling, and swimming) or a sport that requires repetition of a specialized skill (tennis, basketball, and baseball) (Hess et al, 1989).

The athlete will frequently note an increase in the duration, frequency, or intensity of the training regimen. The pain is frequently worse after a period of rest following the training period. Changes in footwear, equipment, or training surface may be present.

- The physical examination may reveal swelling or crepitation along the tendon sheath. The degenerative tendon is often tender to palpation or painful with compression (impingement signs). Range of motion may be restricted (Almekinders, 1998).
- Diagnostic tests include radiographs to exclude stress fractures or osteoarthritis. Ultrasound or magnetic resonance imaging can be useful in tendons that are not easily palpated (rotator cuff).

TREATMENT

- Removing or modifying the mechanical overload (relative rest) is the most important component of treating chronic tendon injuries. Correcting training errors and equipment problems should also be accomplished.
- Prolonged immobilization should be avoided. Immobilization results in deceased tendon strength and stiffness owing to proteolytic degradation of collagen (Hyman and Rodeo, 2000).
- Physical therapy is often prescribed for chronic tendon disorders. Stretching and strengthening (particularly eccentric exercises) are thought to be beneficial but there are few good studies that support this assertion. Modalities such as heat, ice, and ultrasound may also improve the patient's symptoms but there is little evidence that these techniques accelerate tendon healing.
- NSAIDs are frequently taken for chronic tendon disorders. A recent review of the literature stated that five of nine placebo-controlled studies demonstrated the efficacy of NSAIDs in the treatment of tendinopathy (Almekinders and Temple, 1998). There is no evidence that NSAIDs improve the healing process in tendon degeneration and there is evidence in muscle injury that NSAIDs may be harmful to tissue healing (Mishra et al, 1995). Short-term use of NSAIDs may be indicated to provide analgesia for the athlete.
- The use of corticosteroids injections in the treatment of tendinopathy is controversial. The rationale of using a local anti-inflammatory medication for a disease process that involves tissue degeneration is questionable. Corticosteroids may decrease inflammation in the paratenon, reduce adhesions between the tendon and the peritendinous tissue, or block nociceptors in the damaged tendon (Paavola et al, 2002); however, only three of eight placebo-controlled studies in the literature demonstrate the efficacy of corticosteroid injections (Almekinders and Temple, 1998). Direct injections into the tendon substance should be avoided as they result in elevated tissue pressure and tissue

damage. The use of corticosteroid injections around weight-bearing tendons such as the Achilles tendon and patellar tendon is controversial. There have been case reports of tendon rupture but there are no controlled studies and rupture of the tendon may have occurred without an injection. It is difficult to make recommendations on the use of corticosteroid injections owing to the paucity of scientific evidence regarding their use.

- The surgical treatment of chronic tendon injury is usually reserved for those cases that do not resolve with four to six months of nonsurgical treatment. The surgical procedures usually involve debridement of the degenerative tendon tissue. Occasionally complete resection and repair or grafting is required (Almekinders, 1998). Removal of the involved paratenon or release of the tendon sheath is occasionally necessary. Bony prominences may require removal (Haglunds, acromion). Clinical series in the literature demonstrate the success of surgical management but there are a very few controlled studies.

REFERENCES

Almekinders LC, Temple JD: Etiology, diagnosis, and treatment of tendonitis: An analysis of the literature. *Med Sci Sports Exerc* 8:1183–1190, 1998.

Almekinders LC: Tendinitis and other chronic tendinopathies. *J Am Acad Orthop Surg* 6:157–164, 1998.

Armstrong RB: Mechanisms of exercise-induced delayed onset muscular soreness: A brief review. *Med Sci Sports Exerc* 16:529–537, 1984.

Backman C, Boquist L, Friden J, et al: Chronic Achilles paratenonitis with tendinosis: An experimental model in the rabbit. *J Orthop Res* 8:541–547, 1990.

Beiner JM, Jokl P: Muscle contusion injuries: Current treatment options. *J Am Acad Orthop Surg* 9:227–237, 2001.

Beiner JM, Jokl P, Cholewicki J, et al: The effect of anabolic steroids and corticosteroids on healing of muscle contusion injury. *Am J Sports Med* 27:2–9, 1999.

Best TM: Soft-tissue injuries and muscle tears. *Clin Sports Med* 16:419–434, 1997.

Garrett WE, Jr, Nikolaou PK, Ribbeck BM, et al: The effect of muscle architecture on the biomechanical failure properties of skeletal muscle under passive extension. *Am J Sports Med* 16:7–12, 1988.

Garrett WE, Best TM: Anatomy, physiology, and mechanics of skeletal muscle, in Buckwalter JA, Einhorn TA, Simon Sheldon (eds.): *Orthopaedic Basic Science,* 2nd ed. Chicago, American Academy of Orthopaedic Surgeons, 2000, p 683.

Hess GP, Capiello WL, Poole RM, et al: Prevention and treatment of overuse tendon injuries. *Sports Med* 8:371–384, 1989.

Hyman J, Rodeo SA: Injury and repair of tendons and ligaments. *Phys Med Rehabil Clin N Am* 11:267–288, 2000.

Jackson DW, Feagin JA: Quadriceps contusions in young athletes. Relation of severity of injury to treatment and prognosis. *J Bone Joint Surg Am* 55:95–105, 1973.

Jarvinen M: Healing of a crush injury in rat striated muscle. Part 2. A histological study of the effect of early mobilization and immobilization on the repair processes. *Acta Pathol Microbiol Scand (A)* 83:269–282, 1975.

Jarvinen M: Healing of a crush injury in rat striated muscle. Part 4. Effect of early mobilization and immobilization on the tensile properties of gastrocnemius muscle. *Acta Chir Scand* 142:47–56, 1976.

Jarvinen M, Jozsa L, Kannus P, et al: Histopathological findings in chronic tendon disorders. *Scand J Med Sci Sports* 7:86–95, 1997.

Kannus P: Etiology and pathophysiology of chronic tendon disorders in sports. *Scand J Med Sci Sports* 7:78–85, 1997.

Kannus P, Jozsa L: Histopathological changes preceding spontaneous rupture of a tendon. A controlled study of 891 patients. *J Bone Joint Surg Am* 73:1507–1525, 1991.

Lehto M, Duance VC, Restall, D: Collagen and fibronectin in a healing skeletal muscle injury. An immunohistological study of the effects of physical activity on the repair of injured gastrocnemius muscle in the rat. *J Bone Joint Surg Br* 67:820–828, 1985.

Lehto MK, Jarvinen MJ: Muscle injuries, their healing process and treatment. *Ann Chir Gynaecol* 80:102–108, 1991.

Maffulli N, Kahn KM, Puddu G: Overuse tendon conditions: Time to change a confusing terminology. *Arthroscopy* 14:840–843, 1998.

Mair SD, Seaber AV, Glisson RR, et al: The role of fatigue in susceptibility to acute muscle strain injury. *Am J Sports Med* 24:137–143, 1996.

Mishra DK, Friden J, Schmitz MC, et al: Anti-inflammatory medication after muscle injury. A treatment resulting in short-term improvement but subsequent loss of muscle function. *J Bone Joint Surg Am* 77:1510–1519, 1995.

Nikolaou PK, MacDonald BL, Glisson RR, et al: Biological and histological evaluation of muscle after controlled strain injury. *Am J Sports Med* 15:9–14, 1987.

Noonan TJ, Garrett WE, Jr: Muscle Strain Injury: Diagnosis and treatment. *J Am Acad Orthop Surg* 7:262–269, 1999.

Obremsky WT, Seaber AV, Ribbeck BM, et al: Biomechanical and histologic assessment of a controlled muscle strain injury treated with piroxicam. *Am J Sports Med* 22:558–561, 1994.

Paavola M, Kannus P, Jarvinen TA, et al: Treatment of tendon disorders. Is there a role for corticosteroids injection? *Foot Ankle Clin N Am* 7:501–513, 2002.

Ryan JB, Wheeler JH, Hopkinson WJ, et al: Quadriceps contusions. West Point update. *Am J Sports Med* 19:299–304, 1991.

Safran MR, Garrett WE Jr, Seaber AV, et al: The role of warmup in muscular injury prevention. *Am J Sports Med* 16:123–129, 1988.

Shrier I: Stretching before exercise does not reduce the risk of local muscle injury: A critical review of the clinical and basic science literature. *Clin J Sports Med* 9:221–227, 1999.

Taylor DC, Dalton JD Jr, Seaber AV, et al: Viscoelastic properties of muscle-tendon units: The biomechanical effects of stretching. *Am J Sports Med* 18:300–309, 1990.

Taylor DC, Dalton JD, Jr, Seaber AV, et al: Experimental muscle strain injury: Early functional and structural deficits and the increased risk for reinjury. *Am J Sports Med* 21:190–194, 1993.

Tidball JG: Inflammatory cell response to acute muscle injury. *Med Sci Sports Exerc* 27:1022–1032, 1995.

Walton M, Rothwell, AG: Reactions of thigh tissues of sheep to blunt trauma. *Clin Orthop* 176:273–281, 1983.

Wood SL, An KN, Frank CB, et al: Anatomy, biology, and biomechanics of tendon and ligament, in Buckwalter JA, Einhorn TA, Simon Sheldon (eds.): *Orthopaedic Basic Science,* 2nd ed. Chicago, American Academy of Orthopaedic Surgeons, 2000, p 581.

11 BONE INJURY AND FRACTURE HEALING

Carlos A Guanche, MD

- Bone injury is multifactorial in its effects. The cellular content of bone, the ability of such cells to produce extracellular matrix and the structure and organization of the components of bone are altered.

BONE ANATOMY(RECKER, 1992)

OSTEOGENIC PRECURSOR CELLS
- Present on all nonresorbtive bone surfaces and make up the deep layer of the periosteum and the endosteum.
- The *Periosteum* is a tough vascular layer of connective tissue. It covers the bone but not its articulating surface.
- The *Endosteum* is a single layer of osteogenic cells lacking a fibrous component.

OSTEOBLASTS
- Mature, metabolically active bone forming cells.
  a. Secrete osteoid the unmineralized matrix that subsequently undergoes mineralization.
  b. Some osteoblasts are converted into osteocytes, whereas others remain on the surfaces of bone as lining cells.
  c. Play a role in the activation of bone resorption by osteoclasts.

OSTEOCYTES
- Mature osteoblasts trapped within the bone matrix.
- Form a network of cytoplasmic processes extending through cylindrical canaliculi to blood vessels and other osteocytes.
- Involved in extracellular calcium and phosphorus homeostasis.

OSTEOCLASTS

- Multinucleated bone resorbing cells controlled by hormonal and cellular mechanisms
- Function in groups termed *cutting cones* that attach to bare bone surfaces and dissolve inorganic and organic matrices of bone and calcified cartilage through the use of hydrolytic enzymes.
- Process results in the formation of shallow pits on the bone surface called Howship's Lacunae (Recker, 1992).

HEMATOPOIETIC ELEMENTS

- Cells primarily responsible for the proliferation of the cellular element of blood

TYPES OF BONE

WOVEN BONE

- Formed during embryonic development, during fracture healing and in some pathologic states such as hyperparathyroidism and Paget's disease (Recker, 1992).
- Composed of randomly arranged collagen bundles and irregularly shaped vascular spaces.

CORTICAL BONE (COMPACT OR LAMELLAR BONE)

- Remodeled from woven bone by means of vascular channels that invade the embryonic bone from its periosteal and endosteal surfaces.
- The primary structural unit of cortical bone is an osteon, also known as a Haversian system.
  a. Consists of cylindrical shaped lamellar bone that surrounds longitudinally oriented vascular channels called Haversian canals.
  b. Horizontally oriented canals (Volkmann) connect adjacent osteons.
  c. Mechanical strength of cortical bone is dependent on the concentration of the osteons.

CANCELLOUS BONE (TRABECULAR)

- Lies between cortical bone surfaces and consists of a network of honeycombed interstices containing hematopoietic elements and bony trabeculae.
- Trabeculae are oriented perpendicular to external forces to provide structural support (White and Hirsch, 1971).

BONE BIOCHEMISTRY (RECKER, 1992)

- Bone is composed of organic and inorganic elements.
  a. Inorganic elements: Dry bone is made up of calcium phosphate (65–70% of the weight).
  b. Organic matrix: Fibrous protein and collagen (30–35% of the weight).
  c. Osteoid: (1) Unmineralized organic matrix secreted by osteoblasts. (2) Composed of 90% type I collagen

and 10% ground substance (noncollagenous proteins, glycoproteins proteoglycans, peptides, carbohydrates, and lipids). (3) Mineralization of this substance by inorganic mineral salts provides bone with its strength and rigidity.
  d. Inorganic bone contents: (1) Primarily calcium phosphate and calcium carbonate with small quantities of magnesium, chloride, and sodium. (2) Mineral crystals form hydroxyapatite, an orderly precipitate around the collagen fibers of the osteoid.

REGULATORS OF BONE METABOLISM (BODEN AND KAPLAN, 1990; REICHEL, 1989)

- Three of the calcitropic hormones that have the most effect on metabolism are parathyroid hormone, vitamin D, and calcitonin.
  1. Parathyroid hormone increases the flow of calcium into the calcium pool and maintains the body's extracellular calcium level relatively constant.
    a. Osteoblasts are the only bone cells that have parathyroid hormone receptors.
  2. Vitamin D stimulates intestinal and renal calcium binding proteins and facilitates active calcium transport.
  3. Calcitonin is secreted by the parafollicular cells of the thyroid gland in response to rising plasma calcium level. Calcitonin serves to inhibit calcium dependent cellular metabolic activity.
  4. Miscellaneous proteins: (1) Released from platelets, macrophages, and fibroblasts. (2) Effect healing bone to vascularize, solidify, incorporate, and function mechanically. (3) Induce mesenchymal derived cells such as monocytes and fibroblasts to migrate, proliferate and differentiate into bone cells (Hruska et al, 1993; Hynes, 1992).
- Proteins that enhance bone healing include the *bone morphogenic proteins* (BMPs), insulin-like growth factors, transforming growth factors, platelet derived growth factor, and fibroblast growth factor, among others (Reddi and Sampath, 1996).

BMPs

- A family of glycoproteins derived from bone matrix. These proteins produce mesenchymal cells to differentiate into bone cells.
- Present in only minute quantities in the body.
- Several BMPs have been synthesized using recombinant DNA technology. Clinical trials are currently underway to assess their potential to facilitate bone fusion (Boden et al, 2000; Geesink, Hoefnagels, and Bulstra, 1999).

PHYSIOLOGY OF BONE REPAIR AND INCORPORATION

- Several physiologic properties of bone grafts directly affect the success or failure of graft incorporation.

OSTEOGENESIS (BRIGHTON, 1984; MUSCHLER, LANE, AND DAWSON, 1990)

- The ability of the graft to produce new bone. This process is dependent on the presence of live bone cells in a graft material.
- Contain viable cells with the ability to form bone (osteoprogenitor cells) or the potential to differentiate into bone forming cells.
- Osteogenesis is a property found only in fresh autogenous bone and in bone marrow cells.

OSTEOCONDUCTION (HOLLINGER ET AL, 1996; GAZDAG ET AL, 1995)

- The physical property of the graft to serve as a scaffold for viable bone healing.
- Allows for the ingrowth of neovasculature and the infiltration of osteogenic precursor cells into a graft site.
- Osteoconductive properties are found in cancellous autografts and allografts, demineralized bone matrix, hydroxyapatite, collagen, and calcium phosphate.

OSTEOINDUCTION (CONNOLLY, 1998; MOHAN AND BAYLINK, 1991)

- The ability of graft material to induce stem cells to differentiate into mature bone cells
- Typically associated with the presence of bone growth factors within the graft material
  a. BMPs and demineralized bone matrix are the principal osteoinductive materials.
  b. Autograft and allograft bone also have some osteoinductive properties (Muschler, Lane, and Dawson, 1990).

CREEPING SUBSTITUTION (PROLO, 1990; STEINBERG ET AL, 1989)

- An integrated process in which old necrotic bone is slowly reabsorbed and simultaneously replaced with new viable bone, thus incorporating bone grafts
  a. Permanent mesenchymal cells differentiate into osteoblasts and deposit osteoid around cores of the necrotic bone.
  b. Eventually results in the replacement of necrotic bone within the graft.

BONE HEALING PROCESS

- Fracture healing restores the tissue to its original physical and mechanical properties and is influenced by a variety of systemic and local factors (Kalfas, 2001; Perlman and Thordarson, 1999).
  1. The most critical period of bone healing is the first 1–2 weeks. During this period, inflammation and vascularization occur.
  2. Systemic factors can inhibit bone healing including the following:
     a. Cigarette smoking (Glassman, 1998)
     b. Malnutrition (Mankin, 1990)
     c. Diabetes (Macey et al, 1995)
     d. Rheumatoid arthritis
     e. Osteoporosis (Kelsey and Hoffman, 1987)
     f. Steroid medications: First week has most impact (Jones, 1994)
     g. Cytotoxic agents
     h. Nonsteroidal anti-inflammatory medications (Glassman et al, 2000)
- Healing occurs in three distinct but overlapping stages (McKibbin, 1978; Perren, 1979).

INFLAMMATORY STAGE

- A hematoma develops within the fracture site during the first few hours and days. Inflammatory cells and fibroblasts infiltrate the bone under prostaglandin mediation. This results in the formation of granulation tissue, ingrowth of vascular tissue, and migration of mesenchymal cells.
- Exposed skin cells, bone, and muscle provide the primary nutrients of this early process.
- Anti-inflammatory or cytotoxic medications during this first week are particularly detrimental (Kalfas, 2001).

REPAIR STAGE

- Fibroblasts begin to lay down a stroma that helps support vascular ingrowth.
- At this stage nicotine can inhibit capillary ingrowth (Daftari et al, 1994; Riebel et al, 1995).
- As vascular ingrowth progresses, a collagen matrix is laid down while osteoid is secreted and subsequently mineralized. This leads to the formation of a soft callus around the repair site.
  1. Callus is very weak in the first 4–6 weeks and requires adequate protection (Kenwright and Gardner, 1998).
  2. Eventually, ossified callus forms a bridge of woven bone between the fracture fragments. If proper immobilization is not employed, failure of ossification results in a fibrous union (Burchardt and Enneking, 1978).

REMODELING STAGE

- Healing bone is restored to its original shape, structure, and mechanical strength.
- Remodeling is a long-term process facilitated by mechanical stresses placed on the bone.
  a. Axial loading across the fracture site leads to bone being deposited where it is needed and reabsorbed where it is not (Wolff, 1986). Adequate strength is typically achieved in three to six months.

BIOMECHANICS OF FRACTURES

STRESS FRACTURES (WHITE, PANJABI, AND SOUTHWICK, 1977)

- Cyclic loading repeated over a long period of time may cause disruption of the bony architecture.
- The susceptibility of bone to fracture under stresses of low magnitude is related to its crystal structure and collagen orientation.
- Under each cycle of loading, a small amount of strained energy may be lost through microscopic cracks along the cement lines of bone.
- Fatigue load under certain strain rates can cause progressive accumulation of micro damage in cortical bone.
  a. Prolonged loading may eventually lead to failure through propagation of these cracks.
  b. Bone may be created near the microscopic cracks through periosteal callus formation, thus arresting propagation.

ACUTE FRACTURES (BRIGHTON, 1984)

- Classified according to the magnitude and area of distribution of the force applied and the rate at which the force acts.
  a. Soft tissue injury and fracture comminution directly proportional to the loading rate (Karladani et al, 2001).
  b. Modifies normal healing response by changing concentration of normal reparative mediators.
- Typically force is applied to bone in many directions and generates compressive, tensile, or sheer stress (or some combination).
- The combination of the bone's material strength and anisometric properties dictate when, how, and along which path a fracture will occur.
  a. Cortical bone is generally weak in tension and shear.
  b. Area where tensile stresses arise fails first.
- Transverse fractures are the result of pure tensile forces or bending.
- Fractures from pure tensile force occur progressively across the bone, creating a transverse break without comminution.

- The pattern of fracture arising from pure bending is a simple transverse line.
- Bone undergoing rapid loading must absorb more energy than bone loaded at a slower rate.
  a. At low speed, bending with tensile stress will cause a fracture with a single butterfly fragment.
  b. High speed bending will cause several butterfly fragments.
- The pattern of bone injury also impacts healing capacity (Carter, Blenman, and Beaupre, 1988).
  a. Time to union is greatly prolonged in fractures with more soft tissue stripping.
  b. Larger load under bending failure may cause the surrounding soft tissues and periosteum to sustain more damage and thus may affect the fracture healing potential.

FACTORS INFLUENCING FRACTURE REPAIR

NUTRITION

- Typical diet including all food groups in proper amounts is enough to effect healing in a healthy individual.
  1. Calcium usage is limited by absorption.
     a. Preinjury calcium levels are predictive.
     b. Intake of about 1g/day is optimal, along with supplemental vitamin D up to 1000 IU/day.
  2. True vegans with no alternative proteins risk for nonunion.

AUGMENTATION OF FRACTURE HEALING (EINHORN, 1995)

OSTEOGENESIS

- Naturally occurring material to induce or support the formation of bone

CANCELLOUS GRAFTS

- Cancellous grafts effect vascular ingrowth and progenitor mesenchymal cell invasion, osteoblastic appositional new bone formation, and ultimately, remodeling of the trabecular structure.

CORTICAL GRAFTS

- Slow to vascularize
- Must undergo osteoclastic resorption prior to osteoblastic new bone formation
- Do not demonstrate complete incorporation
- Healing process begins at host–graft cortical junction

Autogenous Bone Marrow
- Independent of cancellous or cortical bone
- Contains osteogenic precursor cells

OSTEOCONDUCTIVE METHODS (HOLLINGER ET AL, 1996)
- Support ingrowth of capillaries, perivascular tissues, and osteoprogenitor cells from host
- Examples: Ceramic materials (Hydroxyapatite), bioactive glasses, and synthetic polymers (poly-lactic and glycolic acid).

OSTEOINDUCTIVE METHODS
- Mitogenesis of undifferentiated mesenchymal cells to form osteoprogenitor cells
- Growth-promoting proteins. Several factors are known to be associated with healing:
  1. TGF-Beta
  2. *Insulin-like growth factor* (IGFs)
  3. *Bone Morphogenetic Proteins* (BMPs)
     a. Glycoproteins known to induce bone.
     b. Several BMPs are known to exist: (1) BMP-3 (Osteogenin) induces rapid differentiation of mesenchymal tissue to bone. (2) Induce endochondral bone formation in segmental defects (Yasko et al, 1992).
- Systemic factors: Injury to bone marrow enhances osteogenesis at distant skeletal sites.
  a. Factors thought to be responsible: (1) IGF-I and IGF-II, (2) parathyroid hormone, and (3) prostaglandins.
  b. Isolation and clinical development of these factors may lead to systemic treatment of fractures.

ELECTROMAGNETIC FIELDS
- Bone has a piezoelectric potential that is load-induced owing to two factors:
  a. Current is induced by deformation of collagen.
  b. Electrokinetic current produced by the strain-induced flow of charged extracellular fluids
- *Pulsed electromagnetic fields* (PEMFs) are intended to noninvasively induce electrical currents to replace endogenous currents in the absence of loading.
- Double-blind trial shown to double the number of healed fractures (tibial nonunions) (Yasko et al, 1992).

LOW-INTENSITY ULTRASOUND (LIU) (DAY ET AL, 1999)
- The sole intervention approved by the Food and Drug Administration (FDA) to augment the healing of fresh fractures.

- Shown to increase calcium incorporation in both differentiating cartilage and bone cell cultures
- Evidence that it can modulate gene expression, influence second messenger activity of chondroblasts and osteoblasts, enhance blood flow, and accelerate and augment fracture healing.
- In a study of distal radius fractures, LIU decreased time to healing by 38% as compared to placebo treatment (Day et al, 1999).

REFERENCES

Boden SD, Kaplan FS: Calcium homeostasis. *Orthop Clin North Am* 21:31–42, 1990.

Boden SD, Zdeblick TA, Sandhu HS, et al: The use of rhBMP-2 in interbody fusion cages: Definitive evidence of Osteoinduction in humans: A preliminary report. *Spine* 25:376–381, 2000.

Brighton CT: Principles of fracture healing: Part I. The biology of fracture repair, in Murray JA (ed.): *Instructional Course Lectures XXXIII*. St. Louis, MO, CV Mosby, 1984, pp 60–82.

Burchardt H, Enneking WF: Transplantation of bone. *Surg Clin North Am* 58:403–427, 1978.

Carter DR, Blenman PR, Beaupre GS: Correlations between mechanical stress history and tissue differentiation in initial fracture healing. *J Orthop Res* 6:736–748, 1988.

Connolly JF: Clinical use of marrow osteoprogenitor cells to stimulate Osteogenesis. *Clin Orthop* 355 (suppl):S257–S266, 1998.

Daftari TK, Whitesides TE, Heller JG, et al: Nicotine on the revascularization of bone graft. An experimental study in rabbits. *Spine* 19:904–911, 1994.

Day SM, Ostrum RF, Chao EY, et al: Bone injury, regeneration and repair, in Buckwalter JA, Einhorn TA, Simon SR (eds.): *Orthopaedic Basic Science*. Rosemont, IL, American Academy of Orthopaedic Surgeons Press, 1999, pp. 392–398.

Einhorn TA: Enhancement of fracture-healing. *J Bone Joint Surg* 77A:940–956, 1995.

Gazdag AR, Lane JM, Glaser D, et al: Alternative to autogenous bone graft: Efficacy and indications. *J Am Acad Orthop Surg* 3:1–8, 1995.

Geesink RG, Hoefnagels NH, Bulstra SK: Osteogenetic activity of OP-1 bone morphogenetic protein (BMP-7) in a human fibular defect. *J Bone Joint Surg* 81B:710–718, 1999.

Glassman SD: The effect of postoperative nonsteroidal anti-inflammatory drug administration on spinal fusion. *Spine* 23:834–838, 1998.

Glassman SD, Anagnost AC, Parker A, et al: The effect of cigarette smoking and smoking cessation on spinal fusion. *Spine* 25:2608–2615, 2000.

Hollinger JO, Brekke J, Gruskin E, et al: Role of bone substitutes. *Clin Orthop* 324:55–65, 1996.

Hruska KA, Rolnick F, Duncan RL, et al: Signal transduction in osteoblasts and osteoclasts, in Noda M (ed.): *Cellular and Molecular Biology of Bone*. San Diego, CA, Academic Press, 1993, pp 413–444.

Hynes RO: Integrins: Versatility, modulation and signaling in cell adhesion. *Cell* 69:11–25, 1992.

Jones JP: Concepts of etiology and early pathogenesis of osteonecrosis, in Schafer M (ed.): *Instructional Course Lectures 43*. Rosemont, IL, American Academy of Orthopaedic Surgeons, 1994, pp 499–512.

Kalfas IH: Principles of bone healing. *Neurosurg Focus* 10:1–4, 2001.

Karladani AH, Granhed H, Karrholm J, et al: The influence of fracture etiology and type of fracture healing: A review of 104 consecutive tibial shaft fractures. *Arch Orthop Trauma Surg* 121:325–328, 2001.

Kelsey JL, Hoffman SL: Risk factors for hip fracture. *N Engl J Med* 316:404–406, 1987.

Kenwright J, Gardner T: Mechanical influences on tibial fracture healing. *Clin Orthop* 355 (suppl): S179–S190, 1998.

Macey LR, Kana SM, Jingushi S, et al: Defects of early fracture healing in experimental diabetes. *J Bone Joint Surg* 77A:940–956, 1995.

Mankin HJ: Rickets, osteomalacia and renal osteodystrophy: An update. *Orthop Clin North Am* 21:81–96, 1990.

McKibbin B: The biology of fracture healing in long bones. *J Bone Joint Surg* 60B:150–162, 1978.

Mohan S, Baylink DJ: Bone growth factors. *Clin Orthop* 263:30–48, 1991.

Muschler GF, Lane JM, Dawson EG: The biology of spinal fusion, in Cotler JM, Cotler HP (eds.): *Spinal Fusion: Science and Technique*. Berlin, Springer-Verlag, 1990, pp 9–21.

Perlman MH, Thordarson. Ankle fusion in a high-risk population: An assessment of nonunion risk factor. *Foot Ankle Int* 20:491–496, 1999.

Perren SM: Physical and biological aspects of fracture healing with special reference to internal fixation. *Clin Orthop* 232:139–151, 1979.

Prolo DJ: Biology of bone fusion. *Clin Neurosurg* 36:135–146, 1990.

Recker RR: Embryology, anatomy and microstructure of bone, in Coe FL, Favus MJ (eds.): *Disorders of Bone and Mineral Metabolism*. New York, NY, Raven, 1992, pp 219–240.

Reddi AH, Sampath TK: Bone morphogenetic proteins: Potential role in osteoporosis, in Marcus R, Feldman D, Kelsey J (eds.): *Osteoporosis*. San Diego, CA, Academic Press, 1996, pp 281–287.

Reichel H, Koeffler HP, Norman AW: The role of the vitamin D endocrine system in health and disease. *N Engl J Med* 320:980–991, 1989.

Riebel ED, Boden SD, Whitesides TE, et al: The effect of nicotine on incorporation of cancellous bone graft in an animal model. *Spine* 20:1549–1553, 1995.

Steinberg ME, Brighton CT, Corces A, et al: Osteonecrosis of the femoral head: Results of core decompression and grafting with and without electrical stimulation. *Clin Orthop* 249:199–208, 1989.

White AA III, Hirsch C: An experimental study of the immediate load bearing capacity of some commonly used iliac bone grafts. *Acta Orthop Scand* 42:482–490, 1971.

White AA III, Panjabi MM, Southwick WO: The four biomechanical stages of fracture repair. *J Bone Joint Surg* 59A:188–192, 1977.

Wolff J: *The Law of Bone Remodeling*. Translated by Maquet P, Furlong R. Berlin, Springer-Verlag, 1986.

Yasko AW, Lane JM, Fellinger EJ, et al: The healing of segmental bone defects, induced by recombinant human bone morphogenetic protein: A radiographic, histologic and biomechanical study in rats. *J Bone Joint Surg* 74A:659–670, 1992.

BIBLIOGRAPHY

Dee R: Bone healing, in Dee R, Mango E, Hurst E, (eds.): *Principles of Orthopaedic Practice*. New York, NY, McGraw-Hill, 1988, pp 68–73.

Dee R: Bone healing, in Dee R, Mango E, Hurst E, (eds): *Principles of Orthopaedic Practice*. New York, McGraw-Hill, 1988; pp 68–73, 1988.

12 THE PREPARTICIPATION PHYSICAL EXAMINATION

Robert E Sallis, MD, FAAFP, FACSM

INTRODUCTION

- It is estimated that well over one million physician hours are consumed annually in examining over six million youth athletes.
- The cost effectiveness of yearly *preparticipation examinations* (PPEs) has been questioned: Risser et al, looked at 763 adolescent athletes screened and found only 16 athletes were identified with significant problems. Two were disqualified and one received treatment prior to participation. The cost of identifying these three problems was $4,537.00 per problem.
- Various studies show *preparticipation evaluations* (PPEs) disqualified only 0.3 to 1.3% of athletes, and only 3.2 to 13.5% required consultation.

GOALS

- Detect any condition that may limit an athlete's participation.
- Detect any condition that may predispose an athlete to injury or lead to sudden death during competition.
- Meet legal or insurance requirements. (49 of 50 states require yearly examinations.)

- Determine general health of the athlete.
  a. Assess fitness level for specific sports.
  b. Counsel on life-style issues and high-risk behaviors.
  c. Answer health related questions.

FORMAT

- Private office with primary care physician.
  a. Advantages: better continuity of care and easier to do counseling
  b. Disadvantages: higher cost and less communication with school athletic staff
- Group examination (Usually done as a station-based examination)
  a. Advantages: more cost effective, usually done at school with athletic staff present
  b. Disadvantages: lack of privacy and poor follow-up

FREQUENCY AND TIMING OF EXAMINATION

- Most states require the examination to be done yearly. However, every 3–4 years with yearly updates as needed, is probably adequate.
- Optimal timing for the examination is 4–6 weeks before the season starts to allow sufficient time for further evaluation and treatment of any problems that are uncovered.

CONTENT

- Since the stress of sports and exercise falls primarily on the cardiovascular and musculoskeletal systems, these areas are essential for assessment as part of the preparticipation physical examination. This evaluation should begin with a thorough history, followed by a focused physical examination.
- Many schools provide a specific form. If not, one such as the "preparticipation physical evaluation" form is recommended (see Fig. 12-1). These forms ask specific questions about the athletes past medical history and guide a physical examination.

MEDICAL HISTORY

- Medical history has been shown to identify approximately 75% of problems affecting athletes.
  a. The easiest method for obtaining an athlete's history is to make medical history forms available before the examination (see Fig. 12-1). These forms are probably best completed by the parents of adolescent athletes.
  b. Key questions include asking about any major pre-existing medical problems or injuries, if they are taking any medicines or supplements, their current state of health, and family history of early death (before age 50).

CARDIOVASCULAR ASSESSMENT

- Critical history question "Have you ever felt dizzy, fainted, or actually passed out while exercising?" may be a sign of a structural heart problem.
- Benign systolic murmurs are common in athletes. If a murmur is grade III or louder and/or diastolic, further evaluation is recommended. Accentuation with Valsalva should alert to possible outflow tract obstruction such as hypertrophic cardiomyopathy.
- Ectopic beats are also common. Those that disappear with exercise are usually benign, while those brought on with exercise are more worrisome. Ventricular ectopy in young athletes should raise suspicion for cocaine use.
- Simultaneous palpation of the radial and femoral pulses for asymmetry is a simple screen for coarctation of the aorta.

BLOOD PRESSURE

- Readings that indicate hypertension vary for different age ranges (see Table 12-1). Should have three separate elevated *blood pressure* (BP) readings to diagnose hypertension.
- *Mild to moderate* hypertension without end organ damage need not be restricted from competitive sports.
- *Severe to very severe* hypertension should be restricted from high static sports until BP controlled.
- Systolic hypertension in young athletes is frequently related to anxiety or inappropriate cuff size in husky individuals.

MUSCULOSKELETAL ASSESSMENT

- Look for preexisting injuries, as they are likely to recur. The knees, shoulders, and ankles are most at risk.
- The "Two–minute musculoskeletal examination" can be a useful screen (see Table 12-2).
- Keep in mind the demands of the particular sport the athlete will be playing, and focus on areas of the body that will be under stress and prone to injury from that sport.

Preparticipation Sports Evaluation

School _____
Age _____ Grade _____ Sex _____
Sports _____

Health History
Athlete/Parent or Guardian*
Provide the following Information

	YES	NO
Chronic/recent illness?		
Hospitalization?		
Surgery?		
Injury?		
Bone/joint injuries?		
Missing organs?		
Dizziness, fainting convulsions?		
Frequent headaches?		
Knocked out/concussion?		
Wear glasses/contacts?		
Hearing problems?		
False teeth/braces?		
High blood pressure?		
Heart problems/murmurs?		
Asthma/chronic cough?		
Hernia?		
Recurrent skin disease?		
Current medications List		
Family history of heart disease or unexpected death at young age?		
Other family history of disease?		
Allergy to medication? List		
Immunizations current?		
Date of last tetanus		
Date of last measles		
Other		
For women only Has menses started?		
Age at first menses		
Are periods regular?		

The above is correct and current to the best of my knowledge.

_____ _____
Athlete/parent or guardian*   Date

*Parent or guardian if less than 18 years old

Family Physician _____ Phone _____
Address _____

	Satisfactory			Comments
	Yes	No	NE	
Ht.				
Wt				
BP				
General				
Head				
Eyes				
ENT				
Dental				
Chest				
Heart				
Abdomen				
Genitalia				
Skin				
Ortho				
Flex/Strength				

Follow-up recommendations:

Sports participation approved: Yes _____ No _____ Restricted _____
Limitations:

_____
Physician   Date   ar9/90

KAISER PERMANENTE
Southern California Permanente
Medical Group

FIG. 12-1 Sample preparticipation physical evaluation form.

• Musculoskeletal problems found during the preparticipation examination should be treated with appropriate rehabilitation and conditioning programs.

OTHER AREAS FOR ASSESSMENT (SEE TABLE 12-3)
• Height/Weight (eating disorders, ideal body weight)
• Lungs (asthma)

• Abdominal (hepatosplenomegaly, masses)
• Skin (infectious diseases, acne)
• Neuro (history of concussion)
• Genitourinary (single testicle, hernia, testicular mass)
• Tanner staging (to assess physical maturity) *is no longer recommended*

TABLE 12-1   Classification of Blood Pressure by Age in Children, Adolescents, and Adults

| AGE GROUP | MAGNITUDE OF HYPERTENSION* | | | |
	MILD (STAGE 1) (MMHG)	MODERATE (STAGE 2) (MM HG)	SEVERE (STAGE 3) (MM HG)	VERY SEVERE (STAGE 4) (MM HG)
Children				
6–9 years				
Systolic BP	120–124	125–129	130–139	>140
Diastolic BP	75–79	80–84	85–89	>90
10–12 yr				
Systolic BP	125–129	130–134	135–144	>145
Diastolic BP	80–84	85–89	90–94	>95
Adolescents				
13–15 years				
Systolic BP	135–139	140–149	150–159	>160
Diastolic BP	85–89	90–94	95–99	>100
16–18 yr				
Systolic BP	140–149	150–159	160–179	>180
Diastolic BP	90–94	95–99	100–109	>110
Adults				
>18 years				
Systolic BP	140–159	160–179	180–209	>210
Diastolic BP	90–99	100–109	110–119	>120

SOURCE: Aadapted from the 26th Bethesda Conference on Recommendations for Determining Eligibility for Competition in Athletes with Cardiovascular Abnormalities.
ABBREVIATION: BP = blood pressure.
*Applies to patients who are not receiving antihypertensive drugs and who are not acutely ill. When the systolic and diastolic BP measurements fall into different categories, the higher category should be selected to classify that patient's BP status. In adults, isolated systolic hypertension is defined as systolic BP = 140 mmHg and a diastolic BP <90 mmHg and staged appropriately. Blood pressure values are based on the average of three or more readings taken at each of two or more visits after the initial screening

TABLE 12-2   The Two-Minute Musculoskeletal Examination for Screening Athletes During the Preparticipation Examination

INSTRUCTIONS	OBSERVATION
Stand facing examiner	Acromioclavicular joints, General habitus
Look at ceiling, floor, over both shoulders; touch ears to shoulders	Cervical spine motion
Shrug shoulders (examiner resists at 90°)	Trapezius strength
Abduct shoulders 90° (examiner resists at 90°)	Deltoid strength
Full external rotation of arms	Shoulder motion
Flex and extend elbows	Elbow motion
Arms at sides, elbows 90° flexed; pronate and supinate wrists	Elbow and wrist motion
Spread fingers; make fist	Hand or finger motion and deformities
Tighten (contract) quadriceps	Symmetry and knee effusion; ankle effusion
"Duck walk" four steps (away from examiner with buttocks on heels)	
Back to examiner	Shoulder symmetry, scoliosis
Knees straight, touch toes	Scoliosis, hip motion, hamstring tightness
Raise up on toes, raise heels	Calf symmetry, leg strength

SOURCE: *Sports Medicine: Health Care for Young Athletes.* Evanston, IL, American Academy of Pediatrics, 1983.

TABLE 12-3   Areas for Emphasis During the Preparticipation Physical Examination of Youth Athletes

General	*Skin*	*Visual acuity*
Height	Jaundice	Severe myopia
Weight	Herpetic lesions	Amblyopia
Body habitus (especially for weight-determined sports)	Impetigo Severe acne	Single eye
Funduscopic	*Lungs*	*Cardiovascular*
Detached retina Early atherosclerotic changes	Asthma Bronchitis	Murmurs Uncontrolled Hypertension
Diabetic Retinopathy		Cyanosis
Abdomen	*Back*	*Genitourinary*
Hepatosplenomegaly Masses	Scoliosis Kyphosis Lordosis	Single testicle Hernia Testicle mass
Neurologic	*Musculoskeletal*	
Gross coordination Gait abnormalities	Knee and ankle ligaments Shoulder instability Elbow stability Anterior Knee Pain Muscular Development Marfan's Syndrome	

SOURCE: Tanji JL: *Am Fam Physician* 42(2), 397–402, Aug 1990.

DIAGNOSTIC TESTS

LAB TESTS
- The most commonly used lab tests are the *complete blood count* (CBC) and urinalysis. Consensus is that they should not be done routinely during the preparticipation examination.
- Consider routine hematocrit in female athletes.
- Cholesterol testing if indicated by history.
- Consider testing for sickle cell trait in black athletes.

CARDIAC TESTING
- Routine *electrocardiogram* (EKG) and/or *echocardiogram* are not cost effective as screening tests.
- Exercise stress testing may be indicated in the adult athlete with cardiac risk factors, prior to starting an exercise program.

CLEARANCE

- After a problem is found, the following factors should be considered in deciding whether to clear an athlete to participate:
  a. Does the problem place the athlete at increased risk of injury?
  b. Is any other participant at risk of injury because of the problem?
  c. Can the athlete safely participate with treatment (medication, rehabilitation, bracing, or padding)?
  d. Can limited participation be allowed while treatment is being initiated?
  e. If clearance is denied only for certain activities, in what activities can the athlete safely participate?
- The American Academy of Pediatrics Recommendations for Participation in Competitive Sports is a useful guide to help decide about clearance (see Tables 12-4(*a*), 12-4(*b*), and 12-5).
- The "26th Bethesda Conference: Recommendations for Determining Eligibility for Competition in Athletes With Cardiovascular Abnormalities" covers guidelines for clearance in athletes who have congenital heart disease and other cardiovascular abnormalities.
- A clearance form (see Fig. 12-2) is a useful tool to clearly express recommendations regarding clearance.

SCREENING TO PREVENT EXERCISE RELATED SUDDEN DEATH

- Preparticipation screening is the primary preventive tool. The incidence of exercise related sudden death rate is rare—around 0.2–0.5 per 100,000 adolescents per year.
- The cause is usually cardiac: under 30 years, usually structural heart problem; over 30 years, usually coronary artery disease. Causes include the following:

HYPERTROPHIC CARDIOMYOPATHY
- Symptoms: palpitations, syncope, chest pain, and dyspnea on exertion. Most are asymptomatic until the time of death.
- Examination: may have high frequency systolic ejection murmur at the left lower sternal border, increased with Valsalva, decreased with squatting.
- Diagnosis: echocardiogram (ventricular septum >15-mm thick). The presence of the "athletic heart syndrome" may complicate screening.

CONGENITAL CORONARY ARTERY ANOMALIES
- Types:
  a. Origin of left coronary artery from right of sinus of Valsalva
  b. Single coronary artery

TABLE 12-4(*a*)   The Classification of Sports by Strenuousness

HIGH TO MODERATE DYNAMIC AND STATIC DEMANDS	HIGH TO MODERATE DYNAMIC AND LOW STATIC DEMANDS	HIGH TO MODERATE STATIC AND LOW DYNAMIC DEMANDS	LOW DYNAMIC LOW STATIC AND DEMANDS
Boxing	Badminton	Archery	Bowling
Crew/rowing	Baseball	Auto racing	Cricket
Cross-country skiing	Basketball	Diving	Curling
Downhill skiing	Field hockey	Equestrian	Golf
Fencing	Orienteering	Field events (jumping)	Riflery
Football	Ping-pong	Field events (throwing)	—
Ice hockey	Racquetball	Gymnastics	—
Ice hockey	Soccer	Karate or judo	—
Rugby	Squash	Motorcycling	—
Running (sprint)	Swimming	Rodeoing	—
Speed skating	Tennis	Sailing	—
Water polo	Volleyball	Ski jumping	—
Wrestling	—	Water skiing	—
—	—	Weight lifting	—

TABLE 12-4(*b*)   The Classification of Sports by Contact

CONTACT/COLLISION	LIMITED CONTACT	NONCONTACT
Basketball	Baseball	Archery
Boxing	Bicycling	Badminton
Diving	Cheerleading	Body building
Field hockey	Canoeing/kayaking (white water)	Bowling
Football (flag or tackle)	Fencing	Canoeing/kayaking (flat water)
Ice hockey	Field	Crew/rowing
Lacrosse	High jump	Curling
Martial arts	Pole vault	Dancing
Rodeo	Floor hockey	Field
Rugby	Gymnastics	Discus
Ski jumping	Handball	Javelin
Soccer	Horseback riding	Shot put
Team handball	Racquetball	Golf
Water polo	Skating	Orienteering
Wrestling	Ice	Power lifting
—	Inline	Race walking
—	Roller	Riflery
—	Skiing	Rope jumping
—	Cross country	Running
—	Downhill	Sailing
—	Water	Scuba diving
—	Softball	Strength training
—	Squash	Swimming
—	Ultimate Frisbee	Table tennis
—	Volleyball	Tennis
—	Windsurfing/surfing	Track
—	—	Weight lifting

SOURCE: American Academy of Pediatrics, Committee on Sports Medicine, Recommendations for Participation in Competitive Sports, *Pediatrics* 1998.

    c. Origin of coronary artery from pulmonary artery
    d. Coronary artery hypoplasia
- Symptoms: exertional chest pain or syncope
- Diagnosis: angiogram

MARFAN'S SYNDROME
- Diagnosis: need two of four major features
    a. Family history.
    b. Cardiovascular abnormality (aortic aneurysm, mitral valve prolapse, congestive heart failure symptoms)
    c. Musculoskeletal abnormality (arm span more than height, kyphoscoliosis, anterior thoracic deformity)
    d. Ocular abnormality (ectopic lens, myopia)
- If suspected, should get genetic and cardiology consults (include echocardiogram). See suggested screening formal for Marfan's syndrome (Table 12-6).

CORONARY ARTERY DISEASE
- Consider exercise stress testing for the following:
    a. Male over 45; female over 55
    b. Those with risk factors: diabetic, smoker, family history of heart disease, total cholesterol over 250, *high-density lipoprotein* (HDL) cholesterol under 30
    c. Anyone with exertional chest pain, syncope, or palpitations

VALVULAR DISORDERS
- Aortic stenosis: This often results in sudden death, with or without exercise.
- Mitral valve prolapse: this is not a risk factor for sudden death.

CARDIAC CONDUCTION SYSTEM ABNORMALITIES
- Idiopathic long QT syndrome
    a. QT interval greater than 440 ms
    b. Frequently suspected in cases of sudden death in which no structural heart problems are found
    c. May produce syncope or near syncope

SCREENING FOR SUDDEN DEATH

- *History:* family history; syncope, exertional chest pain or dyspnea on exertion.
- *Examination:* Marfan's habitus; murmur.
- *EKG/CXR:* reassuring if both normal
- *Exercise stress test, Holter, and angiogram* should be done as indicated by history and examination findings.

ATHLETIC HEART CAN COMPLICATE SCREENING
- Athletic heart is the normal adaptation of a healthy heart to exercise.

Table 12-5 Recommendations Regarding Sports Participation with Common Medical Conditions

CONDITION	MAY PARTICIPATE
Atlantoaxial instability (instability of the joint between cervical vertebrae 1 and 2)	Qualified yes
Explanation: Athlete needs evaluation to assess risk of spinal cord injury during sports participation.	
Bleeding disorder	Qualified yes
Explanation: Athlete needs evaluation.	
Cardiovascular disease	
Carditis (inflammation of the heart)	No
Explanation: Carditis may result in sudden death with exertion.	
Hypertension (high blood pressure)	Qualified yes
Explanation: Those with significant essential (unexplained) hypertension should avoid weight and power lifting, body building, and strength training. Those with secondary hypertension (hypertension caused by a previously identified disease) or severe essential hypertension need evaluation. The National High Blood Pressure Education Working Group (American College of Sports Medicine and American College of Cardiology, 1994) defined significant and severe hypertension.	
Congenital heart disease (structural heart defects present at birth)	Qualified yes
Explanation: Those with mild forms may participate fully; those with moderate or severe forms or who have undergone surgery need evaluation. The 26th Bethesda Conference (Franklin, 1997) defined mild, moderate, and severe disease for common cardiac lesions.	
Dysrhythmia (irregular heart rhythm)	Qualified yes
Explanation: Those with symptoms (chest pain, syncope, dizziness, shortness of breath, or other symptoms of possible dysrhythmia) or evidence of mitral regurgitation (leaking) on physical examination need evaluation. All others may participate fully (Koester and Amundson, 2003).	
Heart murmur	Qualified yes
Explanation: If the murmur is innocent (does not indicate heart disease), full participation is permitted. Otherwise, the athlete needs evaluation (see congenital heart disease and mitral valve prolapse) (Koester and Amundson, 2003).	
Cerebral palsy	Qualified yes
Explanation: Athlete needs evaluation.	
Diabetes mellitus	Yes
Explanation: All sports can be played with proper attention to diet, blood glucose concentration, hydration, and insulin therapy. Blood glucose concentration should be monitored every 30 min during continuous exercise and 15 min after completion of exercise.	
Diarrhea	Qualified no
Explanation: Unless disease is mild, no participation is permitted, because diarrhea may increase the risk of dehydration and heat illness. See fever.	
Eating disorders	Qualified yes
Anorexia nervosa	
Bulimia nervosa	
Explanation: Patients with these disorders need medical and psychiatric assessment before participation.	
Eyes	Qualified yes
Functionally one-eyed athlete	
Loss of an eye	
Detached retina	
Previous eye surgery or serious eye injury	
Explanation: A functionally one-eyed athlete has a best-corrected visual acuity of less than 20/40 in the eye with worse acuity. These athletes would suffer significant disability if the better eye were seriously injured, as would those with loss of an eye. Some athletes who previously have undergone eye surgery or had a serious eye injury may have an increased risk of injury because of weakened eye tissue. Availability of eye guards approved by the American Society for Testing and Materials and other protective equipment may allow participation in most sports, but this must be judged on an individual basis (Kurowski and Chandran, 2000; Maron et al, 1996).	
Fever	No
Explanation: Fever can increase cardiopulmonary effort, reduce maximum exercise capacity, make heat illness more likely, and increase orthostatic hypertension during exercise. Fever may rarely accompany myocarditis or other infections that may make exercise dangerous.	
Heat illness, history of	Qualified yes
Explanation: Because of the increased likelihood of recurrence, the athlete needs individual assessment to determine the presence of predisposing conditions and to arrange a prevention strategy.	
Hepatitis	Yes
Explanation: Because of the apparent minimal risk to others, all sports may be played that the athlete's state of health allows. In all athletes, skin lesions should be covered properly, and athletic personnel should use universal precautions when handling blood or body fluids with visible blood (Risser et al, 1985).	
Human immunodeficiency virus infection	Yes

(continued)

Table 12-5 (*Continued*)

CONDITION	MAY PARTICIPATE

Explanation: Because of the apparent minimal risk to others, all sports may be played that the athlete's state of health allows. In all athletes, skin lesions should be covered properly, and athletic personnel should use universal precautions when handling blood or body fluids with visible blood (Risser et al, 1985).

Kidney, absence of one	Qualified yes

Explanation: Athlete needs individual assessment for contact, collision, and limited-contact sports.

Liver, enlarged	Qualified yes

Explanation: If the liver is acutely enlarged, participation should be avoided because of risk of rupture. If the liver is chronically enlarged, individual assessment is needed before collision, contact, or limited-contact sports are played.

Malignant neoplasm	Qualified yes

Explanation: Athlete needs individual assessment.

Musculoskeletal disorders	Qualified yes

Explanation: Athlete needs individual assessment.

Neurologic disorders

History of serious head or spine trauma, severe or repeated concussions, or crainotomy (Sallis, 1996; Smith and Laskowski, 1998).	Qualified yes

Explanation: Athlete needs individual assessment for collision, contact, or limited-contact sports and also for noncontact sports if deficits in judgment or cognition are present. Research supports a conservative approach to management of concussion (Sallis, 1996; Smith and Laskowski, 1998).

Seizure disorder, well-controlled	Yes

Explanation: Risk of seizure during participation is minimal

Seizure disorder, poorly controlled	Qualified yes

Explanation: Athlete needs individual assessment for collision, contact, or limited-contact sports. The following noncontact sports should be avoided: archery, riflery, swimming, weight or power lifting, strength training, or sports involving heights. In these sports, occurrence of a seizure may pose a risk to self or others.

Obesity	Qualified yes

Explanation: Because of the risk of heat illness, obese persons need careful acclimatization and hydration.

Organ transplant recipient	Qualified yes

Explanation: Athlete needs individual assessment.

Ovary, absence of one	Yes

Explanation: Risk of severe injury to the remaining ovary is minimal.

Respiratory conditions

Pulmonary compromise, including cystic fibrosis	Qualified yes

Explanation: Athlete needs individual assessment, but generally, all sports may be played if oxygenation remains satisfactory during a graded exercise test. Patients with cystic fibrosis need acclimatization and good hydration to reduce the risk of heat illness.

Asthma	Yes

Explanation: With proper medication and education, only athletes with the most severe asthma will need to modify their participation.

Acute upper respiratory infection	Qualified yes

Explanation: Upper respiratory obstruction may affect pulmonary function. Athlete needs individual assessment for all but mild disease. See fever.

Sickle cell disease	Qualified yes

Explanation: Athlete needs individual assessment. In general, if status of the illness permits, all but high exertion, collision, and contact sports may be played. Overheating, dehydration, and chilling must be avoided.

Sickle cell trait	Yes

Explanation: It is unlikely that persons with sickle cell trait have an increased risk of sudden death or other medical problems during athletic participation, except under the most extreme conditions of heat, humidity, and possibly increased altitude (Tanner, 1994). These persons, like all athletes, should be carefully conditioned, acclimatized, and hydrated to reduce any possible risk.

Skin disorders (boils, herpes simplex, impetigo, scabies, molluscum contagiosum)	Qualified yes

Explanation: While the patient is contagious, participation in gymnastics with mats; martial arts; wrestling; or other collision, contact, or limited-contact sports is not allowed.

Spleen, enlarged	Qualified yes

Explanation: A patient with an acutely enlarged spleen should avoid all sports because of risk of rupture. A patient with a chronically enlarged spleen needs individual assessment before playing collision, contact, or limited-contact sports.

Testicle, undescended or absence of one	Yes

Explanation: Certain sports may require a protective cup.

SOURCE: American Academy of Pediatrics, Committee on Sports Medicine, Recommendations for Participation in Competitive Sports, *Pediatrics* 1998. Those listed with a "Qualified" yes or no require individual assessment.

Preparticipation Physical Evaluation

CLEARANCE FORM

❏ **Cleared**

❏ **Cleared after completing evaluation/rehabilitation for:** _____

_____

_____

_____

❏ **Not cleared for:** _____ **Reason:** _____

Recommendations: _____

_____

_____

_____

Name of physician (print/type) _____ **Date** _____

Address _____ **Phone**_____

Signature of physician _____, **MD or DO**

FIG. 12-2 Sample clearance form, used to communicate findings on the preparticipation examination to parents and team officials. (From *Preparticipation Physical Evaluation*, 2nd ed. American Academy of Family Physicians, The Physician and Sportsmedicine, McGraw-Hill Healthcare Minneapolis, Minnesota, 1997)

a. Physiologic hypertrophy of an athlete's heart in response to exercise can approach that seen with HCM (but left ventricle or LV end diastolic cavity dimensions remain normal).
b. These changes reverse when exercise intensity decreased.
• Will see EKG, radiographic and Echo changes of cardiac enlargement and enhanced vagal tone.

Table 12-6 Suggested Screening Format to Look for Marfan's Syndrome

Screen men over 6 ft and women over 5 ft 10 in. in height with an echocardiogram and slit-lamp examination when any two of the following are found:

1. Family history of Marfan's syndrome*
2. Cardiac murmur or mid-systolic click
3. Kyphoscoliosis
4. Anterior thoracic deformity
5. Arm span greater than height
6. Upper to lower body ratio more than one standard deviation below the mean
7. Myopia
8. Ectopic lens

*This finding *alone* should prompt further investigation.
SOURCE: Hara JH, Puffer JC: in Mellion MB: *Sports Injuries & Athletic Problems*. Philadelphia. Hanley & Belfus, 1988.

a. EKG often shows resting bradycardia, sinus arrhythmia, 1° *atrioventricular* (AV) block, Mobitz type 1 (Wenkebach) 2° AV block, and junctional rhythms. These changes reverse during exercise and increased sympathetic tone.
b. Clinical examination often shows bradycardia, S3 or S4 heart sounds, and innocent flow murmurs.

REFERENCES

American College of Sports Medicine, American College of Cardiology. 26th Bethesda Conference: Recommendations for determining eligibility for competition in athletes with cardiovascular abnormalities. *Med Sci Sports Exerc* 26(10): 5223–5283, 1994.

Franklin BA, Fletcher GF, Gordon NF, et al: Cardiovascular evaluation of the athlete. *Sports Med* 24:97–119, 1997.

Koester KC, Amundson CL: Preparticipation screening of high school athletes. *Phys Sportsmed* 31(8):35–38, 2003.

Kurowski K, Chandran S: The preparticipation athletic evaluation. *Am Fam Physician* 61(9):2683–2690, 2000.

Maron BJ, Thompson PD, Puffer JC, et al: Cardiovascular preparticipation screening of competitive athletes. *Circulation* 94:850–856, 1996.

Risser WL, et al: A cost benefit analysis of pre-participation examinations of adolescent athletes. *J Sch Health* 55(7):270, 1985.

Sallis RE. The preparticipation exam, in Sallis RE (ed.): *Essentials of Sports Medicine.* Philadelphia, PA, Mosby-Yearbook, 1996, pp 151–160.

Smith J Laskowski ER: The preparticipation physical examination: Mayo clinic experience with 2739 examinations. *Mayo Clin Proc* 73:419–429, 1998.

Tanner SM. Preparticipation examination targeted for the female athlete. *Clin Sports Med* 13(2):337–353, 1994.

BIBLIOGRAPHY

American Academy of Pediatrics. Committee on Sports Medicine and Fitness: Medical conditions affecting sports participation. *Pediatrics* 107(5):1205–1209, 2001.

Preparticipation Physical Evaluation, 2nd ed. American Academy of Family Physicians, American Academy of Pediatrics, American Medical Society for Sports Medicine, American Orthopedic Society for Sports Medicine, and American Osteopathic Academy of Sports Medicine. *The Physician and Sportsmedicine,* Minneapolis, MN, McGraw-Hill Healthcare, 1997.

13 BASIC PRINCIPLES OF EXERCISE TRAINING AND CONDITIONING
Craig K Seto, MD, FAAFP

INTRODUCTION

- Regular physical activity is an important component of a healthy lifestyle. Increases in physical activity and cardiorespiratory fitness have been shown to reduce the risk of death from coronary heart disease as well as from all causes. There is increasing evidence showing that regular participation in moderate-intensity physical activity is associated with health benefits, even when aerobic fitness remains unchanged. To reflect this evidence, the Centers for Disease Control and Prevention (CDC) and the American College of Sports Medicine (ACSM) are now recommending that every US adult accumulate 30 min or more of moderate-intensity physical activity on most—and preferably all—days of the week. Those who follow these recommendations will experience many of the health-related benefits of physical activity, and if they are interested in achieving higher levels of fitness, will be ready to do so (Whaley and Kaminsky, 2001; Franklin et al, 2000*a*; 2000*b*).

OVERVIEW OF EXERCISE PHYSIOLOGY

METABOLIC ENERGY SYSTEMS

- At rest, a 70-kg human has an energy expenditure of about 1.2 kcal/min with less than 20% of resting energy expenditure attributed to skeletal muscle; however, during intense exercise, total energy expenditure may increase 15–25 times above resting values, resulting in a caloric expenditure between 18 and 30 kcal/min. Most of this increase is used to provide energy to the exercising muscles, which may increase energy requirements by a factor of 200 (Demaree et al, 2001; Rupp, 2001).

ROLE OF ADENOSINE TRIPHOSPHATE
- The energy used to fuel biological processes comes from the breakdown of *adenosine triphosphate* (ATP), specifically from the chemical energy stored in the bonds of the last two phosphates of the ATP molecules. When work is performed, the bond between the last two phosphates is broken, producing energy and heat.

$$ATP \xrightarrow{\text{ATPase}} ADP + Pi + energy$$

- The limited stores of ATP in skeletal muscles can fuel approximately 5–10 s of high-intensity work. Therefore, ATP must be continuously resynthesized from *adenosine diphosphate* (ADP) to allow exercise to continue (Demaree et al, 2001; Rupp, 2001). Muscle fibers contain three metabolic pathways for producing ATP: creatine phosphate, rapid glycolysis, and aerobic oxidation (Demaree et al, 2001; Rupp, 2001).

THREE ENERGY SYSTEMS ARE RESPONSIBLE FOR THE RESYNTHESIS OF ATP

Creatine Phosphate System
- When limited stores of ATP are nearly depleted during high-intensity exercise (5–10 s), the *creatine phosphate* (CP) system transfers a high-energy phosphate from CP to rephosphorylate ATP from ADP. Since it involves a single reaction, this system can provide ATP at a very rapid rate; however, as there is a limited supply of CP in the muscle the amount of ATP that can be produced is also limited.

$$ADP + CP \xrightarrow{\text{creatine kinase}} ATP + C$$

- There is enough CP stored in skeletal muscle for approximately 25 s of high-intensity work. Therefore, the ATP-CP system will last for about 30 s (5 s for the stored ATP, and 25 s for CP). This will provide energy for activities such as sprinting and weight lifting. The CP system is considered an anaerobic system since oxygen is not required (Demaree et al, 2001; Rupp, 2001).

Rapid Glycolysis (Lactic Acid System)

- Glycolysis uses carbohydrate, primarily muscle glycogen as a fuel source. When glycolysis is rapid, it is capable of producing only a few ATP without involvement of oxygen. Lactic acid is also produced as a by-product of this reaction. The accumulation of excessive amounts of lactic acid in muscle tissue is associated with fatigue. The lactic acid system produces enough energy to last approximately 1–2 min before the accumulation of excessive lactic acid would produce fatigue. It would fuel activities such as middle distance sprints (400-, 600-, and 800-m runs). Although glycolysis is considered an anaerobic pathway, it can readily participate in aerobic metabolism when oxygen is available, and it is considered the first step in the aerobic metabolism of carbohydrate (Demaree et al, 2001; Rupp, 2001).

Aerobic Oxidation System

- The final metabolic pathway for ATP production combines two complex metabolic processes, the Krebs cycle and the electron transport chain. This system resides in the mitochondria. It is capable of using carbohydrates, fat, and small amounts of protein to produce energy (ATP) during exercise through a process called oxidative phosphorylation. During exercise this pathway uses oxygen to completely metabolize the carbohydrates to produce energy (ATP) leaving only carbon dioxide and water as by-products. The aerobic oxidation system is complex, and thus requires 2–3 min to adjust to a change in exercise intensity; however, it has an almost unlimited ability to regenerate ATP, limited only by the amount of fuel and oxygen that is available to the cell. *Maximal oxygen consumption,* also known as VO_2max, is a measure of the power of the aerobic energy system and is generally regarded as the best indicator of aerobic fitness (Demaree et al, 2001; Rupp, 2001).

FUEL USAGE DURING EXERCISE

- All the energy-producing pathways are active during most exercise; however, different types of exercise place greater demands on different pathways. The contribution of the anaerobic pathways (CP system and glycolysis) to exercise energy metabolism is inversely related to the duration and intensity of the activity. The shorter and more intense the activity, the greater the contribution of anaerobic energy production; whereas the longer the activity and the lower the intensity, the greater the contribution of aerobic energy production. In general, carbohydrates are used as the primary fuel at the onset of exercise and during high-intensity work; however, during prolonged exercise of low to moderate intensity (longer than 30 min), a gradual shift from carbohydrate toward an increasing reliance on fat as a substrate occurs. The greatest amount of fat use occurs

at about 60% of *maximal aerobic capacity* (VO_{2max}) (Demaree et al, 2001; Rupp, 2001).

MUSCLE PHYSIOLOGY

CLASSIFICATION OF MUSCLE FIBERS

- Muscle fibers possess certain characteristics that result in relative specialization and can be classified broadly as Type I (slow-twitch) or Type II (fast-twitch) with differing functional and metabolic characteristics. The type of muscle fiber recruited to perform a specific activity depends on intensity and duration of exercise. Most muscles contain both fast-twitch and slow-twitch muscle fibers; however, the ratio of fast-twitch to slow-twitch muscle fibers varies in an individual. The ratio also differs within the same muscle from one individual to another (Rupp, 2001; Humphrey, 2001).

Type I (Slow-Twitch) Muscle Fibers

- Type I fibers are those that resist fatigue and thus are recruited for lower intensity, longer duration activities. Sedentary persons have approximately 50% Type I, and this distribution is generally equal throughout the major muscle groups of the body. Endurance athletes have a greater percentage of Type I fibers thought to be the result of genetic predisposition (Rupp, 2001; Humphrey, 2001).

Type II (Fast-Twitch) Muscle Fibers

- Type II fibers are muscle fibers that can generally generate a great deal of force very rapidly. These fibers are recruited when a person is performing high-intensity activities. These fibers can produce large amounts of tension in a very short time period, but the accumulation of lactic acid from anaerobic glycolysis causes them to fatigue quickly. Type II fibers are subdivided into Type IIa and IIb fibers.
- **Type IIa fibers:** Type IIa fibers represent a transition type of fiber. While these fibers are capable of generating a moderately large amount of force, they also have some aerobic capacity, although not as much as the Type I fibers. These fibers represent a logical and necessary bridge between the two types of muscle fibers allowing one to meet the energy demands for a variety of physical tasks (Rupp, 2001; Humphrey, 2001).
- **Type IIb fibers:** Type IIb fibers are the classic fast-twitch fibers that are predominately anaerobic since they rely on energy sources intrinsic to the muscle.

CARDIORESPIRATORY PHYSIOLOGY

- The cardiorespiratory system consists of the heart, lungs, and blood vessels. The purpose of this system is for the delivery of oxygen and nutrients to the cells as well as the removal of metabolic waste products in order to maintain the internal equilibrium (Rupp, 2001; Holly and Shaffrath, 2001).

CARDIAC FUNCTION

Heart Rate

- Normal *resting heart rate* (HR_{rest}) is approximately 60–80 beats/min. With the onset of dynamic exercise, HR increases in proportion to the relative workload. The *maximal HR* (HR_{max}) decreases with age, and can be estimated in healthy men and women by using the formula: $HR_{max} = 220 − Age$. There is considerable variability in this estimation for any fixed age with a standard deviation of ±10 beats/min (Rupp, 2001; Holly and Shaffrath, 2001).

Stroke Volume

- *Stroke volume* (SV) is the amount of blood ejected from the left ventricle in a single beat. SV is equal to the difference between end diastolic volume (EDV) and *end systolic volume* (ESV). Greater *diastolic filling* (preload) will increase SV. Factors that resist *ventricular outflow* (afterload) will result in a reduced SV.
- During exercise, SV increases curvilinearly with the work rate until it reaches near maximum at a level equivalent to approximately 50% of aerobic capacity. Thereafter, SV starts to plateau and further increases in workload do not result in increased SV primarily owing to reduced filling time during diastole.
- SV is also affected by body position, with SV being greater in the supine or prone position and lower in the upright position. *Static exercise* (weight training) may also cause a slight decrease in SV owing to increased intrathoracic pressure (Rupp, 2001; Holly and Shaffrath, 2001).

Cardiac Output

- *Cardiac output* (Q) is the amount of blood pumped by the heart each minute. It is calculated by the following formula:

$$Q \text{ (L/min)} = \text{Heart Rate (beats/min)} \times \text{Stroke Volume (mL/beat).}$$

- Resting cardiac output in both trained and sedentary individuals is approximately 4–5 L/min; however, during exercise maximal cardiac output can reach 20 L/min. During dynamic exercise, cardiac output increases with increasing exercise intensity by increases in SV and HR; however, increases in cardiac output beyond 40–50% of VO_{2max} are accounted for only by increases in HR (Rupp, 2001; Holly and Shaffrath, 2001).

Blood Flow

- At rest, 15–20% of the cardiac output is distributed to the skeletal muscles with the remainder going to visceral organs, the brain and the heart; however, during exercise, 85–90% of the cardiac output is selectively delivered to working muscles. Myocardial blood flow may increase four to five times with exercise, whereas blood supply to the brain is maintained at resting levels. The difference between the oxygen content of arterial blood and the oxygen content of venous blood year is termed the *arteriovenous oxygen difference* (a-vO_2 Diff.). It reflects the oxygen extracted from arterial blood by the tissues. At rest the oxygen extraction is approximately 25%, but at maximal exercise the oxygen extraction can reach 75% (Rupp, 2001; Holly and Shaffrath, 2001).
- *Venous return* is maintained and/or increased during exercise by the following mechanisms: (1) Contracting skeletal muscle acts as a *pump*. (2) Smooth muscle around the venules contract, increasing the pressure on the venous side. (3) Diaphragmatic contraction during exercise creates lowered intrathoracic pressure, facilitating blood flow (Rupp, 2001; Holly and Shaffrath, 2001).

Blood Pressure

- *Blood pressure* (BP) is the driving force behind blood flow.
- *Systolic blood pressure* (SBP): SBP increases linearly with increasing work intensity, by 8–12 *mm-Hg per metabolic equivalent* (MET), where 1 MET = 3.5 mL-O_2/kg/min. Maximal values typically reach 190 to 220 mm-Hg. Maximal SBP should not be greater than 260 mm-Hg. *Diastolic blood pressure* (DBP) either remains unchanged or only slightly increases with exercise (Rupp, 2001; Holly and Shaffrath, 2001).
- Failure of SBP to rise or decreased SBP with increasing work rates or a significant increase in DBP is an abnormal response to exercise and indicates either severe exercise intolerance or underlying cardiovascular disease (Rupp, 2001; Holly and Shaffrath, 2001).
- *Postural considerations:* In the supine position, SBP is lower. When the body is upright, SBP increases. DBP does not change significantly with body position in healthy individuals (Franklin, 2001).
- *Effects of arm versus leg exercise:* At similar oxygen consumptions, HR, SBP, and DBP are higher during arm work than during leg work (Rupp, 2001; Holly and Shaffrath, 2001).

PULMONARY VENTILATION

- *Pulmonary ventilation* (Ve) is the volume of air exchanged per minute, and generally is approximately 6 L/min at rest in an average sedentary adult male; however, at maximal exercise, Ve increases 15- to 25-fold over resting values. During mild to moderate exercise Ve increases primarily by increasing tidal volume, but during vigorous activity increases in the respiratory rate are the primary way Ve increases (Franklin, 2001).

- Generally, increases in Ve are directly proportional to an increase in *oxygen consumption* (VO_2) and *carbon dioxide produced* (VCO_2); however, at a critical exercise intensity (usually 47–64% of the VO_{2max} in healthy untrained individuals and 70–90% VO_{2max} in highly trained individuals), Ve increases disproportionately relative to the VO_2, paralleling an abrupt increase in serum lactate and VCO_2. This is called the *anaerobic* (ventilatory) *threshold* (AT) (Franklin, 2001).

- AT signifies the onset of metabolic acidosis during exercise, and traditionally has been determined by serial measurements of blood lactate. It can be non-invasively determined by assessment of expired gases during exercise testing, specifically Ve and VCO_2. AT signifies the peak work rate or oxygen consumption at which the energy demands exceed circulatory ability to sustain aerobic metabolism (Franklin, 2001).

MAXIMAL OXYGEN CONSUMPTION

- The most widely recognized measure of cardiopulmonary fitness is the aerobic capacity, or VO_{2max}. This variable is defined physiologically as the highest rate of oxygen transport and use that can be achieved at maximal physical exertion (Franklin, 2001).

EFFECTS OF EXERCISE TRAINING

CARDIOVASCULAR SYSTEM

- The effects of regular exercise on the cardiovascular system can be grouped into changes that occur at rest, during submaximal exercise and during maximal work (Rupp, 2001).

Changes at Rest

- Heart rate (HR) decreases likely secondary to decreased sympathetic tone, increased parasympathetic tone, and a decreased intrinsic firing rate of the SA node.
- SV increases secondary to increased myocardial contractility.
- Cardiac output is unchanged at rest.
- Oxygen consumption does not change at rest (Rupp, 2001).

Changes at Submaximal Work

- Submaximal work is defined as a workload during which a steady state is achieved.
  a. HR decreases at any given workload owing to the increased SV and decreased sympathetic drive.
  b. SV increases owing to increased myocardial contractility.

  c. Cardiac output does not change significantly for a fixed workload; however, the same cardiac output is generated with a lower HR and higher SV.
  d. Submaximal oxygen consumption does not change significantly since oxygen requirement is the similar for a fixed workload.
  e. a-vO_2 Diff. increases during submaximal work.
  f. Lactate levels are decreased owing to metabolic efficiency and increased lactate clearance rates (Rupp, 2001).

Changes at Maximal Work

- *Maximal heart rate* (HR_{max}) does not change with exercise training.
- SV increases owing to increased contractility and/or increased heart size.
- Maximal cardiac output increases owing to increased SV.
- Maximal oxygen consumption (VO_{2max}) increases owing to increased SV and a-vO_2 Diff.
- a-vO_2 Diff. increases owing to improved ability of the mitochondria to use oxygen (Rupp, 2001).

Blood Pressure

- In normotensive individuals, regular exercise does not appear to have a significant impact on resting or exercising blood pressure.
- In hypertensive individuals there may be a modest reduction in resting blood pressure as a result of regular exercise (Rupp, 2001).

BLOOD LIPIDS

- Total cholesterol may be decreased in individuals with hypercholesterolemia.
- *High-density lipoprotein cholesterol* (HDL) increases with exercise training.
- *Low-density lipoprotein cholesterol* (LDL) may remain the same or decrease with regular exercise.
- Triglycerides may decrease in those with elevated triglycerides initially. This change is facilitated by weight loss (Rupp, 2001).

BODY COMPOSITION

- Total body weight usually decreases with regular exercise.
- Fat-free weight does not normally change.
- Percent body fat declines (Rupp, 2001).

BLOOD VOLUME CHANGES

- Total blood volume increases owing to an increased number of red blood cells and expansion of the plasma volume (Rupp, 2001).

BIOCHEMICAL CHANGES

- Stored muscle glycogen increases.
- The percentage of fast- and slow-twitch fibers does not change, but the cross sectional area occupied by these fibers may change owing to selective hypertrophy of either fast- or slow-twitch fibers (Rupp, 2001).

DETRAINING

- The changes induced by regular exercise training generally are lost after 4–8 weeks of detraining. If training is reestablished, the rate at which the training effects occur do not appear to be faster (Rupp, 2001).

OVERTRAINING

- Overtraining refers to a condition usually induced after prolonged heavy exercise over an extended period of time. Symptoms of overtraining may include the following:
  1. Sudden decline in quality of work or exercise performance
  2. Extreme fatigue
  3. Elevated HR_{rest}
  4. Early onset of blood lactate accumulation
  5. Altered mood states
  6. Unexplained weight loss
  7. Insomnia
  8. Injuries related to overuse
- Overtraining may require weeks to months of complete rest in order to recover (Rupp, 2001).

THE EXERCISE PRESCRIPTION AND PROGRAM

EXERCISE PRESCRIPTIONS

ACSM RECOMMENDATIONS FOR CARDIORESPIRATORY ENDURANCE TRAINING

Mode

- The best improvements in cardiorespiratory endurance occur when large muscle groups are engaged in rhythmic aerobic activity.
- Various activities can be incorporated into an exercise program to increase enjoyment and improve compliance.
- Appropriate activities include—walking, jogging, cycling, rowing, stair climbing, aerobic dance (aerobics), water exercise, and cross-country skiing (Franklin et al, 2000b).

Intensity

- The ACSM recommends that exercise intensity be prescribed within a range of 70–85% of HR_{max}, 50–85% of VO_{2max}, or 60–80% of max METs, or *HR reserve* (HRR).
  1. Owing to the variability in estimating HR_{max} from age, whenever possible use an actual HR_{max} from a graded exercise test.
  2. Lower intensities (40–50% of VO_{2max}) elicit a favorable response in individual with very low fitness levels (Franklin et al, 2000b).
- *Rating of perceived exertion* (RPE) may be used with HR for regulating intensity.
  1. ACSM recommends an intensity that will elicit an RPE within a range of 12–16 on the original 6–20 Borg scale.
  2. RPE is considered a reliable indicator of exercise intensity and is particularly useful when a participant is unable to monitor their pulse or when HR response to exercise has been altered by medications (Franklin et al, 2000b).
- **Calculating intensity:** Owing to limitations in using VO_2 calculations for prescribing intensity, the most common methods of setting the intensity of exercise to improve or maintain cardiorespiratory fitness use HR and RPE (Franklin et al, 2000b; Pollock et al, 1998).
- **Heart rate methods:** HR is used as a guide to set exercise intensity because of the relatively linear relationship between HR and *percentage of VO_{2max}* (%VO_{2max}). It is best to measure HR_{max} during a progressive exercise test whenever possible since HR_{max} declines with age. HR_{max} can be estimated by using the following equation: ($HR_{max} = 220 -$ age). This estimation has significant variance with a standard deviation of 10–12 beats per minute (SD = 10 – 12 bpm) (Franklin et al, 2000b; Pollock et al, 1998).
- **HR_{max} method:** One of the oldest methods of setting the target HR range uses a straight percentage of the HR_{max}. Using 70–85% of an individual's HR_{max} approximates 55–75% VO_{2max} and provides the stimulus needed to improve or maintain cardiorespiratory fitness (Franklin et al, 2000b; Pollock et al, 1998). Example: If $HR_{max} = 180$ bpm then target HR (70–85% HR_{max}) would range 126–152 bpm.
- **Heart rate reserve method:** The *HR reserve* (HRR) method is also known as the Karvonen method. Target HR range = $[(HR_{max} - HR_{rest}) \times 0.50$ and $0.85] + HR_{rest}$. Using the HR method allows a more direct correlation between HR and % VO_2 max. (Franklin et al, 2000b; Pollock et al, 1998).
- **Rating of perceived exertion:** Use of RPE is considered an adjunct to monitoring HR. It has proven to be

a valuable aid in prescribing exercise for individuals who have difficulty with HR palpation, and in cases where the HR response to exercise may have been altered owing to a change in medication. The average RPE range associated with physiologic adaptation to exercise is 12–16 ("somewhat hard" to "hard") on the category Borg scale. One should suit the RPE to the individual on a specific mode of exercise and not expect an exact matching of the RPE to a $\%HR_{max}$ or $\%HRR$. It should be used only as a guideline in setting the exercise intensity (Franklin et al, 2000*b*; Pollock et al, 1998).

- Finally, the appropriate exercise intensity is one that is safe and compatible with a long-term active lifestyle for that individual and achieves the desired outcome given the time constraints of the exercise session.

Duration

- The ACSM recommends 20–60 min of continuous aerobic activity.
- However, deconditioned individuals may benefit from multiple, short-duration exercise sessions <10 min with frequent interspersed rest periods.
- An inverse relationship exists between the intensity and duration of training. There may be greater musculoskeletal and cardiovascular risk with exercise performed at high intensities for short durations as compared with lower intensity exercise for a longer duration (Franklin et al, 2000*b*; Pollock et al, 1998).

Frequency

- The ACSM recommends that aerobic exercise be performed 3–5 days per week for most individuals.
- Less conditioned people may benefit from lower intensity, shorter duration exercise performed at higher frequencies per day and/or per week (Franklin et al, 2000*b*).

Progression (Overload)

- The rate of progression depends on health/fitness status, individual goals, and compliance rate.
- Frequency, intensity, and/or duration can be increased to provide overload.
- The goal for most healthy individuals is 30 min, 3–4 days per week at 85% HRR (Franklin et al, 2000*b*).

MUSCULAR STRENGTH AND ENDURANCE TRAINING

- Overload and specificity are precepts of resistance training. *Overload* occurs when a greater than normal physical demand is placed on muscles or muscle groups. Muscular strength and endurance are developed by increasing the resistance to movement or the frequency or duration of activity to levels above those normally experienced. A training intensity of approximately 40–60% of one repetition maximum appears to be sufficient for the development of muscular strength in most normally active individuals (Franklin et al, 2000*b*; Bryant and Peterson, 2001).

- *Specificity* relates to the nature of changes (structural and functional, systemic and local) that occur in an individual as a result of training. These adaptations are specific and occur only in the overloaded muscle groups or muscles (Durstine and Davis, 2001).

The ACSM Provides the Following Guidelines for Resistance Training:

- A 5–10-min warm-up period consisting of aerobic activity or a light set (50–75% of training weight) of the specific resistance exercise should precede the resistance exercise program. The goal is to develop total body strength and endurance in a time-efficient manner (Franklin et al, 2000b; Bryant and Peterson, 2001).
1. *Mode:* The prescription should include a minimum of 8 to 10 separate exercises that target major muscle groups (arms, shoulder, chest, abdomen, back, hips, and legs). Free weights and weight machines are commonly used; however, springs, surgical or rubber tubing, and electronic devices are also used for resistance training (Franklin et al, 2000b).
2. *Intensity/Duration:* Perform a minimum of one set of 8 to 12 repetition of each of the exercises to the point of volitional fatigue. Volitional fatigue refers to the inability to move a resistance through the appropriate range of motion with proper mechanical form. A set of 10 to 15 repetitions is recommended for developing muscular endurance and for those who are older or frailer (Franklin et al, 2000b).
3. *Frequency:* Perform these exercises 2 to 3 days per week, usually with a day of rest in between (Franklin et al, 2000*b*).
4. *Progression:* Resistance may be increased when 12 repetitions can be completed with good technique (Franklin et al, 2000*b*).
5. *Additional Recommendations*
   a. Perform every exercise through a full range of motion using proper technique and in a controlled manner including the lifting (concentric phase) and lowering (eccentric phase).
   b. Maintain a normal breathing pattern and avoid breath holding (*Valsalva*).
   c. Exercise with a partner when possible to provide feedback, assistance, and motivation (Bryant and Peterson, 2001).

MUSCULOSKELETAL FLEXIBILITY TRAINING

Stretching Techniques

- **Static stretching:** Static stretching involves slowly stretching a muscle to the point of mild discomfort and then holding that position for an extended period of time (usually 10 to 30 s). It is effective, requires little time and the risk of injury is low. It is the most commonly recommended method.

- **Ballistic stretching:** Ballistic stretching uses the momentum created by repetitive bouncing movement to produce muscle stretch. This type of stretch can result in muscle soreness or injury and is generally not recommended (Franklin et al, 2000*b*; Fredette, 2001).
- **Proprioceptive neuromuscular facilitation:** Proprioceptive neuromuscular facilitation (PNF) involves a combination of alternating contraction and relaxation of both agonist and antagonist muscles through a designated series of motions. It is effective, but it is time consuming, requires a partner and may cause residual muscle soreness and has potential for injury if applied too vigorously (Franklin et al, 2000*b*; Fredette, 2001).

ACSM Recommendations for Flexibility Training

- Flexibility exercises should be performed in a slow, controlled manner with a gradual progression to greater ranges of motion. It is recommended that an active warm-up precede vigorous stretching exercises (Franklin et al, 2000*b*; Fredette, 2001).
  1. *Mode:* A general stretching routine that exercises the major muscle and/or tendon groups using static or PNF techniques.
  2. *Intensity:* Stretch the muscle to a position of mild discomfort.
  3. *Duration:* 10 to 30 s for static stretches and a 6-s contraction followed by a 10- to 30-s assisted stretch for PNF. Repeat the stretch 3–4 times.
  4. *Frequency:* Minimum of 2 to 3 days per week (Franklin et al, 2000*b*; Fredette, 2001)

GENERAL COMPONENTS OF AN EXERCISE PROGRAM

- Once the exercise prescription has been formulated, it is integrated into a comprehensive physical conditioning program which consists of the following components:
  1. *Warm-up phase* (10 min): Warm-up phase facilitates the transition form rest to exercise, stretches postural muscles, augments blood flow, and increases the metabolic rate from the resting level (1 MET) to the aerobic requirements for endurance training.
  2. *Endurance phase* (20–60 min): Endurance phase develops cardiorespiratory fitness and includes 20 to 60 min of continuous or intermittent (minimum of 10-min bouts accumulated throughout the day) aerobic activity.
  3. *Cool-down* (5–10 min): This phase provides a period of gradual recovery from the endurance phase and includes exercises of diminishing intensities. It permits appropriate circulatory adjustments and return of the HR and BP to near resting values (Franklin et al, 2000*b*; Wygand, 2001).

- While endurance training activities should be performed 3 to 5 days a week, complementary flexibility and resistance training may be undertaken at a slightly reduced frequency of 2 to 3 days a week. Flexibility training can be included as part of the warm-up or cool-down, or undertaken at a separate time. Resistance training is often performed on alternate days when endurance training is not; however, both activities can be combined into the same workout (Franklin et al, 2000*b*; Wygand, 2001).

RATE OF PROGRESSION

- The recommended rate of progression in an exercise-conditioning program depends on functional capacity, medical and health status, age, individual activity preferences and goals, and an individual's tolerance to the current level of training. For apparently healthy adults, the endurance aspect of the exercise prescription has three stages of progression: initial, improvement, and maintenance (Franklin et al, 2000*b*; Wygand, 2001).

INITIAL CONDITIONING

- The initial stage should include light muscular endurance exercises and moderate level aerobic activities (40–60% of HRR), exercises that are compatible with minimal muscle soreness, discomfort, and injury. The duration of the exercise session during the initial stage may begin with approximately 15 to 20 min and progress to 30 min. It is recommended that individuals who are starting a moderate-intensity conditioning program should exercise 3 to 4 times per week (Franklin et al, 2000*b*; Wygand, 2001).

IMPROVEMENT STAGE

- The goal of this stage of training is to provide a gradual increase in the overall exercise stimulus to allow for significant improvements in cardiorespiratory fitness. This stage typically lasts 4 to 5 months, during which intensity is progressively increased within the upper half of the target range of 50 to 85% of HR reserve. Duration is increased consistently every 2 to 3 weeks until participants are able to exercise at a moderate-to-vigorous intensity for 20 to 30 min continuously (Franklin et al, 2000*b*; Wygand, 2001).

MAINTENANCE STAGE

- The goal of this stage of training is the long-term maintenance of cardiorespiratory fitness developed during the improvement stage. This stage of the exercise program usually begins after the first 5 or 6 months of training, but may begin at any time the participant has reached preestablished fitness goals. During this stage, the participant may no longer be interested in further increasing the conditioning stimulus. Further improvement may be minimal, but continuing the same workout routine enables individuals to maintain their fitness (Franklin et al, 2000*b*; Wygand, 2001).

MEDICAL CLEARANCE
• Exercise training may not be appropriate for everyone. Patients whose adaptive reserves are severely limited by disease processes may be unable to adapt to or benefit from exercise. In this small subpopulation of people with severe or unstable cardiac, respiratory, metabolic, systemic, or musculoskeletal disease—exercise programming may be fatal, injurious, or simply not beneficial, depending on the clinical status and condition of the individual (Franklin et al, 2000*c*).

IDENTIFY CONTRAINDICATIONS TO EXERCISE

• **Absolute**
  1. Recent acute myocardial infarction
  2. Unstable angina
  3. Ventricular tachycardia or other dangerous arrhythmias
  4. Severe aortic stenosis
  5. Acute infection and/or fever
  6. Recent systemic or pulmonary embolus
  7. Thrombophlebitis or intracardiac thrombi
  8. Active or suspected myocarditis or pericarditis
  9. Acute congestive heart failure
  10. Dissecting aortic aneurysm (Franklin et al, 2000*d*)
• **Relative**
  1. Severe hypertension (uncontrolled or untreated)
  2. Complicated pregnancy
  3. Moderate aortic stenosis
  4. Severe subaortic stenosis
  5. Supraventricular dysrhythmias
  6. Ventricular aneurysm
  7. Frequent or complex ventricular ectopy
  8. Cardiomyopathy
  9. Uncontrolled metabolic disease (thyroid or diabetes) or electrolyte abnormality
  10. Chronic or recurrent infectious disease (malaria, hepatitis, and the like)
  11. Neuromuscular, musculoskeletal, or rheumatoid diseases exacerbated by exercise (Franklin et al, 2000*d*)

IDENTIFY THOSE WHO NEED AN EXERCISE STRESS TEST

• Indications for an *exercise stress test* according to American College of Cardiology (ACC) and American Heart Association (AHA) are as follows (Stephens et al, 2002):
  1. To evaluate patients for suspected coronary artery disease (typical and atypical angina pectoris)
  2. To evaluate patients with known coronary artery disease
  3. To evaluate healthy asymptomatic individuals in the following categories:
     a. High-risk occupations, such as pilots, firefighter, law enforcement officer, mass transit operator
     b. Men over age 40 and women over age 50 who are sedentary and plan to start vigorous exercise
     c. Individuals with multiple cardiac risk factors or concurrent chronic diseases
  4. To evaluate exercise capacity in patients with valvular heart disease, except severe aortic stenosis.
  5. Individuals with cardiac rhythm disorders for the following reasons:
     a. Evaluate response to treatment of exercise-induced arrhythmia
     b. Evaluate response of rate-adaptive pacemaker setting
• The ACSM and ACC/AHA guidelines discourage using exercise testing to screen asymptomatic adults unless they are at increased risk (Stephens et al, 2002).

SUMMARY

• Numerous studies have quantified the many health and fitness benefits associated with exercise. Although the optimal dose of physical activity has yet to be defined, significant health benefits can be obtained by including a moderate amount of physical activity on most, if not all, days of the week. With a modest increase in daily activity, most patients will improve their health and quality of life.

REFERENCES

Bryant C, Peterson J: Muscular strength and endurance, in Roitman J, Haver E, Herridge M (eds.): *ACSM's Resource Manual for Guidelines for Exercise Testing and Prescription.* Philadelphia, PA, Lipppincott Williams & Wilkins, 2001.

Demaree S, Powers S, Lawler J: Fundamentals of exercise metabolism, in Roitman J, Haver E, Herridge M (eds.): *ACSM's*

Resource Manual for Exercise Testing and Prescription. Philadelphia, PA, Lipincott Williams & Wilkins, 2001.

Durstine J, Davis P: Specificity of exercise training and testing, in Roitman J, Haver E, Herridge M (eds.): *ACSM's Resource Manual for Guidelines for Exercise Testing and Prescription.* Philadelphia, PA, Lipppincott Williams & Wilkins, 2001.

Franklin B: Normal cardiorespiratory responses to acute aerobic exercise, in Roitman J, Haver E, Herridge M (eds.): *ACSM's Resource Manual for Guidelines for Exercise Testing and Prescription.* Philadelphia, PA, Lippincott Williams & Wilkins, 2001.

Franklin B, Whaley M, Howley E (eds.): Benefits and risks associated with exercise: *ACSM's Guidlines for Exercise Testing and Prescription.* Philadelphia, PA, Lippincott Williams & Willliams, 2000*a*.

Franklin B, Whaley M, Howley E (eds.): General principles of exercise prescription: *ACSM's Guidelines for Exercise Testing and Prescription.* Philadelphia, PA, Lippincott Williams & Wilkins, 2000*b*.

Franklin B, Whaley M, Howley E (eds.): Health screening and risking stratification, in Franklin B, Whaley M, Howley E (eds.): *ACSM's Guidelines for Exercise Testing and Prescription.* Philadelphia, PA, Lippincott Williams & Williams, 2000*c*.

Franklin B, Whaley M, Howley E (eds.): Physical fitness testing and interpretation: *ACSM's Guidelines for Exercise Testing and Prescription.* Philadelphia, PA, Lippincott Williams & Wilkins, 2000*d*.

Fredette D: Exercise Recommendations for Flexibility and Range of Motion, in Roitman J, Haver E, Herridge M (eds.): *ACSM's Resource Manual for Guidelines for Exercise Testing and Prescription*, Philadelphia, PA, Lipppincott Williams & Wilkins, 2001.

Holly R, Shaffrath J: Cardiorespiratory Endurance, in Roitman J, Haver E, Herridge M (Eds.): *ACSM's Resource Manual for Guidelines for Exercise Testing and Prescription.* Philadelphia, PA, Lippincott Williams & Wilkins, 2001.

Humphrey R: Musculoskeletal anatomy, in Roitman J, Haver E, Herridge M (eds.): *ACSM's Resource Manual for Guidelines for Exercise Testing and Prescription.* Philadelphia, PA, Lipincott Williams & Wilkins, 2001.

Pollock M, Gaesser G, Butcher J et al: The recommended quantity and quality of exercise for developing and maintaining cardiorespiratory and muscular fitness and flexibility in healthy adults: *Medicine & Science in Sports and Exercise.* American College of Sports Medicine Position Stand, 1998. *Med Sci Sports Exerc* 30(6):975–991.

Rupp J: Exercise physiology, in Roitman J, Bibi K, Thompson W (eds.): *ACSM's Health Fitness Certification Review.* Philadelphia, PA, Lippincott Williams & Wilkins, 2001.

Stephens M, O'Connor F, Deuster P: *Exercise and nutrition: AAFP Home Study—a self-assessment program.* American Academy of Family Physicians, Leawood, KS, 2002.

Whaley M, Kaminsky L: Epidemiology of physical activity, physical fitness and selected chronic diseases, in Roitman J, Haver E, Herridge M, (eds.): *ACSM's Resource Manual for Guidelines for Exercise Testing and Prescription.* Philadephia, PA, Lipincott Williams & Wilkins, 2001.

Wygand J: Exercise programming, in Roitman J, Bibi K, Thompson W, (eds.): *ACSM's Health Fitness Certification Review.* Philadelphia, PA, Lippincott Williams & Wilkins, 2001.

14 NUTRITION

Nancy M DiMarco, PhD, RD, LD
Eve V Essery, BS, PhDc

INTRODUCTION

- Athletes who eat a healthy diet and practice good lifestyle habits perform at peak output, recover more quickly, and reach goals faster.
- This chapter focuses on fuel utilization during exercise, the general dietary needs of competitive individuals, carbohydrate loading for glycogen resynthesis, maintenance of muscle mass, beneficial ergogenic aids, and some dietary supplements, including energy bars.

FUEL UTILIZATION

- Duration, frequency, and intensity of exercise determine the amount of energy expended during activity, and the type of activity performed determines the predominant energy pathway used (Romijn et al, 1993; Weber, 1996).
- Three energy pathways are used for muscular work, including two anaerobic and one primarily aerobic pathways (Powers and Howley, 1990):
1. The *power pathway* is used during high intensity events lasting no longer than 4 s. *Adenosine triphosphate* (ATP) and creatine phosphate within the muscle provide the readily available energy for activity. Examples of activities that use the power pathway include the lean and jerk in weight lifting or a fast break in basketball.
2. The *speed pathway* is used for events lasting 4 to 60 s. The major substrates used in this pathway are glucose and muscle glycogen, which are rapidly metabolized anaerobically through the glycolytic cascade. Typical events include track events of less than 400 m or swimming events less than 100 m. Approximately 25–35% of muscle glycogen stores are used during a single 30-s sprint or resistance exercise bout. Further, if an individual is participating in repeated sprints, muscle glycogen is depleted with each sprint.
3. Neither the power nor the speed pathways can provide sufficient energy for the muscles to contract at a very high rate for events lasting longer than ~2 min.
4. The *endurance pathway* is used for events lasting longer than 2 min. The major substrates for this pathway include glycogen (from the muscle and liver), fat (from the muscle, blood, and adipose tissue), as

well as amino acids (from the muscle, blood, and liver). Examples of events that use the endurance pathway include a 1500-m run, marathon, half-marathon, and all-day cycling or swimming events. As oxygen becomes more available to the working muscle, the body begins to switch from anaerobic systems to more aerobic ones. Only the aerobic endurance pathway can produce large amounts of ATP over extended periods of time via the Krebs cycle and the electron transport system.

5. The changeover from anaerobic to aerobic pathways is not abrupt, nor is there ever a time when one pathway is used exclusively. The intensity, duration, frequency, type of activity, and fitness level of the participant determines when the crossover from primarily anaerobic to aerobic pathways occurs. After 2 h of activity, most of the energy is derived from the endurance pathway (~99%) and only a trace from the anaerobic system (~1%).

• The more energy used in activity, the more calories need to be consumed in the diet. Energy expenditure must balance energy intake.

• Individuals training for an athletic event will require more kilocalories than a sedentary individual. The reference sedentary man weighs 154 lb and expends 2700 to 3500 kcals a day (average 3025) between the ages of 20 and 29 years. The reference sedentary woman weighs 125 lb and expends 1890 to 2000 kcal a day (average 1957) between the ages of 20 and 29 (Briefel et al, 1995).

• The cost of the iron man triathlon (consisting of a 2.4 mi open ocean swim, 112 mi bike race, and 26.2 mi marathon) is approximately 4800 kcals for a male athlete. The cost of training alone ranges from 3000 to 6000 kcals a day for a male athlete (Erp-Baart et al, 1989).

CONVERSION OF ENERGY SOURCES OVER TIME

• Approximately 50–60% of energy during 1 to 4 h of continuous exercise at 70% of maximal oxygen capacity is derived from carbohydrates and the remaining energy is derived from fat (Coyle et al, 1986).

• As the intensity of exercise decreases, a greater proportion of energy comes from the oxidation of free fatty acids (Erp-Baart et al, 1989; Coyle et al, 1997; Martin, III, 1997).

• Training does not alter the total amount of energy expended (during activity of the same intensity and duration) but rather changes the proportion of energy expended from carbohydrates and fat. As a result of training, the energy derived from fat increases and the energy from carbohydrates decreases. A trained individual uses a higher percentage of fat than an untrained person at the same workload (Hurley et al, 1986).

• Long-chain fatty acids derived from stored muscle triglycerides are the preferred fuel for aerobic exercise for individuals involved in mild- to moderate-intensity exercise (Nicklas, 1997; Turcotte, 1999).

GENERAL DIETARY NEEDS OF ACTIVE INDIVIDUALS

CALORIES

• The dietary guidelines are predicated on consumption of adequate calories to sustain daily energy expenditure and should be provided on an individual basis (see Table 14-1).

• The average endurance athlete should consume approximately 55 kcal/kg body weight (Houtkooper, 1992). Energy needs for strength trainers and bodybuilders depend on their training schedule and gender. Energy needs range from 33 to 60 kcal/kg a day for males and 30 to 44 kcal/kg a day for females (Kleiner et al, 1990; 1994).

PROTEINS

• Protein requirements for both endurance and strength athletes should be individualized to determine adequacy of intake. The majority of athletes are consuming adequate amounts of protein.

TABLE 14-1 Estimated Energy Expenditure at Various Levels of Physical Activity

LEVEL OF INTENSITY	TYPE OF ACTIVITY	ENERGY EXPENDITURE (KCAL/KG/DAY)	
Moderate	Walking 3.5 to 4 mph, cycling, skiing, tennis, dancing	Male	41
		Female	37
Heavy	Basketball, climbing, football, soccer	Male	50
		Female	44
Exceptional	Training in professional or world-class athletic events	Male	58
		Female	51

SOURCE: National Academy of Sciences (1989).

- High quality protein intake for the male endurance athlete performing at intensities above 65–85% of VO_{2peak} should be 1.0–1.6 g/kg body weight per day or 150–175% of the current *recommended dietary allowances* (RDA) for protein. This protein intake is required to provide for the oxidation of amino acids during high intensity exercise (Snyder and Naik, 1998). For example, a 150-lb man would need about 75 to 113 g of protein per day. Female athletes may require 10–20% less protein than male athletes.
- There does not appear to be an increased protein requirement for individuals engaged in moderate-intensity endurance exercise or <50% VO_{2peak} (Butterfield and Calloway, 1984).
- Protein intake for strength athletes must be provided to enhance muscle hypertrophy but must also be individualized to the duration, frequency, and intensity of the activity. In early stages of resistance training, the estimated protein requirement is 1.5–1.7g/kg body weight per day, but when training enters the maintenance phase, the protein requirement decreases to 1.0–1.2 g/kg body weight per day (Lemon and Tarnopolsky, 1992; Tarnopolsky et al, 1992).
- Protein intakes above 2.0 g/kg body weight per day are probably oxidized for energy and thus do not enhance muscle mass or performance.
- In general, animal proteins are higher quality proteins than plant proteins. Animal proteins are complete proteins providing all the essential amino acids in amounts necessary for production of body proteins. Plant proteins are incomplete and are not digested as completely as animal proteins. Furthermore, animal foods generally provide more protein per serving than plant foods. Good sources of animal protein include meat, eggs, and dairy products. Plant proteins include grains, legumes, and vegetables. Soy protein is a plant protein; however, soy protein is a higher quality protein than other plant proteins (Jeejeebhoy, 2000).

FATS

- Dietary fat intake should provide no more than 30% of total kilocalories. For example, a 150-lb athlete who consumes 3750 kcals a day would need 125 g of fat. Endurance athletes in training may decrease their intake to 20–25% of total kilocalories to enable them to consume the larger quantities of carbohydrate required to prevent staleness (Houtkooper, 1992; Coleman, 1998).
- Adaptation to a high-fat diet (>60% kcals from fat) will increase the contribution of fatty acid oxidation by 40% to total energy expenditure of exercise; however, neither the rate of use of glycogen nor an

increased performance during moderate intensity exercise has been observed (Helge et al, 1996).

CARBOHYDRATES

- The general guidelines for the endurance athlete are that between 60 and 70% of total kilocalories, or 8 and 10 g/kg body weight should be in the form of carbohydrates, especially for those participating in training or events lasting longer than 1 h (Houtkooper, 1992; Coleman, 1998; Joint position statement: Nutrition and athletic performance, 2000).
- A 150-lb individual who requires 3750 kcals per day of which 1920 to 2700 kcals should be carbohydrate will need 480–675 g carbohydrate/day.
- Endurance athletes training for less than 1 h a day can resynthesize glycogen adequately on dietary intakes of 6 g/kg body weight (Walberg-Rankin, 1995).

WATER/FLUID

- In any event lasting longer than 30 min, fluid and nutrient needs take on greater importance and can influence performance.
- Water is the most important nutrient for regulating hydration status in individuals.
- Water loss during exercise occurs primarily through sweat. Sweat rate is influenced by ambient temperature, humidity, exercise intensity, and rate of exogenous fluid intake. Water loss occurs in both the intra- and extracellular fluid compartments, which can lead to changes in electrolyte balance of both sodium and potassium, particularly, and may influence cardio respiratory function.
- The average person does not consume enough fluid to offset sweat losses during exercise. Average losses during exercise can amount to 2–6% of a person's body weight. Physical performance is impaired when 3–4% body weight is lost (Noakes, 1993).
- Physiologic changes accompanying dehydration include impaired heat dissipation, decreased plasma volume, and impaired skin blood flow, which can lead to decreased stroke volume, increased heart rate, cardiac drift, and ultimately heat stroke (Montain and Coyle, 1992).
- Fluid intake prior to exercise is necessary to offset risk of dehydration during exercise. Drinking throughout the day can ensure a euhydrated state. Consumption of 400 to 600 mL of fluid 2 h prior to competition is recommended (Latzka and Montain, 1999).
- Fluid intake during exercise is necessary to replace fluid lost through sweat at an equivalent rate. The practical recommendation is to consume 150 to 350 mL

TABLE 14-2 Dietary Reference Intakes for Selected Vitamins

NUTRIENT	LIFE STAGE GROUP	RDA*	UL†	SELECTED FOOD SOURCES
Folate	Male			Enriched cereal grains, dark leafy vegetables, enriched and whole-grain breads and bread products, fortified ready-to-eat cereals
	19–50 y	400 µg/d	1000 µg/d	
	Female			
	19–50 y	400 µg/d	1000 µg/d	
Niacin	Male			Meat, fish, poultry, enriched and whole-grain breads and bread products, fortified ready-to-eat cereals
	19–50 y	16 mg/d	35 mg/d	
	Female			
	19–50 y	14 mg/d	35 mg/d	
Riboflavin	Male			Organ meats, milk, bread products and fortified cereals
	19–50 y	1.3 mg/d	ND	
	Female			
	19–50 y	mg/d	ND	
Thiamin	Male			Enriched, fortified, or whole-grain products, bread products and ready-to-eat cereals
	19–50 y	1.2 mg/d	ND	
	Female			
	19–50 y	1.1 mg/d	ND	
Vitamin B_6	Male			Fortified cereals, organ meats
	19–50 y	1.3 mg/d	100 mg/d	
	Female			
	19–50 y	1.3 mg/d	100 mg/d	
Vitamin B_{12}	Male			Meat, fish, poultry, fortified cereals
	19–50 y	2.4 µg/d	ND	
	Female			
	19–50 y	2.4 µg/d	ND	

SOURCE: National Academy of Sciences (1998).
ABBREVIATION: ND = not determined.
Recommended dietary allowances are set to meet the needs of most (97%) individuals in an age and gender group.
†*Tolerable upper Intake level* is the maximum level of daily nutrient intake that is likely to pose no risk of adverse effects.

of water every 15 to 20 min of exercise (Convertino et al, 1996). If the activity lasts less than 1 h, water is generally the recommended fluid. When the exercise lasts more than 1 h, addition of 4–8% carbohydrate (glucose, sucrose, fructose, glucose polymers, and the like) and/or electrolytes can be beneficial (Murray et al, 1989). This amount of carbohydrate with the addition of electrolytes ensures maximal stimulation of fluid absorption because of increased palatability and aids in gastric emptying.

• Fluid intake after exercise is necessary to replace losses incurred during the activity. Body weight changes are the best method of determining fluid replacement amounts after exercise. Five hundred milliliters of fluid should be consumed for every 1 lb of weight lost (Shirreffs et al, 1996). Foods consumed should be rich sources of sodium and potassium, such as fruits and vegetables, particularly if the sweat loss was high (Burke, 1997).

VITAMINS

• Most sedentary adults in the United States meet the Dietary Reference Intakes (DRIs) for the B vitamins involved in energy metabolism (vitamin B_{12}, folate,

niacin, riboflavin, and thiamin) (Alaimo et al, 1994) (see Table 14-2).

• Active individuals expend energy in exercise that elevates both caloric and nutrient needs; however, for the most part, increased nutrient needs are met when athletes consume more calories. Athletes who restrict their intake for the purpose of maintaining a lower body weight may be at increased risk for nutrient deficiencies and may not be meeting DRI recommendations (Janelle and Barr, 1995).

• The majority of research has indicated that athletes are consuming adequate amounts of these micronutrients; however, more research is necessary to adequately evaluate the B_{12} and folate status of athletes (Fogelholm, 1995).

• Deficiencies of the B vitamins have been shown to compromise performance, and when individuals with documented deficiencies are provided supplemental B vitamins, noted increases in performance are observed (van der Beek et al, 1988; 1994).

MINERALS

• Active individuals are encouraged to consume calcium in amounts consistent with the DRI for their age

TABLE 14-3 Dietary Reference Intakes for Selected Minerals

NUTRIENT	LIFE STAGE GROUP	RDA†/AI‡	UL§	SELECTED FOOD SOURCES
Calcium	Males			Milk, cheese, yogurt, calcium-fortified foods
	19–50 y	1000* mg/d	2500 mg/d	
	Females			
	19–50 y	1000* mg/d	2500 mg/d	
Iron	Males			Meat and poultry (heme iron); fruits, vegetables,
	19–50 y	8 mg/d	45 mg/d	fortified grain products (nonheme iron)
	Females			
	19–50 y	18 mg/d	45 mg/d	
Zinc	Males			Red meats, fortified cereals
	19–50 y	11 mg/d	40 mg/d	
	Females			
	19–50 y	8 mg/d	40 mg/d	

SOURCE: National Academy of Sciences (1997; 2001).

†*Recommended dietary allowances* are set to meet the needs of most (97%) individuals in an age and gender group.

‡*Adequate intakes* are believed to meet the needs of all individuals in a life stage group, but lack of data prevent being able to specify an RDA—indicated with asterisk (*).

§*Tolerable upper intake level* is the maximum level of daily nutrient intake that is likely to pose no risk of adverse effects.

and sex. Athletes who perspire heavily or engage in physical activity in hot conditions may be prone to increased losses of calcium in sweat. If an individual consumes calcium supplements, no more than 500 mg should be consumed at any one time to enhance absorption (Bergeron et al, 1998) (see Table 14-3).

• During and immediately following exercise, there is a transient shift in potassium from the intracellular to the extracellular fluid space, which returns to normal approximately 1 h after exercise. Transient shifts in potassium may indicate that athletes need more potassium in their diets than what is recommended (Millard-Stafford et al, 1995).

• Increased intake of sodium is recommended, especially for individuals exercising in hot, humid environments. Adequate sodium intakes are necessary to maintain fluid balance and prevent muscle cramping; however, sodium needs can typically be met by adding salt while eating or eating foods that are known to be high in sodium. Chloride needs of athletes may also be increased compared to sedentary individuals. Foods containing sodium often also contain chloride (Convertino et al, 1996).

• Iron deficiency is a common nutrient deficiency, and 30–50% of athletes, especially female athletes, may be at risk of poor iron status. Females are at increased risk of iron depletion and even iron deficiency anemia because of menstruation, sweat losses, low consumption of iron-containing foods, and myoglobinuria from muscle stress during exercise. Iron deficiency, as a result of decreased iron stores, negatively impacts exercise performance as a result of decreased maximal oxygen consumption. Adequate intake of iron daily will help to ensure optimal performance (Schena, 1995).

• Zinc intake is less than optimal for approximately 25% of females in the United States (CSFII, 1994–1996) (Ma and Betts, 2000), and it has been estimated that about 50% of female distance runners also have less than optimal intakes (Deuster et al, 1989); however, few studies have been conducted that assess long-term changes in zinc status as a result of exercise training.

CARBOHYDRATE LOADING, GLYCOGEN RESYNTHESIS, MUSCLE MAINTENANCE—CHO/PRO RATIO

• Individuals training for any sport must replace carbohydrate on a regular basis.

1. The modified carbohydrate loading regimen still used today involves consumption of a diet initially consisting of 60% carbohydrate. The athlete also manipulates the amount of exercise they perform on a daily basis in a downward fashion (from 90 min down to 20 min) until the day before the event. The day before the event, the individual rests and consumes a diet containing 70% carbohydrate. This method is typically advocated for individuals participating in events lasting longer than approximately 90 min (Sherman et al, 1981).

2. Recent studies have observed improved performance when carbohydrate has been ingested before high intensity and intermittent exercise lasting less than 60 min (Below et al, 1995; Davis et al, 1997; Jeukendrup et al, 1997).

3. Following exercise, carbohydrate should be ingested immediately to ensure rapid muscle glycogen resynthesis. Athletes should consume

~1.2 g of carbohydrate/kg body weight at 2-h intervals up to 4 h (van Loon et al, 2000). The athlete should also maintain a daily carbohydrate intake of 8–11 g/kg body weight per day to ensure optimal muscle glycogen for repeated training bouts (Burke, 1997; 2001).

4. Some research has indicated that consuming carbohydrate and protein following exercise increases muscle glycogen synthesis rates more so than carbohydrate consumption alone (Ivy et al, 2002; Zawadzki et al, 1992); however, other studies have not confirmed this finding (Jentjens et al, 2001; van Hall et al, 2000; Carrithers et al, 2000).

5. Adding protein to carbohydrate probably does not increase muscle glycogen resynthesis but may stimulate muscle protein synthesis. Data does indicate that the optimal amount of carbohydrate required to promote glycogen repletion is ~1.2 g/kg body weight. The addition of protein to carbohydrate may allow athletes to recover faster and perform better during multiple training or competition bouts and may help to repair damaged muscle fibers.

FLUID REPLACEMENT BEVERAGES

- During and after exercise of ~1-h duration, a fluid replacement beverage containing 4–8% carbohydrate (consisting of glucose, sucrose, glucose polymers, fructose), sodium (10–20 mmol/L), and potassium (3–5mmol/L) will provide both fluid and energy (Convertino et al, 1996).
- Fluid replacement beverages exhibit high rates of gastric emptying compared to water and their taste facilitates increased consumption compared to water (Tsintzas et al, 1995).
- Urinary losses are less and fluid retention is greater after training or exercise when consuming fluid replacement beverages because of the increased drive to drink owing to electrolyte content, particularly sodium (Burke, 1997).
- Some research suggests that even for intermittent, high intensity, short duration type activities such as sprinting, running, or jogging, there may be benefit in use of fluid replacement beverages compared to water (Sugiura and Kobayashi, 1998).
- Carbonated beverages and fruit juices are not optimal fluid replacement beverages because the carbohydrate content is typically between 10 and 11%, too high to ensure rapid fluid absorption, and the low electrolyte content will not increase the drive to drink or maintain fluid balance. In addition, carbonation will increase the carbon dioxide content in the stomach and can lead to gastric distress. Caffeinated products can increase fluid loss, as well, but not all studies support this view (Wemple et al, 1997).

- Fructose as the sole carbohydrate source in fluid replacement beverages should be avoided because fructose absorption is considerably slower than glucose and sucrose absorption which can contribute to gastrointestinal distress (Murray et al, 1989).
- The American College of Sports Medicine and the National Athletic Trainers' Association both recommend drinking 400 to 600 mL (17–20 oz) of fluid 2–3 h before exercise, another 7–10 oz, 10–20 min before the event and then 150 to 350 mL (6–12 oz) every 15–20 min during exercise, beginning at the start of the activity (Convertino et al, 1996).
- Following training or competition, it is necessary to rehydrate with ~150% of fluid lost to completely rehydrate (Burke, 1997).

ERGOGENIC AIDS

- Ergogenic aids are products that have work-enhancing effects (Burke and Read, 1993). Although many products are advertised as nutritional ergogenic aids, few products are actually supported by research. Many purported ergogenic aids provide no benefit (but are harmless, e.g., coenzyme Q_{10}, pyruvate, and the like), while others may be harmful (bee pollen, dehydroepiandrosterone (DHEA), *ma huang*, and the like).
- The use of creatine and caffeine as ergogenic aids has been supported by research in some instances. Some research does support creatine supplementation in high-intensity strength activities such as resistance exercise (Kreider et al, 1998). A common side effect of this product is weight gain. Most studies that have investigated creatine have used creatine phosphate supplementation for 5 to 7 days (20 g/day) followed by a maintenance dose of 2 g/day.
- Caffeine is a stimulant that may have ergogenic effects in those who respond to supplementation (Bruce et al, 2000). Possible side effects include upset stomach, nervousness, irritability, and diarrhea. Caffeine is a banned substance at college, national, and international competitions; however, ergogenic benefits can be seen with as little as 5–6 mg/kg body weight, and positive drug tests are not likely at this level (Pasman et al, 1995). Tea, coffee, and sodas with caffeine can provide 50–100 mg/serving.
- A careful review of literature is necessary when determining if an ergogenic aid should be consumed. Most advertisements use personal testimonials that may be convincing, but are not based on research that has been duplicated and widely accepted. Some health care professionals oppose the use of all nutritional

ergogenic aids. Those who do recommend their use should examine the safety, efficacy, potency, and legality of the product before discussing the product with clients (Joint position statement: Nutrition and athletic performance, 2000).

DIETARY SUPPLEMENTS/ENERGY BARS

- Dietary supplements can be found as pills, powders, beverages, and bars. As with ergogenic aids, many dietary supplements are advertised with claims that sound appealing, but for the most part are not supported by research.
- Most athletes can meet their nutrient needs by consuming a well-balanced diet. Athletes have increased caloric needs, and if caloric needs are met by the consumption of foods, most nutrient needs are met as well.
- However, supplements may be necessary for athletes who restrict energy intake, use severe weight-loss practices, or eliminate food group(s) from the diet (Bruce et al, 2000). Also some supplements may be beneficial when a compact source of energy is required. For example, when athletes train in intensely, they may expend 3000–6000 kcal in training alone. Consumption of an energy dense beverage or bar may help athletes meet calorie needs. Products that provide carbohydrate and protein are recommended. Supplementation with individual amino acids has not been supported by research.
- When choosing supplements, look for the U.S. Pharmacopoeia (USP) seal. The USP establishes standards for quality and purity of supplements. Also, it is generally recommended that supplements provide no more than 150% of the daily value of nutrients.

SUMMARY

- A balanced diet that provides the proper amounts of all required nutrients is essential for peak performance and a healthy lifestyle. This is especially important for the athlete who might be training intensely or competing on successive days. The three primary energy systems used during running are the power, speed, and endurance systems. The energy systems used and energy requirements will vary for each individual depending on such factors as mode of activity, intensity, duration, height, weight, and gender. To aid in peak performance it is recommended that the athlete pay special attention to preevent, event, and postevent nutrient consumption. This will help ensure adequate hydration, glucose intake, and recovery. Finally, the use of such methods as glycogen loading

and creatine intake may help increase performance and power output for both long-distance runners and sprinters, respectively.

REFERENCES

Alaimo K, McDowell MA, Briefel RR, et al: Dietary intake of vitamins, minerals, and fiber of persons ages 2 months and over in the United States. Third National Health and Nutrition Examination Survey, Phase 1, 1988–91. *Adv Data* 1–28, 1994.

Below PR, Mora-Rodriguez R, Gonzalez-Alonso J, et al: Fluid and carbohydrate ingestion independently improve performance during 1 h of intense exercise. *Med Sci Sports Exerc* 27:200–10, 1995.

Bergeron M, Volpe S, Gelinas Y: Cutaneous calcium losses during exercise in the heat: A regional sweat patch estimation technique. *Clin Chem* 44S, 1998.

Briefel RR, McDowell MA, Alaimo K, et al: Total energy intake of the US population: The third national health and nutrition examination survey, 1988–1991. *Am J Clin Nutr* 62:1072S–80S, 1995.

Bruce CR, Anderson ME, Fraser SF, et al: Enhancement of 2000-m rowing performance after caffeine ingestion. *Med Sci Sports Exerc* 32:1958–63, 2000.

Bruce CR, Anderson ME, Fraser SF, et al: Enhancement of 2000-m rowing performance after caffeine ingestion. *Med Sci Sports Exerc* 32:1958–63, 2000.

Burke LM, Read RS: Dietary supplements in sport. *Sports Med* 15:43–65, 1993.

Burke LM: Nutrition for post-exercise recovery. *Aust J Sci Med Sport* 29:3–10, 1997.

Burke LM: Nutritional needs for exercise in the heat. *Comp Biochem Physiol A Mol Integr Physiol* 128:735–48, 2001.

Butterfield GE, Calloway DH: Physical activity improves protein utilization in young men. *Br J Nutr* 51:171–84, 1984.

Carrithers JA, Williamson DL, Gallagher PM, et al: Effects of postexercise carbohydrate-protein feedings on muscle glycogen restoration. *J Appl Physiol* 88:1976–82, 2000.

Coleman E: Carbohydrate—the master fuel. *Nutrition for Sport and Exercise*. Gaithersburg, MD, Aspen, 1998, p 21.

Convertino VA, Armstrong LE, Coyle EF, et al: American College of Sports Medicine position stand: Exercise and fluid replacement. *Med Sci Sports Exerc* 28:i–vii, 1996.

Coyle EF, Coggan AR, Hemmert MK, et al: Muscle glycogen utilization during prolonged strenuous exercise when fed carbohydrate. *J Appl Physiol* 61:165–72, 1986.

Coyle EF, Jeukendrup AE, Wagenmakers AJ, et al: Fatty acid oxidation is directly regulated by carbohydrate metabolism during exercise. *Am J Physiol* 273:E268–75, 1997.

Davis JM, Jackson DA, Broadwell MS, et al: Carbohydrate drinks delay fatigue during intermittent, high-intensity cycling in active men and women. *Int J Sport Nutr* 7:261–73, 1997.

Deuster PA, Day BA, Singh A, et al: Zinc status of highly trained women runners and untrained women. *Am J Clin Nutr* 49:1295–1301, 1989.

Erp-Baart AM, Saris WH, Binkhorst RA, et al: Nationwide survey on nutritional habits in elite athletes. Part I. Energy, carbohydrate, protein, and fat intake. *Int J Sports Med* 10 Suppl 1:S3–10, 1989.

Fogelholm M: Indicators of vitamin and mineral status in athletes' blood: A review. *Int J Sport Nutr* 5:267–84, 1995.

Helge JW, Richter EA, Kiens B: Interaction of training and diet on metabolism and endurance during exercise in man. *J Physiol* 492 (Pt 1):293–306, 1996.

Houtkooper L: Food selection for endurance sports. *Med Sci Sports Exerc* 24:S349–59, 1992.

Hurley BF, Nemeth PM, Martin WH, III, et al: Muscle triglyceride utilization during exercise: Effect of training. *J Appl Physiol* 60:562–67, 1986.

Ivy JL, Goforth HW, Jr., Damon BM, et al: Early postexercise muscle glycogen recovery is enhanced with a carbohydrate-protein supplement. *J Appl Physiol* 93:1337–44, 2002.

Janelle KC, Barr SI: Nutrient intakes and eating behavior scores of vegetarian and nonvegetarian women. *J Am Diet Assoc* 95:180–6, 189, quiz, 1995.

Jeejeebhoy KN: Vegetable proteins: Are they nutritionally equivalent to animal protein. *Eur J Gastroenterol Hepatol* 12:1–2, 2000.

Jentjens RL, van Loon LJ, Mann CH, et al: Addition of protein and amino acids to carbohydrates does not enhance postexercise muscle glycogen synthesis. *J Appl Physiol* 91:839–46, 2001.

Jeukendrup A, Brouns F, Wagenmakers AJ, et al: Carbohydrate-electrolyte feedings improve 1 h time trial cycling performance. *Int J Sports Med* 18:125–29, 1997.

Joint position statement: Nutrition and athletic performance. American College of Sports Medicine, American Dietetic Association, and Dietitians of Canada. *Med Sci Sports Exerc* 32:2130–145, 2000.

Kleiner SM, Bazzarre TL, Ainsworth BE: Nutritional status of nationally ranked elite bodybuilders. *Int J Sport Nutr* 4:54–69, 1994.

Kleiner SM, Bazzarre TL, Litchford MD: Metabolic profiles, diet, and health practices of championship male and female bodybuilders. *J Am Diet Assoc* 90:962–67, 1990.

Kreider RB, Ferreira M, Wilson M, et al: Effects of creatine supplementation on body composition, strength, and sprint performance. *Med Sci Sports Exerc* 30:73–82, 1998.

Latzka WA, Montain SJ: Water and electrolyte requirements for exercise. *Clin Sports Med* 18:513–24, 1999.

Lemon PW, Tarnopolsky MA, MacDougall JD, et al: Protein requirements and muscle mass/strength changes during intensive training in novice bodybuilders. *J Appl Physiol* 73:767–75, 1992.

Ma J, Betts NM: Zinc and copper intakes and their major food sources for older adults in the 1994–96 continuing survey of food intakes by individuals (CSFII). *J Nutr* 130:2838–43, 2000.

Martin WH, III: Effect of endurance training on fatty acid metabolism during whole body exercise. *Med Sci Sports Exerc* 29:635–39, 1997.

Millard-Stafford M, Sparling PB, Rosskopf LB, et al: Fluid intake in male and female runners during a 40-km field run in the heat. *J Sports Sci* 13:257–63, 1995.

Montain SJ, Coyle EF: Fluid ingestion during exercise increases skin blood flow independent of increases in blood volume. *J Appl Physiol* 73:903–10, 1992.

Murray R, Paul GL, Seifert JG, et al: The effects of glucose, fructose, and sucrose ingestion during exercise. *Med Sci Sports Exerc* 21:275–82, 1989.

National Academy of Sciences: *Recommended Dietary Allowances*, 10th ed. Washington DC, National Academy Press, 1989.

National Academy of Sciences: Dietary reference intakes for calcium, phosphorus, magnesium, vitamin D, and fluoride. Washington, DC, National Academy Press, 1997.

National Academy of Sciences: Dietary Reference Intakes for thiamin, riboflavin, niacin, vitamin B6, folate, vitamin B12, pantothenic acid, biotin, and choline. Washington, DC, National Academy Press, 1998.

National Academy of Sciences: Dietary reference intakes for vitamin A, vitamin K, arsenic, boron, chromium, copper, iodine, iron, manganese, molybdenum, nickel, silicon, vanadium, and zinc. Washington, DC, National Academy Press, 2001.

Nicklas BJ: Effects of endurance exercise on adipose tissue metabolism. *Exerc Sport Sci Rev* 25:77–103, 1997.

Noakes TD: Fluid replacement during exercise. *Exerc Sport Sci Rev* 21:297–330, 1993.

Pasman WJ, van Baak MA, Jeukendrup AE, et al: The effect of different dosages of caffeine on endurance performance time. *Int J Sports Med* 16:225–30, 1995.

Powers S, Howley E: *Exercise Physiology*. Dubuque, IA, Wm C Brown, 1990.

Romijn JA, Coyle EF, Sidossis LS, et al: Regulation of endogenous fat and carbohydrate metabolism in relation to exercise intensity and duration. *Am J Physiol* 265:E380–91, 1993.

Schena F: Iron status in athletes involved in endurance and in prevalently anaerobic sports, in Kies C, Driskell JA (eds.): *Sports Nutrition: Minerals and Electrolytes*. Philadelphia, PA, CRC Press, 1995, pp 65–79.

Sherman WM, Costill DL, Fink WJ, et al: Effect of exercise-diet manipulation on muscle glycogen and its subsequent utilization during performance. *Int J Sports Med* 2:114–18, 1981.

Shirreffs SM, Taylor AJ, Leiper JB, et al: Post-exercise rehydration in man: Effects of volume consumed and drink sodium content. *Med Sci Sports Exerc* 28:1260–71, 1996.

Snyder AC, Naik J: Protein requirements of athletes, in Berning JR, Steen SN (eds.): *Nutrition for Sport and Exercise*. Gaithersburg, MD, Aspen, 1998, p 45.

Sugiura K, Kobayashi K: Effect of carbohydrate ingestion on sprint performance following continuous and intermittent exercise. *Med Sci Sports Exerc* 30:1624–30, 1998.

Tarnopolsky MA, Atkinson SA, MacDougall JD, et al: Evaluation of protein requirements for trained strength athletes. *J Appl Physiol* 73:1986–95, 1992.

Tsintzas OK, Williams C, Singh R, et al: Influence of carbohydrate-electrolyte drinks on marathon running performance. *Eur J Appl Physiol Occup Physiol* 70:154–60, 1995.

Turcotte LP: Role of fats in exercise: Types and quality. *Clin Sports Med* 18:485–98, 1999.

van der Beek EJ, van Dokkum W, Schrijver J, et al: Thiamin, riboflavin, and vitamins B-6 and C: Impact of combined restricted intake on functional performance in man. *Am J Clin Nutr* 48:1451–62, 1988.

van der Beek EJ, Lowik MR, Hulshof KF, et al: Combinations of low thiamin, riboflavin, vitamin B6 and vitamin C intake among Dutch adults. Dutch Nutrition Surveillance System. *J Am Coll Nutr* 13:383–91, 1994.

van Loon LJ, Saris WH, Kruijshoop M, et al: Maximizing post-exercise muscle glycogen synthesis: Carbohydrate supplementation and the application of amino acid or protein hydrolysate mixtures. *Am J Clin Nutr* 72:106–11, 2000.

van Hall G, Shirreffs SM, Calbet JA: Muscle glycogen resynthesis during recovery from cycle exercise: No effect of additional protein ingestion. *J Appl Physiol* 88:1631–36, 2000.

Walberg-Rankin J: Dietary carbohydrate as an ergogenic aid for prolonged and brief competitions in sport. *Int J Sport Nutr* 5S:S13–28, 1995.

Weber JM, Brichon G, Zwingelstein G, et al: Design of the oxygen and substrate pathways. Part IV. Partitioning energy provision from fatty acids. *J Exp Biol* 199 (Pt 8):1667–74, 1996.

Wemple RD, Morocco TS, Mack GW: Influence of sodium replacement on fluid ingestion following exercise-induced dehydration. *Int J Sport Nutr* 7:104–16, 1997.

Zawadzki KM, Yaspelkis BB, III, Ivy JL: Carbohydrate-protein complex increases the rate of muscle glycogen storage after exercise. *J Appl Physiol* 72:1854–59, 1992.

15 EXERCISE PRESCRIPTION

Mark B Stephens, MD, MS, FAAFP, CAQAM

INTRODUCTION

- Three of every four Americans do not engage in sufficient physical activity on a regular basis (US Department of Health and Human Services, 2000). One of every four Americans is considered to be sedentary.
- Sixty percent of all Americans are either overweight or obese (US Public Health Service, 2001). Physical inactivity and obesity are correlated with increases in heart disease, diabetes, certain cancers and all-cause mortality (Stephens, O'Connor, and Deuster, 2002). Sufficient physical activity protects against these conditions.
- Physical activity has been listed as a leading health indicator for the national public health initiative *Healthy People 2010* (US Public Health Service, 2001).
- Healthcare providers generally do a poor job of counseling patients regarding the benefits of physical activity. Only 20–40% of preventive health care visits document physical activity counseling (Walsh et al, 1999). During these visits, providers include a written physical activity plan (exercise prescription) only 25% of the time.

- While the U.S. Preventive Services Task Force has stated that there is insufficient evidence to recommend for or against routine physical activity counseling (US Preventive Services Task Force, 2002), patients consider such counseling to be an important part of their medical visit and expect physicians to provide them with information regarding physical activity and nutrition.

BENEFITS OF PHYSICAL ACTIVITY

- The benefits of physical activity are well described. Regular physical activity prevents hypertension, hyperlipidemia, osteoporosis, cardiovascular disease, certain cancers and type-2 diabetes (US Department of Health and Human Services, 1996).

THE EXERCISE PRESCRIPTION: COMPONENTS OF PHYSICAL FITNESS

- Physical fitness can be defined as the ability to carry out functional and recreational activities of daily living without undue stress or fatigue.
- There are five primary components included in the definition of physical fitness:
  1. *Cardiorespiratory endurance* represents the ability of the cardiovascular and respiratory systems to take in and transport oxygen to metabolically active tissue.
  2. *Muscular strength* represents the maximal force generated by a muscle group against a fixed resistance.
  3. *Muscular endurance* represents the ability to repetitively move a muscle group against a set resistance before the onset of muscular fatigue.
  4. *Body composition* represents the distribution of fat and lean tissue (bone and muscle) mass within a given individual.
  5. *Flexibility* represents the ability to move a particular joint or series of joints through an entire range of motion.
- To be thorough, an exercise prescription should include specific recommendations targeted toward each component of physical fitness within the context of an individual's preexisting state of health and personal goals.

THE EXERCISE PRESCRIPTION: WHAT TO INCLUDE

- An exercise prescription (also referred to as an activity prescription) should include clear written instructions about the frequency, intensity, type, and duration (time) of activities that they should engage in.

- The mnemonic "FITT" (Frequency, Intensity, Type, Time) is a useful aid for guiding clinicians when writing an exercise prescription.

FREQUENCY

- All patients should be encouraged to engage in at least 30 min of moderate to vigorous physical activities on most and preferably all days of the week (Stephens, O'Connor, and Deuster, 2002).

INTENSITY

- There are many ways to prescribe exercise intensity. The intensity of the exercise session should be tailored to the individual's preexisting state of health and individual goals.
- Individuals wishing to improve health and lower disease-specific risk should be advised that sufficient levels of physical activity can be accumulated through small bouts of activity throughout the day. A dedicated activity or training session is not necessary.
- The target heart rate is the most common method of prescribing exercise intensity. The training heart rate is based on an age-predicted maximal heart rate (based on the formula $HR_{max} = 220 -$ patient age). Patients are instructed to exercise at a range of 40–80% of HR_{max} based on their specific goals.
- A modification of the target heart rate includes calculation of the heart rate reserve. This method takes into account the patient's resting heart rate. To calculate the target heart rate based on this method:
  a. $HR_{reserve} = \{(220 - \text{patient age}) - HR_{resting}\}$
  b. $HR_{target} = \{(HR_{reserve} * \text{training intensity}) + HR_{resting}\}$
- The *talk test* provides another safe and easy way to counsel individuals about exercise intensity. Patients should exercise at an intensity where they are able to carry out a conversation without undue shortness of breath.

TYPE

- The type of activity should be based on the individual's fitness level and interests.
- Activities involving repetitive movement of large muscle groups are recommended. Walking is the easiest activity on which to base an exercise prescription. Non-weightbearing activities, such as swimming, rowing, and cycling should be considered for individuals with orthopedic concerns.

DURATION (TIME)

- All individuals should strive to accumulate 30–60 min of physical activity on each and every day of the week (Stephens, O'Connor, and Deuster, 2002).

THE EXERCISE PRESCRIPTIONS: OVERCOMING BARRIERS TO ACTIVITY

- **Time:** Patients commonly cite lack of time as a significant barrier to physical activity. Small bouts of physical activity scattered through the day help overcome this barrier. An alternative is to remind patients that to achieve the recommended 30 min of daily activity, they need only forego one television show per day.
- **Convenience:** Patients also cite lack of convenience as a common obstacle. Patients should be encouraged to seek alternative forms of physical activity, such as parking farther away from the store, or using the stairs instead of the elevator.
- **Fatigue:** Patients should be reminded that physical activity actually improves their energy level.
- **Boredom:** Exercising with a friend or family member increases accountability and reduces boredom.

THE EXERCISE PRESCRIPTION: ASSESSING READINESS TO CHANGE

- Not all patients are immediately ready to embark on a program of increased physical activity. The likelihood of sustaining an active lifestyle can be quickly assessed using the stages-of-change model (Zimmerman, Olsen, and Bosworth, 2000).

Precontemplation
- Individuals who are in the precontemplative stage have not seriously considered participating in regular physical activity. They are unlikely to significantly change their current pattern of behavior. Informing patients about risks associated with physical inactivity and encouraging them to be more active are useful counseling points for patients who are in the precontemplative stage.

Contemplation
- Patients who are contemplating change are ready for an exercise prescription, but often will present barriers or excuses for not adopting an active lifestyle. Steady encouragement with suggestions for overcoming predictable barriers is helpful for patients in the contemplative stage.

Preparation/Action

- Patients in this stage should have an individualized exercise prescription. Encouragement and support should be offered with specific follow-up to assess progress.

Maintenance

- Individuals in this stage have incorporated physical activity into their regular routine. The exercise prescription should be revised and updated periodically to ensure patients do not extinguish their behaviors. Most individuals incorporating an exercise prescription into their routine lifestyle will progress through predictable phases of *acclimation, improvement,* and *maintenance.*
- **Acclimation:** Acclimation typically lasts several weeks and is often the most psychologically challenging phase. Dropout rates are highest during the acclimation phase. Patients should be encouraged to commit to the frequency of activity first, then to duration, and finally to intensity.
- **Improvement:** Improvement occurs after patients have acclimated to regular activity. Patients experience predictable improvements in self-efficacy, physical fitness, and mood. The exercise prescription can be modified during the improvement phase as well to target patient goals.
- **Maintenance:** In addition to the psychologic characteristics described with the stages-of-change model, maintenance also has physical characteristics as well including heart rate adaptations, and exercise tolerance. The exercise prescription should be modified to account for changes in cardiovascular condition and enhanced muscular performance.

THE EXERCISE PRESCRIPTION: BEYOND CARDIOVASCULAR ENDURANCE

- An exercise prescription should also include specific advice regarding muscular strength and endurance.
- Muscular strengthening exercises should be performed twice weekly (General Principles of Exercise Prescription, 2000). The same FITT principle can be applied to muscular conditioning as well.
- **Frequency:** Activities focused on improving muscular strength should be performed two to three times per week (General Principles of Exercise Prescription, 2000).
- **Intensity:** To develop muscular strength, individuals should perform several sets of exercises using three to five *repetition maximum* (RM) resistance (one RM is the maximum amount of weight that an individual can

lift one time using proper technique). To develop muscular endurance, an individual should perform several sets using lower resistance——typically 8–20 RM.
- **Type:** Muscular strength and endurance can be developed using either free weights or dedicated resistance machines. Household items such as rubber tubing can also serve as creative forms of resistantce.
- **Duration (Time):** For muscular strength and conditioning, time refers to the number of sets of a particular exercise that an individual performs. Typically, two sets are performed for each muscular group.

EXERCISE PRESCRIPTIONS FOR SPECIAL POPULATIONS

ELDERLY

- Regular physical activity helps prevent many common chronic medical conditions associated with aging including obesity, hypertension, diabetes, osteoporosis, stroke, depression, colorectal cancer, and premature death (Stephens, O'Connor, and Deuster, 2002).
- Regular physical activity improves an elderly individual's ability to carry out functional activities of daily living (Nied and Franklin, 2002). Strength training, balance training, and flexibility training are particularly important for elderly patients.
- Elderly patients should accumulate at least 30 min of moderate aerobic activity on most, preferably all days of the week. Elderly patients should also perform strength training activities with single sets of 10–15 repetitions using at least eight different activities two to three times per week. While many elderly patients are fearful that increased levels of physical activity increases their risk of falling and bone fracture, evidence indicates that patients who are physically active have a *reduced* risk of falling and lower rates of fracture (Mazzeo and Tanaka, 2001).
- Elderly patients should also stretch major muscle groups after exercising on a daily basis. Balance training also helps elderly patients reduce the risk of falling.

DIABETES

- Patients with diabetes are four to six times more likely to have a heart attack and are 80% more likely to die from cardiovascular complications than individuals without diabetes (US Dept HHS, 1996). Exercise and proper nutrition are essential components of diabetic disease management.
- To avoid rapid fluctuations in serum glucose levels, diabetic patients should exercise only when feeling well.

Diabetic patients should be familiar with their individual blood glucose patterns and should be taught to recognize symptoms of hypoglycemia and hyperglycemia.

- Exercise is safe when diabetes is under good control (serum glucose of 90–140 mg/dL). Diabetic patients should eat approximately 1–3 h before exercise. The content of the meal should be tailored in accordance with estimated intensity, duration, and energy expenditure of the exercise session.
- Type I diabetic patients should administer insulin in the abdomen (away from exercising muscle groups that delay absorption) 1 h prior to exercise. If the pre-activity serum glucose is less than 100 mg/dL, a supplemental snack should be consumed before exercise. If the serum glucose is greater than 250 mg/dL or the urine is positive for ketones, the exercise session should be postponed.
- During exercise, supplemental snacks should be consumed during particularly strenuous or lengthy exercise. All patients should be advised to consume adequate fluids during their exercise session.
- After exercise, patients should monitor serum glucose levels and be alert for signs and symptoms of either hypoglycemia or hyperglycemia.

CORONARY ARTERY DISEASE

- An individualized exercise prescription is an important secondary preventive tool for patients with documented coronary artery disease. All-cause mortality is reduced in patients suffering a myocardial infarction who participate in a program of cardiac rehabilitation (Franklin BA, 2000).
- The level of supervision for patients with known coronary artery disease should be based on the patient's clinical status, vocational demands, and personal goals.
- The American Heart Association has published specific guidelines regarding staffing, supervision, and progression of cardiac rehabilitation programs for patients with known coronary artery disease (Balady et al, 2000).

PREGNANCY

- Physical activity is safe for pregnant patients and should be routinely encouraged. Pregnant women should accumulate 30–60 min of moderate physical activity at least three times per week (American College of Obstetricians and Gynecologists, 1994). Vigorous sustained exercise should be avoided during pregnancy.
- As pregnancy progresses, a pregnant woman's center of gravity changes, and she should be counseled to avoid activities with a high risk of falling.

- Pregnant women should avoid saunas, hot tubs, or prolonged exercise that consistently elevates core body temperature.
- Pregnant women should be encouraged to consume adequate amounts of fluid during exercise. Pregnancy-induced hypertension, preterm, or premature rupture of membranes, preterm labor, persistent, or unexplained vaginal bleeding or intrauterine growth restriction are all contraindications to exercise during pregnancy (American College of Obstetricians and Gynecologists, 1994).

REFERENCES

American College of Obstetricians and Gynecologists: Exercise during pregnancy and the postpartum period. *ACOG Tech Bull* 189(45):1–5, 1994.

Balady GJ, Ades PA, Comoss P, et al: Core components of cardiac rehabilitation/secondary prevention programs: A statement for healthcare professionals from the American Heart Association and the American Association of Cardiovascular and Pulmonary Rehabilitation Writing Group. *Circulation* 102(9):1069–1073, 2000.

Evidence-based nutrition principles and recommendations for the treatment and prevention of diabetes and related complications. *Diabetes Care* 25:S50–S60, 2002.

Exercise prescription for cardiac patients, in Franklin BA, Whaley MH, Howley ET (eds.): *ASCM's Guidelines for Exercise Testing and Prescription,* 6th ed. Philadelphia, Lippincott, Williams & Wilkins, 2000, pp 165–199.

General principles of exercise prescription, in Franklin BA, Whaley MH, Howley ET (eds.): *ASCM's Guidelines for Exercise Testing and Prescription,* 6th ed. Philadelphia, Lippincott, Williams & Wilkins, 2000, pp 137–164.

Mazzeo RS, Tanaka H: Exercise prescription for the elderly: Current recommendations. *Sports Med* 31:809–818, 2001.

Nied RJ, Franklin B. Promoting and prescribing exercise for the elderly. *Am Fam Phys* 65:419–426, 2002.

Stephens MB, O'Connor FC, Deuster PA. Exercise and Nutrition. *Mongraph,* 283 ed., AAFP Home Study. Leawood, KS, American Academy of Family Physicians, December 2002.

US Department of Health and Human Services. Physical activity and health: A report of the surgeon general. Atlanta, GA, US Department of Health and Human Services, Centers for Disease Control and Prevention, National Center for Chronic Disease Prevention and Health Promotion, 1996.

US Department of Health and Human Services. *Healthy People 2010: Understanding and Improving Health.* Washington, DC, US Department of Health and Human Services, Government Printing Office, 2000.

US Preventive Services Task Force. Behavioral counseling in primary care to promote physical activity: Recommendations and rationale. *Guide to Clinical Preventive Services,* 3rd ed. Rockville, MD, 2002.

US Public Health Service. *The Surgeon General's Call to Action to Prevent and Decrease Overweight and Obesity*. Rockville, MD, US Department of Health and Human Services, Public Health Service; Washington, DC, Office of the Surgeon General, 2001.

Walsh JM, Swangard DM, Davis T, et al: Exercise counseling by primary care physicians in the era of managed care. *Am J Prev Med* 16(4):307–313, 1999.

Zimmerman GL, Olsen CG, Bosworth MF. A "stages of change" approach to helping patients change behavior. *Am Fam Phys* 61:1409–1416, 2000.

16 EXERCISE AND CHRONIC DISEASE

Karl B Fields, MD
Michael Shea, MD
Rebecca Spaulding, MD
David Stewart, MD

INTRODUCTION

- Medical problems are common in athletes and lead to approximately 70% of the visits that athletes make to doctors.
- Chronic medical problems are common in athletes greater than 35 years of age.
- Certain conditions such as obesity, hypertension, asthma and thyroid disease occur in all age groups.
- This chapter addresses principles of healthy exercise in individuals who remain athletic but have chronic disease.
- Details of diagnosis, evaluation, and treatment are reserved for later chapters.

OBESITY

- According to 1998 estimates from NHLBI estimated 97 million U.S. adults were overweight (BMI > 25) or met the definition of true obesity (BMI > 30) (NIH).
- Pediatric obesity has become a major public health issue with estimates of 25% of children being overweight and as many as 15% having true obesity (NIH).
- Obesity contributes to excess mortality from hypertension, type-2 diabetes, coronary artery diseases, stroke, gallbladder disease, sleep apnea, and *osteoarthritis* (OA) (NIH; Perry et al, 1998). Cancers occurring more commonly in these individuals include endometrial, breast, prostate, and colon cancers.

- Centripetal obesity in which the waist-to-hip ratio is high indicates a subset of individuals at much higher risk of cardiovascular diseases (Perry et al, 1998).
- In spite of the health risks of obesity, a number of overweight athletes have achieved high levels of sports success. In some sports, including football, weight throws in track and field, heavyweight wrestling, and power lifting, excessive weight has generally been considered advantageous.
- Athletes often pursue strategies that lead to dietary excess and pose health risks when they're trying to gain excessive weight. These may include diets with excessive high fat and high glycemic foods.
- Obesity has direct consequences in sport in that overweight athletes experience a much greater risk of heat illness during competition, and injury rates in physical training programs have been shown to parallel body fat measurement (Jones et al, 1993).
- Highly competitive athletes may need to consume 1500 to 2000 access calories per day to account for the calorie expenditure of intense training. Dietary calorie consumption appears to be a learned behavior and appetite often does not decline with a reduction in activity levels (King, Tremblay, and Blundell, 1997).
- Injured athletes and athletes who retire from a sport have a tendency to continue to ingest excessive calories. This may lead to weight gain during injury recovery, the off-season, or after retirement in those who do not maintain high levels of physical activity. This can quickly lead to obesity.
- All forms of muscular activity burn calories and contribute to weight loss with aerobic activity generally serving as the backbone of a weight-loss program. Individuals on a strength-training program or on a mixed exercise program may show comparable weight loss with a well-designed, vigorous program.
- Athletes who are used to training may be more efficient at losing weight through exercise.
- Nonathletes have trouble losing weight on an exercise program alone perhaps because effective weight-loss through exercise requires a consistent moderate-to-high level of activity.
- While almost all successful weight-loss programs require dietary adjustments if individuals are to succeed at maintaining weight loss they must begin an exercise program. A combination of a reduced calorie diet and increased physical activity has been given an evidence category A rating based on meta-analysis of 15 RCTs as an effective way to achieve weight loss (National Heart, Lung, and Blood Institute *(b)*).
- Epidemiologists have pointed out that we have seen a dramatic gain in weight of Americans in the last two decades, a period in which calorie consumption has

increased modestly but the decline in physical activity has been dramatic.

HYPERTENSION

- Blood pressure above the 95th percentile for age-adjusted norms is considered hypertension (National Heart, Lung, and Blood Institute (a)). Blood pressures above the 99th percentile of age-adjusted norms are considered severe hypertension.
- For adults any levels above 140 systolic or 90 diastolic indicate hypertension.
- JNC 7 report defined levels above 120 systolic or 80 diastolic as pre hypertension (National Heart, Lung, and Blood Institute (a)).
- Blood pressure is a product of cardiac output multiplied by peripheral resistance. Peripheral resistance must fall dramatically or else blood pressure rises excessively during exercise since the cardiac output must remain high to support activity.
- In patients whose blood pressure rises too dramatically during dynamic exercise the relative risk of subsequent hypertension is higher (Wilson et al, 1990; Tanji et al, 1989).
- Heavy resistance exercise can cause dramatic rises in blood pressure (MacDougall ct al, 1985).
- The effect of exercise on hypertension has been studied extensively. A Meta-analysis of 54 clinical trials of aerobic exercise showed reductions of systolic and diastolic blood pressure in both hypertensive and normotensive individuals (Whelton et al, 2002).
- The Osaka Health Survey demonstrated that a daily walk of 20 min or more reduced the risk of hypertension in men. In fact, for every 26 men who walked, one case of hypertension was prevented (Hayashi et al, 1999). Vigorous exercise for as little as 30 min, just once weekly, also reduced risk.
- Hypertensive patients do best by starting with a low intensity warm-up and pursuing aerobic exercise at about 55–70% of maximum heart rate (ACSM, 2000).
- Most resistance exercise seems to benefit hypertensive athletes, although maximal resistance efforts pose theoretical risks.
- The American College of Sports Medicine recommends that resistance training in hypertensive patients be mixed with aerobic activity (ACSM, 2000).

CORONARY ARTERY DISEASE

- Patients with known coronary artery disease can reduce their risk of coronary events by maintaining high fitness levels (Myers et al, 2002).

- Moderate exercise is recommended for individuals with coronary artery disease and the individual's exercise capacity should be measured by exercise tolerance testing.
- Formal cardiac rehabilitation programs help coronary artery disease patients get started on a therapeutic exercise regimen.
- Patients with coronary artery disease who develop the fitness to achieve a 10.7 MET level workload have a normal age adjusted mortality rate (Myers et al, 2002).
- Recent research suggests that exercise lowers C-reactive protein (CRP) levels. Athletes such as swimmers and runners have significantly lower CRP levels than the average individual and the more intensely they train, the greater the decline in their CRP level. Speculation centers as to whether this may be one of the mechanisms by which exercise lowers the risk of cardiovascular disease (Zebrack and Anderson, 2002).

DIABETES

- There are 16 million Americans with diabetes mellitus, with approximately 10% having type-1 diabetes.

CARDIOVASCULAR BENEFITS

- Cardiovascular disease is high in diabetics. Maintaining a good fitness level lowers the risk of cardiac death and is associated with longevity (Blair et al, 1989).
- Diabetics improve fitness levels with training (VO_{2max}) (Wallberg-Henriksson, 1992).
- Blood pressure (BP) is improved with moderate aerobic exercise (Uusitupa, 1992).
- Exercise may improve hyperlipidemia by reducing total cholesterol, triglyceride, LDL, and VLDL; and increasing HDL concentration. These changes inhibit the development and progression of atherosclerotic plaques and ultimately, adverse cardiovascular events (Schneider, Vitug, and Ruderman, 1996; Laaksonen et al, 2000).
- Lehmann et al demonstrated that type-1 diabetics reduced abdominal fat content, blood pressure, and adverse lipid levels by exercising 135 min/week (Lehmann et al, 1997).

IMPROVED METABOLIC CONTROL

- Metabolic control usually improves with exercise, although improvements in FBG or A1C in type-1 diabetics has not consistently been shown in studies (Tanji, 1995).

- Exercise does improve insulin sensitivity in liver, muscle, and fat cells (Wallberg-Henriksson, 1992).
- A single exercise session has been shown to increase insulin sensitivity for 16 h (Landry and Allen, 1992).

REDUCED MORBIDITY AND MORTALITY

- Epidemiologic studies demonstrate the benefits of exercise. One study following male type-1 diabetics for 20 years shows those who participated in High School or college sports had lower mortality and lower incidence of macro vascular disease than sedentary counterparts (LaPorte et al, 1986).

IMPROVED SELF ESTEEM

- Exercise has a positive effect on the self-esteem of diabetic patients and allows many to cope better with physical and emotional stress.

RENAL DISEASE IN ATHLETES

KIDNEY PROBLEMS ASSOCIATED WITH EXERCISE

- Dehydration, hyperpyrexia, hyperkalemia, and rhabdomyolysis may all occur as a result of exercise and may lead to renal damage (Fields and Fricker, 1997).
- Rhabdomyolysis, especially in untrained athletes, can lead to renal ischemia and nephrotoxins (Olerud, Homer, and Carrol, 1994).

PREVENTION OF RENAL DISEASE

- Fluids are important in minimizing muscle damage, promoting myoglobin elimination, and maintaining renal blood flow.
- Prevent rhabdomyolysis through adequate fluid intake, appropriate carbohydrate intake to avoid glycogen depletion and avoiding exercising to exhaustion.

THYROID DISEASE IN ATHLETES

HYPOTHYROIDISM

- Hypothyroidism is associated with decreased exercise tolerance (McAllister, Sansone, and Laughlin, 1995).
- Replacement of thyroxin is the mainstay of treatment.
- Exercise is safe when adequate replacement is maintained.

HYPERTHYROIDISM

- Hyperthyroidism is associated with decreased exercise tolerance (McAllister, Sansone, and Laughlin, 1995).
- Higher blood lactate, depletion of glycogen, and relative hyperthermia may all contribute to decreased performance (Nazar et al, 1978).
- Beta-blockers can be helpful in the treatment of hyperthyroidism but may have a negative effect on performance and are banned under Olympic regulations.
- Exercise is safe after appropriate treatment and close supervision.

OSTEOPOROSIS

- The National Osteoporosis Society estimates one in three women and one in 12 men over the age of 50 will be affected by osteoporosis (Boutaiuti et al, 2000). Additionally, 1.5 million fractures are attributable to osteoporosis each year.
- Exercise at an early age is important to develop adequate bone density. Multiple studies on young men and women have shown that both resistance and endurance exercise programs can lead to site-specific increases in *bone mineral density* (BMD) (Snow-Harter et al, 1992; Margulies et al, 1986). BMD is reported to be higher in athletic young adults than in their sedentary peers (Kirchner, Lewis, and O'Conner, 1996).
- Bone loss in the postmenopausal period can be slowed by weight bearing and resistance exercise. In a Cochrane meta-analysis, aerobic exercise, resistance exercise, and walking were all shown to be more effective at slowing bone loss at 1 year when compared to no exercise (Boutaiuti et al, 2000). A majority of studies show that weight-bearing exercise mainly prevents bone loss of the lumbar spine but suggest that this may occur at the femur and forearm as well (Boutaiuti et al, 2000; Wolff et al, 1999; Michel et al, 1991).
- A few studies suggest exercise may increase BMD even in the postmenopausal state when combined with other therapy for osteoporosis (Michel et al, 1991). Multiple studies suggest even if BMD is not increased, exercise lessens the risk of osteoporotic fractures by improving balance and muscular strength (Nelson et al, 1994).
- Exercise goals for individuals with osteoporosis should include reducing pain, increasing mobility, improving muscle endurance, balance, and stability in order to improve the quality of life and reduce the risk of falling.

- The role of exercise in preventing and treating osteo-porosis can be summarized by five points in the American College of Sports Medicine position statement (ACSM Post Stand, 1995):
  1. Weight-bearing physical activity is essential for developing and maintaining a healthy skeleton.
  2. Strength exercises may also be beneficial, particularly for non-weight-bearing bones.
  3. If sedentary women increase their activity, they may avoid the further loss of bone that inactivity can cause and may even slightly increase bone mass.
  4. Exercise is not a substitute for postmenopausal hormone replacement therapy.
  5. An optimal exercise program for older women includes activities for improving strength, flexibility, and coordination, since improvement in these areas lessens the likelihood of falls and fractures.

EPILEPSY

- It is estimated that less than 5% of individuals with epilepsy participate in a regular exercise program (Nakken, Lyning, and Tauboll, 1985). Parents, coaches, physicians, and epileptics themselves often limit participation in exercise for fear of uncontrolled seizures, embarrassment, or because of ignorance about the disease.
- Contrary to common fears, it is rare for seizures to occur during exercise. Multiple studies show that exercise decreases seizure frequency (Nakken, Lyning, and Tauboll, 1985; Horyd et al, 1981). The cause of this is under debate but is thought to be possibly from beta-endorphin release, lowered blood pH after lactic acid release, increased *gamma-aminobutyric acid* (GABA) concentration, or possibly increased mental alertness and attention.
- Some studies have shown that seizure frequency can increase in the post exercise period (Nakken et al, 1990; Horyd et al, 1981).
- Exercise has been shown to improve self-esteem and the overall sense of well being in epileptics (Nakken, Lyning, and Tauboll, 1985-Nakken et al, 1990). In a population where isolation and depression are common, participation in exercise may be a way to improve self worth and social integration.

EXERCISE POST CEREBRAL VASCULAR ACCIDENT

- Exercise is important in primary and secondary prevention of cardiovascular and stroke risk. A study of over 16,000 men found an inverse relationship between cardiovascular fitness and stroke mortality (Lee and Blair, 2002).
- Poststroke patients often suffer from weakness, paralysis, sensory loss, and decreased overall exercise capacity. A study by Mackay-Lyons revealed in less than 1 month after stroke, patients developed a significant compromise in exercise capacity (MacKay-Lyons and Makrides, 2002).
- A study by Fujitani showed that poststroke patients who exercised by increasing activities of daily living, showed a significant increase in peak oxygen intake (Fujitani et al, 1999). Additionally, poststroke patients' training on treadmills showed significant improvements of VO_{2max}, gait, and overall functional mobility, balance, and muscular activity (Macko et al, 2001; Laufer et al, 2001). A supervised exercise program for stroke survivors with multiple comorbidities is effective at improving fitness while potentially decreasing risk of further disease and disability (Rimmer et al, 2000).
- Strength training can safely be used in most post-stroke rehabilitation to improve muscle strength and overall balance (Rimmer et al, 2000). Caution should be used in patients with uncontrolled hypertension as well as avoidance of excessive weight and valsalva.

CEREBRAL PALSY (CP)

- In patients with cerebral palsy and other chronic neuromuscular syndromes, physical therapy has become a mainstay in treatment. The purpose of therapy is to enhance motor development and minimize the development of contractures. Emphasis is generally placed on range of motion, both passive and active. Neuromuscular electric stimulation has been added to improve mobility, control muscular movements, increase strength, and to decrease spasticity.
- Strength training has been avoided in cerebral palsy owing to a theory that it can lead to increased spasticity in antagonist muscles; however, multiple studies have shown that in mild-moderate spastic CP strength training can improve motor skills and strength without decreased range of motion or increased spasticity (Dodd, Taylor, and Damiano, 2002; Haney, 1998). In addition, strength training may lessen the amount of bone loss that frequently occurs in less mobile CP patients (Dodd, Taylor, and Damiano, 2002).
- Aerobic exercise has been studied minimally in CP patients. Horseback riding and swimming are often activities offered for patients with cerebral palsy; however, studies show that many patients with cerebral palsy do not participate in aerobic activities (Darrah et al, 1999). Aerobic exercise in CP has been shown to increase fitness level and VO_{2max} while also improving patient's social skills, behavioral and emotional problems, and overall sense of well being.

- Caution must be used in planning an exercise program for patients with cerebral palsy. Scoliosis, contractures, chronic arthritis, and risk of hip subluxation can limit patient's physical ability. Likewise, patients often suffer from sensory defects, such as poor vision. Lastly, behavioral and emotional maladjustments can be present, so special accommodations may need to be made (Vessey, 1996).

ASTHMA

- The cardiorespiratory fitness of asthmatic patients is frequently suboptimal, either because of symptom-limited exercise tolerance or secondary deconditioning from inactivity (Clark, 1999).
- When physically fit and free from significant airway obstruction, the maximal heart rate, ventilation, blood pressure, and work capacity of asthma patients fall within the normal range (Bundgaard, 1985).
- Sedentary asthmatics produce more lactate and are more subject to acidosis than unfit individuals without asthma who undertake similar physical exertion (McFadden, Jr, 1984).
- Patients who followed aerobic exercise programs have demonstrated reductions in airway responsiveness (Cochrane and Clark, 1990).
- It is not clear if the improvement in fitness translates into a reduction in symptoms or an improvement in the quality of life (Ram, 2000*b*).
- In a systematic review, physical training had no effect on resting lung function but led to an improvement in cardiopulmonary fitness as measured by an increase in maximum oxygen uptake of 5.6 mL/kg/min (95% confidence interval 3.9 to 7.2) (Ram, 2000*a*).
- Asthma sufferers who exercise regularly may have fewer exacerbations, use less medication, and miss less time from school and work (Szentagothai et al, 1987).
- Recommendations for rehabilitation of asthmatic patients include individualized exercise prescription and advice based on objective criteria of exercise capability (Clark, 1999).

CHRONIC LUNG DISEASE IN CHILDREN

CYSTIC FIBROSIS (BRADLEY, 2002; PRASAD, 2002)

- Exercise is believed to be beneficial to patients with cystic fibrosis.

- Decreased breathlessness allows greater mobility and participation with peers in social and sporting activities, improves confidence and self-esteem, and creates a greater pleasure in life for the individual patient.
- Limitations in exercise performance appear related to the extent of lung disease and compromised nutritional status.
- One systematic review found that the small size, short duration, and incomplete reporting of most of the trials limit conclusions about the efficacy of physical training in cystic fibrosis.

BRONCHOPULMONARY DYSPLASIA

- There is limited information concerning the exercise performance of long-term survivors of bronchopulmonary dysplasia.

BRONCHIECTASIS

- A systematic review only found evidence of the benefits of inspiratory muscle training and provided no evidence of the effect of other types of physical training (including pulmonary rehabilitation) in bronchiectasis; however, the review included only two studies.
- Left ventricular diastolic functions are affected in bronchiectasis, and the performance of patients is dependent on their pulmonary status. This is the first study demonstrating the cardiac effects of bronchiectasis according to our survey of the published literature.

COPD IN ADULTS

- Studies consistently demonstrate that peripheral muscles are weak in patients with *chronic obstructive pulmonary disease* (COPD), exhibiting effort-dependent strength scores that are 70–80% of these measures in age-matched healthy subjects (Storer, 2001).
- In COPD patients, up to 40% of total oxygen intake during low-level exercise is devoted to the respiratory muscles, compared to 10–15% in healthy persons (Mink, 1997).
- In a review of 32 studies, 31 showed increased exercise tolerance after a training program (Belman, 1996). The most dramatic improvements are often seen in the most severely impaired patients (Mink, 1997).
- Exercise training improves the fitness of patients with mild or moderate COPD, but has not been shown to significantly benefit quality of life, dyspnea, or long-term disease progression (Chavannes, 2002).

- There is evidence that exercise facilitates tolerance to and delays the appearance of dyspnea to higher levels of exertion. No other intervention is able to produce this desensitization, including medication and supplemental oxygen (Mink, 1997).
- In COPD patients, exercise does not appear to significantly affect lung function directly. In a review of 29 trials that included spirometry, only two showed improved FEV1 (Belman, 1996).
- A review of 18 studies found that VO_{2max} improved in only 10 studies (Belman, 1996).
- Even at very low training levels, aerobic training for COPD patients reduces ventilation at comparable oxygen consumption levels (although only to a third the extent of that seen in normal subjects) (Mink, 1997).
- Exercise tolerance may improve following exercise training because of gains in aerobic fitness or peripheral muscle strength; enhanced mechanical skill and efficiency of exercise; improvements in respiratory muscle function, breathing pattern, or lung hyperinflation; as well as reduction in anxiety, fear, and dyspnea associated with exercise (Bourjeily, 2000).
- Both high- and low-intensity programs produce significant improvements in exercise tolerance and reductions in minute ventilation and dyspnea, even when the disease is severe (Killian et al, 1992).
- *European Respiratory Society* (ERS), *American Thoracic Society* (ATS), and *British Thoracic Society* (BTS) guidelines support the use of pulmonary rehabilitation (Ferguson, 2000).
- Exercise training and pulmonary rehabilitation should be considered for all patients who experience exercise intolerance despite optimal medical therapy (Bourjeily, 2000).
- Before prescribing an exercise program, COPD patients require careful evaluation to assess cardiac risk and exercise capacity (Mink, 1997).

OSTEOARTHRITIS

- Patients with arthritis have substantially worse health-related quality of life than those without arthritis (The Centers for Disease Control and Prevention, 2000).
- Studies show that exercise improves the pain and disability of patients with osteoarthritis (Van Baar et al, 1999).
- Aerobic exercise for patients with OA has been shown to improve cardiovascular fitness, reduce symptoms, and improve functional capacity (DiNubile, 1997).
- Data from the Fitness Arthritis and Seniors Trial suggested that beneficial effects of exercise on functional capacity in OA patients are independent of exercise type (Ettinger et al, 1997).

- Strength training of the whole body appears to be more beneficial than limiting work to the muscles around the affected joint (DiNubile, 1991).
- One review found that available data supports the theory that in the absence of joint abnormalities, physical activity that remains within the limits of comfort and normal range of motion does not lead to OA (Bouchard, Shepard, and Stephens, 1993).
- High-impact activities that include running and jumping may be detrimental for established OA of lower extremity joints (Buckwalter and Lane, 1996).
- Treatment guidelines for OA from the American College of Rheumatology and American Academy of Orthopedic Surgeons advocate exercise as an important therapeutic modality (Hochberg et al, 1995; Pate et al, 1995).

REFERENCES

ACSM: *ACSM's Guidelines for Exercise Testing and Prescription*, 6th ed. Philadelphia, PA, Williams & Wilkins, 2000.

A C S M Position Stand: Osteoporosis and exercise. *Med Sci Sports Exerc* 27(4):i–vii, Apr 1995.

Belman MJ: Therapeutic exercise in chronic lung disease, in Fishman AP (ed.): *Pulmonary Rehabilitation*. New York, NY, Marcel Dekker, 1996, pp 505–521.

Blair SN, Khol HW, Paffenbarger RS, et al: Physical fitness and all-cause mortality: A prospective study of healthy men and women. *JAMA* 262:2395–2401, 1989.

Bouchard C, Shepard RJ, Stephens T: Physical activity, fitness and health consensus statement. Champaign, IL, Human Kinetics Publishers, 1993.

Bourjeily G: Exercise training in chronic obstructive pulmonary disease. *Clin Chest Med* 21(4):763–781, 2000.

Boutaiuti D, Shea B, Iovine R, et al: Exercise for preventing and treating osteoporosis in postmenopausal women (Cochrane Review), in *Cochrane Library* Issue 2 Oxford, Update Software, 2000.

Bradley J: Physical training for cystic fibrosis. *Cochrane Database Syst Rev* (2):CD002768, 2002.

Buckwalter JA, Lane NE: Aging, sports, and osteoarthritis. *Sports Med Arthros Rev* 4(3):276–287, 1996.

Bundgaard A. Exercise and the asthmatic. *Sports Med* 1985;2(4): 254-66.

Chavannes N: Effects of physical activity in mild to moderate COPD: A systematic review. *Br J Gen Pract* 52(480):574–578, 2002.

Clark CJ: Physical activity and asthma. *Curr Opin Pulm Med* 5(1):68–71, 1999.

Cochrane LM, Clark CJ: Benefits and problems of a physical training programme for asthmatic patients. *Thorax* 45(5):345–351, 1990.

Darrah J, Wessel J, Nearingburg P, et al: Evaluation of a community fitness program for adolescents with cerebral palsy. *Ped Phys Ther* 11:18–23, 1999.

DiNubile NA: Strength training. *Clin Sports Med* 10(1):33–62, 1991.

DiNubile NA: Osteoarthritis: How to make exercise part of your treatment plan. *Phys Sports Med* 25(7), 1997.

Dodd KJ, Taylor NF, Damiano DL: A systemic review of the effectiveness of strength-training programs for people with cerebral palsy. *Arch Phys Med Rehabil* 83:1157–1164, 2002.

Ettinger WH, Burns R, Messier SP, et al: A randomized trial comparing aerobic exercise and resistance exercise with a health education program in older adults with knee osteoarthritis: The fitness arthritis and seniors trial (FAST). *JAMA* 277(1):25–31, 1997.

Ferguson GT. Recommendations for the management of COPD. *Chest* 117(2 Suppl):23S–28S, 2000.

Fields KB, Fricker PA: *Medical Problems in Athletes.* Blackwell science, 1997, pp 209–215.

Fujitani J, Ishikawa T, Akai M, et al: Influence of daily activity on changes in physical fitness for people with post-stroke hemiplegia. *Am J Phys Med Rehabil* 78(6) 540–544, 1999.

Haney NB: Muscular strengthening in children with cerebral palsy. *Phys Occup Ther Pediatr* 18:149–157, 1998.

Hayashi T, et al: Walking to work and the risk for hypertension in men: The Osaka Health Survey. *Ann Intern Med* 131:21–26, 1999.

Hochberg MC, Altman RD, Brandt KD, et al: Guidelines for the medical management of osteoarthritis, part II: osteoarthritis of the knee. *Arthritis Rheum* 38(11):1541–1546, 1995.

Horyd W, Gryziak J, Niedzielska K, et al: Effect of physical exertion in the EEG of epilepsy patients. *Neurol Neurochir Pol* 15(5–6):545–552, 1981.

Jones BH, Bovee MW, McA Harris J, et al: Intrinsic risk factors for exercise-related injuries among male and female army trainees. *Am J Sports Med* 21(5):705–710, 1993.

Killian KJ, Leblanc P, Martin DH, et al: Exercise capacity and ventilatory, circulatory, and symptom limitation in patients with chronic airflow limiatation. *Am Rev Respir Dis* 146(4):935–940, 1992.

King NA, Tremblay A, Blundell JE: Effects of exercise on appetite control: implications for energy balance. *Med Sci Sports Exerc* 29(8):1076–1089, 1997.

Kirchner EM, Lewis RD, O'Conner PJ: Effect of past gymnastic participation on adult bone mass. *J Appl Physiol* 80(1):226–232, 1996.

Laaksonen DE, Atalay M, Niskanan LK, et al: Aerobic exercise and the lipid profile in type 1 diabetic men: A randomized controlled trial. *Med Sci Sports Exerc* 32(9):1541–1548, 2000.

Landry GL, Allen DB: Diabetes mellitus and exercise. *Lin Sports Med* 11(2):403–418, 1992.

LaPorte RE, Dorman JS, Tajima N, et al: Pittsburg insulin-dependent diabetes mellitus morbidity and mortality study: Physical activity and diabetic complications. *Pediatrics* 78:1027–1033, 1986.

Laufer Y, Dickstein R, Chefex Y, et al: The effect of treadmill training on the ambulation of stroke survivors in the early stages of rehabilitation: A randomized study. *J Rehabil Res Dev* 38(1):69–78, 2001.

Lee CD, Blair SN: Cardiorespiratory fitness and stroke mortality in men. *Med Sci Sport Exerc* 34:592–595, 2002.

Lehmann R, Kaplan V, Bingisser R, et al: Impact of physical activity on cardiovascular risk factors in IDDM. *Diabetes Care* 20(10):1603–1611, 1997.

MacDougall JD, Tuxen D, Sale DG, et al: Arterial blood pressure response to heavy resistance exercise. *J Appl Physiol* 58:785–790, 1985.

MacKay-Lyons MJ, Makrides L: Exercise capacity early after stroke. *Arch Phys Med Rehabil* 83(12):1697–1702, 2002.

Macko RF, Smith GV, Dobrovolny CL, et al: Treadmill training improves fitness reserve in chronic stroke patients. *Arch Phys Med Rehabil* 82(7):879–884, 2001.

Margulies JY, Simkin A, Leichter I, et al: Effect of intense physical activity on the bone-mineral content in the lower limbs of young adults. *J Bone Joint Surg* 68(7):1090–1093, 1986.

McAllister RM, Sansone JC, Laughlin MH: Effects of hyperthyroidism on muscle blood flow during exercise in the rat. *Am J Physiol* 268:H330–H335, 1995.

McFadden ER, Jr: Exercise performance in the asthmatic. *Am Rev Respir Dis* 129(2 pt 2):S84–S87, 1984.

Michel BA, Lane NE, Bloch DA, Et al: Effect of changes in weight-bearing exercise on lumbar bone mass after age fifty. *Ann Med* 23(4):397–401, Oct 1991.

Mink BD: Exercise and chronic obstructive pulmonary disease: Modest fitness gains pay big dividends. *Phys Sportsmed* 25(11), 1997.

Myers J, Prakash M, Froelicher V, et al: Exercise capacity and mortality among men referred for exercise testing. *N Engl J Med* 346(11):783–801, 2002.

Nakken KO, Bjorhold PG, Johannessen SI, et al: Effect of physical training on aerobic capacity, seizure occurrence and serum level of antiepileptic drugs in adults with epilepsy. *Epilepsia* 31(1):88–94, 1990.

Nakken KO, Lyning T, Tauboll O: Epilepsy and physical fitness. *Tidsskr Nor Laegeforen* 105(16):1136–1138, 1985.

National Heart, Lung and Blood Institute *(a)*: JNC VI: The sixth report of the joint national committee on prevention, detection, evaluation, and treatment of high blood pressure. NIH publication No. 98-4080.

National Heart, Lung, and Blood Institute *(b)*: Clinical guidelines on the identification, evaluation, and treatment of overweight and obesity in adults. NIH publication No. 98-4083 page xxvi.

National Institutes of Health: The practical guide identification, evaluation and treatment of overweight and obesity in adults. NIH publication No. 02–4084.

Nazar K, Chwa;bomsla-Moneta J, Machalla J, et al: Metabolic and body temperature change during exercise in hyperthyroid patients. *Clin Sci Mol Med* 54:323–327, 1978.

Nelson ME, Fiatarone MA, Morganti CM, et al: Effects of high-intensity strength training on multiple risk factors for osteoporotic fractures: A randomized controlled trial. *JAMA* 272:1909–1914, 1994.

Olerud JE, Homer LD, Carrol HW: Incidence of acute exertional rhabdomyolysis. *Ann Emerg Med* 23:1301–1306, 1994.

Pate RR, Pratt M, Blair SN, et al: Physical activity and public health: A recommendation from the Centers for Disease Control and Prevention and the American College of Sports Medicine. *JAMA* 273(5):402–407, 1995.

Perry AC, Miller PC, Allison MD, et al: Clinical predictability of waist-to-hip ratio in assessment of cardiovascular disease risk factors in overweight, premenopausal women. *Am J Clin Nutr* 68:1022–1027, 1998.

Prasad SA: Factors that influence adherence to exercise and their effectivenss: Application to cystic fibrosis. *Pediatr Pulmonol* 34(1):66–72, 2002.

Ram FS: Effects of physical training in asthma: a systematic review. *Br J Sports Med* 34(3):162–167, 2000*a*.

Ram FS: Physical training for asthma. *Cochrane Database Syst Rev.* (2):CD001116, 2000*b*.

Rimmer JH, Riley B, Creviston T, et al: Exercise training in a predominately African-American group of stroke survivors. *Med Sci Sport Exerc* 32(12):1990–1996, 2000.

Schneider SH, Vitug A, Ruderman N: Atherosclerosis and physical activity. *Diabetes Metab Rev* 1(4):513–553, 1996.

Snow-Harter C, Bouxsein ML, Lewis BT, et al: Effects of resistance and endurance exercise on bone minteral status of young women: A randomized exercise intervention trial. *J Bone Miner Res* 7(7):761–769, 1992.

Storer TW: Exercise in chronic pulmonary disease: Resistance exercise prescription. *Med Sci sports Exerc* 33(7 Suppl):S680–S692, 2001.

Szentagothai K, Gyene I, Szocska M, et al: Physical exercise program for children with bronchial asthma. *Pediatr Pulmonol* 3(3):166–172, 1987.

Tanji JL: Exercise and the hypertensive athlete. *Clin Sports Med* 11:291–302, 1995.

Tanji JL, Champlin JJ, Wong GY, et al: Blood pressure recovery curves after submaximal exercise: A predictor of hypertension at ten year follow up. *Am J Hypertens* 2:135–138, 1989.

The Centers for Disease Control and Prevention: Health-related quality of life among adults with arthritis: Behavioral risk factor surveillance system, 11 states, 1996–1998. *MMWR Morb Mortal Wkly Rep* 49(17):366–369, 2000.

Uusitupa M: Hypertension in diabetic patients: Use of exercise-based outpatient life-style modification program in the treatment of diabetes mellitus. *Diabetes Care* 15:1800–1810, 1992.

Van Baar ME, Assendelft WJ, Dekker J, et al: Effectiveness of exercise therapy in patients with osteoarthritis of the hip or knee: A systematic review of randomized clinical trials. *Arthritis Rheum* 42(7):1361–1369, 1999.

Vessey J: Primary care of the child with a chronic condition, 2nd ed. Philadelphia, PA, MosbyYear Book, 1996.

Wallberg-Henriksson H: Exercise and diabetes mellitus. *Exerc Sports Sci Rev* 20:339–368, 1992.

Whelton SP, Chin A, Xin X, et al: Effect of aerobic exercise on blood pressure: A meta-analysis of randomized, controlled trials. *Ann Intern Med* 136(7):493–503, 2002.

Wilson MF, Sung BH, Pincomb GA, et al: Exaggerated pressure response to exercise in men at risk for systemic hypertension. *Am J Cardiol* 66:731–736, 1990.

Wolff I, van Croonenborg JJ, Kemper HC, et al: The effect of exercise training programs on bone mass: A meta-analysis of published controlled trials in pre- and postmenopausal women. *Osteoporos Int.* 9(1):1–12, 1999.

Zebrack JS, Anderson JL: Role of inflammation in cardiovascular disease: How to use C-reactive protein in clinical practice. *Prog Cardiovasc Nurs* 17(4):174–185, 2002.

17 PLAYING SURFACE AND PROTECTIVE EQUIPMENT

Jeffrey G Jenkins, MD
Scott Chirichetti, DO

PLAYING SURFACE

- In many sports, the athlete or event organizer has no choice with regard to playing surface: only one option exists; however, in some sports, different options offer their own advantages and disadvantages. These are addressed below.

TURF SPORTS

- Turf sports (e.g., football, soccer, and field hockey) may be played on either artificial turf or natural grass. Natural grass is generally held to be safer and is associated with lower rates of significant injury owing to the lack of "give" or "cushion" afforded by synthetic turf. The literature, however, has been inconclusive.
- The Stanford Research Institute study found that among National Football League (NFL) players, major ligamentous injuries occurred more frequently on artificial turf (Grippo, 1973). (This study also found that concussions occurred 33% more often on synthetic turf, presumably owing in part to increased player speed and, consequently, increased collision forces.)
- Powell's landmark NFL study confirmed these findings, showing a statistically significantly higher rate of *anterior cruciate ligament* sprains on astroturf among NFL players between 1980 and 1989 (Powell and Schootman, 1992).
- However, two studies of college athletes dispute these results. A national athletic injury/illness reporting system study in 1975 concluded that "artificial turf did not constitute an imminent hazard to the . . . teams using it (Troy, 1977)." Furthermore, a study from the University of Wisconsin in 1980 actually reported a decreased incidence of serious sprains on artificial surface (Keene, 1996).
- A German study by Gaulrapp et al showed no significant increase in rate of injury of soccer players using artificial rather than natural grass fields (Gaulrapp, Siebert, and Rosemeyer, 1999).
- Certain types of minor injuries are exclusive to artificial turf. These include *turf burns*, the common abrasions associated with the surface. These injuries can be accompanied by contamination of the wounds with

"green dust," which can result in secondary infections (Gieck and Saliba, 1988).

- Increased incidence of *turf toe*, a sprain of the plantar capsule ligament complex of the *metatarsophalangeal* (MTP) joint of the great toe, is also associated with this increased traction. Hyperextension of the MTP is the most common mechanism.
- Leg fatigue and shin splints are common on artificial turf. Blisters are more common owing to increased traction.
- Because of the tremendous build-up of heat near the surface of artificial turf, heat exhaustion is a danger to players, particularly in the summer.

TENNIS

- Tennis is another sport with playing surface options, including hard court, clay, composition, grass, and carpet.
- Hard courts are associated with greater stress on the lower extremities as a result of the reduced shock absorbing ability and increased traction between shoe and court.
- With its energy absorbing properties, clay is more forgiving to the upper extremities owing to reduced ball speed (Nicola, 1997).
- During rehabilitation from injury, carpet, composition, and clay offer more cushion and are more forgiving to the lower extremities.

PROTECTIVE EQUIPMENT

- The purpose of protective equipment is to prevent injury and to protect injured areas from further injury. Sanctioning bodies, e.g., the National Collegiate Athletic Association (NCAA), of various sports have rendered certain protective equipment mandatory.

FOOTBALL

- The NCAA mandates the use of a helmet; face mask; four-point chin strap; mouth guard; shoulder pads; and hip, coccyx, thigh, and knee pads during football competition.
- There are two types of helmets currently in use: (1) padded, and (2) air and fluid filled, with combinations of both types.
- All football helmets in use at the high school or college level must be certified by the National Operating Committee on Standards for Athletic Equipment (NOCSAE). This ensures that each helmet has been

tested to withstand repeated blows of high mass and low velocity. A study by Cantu et al attributed in large part a dramatic reduction in brain injury-related fatalities from football to the adoption of NOCSAE helmet standards (Cantu and Mueller, 2003). These standards went into effect in 1978 for colleges and in 1980 for high schools.

- Proper fitting of a helmet is ensured by the following criteria: the frontal crown of the helmet should sit approximately one to two finger breadths above the eyebrows; the back edge of the helmet should not impinge on the neck as it extends; when the head is held straight forward, an attempt to turn the helmet on the head should result in only a slight movement; jaw pads should fit the jaw area snugly to prevent lateral rocking of the helmet; the chin strap should fit snugly with equal tension on both sides; the hair should be cut to normal length prior to fitting.
- Mouth guards include ready-to-wear, mouth-formed, and custom-fitted types. Ready-made guards are the least comfortable and least protective type. Mouth guards have been required equipment for high school football players since 1962 and for their collegiate counterparts since 1973. Mouth injuries, which at one time comprised 50% of all football injuries, have been reduced by more than half since the adoption of face masks and mouth guards for use in the sport.
- Two types of shoulder pads are in use: flat and cantilevered. Flat pads allow greater glenohumeral motion and are appropriate for limited contact positions, such as quarterback and receiver. Cantilevered pads are named for the cantilever bridge that extends over the shoulder, dispersing impact force over a wider area. These pads offer greater protection to the shoulder area and are appropriate for the majority of players.
- A proper shoulder pad fit is achieved when the tip of the inner pad extends just to the lateral edge of the shoulder. The sternum and clavicles should be covered, and the flaps or epaulets should cover the deltoid area.
- Hip and coccyx pads are mandatory equipment and should cover the greater trochanters, the iliac crests, and the coccyx. Snap-in, girdle, and wrap-around pads are available. Girdle pads are the most common type but also the most difficult to keep in place. Care should be taken to ensure coverage of the iliac crest.
- Controversy exists regarding the use of prophylactic knee braces in football. A study by Rovere in 1987 actually showed an increased rate of *anterior cruciate ligament* (ACL) injuries with brace use (Rovere, Haupt, and Yates, 1987). Since then, however, a study carried out at West Point (Sitler et al, 1990) and

another from the Big Ten Conference(Albright et al, 1994) showed a consistent trend toward a reduction of *medial collateral ligament* MCL injuries with use of prophylactic braces. Owing to these inconsistent findings and the lack of demonstrated proof of efficacy, both the American Academy of Pediatrics and the American Academy of Orthopedic Surgeons have recommended against the routine use of prophylactic knee bracing in football.

• ACL functional braces are available for players with ACL-deficient knees. Custom-fit braces have not been shown to perform better or offer more protection than off-the-shelf braces (Wojtys and Huston, 2001).

BASEBALL/SOFTBALL

• The NCAA mandates the use of a double ear-flap helmet for all batters and base-runners as well as a mask and throat guard for catchers.
• Little League Baseball requires protective helmets for batters, catchers, baserunners, first and third base coaches, and on-deck hitters.
• All helmets should be NOCSAE certified to ensure strength and safety, and bear a "Meets NOCSAE Standard" seal on the outside.
• It is recommended that baseball batters age 4 to 14 wear helmets with face protectors to reduce the risk of eye and facial bone injury. This recommendation was originally made in 1984 by the Sports Eye Safety Committee of the National Society to Prevent Blindness.
• Breakaway bases are available which can decrease sliding-associated injuries by approximately 98% (Naftulin and McKeag, 1999).

ICE HOCKEY

• The NCAA mandates the use of helmets with fastened chin straps, face masks, and an internal mouthpiece.
• Shoulder pads, elbow pads, protective gloves, padded pants, and shin guards are also standard equipment.
• Athletic supporter and neck or throat guard are also recommended for goalies.
• The use of full face shields results in a significantly decreased risk of facial or dental injury (Benson et al, 1999).
• Unfortunately, the use of helmets and face shields in hockey and the style of play allowed a player with head protection have contributed to an increase in cervical spine injuries (Reynen and Clancy, Jr, 1994).
• It has been shown that prophylactic knee braces do not significantly reduce the incidence of knee injury among hockey players (Tegner and Lorentzon, 1991).

LACROSSE

• The NCAA requires the use of a NOCSAE certified helmet with face mask, chin strap, and chin pad, as well as protective gloves and a mouthguard for all male lacrosse players. Goalies are additionally required to wear chest and throat protectors.
• Shoulder and rib pads are also standard, but not mandatory, equipment. Many players also wear rib protector vests.

RACQUET SPORTS

• Some clubs require eye protection for badminton, squash, and racquetball players.
• Lenses should be composed of at least a 3-mm thick CR 39 plastic or polycarbonate plastic.
• Glass lenses are discouraged owing to risk of breakage.
• Lenses should be mounted in a nylon sports frame with a steep posterior lip and temples that rotate about 180°. When a lens in a sports frame is struck, it projects forward rather than back and towards the eye. (Kulund, 1988)

BASKETBALL

• Mouth guards are recommended, but not mandatory, to reduce risk of dental trauma.
• High top basketball shoes have been shown not to reduce the incidence of ankle sprains during play (Barret et al, 1993).
• The use of a semi-rigid ankle stabilizing brace does seem to reduce the incidence of ankle injury, but not the severity of such injuries (Sitler et al, 1994).

WRESTLING

• The NCAA requires use of ear protectors, which protect against the formation of auricular hematomas and the cosmetic deformity, *cauliflower ear.*

SOCCER

• Shin guards should be worn to reduce incidence of tibia and fibula fractures, as well as compartment syndrome from anterior leg contusions. Shin guards should protect the entire length of the tibia (Howe, 1999).
• Use of a semirigid ankle orthosis has been shown to decrease the incidence of recurrent ankle sprains in soccer players with previous history of sprains (Surve et al, 1994).

• Mouth guards are recommended, especially for goal-keepers, to protect against not only dental injury but also concussion resulting from head-to-head collisions.

REFERENCES

Albright JP, Powell JW, Smith W, et al: Medial collateral ligament knee sprains in college football: Effectiveness of preventive braces. *Am J Sports Med* 22(1):12–18, 1994.

American Academy of Pediatrics Committee on Sports Medicine: Knee brace use by athletes. *Pediatrics* 85:228, 1990.

Barret JR, Tanji JL, Drake C, et al: High- versus low-top shoes for the prevention of ankle sprains in basketball players. A prospective randomized study. *Am J Sports Med* 21(4):582–585, 1993.

Benson BW, Mohtadi NG, Rose MS, et al: Head and neck injuries among ice hockey players wearing full face shields vs half face shields. *JAMA* 282(24):2328–2332, 1999.

Cantu RC, Mueller FO: Brain injury related fatalities in American football, 1945–1999. *Neurosurgery* 52(4):846–852, 2003.

Gaulrapp H, Siebert C, Rosemeyer B: Injury and exertion patterns in football on artificial turf. *Sportverletz Sportschaden* 13(4):102–106, 1999.

Gieck JH, Saliba EN: The Athletic Trainer and Rehabilitation, in Kulund DN (ed.): *The Injured Athlete,* 2nd ed. Philadelphia, PA, J.B. Lippincott Company, 1988, pp 165–240.

Grippo A: NFL Injury study 1969–1972. *Final Project Report (SRI-MSD 1961).* Menlo Park, CA, Stanford Research Institute, 1973.

Howe WB: Soccer, in Morris MB (ed.): *Sports Medicine Secrets,* 2nd ed. Philadelphia, PA, Hanley & Belfus, 1999, pp 382–385.

Keene JS, Narechania RG, Sachtjen KM: Tartan turf on trial: A comparison of intercollegiate football injuries occurring on natural grass and tartan turf. *Am J Sports Med* 8(1):43–47, 1980.

Kulund DN, Athletic injuries to the head, face, and neck, in Kulund DN (ed.): *The Injured Athlete*, 2nd ed. Philadelphia, PA, J.B. Lippincott Company, 1988, pp 267–299.

Naftulin S, McKeag DB: Protective equipment: Baseball, softball, hockey, wrestling, and lacrosse, in Morris MB (ed.): *Sports Medicine Secrets*, 2nd ed. Philadelphia, PA, Hanley & Belfus, 1999, pp 110–116.

Nicola TL: Tennis, in Mellion MB, Walsh WM, Shelton GL (eds.): *The Team Physician's Handbook,* 2nd ed. Philadelphia, PA, Hanley & Belfus, 1997, pp 816–827.

Powell JW, Schootman M: A multivariate risk analysis of selected playing surfaces in the National Football League: 1980 to 1989. An epidemiologic study of knee injuries. *Am J Sports Med* 20(6):686–694, 1992.

Reynen PD, Clancy WG, Jr: Cervical spine injury, hockey helmets, and face masks. *Am J Sports Med* 22(2):167–170, 1994.

Rovere GD, Haupt HA, Yates CS: Prophylactic knee bracing in college football. *Am J Sports Med* 15(2):111–116, 1987.

Sitler M, Ryan J, Hopkinson W, et al: The efficacy of a prophylactic knee brace to reduce knee injuries in football. A prospective, randomized study at West Point. *Am J Sports Med* 18(3):310–315, 1990.

Sitler M, Ryan J, Wheeler B, et al: The efficacy of a semirigid ankle stabilizer to reduce acute ankle injuries in basketball. A randomized clinical study at West Point. *Am J Sports Med* 22(4):454–461, 1994.

Surve I, Schwellnus MP, Noakes T, et al: A fivefold reduction in the incidence of recurrent ankle sprains in soccer players using the Sport-Stirrup orthosis. *Am J Sports Med* 22(5):601–606, 1994.

Tegner Y, Lorentzon R: Evaluation of knee braces in Swedish ice hockey players. *Br J Sports Med* 25(3):159–161, 1991.

Troy FE: In defense of synthetic turf. *Trial* 13(1):46–47, 1977.

Wojtys EM, Huston LJ: Custom fit versus off the shelf ACL functional braces. *Am J Knee Surg* 14(3):157–162, 2001.

EVALUATION OF THE INJURED ATHLETE

18   DIAGNOSTIC IMAGING

Leanne L Seeger, MD, FACR
Kambiz Motamedi, MD

INTRODUCTION

- There are several modalities available for the imaging evaluation of sports injuries. The strengths and weaknesses of each modality, along with their specific indications are discussed in this chapter.
- The choice of the imaging modality depends on several factors, including the chronicity of the symptoms, the suspected pathology, and potential treatment alternatives.

IMAGING MODALITIES

- Imaging tools that are commonly available are plain radiography (with or without applied stress), conventional arthrography, *magnetic resonance imaging* (MRI), which may be combined with *arthrography* (referred to as MRA), *computed tomography* (CT), which may be combined with arthrography, ultrasonography, and radionuclide bone scans.

MODALITY STRENGTHS AND WEAKNESSES

- *Plain radiography* is widely available, relatively inexpensive, and provides excellent detail of bony structures and soft tissue calcifications. Even though soft tissue resolution has slightly improved with digital radiography (at the cost of loosing some of fine bone details), the ability of radiography to depict soft tissue pathology remains inferior to cross sectional imaging (MRI, CT, and ultrasound).
- *Stress radiography* (e.g., varusor valgus) reveals abnormal laxity of joints and can indirectly diagnose soft tissue injury. Stress must be applied by the referring physician. Disadvantages include availability of the physician, radiation exposure, and subjectivity of the amount of stress needed. In some cases, it may exacerbate underlying pathology.
- *Conventional arthrography* delineates the synovial space and intra-articular structures by joint distention. Although invasive, there are few inherent risks. Arthrography requires patient preparation and cooperation, informed consent and the availability of a radiologist. When arthrography is combined with MRI or CT, coordination is needed for scheduling scanner time to immediately follow the procedure. Arthrography may be contraindicated in patients with coagulopathy.
- *MRI* provides unparalled soft tissue and bone marrow contrast. With acute or subacute injuries, soft tissue or marrow edema is seen. With chronic injuries, structural abnormalities may be seen. It is of limited value for evaluating bone cortex and soft tissue calcification. There are several relative and absolute contraindications to MRI, including claustrophobia, cardiac pacemakers, and certain kinds of neurosurgical aneurismal clips, and inner ear implants. Because of the popularity of MRI, there may be a prolonged wait time for obtaining an examination.
- *CT* is superior to other modalities for fine bone detail, and is an important tool for depicting the anatomy of complex fractures. Three-dimensional CT reformations are extremely useful in the management of trauma patients. This is especially true with the newer generation (multislice) scanners that significantly

diminish artifact and are capable of submillimeter slice thickness. CT is often utilized as a surrogate for MRI, in cases where MRI is contraindicated. A disadvantage of CT is limited soft tissue contrast. With exception of anatomic areas where various positioning is possible, (e.g., ankles, feet, and hands) direct imaging is limited to the axial or near axial plane. Reconstruction artifact is commonly encountered with older generation scanners.

- The strength of *ultrasonography* lies in its ability to acquire dynamic images. It depicts soft tissue pathology of structures while in motion. A normal control is readily available by acquiring images from the contralateral side. There is direct patient contact of the sonographer, facilitating immediate customization of the exam to patient's symptoms. Ultrasound is strongly operator dependant, requiring intense training with extensive hands-on experience for competency. The need to compare to the contralateral side may prolong examination time, and thus decrease patient compliance. Ultrasound does not provide adequate resolution of intra-articular structures.

- *Radionuclide bone scanning* is extremely sensitive for detecting areas of increased bone turnover. It is, however, nonspecific, and traumatic lesions cannot be differentiated from inflammation or neoplasia. Correlation with plain films is usually needed. There is also poor spatial resolution, which may be improved by obtaining oblique projections and *single photon emission computed tomography* (SPECT).

SPECIFIC USES

- *Radiography* should usually be used for the initial assessment of an acute traumatic event to assess for fracture and/or alignment abnormality. In the case of chronic disorders, radiographs can eliminate alternate diagnoses, such as arthritis or neoplasia. Radiography is also the standard method for following fracture healing and alignment corrections (subluxation or dislocation).

- *Stress radiography* finds its niche in cases of chronic trauma with instability and suspected soft tissue injury. It has, however, been widely replaced by MRI.

- *Arthrography* is utilized when joint distention is required for lesion detection. This may include cases of ligamentous injuries, capsular tears, and intra-articular loose bodies.

- *MRI* is used for suspected bone or soft tissue injury, especially when plain radiographs are normal. There are indications for MRA, including chronic glenoid or acetabular labral tears, low grade *superior labrum*

anterior-posterior (SLAP) lesions, evaluating for retear of a repaired knee meniscus, and detection of noncalcified intra-articular loose bodies.

- *CT* is indicated for demonstrating the extent and anatomy of fractures. It is especially useful with complex pelvic trauma, where plain radiography is limited and the pelvic three-dimensional architecture is complex. It is also useful for evaluation complex elbow trauma, another joint that is difficult to depict three-dimensionally with plain film. CT with multiplanar reformations provides an excellent road map for the surgeon in planning the appropriate operation. CT is also used for intra- versus extra-articular localization of peri-articular mineralization seen on plain film, and is well suited for demonstrating calcifications associated with ligaments and tendons. This latter finding is often associated with chronic injury.

- *Ultrasound* is used when dynamic imaging is desired, as in cases with snapping ankle and hip tendons, and rotator cuff impingement. It is sensitive in demonstrating minute calcium deposits and tiny abnormal fluid collections in and around tendons and ligaments. Mobile field side units are now frequently utilized outside the United States of America., and are gaining popularity here. This allows immediate field-side evaluation of injured athletes for tendon tears, muscle strains, and hematomas.

- *Radionuclide bone scans* are useful for localizing the site of bone pathology in cases where symptoms are diffuse. In lesions such as pars defect, a bone scan done with SPECT will show if the lesion is associated with abnormal activity, implying an active and likely symptomatic lesion. It also provides information about the chronicity of an abnormality, as acute lesions show intense tracer accumulation, and more chronic quiescent conditions appear more normal.

CONSIDERATIONS

- Considering that different modalities have differing sensitivity to demonstrate certain pathology, it becomes evident that clinical information is paramount in not only deciding which method to use, but also to tailor the imaging study to the patient's specific needs.

- Clinical information also helps to choose the correct modality for acute versus overuse injury. In both cases, one should usually begin with plain radiography. In cases of normal radiographs and suspected acute bone injury, one may choose to obtain an MRI to evaluate edema and a possible nondisplaced fracture. MRI is also useful for more chronic injuries where a soft tissue abnormality is suspected.

Complex acute fractures should be evaluated with CT if further imaging is needed.

• The choice of imaging modality also depends on the level of patient's activity. In the case of an elite athlete where the decision of return to play is important, one may choose to obtain advanced imaging (usually MRI) immediately after obtaining radiographs.

TISSUE OF INTEREST

• *Bone* is the fundamental scaffolding of the musculoskeletal system, and plays a central role in diagnostic imaging. With MRI, marrow edema in context of an injury indicates at a minimum trabecular trauma and contusion. Specific patterns of marrow edema may prompt a closer search for injury to specific soft tissue structures. In the knee, e.g., marrow edema in the posterior tibia and the lateral femoral condyle at the sulcus terminalis has a high association with an acute anterior cruciate ligament tear.

• *Cartilage* outlines the bony surfaces of the joints. As a shock absorber it is prone to wear and tear as well as acute injuries. Acute chondral fractures, often with an adjacent bone fragment (osteochondral fracture), are common in sports medicine. Cartilage is not directly visible with plain radiography; however, an initial evaluation of cartilage thickness may be performed with plain radiography to assess joint space narrowing. MRI, on the other hand, not only demonstrates acute injuries to the osteochondral unit, but also nicely shows intrinsic signal abnormalities of cartilage owing to wear and tear (chondromalacia). MRI can also evaluate the cartilage for focal areas of thinning, fissuring, and ulceration. One of the more common areas of interest for cartilage evaluation is the anterior knee for chondromalacia patellae.

• Joint stabilizing *ligaments* and *tendons* and the dynamic *muscle* and tendon units are prone to injuries. Certain sports are associated with specific injury patterns. The examples are innumerable, including jumper's knee (patellar tendon), tennis leg (plantaris tendon and/or gastrocnemius muscle), and tennis or golfers' elbow (collateral ligament). If plain films are normal, MRI will provide the necessary soft tissue contrast for diagnosis. The spectrum of findings range from mild edema to hematoma, partial tear, and complete disruption. Ultrasound is gaining popularity for evaluation of the more superficial tendons and muscles, especially around the elbow and ankle.

• *Bursae* are fluid filled structures with synovial linings that act as cushions at foci of increased motion or friction. They are classically found between bones and tendons or muscles and skin, but can form anywhere protection is needed. Inherent to their function, bursae are prone to inflammation, especially in cases with overuse. MRI is excellent for demonstrating inflamed and fluid filled bursal structures. Ultrasound is suitable for detecting superficial fluid collections and possibly hyperemia in an inflamed superficial bursa. Ultrasound may also provide guidance for therapeutic injections.

ACUTE INJURY VS. OVERUSE

• Plain radiography is usually used to evaluate for acute fracture. With chronic complaints or overuse, plain films provide an effective screening tool for arthritis, inflammatory processes, and musculoskeletal tumors. Plain films may be helpful in demonstrating acute or chronic joint effusions (e.g., knee and elbow) by demonstrating a soft tissue density displacing normal fat planes. In cases of chronic injuries, calcifications are easily seen with radiography. Plain films are also used to evaluate for periosteal new bone formation, abnormal bone sclerosis and callus formation.

• If plain films are deemed to be normal and symptoms warrant, MRI is usually the next modality undertaken. With chronic or overuse disorders, stress reaction or fracture will appear on MRI as edema in bone marrow, possibly with immature periosteal new bone formation. Focal abnormalities are also evident in muscles, tendons, and ligaments. When the suspicion of an acute fracture is high and plain films are normal, MRI will detect radiographically occult fractures in weight-bearing bones such the tibial plateau and proximal femur. Early diagnosis is important to avoid fragment displacement with activity.

• If a patient's symptoms persist after adequate conservative treatment or seem out of proportion to the clinical setting, additional imaging is warranted. It is not uncommon for bone and soft tissue tumors to be initially diagnosed as a hematoma or muscle strain. Any palpable mass diagnosed as a hematoma should be followed clinically to maturation or resolution.

CHRONIC SEQUELA TO TRAUMA

• Areas of prior hemorrhage, hematoma, or inflammation may undergo transformation into mature bone. This phenomenon is called heterotopic ossification or myositis ossificans. The former name is preferred, since this is not an inflammatory process of the muscles. Plain radiography and possibly CT play a crucial role in recognizing this entity. The finding of peripheral calcification around a soft tissue mass is the hallmark of this entity. This is contrary to osteogenic sarcoma, where the osteoid is situated centrally. Unfortunately, these two entities may be confused histologically. With maturation, the mineralization of heterotopic ossification will often completely ossify with marrow induction. An area of heterotopic ossification immediately adjacent to bone may result from an avulsion injury. This is termed periostitis ossificans.

- Calcific deposits may be seen not only in tendons and ligaments, but also in chronic inflammation of a bursa (calcific bursitis). These calcifications are usually hydroxyapetite bound, and have a pasty appearance. They may be linear or globular. Depending on the location of the symptoms, radiographs, CT or ultrasound may be utilized for diagnosis.

SITE SPECIFIC PLAIN RADIOGRAPHY: STANDARD AND SPECIAL VIEWS

- Each institution has its own set of plain film series and as such, it is useful to know what views are included in a given radiologic examination. The referring physician may then request a specific view that may be crucial for the diagnosis of the suspected pathology, or the radiologist may add or vary the study according to the initial findings and the pathology suspected. In the setting of acute joint trauma, a three view minimum is usually required. Two perpendicular views suffice for the long bone shafts, and two views are usually adequate for fracture follow-up.

SHOULDER

- Internal and external rotation views in the *anteroposterior* (AP) projection are included in most shoulder series. Axillary or trans-scapular-Y view are common third projections obtained, needed for a perpendicular view of the glenoid. Grashey, outlet (angulated transscapular) and West Point views may be obtained for evaluation of the glenohumeral joint space, anterior acromial shape and subacromial space, and anteroinferior glenoid rim respectively.

ELBOW

- Anteroposterior and lateral views are standard. The lateral view should be obtained with the elbow in 90° of flexion. Bilateral oblique views may be used for soft tissue calcification or acute fracture, and an angulated radial head view may show a nondisplaced fracture.

HAND/WRIST

- Posteroanterior, lateral, and oblique views usually constitute a hand series. The basic wrist series consists of four projections, those above as well as a navicular (scaphoid) view to lay the bone out on its long axis. The carpal tunnel view will show fractures of the hook of the hamate, and the ball catcher view may reveal widening of the scapholunate space, implying a ligament tear.

CERVICAL/LUMBAR SPINE

- Anteroposterior and lateral views are the basic series, and oblique views are obtained to evaluate the facet joints. Flexion and extension views may be added to evaluate for instability. In the cervical spine, the open mouth view shows alignment of the first two vertebral segment lateral masses and the odontoid base. The Fuchs view shows the odontoid tip. The swimmer's view shows the lower cervical and upper thoracic segments that may be obscured by shoulder soft tissues on the conventional lateral projection. A coned lateral view of the L5-S1 disc is often useful, and this level is subject to distortion from beam angulation on the standard lateral lumbar film.

THORACIC SPINE

- Anteroposterior and lateral views are standard. A swimmer's view is frequently obtained to evaluate the upper thoracic segments. The thoracic facets are best assessed with CT.

PELVIS

- The most common view of the pelvis is the AP projection. Inlet/outlet and bilateral Judet (lateral oblique) views may also be obtained, but these are usually reserved for significant acute pelvic trauma. The PA view is preferred over an AP projection for imaging the SI joints because of their oblique orientation.

HIP

- Anteroposterior and frog-leg lateral views are standard. While these provide two views of the proximal femur, they show the acetabulum in only one projection. A true acetabular lateral may be obtained with an axial lateral (Johnson lateral) view.

KNEE

- Anteroposterior and lateral views are standard for the series. Except in the setting of acute trauma where fracture is of clinical concern, these should be obtained in the upright position. In acute trauma, the lateral view should be positioned in a cross-table manner to allow demonstration of a lipohemarthrosis, a sign of fracture. A patellar view (sunrise of Merchant) shows the patellofemoral joint to best advantage. The flexed PA view gives insight into the intercondylar notch, and is more sensitive than the straight upright position for detecting early joint space narrowing. Oblique views may show additional contour abnormalities of the osseous structures or demonstrate a nondisplaced fracture.

ANKLE/FOOT

- Anteroposterior, lateral and oblique views are usually obtained. As with the knee, the films should be taken upright except when an acute fracture is suspected. Alignment abnormalities require weight-bearing for proper evaluation. If a subtle Lisfranc injury is suspected, weight-bearing AP films of both feet may be needed to evaluate for mild widening through comparison with the uninjured side. The Harris view provides a perpendicular projection of the calcaneous. Coalitions are often only seen on an oblique view of the foot.

CONCLUSION

- When dealing with the athlete, plain radiography is usually the first imaging study that should be performed. This holds true whether dealing with an acute injury or overuse.
- MRI is preferred for the diagnosis of radiographically occult bone injury and soft tissue trauma, be it acute or chronic. This is not an urgent examination unless one is dealing with an elite athlete where return to play is an issue, or if there is concern for a radiographically occult fracture in a weight-bearing bone.
- CT is preferred for complex bone trauma.
- The clinical history will effect both image acquisition and interpretation. Open communication between clinician and radiologist is essential for optimal patient care.

BIBLIOGRAPHY

Anderson MW, Greenspan A: State of the art: Stress fractures. *Radiology* 199:1–12, 1996.

Ballinger PW: *Merrills Atlas of Radiographic Positions and Radiographic Procedures,* 3rd, vol 1. St Louis, MO, Mosby, 1986.

Farooki S, Seeger LL: Magnetic resonance imaging in the evaluation of ligament injuries. *Skeletal Radiol* 28:61–74, 1999.

Helms CA: The impact of MR imaging in sports medicine. *Radiology* 224:631–635, 2002.

Imhof H, Fuchsjäger M: Traumatic injuries: Imaging of spinal injuries. *Eur Radiol* 12:1262–1272, 2002.

Lin J, Fessell DP, Jacobson JA, et al: An illustrated tutorial of musculoskeletal sonography: Part I, Introduction and general principles. *Am J Roentgenol* 175:637–645, 2000a.

Lin J, Fessell DP, Jacobson JA, et al: An illustrated tutorial of musculoskeletal sonography: Part II, Upper Extremity. *Am J Roentgenol* 175:1071–1079, 2000b.

Lin J, Fessell DP, Jacobson JA, et al: An illustrated tutorial of musculoskeletal sonography: Part III, Lower Extremity. *Am J Roentgenol* 175:1313–1321, 2000c.

Lund PJ, Nisbet JK, Valencia FG, et al: Current sonographic applications in orthopaedics. *Am J Roentgenol* 166:889–895, 1996.

Rubin DA: MR imaging of the knee menisci. *Radiol Clin North Am* 35:21–44, 1997.

19 ELECTRODIAGNOSTIC TESTING

Venu Akuthota, MD
John Tobey, MD

INTRODUCTION

- *Electrodiagnostic* (EDX) testing can be an important tool in the evaluation of athletes with neurologic problems.
- The thorough EDX consultation integrates the history, physical examination, and selected nerve conduction or needle electromyographic studies into a meaningful diagnostic conclusion (Robinson and Stop-Smith, 1999).
- EDX studies are an extension of the clinical examination.
- Whereas imaging studies identify structural abnormalities, EDX studies evaluate the physiology and function of the peripheral nervous system.
- A negative EDX examination does not rule out the possibility of pathology because electrophysiologic studies are time and severity dependent (Rogers, 1996).
- Clinical judgment is used in EDX, therefore EDX studies are highly dependent on the quality of the electromyographer (Robinson and Stop-Smith, 1999).
- This chapter will describe the pathophysiology of nerve injury and associated chronology of electrophysiologic

findings. A description of the components of an EDX evaluation will be provided.

- EDX are divided into *nerve conduction studies* (NCS) and *needle examination* (NE). The NE is also referred to as *electromyography* (EMG).
- The purpose of the information presented in this chapter will be to provide the clinician a basis of ordering and understanding proper EDX reports.

ANATOMY

- Electrodiagnostic studies evaluate the peripheral nerve system or lower motor neuron pathway.
- The peripheral nervous system includes both the afferent sensory pathway and the efferent motor pathway.

SENSORY (AFFERENT) PATHWAY

- Cutaneous receptors → sensory axons → pure sensory or mixed nerves → nerve plexus (e.g., brachial plexus, lumbosacral plexus) → cell bodies in the dorsal root ganglion (usually within intervertebral foramina) → dorsal roots synapse in dorsolateral spinal cord.
- NCS of pure sensory and mixed nerves evaluate this aspect of the peripheral nervous system.

MOTOR (EFFERENT) PATHWAY

- Anterior horn cell (spinal cord) → spinal nerves → divide into ventral and dorsal rami. Ventral rami → nerve plexus → peripheral motor nerve → neuromuscular junction → muscle. Entire pathway is referred to as a motor unit.

- NCS of the pure motor and mixed nerves evaluate this aspect of the peripheral nervous system.
- Motor units are evaluated during needle EMG with voluntary muscle activation.

PATHOPHYSIOLOGY OF NERVE INJURY

- Peripheral nerves can either be myelinated or unmyelinated.
- Myelinated fibers have nodes of Ranvier, which facilitate saltatory (jumping) conduction along the nerve fiber.
- NCS evaluate the fastest conducting fibers—usually A alpha myelinated fibers.
- Peripheral nerve injury is categorized by injury to the myelin alone or to the axon.

SEDDON CLASSIFICATION

- Divides peripheral nerve injury into neurapraxia, axonotmesis, neurotmesis (Table 19-1).

NEURAPRAXIA

- Neurapraxia is focal conduction slowing or focal conduction block. Myelin is injured; yet, the nerve fibers remain in axonal continuity. This results in impaired conduction across the demyelinated segment; however, impulse conduction is normal in the segments proximal and distal to the injury.
- Demyelination is mostly seen with focal nerve entrapments, e.g., carpal tunnel syndrome. It may also occur in peripheral polyneuropathies as either a patchy process (e.g., Guillain-Barre syndrome) or a diffuse process (e.g., diabetic peripheral neuropathy).

TABLE 19-1 Classification of Nerve Pathophysiology

TYPE	PATHOLOGY	EDX CORRELATION	PROGNOSIS
Neurapraxia	Myelin injury	CV slowing across segment DL prolonged across segment Loss or amplitude proximal but not distal NE normal	Recovery in weeks
Axonotmeses	Axonal injury with endoneurium intact	Loss of amplitude distal and proximal NE show spontaneous activity NE shows abnormal voluntary motor units	Longer recovery
Neurotmeses	Severance of entire nerve	No waveform with proximal or distal stimulation NE shows spontaneous activity NE shows no recruitable motor units	Poor recovery

ABBREVIATIONS: CV = conduction velocity; DL = distal latency; NE = needle examination

- Runners often experience neurapraxic injury of the tibial nerve branches with putative tarsal tunnel syndrome, possibly due to repeated traction injury with the foot in pronation. (Jackson and Haglund, 1991)

AXONOTMESIS AND NEUROTMESIS

- Axonotmesis and neurotmesis refer to axonal injury with wallerian degeneration of nerve fibers disconnected to their cell bodies. There is a loss of nerve conduction at the injury site and distally. Axonotmetic injuries involve damage to the axon with preservation of the endoneurium (Dimitru, 1995).
- Neurotmetic injuries imply a complete disruption of the enveloping nerve sheath (Dimitru, 1995).
- EDX studies typically cannot separate axonotmesis from neurotmesis.
- Athletes can often experience axonal injury with conditions such as a radiculopathy.

SPECIFIC EDX STUDIES

NERVE CONDUCTION STUDIES

- Nerve conduction studies may be performed on motor, sensory, or mixed nerves.
- There are numerous pitfalls with NCS (Table 19-2), therefore it is imperative that a well-trained consultant performs EDX studies (Robinson and Stop-Smith, 1999).
- Both motor and sensory NCS test only the fastest, myelinated axons of a nerve, thus, the lightly myelinated or unmyelinated fibers (C pain fibers) are not examined with EDX (Wilbourn and Shields, 1998).
- Motor nerves are stimulated at accessible sites, and the *compound muscle action potential* (CMAP) is recorded over the motor points of innervated muscles.
- Deep motor nerves and deep proximal muscles are more difficult to study and interpret (Feinberg, 1999).

TABLE 19-2   Sources of Error in Nerve Conduction Studies

- Temperature
- Inadequate or excessive stimulation
- Improper placement of electrodes
- Tape measurement error
- Age
- Anomalous innervation
- Volume conduction of impulse to nearby nerve
- Improper filter settings
- Improper electrode montage setup
- Involuntary muscle contractions

- Sensory nerves can be studied along the physiologic direction of the nerve impulse (orthodromic) or opposite the physiologic direction of the afferent input (antidromic).
- Stimulated and recorded sensory nerves produce a *sensory nerve action potential* (SNAP).
- Frequently, sensory axons are tested within mixed nerves, such as the plantar nerves, and produce a *mixed nerve action potential* (MNAP).
- CMAP, SNAP, and MNAP waveforms are analyzed and interpreted by the clinician.
- Waveform parameters include amplitude, latency, and conduction velocity.
- Amplitude evaluates the number of functioning axons in a given nerve, and for motor studies, the number of muscle fibers activated.
- Latency refers to the time from the stimulus to the recorded action potential.
- With motor NCS, latency takes into account the peripheral nerve conduction (distal to the site of stimulation), neuromuscular junction transmission time, and muscle fiber activation time (Robinson and Stop-Smith, 1999).
- With sensory nerves, latency measures only the conduction of the segment of nerve stimulated.
- Conduction velocity across a segment of nerve can also be calculated when nerves are stimulated at a distal and proximal site.

LATE RESPONSES

H REFLEX

- The H reflex is the electrophysiologic analog to the ankle stretch reflex. It measures afferent and efferent conduction mainly along the S1 nerve root pathway (Fisher, 1992).
- A latency difference of at least 1.5 ms is significant in most laboratories.
- Amplitude of <50% compared with the uninvolved side is also significant.
- Since the amplitude of this reflex is sensitive to contraction of the plantar flexor muscles, amplitude changes without significant latency abnormalities should be interpreted with caution (Press and Young, 1997).
- The H reflex looks at the afferent and efferent pathways, thus, it gives information about the sensory pathway that is not tested by standard needle EMG.
- The S1 nerve injury can be due to S1 radiculopathy from a herniated lumbar disc or lumbar stenosis, peripheral neuropathy (usually with bilaterally abnormal H reflexes), or sciatic/tibial nerve injuries.

F WAVE

- The F wave is a late muscle potential that results from a motor nerve volley created by supramaximally stimulated anterior horn cells (Fisher, 1998).
- Unlike the H reflex, the F wave can be elicited at many spinal levels and from any muscle.
- F wave studies, like H reflexes, look at a long pathway. Consequently, small focal abnormalities tend to be obscured by the longer segments.
- Abnormalities with F wave values may be due to nerve injury anywhere along the long pathway evaluated.

NEEDLE EXAMINATION

- The NE evaluates the entire motor unit (lower motor neuron pathway), but not the sensory pathway.
- The NE includes the evaluation with needle EMG of the muscles at rest (to detect axonal injury) and with volitional activity (to evaluate voluntary motor unit morphology and recruitment).
- The NE needs to be timed such that abnormalities are optimally detected.
- If the NE is performed too early (i.e., less than 2 to 3 weeks after the initial injury), spontaneous muscle fiber discharges (denervation potentials) may not have had time to develop.
- If the NE is performed too late (i.e., more than 6 months after the initial injury), reinnervation via collateral sprouting may have halted spontaneous muscle fiber discharges (Press and Young, 1997).
- At rest, the electrical activity of selected muscles are studied for abnormal waveforms.
- Of these abnormal waveforms, the most common abnormal finding is the presence of fibrillations and positive sharp waves. They are found when the muscle tested has been denervated (Dimitru, 1995).
- Fibrillations and positive sharp waves are graded on a scale from 0 to 4+ (Table 19-3).
- *Complex repetitive discharges* (CRDs) are also common. They represent a group of single muscle fibers that are time-linked because of crosstalk between neighboring muscle fibers.
- Fasciculation potentials can be found in a variety of benign and pathologic conditions. They represent spontaneous discharges of an entire motor unit. Sometimes fasciculations can be grossly observed as muscle twitches.
- Benign fasciculations may be found in athletes following heavy exercise, dehydration, anxiety, fatigue, caffeine consumption, or smoking.
- With activation of the muscle, motor units are analyzed and this offers an opportunity to distinguish between neuropathic and myopathic processes (Robinson and Stop-Smith, 1999).
- NE may also help differentiate acute from chronic neuropathic conditions.
- The amplitude of fibrillations can grade nerve injury as occurring for less than or more than 1 year (Kraft, 1990). This can be particularly helpful in distinguishing an athlete's acute or chronic nerve injury.
- Chronic nerve injuries, without significant ongoing denervation, will additionally show large-amplitude, long-duration, polyphasic motor unit potentials (Press and Young, 1997).

DYNAMIC EDX

- Some authors advocate performing EDX after exercise or with the limbs in provocative positions. These techniques have not been validated with sound research and are subject to measurement error.
- Anecdotally, however, they appear to have a limited use.
- Peroneal nerve entrapments in runners were detected only with EDX testing following exercise (Leach, Purnell, and Saito, 1989).
- Runners diagnosed with compartment syndrome and potential nerve entrapment (e.g., superficial peroneal nerve entrapment as it exits the fascia of the lateral compartment) have also been postulated as needing EDX testing following exercise (Bachner and Friedman, 1995).
- It has been suggested that electrophysiologic evidence of piriformis syndrome is more apparent when an H reflex is performed with sciatic nerve on stretch (hip flexed to 90°, maximally adducted, and knee flexed to 90°) (Fishman and Zybert, 1992).
- These techniques need to be interpreted with caution as many abnormal readings occur based on measurement error alone.

QUANTITATIVE ELECTROMYOGRAPHY

- Demonstrates sequence of muscle recruitment and muscle force.
- Only available in specialized gait laboratories.

TABLE 19-3 Grading of Fibrillations and Positive Waves

GRADING	CHARACTERISTICS
0	No activity
1+	Persistent (longer than 1 s) in 2 muscle regions
2+	Persistent in 3 or more muscle regions
3+	Persistent in all muscle regions
4+	Continuous in all muscle regions

- Surface or needle electrodes placed into muscles to record EMG signals through multiple channels.
- Caution should be used in correlating EMG signal amplitude with muscle force because the relationship is not consistently linear (Basmajian and DeLuca, 1988).
- Has been used to assess the degree of muscle fatigue and biomechanics of sports activities (Feinberg, 1999).
- The kinesiology of the running gait has been elucidated with EMG. The gluteal muscles and hamstrings are more active in running than in walking, particularly at the termination of the swing phase in preparation for foot strike. The quadriceps and posterior calf group also work during a greater percentage of the swing and stance phase during running than in walking. The calf muscle group in particular becomes much more active as the speed of gait increases (Mann, 1995).
- Surface EMG can be used as a biofeedback technique in athletes to improve their sport specific biomechanics (i.e., training the use of the hip extensors).

INDICATIONS FOR EDX TESTING

- The utility of EDX testing in a given athlete may be estimated following a thorough history and physical examination, by a review of supplemental information (e.g., imaging studies), and through an appreciation for the chronology of the electrophysiologic changes that occur following nerve injury.
- Some useful generalizations about the indications for EDX studies are the following (Press and Young, 1997):
1. Establish and/or confirm a clinical diagnosis.
   a. EDX examination can rule in a suspected diagnosis or rule out a competing diagnosis.
   b. EDX studies may alert the possibility of an unsuspected concomitant pathologic process (i.e., an athlete with tarsal tunnel syndrome with superimposed radiculopathy).
2. Localize nerve lesions.
   a. Nerve injury localization often needs to be objectively confirmed prior to contemplating invasive or surgical treatment.
   b. An athlete presenting with plantar foot numbness and tingling may have a sciatic nerve lesion anywhere along the course of the nerve or its branches.
   c. EDX studies can be used to determine if the sciatic nerve injury is occurring at the piriformis or at its terminal branches.
3. Determine the extent and chronicity of nerve injuries.
   a. Properly timed EDX studies can differentiate a neuropraxic injury from axonal degeneration. This may have a significant impact on the aggressiveness of treatment for nerve injury.
   b. The acuteness and chronicity of the nerve lesion may also be assessed using fibrillation amplitude and motor unit analysis, as well as clinical history (Robinson and Stop-Smith, 1999; Kraft, 1990).
4. Correlate findings of anatomic studies.
   a. EDX studies are useful to correlate nerve function to anatomic abnormalities.
   b. This may be particularly useful in the spine because disc herniations effacing nerve roots can be seen in asymptomatic individuals (Jensen et al, 1994).
5. Assist in prognosis and return to play.
   a. By determining the degree of nerve injury, the clinician can predict nerve function recovery.
   b. In general, neuropraxic injuries recover sooner than axonal injuries.
   c. CMAP amplitude measurements of weak muscles (compared with asymptomatic contralateral amplitude) can give an idea of the extent of neuroproxia and of potential recovery.
   d. A side-to-side amplitude difference of greater than 50% is probably significant.
   e. However, EDX studies should not be the *sine qua non* for return to play because they may lag behind clinical recovery.
   f. The best determination of return to play remains the athlete's functional performance in simulated sports activities (Feinberg, 1999).

LIMITATIONS OF EDX TESTING

- Electrodiagnostic testing is not a perfect test and should not be performed in every athlete with neurologic signs or symptoms.
- Some diagnoses are unequivocal and treatment should be initiated without delay (e.g., progressive neurologic deficits following a traumatic posterior knee dislocation, which should be treated emergently).
- When ordering EDX studies, the timing of findings should be kept in mind (Table 19-4).
- NE findings can take from 2 to 6 weeks to manifest.
- With traumatic injuries, serial EDX studies, including an immediate study, may be helpful to thoroughly determine the degree of nerve injury.
- Relative contraindications to EDX include pacemaker (no Erb's point stimulation), defibrillator, arteriovenous fistula, open wound, coagulopathy, lymphedema, anasarca, and pending muscle biopsy.

TABLE 19-4   Timing of EDX Findings with Axonal Injury

TIME	NCS	NE
Day 0	Decreased CMAP/SNAP amplitudes proximally Normal distal to lesion	Decreased recruitment
Day 1-3	Decreased CMAP/SNAP amplitudes proximally Normal distal to lesion	
Day 3-7	Decreasing CMAP then SNAP amplitudes, proximally and distally	
Day 7-9	Decreased or absent CMAP amplitudes, proximally and distally	Increased insertional activity in proximal muscles
Day 10-14	Decreased or absent SNAP amplitudes	Large PSW/Fibs in proximal denervated muscle
Week 3-6	—	Large PSW/Fibs in distal denervated muscle
Week 6-8	Increasing amplitude w/recovery	Nascent reinnervation of proximal muscles (VMUP = polyphasic, low amplitude, increased duration)
Month 3-4	Increasing amplitude w/recovery Proximal CV 80% of normal	
Month 4		Nascent reinnervation of distal muscles Maturing reinnervation of proximal muscles (VMUP = polyphasic, high amplitude, increased duration)
Month 4-5		Maturing reinnervation of distal muscles
Year 1		Smaller PSW/Fibs

ABBREVIATIONS: NCS = nerve conduction studies; NE = needle examination; PSW = positive sharp waves; Fibs = fibrillations; SNAP = sensory nerve action potential; CMAP = compound muscle action potential; VMUP = voluntary motor unit potential; CV = conduction velocity.

SPECIFIC CONDITIONS

- Many pain complaints in athletes present as neurologic signs and symptoms.
- Athletes most frequently complain of numbness or tingling and focal weakness in the foot.
- Although most long distance runners do not complain of symptoms of neuropathy, they do appear to have subclinical changes in quantitative sensory thresholds and nerve conduction velocities (Dyck et al, 1987). Runners may present with focal nerve entrapments (Table 19-5).
- Athletes with nerve pain describe a burning, shooting, tingling, numb, and/or electric quality to their pain.

- Athletes may commonly present with tibial and peroneal nerve problems which can be evaluated by EDX techniques.

TIBIAL NERVE

- There are specific EDX techniques to evaluate the tibial nerve and its terminal branches (Park and Del Toro, 1998).
- The tibial nerve has four terminal branches: (a) medial plantar nerve, (b) lateral plantar nerve, (c) inferior calcaneal nerve, and (d) medial calcaneal nerve.

TABLE 19-5   Focal Entrapment Neuropathies Seen in Runners

SYNDROME/NERVE	SYMPTOMS	ENTRAPMENT SITE
Tarsal tunnel syndrome (tibial nerve proper)	Plantar pain/paresthesias, worse at night and with prolonged standing or walking	Under flexor retinaculum
Medial calcaneal neuritis	Medial heel pain	At medial heel
Inferior calcaneal nerve (first branch of lateral plantar nerve)	Chronic heel pain, no numbness, weakness of ADM	Between AH and QP or calcaneal heel spur
Medial plantar nerve (jogger's foot)	Medial arch pain	At master knot of Henry (hypertrophy of AH)
Morton's toe (interdigital nerve)	N/T in toes	At intermetatarsal ligament
Superficial peroneal nerve	Lateral ankle pain Fascial herniation	At deep crural fascia as exits lateral compartment
Deep peroneal nerve	Dorsum of foot pain Tightly laced shoes	At inferior extensor retinaculum
Common peroneal nerve	N/T in lateral leg, dorsum of foot	Compression in fibular tunnel by fibrous edge of peroneus longus Traction from ankle sprains

ABBREVIATIONS: N/T = numbness/tingling; AH = abductor hallucis; QP = quadratus plantae; ADM = abductor digiti minimi

- The medial plantar nerve is easily tested as a motor nerve conduction study, stimulating at the tibial nerve proximal to the medial malleolus and recording over the abductor hallucis.
- The lateral plantar motor nerve study is performed by stimulating the tibial nerve proximal to the medial malleolus and recording over the flexor digit minimi brevis.
- The inferior calcaneal motor nerve study is performed to the abductor *digiti minimi pedis.*
- The medial calcaneal nerve can be studied as a sensory nerve antidromic study, where the recording electrode is placed over the skin of the medial calcaneus.
- The sensory components of the medial and lateral plantar nerves may be practically tested with an antidromic mixed nerve study.
- The medial and lateral plantar nerves are stimulated individually at the plantar aspect of the foot and the SNAP is recorded under the medial malleolus.

PERONEAL NERVE

- The peroneal nerve's motor and sensory components can be consistently studied with nerve conduction studies.
- The motor nerve study is performed by stimulating the peroneal nerve at multiple sites, including the anterior ankle, the fibular head, and the popliteal fossa.
- Recording is usually over the extensor digitorum brevis; however, the anterior tibialis can be used as an alternative muscle.
- The sensory nerve study is performed by stimulating the superficial peroneal branch as it exits the lateral compartment and recording over the ankle.

EMG REPORT

- The electrophysiologic report should include a number of important pieces of data for the referring physician.
- The report should correlate with physical finding and any discrepancies identified. Inconsistencies may have as much importance in the clinical treatment of the patient as consistent results.
- Also, the degree of definitiveness of findings needs to be conveyed to the referring physician. A diagnosis of S1 radiculopathy by H reflex changes alone will carry different weight than abundant spontaneous activity in the S1 myotomal distribution.
- One abnormal finding does not make the diagnosis if all other evidence is pointing to a different diagnosis (Rogers, 1996).
- Sufficient evidence to rule out alternative possibilities and to identify superimposed conditions
- Degree of injury and chronicity, if possible

- Prognosis is critical if obtainable
- Comparison with previous EDX data whenever possible

SUMMARY

- Effectiveness and reliability of EDX in detecting pathology in athletes is high, but it must always be understood in light of its capabilities and limitations.
- EDX studies are examiner-dependent and when possible, should be performed by a physician who is a specialist in EDX medicine.
- EDX studies evaluate the degree and location of nerve injury but do not measure pain.
- When performed at the appropriate time, athletes with neurologic symptoms may be aided by EDX studies.

REFERENCES

Bachner EJ, Friedman MJ: Injuries to the leg, in Nicholas JA, Hershman EB (eds.), *The Lower Extremity and Spine in Sports Medicine*, St. Louis, MO, Mosby, 1995.

Basmajian JV, DeLuca CJ: *Muscles Alive: Their Functions Revealed by Electromyography,* 5th ed. Baltimore, MD, Williams & Wilkins, 1988.

Dimitru D: *Electrodiagnostic Medicine*. Philadelphia, PA, Hanley & Belfus, 1995.

Dyck PJ, Classen SM, Stevens JC, et al: Assessment of nerve damage in the feet of long-distance runners. *Mayo Clin Proc* 62:568, 1987.

Feinberg JH: The role of electrodiagnostics in the study of muscle kinesiology, muscle fatigue and peripheral nerve injuries in sports medicine. *J Back Musculoskelet Med* 12;73, 1999.

Fisher MA: AAEM Minimonograph: Part 13: H reflexes and F waves: Physiology and clinical indications. *Muscle Nerve* 15:1223, 1992.

Fisher MA: The contemporary role of F-wave studies. F-wave studies: Clinical utility (see comments). *Muscle Nerve* 21: 1098, discussion 1105, 1998.

Fishman LM, Zybert PA: Electrophysiologic evidence of piriformis syndrome. *Arch Phys Med Rehabil* 73:359, 1992.

Jackson DL, Haglund B: Tarsal tunnel syndrome in athletes. Case reports and literature review. *Am J Sports Med* 19:61, 1991.

Jensen MC, Brant-Zawadzki MN, Obuchowski N, et al: Magnetic resonance imaging of the lumbar spine in people without back pain. *N Engl J Med* 331:69, 1994.

Kraft GH: Fibrillation potential amplitude and muscle atrophy following peripheral nerve injury. *Muscle Nerve* 13:814, 1990.

Leach RE, Purnell MB, Saito A: Peroneal nerve entrapment in runners. *Am J Sports Med* 17:287, 1989.

Mann RA: Biomechanics of running, in Nicholas JA, Hershman EB, (eds.), *The Lower Extremity and Spine in Sports Medicine*, St. Louis, MO, Mosby, 1995, p 335.

Park TA, Del Toro DR: Electrodiagnostic evaluation of the foot. *Phys Med Rehabil Clin North Am* 9(87):vii, 1998.

Press JM, Young JL: Electrodiagnostic evaluation of spine problems, in Gonzalez G, Materson RS (eds.): *The Nonsurgical Management of Acute Low Back Pain.* New York, NY, Demos Vermande, 1997, p 191.

Robinson LR, Stop-Smith KA: Paresthesiae and focal weakness: The diagnosis of nerve entrapment, in AAEM Annual Assembly. Vancouver, British Columbia, Johnson Printing Company, 1999.

Rogers CJ: *Electrodiagnostic Medicine Handbook.* San Antonio, TX, University of Texas Health Science Center-San Antonio, 1996.

Wilbourn AJ, Shields RW: Generalized polyneuropathies and other nonsurgical peripheral nervous system disorders, in Omer GE, Spinner M, Beek ALV (eds.), *Management of Peripheral Nerve Problems.* Philadelphia, PA, Saunders, 1998, p 648.

20   EXERCISE TESTING

David E Price, MD
Kevin Elder, MD
Russell D White, MD

INTRODUCTION

- Various anatomic, electric, and physiologic tests are used in evaluation of the heart. The *exercise stress test* (EST) endures as one of the few valuable and practical physiologic tools to evaluate cardiac perfusion and function under controlled conditions. Many primary care physicians have moved away from this traditional physiologic test thinking it less practical with the advent of newer cardiovascular imaging techniques. But numerous evidence-based guidelines as established by the American College of Cardiology (ACC) as well as the American College of Sports Medicine (ACSM) have shown that many of the new technologies do not necessarily have better diagnostic characteristics than the standard exercise test (Froelicher et al, 1999).
- EST is useful for diagnosis of ischemia (sensitivity of 50–70%, specificity 80–90%), prognosis of known cardiac disease, and exercise prescription (Froelicher et al, 1999; Evans and Karunarante, 1992a).
- When performing an EST, one should understand its physiology, indications, contraindications, and interpretation, with special consideration given to athletes whose abnormal responses may, in fact, be normal variations.

EXERCISE TEST TERMINOLOGY

- It is essential to understand the basic EST terminology prior to performing the test (Fig. 20-1):
- **PR segment:** The isoelectric line from which the ST segment and the J point are measured at rest. With

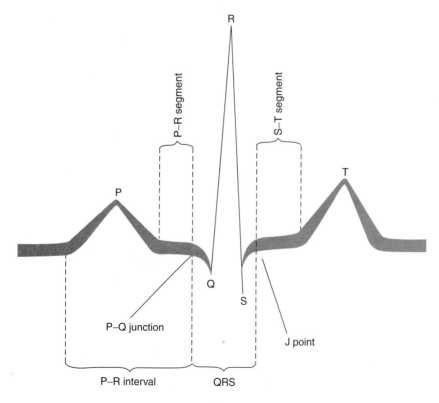

FIG. 20-1   Exercise stress test terminology.

exercise, the PR segment slopes downward and shortens in duration at which point the *PQ junction* becomes the point of reference for the ST segment.

- **J point:** The point that distinguishes the QRS complex from the ST segment; the point at which the ST segment depression is measured.

- **ST segment:** ST segment level is measured relative to the PQ junction. If the baseline is depressed, the deviation from that level to the level during exercise or recovery is measured. The ST segment is measured at 60 or 80 ms after the J point. [At ventricular rates >145 bpm (beats per minute), it is measured at 60 ms after the J point (ACC/AHA Guidelines for Exercise Testing, 1997; American Heart Association Scientific Statement, 2001)].

- **VO_{2max}:** The greatest amount of oxygen a person can use while performing dynamic exercise involving a large part of their muscle mass. This is a function of a person's functional aerobic capacity and defines the limits of the cardiopulmonary system. It is defined by the Fick Equation which incorporates both heart rate (HR) and stroke volume (SV):

$$VO_{2\,max} = (HR_{max}) \times (SV_{max}) \times (CaO_{2\,max} - CvO_{2\,max})$$

$$VO_{2max} = \text{Max Cardiac Output} \times \text{Max Arteriovenous } O_2 \text{ diff.}$$

- $VO_{2\,max}$ then is defined by a central component (cardiac output), which describes the capacity of the heart to function as a pump, and by peripheral factors (arteriovenous-oxygen difference), which describes the capacity of the lungs to oxygenate the blood delivered to it and the capacity of the working muscles to extract this oxygenated blood (Myers, 2001). Many factors affect each of these variables (Mellion, 1996):
  a. HR is affected most importantly by age (220 − age ±12 beats gives a good estimate of maximum HR or HR_{max}). HR is also affected by activity type, body position, fitness, presence of heart disease, medications, blood volume, and environment (Hammond and Froelicher, 1985).
  b. SV is affected by factors such as genetics, conditioning (heart size), and cardiac disease. In normal subjects, an increase in both end-diastolic and end-systolic volume occurs in response to moving from an upright, at rest position to a moderate level of exercise. End-systolic volume decreases progressively as exercise intensifies, in order to maintain SV. At peak exercise, end-diastolic volume may even decline.
  c. Arterial oxygen content is related to the partial pressure of arterial oxygen, which is determined in the lung by alveolar ventilation and pulmonary diffusion capacity and in the blood by hemoglobin

content. In the absence of pulmonary disease, arterial oxygen content, and saturation generally remain similar to resting values throughout exercise, even at high levels (Myers, 2001).
  d. Venous oxygen content is determined by the amount of blood flow directed to the muscle and by capillary density. Muscle blood flow increases with exercise not only because of increased cardiac output, but also by the preferential redistribution of the cardiac output (>85% of total CO) to the exercising muscle. A decrease in local and systemic vascular resistance also facilitates greater skeletal muscle flow. Finally, there is an increase in the overall number of capillaries with training (Myers, 2001).

- **Metabolic equivalents (METs):** A convenient measure for expressing oxygen uptake. One MET is a unit of sitting, resting oxygen requirements (3.5 mL O_2/ kg body weight/min).
  a. 1 MET = Basal O_2 requirements (e.g., sitting)
  b. 5 METs = Energy cost for *activities of daily living* (ADLs), poor prognosis for anginal patients, consider catheterization
  c. 10 METs = Same prognosis with medical treatment versus *coronary artery bypass grafting* (CABG)
  d. 13 METs = Excellent prognosis regardless of other exercise responses
  e. 18 METs = Elite athletes

- **Myocardial oxygen consumption:** The "double product," an indirect measurement of myocardial oxygen consumption, measures the product of maximum or peak HR and systolic blood pressure. Angina normally occurs at the same double product rather than the same external workload. A normal value is considered greater than 25,000.

PERFORMING THE EXERCISE STRESS TEST

INDICATIONS

- The three major cardiopulmonary reasons for EST relate to diagnosis, prognosis, and therapeutic prescription (ACC/AHA Guidelines for Exercise Testing, 1997; White and Evans, 2001).

CLASS I
- Conditions for which there is general consensus that EST is justified
  a. To assist in the diagnosis of *coronary artery disease* (CAD) in those adult patients with an intermediate (20–80%) pretest probability of disease

b. To assess functional capacity and to aid in the prognosis of patients with known CAD

c. To evaluate the prognosis and functional capacity of patients with known CAD soon after an uncomplicated *myocardial infarction* (MI)

d. To evaluate patients with symptoms consistent with recurrent, exercise-induced cardiac arrhythmias

CLASS II

• Conditions which are frequently used but in which there is a divergence of opinion regarding medical effectiveness of EST

a. To evaluate asymptomatic males >45 years (females >55 years) with special occupations

b. To evaluate asymptomatic males >45 years (females >55 years) with two or more cardiac risk factors.

c. To evaluate asymptomatic males >45 years (females >55 years) who plan to enter a vigorous exercise program

d. To assist in the diagnosis of CAD in adult patients with a high or low pretest probability of disease

e. To evaluate patients with a class I indication who have baseline *electrocardiogram* (EKG) changes

CLASS III

• Conditions for which there is general agreement the EST is of little to no value, inappropriate, or contraindicated

a. To assist in the diagnosis of CAD in patients with *left bundle-branch-block* (LBBB) or *Wolff Parkinson White* (WPW) on a resting EKG

b. To evaluate patients with simple *premature ventricular complexes* (PVCs) on a resting EKG with no other evidence for CAD

c. To evaluate men or women with chest discomfort not thought to be cardiac

• The above classes group the indications based on risk according to ACSM guidelines. Patients are categorized into low, moderate, and high-risk groups prior to beginning an exercise program. Risk stratification is based on age, sex, presence of CAD risk factors, major symptoms of disease, or known heart disease (NECP, 2001; American College of Sports Medicine, 2000*a*) (see Tables 20-1 and 20-2).

• **Low risk:** Asymptomatic younger individuals (men < age 45 years; women < age 55 years) and no more than 1 risk factor from Table 20-1.

TABLE 20-1   Coronary Artery Risk Factors Used for Risk Stratification

Positive Factors	
Family History	1. Myocardial infarction or
	2. Coronary revascularization or
	3. Sudden death
	(History of above occurring in male first-degree relative before age 55 years; history of above occurring before age 65 in female first-degree relatives)
Cigarette Smoking	1. Current smoker or
	2. Those who quit smoking in previous six months
Hypertension	1. Currently on antihypertensive medication or
	2. Systolic blood pressure ≥140 mm Hg.* or
	3. Diastolic blood pressure ≤90 mm Hg.*
	(*confirmed on two separate occasions)
Hypercholesterolemia	1. Total serum cholesterol >200 mg/dl or
	2. High-density lipoprotein cholesterol <40 mg/dl or
	3. Low-density lipoprotein cholesterol >100 mg/dl if CHD or CHD risk equivalent
	≥130 mg/dl if ≥2 risk factors
	≥160 mg/dl if 0-1 risk factors
Impaired Fasting Glucose	Fasting blood glucose ≥110 mg/dl
Obesity	1. Waist girth >102 cm (men) or >88 cm (women)
Sedentary Lifestyle	1. Persons not participating in regular exercise program or
	2. Not meeting the minimal physical activity recommendations from the U.S. Surgeon General's report
Negative Factors	
High Serum High-Density Lipoprotein Cholesterol	>60 mg/dL

SOURCE: Expert Panel, on Detection, Evaluation, and Treatment of High Blood Cholesterol in Adults. Summary of the third report of the national Cholesterol Education Program (NCP) expert panel on detection, evaluation, and treatment of high blood cholesterol in adults (Adult Treatment Panel III). *JAMA* 285:2486–2497, 2001.
ABBREVIATION: CHD = Coronary heart disease.

TABLE 20-2 Major Signs/Symptoms Suggestive of Cardiovascular and Pulmonary Disease

1. Pain or discomfort (or other anginal equivalent) in the chest, neck, jaw, arms, or other areas that may be caused by ischemia.
2. Dizziness, near-syncope or syncope
3. Palpitations or tachycardia
4. Shortness of breath at rest or with exertion
5. Orthopnea or paroxysmal nocturnal dyspnea
6. Ankle edema
7. Unusual fatigue with usual activities
8. Known heart murmur
9. Intermittent claudication

SOURCE: American College of Sports Medicine: *Guidelines for Exercise Testing and Prescription*, 6th ed. Baltimore, MD, Lippincott Williams & Wilkins, 2000, p 25.

- **Moderate risk:** Older individuals (men ≥ age 45 years; women ≥ age 55 years) or those individuals with ≥2 risk factors from Table 20-1.
- **High risk:** Individuals with one or more signs/symptoms from Table 20-2 or known cardiovascular, pulmonary, or metabolic disease.
- In addition, level of activity is divided into moderate (3–6 METS or 40–60% of $VO_{2\,max}$) and vigorous (>6 METS or >60% of $VO_{2\,max}$) exercise. Clinicians use these factors to recommend which patients need a stress test (American College of Sports Medicine, 2000a):
  a. Low risk individuals do not need an EST regardless of level of activity.
  b. Moderate risk individuals should have a stress test prior to beginning vigorous exercise only.
  c. High risk individuals need a stress test before any moderate or vigorous activity.
- Risk stratification of patients for diagnosis of CAD divides patients into those with typical angina, atypical angina, nonanginal chest pain, or no chest pain. There are also special disease groups (e.g., diabetes mellitus) that have specific indications for testing (American Diabetes Association, 2003).

CONTRAINDICATIONS

- In some individuals there may be contraindications to performing the procedure.

ABSOLUTE CONTRAINDICATIONS
  a. Acute MI
  b. A recent significant change in EKG
  c. Unstable angina
  d. Rapid ventricular or atrial arrhythmias
  e. History suggesting medicine toxicity
  f. Severe aortic stenosis
  g. Uncontrolled congestive *heart failure* (CHF)
  h. Suspected dissecting aortic aneurysm

  i. Active myocarditis or pericarditis
  j. Active thrombophlebitis
  k. Recent embolism
  l. Active infection
  m. Uncooperative patient

RELATIVE CONTRAINDICATIONS
- Risks of performing procedure may outweigh benefits.
  a. Uncontrolled tachyarrhythmias or bradyarrhythmias
  b. Frequent ventricular ectopic activity
  c. Untreated pulmonary hypertension
  d. Systemic *blood pressure* (BP) >200/110
  e. Ventricular aneurysm
  f. Moderate aortic stenosis/ Hypertrophic cardiomyopathy
  g. Marked cardiac enlargement
  h. Uncontrolled metabolic disease
  i. Chronic infectious disease
  j. Known left main artery disease
  k. Electrolyte abnormalities
  l. Neuromuscular, musculoskeletal disorders that prohibit exercise or are exacerbated by exercise

SPECIAL CONSIDERATIONS

- There are special situations in which the physician must evaluate the patient carefully before doing an EST. These patients are usually put into one of three groups: conduction disturbances (AV blocks, LBBB, WPW), medication effects (beta blockers, calcium channel blockers), and special clinical situations (unstable hypertension, previous MI, known CAD). In these situations, consultation with a cardiologist and/or referral for an imaging study may be warranted (White and Evans, 2001).

PHYSICIAN RESPONSIBILITIES

- During exercise testing, the physician's responsibilities include the following:

PRETEST PATIENT EVALUATION AND CLEARANCE
  a. Review of medical history
  b. Performance of a cardiac exam to evaluate for murmurs or gallops
  c. Clarification of EST indications and exclusion of those with contraindications
  d. Consent of patient and documentation of risks versus benefits
  e. Obtaining a resting baseline EKG and evaluation for abnormalities

PROTOCOL SELECTION

- The physician must decide whether the patient needs a maximal or submaximal test. Most information is obtained from the maximal test, as a true peak maximal HR is achieved, rather than an age-predicted maximal heart rate. If one chooses a symptom-limited maximal test, the patient is in control and the most information is gained. Submaximal testing is generally reserved for patients being discharged from the hospital after an MI. Examples of tests include the following:
  a. Bruce (most common, each stage changes in both speed and grade)
  b. Modified Bruce (less rigorous)
  c. Balke-Ware (smaller workloads, used in cardiac/older patients)
  d. Ramp (most accurate and physiologic in predicting measured oxygen uptake; slow, continuous increase in workload)
  e. Cycle or arm ergometry (if unable to use treadmill)

RUNNING THE TEST

- A pretest checklist should be instituted which includes an equipment and safety check, consent and pretest assessment, supine and standing EKGs, blood pressure measurements, treadmill protocol selection, and indications for termination. During the exercise test, the patient should be monitored continuously along with EKG and BP readings at each stage. The patient should be alerted to stage changes, and the test should be terminated when the patient reaches maximal effort or exhibits clinical signs requiring termination of the test:
  a. Absolute indications for termination of EST
    1. Patient's request
    2. Decreasing systolic blood pressure with increased work
    3. Severe chest pain, vertigo, ataxia, and/or mental confusion
    4. Serious dysrhythmias (e.g., ventricular tachycardia)
    5. Evidence of an acute MI
    6. Malfunction of equipment
    7. Failure of increasing heart-rate response
  b. Relative indications for termination of EST
    1. Moderate chest pain, claudication, or dyspnea
    2. Marked >2-mm horizontal or downsloping ST depression
    3. Hypertensive BP response >250/115
    4. BP failing to rise at least 22 mm Hg during the first 3 stages
    5. Acute onset of bundle branch block
    6. Less serious dysrhythmias such as supraventricular tachycardia

- Recovery includes immediately placing the patient in the supine position or allowing a "cool-down walk" and then placing the patient in a chair. Maximal test sensitivity is achieved with the patient supine postexercise. Auscultate for abnormal heart sounds and obtain BP and EKG every 1 to 2 min. Monitor until clinically stable and EKG has returned to normal.

INTERPRETATION OF THE TEST

- Interpreting the exercise test involves much more than describing whether the test was "positive" or "negative" for ischemia. The written report should include the HR and blood pressure response, the presence or absence of symptoms, any dysrhythmias, the functional aerobic capacity, EKG changes, and the presence or absence of myocardial ischemia (Evans, Harris, and Ellestad, 2001).

HEART RATE RESPONSE

- An increase in HR occurs with aerobic exercise secondary to a withdrawal of vagal tone and an increase in sympathetic tone. The increase is linear and correlates with workload and oxygen uptake. The maximum HR should be reported as a percentage of the predicted maximal HR (220-age). The failure of the HR to elevate above 120 with maximum exercise is defined as chronotropic incompetence and suggests possible underlying CAD. Chronotropic incompetence is an independent predictor of mortality (Ellestad, 1996b; Lauer et al, 1999). Abnormal HR recovery (HRR), defined as the failure of the HR to decrease by 12 beats/min during the first minute of recovery, portends an increased mortality for the patient (Cole et al, 1999).

BLOOD PRESSURE RESPONSE

- As work increases, there is a corresponding increase in the systolic BP that peaks at maximum exercise. A drop in systolic BP during exercise is very suggestive of associated ischemic dysfunction of the myocardium (Froelicher and Myers, 2000). Diastolic BP remains the same or decreases. An increase in diastolic BP of >10 mmHg is abnormal and can be considered a hypertensive response to exercise. The post-exercise systolic BP response (SBPR) has also been described. A three minute systolic BP/peak systolic BP > 0.90 is considered abnormal with a diagnostic accuracy of 75% for CAD (Taylor and Beller, 1998).

SIGNS AND SYMPTOMS

- The presence or absence of symptoms such as chest pain, claudication, or exercise-induced wheezing needs to be mentioned in the report. Patients with exercise-induced angina have been shown to have a worse prognosis than patients with only ST depression (Ellestad, 1996c). Therefore, these patients, even in the absence of EKG ischemic changes, should be regarded as having a test "suggestive of myocardial ischemia." Another parameter worth mentioning is the *rate of perceived exertion* (RPE). It is valuable to measure during exercise testing as it correlates well with HR and VO_2. The Borg scale assigns a number 0–10 to the RPE with a higher number indicative of more difficult exertion (Borg, Holmgren, and Lindblad, 1981).

DYSRHYTHMIAS/CONDUCTION DISTURBANCES

- Ectopy or dysrhythmias that occur during the exercise test should be mentioned on the report. Unifocal pre-*mature ventricular contractions* (PVCs) are seen frequently during testing and are not specific for myocardial ischemia, although if frequent may increase the long-term risk of cardiovascular death in asymptomatic patients (Evans and Froelicher, 2001; Jouven et al, 2000). High-grade ectopy (couplets, mutiforme/ multifocal PVCs, ventricular tachycardia) is more suggestive of severe ischemic heart disease and higher mortality than those without ectopy (Califf et al, 1983). Supraventricular dysrhythmias (atrial-fibrillation/flutter) require termination of the test and further intervention. Intracardiac blocks can occur before, during, or after testing and advanced forms of AV block (Mobitz II and higher) are abnormal. Bundle branch blocks occur very infrequently with exercise and require further evaluation, especially LBBB which may portend an increased mortality if there is structural heart disease (Evans and Froelicher, 2001).

AEROBIC CAPACITY

- The EST can either measure the maximal functional aerobic capacity (VO_{2max}) by direct gas analysis or estimate from workload performed in a maximal test. A nomogram is used to convert minutes (or METs) into VO_{2max}. The results can then be compared with standard tables of fitness levels for age and sex (American College of Sports Medicine, 2000b).

ELECTROCARDIOGRAPHIC RESPONSES TO EXERCISE TESTING

- ST segment changes are the most common signs of ischemia. ST segment depression is subendocardial, and one cannot localize ischemia based on EKG location of the ST depression. ST segment elevation is transmural, and the location of the anatomic obstruction correlates with the associated EKG changes.

NORMAL RESPONSES WITH EXERCISE
- The PR segment shortens and slopes downward in the inferior leads. The QRS complex may show increased Q wave negativity and a decrease in R wave amplitude with an increased S wave depth. The J point becomes depressed with exercise. If already elevated at rest, it will commonly normalize. The T wave decreases in amplitude and the ST segment develops a positive upslope that returns to baseline within 60–80 m.

ABNORMAL RESPONSES WITH EXERCISE (FARDY, YANOWITZ, AND WILSON, 1988)
- ST segment depression: This is the hallmark of ischemia and a positive treadmill (see next section).
- ST segment normalization: ST segments that are depressed and return to normal (pseudonormalization) are suggestive of ischemia.
- ST segment elevation: In patients without a prior history of MI, consider acute MI (if accompanied by chest pain), or serious transmural ischemia. ST elevation over Q waves in patients with a previous history of an MI suggests areas of dyskinesis or ventricular aneurysm (Evans and Karunarante, 1992b).
- U wave inversion: U wave inversion during exercise is suggestive of ischemia.

FINAL DETERMINATION FOR MYOCARDIAL ISCHEMIA

- One of four descriptions should appear in the patient's written report to represent the final determination for myocardial ischemia (American Heart Association Scientific Statement, 2001; Ellestad, 1996b; Evans and Karunarante, 1992b; Lachterman et al, 1990):
  a. Positive
    1. Horizontal or downsloping ST segment depression that is ≥1mm at 60 ms past the J point
    2. Horizontal or upsloping ST segment elevation that is ≥1mm at 60 ms past the J point
    3. Upsloping ST depression that is ≥1.5 mm depressed at 80 ms past the J point

b. Suggestive
   1. Horizontal or downsloping ST segment depression between 0.5 mm and 1 mm at 60 s past the J point
   2. ST elevation b/w 0.5–1.0 mm
   3. Upsloping ST segment depression that is greater than 0.7 mm but less than 1.5 mm at 80 ms past J point
   4. Exercise-induced hypotension
   5. Chest pain occurring with exercise typical of angina
   6. Frequent, high grade, ventricular ectopy
   7. A new third heart sound or murmur at peak exercise
   8. Abnormal 1-min HRR or 3-min systolic BP response
   9. ST-segment depression in recovery only
   10. Normalization of abnormal ST-segments/ T-wave inversion
c. Negative
   1. Above criteria not met and the patient exercised to at least 85% of predicted HR_{max}
d. Inconclusive
   1. The patient does not reach 85% of maximum predicted HR and there is no evidence of ischemia based on the above criteria. (Be sure the patient is not on B-Blockers or has chronotropic incompetence.)

CLINICAL DECISION MAKING

• Physicians can use the results of the exercise test to guide them in the management of their patients. This approach should include a probability statement of CAD and a prediction of severity of CAD, prognosis of the likelihood of future adverse events in a patient based on the *exercise treadmill score* (ETS), and exercise prescription.

PROBABILITY OF CAD

• The exercise test has a role in the diagnosis of CAD with an overall 75% sensitivity and 80% specificity. The predictive value, however, depends on the prevalence of CAD in the population tested. It is therefore imperative to determine a pretest probability of CAD in a patient, and then use the results of the treadmill to determine a new posttest likelihood. Exercise stress testing has the greatest value in those individuals who have a pretest probability between 20 and 80%. Diamond and Forrester have created tables to predict the pretest/posttest likelihood of disease based on age,

sex, and clinical symptoms (Diamond and Forrester, 1979). Two examples serve to illustrate this point:
a. A 40-year old male with atypical angina has a pretest probability of about 35%. If he has between 1 and 2 mm of ST depression on EST, his posttest probability of CAD becomes nearly 70%, a much more significant risk elucidated by EST.
b. A 40-year old female with atypical angina has a pretest probability of less than 10%. If she has between 1 and 2 mm of ST depression, her posttest probability of CAD still is less than 20%, and little is gained from the EST.

PREDICTION OF SEVERITY OF CAD

• A suggestive or positive written report may be used to further manage patients by predicting the severity of CAD. Upsloping, horizontal, and downsloping ST depression correlate respectively with a worsening extent of CAD. The following are important exercise test predictors of severe CAD (Goldschlager, Selzer, and Cohn, 1976):
a. ST depression, >2.5 mm
b. ST depression beginning at low workload, <5 METS
c. Downsloping configuration (99% predictive of CAD) or ST elevation
d. Prolonged ST depression lasting >8 min into rest
e. Global ST depression
f. Serious dysrhythmias at low HR (<130 bpm)
g. U wave inversion
h. Low workload ability, <5 METs
i. Exercise induced hypotension
j. Chronotropic incompetence
k. Anginal symptoms
• ST depression only at high workloads (HR >160 bpm or changes only after Stage IV—Bruce protocol at 12 min) correlates with a low mortality and good prognosis in patients. In fact, the ability to exercise >13 METs has a good prognosis regardless of the EKG changes. Many cardiologists recommend repeating the exercise test in 6 months without further workup in these patients (Goldschlager, Selzer, and Cohn, 1976).

EXERCISE TREADMILL SCORE

• This tool supports the above concepts by assigning a score to determine prognosis (Mark et al, 1987; 1991):

Treadmill score = Exercise duration (min) − 5 × ST deviation (mm) − 4 × treadmill angina index. (TM angina index = 0 if no exercise angina, 1 for exercise angina, and 2 for exercise-limiting angina)

- If score is up to +5, the patient has a very good prognosis and can be followed safely with regular exercise testing. The 5-year survival for this group was 97%. A patient in the high-risk group (TM score ≤11) has a poor prognosis with a 5-year mortality >25%. The ET score is thus valuable for prognosis and should be calculated in all patients undergoing CAD evaluation.

EXERCISE PRESCRIPTION (ACC/AHA GUIDELINES FOR EXERCISE TESTING, 1997; AMERICAN COLLEGE OF SPORTS MEDICINE, 2000a)

- The exercise test can assist in writing the exercise prescription. A symptom-limited test establishes a baseline fitness level and establishes a parameter for improving fitness. The ACSM recommends exercise intensities between 55 and 90% of HR_{max}, or 50–85% of $VO_{2\,max}$. The conditioning range for most adults to improve cardiorespiratory fitness is between 70 and 85% of HR_{max} (65–80% $VO_{2\,max}$).

SPECIAL CONSIDERATIONS IN ATHLETES

- There are no specific indications for testing athletes, although they are tested occasionally for fitness and exercise prescription. The Bruce protocol, with gas exchange to establish a $VO_{2\,max}$, is most often employed. The Astrand, Costill, or ramp protocols may also be used (Marolf, Kuhn, and White, 2001).
- Athletes manifest many differences than the general population both clinically and on EKG. They commonly have increased ventricular volume and mass, along with sinus bradyarrhythmias. It is not uncommon to see certain EKG findings such as 1st degree AV blocks, right axis deviation, ventricular hypertrophy with repolarization abnormalities, or incomplete right bundle branch block. All these findings are normal variants known as the athletic heart syndrome (Hughston, Puffer, and Rodney, 1985).
- Interpretation of the exercise test in this population incorporates the same criteria as the general population; however, because of the variants stated above, there is a greater probability of a false positive test.

SUMMARY

- The EST remains a valuable tool for diagnosing coronary artery disease, evaluating prognosis, and developing an exercise prescription. By implementing the

test appropriately, the primary care physician can enhance its validity and usefulness in clinical decision making.

REFERENCES

ACC/AHA Guidelines for Exercise Testing: A Report of the American College of Cardiology/American Heart Association Task Force on Practice Guidelines (Committee on Exercise Testing). *JACC* 30(3):260–311, July 1997.

American College of Sports Medicine: *Guidelines for Exercise Testing and Prescription,* 6th ed. Baltimore, MD, Lippincott Williams & Wilkins, 2000a, pp 22–32.

American College of Sports Medicine: *Guidelines for Exercise Testing and Prescription,* 6th ed. Philadelphia, PA, Lippincott Williams & Wilkins, 2000b, pp 308–309.

American Diabetes Association: Clinical practice recommendations 2003: Physical activity/exercise and diabetes mellitus. *Diabetes Care* 26(Suppl 1):S73–S77, 2003.

American Heart Association Scientific Statement: Exercise standards for testing and training. *Circulation* 104:1694–1740, 2001.

Borg G, Holmgren A, Lindblad I: Quantitative evaluation of chest pain. *Acta Med Scand* 644:43–45, 1981.

Califf RKM, McKinnis RA, McNeer M, et al: Prognostic value of ventricular arrhythmias for suspected ischemic heart disease. *J Am Coll Cardiol* 2:1060–1067, 1983.

Cole CR, Blackstone EH, Pashkow EJ, et al: Heart rate recovery immediately after exercise as a predictor of mortality. *N Engl J Med* 341:1351–1357, 1999.

Diamond GA, Forrester JS: Analysis of probability as an aid in the clinical diagnosis of coronary artery disease. *N Engl J Med* 300:1350–1358, 1979.

Ellestad MH: *Stress Testing: Principles and Practice,* 4th ed. Philadelphia, PA, FA Davis, 1996a, pp 327–328.

Ellestad MH: *Stress Testing: Principles and Practice,* 4th ed. Philadelphia, PA, FA Davis, 1996b, pp 337–339.

Ellestad MH: *Stress Testing: Principles and Practice,* 4th ed. Philadelphia, PA, FA Davis, 1996c, pp 565–569.

Evans CH, Froelicher VF: Some common abnormal responses to exercise testing: What to do when you see them. *Prim Care* 28:219–231, 2001.

Evans CH, Harris G, Ellestad MH: A basic approach to the interpretation of the exercise test. *Prim Care* 28:73–98, 2001.

Evans CH, Karunarante HB: Exercise stress testing for the family physician. Part I, Performing the Test. *Am Fam Physician* 45:121–132, 1992a.

Evans CH, Karunarante HB: Exercise stress testing for the family physician. Part II, Interpretation of the results. *Am Fam Physician* 45:679–688, 1992b.

Fardy PS, Yanowitz FG, Wilson PK: *Cardiac Rehabilitation, Adult Fitness, and Exercise Testing,* 2nd ed. Philadelphia, PA, Lea & Febiger, 1988.

Froelicher VF, Myers J: *Exercise and the Heart,* 4th ed. St. Louis, MO, Mosby-YearBook, 2000, pp 113–117.

Froelicher VF, Fearon W, Ferguson C, et al: Lessons learned from studies of the standard exercise test? *Chest* 116:1442–1451, 1999.

Goldschlager N, Selzer A, Cohn K: Treadmill stress tests as indicators of presence and severity of coronary artery disease. *Ann Intern Med* 85:277–286, 1976.

Hammond HK, Froelicher VP: Normal and abnormal heart rate responses to exercise. *Prog Cardiovasc Dis* 27:271–296, 1985.

Hughston TP, Puffer JC, Rodney WM: The athletic heart syndrome. *N Engl J Med* 313:24–32, 1985.

Jouven X, Zuriek M, Desnos M, et al: Long-term outcome in asymptomatic men with exercise-induced premature ventricular depolarizations. *N Engl J Med* 343:826–833, 2000.

Lachterman B, Lehmann KG, Abrahamson D, et al: "Recovery only" ST segment depression and the predictive accuracy of the exercise test. *Ann Intern Med* 112:11–16, 1990.

Lauer MS, Francis GS, Okim PM, et al: Impaired chronotropic response to exercise stress testing as a predictor of mortality. *JAMA* 281:524–529, 1999.

Mark DB, Hlathy MA, Harrell FE, Jr, et al: Exercise treadmill score for predicting prognosis in coronary artery disease. *Ann Intern Med* 106:793–800, 1987.

Mark DB, Shaw L, Harrell FE, Jr, et al: Prognostic value of a treadmill exercise score in outpatients with suspected coronary artery disease. *N Engl J Med* 325:849–853, 1991.

Marolf GA, Kuhn A, White RD: Exercise testing in special populations: Athletes, women, and the elderly. *Prim Care* 28:55–72, 2001.

Mellion MB: *Office Sports Medicine*, 2nd ed. Philadelphia, PA, Hanley & Belfus, 1996.

Myers JN: The physiology behind exercise testing. *Prim Care* 28:5–24, 2001.

NCEP: Executive summary of the third report of the National Cholesterol Education Program (NCEP) Expert Panel on Detection, Evaluation, and Treatment of High Blood Cholesterol in Adults (Adult Treatment Panel III). *JAMA* 285:2486–2497, 2001.

Taylor AJ, Beller GA: Postexercise systolic blood pressure response: Clinical application to the assessment of ischemic heart disease. *Am Fam Physician* 58:1126–1130, 1998.

White RD, Evans CH: Performing the exercise test. *Prim Care* 28:29–37, 2001.

21 GAIT ANALYSIS

D Casey Kerrigan, MD
Ugo Della Croce, PhD

INTRODUCTION

- Gait, referring to humans walking and running, is one of the most obvious and fundamental actions in life.
- Recognizing and describing gait patterns is just the first step toward appreciating the complexity of gait

physiology. When trying to improve upon a person's gait pattern, the complexity of gait becomes evident.

- The ultimate goal of gait analysis is to understand the complex relationships between an individual's capabilities/impairments and the person's gait pattern, so as to enhance performance while preventing injury (Birrer et al, 2001).
- Gait analysis is also used to understand the effects of external biomechanical factors such as shoes or orthoses.

GAIT CYCLE

- The basic unit of walking and running is the *gait cycle*, or *stride*. Perry and colleagues described various temporal and functional variables within the gait cycle (Kerrigan and Edelstein, 2001), which have become a standard reference to describe gait (Fig. 21-1).
- Walking gait cycle timing is primarily divided into *double support* and *single support* phases.
- When focusing on each leg's activity, the cycle is divided into the *stance* and *swing* periods which begin at initial and final contact of the foot, respectively.
- When focusing on functional aspects of gait, the walking gait cycle can be divided into three functional tasks: *weight acceptance*, *single limb support* and *limb advancement*; the first two occurring during stance and the third occurring primarily during swing. The tasks are further subdivided into eight phases: weight acceptance comprises *initial contact* and *loading response*, single limb support comprises *midstance*, *terminal stance* and *preswing*, and limb advancement comprises *initial swing*, *mid-swing*, and *terminal swing*.
- *Temporal-spatial gait parameters consist of the following: Stride time* refers to the time from initial contact of one foot to initial contact of the same foot, *step time* refers to the time from initial contact of one foot to initial contact of the opposite foot, *stride length* and *step length* refer to the distances traversed during the respective times. *Gait velocity* is the ratio between stride length and stride time. *Cadence* of gait refers to the stride (or step) frequency, i.e., the number of strides (or steps) per unit of time.
- Temporal-spatial parameters can be effectively measured during either walking or running with pressure mats (cellular mats measuring foot pressure), force platforms (dynamometers sensing ground reaction forces in time), and motion analysis (system of stereophotogrammetric cameras for 3D reconstruction of body motion,

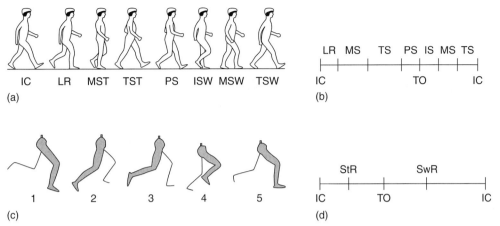

FIG. 21-1   The gait cycle. (a) Walking figure. (b) Walking gait cycle: IC, initial contact; LR, loading response; TO, toe off; MS, midstance; TS, terminal stance; PS, preswing; IS, initial swing; MS, midswing; TS, terminal swing. (c) Running figure: 1. Stance phase absorption. 2. Stance phase generation. 3. Swing phase generation. 4. Swing phase reversal. 5. Swing phase absorption. (d) Running gait cycle: IC, initial contact; TO, toe off; StR, stance phase reversal; SwR, swing phase reversal; absorption, from SwR through IC to StR; generation, from StR through TO to SwR. (From Novacheck, 1998).

including foot contact timing). Temporal, but not spatial parameters can be measured with footswitches (on/off devices detecting foot contact timing).

• Temporal-spatial features of walking and running differ substantially. During walking, at least one foot is always on the ground while during the majority of running neither foot is in contact with the ground. While walking has two double-support phases, running has two phases of *double float* during the swing period. The percentages of time in stance and swing are reversed in walking and running: about 60% and 40% respectively for walking and about 40% and 60%, respectively for running (Fig. 21-2) (Novacheck, 1998; Perry, 1992). During normal walking at an average walking speed, each double-limb support time comprises approximately 10% of the gait cycle while single-limb support comprises about 40%. Typical values (Kerrigan and Edelstein, 2001) of temporal gait parameters in healthy young adults, walking comfortably on a level surface, are summarized in Table 21-1.

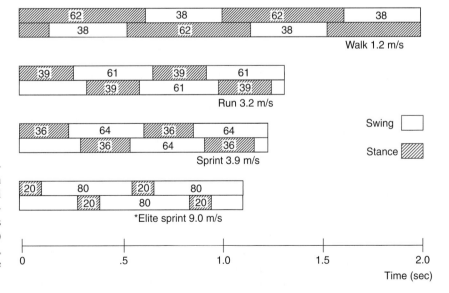

FIG. 21-2   Variation in gait cycle parameters with speed of movement. For each condition, the bar graph begins at initial contact on the left and represents two complete gait cycles or strides. Note that as speed increases, time spent in swing (clear) increases, stance time (shaded) decreases, double float increases, and cycle time shortens (From Novacheck, 1998).

TABLE 21-1   Typical Values of Some Temporal and Spatial Walking Gait Variables

TEMPORAL/SPATIAL VARIABLE	AVERAGE VALUE
Velocity (m/min)	~80
Cadence (steps/min)	113
Stride length (m)	1.41
Stance (percent of gait cycle)	~60
Swing (percent of gait cycle)	~40
Double support (percent per leg per gait cycle)	~10

At slower walking speeds, double-limb support times are greater. Conversely, with increasing walking speeds, double-limb support time intervals decrease. Walking becomes running when there is no longer an interval of time in which both feet are in contact with the ground.

KINEMATICS

- The kinematics (motion) of an individual while walking or running can be effectively assessed by modeling the individual's body as a multibody system. A multibody system is composed of links (body segments) and joints between the links. The kinematics of the system is completely known when orientation and position of each of its segments is known. Joint angles are obtained from the kinematics of both joint distal and proximal segments. Joint angular velocities are obtained from the joint angles and refer to the rapidity of variation of such angles. Joint accelerations are similarly obtained from joint velocities.

- Each segment possesses a *center of mass* (CoM). A whole body CoM can also be defined as the point at the center of the body mass distribution. As segments move, the whole body CoM moves. Its position in time is important for both balance and energy related issues (Birrer et al, 2001).

- With quantitative 3D gait analysis, joint angles throughout the gait cycle are described with respect to flexion/extension, ab/adduction and internal/external rotation. CoM position in time is expressed in vertical, anterior–posterior and mediolateral time histories.

- Both joint and CoM kinematics are obtained from the instantaneous 3D position of markers attached on the individual's body segments.

- Joint kinematics patterns during running differ somewhat from the patterns during walking. Hip flexion/extension and ab/adduction ranges are wider in running (about 60° and 15°, respectively) than in walking (about 40° and 10°, respectively) (Novacheck, 1998; Perry, 1992). Hip and knee full extension is reached only during walking. Maximum knee flexion is higher in running (about 90°) than walking (about 60°). Ankle joint angle ranges are greater in running (about 50°) than in walking (about 30°).

- During walking the CoM trajectory reaches its highest point in stance when its speed is minimum. During running the CoM trajectory reaches its maximum height during the double floating phase at which time its velocity is maximum.

KINETICS

- *Kinetics* is defined as the study of forces and moments that cause movement.

- *Ground reaction forces* refer to the forces exerted on the foot during foot contact. They are measured with force platforms embedded in the ground, over which the individual walks or runs. The center of the distribution of these forces is called *center of pressure*. Knowing segment kinematics and ground reaction forces, in addition to some segment characteristics such as mass and CoM location, it is possible to estimate joint kinetics (*joint forces* and *moments*). Joint moments refer to forces applied at a distance from a joint and are expressed as either external (due to the ground reaction force, gravity, and inertia) or internal due to internal structures including muscle, ligamentous, and bony structures. Joint *powers* indicate the rate of work operated by the joint muscles, and are obtained by multiplying the joint moment by the joint angular velocity.

- To measure ground reaction forces and center of pressure trajectory, one force platform per foot contact is sufficient. To measure joint kinetics, a combination of measurements synchronously obtained from force platforms and a motion analysis system is necessary.

- The vertical ground reaction force typically demonstrates an initial peak at the very first contact of the heel, and then a force absorption and a force generation phase. During walking, in addition to a peak at initial contact at the heel, the pattern of the vertical reaction force shows two maxima—one during the force absorption phase and another during the force generation phase. During running, a single maximum is present which divides absorption from generation. In running, maximum and minimum values are dependent on the speed of the runner. The amplitude of the pattern during running can be threefold the amplitude during walking (Novacheck, 1998).

- Sagittal ankle joint moment (flexion/extension moment) patterns in running and walking are similar. In running the joint moment activity is faster (shorter stance phase) and more intense (greater maximum amplitude). Knee sagittal moment in running demonstrates higher amplitude after initial contact than during walking. Hip sagittal moments patterns are similar during walking and running, except for the amplitude which is greater in running (Novacheck, 1998).

- Ankle, knee, and hip power patterns during walking are very similar to those obtained during running; however, the amplitudes of power absorption and generation are directly related to the individual speed (greater powers for higher speeds).

DYNAMIC ELECTROMYOGRAPHY

- Knowledge of the activation phases of the main lower limb muscles, in association with the joint moment patterns, can provide an effective description of overall gait function. While joint moments provide information regarding the effect of action of all the muscles involved, the knowledge of the activation patterns allows us to discriminate in time the muscle groups that are responsible for the observed joint moment (Perry, 1992).
- Surface *electromyography* (EMG) is the most common method for detecting muscle activity during gait. Current dynamic EMG systems allow one to detect EMG signals from up to 16 muscles at a time, which can be synchronized to both motion analysis systems and force platforms.
- Activation patterns of lower limb muscles during a running gait cycle are different from those observed during a walking gait cycle with respect to both timing and duration of activity. Figure 21-3 illustrates the phases of muscle activity during running. In general, muscle activity during running begins earlier in the swing period and lasts for a relatively longer time during the stance period. During walking the quadriceps are active at the end of swing through 25% of the stance period while during running and sprinting they continue to be active through 50 to 100% of the stance period. Similarly, the hamstrings are active earlier in swing during running and continue nearly to the end of the stance period while in walking they cease activity early

in stance. The ankle dorsiflexors during walking are active from late stance until early stance; while during running they continue to be active through midstance. During walking the ankle plantarflexors are active only during stance from loading response or midstance to terminal stance; while in running they are active in terminal swing through mid to terminal stance (Perry, 1992).

OXYGEN CONSUMPTION

- Measurement of oxygen consumption is typically obtained with pulmonary gas exchange devices, which are usually wearable and can be used outside a laboratory. Respiratory volumes of O_2 and CO_2 can be monitored during the execution of the motor task.
- The measurement of oxygen consumption provides information regarding the economy of gait. Walking energy expenditure per unit of distance is highly dependent on walking speeds. At natural walking speed, energy expenditure is lower than at both lower and higher speeds. In running, this dependency is not as evident. In both running and walking the highest energy expenditure per distance unit occurs at slower speed.

OVERALL GAIT EVALUATION

- Clinically meaningful information can be obtained from the wealth of data gathered from the measurement instruments and analysis techniques reported here. By relating EMG, kinetic, and kinematic patterns, it is possible to describe and evaluate the function of gait at a local level (i.e., the joint). By combining CoM time histories and more complete segmental kinematic information with oxygen consumption measurements, an overall evaluation of the energetics of gait at a global level is possible.
- While during walking the total energy (kinetic plus potential) is almost constant throughout the cycle, in

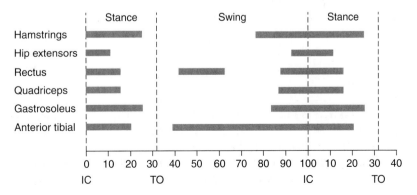

FIG. 21-3 Solid bars representing the timing of active muscles in various phases of the gait cycle. (From Novacheck, 1998).

running the potential and the kinetic energies are in phase (i.e., when one is minimum or maximum, so is the other), which means that energy is periodically stored and released. This action is performed mainly by the muscle tendons, which behave as springs activated by the relevant muscles.

- In analyzing gait (in particular, an atypical gait pattern or an effect of a shoe-type, brace, musculoskeletal injury or impairment), at least two distinct qualities need to be considered. The first is energetics, i.e., how does the pattern, shoe, etc., affect energetics—this can be measured directly with oxygen consumption and indirectly with CoM calculations and by observing if EMG activities are consistent with kinetic needs. The second is risk for biomechanical injury, i.e., how does the pattern affect risk over time, for ligamentous, muscle, tendon, cartilage, or bone injury—this is best estimated with joint kinetics, in particular joint moments, which may be higher than normal indicating a greater risk for biomechanical injury.

REFERENCES

Birrer RB, Buzermanis S, DellaCorte MP, et al: Bio-mechanics of running, in O'Connor F, Wilder R (eds): *The Textbook of Running Medicine.* New York, NY, McGraw-Hill, 2001, pp 11–19.

Kerrigan DC, Edelstein JE: Gait, in Gonzalez EG, et al (eds.): *The Physiological Basis of Rehabilitation Medicine.* Boston, MA, Butterworth-Heinemann, 2001, pp 397–416.

Novacheck TF: The biomechanics of running. *Gait Posture* 7:77–95, 1998.

Perry J: *Gait Analysis: Normal and Pathological Function.* Thorofare, NJ, SLACK, 1992.

22 COMPARTMENT SYNDROME TESTING

John E Glorioso, MD
John H Wilckens, MD

INTRODUCTION

- Exertional leg pain is a common complaint in the running athlete. The differential diagnosis includes stress fracture, tibial stress reaction such as periostitis or medial tibial stress syndrome (shin splints), tendonitis, nerve compression or entrapment, and *chronic exertional compartment syndrome* (CECS).
- Though a classic history may suggest the diagnosis of CECS, an exercise challenge and measurement of compartmental pressures is essential to confirm the diagnosis.
- Intracompartmental pressure measurement is the most clinically useful test to rule out or confirm CECS as the etiology of exertional leg pain.

COMPARTMENT SYNDROMES

- Compartment syndrome exists when tissue pressures are elevated in a restricted fascial space resulting in decreased perfusion causing nerve and muscle ischemia.
- Compartment syndromes in the athlete can occur in two forms, acute and chronic. The distinction between the two is in the reversibility of the ischemic insult.
- In acute compartment syndrome, the ischemia is irreversible and rapidly leads to tissue necrosis unless emergently decompressed via fasciotomy.
  - Most commonly occurs with acute trauma (fracture) or soft tissue/muscle injury (crush injury, rhabdomyolysis)
  - A clinical diagnosis made by historical and physical examination findings. Characteristic findings include pain out of proportion to injury, presence of paresthesias and sensory deficits, tense and swollen compartment on palpation, decreased or loss of active motion, and severe pain with passive stretch.
- Treatment is emergent surgical decompression via fasciotomy.
- If doubt exists as to the diagnosis in the acute presentation, intracompartmental pressure measurements may be indicated prior to emergent fasciotomy.
- Resting intracompartmental pressures of greater than 30 mmHg is the generally accepted level that can be associated with decreased blood flow and resultant muscle and nerve ischemia (Andrish, 2003).
- CECS involves reversible ischemia that is exercise induced and occurs at a predictable distance/intensity of exertion.
  - This form is much more common in athletes.
  - The reversible ischemia of exertional compartment syndrome occurs secondary to a noncomplaint osseofascial compartment that is not responsive to the expansion of muscle volume that occurs with exercise.

- Characterized by recurrent episodes of a transient elevation in the intracompartmental pressure, which subsides with rest or cessation of activity.
  - Any athlete can develop CECS; however, runners are most commonly affected (Martens and Moeyersoons, 1990; Detmer et al, 1985; Pedowitz et al, 1990).
- Although compartment syndrome testing is useful in the diagnosis of acute compartment syndrome, the following discussion applies to the use of intracompartmental pressure measurements for the chronic exertional form of compartment syndrome.

THE LEG COMPARTMENTS

- The leg contains four anatomically distinct muscle compartments with structural support provided by the tibia and fibula. Each compartment is covered by a tight fascia.
- The anterior compartment contains muscles used for extension of the toes and dorsiflexion of the ankle: the tibialis anterior, the extensor hallucis longus, and the extensor digitorum longus. Blood supply to the anterior compartment is from the anterior tibial artery. The deep peroneal nerve provides innervation as it passes through the compartment.
- The lateral compartment contains the evertors of the foot: the peroneus longus and the peroneus brevis. Nerve supply is via the superficial peroneal nerve. Blood supply is from branches of the peroneal artery.
- The superficial posterior compartment contains the plantarflexors of the foot: the gastrocnemius, soleus, and plantaris. These muscles are supplied by branches of the tibial nerve.
- The deep posterior compartment contains the muscles of toe flexion, ankle plantarflexion and inversion, the flexor hallicus longus, the flexor digitorum longus, and the tibialis posterior. These muscles are supplied by the tibial nerve and posterior tibial artery.
- A 5th compartment has been described. The fascia surrounding the posterior tibialis has been described as a separate and distinct compartment (Davey, Rorabeck, and Fowler, 1984).

PATHOPHYSIOLOGY
- Four factors have been identified that may contribute to an increase in the intracompartmental pressure seen during exercise (McDermott et al, 1982):
  1. Enclosure of compartmental contents in an inelastic fascial sheath
  2. Increased volume of the skeletal muscle with exertion resulting from blood flow and edema
  3. Muscle hypertrophy as response to exercise
  4. Dynamic contraction factors due to the gait cycle

- The transient increase in pressure within the myofascial compartment compromises blood flow. When tissue perfusion is not adequate to meet the metabolic demands, the result is traversing neurologic and muscular ischemia, pain, and impairment of muscular function.

CLINICAL PRESENTATION
- In chronic exertional compartment syndrome, the characteristic complaint is recurrent exercise induced leg discomfort that occurs at a well-defined and reproducible point of activity and increases if the training persists.
- The quality of pain is described as a tight, cramplike, or squeezing ache over a specific compartment of the leg. Relief of symptoms occurs only with discontinuation of activity.
- Neurologic complaints such as paresthesias of the leg or foot with exertion may indicate involvement of the nerve traversing the compartment.
  - Nerve entrapment syndromes of the lower extremity often present with similar complaints and should be included in the differential diagnosis.
- At rest, the physical examination is commonly unremarkable with a normal gait and normal lower extremity examination. A muscle herniation through a fascial defect may be the only clinical abnormality noted.
- An exercise challenge followed by post exercise clinical examination is helpful in establishing the diagnosis (Glorioso and Wilckens, 2001a).
  - After reproduction of discomfort, the athlete should be assessed for tenderness, tightness, and swelling over the involved compartment.
  - The tenderness noted should involve the muscle mass and not the bone or muscle–tendon junction.
  - Neurologic and vascular examination should be completed.
- Though history may be suggestive of CECS, no physical examination finding can firmly establish the diagnosis (Styf and Korner, 1987; Kiuru et al, 2003). Diagnosis based solely on clinical presentation can lead to misdiagnosis, inappropriate therapy, and/or delay of proper therapy (Pedowitz et al, 1990).

INDICATIONS FOR INTRACOMPARTMENTAL PRESSURE MEASUREMENTS
- Any patient with clinical evidence of CECS should be considered for intracompartmental testing.
  - Significant historical features include a recurrent, exercise induced leg discomfort which increases as the training persists and dissipates on cessation of activity.

- Pain quality described as a tight, cramplike, or squeezing ache over a specific compartment of the leg.
- Paresthesias of the leg or foot with exertion.
- An exercise challenge with detailed physical examination immediately after reproduction of symptoms will lead to a more judicious use of invasive techniques (Glorioso and Wilckens, 2001a).

TECHNIQUES TO MEASURE COMPARTMENT PRESSURES

- Multiple techniques have been described for measuring both static and dynamic intramuscular pressures. Techniques include the needle manometer (Whitesides et al, 1975), the wick catheter (Mubarak et al, 1976), slit catheter (Rorabeck et al, 1981), continuous infusion (Matsen et al, 1976), and a solid-state transducer intracompartmental catheter (McDermott et al, 1982).
- The Stryker Intracompartmental Pressure Monitor (Stryker Corporation, Kalamazoo, Michigan) is a battery operated, hand-held, digital, fluid pressure monitor. This device has been found to be more accurate, versatile, convenient, and much less time consuming in the clinical setting (Hutchinson and Ireland, 1999; Awbrey, Sienkiewicz, and Mankin, 1988).

PERFORMANCE OF THE PROCEDURE

- As intracompartmental pressure measurement is an invasive procedure, proper technical performance as well as patient safety demands a thorough knowledge of the anatomy of the leg. Prior to attempting to measure compartment pressures, the physician should ensure an understanding of the anatomical structures in each compartment so as to avoid damage to neurovascular structures.
- The athlete must be made aware of the indications of the procedure, and consent should be obtained and the athlete counseled on the risk of infection, scarring, damage to nerve and vascular structures, and reaction to local anesthesia.
- Two types of measurements may be obtained during the procedure, *static* or *dynamic*.
  1. Static, or intermittent, pressures are performed with a straight needle. Here, intracompartmental pressures are determined with a needle stick at rest and then again after exertion. The benefits of this procedure are that the athlete can perform activity causing symptoms without the measuring device attached to the leg and without an indwelling catheter in the compartment. Also, several compartments can be measured. A negative aspect of this technique is that it requires at least two needle stick into each compartment being evaluated (one

pre- and one postexertion). This procedure is most commonly used.
  2. Dynamic monitoring is performed with the use of a slit catheter inserted prior to exertion and taped/attached to the athlete's leg for continuous measurements. The benefit of this procedure is that the clinician can monitor the pressure changes during exertion without halting activity and that pressure monitoring during activity may be a more precise indicator of pathology (McDermott et al, 1982). There are several negative aspects of this technique. Problems include maintaining the placement of catheter in the compartment during activity, attachment of the system to the athlete, and restrictions of the athlete's gait as they run to reproduce symptoms. The procedure must be performed on a treadmill in order to continuously monitor pressure changes. Thus, the athlete cannot run outdoors on their usual training surface. In addition, only one compartment can be measured at a time. Some believe that with this technique, the results are inconsistent and difficult to obtain and interpret (Rorabeck et al, 1988; Rorabeck, Fowler, and Nott, 1988).
- With the static technique, measurements should be obtained at rest (prior to exertion), immediately after (1 min) the reproduction of symptoms, and 5–10 min into rest.
- To properly reproduce symptoms, athletes should perform the specific activity that causes pain/discomfort.
- Three factors may alter the pressure measurements:
  1. Proper calibration of the monitor is essential for reliable readings. The monitor must be zeroed at the same angle that will be used to penetrate the skin, and this angle must be maintained with repeated sticks.
  2. Joint position at both the knee and ankle affect pressures (Gershuni et al, 1984).
  3. Compression or squeezing the leg can alter pressures. Externally applied pressure is additive to any pressure already existing within the compartment (Matsen et al, 1976).
- Each compartment should be approached with an understanding of the anatomical contents of each compartment so as to avoid injury to neurovascular structures.

APPROACH TO EACH LEG COMPARTMENT

- Measurement of intracompartmental pressures is an invasive procedure. To avoid damage to neurovascular structures, each compartment should be approached with an understanding of the anatomical contents (Glorioso and Wilckens, 2001a).

Anterior Compartment

- Identify the muscle belly of the anterior tibialis just lateral to the anterior tibial border. Approach should have needle penetrate through fascia and into muscle belly of anterior tibialis at the level of the mid third of the tibia.
- Anatomical structures to avoid include the neurovascular bundle containing the deep peroneal nerve, anterior tibial artery, and veins. This neurovascular bundle sits just above the interosseous membrane.

Lateral Compartment

- The muscle bellies of the peroneus longus and brevis are palpable on the lateral surface of the leg just superficial to the shaft of the fibula.
- Helpful technique to enter this compartment involves palpation of the head of the fibula and lateral malleolus and palpating the muscle bellies at the midpoint between these two bony landmarks.
- The superficial peroneal nerve resides within this compartment and provides innervation. The lateral compartment receives it blood supply from branches of the peroneal artery, but does not itself run through the lateral compartment.

Posterior Superficial Compartment

- The muscle bellies of the gastrocnemius and soleus muscles are easily identified and palpated.
- Approach to this compartment just medial to the midline will avoid the small saphenous vein and the medial and lateral sural cutaneous nerves.
- Branches of the tibial nerve innervate these muscles.

Posterior Deep Compartment

- The approach to the posterior deep is technically more difficult because of the proximity of neurovascular structures.
- Two bundles are contained within this compartment that should be understood anatomically prior to needle insertion. A vascular bundle consisting of the peroneal artery and veins lies medial to the posterior aspect of the fibula. A neurovascular bundle consisting of the tibial nerve, posterior tibial artery, and veins lies in the posterior aspect of this compartment behind the mass of the tibialis posterior muscle.
- The posterior medial aspect of the mid tibia must first be palpated. The needle should then be inserted just posterior to the tibia, closely approximating the posterior border of the bone. The needle will first enter the flexor digitorum longus muscle and if guided deeper will enter the posterior tibialis muscle. As long as not driven too deeply, this approach will keep the needle anterior and medial to the neurovascular structures.

DIAGNOSTIC CRITERIA

- Compartment pressure must be obtained both preexercise and postexercise. Postexercise pressures should be performed immediately after an exercise challenge that reproduces the patient's symptoms.
- Findings consistent with the diagnosis of CECS include an elevated resting pressure, and increased postexertion pressure, and/or a delayed return to normal pressure after exertion.
- For chronic exertional compartment syndrome, the diagnostic criteria described by Pedowitz and colleagues are commonly used (Pedowitz et al, 1990). One or more of the following criteria must be met in addition to an appropriate history and physical examination:
  1. Preexercise ≥15 mmHg
  2. 1 min postexercise ≥30 mmHg
  3. 5 min postexercise ≥20 mmHg

DIFFERENTIAL DIAGNOSIS

- Stress fractures, periostitis/medial tibial stress syndrome, and tendonitis can usually be differentiated from CECS by clinical presentation; however, several syndromes present very similar to CECS and must be suspected when intracompartmental pressures are found to be normal.
- Nerve entrapment and compression may cause exertional leg pain. This diagnosis should always be suspected when patient presents with symptoms consistent with CECS, but who has normal pressures.
  - Common peroneal nerve entrapment presents as activity related pain, paresthesias, and/or numbness in the anterolateral aspect of the leg.
  - Superficial peroneal nerve entrapment presents with a history very similar to that of CECS of the lateral compartment.
  - Saphenous nerve entrapment presents as medial knee and medial leg pain.
  - Sural nerve entrapment will present with posterior calf symptoms and can be almost indistinguishable from CECS of the superficial posterior compartment.
  - Proximal tibial nerve entrapment also presents similar to CECS of the posterior compartment.
- Lumbosacral radiculopathy should be suspected in athletes with the complaints of leg pain, especially if associated with back or buttock discomfort.
- Popliteal artery entrapment is often misdiagnosed as chronic posterior exertional compartment syndrome, because of the ischemic etiology in the pathogenesis of symptoms in both syndromes (Glorioso and Wilckens, 2001b).

RADIOLOGIC MODALITIES TO DIAGNOSE CHRONIC EXERTIONAL COMPARTMENT SYNDROME

- **Nuclear medicine:** Scintigraphy has recently been investigated in the diagnosis of CECS (Samuelson and Cram, 1996; Edwards et al, 1999; Owens et al, 1999). The utility of this study is based on the detection of abnormalities in tracer uptake in muscle compartments. Specifically, the identification of decreased postexertional muscle perfusion and radionuclide concentration in the compartment with increased pressure when compared to resting images (Edwards et al, 1999; Owens et al, 1999).
- **MRI:** Recent interest has focused on the use of *magnetic resonance* (MR) imaging in the evaluation and diagnosis of CECS (Eskelin, Lotjonen, and Mantysaari, 1998; Verleisdonk, van Gils A, and van der Werken, 2001). The theory behind use of MR imaging is based on the fact that MR imaging is sensitive to changes in water distribution in skeletal muscle. In CECS, if tissue edema causes pressure elevations in muscle compartments, theoretically postexercise MR imaging should be able to detect the increased water content (Kiuru et al, 2003; Eskelin, Lotjonen, and Mantysaari, 1998).

REFERENCES

Andrish JT: The leg, in DeLee JC, Drez DD, Miller MD (eds.): *DeLee and Drez's Orthopaedic Sports Medicine: Principles and Practice,* 2nd ed. Philadelphia, PA, Saunders, 2003, p 2155.

Awbrey BJ, Sienkiewicz PS, Mankin HJ: Chronic exercise induced compartment pressure elevation measured with a miniaturized fluid pressure monitor: A laboratory and clinical study. *Am J Sports Med* 16(6): 610–615, 1988.

Davey JR, Rorabeck CH, Fowler PJ: The tibialis posterior muscle compartment—An unrecognized cause of exertional compartment syndrome. *Am J Sports Med* 12(5):391–397, 1984.

Detmer DE, Sharpe K, Sufit RL, et al: Chronic compartment syndrome: Diagnosis, management, and outcomes. *Am J Sports Med* 13(3):162–170, 1985.

Eskelin MK, Lotjonen JM, Mantysaari MJ: Chronic exertional compartment syndrome: MR imaging at 0.1 T compared with tissue pressure measurement. *Radiology* 206(2):333–337, 1998.

Edwards PD, Miles KA, Owens SJ, et al: A new non-invasive test for the detection of compartment syndromes. *Nucl Med Commun* 20(3):215–218, 1999.

Gershuni DH, Yaru NC, Hargens AR, et al: Ankle and knee position as a factor modifying intracompartmental pressure in the human leg. *J Bone Joint Surg* 66-A (9):1415–1420, 1984.

Glorioso JE, Wilckens JH: Compartment syndrome testing, in O'Connor FG, Wilder RP (eds.): *Textbook of Running Medicine.* New York, NY, McGraw-Hill, 2001a, p 95.

Glorioso JE, Wilckens JH: Exertional leg pain, in O'Connor FG, Wilder RP (eds.): *Textbook of Running Medicine.* New York, NY, McGraw-Hill, 2001b, p 95.

Hutchinson MR, Ireland ML: Chronic exertional compartment syndrome—Gauging pressure. *Phys Sportsmed* 27(5):101–102, 1999.

Kiuru MJ, Mantysaari MJ, Pihlajamaki HK, et al: Evaluation of stress related anterior lower leg pain with magnetic resonance imaging and intracompartmental pressure measurement. *Mil Med* 168:48–52, 2003.

Martens MA, Moeyersoons JP: Acute and recurrent effort-related compartment syndrome in sports. *Sports Med* 9(1):62–68, 1990.

Matsen FA, Mayo KA, Sheridan GW, et al: Monitoring of intramuscular pressure. *Surgery* 79(6):702–709, 1976.

McDermott AGP, Marble AE, Yabsley RH, et al: Monitoring dynamic anterior compartment pressures during exercise—A new technique using the STIC catheter. *Am J Sports Med* 10(2):83–89, 1982.

Mubarak SJ, Hargens AR, Owen CA, et al: The wick catheter technique for measurement of intramuscular pressure. *J Bone Joint Surg* 58-A(7):1016–1020, 1976.

Owens S, Edwards P, Miles K, et al: Chronic compartment syndrome affecting the lower limb: MIBI perfusion imaging as an alternative to pressure monitoring: two case reports. *Br J Sports Med* 33(1):49–51, 1999.

Pedowitz RA, Hargens AR, Mubarak SJ, et al: Modified criteria for the objective diagnosis of chronic compartment syndrome of the leg. *Am J Sports Med* 18(1): 35–40, 1990.

Rorabeck CH, Fowler PJ, Nott L: The results of fasciotomy in the management of chronic exertional compartment syndrome. *Am J Sports Med* 16(3):224–227, 1988.

Rorabeck CH, Castle GSP, Hardie R, et al: Compartmental pressure measurements: An experimental investigation using the slit catheter. *J Trauma* 21(6):446–449, 1981.

Rorabeck CH, Bourne RB, Fowler PJ, et al: The role of tissue pressure measurement in diagnosing chronic anterior compartment syndrome. *Am J Sports Med* 16(2):143–146, 1988.

Samuelson DR, Cram RL: The three phase bone scan and exercise induced lower leg pain: The tibial stress test. *Clin Nucl Med* 21(2):89–93, 1996.

Styf JR, Korner LM: Diagnosis of chronic anterior compartment syndrome in the lower leg. *Acta Orthop Scand* 58:139–144, 1987.

Verleisdonk EJ, van Gils A, van der Werken C: The diagnostic value of MRI scans for the diagnosis of chronic exertional compartment syndrome of the lower leg. *Skeletal Radiol* 30(6):321–325, 2001.

Whitesides TE, Haney TC, Harada H, et al: A simple method for tissue pressure determination. *Arch Surg* 110:1311–1313, 1975.

23 EXERCISE-INDUCED ASTHMA TESTING

Major Fred H Brennan, Jr, DO

EXERCISE-INDUCED ASTHMA TESTING

EPIDEMIOLOGY

- *Exercise-induced asthma* (EIA) is a common medical condition that affects at least 10 to 15% of athletes (Eliasson, Phillips, and Rajagopal, 1992).
- Respiratory symptoms alone are insensitive in predicting bronchospasm in athletes (Holzer, 2002).
- Common respiratory symptoms suggestive of asthma (coughing, wheezing etc.) have only a 60–70% positive predictive value for EIA (Rundell et al, 2001; Rice et al, 1985).

INDICATIONS FOR EIA TESTING

- An athlete with signs or symptoms suggestive of exercise-induced asthma
- An athlete with known chronic asthma may be tested for an exercise-triggering event.
- An athlete with exertional dyspnea, once cardiac etiologies have been clinically and/or diagnostically eliminated.

CONTRAINDICATIONS FOR EIA TESTING

- Active or recent pulmonary infection within past 30 days
- Ongoing or recent exacerbation of asthma
- Known allergy to methacholine (methacholine challenge)
- An athlete using inhaled corticosteroids may still be tested; however, the provocation test may be falsely negative in up to 50% of patients (Anderson et al, 2001; Waalkans et al, 1993).

EIA PROVOCATIVE TESTING

EXERCISE CHALLENGE

- A baseline *pulmonary function test* (PFT) should be performed and results recorded prior to this provocative test.
- The sensitivity and specificity of this test for identifying EIA in athletes is approximately 65% (Eliasson, Phillips, and Rajagopal, 1992; Avital, 2000).
- The challenge should be sport-specific and conducted in the environment in which athletes most commonly experience their symptoms (Brennan, Jr, 2001).
- An exercise challenge may be used as a first-line diagnostic study.

CONDUCTING AN EXERCISE CHALLENGE
- Allow athletes to stretch but do not allow them to exercise or warm up prior to the challenge. A warm-up period may result in a false negative result.
- Obtain a baseline PFT or *peak expiratory flow rate* (PEFR). Record FEV1 and FEF 25-75, or PEFR.
- The sport-specific exercise should be conducted for 8–10 min at a heart rate of 85–90% maximum calculated heart rate (220 − age in years = calculated maximum heart rate).
- After 10 min of exercise allow a 1-min rest. Check PFT or PEFR three times and record the best result.
- Repeat these at 3, 5, 10, 15 and 20 min post termination of the exercise challenge.
- A decrease of >10% in the FEV1 or PEFR, and/or a decrease in FEF 25–75 of >20% are diagnostic for EIA (Mannix, Manfredi, and Farber, 1999; Provost, et al, 1996).

METHACHOLINE CHALLENGE

- Methacholine stimulates muscarinic receptors located in the airway smooth muscle (Lin et al, 1991).
- The sensitivity of this test is estimated to be 55% and up to 100% specific (Eliasson, Phillips, and Rajagopal, 1992).
- The positive predictive value may be as high as 100%, with a negative predictive value of 61% (Holzer, 2002).

CONDUCTING THE METHACHOLINE CHALLENGE
- Obtain a baseline PFT. Record the best FEV1.
- Solutions of methacholine are prepared in the following concentrations: 0.025, 0.25, 2.5, 10, and 25 mg/mL.
- The athlete inhales five breaths of the lowest concentration solution via nebulizer. A PFT is performed 3 min post inhalation of the methacholine.
- The concentration of methacholine solution is increased to the next highest concentration and a PFT performed 3 min post inhalation.
- This provocative test is concluded and considered positive if there is a decline in the FEV1 of at least

20%. The test is concluded but considered negative if the maximum solution concentration of 25 mg/mL is administered without the diagnostic drop in FEV1 (Eliasson, Phillips, and Rajagopal, 1992).

- Albuterol may be given 3 min after a positive test to demonstrate airway bronchospasm reversibility that is consistent with asthma.

EUCAPNIC VOLUNTARY HYPERVENTILLATION (EVH) TEST

- Used by the International Olympic Committee-Medical Committee (IOC-MC) to verify EIA and the need for precompetition beta agonist (Anderson et al, 2003).
- Sensitivity in athletes has been shown to be 50% sensitive and up to 100% specific (Eliasson, Phillips, and Rajagopal, 1992).
- EVH is a well-known and accepted provocative test for EIA (Holzer, 2002; Mannix, Manfredi, and Farber, 1999).
- This test is more sensitive than an exercise challenge in the field or in the lab (Holzer, 2002; Mannix, Manfredi, and Farber, 1999).
- EVH is more sensitive than methacholine in response to dry air hyperpnea (Holzer, 2002).

CONDUCTING THE EVH TEST
- Obtain a baseline PFT. Record the best FEV1.
- Argyros and colleagues (Anderson et al, 2001; Argyros et al, 1995) protocol based on single-level ventilation of 85% of the *maximum voluntary ventilation* (MVV) is used. MVV is calculated as 35 times the best recorded pretest FEV1 and is used to calculate the volume of dry gas ventilated per minute.
- The athlete inhales dry gas consisting of 5% carbon dioxide, 21% oxygen, and the remainder nitrogen gas. The volume of ventilated gas is measured by a metered instrument. The athlete gauges and adjusts the rate of ventilation based on the volume of dry gas ventilated.
- The athlete breaths at a rate of 85% MVV for 6 min.
- At the completion of the 6 min the FEV1 is measured twice at 1, 3, 5, 7, and 8 min post challenge. The best FEV1 value is used.
- A drop in FEV1 of at least 20% is diagnostic for EIA (Holzer, 2002).
- A bronchodialator may be administered at the conclusion of the study to decrease the patient's symptoms and document reversibility of airway hyperresponsiveness.

EVALUATING ATHLETES WITH SUSPECTED EIA

- The most appropriate provocative test for identifying EIA remains controversial (Rundell et al, 2001; Anderson et al, 2001; Eliasson, 1999).
- EVH may be the preferred method of laboratory provocative testing because of its relative ease and excellent sensitivity. It is also more sensitive than an exercise challenge in a lab or field environment (Holzer, 2002; Mannix, Manfredi, and Farber, 1999). EVH provocative testing is the preferred diagnostic study of the IOC-MC.
- If EVH testing is unavailable, a sport and climate-specific exercise challenge is an acceptable alternative. A methacholine challenge is also an acceptable option.
- Avoid empirically treating for EIA without formal provocative testing. Classic symptoms alone are unreliable and may lead to over- or underusage of the appropriate medical therapy.

REFERENCES

Anderson SD, Argyros GJ, Magnussen H, et al: Provocation by eucapnic voluntary hyperpnea to identify exercise-induced bronchoconstriction. *Br J Sports Med* 35:344–347, 2001.

Anderson SD, Fitch K, Perry CP, et al: Response to bronchial challenge submitted for approval to use inhaled beta 2 agonists before an event at the 2002 winter Olympics. *J Allergy Clin Immunol* 111(1):45–50, 2003.

Anderson SD, Lambert S, Brannan JD, et al: Laboratory protocol for exercise asthma to evaluate salbutamol given by two devices. *Med Sci Sports Exerc* 33:893–900, 2001.

Argyros GJ, Roach JM, Hurwitz KM, et al: The refractory period after eucapnic voluntary hyperventilation challenge and its effect on challenge technique. *Chest* 108:419–424, 1995.

Avital A: Exercise, methacholine, and adenosine 5' monophosphate challenges in children with asthma: relation to decreased severity of disease. *Pediatr Pulmonol* 30(3):207–214, 2000.

Brennan Fred H, Jr: Exercise-induced asthma testing, in O'Connor FG, Wilder R (eds.): *Textbook of Running Medicine.* New York, NY, McGraw-Hill, 2001, p 101–107.

Eliasson AH: Blow dry your asthma. *Chest* 115:608–609, 1999.

Eliasson AH, Phillips YY, Rajagopal KR: Sensitivity and specificity of bronchial provocation testing. An evaluation of four techniques in exercise-induced bronchospasm. *Chest* 102:347, 1992.

Holzer K: Exercise in elite summer athletes: challenges for diagnosis. *J Allergy Clin Immunol* 110(3):374–380, 2002.

Lin CC, Wu JL, Huang WC, et al: A bronchial response comparison of exercise and methacholine in asthmatic subjects. *J Asthma* 28:31–35, 1991.

Mannix ET, Manfredi F, Farber MO: A comparison of two challenge tests for identifying exercise-induced bronchospasm in figure skaters. *Chest* 115:649–653, 1999.

Provost CM, Arbour KS, Sestili DC, et al: The incidence of exercise-induced bronchospasm in competitive figure skaters. *J Asthma* 33:67–71, 1996.

Rice SG, Bierman CW, Shapiro GG et al: Identification of exercise-induced asthma among intercollegiate athletes. *Ann Allergy* 55:790–793, 1985.

Rundell KW, Im J, Mayers LB, et al: Self-reported symptoms and exercise-induced asthma in elite athletes. *Med Sci Sports Exerc* 33:208–213, 2001.

Waalkans HJ, vanEssen-Zandvliet EEM, Gerritsen J, et al: The effect of inhaled corticosteroid (budesonide) on exercise-induced asthma in children. *Eur Respir J* 6:652–656, 1993.

24 DRUG TESTING

Aaron Rubin, MD, FAAFP, FACSM

INTRODUCTION

- Drug testing of the athlete is an ethical, moral, legal, and occasionally medical issue.
- Team physicians, athletic trainers, team psychologists, coaches, administrators, and others dealing with the care of the athlete may be asked to become involved with drug testing.
- Care should be exercised to keep the punitive aspect of drug testing separate from the therapeutic care for athlete's problems.
- Drug testing is performed for many reasons:
  a. To prevent cheating by use of drugs and chemicals
  b. To level the playing field by keeping clean athletes from having to compete with anabolic using athletes
  c. To prevent drug-induced illness and death
  d. To prevent public-relations problems for teams and organizations

SCOPE OF PROBLEM

- Olympic drug testing began in the 1964 Tokyo Olympics.
- Between the 1968 and 1994 Olympics, over 14,000 athletes were tested at competition and 56 tested positive.

- Various studies suggest that 5–11% of high school males and 0.5–2.5% of high school females had tried anabolic steroids.
- This is not merely a problem of athletes: of the high school students, 33% using anabolic steroids were not athletes.

REGULATING AGENCIES

- **United States Anti-doping Agency (USADA)—www.usantidoping.org:** USADA is an independent antidoping agency for Olympic sports in the United States.
- **World Anti-doping Agency (WADA)—www.wada-ama.org:** The mission of WADA is to promote and coordinate at international level the fight against doping in sport in all forms.
- **National Collegiate Athletic Association (NCAA)—www1.ncaa.org/membership/ed_outreach/health-safety/drug_testing/index.html:** NCAA regulates and provides safety guidelines for student athletes from member colleges in the United States.

DRUGS, MEDICATIONS, AND OTHER SUBSTANCES

- There are no inherently good, bad, dangerous, legal, or illegal substances.
- In terms of athletic use, it is best to consider *allowed* or *not allowed* substances.
- Illegal substances are determined by rule of law and may vary from jurisdiction to jurisdiction. Use of illegal substance can be punished by criminal law. (Marijuana and crack cocaine are illegal substances in most jurisdictions in the United States.)
- Components of these substances may be legal. (Dronabinol is a derivative of marijuana and legal under prescription of a licensed physician. Cocaine is a legal medicine for specific indications.)
- Some legal substances can be used illegally. (Anabolic steroids are legal substances but can be obtained and used illegally.)
- Over the counter medications are generally legal, but may not be allowed for athletic competitions (such as high dose caffeine).
- Some substances are legal but not allowed under certain circumstance. (Alcohol may not be allowed for some events.)
- The ultimate decision regarding allowed or not allowed substances falls to the regulating agencies responsible for establishing the rules for the various sports teams, leagues, and organizations.

THERAPEUTIC DRUGS

- *Prescribed drugs* are those given to the athlete under the direction (prescription) of a licensed physician or dentist. Just because a medication is prescribed does not exempt an athlete from sanctions.
- *Over the counter medications* may be taken by the athlete on their own or by direction of a physician or other health care provider. Again, this does not exempt and athlete from sanctions if products are not allowed.
- *Natural products* are often a misnomer. Many drugs (legal and illegal, prescription and nonprescription) are based in natural products. To complicate matters even more, these products may not be fully labeled with all ingredients. Again, the athlete is ultimately responsible for what they put in their body.

RECREATIONAL DRUGS

- *Alcohol* is banned by the NCAA for rifle competition and by the Olympic movement "where the rules of the governing body so provide. . . ." Keep in mind that use of alcohol in minors is illegal.
- *Tobacco* is generally not tested, though use of tobacco is not allowed at NCAA events.
- *Marijuana* is not allowed and is tested by the NCAA at any concentration and Olympics at set concentrations.
- *Stimulants* such as amphetamine, cocaine, ephedrine, caffeine (at set concentrations), *methylene-dioxyme-thamphetamine* (MDMA or Ecstasy), and related products are banned.
- *Hallucinogens* such as *lysergic acid diethylamide* (LSD) are not listed as banned substances but are illegal.

PERFORMANCE ENHANCEMENTS

- Stimulants as discussed above are prohibited.
- Androgenic/anabolic agents, such as anabolic steroids, testosterone, clenbuterol and related compounds are banned by the NCAA and Olympic movement.
- Epogen and related compounds and blood doping are not allowed.
- In addition, techniques to mask drug testing or fool drug testers are not allowed. These include diuretics, urine substitution, masking agents, and other techniques.

TESTING PROCEDURES (BASED ON THE NCAA DRUG TESTING PROGRAMS)

- Selection process must be fair and based on random testing, universal testing, or testing based on probable cause (evidence of drug use or previous positive test).
- Testing may be done out-of-competition (year round) or in-competition (postseason championship).

POSTSEASON TESTING

- Facilities and procedures are fully outlined in the NCAA Drug-Testing Programs Site Coordinators Manual.
- The athlete is notified of testing by a drug-testing courier and given a written notification form instructing the athlete to accompany the courier to the collection station. The athlete must report within 1 h and remain in visual contact with the courier until the athlete signs in at the testing center. Only authorized agents for testing and the athletes are allowed in the testing center.
- Sealed beverages without caffeine or other banned substances are allowed at the testing center.
- The athlete selects a sealed beaker to provide their specimen. Sample will be given as an observed specimen.
- Specimen must be at least 85 mL. If the specimen is not sufficient, it is discarded and the athlete is asked to provide another specimen. The athlete is not allowed to leave the test center till adequate specimen is provided.
- Specific gravity and pH is checked. If the specific gravity is less than 1.005 (1.010 if checked with a reagent strip), the specimen is discarded. If the pH is greater than 7.5 or less than 4.5, the specimen is discarded.
- The specimen is processed if the specific gravity is above 1.005 (1.010 if using a reagent strip) and the pH between 4.5 and 7.5.
- The athlete selects containers and unique bar-coded labels.
- The crew member pours approximately 60 mL of the specimen into the "A vial" and 25 mL into the "B vial." The vials are sealed, forms filled out, and the specimens prepared for shipping. All is done in the presence of the athlete.
- Chain of evidence must be maintained. The specimen must be controlled and signed every step in the process.
- The specimens are sent to an approved laboratory for testing. Specimen A is tested.
- Results of positive tests are reported to the National Center for Drug Free Sport who breaks the number code and identifies the athlete. The athletics director or designate is notified by overnight mail marked confidential, who in turn must notify the athlete.
- The athlete may be represented at the laboratory when testing specimen B. Different lab personnel will test specimen B.
- The results of specimen B is considered final.

INSTITUTIONAL DRUG TESTING

- Extreme care must be taken to protect the rights of the athlete.
- Goals of testing, education program, punishment, selection process, procedures for testing, notification, confidentiality, appropriate follow-up, and legal issues must be carefully thought out and put into writing.
- Multiple individuals may be involved in creating such a policy including, but not limited to, administrators, legal counsel, medical advisors, psychologists, and representatives of the athletes.
- Selection of athletes for testing may not be arbitrary.
- After notification, the athlete must present to a testing center within a set amount of time.
- Testing may be performed at an on-campus center or a designated industrial clinic for drug testing. If sent to an outside facility, the school or organization must assure that proper conduct and procedures are followed.
- Testing procedures should be similar to that discussed above under the end of season testing.
- Lists of substances that are not allowed must be published and the athletes educated regarding the substances, health risks, treatment options, and sanctions for positive tests.

TESTING TECHNIQUES

- Initial screening may be done by the relatively lower cost thin-layer chromatography or *Radioimmunassay* (RIA) methods.
- Confirmation and definitive testing should be performed by gas chromatography and mass spectroscopy.

LEGAL ISSUES

- Expect legal challenges to testing procedures and especially to positive tests.
- Athletes should be afforded due process of law.
- One should consider outlining rights of appeal.

PUBLIC RELATIONS

- Privacy of the athlete must be maintained.
- The public and press often feel they have a "right-to-know" about the dealings of their teams, schools, and athletes.
- The loss of an athlete from a team for disciplinary reasons is often assumed to be for positive drug tests.

BIBLIOGRAPHY

Bowers LD: Athletic drug testing. *Clin Sports Med* 17(2): 299–319, April 1998.

Greydanus DE, Patel DR: Sports doping in the adolescent athlete the hope, hype, and hyperbole. *Pediatr Clin North Am* 49(4):829–855, Aug 2002.

Knopp WD, Wang TW, Bach BR: Ergogenic drugs in sports. *Clin Sports Med* 16(3):375–393, July 1997.

MacAuley D: Drugs in sport. *BMJ* 313(7051):211–215, Jul 27, 1996.

National Collegiate Athletics Administration: Drug testing program, http://www1.ncaa.org/membership/ed_outreach/health-safety/drug_testing/index.html

United States Anti-doping Agency (USADA): www.usantidoping.org World Anti-doping Agency (WADA): www.wada-ama.org

25 CARDIOVASCULAR CONSIDERATIONS

Francis G O'Connor, MD, FACSM
John P Kugler, MD, MPH
Ralph P Oriscello, MD, FACC

INTRODUCTION

- Enhanced cardiovascular health is one of the key benefits of most forms of consistent athletic endeavors throughout life. Regular physical activity promotes cardiovascular fitness and lowers the risk of disease.
- While there is generally a net cardiovascular benefit from athletic activity, there is also an increased cardiovascular risk for certain susceptible individuals. These individuals may be known with identified cardiovascular disorders or they may be unrecognized until the adverse event occurs.
- Cardiovascular conditions are the leading cause of sudden death in high school and college athletes, with the majority of sudden deaths occurring during or immediately after a training session or a formal competition.

CARDIOVASCULAR BENEFITS OF EXERCISE

- Numerous studies (Williams, 1998; Paffenbarger et al, 1993; Powell et al, 1987; Leon et al, 1987; Berlin and Colditz, 1990) have clearly identified physical inactivity and a sedentary lifestyle as significant risk factors for the development and progression of coronary heart disease. Moreover, studies (Pate et al, 1995; Williams, 1997; Villeneuve et al, 1998; Kohl et al, 1992; Blair et al, 1995) have consistently confirmed the cardiovascular benefit of aerobic exercise with a reduction in the number of adverse events and a reduction in mortality.
- While there is a definite increased risk for certain susceptible individuals, particularly middle-aged persons with *coronary artery disease* (CAD) and a sedentary lifestyle, there is abundant evidence (Maron, 2000) of net cardiovascular benefits from consistent exercise as a primary-prevention recommendation for coronary disease in asymptomatic middle-aged and older persons.

THE ATHLETIC HEART SYNDROME

- Vigorous athletic training is associated with specific physiologic and structural cardiovascular change (Murkerji, Albert, and Mukerji, 1989), which comprises what has been termed the *athletic heart syndrome*. These changes are nonpathologic and represent appropriate adaptations to physical training.
- It is important to remember that the adaptive structural and physiologic response of the normal athletic heart do not rule out the presence of an underlying pathologic condition. In fact, it makes the task of diagnosing that condition more challenging for the primary care physician and cardiologist. Of note, detraining for 2–3 months can result in a reversal of athletic heart syndrome changes, which is not seen in pathologic conditions.
- Studies (Pluim et al, 2001) have suggested that there is a continuum of athletic adaptations depending on the training stress of the athlete.
  - For endurance-trained athletes, the heart has to adapt to principally a chronic volume overload that results in an increase in both left ventricular end-diastolic diameter and left ventricular wall thickness.

This results in eccentric hypertrophy with a more pronounced increase in wall thickness than expected.
• The strength-trained athlete adapts by developing a concentric hypertrophy with an increase in absolute and relative wall thickness without significant changes in end-diastolic diameter.

PHYSICAL EXAMINATION

• The heart rate of well-conditioned athletes is usually between 40 and 60 bpm, secondary to enhanced vagal tone and decreased sympathetic tone. Normal sinus arrhythmia may be more noticeable.
• The physiologic splitting of S2 may be slightly delayed during inspiration. An S3 may be noted in endurance-trained athletes secondary to the increased rate of left ventricular filling associated with the relative left ventricular dilatation (Zeppilli, 1988).
• While an S4 may be noted in strength-trained athletes secondary to concentric hypertrophy, its presence always warrants clinical evaluation. Functional murmurs may be noted in 30–50% of athletes on careful examination (Huston, Puffer, and Rodney, 1985).

ELECTROCARDIOGRAPHIC CHANGES

• Several minor electrocardiogaphic variations have been commonly noted in highly trained athletes and are considered to be consistent with the athlete's heart syndrome (Huston, Puffer, and Rodney, 1985; Oakley and Oakley, 1982) (Tables 25-1 and 25-2).
• More significantly abnormal appearing *electrocardiogram* (EKG) patterns have also been identified in otherwise normal athletic hearts. In a recent Italian study (Pelliccia et al, 2000), 1005 athletes were consecutively assessed with EKGs and echocardiograms. The study found that 40% of the athletes had abnormal EKGs, not including the minor alterations associated with the athlete's heart syndrome mentioned above. Of these athletes, 36% had *distinctly* abnormal patterns. Of those with the distinctly abnormal patterns, only 10% actually had evidence of structural cardiac disease, suggesting that the EKG manifestation of the normal athletic heart is much more variable than previously believed.

TABLE 25-1   Common ECG Findings in Athletic Heart Syndrome

Sinus bradycardia	Sinus arrhythmia
First-degree AV block	Wenckebach AV block
Incomplete RBBB	Notched P waves
RVH by voltage criteria	LVH by voltage criteria
Repolarization changes	QTc interval at upper limit
Tall, peaked and inverted t waves	

TABLE 25-2   Rhythm Disturbances on Resting Electrocardiograms of the General Population and Athletes

ARRHYTHMIA	GENERAL POPULATION (%)	ATHLETES (%)
Sinus bradycardia	23.7	50–85
Sinus arrhythmia	2.4–20	13.5–69
Wandering atrial pacemaker	—	7.4–19
First degree block	0.65	6–33
Second degree block	—	—
Mobitz I	0.003	0.125–10
Mobitz II	0.003	Not reported
Third degree block	0.0002	0.017
Nodal rhythm	0.06	0.031–7
Ventricular pre-excitation	0.1–0.15	0.15–2.5
Atrial fibrillation	0.004	0–0.063

SUDDEN DEATH IN EXERCISE

• While there is considerable net cardiovascular benefit to exercise, there is also a clear risk for susceptible individuals. Indeed, as Barry J. Maron (Maron, 2000) has clearly shown, there is a "paradox of exercise" that requires a clinical assessment of risk prior to the initiation of a vigorous program.
• Overall risk of sudden death during exercise is low. Estimates from various studies (Siscovick et al, 1984; Ragosta et al, 1984; Thompson et al, 1982; Maron, Poliac, and Roberts, 1996; Van et al, 1995; Maron, Gohman, and Aeppli, 1998) range from 1:15,000 joggers per year (Siscovick et al, 1984; Thompson et al, 1982) to 1:50,000 marathon participants (Maron, Poliac, and Roberts, 1996). For high school and college-aged athletes the range is estimated at 1:200,000 to 1:300,000 per academic year (Van camp et al, 1995; Maron, Gohman, and Aeppli, 1998).
• The specific etiologies contributing to sudden cardiac death are most closely related to age. Generally, the dividing age is 35 (Basilico, 1999). This primarily stems from the observation that for sudden deaths over age 35, over 75% are associated with coronary artery disease. The high prevalence of atherosclerosis in this age group clearly predominates as an etiology.
• In younger athletes, nonobstructive *hypertrophic cardiomyopathy* (HCM) is the most common etiology. Coronary artery anomalies, myocarditis, premature atherosclerotic disease, and dilated cardiomyopathy are next most common, at least in the United States. In European studies (Tabib et al, 1999; Firoozi et al, 2002; Priori et al, 2002), *arrhythmogenic right ventricular cardiomyopathy* (ARVC) is more commonly recognized as an etiology than it is in the United States. Other less common etiologies include aortic rupture from Marfan's syndrome, genetic conductive system abnormalities, idiopathic concentric left ventricular hypertrophy, substance abuse (cocaine or steroids), aortic stenosis, mitral valve prolapse,

sickle cell trait, and blunt chest trauma (commotio cordis).

SCREENING FOR SUDDEN DEATH

- The American Heart Association (AHA) Science and Advisory Committee published consensus guidelines for preparticipation cardiovascular screening for high school and college athletes in 1996 (Maron et al, 1996). It is recommended that a complete personal and family history and physical examination be done for all athletes. It should focus on identifying those cardiovascular conditions known to cause sudden death. It should be done every 2 years with an interim history between examinations. The 26th Bethesda Conference specifies participation guidelines for different conditions (Maron and Mitchell, 1994). These are summarized in Table 25-3.
  - Family history should include a specific inquiry for a family history of premature coronary artery disease, diabetes mellitus, hypertension, sudden death, syncope, significant disability from cardiovascular disease in relatives younger than age 50, HCM, ARVC, Marfan's syndrome, prolonged QT syndrome, or significant arrhythmias.
  - Personal past history should include specific inquiries on the detection of heart murmur, diabetes mellitus, hypertension, hyperlipidemia, smoking, or on the presence of HCM, ARVC, Marfan's syndrome, prolonged QT syndrome, or significant arrhythmias. Recent

TABLE 25-3   Guidelines on Restriction of Exercise for Cardiovascular Disease

Contraindications to Vigorous Exercise

Hypertrophic cardiomyopathy
Idiopathic concentric left ventricular hypertrophy
Marfan's syndrome
Coronary heart disease
Uncontrolled ventricular arrhythmia's
Severe valvular heart disease (especially aortic stenosis and pulmonic
  stenosis)
Coarctation of the aorta
Acute myocarditis
Dilated cardiomyopathy
Congestive heart failure
Congenital anomalies of the coronary arteries
Cyanotic congenital heart disease
Pulmonary hypertension
Right ventricular cardiomyopathy
Ebstein's anomaly of the tricuspid valve
Idiopathic long Q-T syndrome

Require Close Monitoring and Possible Restriction

Uncontrolled hypertension
Uncontrolled atrial arrhythmia's
Hemodynamic significant valvular heart disease (aortic insufficiency,
  mitral stenosis, mitral regurgitation)

SOURCE: (Maron and Mitchell, 1994; Kugler and O'Connor, 1999)

TABLE 25-4   Features of Marfan Syndrome on Physical Examination

Musculoskeletal

Tall stature
Thin body habitus (armspan to height ratio >1.05)
Arachnodactly (long thin fingers; able to wrap hand around opposite
  wrist and overlap thumb and small finger)
Pectus deformity
High arched palate
Kyphoscoliosis
Joint laxity

Cardiovascular

Systolic murmur (mitral valve prolapse)
Evidence of easing bruising
Diastolic murmur (aortic regurgitation)

Ocular

Myopia
Retinal detachment
Lens subluxation

history inquiries must include a history of syncope, near syncope, profound exercise intolerance, exertional chest discomfort, dyspnea, or excessive fatigue.

- Physical examination should specifically address hypertension, heart rhythm, cardiac murmur, and the findings of unusual facies or body habitus associated with a congenital cardiovascular defect, especially Marfan's syndrome (Table 25-4) (Pyeritz, 1986). Cardiac auscultation should be performed in the supine and standing positions and murmurs should be assessed with Valsava and position maneuvers when indicated.
- The classic murmur of obstructive HCM accentuates with Valsalva, this may also be seen in mitral valve prolapse. The murmur of aortic stenosis intensifies with squatting, and decreases with Valsalva.
- Femoral pulses should be assessed and blood pressure measured with the appropriately sized cuff in the sitting position.
- Ancillary testing should be directed by the patient's history, physical, and age. Lipid profiles should be checked in the older athlete and should be considered in athletes of any age. Exercise stress testing is not recommended as a routine screening device for the detection of early coronary artery disease because of low predictive value and high rates of false positive and false negative results. Exercise testing may be required prior to beginning an exercise program in select cases (see chapters 15 and 20)
- EKG and echocardiograms are not currently recommended as screening tools (Basilico, 1999; Kugler and O'Connor, 1999; Kugler, O'Connor and Oriscello, 2001). As mentioned above, the normal adaptations of the "athletic heart" make interpretation of the routine EKG and echocardiogram problematic (Pelliccia et al, 2000). High rates of false positivety, high relative costs, limited availability, and low prevalence of disease make

these modalities impractical as screening devices, at this point in time.

- Despite the fact that many conditions that cause sudden death in young athletes are familial (hypertrophic cardiomyopathy-autosomal dominant defect in sarcomere formation; Long QT syndrome-autosomal dominant sodium channel defect; Marfan's Syndrome-autosomal dominant mutation of FBN1 fibrilin gene; Brugada Syndrome-autosomal dominant SCN5A channelopathy; ARVC-autosomal dominant defect), genetic testing is not routinely recommended.

SYNCOPE-AND EXERCISE-ASSOCIATED COLLAPSE

- Syncope is most often defined as a sudden loss of consciousness for a brief duration, not secondary to head trauma but usually secondary to a sudden drop in cerebral blood flow or metabolic change (e.g., hypoglycemia and hypoxia). *Exercise-associated collapse* (EAC) refers to athletes who are unable to stand or walk unaided because of lightheadedness, faintness, dizziness, or outright syncope. The potential differential diagnosis is extensive and includes multiple cardiovascular and neurologic etiologies (Kapoor, 1992; Manolis et al, 1990). Athletes who present with a history of "passing out with exercise" require a careful history and physical to differentiate benign from life threatening etiologies (Kugler, O'Connor, and Oriscello, 2001) (see Table 25-5).

- The first step involves determining if the event was a brief, true syncopal episode versus the more common and generally benign EAC event which involves a longer time period of "being out of it" even in the supine position with normal vital signs. The second step is to differentiate between syncope that occurs during the event (suggesting a more ominous arrhythmic etiology) and syncope that occurs following the event, usually associated with orthostatic hypotension on exercise cessation (suggesting a less ominous etiology). It is also critical to identify prodromal symptoms that may have occurred during exercise such as palpitations (arrhythmia), chest pain (ischemia or aortic dissection), nausea (ischemia or vagal activity), wheezing, or pruritus (anaphylaxis).

- The physical examination should include a careful assessment of orthostatic vital signs, precordial auscultation especially focusing on ruling out the murmurs of aortic stenosis and HCM, and a careful search for the morphologic features of Marfan's syndrome. An EKG should be ordered in most cases and should be evaluated closely for rate, rhythm, QT interval, repolarization abnormalities, left or right hypertrophy, preexcitation evidence, and complications of ischemic heart disease. Further testing, including blood work, echocardiogram, and stress testing may be done depending on whether a diagnosis has been made, suggested, or remains unexplained.

- See Fig. 25-1 for a suggested algorithm for the primary care evaluation of exertional syncope in the young athlete (Kugler, O'Connor, and Oriscello, 2001).

TABLE 25-5 Clinical Clues to Common Etiologies Presenting with Exertional Syncope

DIAGNOSIS	CLINICAL CLUES	ELECTROCARDIOGRAM	SUGGESTED DIAGNOSTIC TESTING
Neurocardiogenic syncope	Noxious stimulus, prolonged upright position	Normal	Exercise testing
Supraventricular tachyarrhythmias	Palpitations, response to carotid sinus pressure	Preexcitation	Electrophysiologic study and definitive therapy
Hypertrophic cardiomyopathy	Grade III/VI systolic murmur, louder with valsalva, when present	Normal, pseudoinfarction pattern, left ventricular hypertrophy with strain	Echocardiography with doppler
Myocarditis	Prior upper respiratory tract infection, pneumonia, shortness of breath, recreational drug use	Simulating a myocardial infarction with ectopy	Viral studies, echocardiogram, drug screening
Aortic stenosis	Exertional syncope, grade III/VI harsh systolic crescendo-decrescendo murmur	Left ventricular hypertrophy	Echocardiography with doppler
Mitral valve prolapse	Thumping heart, midsystolic click with or without a murmur	QT interval may be prolonged	Echocardiography with doppler
Prolonged QT syndrome	Recurrent syncope with family history of sudden death	Prolonged corrected QT interval (>0.44)	Family history; exercise stress test with ECG after exercise
Coronary anomalies	Usually asymptomatic, sudden death event	Normal rest electrocardiogram	Coronary angiography, cardiac MRI
Acquired coronary artery diseases	Chest pain syndrome, family history	Ischemia, may be normal	Exercise testing with or without perfusion or contractile imaging
Right ventricular dysplasia	Asymptomatic until syncope, tachyarrhythmias	T-wave inversion v1-v3 PVCs with LBBB configuration	Echo/doppler study electrocardiography

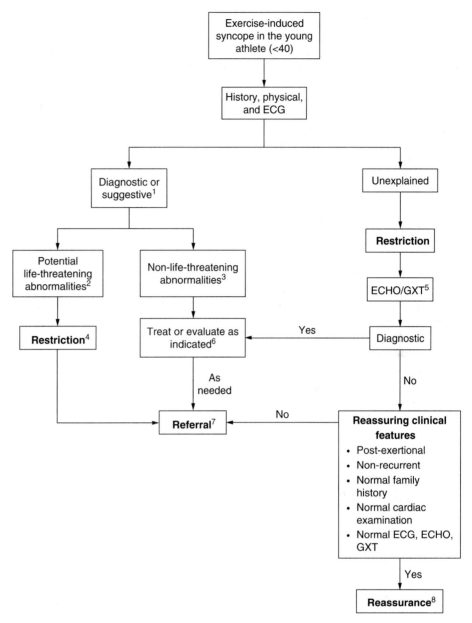

FIG. 25-1 Algorithm for the primary care evaluation of exertional syncope in the athlete under 40 years of age.

¹ Diagnostic or Suggestive: the history, physical examination, and electrocardiographic analysis result in a definitive or presumptive diagnosis, e.g., hypertrophic cardiomyopathy, exertional hyponatremia.

² Potential life-threatening diagnoses may include hypertrophic cardiomyopathy, arrhythmogenic right ventricular dyslpasia, and heat stroke.

³ Non-life-threatening diagnose may include hypoglycemia, mild hyponatremia, and mild heat exhaustion.

⁴ Restriction: this individual should be restricted from strenuous/vigorous exercise pending completion of the syncope evaluation.

⁵ An echocardiogram and exercise stress test is warranted in all cases of unexplained exertional syncope to include postexertional syncope. Echocardiography should precede exercise stress testing.

⁶ The diagnostic evaluation should be ordered as indicated according to the diagnosis being entertained. This may be in consultation with a cardiologist, neurologist and/or psychiatrist. Temporary restriction from vigorous activity should be considered on an individual basis.

⁷ Referral: Consultation is warranted and may include Holter or event monitoring, tilt-table testing, electrophysiologic studies, coronary angiography, electrophysiologic studies, cardiac and/or brain MRI, electroencephalography, and/or psychiatric testing.

⁸ Reassurance: The athlete may return to vigorous activity with an appropriate follow-up plan.

HYPERTENSION IN ATHLETES

- Systemic hypertension remains one of the most common life-threatening cardiovascular disorders in the United States and affects athletes of all ages and sports. The diagnosis, work-up, and the initial non-pharmacologic approach to treatment does not differ between athletes and nonathletes. This approach is well described in the JNC-VII recommendations (Joint National Committee on Prevention, Detection, Evaluation, and Treatment of High Blood Pressure, 2003).
- Care must be taken not to overdiagnose the condition in young athletes and to use proper fitting cuffs with three different measures on three different days, adjusting for norms for age, and height (Luckstead, 2002) (see Table 25-6).
  - An appropriate search for secondary etiologies and target organ damage assessment should guide the history, physical, and laboratory evaluation.
  - History should include an inquiry about performance enhancing substances (e.g., anabolic steroids) and lab should include EKG, urinalysis, *complete blood count* (CBC), electrolytes, fasting glucose, lipid profile, *blood urea nitrogen* (BUN), creatinine, and uric acid. It often includes a chest X-ray and echocardiogram to assess for left ventricular hypertrophy as well as a stress test to assist in determining the intensity level of activity participation (Maron and Mitchell, 1994; Strong and Steed, 1982).
- Nonpharmacologic treatment should be properly initiated with enthusiastic physician endorsement (Whelton et al, 2002; Niedfeldt, 2002). It includes engagement in moderate physical activity, maintenance of ideal body weight, limitation of alcohol (1 oz/day), reduction in sodium intake (100 mmol/day), maintenance of adequate potassium intake (90 mmol/day), and consumption of a diet high in fruit and vegetables and low in total and saturated fat.
- When indicated, pharmacologic treatment should be initiated. Generally, *angiotensin converting enzyme* (ACE) inhibitors, calcium channel blockers, and angiotensin-II receptor blockers are excellent choices for athletes with hypertension. Their low side effect profile and favorable physiologic hemodynamics make them generally safe and effective. It is preferable to avoid diuretics and beta-blockers in young athletes. Volume and potassium balance issues limit diuretic use and beta-blockers adversely impact the cardiovascular training effect of exercise (Kugler and O'Connor, 1999; Kugler, O'Connor, and Oriscello, 2001). Both substances, as well as a number of other antihypertensives are banned by the National Collegiate Athletic Association and the

TABLE 25-6 Classification of Hypertension (Boys and Girls Combined) (mmHg)

AGE (YEARS)	HIGH NORMAL BP (90TH–94TH PERCENTILE)	SIGNIFICANT HTN (95TH–98TH PERCENTILE)	SEVERE HTN (99TH PERCENTILE)
6–9			
Systolic	111–121	122–129	>129(129)*
Diastolic	70–77	70–85	>85(84)
10–12			
Systolic	117–125	126–133	>133(134)
Diastolic	75–81	82–89	>89(89)
13–15			
Systolic	124–135	136–143	>143(149)
Diastolic	77–85	86–91	>91(94)
16–18			
Systolic	127–141	142–149	>149(159)
Diastolic	80–91	92–97	>97(99)
>18			
Systolic	not given	[140–179]†	>(179)
Diastolic	not given	[90–109]	>(109)

SOURCE: (Committee on Sports Medicine and Fitness, 1997)
*The values in parentheses are those used for the classification of severe hypertension by the 26th Bethesda Conference on cardiovascular disease and atheletic participation (Maron and Mitchell, 1994).
†The values in brackets are those for mild and moderate hypertension given by the 26th Bethesda Conference (Maron and Mitchell, 1994).

U.S. Olympic Committee (Fuentes, Rosenberg, and Davis, 1996).

• Restriction of activity for athletes with hypertension depends on the degree of target organ damage and on the overall control of the blood pressure (Maron and Mitchell, 1994; Committee on Sports Medicine and Fitness, 1997).

• The presence of mild to moderate hypertension with no target organ damage or concomitant heart disease should not limit eligibility for competitive sports (Maron et al, 2001). Athletes with severe degrees of hypertension should be restricted, particularly from static sports, until their hypertension is controlled. When hypertension coexists with other cardiovascular diseases, eligibility for competitive sports is usually based on the severity of the other associated condition. In children and adolescents, the presence of severe hypertension or target organ disease warrants restriction until hypertension is under adequate control. The presence of significant hypertension should not limit a young athlete's eligibility for competitive athletics.

CORONARY ARTERY DISEASE IN ATHLETES

• Vigorous exercise represents a dangerous paradox for cardiovascular disease (Maron, 2000). While it may be a potent preventive tool, it can also represent substantial risk for the susceptible individual. This is particularly poignant for the athlete with an established diagnosis of CAD.

• These individuals will absolutely require careful risk

TABLE 25-7 Stratification Categories for Cad Patients by 26th Bethesda Conference

mildly increased risk	substantially increased risk
LVEF >50%	LVEF <50% at rest
Normal exercise tolerance for age, i.e., >10 METS if < age 50 >9 METS if age 50–59 >8 METS if age 60–69 >7 METS if > age 70	Evidence of exercise-induced myocardial ischemia
Absence of exercise-induced ischemia by exercise testing	
Absence of exercise-induced complex ventricular arrhythmia	Evidence of exercise-induced complex ventricular arrhythmias
Absence of hemodynamically significant stenosis in all major coronary arteries if angiography performed or successful myocardial revascularization by surgical or percutaneous techniques	Evidence of hemodynamically significant stenosis of a major coronary artery (>50%) if angiography performed

SOURCE: (Maron and Mitchell, 1994; Kugler and O'Connor, 2001)

TABLE 25-8 Summary of 26th Bethesda Conference Recommendations for Patients with Coronary Artery Disease

General

1. All athletes should understand that the risk of a cardiac event with exertion is probably increased once coronary artery disease is present.
2. Athletes should be informed of the nature of prodromal symptoms and should be instructed to promptly cease their sports activity and contact their physician if symptoms appear.

Specific

1. Mildly increased risk. May participate in low and moderate static and low dynamic competitive sports (IA and IIA) and avoid intensely competitive situations.
2. Substantially increased risk. May participate in low intensity competitive sports (IA) after careful assessment and individualization. These patients should be reevaluated every 6 months and should undergo repeat exercise testing at least yearly.

SOURCE: (Maron and Mitchell, 1994; Kugler and O'Connor, 2001)

stratification prior to returning to their active lifestyle (Kugler, O'Connor, and Oriscello, 2001). They will require procedures for left ventricular assessment, maximal treadmill testing to determine functional capacity, and testing for inducible ischemia. Patients should be tested on their medications.

• The 26th Bethesda Conference (Maron and Mitchell, 1994) defines clear stratification criteria (Table 25-7) accompanied by activity recommendations (Table 25-8). This provides a general and conservative approach to the individual in regards to competitive sports.

• The American College of Sports Medicine has recently published guidelines that assist the primary care physician in guiding the level of aerobic intensity (American College of Sports Medicine, 2000) (Table 25-9).

TABLE 25-9 Signs and Symptoms Below which an Upper Limit for Exercise Intensity Should be Set*

Onset of angina or other symptoms of cardiovascular insuffciency
Plateau or decrease in systolic blood pressure, systolic blood pressure of >240 mm Hg, or diastolic blood pressure of >110 mmHg
Greater than or equal to 1 mm ST-segment depression, horizontal, or downsloping
Radionuclide evidence of left ventricular dysfunction or onset of moderate-to-severe wall motion abnormalities during exertion
Increased frequency of ventricular arrhythmias
Other significant ECG disturbances (e.g., second degree or third degree AV block, atrial fibrillation, supraventricular tachycardia, complex ventricular ectopy)
Other signs/symptoms of intolerance to exercise

SOURCE: (Americal College of Sports Medicine, 2000)
*The peak exercise rate should generally be at least 10 bpm below the heart rate associated with any of the above-referenced criteria. Other variables (e.g., the corresponding systolic blood pressure response and perceived exertion), however, should also be considered when establishing the exercise intensity.

ARRHYTHMIAS IN ATHLETES

• Lethal cardiac arrhythmias represent the most serious risk for sudden death in athletes. Symptoms of a potential arrhythmia may include syncope, near syncope, palpitations, exertional chest discomfort, severe dyspnea, or uncommon exertional fatigue.

EVALUATION

• Structural heart disease must be ruled out before the athlete is allowed to return to sports (Maron and Mitchell, 1994; Kugler and O'Connor, 1999; Luckstead, 2002). This will include a meticulous history, physical examination, and EKG and may be followed by chest X-ray, echocardiogram, stress test, Holter monitoring, electrolytes, and other laboratory testing.
• It may very well include early referral to a cardiologist for electrophysiologic study and/or ongoing management.

TABLE 25-10 Activity Recommendations for the Common Dysrhythmias

ACTIVITY	RECOMMENDATIONS
Disturbances of sinus node function (includes sinus bradycardia, tachycardia, arrhythmia, arrest, exit block; sick sinus syndrome)	No symptoms, no treatment; if symptoms require pacemaker, then no collision sports
Premature atrial complexes	No restrictions
Atrial flutter and atrial fibrillation	If no structural heart disease and rate controlled by drugs, then low-intensity sports; if no flutter or fibrillation for 6 months, then full participation
Supraventricular tachycardia	If episodes are prevented by drugs, then full participation; if structural disease and if syncope or pre-syncope, no competitive sports; reconsider after 6 mos without recurrence
Ventricular pre-excitation (WPW)	If no structural heart disease and no symptoms, then no limit; if structuralheart disease and PVCs worsen with exercise, restrict; PVCs plus prolonged QT interval should be restricted (high risk for sudden death)
Heart blocks (first-degree or Mobitz I second-degree)	If no symptoms and no structural disease, then no restrictions
Heart blocks (Mobitz II second degree or third degree)	If no symptoms and no structural disease, then no restrictions if rate 40–80; if symptoms then pacer and avoid collision sports
Congenital long Q-T Syndrome	Restrict from all competitive sports (High risk for death)

SOURCE: (Maron and Mitchell, 1994; Kugler and O'Connor, 1999)

SPORTS PARTICIPATION

• Various arrhythmias are compatible with competitive sports once they are diagnosed and controlled. See Table 25-10 for a summary of the common dysrhythmias and the recommendations from the 26th Bethesda Conference (Maron and Mitchell, 1994).
• The Committee on Sports Medicine and Fitness for the American Academy of Pediatrics specifically recommends that the presence of a symptomatic dysrhythmia requires exclusion from physical activity until the athlete's problem can be adequately evaluated by a cardiologist and controlled (Committee on Sports Medicine and Fitness, 1995).

REFERENCES

American College of Sports Medicine: *ACSM's Guidelines for Exercise Testing and Prescription,* 6th ed. Philadelphia, PA, Lippincott Williams, and Wilkins, 2000, pp 165–199.

Basilico FC: Cardiovascular disease in athletes. *Am J Sports Med* 27:108–121, 1999.

Berlin JA, Colditz GA: A meta-analysis of physical activity in the prevention of coronary heart disease. *Am J Epidemiol* 132:612–628, 1990.

Blair SN, Kohl HW III, Barlow CE, et al: Changes in physical fitness and all-cause mortality: A prospective study of healthy and unhealthy men. *JAMA.* 273:1093–1098, 1995.

Cantu RC: Congenital cardiovascular disease: The major cause of athletic death in high scool and college. *Med Sci Sports Exerc* 24:279–280, 1992.

Committee on Sports Medicine and Fitness: Cardiac dysrhythmias and sports. *Pediatrics* 95:786–789, 1995.

Committee on Sports Medicine and Fitness: Athletic participation by children and adolescents who have systemic hypertension. *Pediatrics* 99(4), 1997.

Firoozi S, Sharma S, Hamid MS, et al: Sudden death in young athletes: HCM or ARVC? *Cardiovasc Drugs Ther* 16:11–17, 2002.

Fuentes RJ, Rosenberg JM, Davis A (eds.): Athletic Drug reference '96. Durham, NC, Clean Data, 1996.

Huston TP, Puffer JC, Rodney WM: The athletic heart syndrome. *N Engl J Med* 313:24–32, 1985.

Joint National Committee on Prevention, Detection, Evaluation, and Treatment of High Blood Pressure: The seventh report of the Joint National Committee on Prevention, Detection, Evaluation, and Treatment of High Blood Pressure. *JAMA* 289:2560–2572, 2003.

Kapoor WN: Evaluation and management of the patient with syncope. *JAMA* 268:2553–2560, 1992.

Kohl HW III, Powell KE, Gordon NF, et al: Physical activity, physical fitness, and sudden cardiac death. *Epidemiol Rev* 14:37–58, 1992.

Kugler JP, O'Connor FG: Cardiovascular problems, in Lillegard WA, Butcher JD, Rucker KS, (eds.): *Handbook of Sports Medicine,* 2nd ed. Boston, MA, Butterworth/Heinemann, 1999, p 339.

Kugler JP, O'Connor FG, Oriscello RG: Cardiovascular considerations in the runner, in O'Coonor FG, Wilder RP, (eds.): *Textbook of Running Medicine.* New York, NY, McGraw-Hill, 2001, p 341.

Leon AS, Connett J, Jacobs DR Jr, et al: Leisure-time physical activity levels and risk of coronary heart disease and death: the Multiple Risk Factor Intervention Trial. *JAMA* 258:2388–2395, 1987.

Luckstead EF, Sr: Cardiac risk factors and participation guidelines for youth sports. *Pediatr Clin North Am* 49:681–707, 2002.

Manolis AS, Linzer M, Salem D, et al: Syncope: Current diagnostic evaluation and management. *Ann Intern Med* 112:850–863, 1990.

Maron BJ: The paradox of exercise. *N Engl J Med* 343:1409–1411, 2000.

Maron BJ, Araujo CG, Thompson PD, et al: AHA science advisory: Recommendations for preparticipation screening and the assessment of cardiovascular disease in master athletes, an advisory for healthcare professionals from the working groups of the World Heart Federation, the International Federation of Sports Medicine, and the AHA Committee on Exercise, Cardiac Rehabilitation, and Prevention. *Circulation* 103:327, 2001.

Maron BJ, Gohman TE, Aeppli D: Prevalence of sudden cardiac death during competitive sports activities in Minnesota high school athletes. *J Am Coll Cardiol* 32:1881–1884, 1998.

Maron BJ, Mitchell JH (eds): 26th Bethesda Conference. Recommendations for determining eligibility for competition in athletes with cardiovascular abnormalities. *Am J Cardiol* 24:845–899, 1994.

Maron BJ, Poliac LC, Roberts WO: Risk for sudden cardiac death associated with marathon running. *J Am Coll Cardiol* 28:428–431, 1996.

Maron BJ, Thompson PD, Puffer JC, et al: Cardiovascular preparticipation screening of competitive athletes: a statement for health professionals from the Sudeen Death Committee (Clinical Cardiology) and Congenital Cardiac Defects Committee (Cardiovascular Disease in the Young), American Heart Association. *Circulation* 94:850–856, 1996.

Murkerji B, Albert MA, Mukerji V: Cardiovascular changes in athletes. *Am Fam Physician* 40:169–175, 1989.

Niedfeldt MW: Managing hypertension in athletes and physically active patients. *Am Fam Physician* 66:445–452, 2002.

Oakley DG, Oakley CM: Significance of abnormal electrocardiograms in highly trained athletes. *Am J Cardiol* 50:985–989, 1982.

Paffenbarger RS, Hyde RT, Wing AL, et al: The association of changes in physical activity level and other lifestyle characteristics with mortality among men. *N Engl J Med* 328:538–545, 1993.

Pate RR, Pratt M, Blair SN, et al: Physical activity and public health. *JAMA* 273, 402, 1995.

Pelliccia MD, Maron BJ, Culasso F, et al: Clinical significance of abnormal electrocardiographic patterns in trained athletes. *Circulation* 102:278, 2000.

Pluim BM, Zwinderman AH, van der Laarse A, et al: The athlete's heart. A meta-analysis of cardiac structure and function. *Circulation* 101:336–344, 2001.

Powell KE, Thompson PD, Caspersen CJ, et al: Physical activity and the incidence of coronary heart disease. *Annu Rev Public Health* 8:253–287, 1987.

Priori SG, Aliot E, Blomstrom-Lundqvist C, et al: Task force on sudden cardiac death, European Society of Cardiology. Summary of recommendations. *Europace* 4:3–18, 2002.

Pyeritz RE: The Marfan syndrome. *Am Fam Physician* 34:83–94, 1986.

Ragosta M, Crabtree J, Sturner WQ , et al: Death during recreational exercise in the State of Rhode Island. *Ned Sci Sports Exerc* 16:339–342, 1984.

Siscovick DS, Weiss NS, Fletcher RH, et al: The incidence of primary cardiac arrest during vigorous exercise. *N Engl J Med* 311:874–877, 1984.

Strong WB, Steed D: Cardiovascular evaluation of the young athlete. *Pediatr Clin North Am* 29:1325–1339, 1982.

Tabib A, Miras A, Taniere P, et al: Undetected cardiac lesions cause unexpected sudden cardiac death during occasional sport activity. A report of 80 cases. *Eur Heart J* 20:900–903, 1999.

Thompson PD, Funk EJ, Carleton RA, et al: Incidence of death during jogging in Rhode Island from 1975 through 1980. *JAMA* 247:2535–2538, 1982.

Van camp SP, Bloor CM, Mueller FO, et al: Nontraumatic sports death in high school and college athletes. *Med Sci Sports Exerc* 27:641–647, 1995.

Villeneuve PJ, Morrison HI, Craig CL, et al: Physical activity, physical fitness, and risk of dying. *Epidemiology* 626–631, 1998.

Whelton PK, He J, Appel LJ, et al: Primary prevention of hypertension. *JAMA* 288:1882–1888, 2002.

Williams PT: Relationship of distance run per week to coronary heart disease risk factors in 8283 male runners. *Arch Intern Med* 157, 191, 1997.

Williams PT: Relationships of heart disease risk factors to exercise quantity and intensity. *Arch Intern Med* 158, 237, 1998.

Zeppilli P: The athlete's heart: Differentiation of training effects from organic heart disease. *Pract Cardiol* 14:61–84, 1988.

26 DERMATOLOGY
Kenneth B Batts, DO

INTRODUCTION

- Skin serves as a protective barrier against mechanical, environmental, and infective forces.
- Sport-specific dermatoses may incapacitate an athlete or expose a teammate to a potential infection placing him or her at risk for disqualification or impede his or her performance.

MECHANICAL INJURY

ABRASIONS

- Commonly known as *rug burn, strawberries,* or *road rash,* occur on artificial turf, floor mats, synthetic courts, and asphalt roads.

- Treatment consists of cleaning and debriding the tissue with warm, soapy water and applying a topical antibacterial ointment.
- Thin covering of antibacterial ointment (mupirocin) or an adhesive dressing (DuoDerm, Op-Site) promotes healing.
- Because of the risk of blood-borne pathogens and subsequent disease transmission, all wounds should be covered with an occlusive dressing during participation.
- National Collegiate Athletic Association (NCAA) mandates athletes be removed from competition if active bleeding exists, the bleeding stopped and a dressing applied to withstand the rigors of competition (Bubb, 2002).

ACNE MECHANICA

- An occlusive obstruction of the follicular pilosebaceous units
- The papulopustular eruption commonly affects areas include the forehead, cheek, chin, shoulders, back, and hips.
- Preventive measures include wearing a clean, cotton T-shirt against the skin to absorb the perspiration, reduce friction, and prevent follicular occlusion (Basler, 1989).
- The equipment should be routinely cleaned with soap and water or an alcohol solution to prevent bacterial formation.
- Acne mechanica in dark-skinned athletes may evolve into acne keloidalis on the nape of the neck (Pharis, Teller, and Wolf, Jr, 1997).
- The athlete can treat the condition with various topical acne keratolytics with astringents (3% salicylic acid, 70% resorcinol) and antibiotics (tetracycline, clindamycin) (Basler, 1989). Athletes should be well informed and educated prior to the use isotretinoin for severe pustular acne because of the side effects of muscle soreness, joint pain, and lethargy (Basler, 1989).

ATHLETIC NODULES

- Fibrotic connective tissue (collagenomas) because of repetitive pressure, friction, or trauma over bony prominences (Cohen, Eliezri, and Silvers, 1992).
- Commonly located on knuckles (boxers, football players), tibial tuberosity (surfers), dorsal feet (hockey, skate bites. runners. hikers) (Pharis, Teller, and Wolf, Jr, 1997; Erickson, 1967).
- Treatment includes intralesional steroids and protective taping and padding (Cohen, Eliezri, and Silvers, 1992).

BLACK HEEL

- Black heel, or *talon noir,* refers to a bluish-black plaque formation of horizontally arranged dots or calcaneal petechiae within the stratum corneum on the posterior or posterolateral aspect of the heel (Wilkinson, 1977).
- The condition occurs more frequently in adolescent and younger adults playing basketball, tennis, track, and field events where athletes are changing direction suddenly.
- A similar condition, mogul's palm, has been described on the hypothenar eminence of mogul skiers' palms that are constantly planting their poles and shifting direction (Swinehart, 1992).
- Self-limiting and will resolve spontaneously once the season ends.
- The use of heel cups, felt pads, cushioned athletic socks, and properly fitted footwear may help to prevent black heel formation.

BLACK TOENAIL

- Rapid deceleration of the forefoot against the shoe toe box may produce subungual hemorrhages of the first and second toenail beds.
- The condition occurs with greater frequency in sports requiring quick stops, such as tennis, skiing, hiking, and rock climbing (Pharis, Teller, and Wolf, Jr, 1997).
- The hematoma can be drained by carefully boring a hole through the nail with an 18-gauge needle or electrocautery unit.
- Appropriate running shoes (2 cm from the longest toe to the end of the shoe) and properly trimming the distal nail to its shortest length in a straight-cut line will reduce the likelihood of developing this condition (Adams, 2002*a*).
- Notable exceptions are the persistence of a linear black band or streak running the entire length of the nail representing a melanocytic nevus or the more serious involvement of the proximal nail fold in malignant melanoma (Crowe and Sorensen, 1999).

BLISTERS

- Vesicles or bulla filled with either serosanguinous fluid or blood.
- Repeated pressure or friction over boney prominences associated with excessive perspiration and improperly fitted equipment leads to the formation of blisters.
- Treat early with moleskin donuts and nylon foot stockings to decrease friction, talcum powder to absorb perspiration, and benzoin to harden the epidermis (Levine, 1980).

- Bullous blisters should be drained at the edge with a small needle leaving the roof of the blister as a protective layer.
- Ruptured and deroofed blisters may require the application of a hydrocolloidal dressing (Duoderm) or an adhesive polyurethane dressing (Op-Site) as a second-skin layer to reduce discomfort and enhance healing (Bergfeld and Elston, 1994).
- Primary prevention includes wearing properly fitted and broken-in footwear, use of absorbent socks, and applying petrolatum jelly over bony prominences.

CORN AND CALLUSES

- Corns are small, soft or hard, deep painful conical lesions with a translucent central core in the web spaces of the toes and the plantar surface of a malaligned distal metatarsal head.
- Calluses tend to be larger, hyperkeratotic nonpainful lesions that serve as a protective skin layer and are considered an advantage in gymnastics, racquet sports, and rowing.
- The development of small black dots representing thrombosed capillaries implies the presence of plantar warts, compared to calluses that display a thickened epidermis with intact dermatoglyphics.
- The most important factor for successful recovery and prevention of the condition is redistributing the source of pressure (Conklin, 1990).
- The shaping of a metatarsal pad to the plantar surface, creating a wider shoe toebox, adding cotton or foam padding between the toes, and applying moleskin will all aid in decreasing the pressure over the existing lesion and prevent further injury.
- Keratolytic agents such as 5–10% salicylic acid in collodian, 40% salicylic acid plaster, and 12% lactic acid will eliminate the lesions (Kantor and Bergfeld, 1988).

FOLLICULAR KELOIDITIS

- An inflammatory proliferation of fibrous tissue—usually painless and more prevalent in dark-skinned African athletes.
- Multiple, small keloids commonly develop where the headgear comes in contact with the forehead, cheeks, and posterior neck or where the undergarment pads cover the thighs, knees, and shoulders (Basler, 1983).
- Treatment involves gradual reduction of the lesion with intralesional injections of steroids or topical application of a steroid-impregnated adhesive tape (Dover, 1993).

INGROWN TOENAIL

- The condition is caused by nailbed pressure forcing the lateral edge of the nailplate into the lateral nail fold.
- The distal nail should be trimmed straight across and at least one thumbnail in distance should exist from the longest distal toenail to the end of the shoe to prevent reoccurrence.
- Acute treatment options include Epsom salt water bath, gentle manual nail elevation, placing a small piece of cotton under the corner of the nail to elevate the lateral margin to alleviate inflammation, use of antibiotics, and excision of the lateral one-third of the nail (Williams and Batts, 2001).

JOGGER'S NIPPLES

- Irritation and friction between coarse, cotton fabrics and the unprotected nipple and areola lead to painful, bleeding nipples (Levit, 1977).
- The majority of jogger's nipples occur in male athletes, especially long-distance runners and triathletes (Basler, 1989).
- Preventive measures include wearing of soft, natural, silk fiber shirts, and the application of breast padding, electrocardiographic lead pads, band-aids, or a double coat of fingernail polish over the nipples prior to running.

PIEZOGENIC PAPULES

- Painful herniations of subdermal fat into the dermis on the lateral or medial heel surface (Shelly and Raunsley, 1968).
- Flesh-colored papules noticeable only on weight-bearing are found in up to 20% of the general population (Dover, 1993).
- More common in endurance athletes.
- Padding, taping for support and/or heel cups may help reduce the pain.

ROWER'S RUMP

- Rower's rump develops in the gluteal cleft of rowers training on small, unpadded scull seats, and metal rowing machines (Tomecki and Mikesell, 1987).
- Repeated friction produces a lichen simplex chronicus of the buttocks.
- Treatment consists of padding the rowing seat and the use of potent, fluorinated topical steroids.

RUNNER'S RUMP

- A collection of ecchymotic lesions on the superior portion of the gluteal cleft of long-distance runners (Basler, 1989).
- Results from constant friction between the gluteal folds with each running stride.
- The hyperpigmentation will spontaneously resolve with rest.

ENVIRONMENTAL INJURY

HEAT

SUNBURN
- Exposure to *ultraviolet B* or UVB (290–320 nm) light during the hours of 10 a.m. and 2 p.m. for 2–6 h will produce mild erythema to intense blistering, edema, and pain (Kantor and Bergfeld, 1988).
- A rise in altitude from sea level to 5,000 feet intensifies sunlight by 20% (Levine, 1980).
- The *ultraviolet A* (UVA) light range of 320–400 nm is 1000-fold less burning to the skin than UVB. UVA is more penetrating and produces chronic damage to the skin (Conklin, 1990).
- Preventive measures include avoiding exercise between 10 a.m. and 2 p.m., applying *sun protective factor* (SPF) 15 or greater sunscreens with *para-aminobenzoic acid ester* (PABA) at least 20 min prior to sun exposure and recoating after water exposure (Levine, 1980).

MILIARIA
- Miliaria rubra, or prickly heat, occurs in hot, humid summer environments.
- Fine, diffuse erythematous vesiculopapular rash develops over the occluded eccrine sweat glands (spares the palms and soles) (Habif, 1996).
- Application of hydrophilic ointments (Eucerin) and mild topical corticosteroids can open the occluded ducts (Bergfeld and Elston, 1994).

SOLAR URTICARIA
- Solar urticaria is an uncommon cause of urticaria in athletes (Kantor and Bergfeld, 1988).
- The dermatoses manifest by itching and burning of the skin within minutes after exposure to UVA, UVB, or both wavelengths (Mikhailov, Berova, and Andreev, 1977).
- Erythema and wheal formation will follow and clear within 1 h after exposure (Pharis, Teller, and Wolf, Jr, 1997).
- Normally unexposed skin areas of the trunk will be more prone to develop an urticarial reaction than the previously exposed face or distal extremities.

- Phototesting is recommended to determine the type and treatment of solar urticaria.
- Desentization and *combination of psoralen and long-wave ultraviolet light* (PUVA) have been successful in minimizing symptoms (Fitzpatrick et al, 1992).
- Antimalarials have been found effective (Mikhailov, Berova, and Andreev, 1977).

CHOLINERGIC URTICARIA
- Cholinergic urticaria is an acetylcholine-mediated, pruritic dermatosis that occurs commonly on the chest and back during exercise or emotional stress (Houston and Knox, 1997).
- The condition is characterized by the eruption of pinpoint papular wheals with a surrounding subcutaneous erythematous flare during and after heat exposure or exercise.
- The most reliable and safe test is to have the athlete perform exercise for 15 min on a treadmill or bike to reproduce the lesions.
- Treatment with H_1 antihistamines and danazol has been found to be effective if taken 1 h prior to exercise (Elston, 1999).
- A hot shower the night prior may deplete histamine and provide a refractory period for the athlete to compete (Habif, 1996).
- The condition can be exacerbated with the use of aspirin.

COLD

CHILBLAIN
- Chilblain or pernio is the mildest form of cold injury and develops on the feet, hands, and face.
- Athletes participating in winter sports are initially unaware of the injury, but later complain of reddish-blue patches that burn, itch, and may later develop blisters (Kantor and Bergfeld, 1988).
- The injured area should be rewarmed, massaged gently to increase circulation, and protected from further environmental exposure.
- Topical corticosteroids or a short burst of oral corticosteroids may be utilized to minimize the painful, inflammatory skin lesions.
- The use of moisture-wicking socks and gloves, frequent sock and glove changes, and protective covering over the face aid in preventing this injury.

FROSTNIP
- Frostnip or superficial frostbite occurs as temperatures drop below 50°F (10°C) (Williams and Batts, 2001).
- The skin and superficial subcutaneous tissue of the fingertips, toes, nose, cheeks, and ears will blanche or

turn grayish-white, develop paresthesias, and finally lose sensation.

- Penile frostnip has been reported in joggers wearing polyester trousers and cotton undershorts (Hershkowitz, 1977).
- Frostnip can be reversed with immediate self-rewarming of the exposed area.
- Paresthesias and a burning sensation may persist for several months after the injury.
- Prevention includes insulation and skin protection from both wind and cold, not shaving prior to participation to preserve the natural skin oils and application of a sunscreen. (D'Ambrosia, 1977)

FROSTBITE

- Frostbite occurs as living tissue ceases cellular metabolism from exposure to temperatures below 28°F (–2°C) (D'Ambrosia, 1977).
- Muscles, nerves and blood vessels are damaged earlier than tendons and bone (D'Ambrosia, 1977).
- The tissue appears cold, white, and hard and will not exhibit pain or sensation to tactile stimulation until thawing occurs.
- Rewarming of the tissue should be attempted only when the environment can be controlled and risk of refreezing of the affected part is eliminated.
- Frozen areas should be rewarmed as rapidly as possible in a warm-water, circulating bath of 110–112°F (38–44°C) to prevent mechanical trauma (D'Ambrosia, 1977).
- Tissue necrosis may occur for weeks to months as reepithelialization replaces the denuded areas (Levine, 1980).

COLD URTICARIA

- Cold urticaria is rare but the most common form of acquired physical urticaria in winter athletics and cold water swimming (Mikhailov, Berova, and Andreev, 1977).
- Wheals or hives are usually confined to the exposed area.
- Athletes with cold urticaria are likely to have recurrent, severe episodes during similar circumstances because of the antigen–antibody reaction resulting in the release of histamine (D'Ambrosia, 1977).
- To confirm the diagnosis, provocative testing of the forearm with ice cubes for 5 min or submerging the forearm in cold water for 5–15 min will produce wheals (Pharis, Teller, and Wolf, Jr, 1997).
- The prophylactic use of cyproheptadine (Periactin), 2 mg once or twice a day, or doxepin (Sinequan), 10 mg two or three times daily have been useful in preventing reoccurrence (Williams and Batts, 2001).

INFECTIOUS INJURY

BACTERIAL

FURUNCULOSIS

- Erythematous, nodular abscesses found in the hairy areas of the axilla, buttocks, and groin.
- Highly contagious and known outbreaks have occurred in team sports, implicating close contact and poor hygiene practices (Sosin et al, 1989).
- Staphyloccocci are the most common bacteria and the nares should be cultured because of the predisposition of the nares to harbor the staphylococcus species (Adams, 2002a).
- Acute treatment consists of warm compresses and a 10-day course of a cephalosporin, erythromycin, or penicillinase-resistant penicillin derivative (Bergfeld and Helm, 1991).
- A prophylactic dose of rifampin, 600 mg for 10 days, has been utilized in resistant cases (Williams and Batts, 2001).
- Incision and drainage is necessary because of the poor hematogenous antibiotic penetration.
- The NCAA requires all wrestlers to be without new lesions for 48 h before a meet, have completed 72 h of antibiotic therapy, and have no moist or draining lesions prior to competition (Bubb, 2002).

PITTED KERATOLYSIS

- A scalloped-bordered plaque with sculpted pits of variable depth forms on the weight-bearing plantar surfaces (heel and toes) and is often misdiagnosed as tinea pedis.
- Hyperhidrosis and gram-positive bacteria, most commonly *Corynebacterium* and *Micrococcus* species, found in the stratum corneum have been implicated in producing the pungent foot odor (Schissel, Aydelotte, and Keller, 1999).
- Application of topical antibiotics for 2–4 weeks (5% erythromycin in 10% benzoyl peroxide) will reduce the bacterial inflammatory component and result in clearing (Kantor and Bergfeld, 1988).
- Prophylactic therapy includes washing with benzoyl peroxide soap and adding topical foot powders with 20% aluminum chloride (Drysol) to control hyperhidrosis (Schissel, Aydelotte, and Keller, 1999).

IMPETIGO

- Serosanguinous, honey-crusted pustules on an erythematous base.
- Beta-hemolytic streptococci more commonly produce impetigo, but staphylococcal species have been isolated from cultured wounds.
- Athletes participating in contact sports or swimming are highly contagious and should not participate in

competition until all lesions have resolved (Bergfeld and Elston, 1994).

- Less extensive lesions may respond to twice-daily mupirocin ointment with aluminum acetate compresses (Burow's solution) in a 1:40 dilution three times daily (Bergfeld and Elston, 1994).
- A 10-day course of an oral cephalosporin or penicillinase-resistant penicillin promotes rapid healing.
- The NCAA guidelines for participation of wrestlers with bacterial infections are described in furunculosis (Bubb, 2002).

ERYTHRASMA

- Chronic, bacterial infection affecting the intertriginous areas.
- The causative organism is a gram-positive rod, *Corynebacterium minutissimum.*
- The sharply, demarcated reddish-brown plaques are similar in appearance to tinea cruris (Bergfeld, 1984).
- Under a wood's lamp (black light), the lesions will fluoresce coral-red; while tinea cruris does not fluoresce (Bergfeld and Elston, 1994).
- Treatment options include a topical erythromycin cream or gel and oral erythromycin 250 mg four times a day for 14 days.
- The areas should be covered for athletes to participate in close contact drills or events.

VIRAL

VERRUCAE

- The human papilloma virus induces warts, or verrucae vulgaris.
- Plantar warts disrupt the normal dermatoglyphics of the pressure points of the feet and often coalesce to form a gyrate or mosaic pattern.
- Small black dots representing thrombosed capillaries within a hyperkeratotic plaque confirm the diagnosis (Adams, 2002*a*).
- The NCAA requires wrestlers to be able to cover multiple digitate verrucae of the face with a mask and verrucae plana or vulgaris must be adequately covered to compete (Bubb, 2002).
- Salicylic acid solutions (Duofilm, Compound W) and 40% plaster compounds (Mediplast) can be applied overnight with an occlusion wrap during the season (Bergfeld and Elston, 1994).
- Liquid nitrogen cryotherapy can be done concurrently or separately every 2 weeks.

MOLLUSCUM CONTAGIOSUM

- Characterized by small umbilicated, flesh-colored, and dome-shaped papules.

- The poxvirus is highly contagious and spread by direct skin transmission from person to person, autoinnoculation, water transmission, and gymnastic equipment (Kantor and Bergfeld, 1988).
- The papules are self-limiting and resolve over weeks to months.
- To compete the lesions must be removed by sharp curettage or liquid nitrogen and any solitary lesions must be covered with a gas permeable dressing (Op-Site, Bioclusive) and ProWrap and tape (Bubb, 2002).
- Liquid nitrogen, cantharidin (0.7% in collodion), topical tretinoin (Retin-A), electrodessication and the use of imiquimod 5% cream have been successful but may require several treatments (Buescher, 2002).

HERPES GLADIATORUM

- Herpes gladiatorum or rugbeiorum refers to a *herpes simplex virus* (HSV-1) outbreak on the face of wrestlers or rugby players during "lock-up" or in a scrum.
- Classic lesions appear as a cluster of painful vesicles on an erythematous base.
- The virus is passed by direct face-to-face transmission between athletes, and headgear does not decrease the risk of transmission (Belongia et al, 1991).
- Famciclovir, 250 mg three times a day for 5 days and valaciclovir 1 gm twice a day for 5 days are recommended for initial therapy (Buescher, 2002).
- Famciclovir and valaciclovir have not been approved for use in children less than 18 years of age.
- Valacyclovir, 500 mg once daily has been prescribed for prophylaxis during the season (Adams, 2002*a*).
- In the pediatric population, 40–80 mg/kg/day in three or four does for 7–10 days remains the standard of care (Buescher, 2002).
- The NCAA will allow a wrestler to participate if free of systemic systems, not developed new lesions during the last 72 h, all lesions have a firm adherent crust and the wrestler had been on antiviral therapy for 120 h (Bubb, 2002).

FUNGAL

TINEA PEDIS

- A papulosquamous fungal infection producing a pruritic, red, scaly rash on the lateral soles of the feet and between the toes.
- The superficial dermatophytic fungal infection is caused by *Trichophyton rubrum, Trichophyton mentagrophytes* or *Epidermophyton floccusum* (Buescher, 2002).
- The majority of cases respond promptly to topical antifungal creams, such as miconazole, clotrimazole, and econazole.

TINEA CORPORIS

- Annular lesion having a sharply demarcated, reddened border with central clearing.
- The dermatophyte infection produces concentric rings along its annular margins.
- Tinea corporis gladiatorum has been more frequently isolated and reported in wrestlers on their head, neck, and upper arms (Adams, 2002*b*).
- In the majority of cases, *Trichophyton tonsurans* is the causative fungus (Adams, 2002*b*).
- Recent studies reveal oral fluconazole, 200 mg, taken once weekly for 4 weeks had negative cultures after 7 days in 60% of the wrestlers (Adams, 2002*b*).
- The NCAA requires a minimum of 72 h of topical terbinafine or naftifine to skin lesions, a minimum of 2 weeks of oral therapy for scalp lesions, and all lesions to be adequately covered with an antifungal cream, gas-permeable dressing, and ProWrap with stretch tape prior to wrestling (Bubb, 2002).

TINEA CRURIS

- An erythematous, pruritic plaque with well-demarcated, scaly borders that extends to the groin, upper thighs, abdomen, and perineum, but spares the scrotum (Freeman and Bergfeld, 1977).
- The scrotum is spared because of the fungistatic sebum produced by the scrotal skin (Basler, 1983).
- The appearance of an inflammatory, red rash with satellite lesions involving the scrotum is candidiasis and requires treatment with imadazole creams.
- Diagnosis can be confirmed by the presence of fungal hyphae on a KOH slide.
- Oral antifungal agents may be required in recalcitrant cases, if the hair roots are involved.
- Tinea cruris must also be differentiated from candidia intertrigo (scrotal involvement and satellite lesions), erythrasma (brown and scaly, fluoresces coral red), psoriasis (silvery scale, pitted nails, and scalp lesions), folliculitis (punctate pustules), or a chronic irritant dermatitis from elasticized undergarments (Hainer, 2003).

TINEA VERSICOLOR

- A chronic, asymptomatic pigmented scaling macular dermatosis associated with the overgrowth of the active fungal form of *Pityrosporum orbiculare* known as *Malasseziafurfur* (Kantor and Bergfeld, 1988).
- Wood's lamp reveals a yellow-green flourescence of the skin scales (Conklin, 1990).
- Tinea versicolor is treated with topical 2.5% selenium sulfide shampoo (Selsun) for 15 to 30 min over 5 to 10 days or by applying the lotion from the neck down to the thighs overnight (6 to 12 h) and rinsed off the next morning (Bergfeld and Helm, 1991).

- In extensive disease, oral ketoconazole 200 mg daily for 5 days or 400 mg once a month has been shown to be an effective alternative therapy (Conklin, 1990).
- The athlete needs to continue to exercise and perspire for at least 1 h after taking ketoconazole to promote absorption into the hair root (Bergfeld and Elston, 1994).
- Griseofulvin is not an effective treatment.

ONYCHOMYCOSIS

- Onychomycosis is a common toenail fungal infection known as tinea unguium and can be attributed to either of two dermataphytes, *trichophyton rubrum* or *trytophytum mentagrophytes*, in 80% of cases (Scher, 1999).
- Itraconazole (Sporanox) and terbinafine (Lamisil) are the therapeutic agents of choice for both toenail and fingernail therapy in adults (Rodgers and Basler, 2001).
- Itraconazole can be given in either a continuous dose of 200 mg daily for 12 weeks for toenails and 6 weeks for fingernails or a pulsed dose of 400 mg daily for the first full week of 3–4 successive months (toenails) and two successive months (fingernails) (Scher, 1999; Rodgers and Basler, 2001).
- Terbinafine 250 mg, is taken daily for 12 weeks for toenails and 6 weeks for fingernails (Scher, 1999; Rodgers and Basler, 2001).
- Laboratory analysis for hepatotoxicity and pancytopenia must be performed during therapy.

MISCELLANEOUS

CONTACT DERMATITIS

- Primary irritant dermatitis is a nonallergic reaction that leads to symptoms within minutes of the exposure (Bergfeld, 1984). The dermatitis is localized to the contact site and exhibits erythema and a burning sensation. Common irritants are detergents and soaps, adhesive pretape sprays, sunscreens, and fiberglass (Adams, 2002*a*).
- Allergic contact dermatitis is an acquired immune response that develops hours to days after recurrent exposure to an allergen. The dermatitis exhibits patches of erythema, edema, vesicle formation, and extreme pruritus. Equipment with protective rubber coverings (golf clubs) and black rubber seals (swim gear), tanned leather straps, latex products, iodine preparations, topical antibiotic ointments, adhesive tape, shoe dyes, and poison ivy or oak have all produced allergic reactions (Bergfeld and Helm, 1991).
- Initial treatment includes avoidance, washing with water in an attempt to physically remove the irritant and prevent further systemic progression.

- Alternative equipment has been manufactured using polyurethane, neoprene, and silicone to alleviate allergic reactions.
- Antihistamines, corticosteroids, analgesics, and H₂-antagonists are commonly utilized for moderate to severe systemic hypersensitivity reactions by either oral or intravenous routes.
- Patch testing can often help identify the allergan triggering the dermatitis.

ENVENOMATION

- Most of the allergic reactions are from hornets and wasps (Frazier, 1977).
- The venom can be neutralized with meat tenderizer or shaving cream at the site.
- Ice packs will reduce the swelling and slow the absorption of the venom.
- Antihistamines and nonsteroidal anti-inflammatory agents are commonly prescribed.
- Participants with known allergic reactions to hymenoptera should be advised to use sunscreens with insect repellent formulas.
- Athletic trainers or physicians covering events should always carry an Epi-Pen kit.

SWIMMER'S ITCH

- Parasitic dermatitis produced by the cercariae form of the schistosomes commonly found in freshwater lakes of the United States (Hoeffler, 1977).
- One- to two-millimeter macules develop into papules on exposed areas, not under the bathing suit.
- Acute symptomatic therapy with antihistamines and topical steroids.

SEABATHER'S ERUPTION

- Pruritic, papules, and wheals primarily occur in scuba divers off the East Coast of the United States from Long Island, New York down into the Caribbean (Freudenthal and Joseph, 1993).
- Free-swimming, larval forms of *Edwardsiella lineata* and *Linuche unguiculata* contain stinging nematocysts (Freudenthal and Joseph, 1993).
- Prolonged wearing of the bathing suit, washing off with freshwater and strenuous exercise activate the nematocysts (Freudenthal and Joseph, 1993).
- Meat tenderizer, baking soda, warm saltwater, vinegar or shaving cream denature the nematocysts (Freudenthal and Barbagallo, 2002).

GREEN HAIR

- Regular swimmers with natural or tinted blonde, gray or white hair may develop a green tint to their hair from the release of copper from pipes or algicides in swimming pools (Basler et al, 2000).
- Immediately washing the hair and maintaining the pool pH between 7.4 and 7.6 will prevent this condition (Pharis, Teller, and Wolf, Jr, 1997).
- Washing the hair with copper-chelating shampoos (ultraswim) for 30 min or 3% hydrogen peroxide for 3 h will return the hair to its previous color (Basler, 1989).

EXERCISED-INDUCED ANAPHYLAXIS

- The most severe form of urticaria is *exercised-induced anaphylaxis* (EIA) (Pharis, Teller, and Wolf, Jr, 1997).
- Pruritus with large wheals may progress to systemic symptoms of wheezing, nausea, diarrhea, angioedema, hypotension, and shock.
- Running has been found to be the most common exercise predisposed to EIA (Adams, 2002a).
- Three distinct patterns of cutaneous involvement may be seen: cholinergic urticaria, giant urticaria, and angioedema without urticaria (Lewis et al, 1981).
- EIA lesions are large and are not produced by hot showers, pyrexia, or anxiety.
- Plasma histamine levels are elevated in all forms of EIA.
- Preventive measures include not exercising in extremes of either hot or cold weather and the use of nonsedating antihistamines 1 h prior to exercise (Fisher, 1992).
- Athletes who want to continue vigorous exercise should be instructed to exercise with someone (jogging partner) who has knowledge of their condition and can administer an injectable subcutaneous 1:1000 epinephrine syringe (EpiPen kit) (Bergfeld and Elston, 1994).

REFERENCES

Adams BB: Dermatologic disorders of the athlete. *Sports Med* 32:309, 2002a.

Adams BB: Tinea corporis gladiatorum. *J Am Acad Dermatol* 47:286, 2002b.

Basler RSW: Skin injuries in sports medicine. *J Am Acad Dermatol* 21:1257, 1989.

Basler RSW: Skin lesions related to sports activity, in Callen JP (ed.): *Primary Care.* Philadelphia, PA, Saunders, 1983, p 479.

Basler RSW et al: Special skin symptoms seen in swimmers. *J Am Acad Dermatol* 43:299, 2000.

Belongia EA et al: An outbreak of herpes gladiatorum at a high-school wrestling camp. *N Engl J Med* 325:906, 1991.

Bergfeld WF: Dermatologic problems in athletes, in Lombardo JA (ed.): *Primary Care,* Philadelphia, PA, Saunders, 1984, p 151.

Bergfeld WF, Elston DM: Diagnosis and treatment of dermatologic problems in athletes, in Fu FH, Stone DA (eds.): *Sports Injuries: Mechanisms, Prevention, Treatment.* Baltimore, MD, Williams & Wilkins, 1994, p 781.

Bergfeld WF, Helm TN: Skin disorders in athletes, in Grana WA, Kalenak A (eds.): *Clinical Sports Medicine.* Philadelphia, PA, Saunders, 1991, p 100.

Bubb RG: Appendix D: Skin infections, in Halpin T (ed.): *NCAA 2003: Wrestling Rules and Interpretations.* USA, NCAA, 2002.

Buescher SE: Infections associated with pediatric sport participation, in Luckstead EF (ed.): *Ped Clinic of North America.,* Philadelphia, PA, Saunders, 2002, p 743.

Cohen PR, Eliezri YD, Silvers DN: Athlete's nodules: Sports-related connective tissue nevi of the collagen type (collagenomas). *Cutis* 50:131, 1992.

Conklin RJ: Common cutaneous disorders in athletes. *Sports Med* 9:100, 1990.

Crowe MA, Sorensen GW: Dermatologic problems in athletes, in Butcher JD, Rucker KS, (eds.): *Handbook of Sports Medicine: A Symptom-Oriented Approach, Lillegard, WA.* Boston, MA, Butterworth-Heinemann, 1999, chap. 27.

D'Ambrosia RA: Cold injuries encountered in a winter resort. *Cutis* 20:365, 1977.

Dover JS: Sports dermatology, in Fitzpatrick TB et al (eds.): *Dermatology in General Medicine.* New York, NY, McGraw-Hill, 1993, chap. 129.

Elston DM: Sports dermatology, in Freedberg IM et al (eds.): *Fitzpatrick's Dermatology in General Medicine.* New York, NY, McGraw-Hill, 1999, chap. 132.

Erickson JG, von Gemmingen G R: Surfer's nodules and complications of surfboarding. *JAMA* 201:148, 1967.

Fisher AA: Sports related allergic dermatology. *Cutis* 50:95, 1992.

Fitzpatrick TB et al: *Color Atlas and Synopsis f Clinical Dermatology: Common and Serious Diseases,* 2nd ed. New York, NY, McGraw-Hill, 1992, p 238.

Frazier CA: Insect reactions related to sports. *Cutis* 19:439, 1977.

Freeman MJ, Bergfeld WF: Skin diseases of football and wrestling participants. *Cutis* 20:333, 1977.

Freudenthal AR, Barbagallo JS: Ghost anemone dermatitis. *J Am Acad Dermatol* 47:722, 2002.

Freudenthal AR, Joseph PR: Seabather's eruption. *N Engl J Med* 329:542, 1993.

Habif TP: *Clinical Dermatology: A Color Guide to Diagnosis and Therapy,* 3rd ed. St. Louis, MO, Mosby, 1996, chap. 7.

Hainer BL: Dermatophyte infections. *Am Fam Physician* 67:101, 2003.

Hershkowitz M: Penile frostbite, an unforeseen hazard of jogging. *N Engl J Med* 292:178, 1977.

Hoeffler DF: Swimmer's itch (cercarial dermatitis). *Cutis* 19:461, 1977.

Houston SD, Knox JM: Skin problems related to sports and recreational activities. *Cutis* 19:487, 1977.

Kantor GR, Bergfeld WF: Common and uncommon dermatologic diseases related to sports activities, in Pandolf KB (ed.): *Exercise and Sport Sciences Reviews.* New York, NY, Macmillan, 1988, chap. 7.

Levine N: Dermatologic aspects of sports medicine. *J Am Acad Dermatol* 3:415, 1980.

Levit F: Jogger's nipples. *N Engl J Med* 297:1127, 1977.

Lewis J et al: Exercise-induced urticaria, angioedema and anaphylactoid episodes. *J Allergy Clin Immunol* 68:432, 1981.

Mikhailov P, Berova N, Andreev VC: Physical urticaria and sport. *Cutis* 20:381, 1977.

Pharis DB, Teller C, Wolf JE, Jr: Cutaneous manifestations of sports participation. *J Am Acad Dermatol* 36:448, 1997.

Rodgers P, Basler M: Treating onychomycosis. *Am Fam Physician* 63:663, 2001.

Scher RK: Onychomycosis: therapeutic update. *J Am Acad Dermatol* 40:S21, 1999.

Schissel DJ, Aydelotte J, Keller R: Road rash with a rotten odor. *Mil Med* 164:65, 1999.

Shelly WB, Raunsley AM: Painful feet due to herniation of fat. *JAMA,* 205:308, 1968.

Sosin DM et al: An outbreak of furunculosis among high school athletes. *Am J Sports Med.* 17:828, 1989.

Swinehart JM: Mogul skier's palm: traumatic hypothenar ecchymosis. *Cutis* 50:117, 1992.

Tomecki KJ, Mikesell JF: Rower's rump (letter to editor). *J Am Acad Dermatol* 16:890, 1987.

Wilkinson DS: Black heel: A minor hazard of sport. *Cutis* 20:393, 1977.

Williams MS, Batts KB: Dermatological disorders, in O'Connor FG, Wilder RP, Nirschl R (eds.): *Textbook of Running Medicine.* New York, NY, McGraw-Hill, 2001, chap. 21.

27 GENITOURINARY

Michael W Johnson, MD

EPIDEMIOLOGY

- Hematuria and proteinuria are the most common urinary findings in athletes. In a study of 383 runners, 17% developed hematuria and 30% developed proteinuria following the completion of a marathon regardless of gender (Boileau et al, 1980).
- Acute renal failure in athletes is a rare event and is usually associated with volume depletion, rhabdomyolysis, or the nephrotoxic effects of *nonsteroidal antiinflammatory drugs* (NSAIDs).
- Though uncommon, acute genitourinary tract injuries occur. Contusion is the most frequent

kidney and bladder injury while laceration and rupture may be life threatening. Individual sports rather than team sports account for the majority renal injuries (McAleer, Kaplan, and Lo, 2002). Bicycle riding is the most common sports-related cause of renal injury (Gerstenbluth, Spirnak, and Elder, 2002).

- The male genitalia are often subjected to trauma ranging from testicular contusions to penile frostbite. Bikers are at risk for overuse pudendal nerve injury and straddle injuries.

- The prevalence of *sexually transmitted diseases* (STDs) in athletes is similar to that of the general population, although a study of college athletes showed they tend to be at higher risk for certain lifestyle behaviors. These maladaptive behaviors include less safe sex, greater number of sexual partners, and less contraceptive use when compared with their nonathlete peers (Nattiv, Puffer, and Green, 1997).

PATHOPHYSIOLOGY

ANATOMY

- The genitourinary system is comprised of the kidneys, ureters, bladder, urethra, and genital organs and is located in the lower abdomen and pelvis.

- The kidneys can be found high in the retroperitoneum bilaterally and are well protected. A solitary or malpositioned kidney is prone to injury. The urinary bladder is located in the anterior pelvis and is rarely acutely injured.

PHYSIOLOGY

- The kidneys receive more blood flow per unit weight than any other organ in the body. Renal blood travels to the glomerulus via the afferent arteriole and exits through the efferent arteriole. With afferent arteriole constriction, a pressure drop occurs within the glomerulus and filtration fraction decreases. With efferent arteriole vasoconstriction, pressure increases within the glomerulus thereby increasing the filtration fraction.

- Exercise causes acute changes in a variety of organ systems, as exercising muscle requires a significantly larger proportion of cardiac output. Blood flow is shunted away from the kidney to meet the demands of working muscle. Studies have noted a drop in renal blood flow from 1000 mL/min to as little as 200 mL/min with exercise (Jones, 1997).

- In an attempt to maintain glomerular filtration rate, the efferent arteriole constricts to a greater degree than the afferent arteriole creating a "pressure-head" at the glomerulus. This increases filtration fraction accounting for many of the renal changes seen with exercise.

- The increase in filtration fraction is proportional to the intensity of exercise and is attenuated by improving the runner's hydration status. Poorly hydrated individuals have a significantly larger decrease in renal blood flow compared with normally hydrated individuals.

- With moderate exercise (50% VO_{2max}) renal plasma flow decreases by 30% while with heavy exercise (65% VO_{2max}) renal plasma flow decreases by 75%. These changes are temporary as renal blood flow typically returns to preexercise levels within 60 min of exercise cessation (Cianflocco, 1992).

HEMATURIA

CLINICAL FEATURES

- Exercise-induced hematuria is known by a variety of names to include *sports hematuria, stress hematuria* and *10,000-m hematuria*. Sports hematuria is defined as hematuria, gross or microscopic, that occurs following vigorous exercise and resolves promptly with rest.

- The longer and more strenuous the event, the more prominent the hematuria. Sports hematuria is most common in swimmers and runners. Sports hematuria does not appear to be gender specific (Boileau et al, 1980).

- A thorough history should be obtained in athletes who present with gross hematuria, to include the presence of urinary urgency, dysuria, frequency, or clots. Further history includes trauma, penile discharge, or a history of nephrolithiasis. General historical questions include the presence of bleeding disorders, ongoing menses, recent streptococcal infection, generalized swelling, or risk factors for urologic cancer, such as tobacco use, age greater than 40, and pelvic irradiation. Other important questions include prescription and over-the-counter drug use, dietary supplement use, family history, and diet history.

- A complete exercise history should be obtained when microscopic hematuria is discovered incidentally.

- The timing of gross hematuria is an important historical feature. Presence of blood on initiating urination is likely urethral in origin. Hematuria on termination of urination originates from the bladder or posterior urethra. Continuous hematuria likely originates from the upper urinary tract.

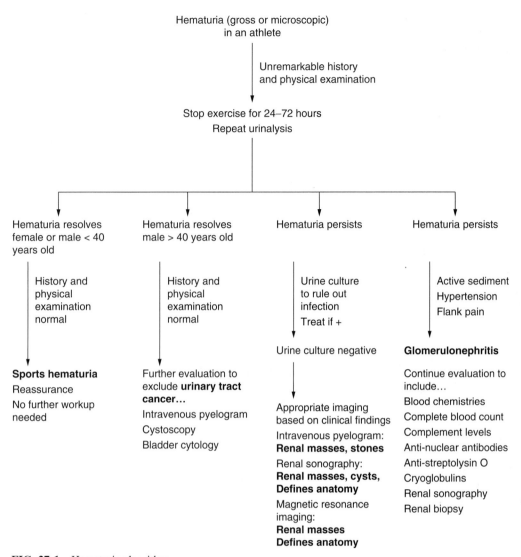

Hematuria (gross or microscopic)
in an athlete

Unremarkable history
and physical examination

Stop exercise for 24–72 hours
Repeat urinalysis

| Hematuria resolves female or male < 40 years old | Hematuria resolves male > 40 years old | Hematuria persists | Hematuria persists |

Hematuria resolves
female or male < 40
years old

History and
physical
examination
normal

Sports hematuria
Reassurance
No further workup
needed

Hematuria resolves
male > 40 years old

History and
physical
examination
normal

Further evaluation to
exclude **urinary tract
cancer...**
Intravenous pyelogram
Cystoscopy
Bladder cytology

Hematuria persists

Urine culture
to rule out
infection
Treat if +

Urine culture negative

Appropriate imaging
based on clinical findings
Intravenous pyelogram:
Renal masses, stones
Renal sonography:
**Renal masses, cysts,
Defines anatomy**
Magnetic resonance
imaging:
**Renal masses
Defines anatomy**

Hematuria persists

Active sediment
Hypertension
Flank pain

Glomerulonephritis

Continue evaluation to
include...
Blood chemistries
Complete blood count
Complement levels
Anti-nuclear antibodies
Anti-streptolysin O
Cryoglobulins
Renal sonography
Renal biopsy

FIG. 27-1   Hematuria algorithm.

- A thorough and meticulous physical examination should be completed. Vital signs—especially blood pressure—should always be obtained. The back, flank, abdomen and genitalia are examined paying particular attention to signs of trauma or infection.

DIFFERENTIAL DIAGNOSIS AND TREATMENT

- Differential diagnosis includes urinary tract infection, nephrolithiasis, urethritis, prostatitis, glomerulonephritis, bladder cancer, and medications.
- Grossly bloody urine should always be dipstick tested for blood and red blood cells confirmed by microscopy. When myoglobin or hemoglobin is present, urine will test positive for blood but red blood cells are absent on microscopic examination. Medications, dyes, and food

coloring often discolor urine. In this case, dipstick testing and microscopy will be negative for blood.
- See "hematuria algorithm" (Figure 27-1) for evaluation and treatment.

PROTEINURIA

CLINICAL FEATURES

- Proteinuria is defined as more than 150 mg of protein excreted in a 24-h period. Normal urine protein is composed of 30% albumin, 30% serum globulins, and 40% tissue proteins. Post-exercise proteinuria is relatively common and has been described for well over 120 years. It occurs in a variety of sports, both contact and noncontact and is associated with strenuous activity,

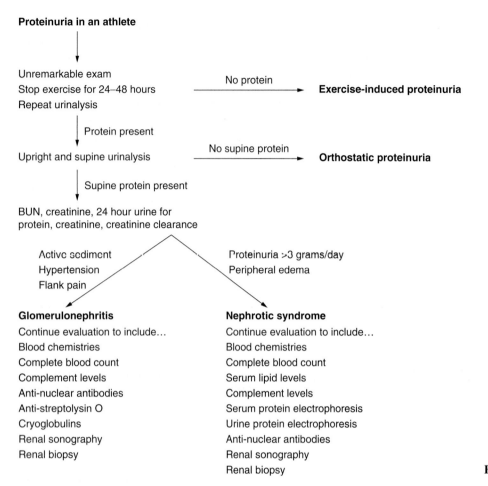

Proteinuria in an athlete

Unremarkable exam
Stop exercise for 24–48 hours   No protein → **Exercise-induced proteinuria**
Repeat urinalysis

Protein present

Upright and supine urinalysis   No supine protein → **Orthostatic proteinuria**

Supine protein present

BUN, creatinine, 24 hour urine for
protein, creatinine, creatinine clearance

Active sediment   Proteinuria >3 grams/day
Hypertension   Peripheral edema
Flank pain

Glomerulonephritis   **Nephrotic syndrome**
Continue evaluation to include...   Continue evaluation to include...
Blood chemistries   Blood chemistries
Complete blood count   Complete blood count
Complement levels   Serum lipid levels
Anti-nuclear antibodies   Complement levels
Anti-streptolysin O   Serum protein electrophoresis
Cryoglobulins   Urine protein electrophoresis
Renal sonography   Anti-nuclear antibodies
Renal biopsy   Renal sonography
                                    Renal biopsy

FIG. 27-2 Proteinuria algorithm.

such as maximal short-term effort, rather than prolonged activity.
- Important historical questions include exposure to nephrotoxic drugs, IV drug use, and chronic conditions, such as diabetes, systemic lupus erythematosus, or chronic active hepatitis. A family history of hereditary nephritis or polycystic kidney disease is important.
- Often, the proteinuria is an incidental finding and the patient should be questioned about prior exercise, its duration and, more importantly, its intensity.
- A meticulous physical examination should be completed. Vital signs, especially blood pressure, should always be obtained. The back, flank, abdomen, skin, and genitalia are examined in routine fashion. The extremities are evaluated for any signs of edema.

DIFFERENTIAL DIAGNOSIS AND TREATMENT

- Differential diagnosis includes exercise-induced proteinuria, orthostatic proteinuria, glomerulonephritis, nephrotic syndrome, and multiple myeloma.
- Proteinuria is usually identified through dipstick testing and, when exercise-induced, is usually 2+ to 3+.

- False positives occur because of very concentrated urine, gross hematuria, alkaline urine, or phenazopyridine.
- See "proteinuria algorithm" (Figure 27-2) for evaluation and treatment.

ACUTE RENAL FAILURE

CLINICAL FEATURES

- Acute renal failure in athletes is typically caused by complications associated with strenuous exercise such as rhabdomyolysis, dehydration, or hyperpyrexia. Increased magnitude and duration of dehydration can lead to acute tubular necrosis. Hemolysis due to hyperpyrexia contributes to *acute tubular necrosis* (ATN) and renal failure.
- Nonsteroidal anti-inflammatory agents inhibit prostaglandins thereby decreasing renal blood flow and contribute to acute renal failure in athletes who premedicate in the hopes of decreasing postexercise muscle soreness. Experienced athletes are at much lower risk to develop acute renal failure than untrained athletes.

- The athlete in acute renal failure often presents with nonspecific complaints, such as malaise, weakness, loss of appetite, nausea, anuria or oliguria, and symptoms of dehydration.

DIFFERENTIAL DIAGNOSIS AND TREATMENT

- Kidney failure in athletes is most often caused by renal hypoperfusion or ATN. Obstructive uropathy is rarely a source of renal failure.
- Serum laboratory tests include a complete blood count, *blood urea nitrogen* (BUN), creatinine, and basic chemistry panel. Urine tests include osmolality, sodium, and creatinine. With this data, a *fractional excretion of sodium* (FE_{Na}) can be calculated to differentiate between prerenal azotemia and ATN as the cause of kidney failure.
- Treatment of prerenal azotemia involves rapid and aggressive volume replacement.
- Identification of the endogenous nephrotoxin such as myoglobin in rhabdomyolysis or the exogenous nephrotoxin as in NSAID-induced renal failure is crucial. All reversible causes must be sought and treated.
- Treatment involves appropriate intravenous fluid hydration, electrolyte management, and cardiovascular monitoring. Diuretics are only indicated in fluid overload states. Indications for dialysis include the need for ultrafiltration of a volume-overloaded state or the need for solute clearance.

GENITOURINARY TRAUMA

RENAL

- The kidneys are normally well protected by surrounding muscles, ribs, and pericapsular fat. A blow to the flank or abdomen produces a coup or countercoup mechanism of injury. Abnormally located or anomalous kidneys are more prone to injury.
- Flank pain and hematuria are the most common presenting complaint.
- Kidney injuries are divided into 5 classes based on severity and type of injury:
  Class I: Contusion—most common renal sports injury
  Class II: Cortical laceration
  Class III: Caliceal laceration
  Class IV: Complete renal fracture—rare sports injury
  Class V: Vascular pedicle injury—again, rare in sports
- Flank pain or gross hematuria after blunt trauma in an athlete requires consideration of possible renal injury. Physical examination may reveal flank echymosis and tenderness. Gross or microscopic hematuria is present in greater than 95% of renal trauma.

- Athletes with severe renal injuries (Class IV and V) often present in hypovolemic shock. Aggressive intravascular volume replacement, transfusion, and surgical exploration to control life-threatening bleeding are required for these injuries.
- Evaluation of renal injuries in hemodynamically stable athletes may use *intravenous pyelogram* (IVP), computed tomography, or magnetic resonance imaging. Treatment of Class I–III injuries involve observation, bed rest, and repeat urinalysis to assess for resolution of hematuria. The athlete is restricted from contact sports and a repeat IVP is obtained at 3 months.

URETERS

- Ureteral injury is associated with severe trauma, such as pelvic fractures and lower lumbar vertebrae fractures.
- Trauma to flank or pelvis raises the possibility of ureteral injury. Hematuria is present in 90% of ureteral trauma. The diagnosis is best established utilizing IVP and retrograde pyelogram.
- Treatment is accomplished with placement of a ureteral stent in a partially intact ureter or, as is often the case, open surgical repair.

BLADDER

- Injury often occurs with blunt trauma to a distended bladder resulting in contusion or rupture. Patients with bladder contusion present with a history of trauma, suprapubic pain, guarding, hematuria, and possibly dysuria.
- Bladder rupture may be intra- or extra-peritoneal and is usually associated with pelvic fracture.
- *Biker's bladder* is a complication of aggressive bicycling and presents with abrupt onset of urinary frequency, diminished urinary stream, nocturia, and terminal dribbling.
- Cystography is the definitive study for the diagnosis of bladder rupture. If bladder rupture is present, assessment for pelvic fracture is mandatory. Bladder contusions are treated with catheter drainage for a few days. Bladder rupture is surgically repaired (Sagalowsky and Peters, 1998).

GENITALIA

- Genital trauma may occur in any sport, though it's often seen in gymnastics, cycling, martial arts, and contact sports.
- Testicular injuries result from direct trauma and include contusion, torsion, or fracture.

- The extent of testicular trauma and testicular blood flow can be evaluated by ultrasound. Testicular rupture is a urologic emergency requiring surgical management if the testis is to be salvaged. Testicular contusions are treated symptomatically.
- Penile injuries are unusual in athletes. The penis may be injured in straddle-type injuries or by direct blow. Irritation of the pudendal nerve in bicycle racers can cause priapism or ischemic neuropathy of the penis. Symptoms usually resolve once the race is over.
- Penile frostbite occurs in runners who wear inadequate clothing in extremely cold conditions.
- Female genitalia may be injured by direct trauma and results in contusion, lacerations, or vulvar hematoma.

REFERENCES

Boileau M, Fuchs E, Barry JM, et al: Stress hematuria: Athletic pseudonephritis in marathoners. *Urology* 15:471, 1980.

Cianflocco AJ: Renal complications of exercise. *Clin Sports Med* 11:437, 1992.

Gerstenbluth RE, Spirnak JP, Elder JS: Sports participation and high grade renal injuries in children. *J Urol* 168(6):2575, 2002.

Jones GR, Newhouse I: Sports-related hematuria: A review. *Clin J Sport Med* 7:119, 1997.

McAleer IM, Kaplan GW, Lo Sasso BE: Renal and testis injuries in team sports. *J Urol* 168(4 Pt 2): 1805, 2002.

Nattiv A, Puffer JC, Green GA: Lifestyle and health risks of collegiate athletes: A multi-center study. *Clin J Sport Med* 7:262, 1997.

Sagalowsky AI, Peters PC: Genitourinary Trauma, in Walsh PC, Retik, AB, Vaughan ED, Jr, et al (eds.): *Campbell's Urology*, 7th ed. Philadelphia, PA, Saunders, 1998, pp 3085–3108.

28   OPHTHALMOLOGY
Ronica A Martinez, MD
Kayvan A Ellini, MD

EPIDEMIOLOGY

- There are over 40,000 sports-related eye injuries in the United States annually, with blunt ocular trauma being the most common form of injury.
- Nearly 90% of these are considered preventable (Erie, 1991; Jeffers, 1990; Cassen, 1997).

- As a general rule, sports involving a stick, racquet, or ball are considered high-risk for eye injuries. Other sports to include in this category are basketball, boxing, and wresting.
- Hockey, baseball, and racquet sports account for the majority of sports-related eye injuries (Napier et al, 1996).

PREPARTICIPATION PHYSICAL EXAMINATION

- An eye examination is an important part of any sports physical.
- The ocular history should be sure to include the presence of severe myopia, prior eye injuries or surgeries, and any history of retinal detachments, as these may predispose the athlete to more threatening eye injuries (Vinger, 1998).
- Athletes with any of these predisposing risks should be evaluated by an ophthalmologist prior to being cleared for any high-risk sports.
- Monocular athletes must wear protective eyewear at all times. They should also understand that despite using protective eyewear, participating in sports places the good eye at risk for injury.

BASICS OF THE EYE EXAMINATION

HISTORY

- The history should include a detailed description of the mechanism of injury. Also obtain an estimate of visual acuity immediately before and after the injury, along with the timing of visual loss, if any.
- Ask regarding pain, photophobia, diplopia, floaters, flashing lights, tearing, headache, and nausea.

PHYSICAL EXAMINATION

- The eye examination should be performed in a systematic fashion, using the uninvolved eye as a baseline for comparison. Any asymmetry suggests a problem that needs further investigation. It is also critical to perform a thorough examination, and not solely focus on the obvious area of involvement.
- **Visual acuity:** This is the first and most important step of any eye examination. Document best corrected visual acuity using a Snellen card or other text source. If vision is too poor for text, check count fingers and light perception.

- **Pupils:** Using a bright light source, check to ensure pupils are round, symmetric, and reactive.
- **Extraocular muscles:** Ensure full range of motion, especially looking for significant asymmetry.
- **External Examination:** This includes examination of the bony orbits, eyelids, adnexal structures, periorbital skin, and conjunctiva, cornea, *anterior chamber* (AC), and iris.
  1. Conjunctiva and sclera: Here pay close attention for signs that suggest a ruptured globe, including lacerations, 360° subconjunctival hemorrhage, or extruding pigment (uveal tissue) or gel (vitreous humor).
  2. Cornea: Assess for clarity, then apply fluorescein to identify epithelial defects or foreign bodies.
  3. Anterior chamber: Ensure the chamber is well-formed, comparing to unaffected side. Look closely for any blood present in the anterior chamber.
- **Fundoscopic examination:** This should be performed in all cases of eye trauma, paying special attention to the red reflex. Asymmetry in the red reflex is often a subtle clue to the presence of significant pathology.
- **Other:** Although slit-lamp examination is ideal for all cases of ocular injury, it is generally not available. As such, it is often deferred for more serious cases that require evaluation by an ophthalmologist.

COMMON EYE INJURIES

EYELID LACERATIONS

- Seen after blunt or sharp trauma to the area. May also be indirect from broken spectacles.

SYMPTOMS
- Localized pain and bleeding around the eye

EXAMINATION
- Check for involvement of the lid margin. Assess the depth of the laceration, to see if orbital fat is exposed. If lesion is medial, assess if it involves the lacrimal drainage system.
- Perform thorough eye examination to ensure globe is not injured.

TREATMENT
- Clean area with betadine and inject lidocaine for local anesthesia. Then explore wound for foreign body, irrigate with normal saline or Lactated Ringer's solution and suture using 5-0 nylon. Apply antibiotic ointment to area and apply protective eye shield. Remove suture in 7–10 days.

- Lacerations suspected of involving the lacrimal drainage system, full-thickness lacerations, exposure of orbital fat, and those involving the lid margin require immediate ophthalmology referral.

CORNEAL ABRASIONS

- One of the most common sports-related eye injuries (Zagelbaum, 1997), accounting for 33% of all eye injuries seen in Major League Baseball and 12% of these seen in the National Basketball Association (Zagelbaum et al, 1994; Zagelbaum et al, 1995).

SYMPTOMS
- Sharp pain, photophobia, foreign body sensation, and tearing

EXAMINATION
- Check visual acuity. Then apply fluorescein stain, preferably with topical anesthetic and assess using a cobalt blue light. The pain should improve with the topical anesthetic. Any epithelial staining confirms the diagnosis.
- Flip upper and lower lid to search for foreign body, if suspected from mechanism.

TREATMENT
- Apply topical broad-spectrum antibiotic and follow daily until epithelial defect resolved. For larger lesions, a pressure patch can be applied overnight.
- For patients with significant photophobia, prescribe 1% cyclopentolate tid for 2–3 days.

CORNEAL/CONJUNCTIVAL LACERATIONS

SYMPTOMS
- Mild pain and foreign body sensation for conjunctival lacerations.
- Severe pain, tearing, and blurry vision for corneal lacerations.

EXAMINATION
- **Conjunctival:** Often see area of subconjunctival hemorrhage. Fluorescein stain may show area of tear. Perform complete eye examination, especially looking for scleral laceration, other evidence for ruptured globe, or a conjunctival foreign body.
- **Cornea:** Best viewed with a slit-lamp, but may suspect from penlight examination. Especially look for a flat AC, irregularities of the iris, or fold in the cornea.

TREATMENT

- Apply topical broad-spectrum antibiotic and overnight pressure patch for conjunctival lacerations without evidence for a ruptured globe. Large lacerations may need suturing, best done by an ophthalmologist.
- In cases of suspected corneal laceration, a rigid eye shield should be placed and the athlete sent for immediate ophthalmology evaluation.

SUBCONJUNCTIVAL HEMORRHAGE

- Very common finding after blunt trauma.

SYMPTOMS

- Generally asymptomatic, but occasionally mild irritation

EXAMINATION

- Mainly assess for foreign body and ensure no ruptured globe present.

TREATMENT

- Reassurance. Most resolve within 2–3 weeks.
- Urgent ophthalmology referral only if extensive hemorrhage (nearly 360° around the cornea).

HYPHEMA

- Bleeding into the AC that can occur after any type of significant blunt trauma.

SYMPTOMS

- Severe pain and photophobia. Blurry vision if larger hyphema or associated traumatic iritis.

EXAMINATION

- Perform complete eye examination, including intraocular pressure.
- The blood generally layers, but may see clots or stranding. With slit lamp, can see actual red cells floating, enabling the identification of a microhyphema.

TREATMENT

- Obtain ophthalmologic consultation, as many will admit for observation. Emphasize strict bed rest, elevate head of bed to 30°, and eyeshield at all times to help avoid rebleeding, seen in up to 30%.
- Cyclopentolate 1% or atropine 1% tid for pain.
- Daily follow-up by an ophthalmologist to assess for elevated intraocular pressure and evidence of rebleeding.

TRAUMATIC IRITIS

- Inflammation in the AC that can occur days to weeks after blunt trauma to the eye.
- Same presentation and examination as for hyphema, but no blood present in AC.
- Requires slit-lamp examination to diagnose. If suspected, send for urgent ophthalmologic evaluation. Definitive treatment involves topical steroid drops.

RETINAL DETACHMENT

- May occur after any direct trauma to the orbit, or even from significant head trauma. More common among myopic athletes.

SYMPTOMS

- Often presents with blind spot in edge of visual field. Ask about "flashing lights" or new "floaters," as often dismissed by the patient. This is important for treatment and prognosis.

EXAMINATION

- Check confrontational visual field for defect. Check for afferent pupillary defect (present with larger detachments).
- Perform fundoscopic examination, but identification is difficult because it generally begins peripherally.

TREATMENT

- Urgent ophthalmologic consultation for dilated fundoscopic examination. Laser treatment for certain retinal tears or holes, while surgery for detachments.

RUPTURED GLOBE/PENETRATING INJURIES

- These injuries may occur after any direct trauma to the orbit, or even from significant head trauma. More common among myopic athletes.

SYMPTOMS

- Vary with area of involvement. May be asymptomatic for occult ruptures, present similar to retinal detachment, or with complaints of eye pain or blurry vision.

EXAMINATION

- A thorough eye examination is important, but do not apply pressure to the globe.
- Look for a flattened AC, an area leaking gel or fluid (vitreous or aqueous humor), or darkly pigmented tissue exposed (uveal tissue).
- Presence of 360° subconjunctival hemorrhage strongly suggests a ruptured globe.

TREATMENT
- Place an eye shield over area and send for immediate ophthalmologic consultation.
- Keep NPO as may require surgical exploration and repair.

ORBITAL WALL FRACTURES

- Most often seen after significant blunt trauma.

SYMPTOMS
- Mainly localized pain and swelling to the area. May have pain with eye movements or diplopia (suggests extraocular muscle entrapment). If infraorbital nerve involved, may have numbness on the cheek.

EXAMINATION
- A complete eye examination, with special focus on extraocular motility, facial numbness, and palpation of the bony orbits. Rule out ruptured globe.
- Order a *computed tomography imaging* (CT scan) of the orbits for definitive diagnosis.

TREATMENT
- Give cefalexin 500 mg qid and oxymetazoline nasal spray bid for 14-day course (to prevent orbital cellulitis).
- Set up for ophthalmologic evaluation within 7 days. May require surgical repair if any extraocular muscle entrapment present.
- Hold athlete from any contact until released by ophthalmology.

PREVENTION OF EYE INJURIES

PROTECTIVE EYEWEAR

- Eyewear should be made of polycarbonate lenses, which are up to 20 times stronger than regular prescription glasses (Cassen, 1997; Rodriguez and Lavina, 2003; American Academy of Pediatrics, 1996).
- Should meet American Society for Testing and Materials (ASTM) standards for specific high-risk sports (i.e., racquetball, lacrosse, or baseball) (International Federation of Sports Medicine, 1998).
- If a helmet is required for the sport, then protective shield may need to be integrated.
- Contact lenses offer no protection whatsoever.
- Eye protection can reduce the risk of eye injury by 90% (Rodriguez and Lavina, 2003).
- Sports goggles with polycarbonate lenses are recommended for all athletes participating in sports with higher risk for ocular injury.

- Higher risk sports include activities of small, fast projectiles, hard projectiles, fingers, close contact, and *sticks.*
- All include sports causing intentional injury such as boxing, and full contact martial arts.

CHOOSING EYE PROTECTION

- It is important to know athlete's vision and eye history.
- Use only eye protectors that have been national certified and are up to standard.
- Always have professionals assist the athlete in selecting proper eye protection
  - Professionals include an ophthalmologist, optometrist, athletic trainer, or optician.

THE MONOCULAR ATHLETE

- Encompasses any athlete with best corrected visual acuity less than 20/40 in one eye.
- Should have thorough ophthalmologic evaluation prior to allowing participation in sports.
- Must be required to wear ASTM approved eye protection for all practices and games that carry risk for eye injury.
- They should not be allowed to participate in sports in which no type of eye protection is sufficient (i.e., wrestling or boxing).
- Monocular athletes should wear polycarbonate lenses at all times to prevent eye injuries outside of sports.

REFERENCES

American Academy of Pediatrics: Protective eyewear for young athletes. *Pediatrics* 98:311, 1996.

Cassen JH: Ocular trauma. *Hawaii Med J* 56:292–294, 1997.

Erie JC: Eye injuries: Prevention, evaluation and treatment. *Phys Sportsmed* 19:108–122, 1991.

International Federation of Sports Medicine: Eye injuries and eye protection in sports. *Br J Sportsmed* 23, 1998.

Jeffers JV: An ongoing tragedy: Pediatric sports-related eye injuries. *Semin Ophthalmol* 5:216–223, 1990.

Napier SM, Baker RS, et al: Eye injuries in athletics and recreation. *Surv Ophthalmol* 40:229–244, 1996.

Rodriguez JO, Lavina AM: Prevention and treatment of common eye injuries in sports. *Am Fam Phys* 67:1481–1488, 2003.

Vinger PF. Sports medicine and the eye care professional. *J Am Optom Assoc* 69:395–413, 1998.

Zagelbaum BM: Treating corneal abrasions and lacerations. *Phys Sportsmed* 25, 1997.

Zagelbaum BM, Hersh PS, Donnenfeld ED, et al. Ocular trauma in Major League baseball players. *N Engl J Med* 330:1021–1023, 1994.
Zagelbaum BM, Starkey C, et al. The National Basketball Association (NBA) eye injury study. *Arch Ophthalmol* 113:749–752, 1995.

BIBLIOGRAPHY

Diamond GR, Quinn GE, et al: Ophthalmologic injuries. *Prim Care* 11:161, 1984.
Easterbrook M, Johnston RH, Howcroft MJ: Assessment of ocular foreign bodies. *Phys Sportsmed* 25, 1997.
Rhee DJ, Pyfer MF, Rhee DM: *The Wills Eye Manual.* Pennsylvania, IN, Lippincott, Williams, & Wilkins, 1999.
Tucker JB, Marron JT: Fieldside management of athletic injuries. *Am Fam Phys* 34:137–142, 1996.
Vaughan D, Asbury T, Riordan-Eva P: *General Ophthalmology.* Norwalk, CT, Appleton & Lange, 1999.
Vinger PF: A practical guide for sports eye protection. *Phys Sportsmed* 28, 2000.

29 OTORHINOLARYNGOLOGY
Charles W Webb, DO

INTRODUCTION

• Facial injuries are among the most common injuries in athletics. They comprise 4–19% of all sports related injuries depending on age and gender. One-third of all dental injuries are sports related (Truman et al, 2002). In the pediatric age ranges, one-third of injuries are sports related (Luke and Micheli, 1999). The gender difference increases with age from 1.5:1 male to females during the ages of 1–10 years, to 12:1 in the 16–18 year olds (Truman et al, 2002; Shaikh and Worrall, 2002). With the addition of face-masks and mouth guards in football and hockey (1950s and 1970s respectively), the number of severe facial injuries has declined dramatically (Hart, 2002). Baseball now accounts for the majority (40%) of all sports related facial injuries in the United States.

ASSESSMENT OF INJURIES ON THE SIDELINE

• Sideline management of the athlete with a facial injury begins with the ABCs (*airway, breathing, circulation*).

Blood, avulsed teeth, mouth guards, or other objects are airway hazards. Cervical spine precautions must be observed in all head injuries, especially when the player is unconscious.
• The history should include the mechanism of injury, and the presence of any other injuries past or present. An important question to ask is, "Does it feel the same when you (the athlete) bite down?" If not, then there is a question of mandibular dislocation, fracture, or tooth injury (Douglass and Douglass, 2003).
• Physical examination includes observation, palpation, and imaging (if there is any question about the diagnosis). Observation includes evaluation of facial symmetry, bruising, and swelling. Palpation includes the orbital rim, nasal bones, maxillary bones, mandible, temporal mandibular joint, and the upper and lower jaws intra- and extraorally.
• The nares should be inspected for any type of fluid drainage. This may be blood or *cerebral spinal fluid* (CSF). The "ring test" is a method of detecting CSF on the sideline. It is done by placing a drop of blood from the nares on a piece of paper or gauze, CSF will form a halo (clear fluid ring) around the drop of blood. This represents a severe facial fracture and requires immediate transport.
• Imaging is usually of limited value. X-rays may be helpful in determining the presence of a facial fracture; however, *computed tomography* (CT) is the gold standard.
• Return to play guidance is based on the history and physical examination. Suspected fractures, airway obstruction or impending obstruction, bleeding, loss of consciousness, and changes in vision are contraindications for return to play.

EAR INJURIES

EAR LACERATION

• **Signs and symptoms:** Pain and bleeding around the ear with history of trauma.
• **Examination:** Must evaluate for cartilage involvement and for radial extension to the scalp.
• **Treatment:** Cartilage tear, repair with absorbable 5-O suture prior to closing the skin. Laceration should be irrigated and debrided prior to suturing. Prophylactic antibiotics are recommended to prevent chondritis.

AURICULAR HEMATOMA

• "Wrestler's Ear" or "Cauliflower Ear" is caused by bleeding between the skin (perchondrium) and the auricular cartilage. This occurs secondary to repetitive contusions to the pinna. This can evolve into a permanent cosmetic deformity with chronic hematomas, secondary to an increased pressure and eventual necrosis of the pinna and cartilage.

- **Signs and symptoms:** Acute throbbing pain, tenderness and edema
- **Examination:** Soft hematoma within the auricle
- **Treatment:** Recommended treatment is ice and prompt aspiration with an 18–20-gauge needle using sterile technique, prophylactic antibiotics, and pressure dressing (collodium splint or tie through suture with dental row or button). Compression prevents hematoma from reforming and should be left in place for 7–10 days. The athlete should not return to play until after the removal of the compression device, and should always wear proper ear protection (head gear).
- An alternative treatment method is repeated aspiration of the hematoma. This allows the athlete to return to play quickly (same day with head gear); however, this treatment method usually leads to a permanent cauliflower ear. Both the athlete and the parents should be informed of the risk and the permanence of this defect (Swinson and Lloyd, 2003).

OTITIS EXTERNA

- Infection of the external auditory canal is most commonly caused by *Pseudomonas spp., Proteus spp., E. coli,* or fungi. It is mostly seen in water sports and has an increased incidence in poorly chlorinated pools and fresh water.
- **Signs and symptoms:** Pain with movement of the auricle is the classic finding with or without a watery discharge and/or a mild hearing loss.
- **Examination:** Erythematous and edematous auditory canal with a normal or mildly erythematous tympanic membrane. Fungal infections typically have a white to gray appearance with spots that resemble cheese, and pseudomonal infections will usually have a sweet odor.
- **Treatment:** Irrigating the canal allows the medication to enter the canal. Cortisporin otic suspension (solution if the *tympanic membrane* (TM) is perforated) should be applied (5 drops in the ear qid) for 7 days. If the canal is swollen, a cotton wick may be used to help deliver the antibiotic. Tolnaftate drops applied twice a day for 7 days is the drug of choice for most fungal infections. Swimmers will use a mixture of 50% white vinegar and 50% rubbing alcohol after swimming and showering to prevent this from occurring (Blanda and Gallo, 2003).

TYMPANIC MEMBRANE RUPTURE

- This usually occurs secondary to a diving, water skiing, surfing, or slap injury.
- **Signs and symptoms:** Acute pain, sudden unilateral hearing loss, nausea, and vertigo.
- **Examination:** Visualization of the defect with an otoscope.
- **Treatment:** Observation and reassurance are the treatments of choice, as 90% will heal in 8 weeks. Antibiotic otic drops are recommended when an infection develops or the injury occurred in water sports. Hearing tests are recommended if greater than 25% of the TM is involved to rule out nerve injury (Blanda and Gallo, 2003).

NASAL INJURIES

NASAL FRACTURES

- Most common sports-related facial fracture as well as the most common facial structure injured. Direct end-on blows usually result in comminuted fractures of both the bone and the cartilage. Side blows usually result in simple fractures with deviation to the opposite side.
- **Signs and symptoms:** Acute pain, tearing, epistaxis, facial swelling, and ecchymosis.
- **Examination:** Crepitus over the nasal bridge and observation of nasal deformity. If bleeding is present a ring test should be performed.
- **X-rays:** Seldom helpful for treatment decisions in the clinic or emergency room, but may be useful in documentation.
- **Treatment:** If done immediately, reduction of the displaced nasal fracture is semipainless. Swelling makes adequate assessment of nasal deformity difficult. If unable to reduce an otorhinolaryngology referral is required in 5–7 days for reduction. Athletes should not return to play the same day unless there are absolutely no other associated injuries and the nose can be protected. Return to play is typically not advised for at least the first week postreduction. External protective devices are recommended for the first 4 weeks postinjury.

SEPTAL HEMATOMA

- This is an accumulation of blood between the septal cartilage and the overlying mucoperichondrium. Septal hematomas are prone to abscess formation, leading to pressure necrosis of the underlying bone and cartilage (saddle nose deformity) if not treated.

- **Signs and symptoms:** Acute pain, facial swelling, and nasal obstruction.
- **Examination:** A bluish bulge is seen on the nasal septum.
- **Treatment:** Prompt aspiration is the key to successful treatment. Aspiration is done using an 18–20-gauge needle; then packing the nose with bilateral nasal packing for 4–5 days to prevent recurrence. Prophylactic antibiotics are used for 10–14 days to prevent abscess formation (Norris and Peterson, 2001*a*).

EPISTAXIS

ANTERIOR EPISTAXIS
- Ninety to ninety-five percent of all nosebleeds are anterior. The most common site for bleeding is from the Kiesselbach's plexus in Little's area on the anterior septum.
- **Signs and symptoms:** Dripping blood from the nostrils.
- **Treatment:** Ice and compression of the nose are the mainstays of treatment. Cautery may be considered if pressure fails and the bleeding site can be identified (silver nitrate or electrocautery pen). Nasal packing may also be used for compression if bleeding site cannot be identified. Strenuous activity should be restricted if nasal packing is required, until the packing can be removed. Return to play should not be allowed with nasal packing in place as the potential for airway obstruction exists. If no packing is required and the bleeding is controlled with ice and compression, the athlete may return to play as soon as the bleeding has ceased.

POSTERIOR EPISTAXIS
- Five to ten percent of nosebleeds.
- **Signs and symptoms:** Bleeding that drains mainly through the posterior pharynx.
- **Examination:** The bleeding cannot be directly visualized. Must evaluate for other facial trauma to include orbital fracture and nasal fracture.
- **Treatment:** Failure of bleeding to stop with compression is a sign that it may be of posterior origin. Most posterior bleeds require more than an on-the-field assessment. These athletes should be evacuated to a hospital for *ear, nose, throat* (ENT) consultation. Emergent hemostasis can be achieved with a small Foley catheter, inserted through the nare, inflated in the posterior pharynx, then pulled snug against the posterior nare, tamponading the bleeding and protecting the airway (Norris and Peterson, 2001*a*; 2001*b*).

TRACHEAL INJURIES

- Blunt trauma to the anterior neck can have devastating effects on the larynx and the trachea, causing serious airway compromise. Hockey (ice, field, roller), football, softball, baseball, wrestling, soccer, lacrosse, and gymnastics are the sports more commonly associated with tracheal/laryngeal injury. Hockey, baseball, softball, lacrosse, and fencing all require the athlete to wear neck protecting extensions or masks to protect the anterior neck. Blunt trauma to this region can produce both contusions and fractures of the larynx and the trachea, causing laryngospasm.

LARYNGOSPASM

- Laryngospasm is a spasmodic closure of the glottic aperture. This occurs when the muscles of the vocal cords contract and pull the cords together and the upper surface of the cords overlap—causing obstruction of the airway.
- **Signs and symptoms:** Bruising, shortness of breath, hoarseness, loss of voice, pain, point tenderness, cough, dysphagia, cyanosis, and loss of consciousness.
- **Examination:** Ensure an open airway, palpate for subcutaneous emphysema, and fracture of the thyroid cartilage (Adam's apple). Observe respiratory rate and monitor for signs of respiratory compromise.
- **Treatment:** Laryngospasm causes a sudden inability to breathe; causing immediate anxiety and even panic in the athlete. The athlete needs reassurance and careful maintenance of the cervical spine in a neutral position. The jaw thrust maneuver should be used to pull the hyoid bone and the surrounding tissues away from the larynx, thereby opening the airway. As the spasm relaxes a loud inspiratory crowing sound is heard. The spasm usually relaxes in less than 1 min. A responsible adult should observe this individual for the next 48 h, as future swelling may occur. Laryngeal swelling usually maximizes in 6 h postinjury but may occur as late a 48 h postinjury. This swelling of the larynx can lead to airway obstruction and fatality if not monitored for signs of respiratory compromise. The athlete should not be allowed to return to play for at least 48 h, to ensure the swelling has resolved (Swinson and Lloyd, 2003; Blanda and Gallo, 2003; Norris and Peterson, 2001*a*).

LARYNGEAL FRACTURE

- Laryngeal and tracheal fractures are also caused by blunt anterior neck trauma; however, the blow is usually much greater in force. The signs and symptoms are the same as that for laryngeal spasm; however, there is associated subcutaneous crepitus, loss of thyroid cartilage contour, and cyanosis from damage to the airway. It is of the upmost importance to establish an airway, protect it, then transport the athlete to the nearest health care facility. If there is an associated facial injury, it may be impossible to place an orotracheal tube or a nasotracheal tube. In these cases the surgical airway of choice is the cricothyroidotomy.

CRICOTHYROIDOTOMY

- Percutaneous transtracheal ventilation or needle cricothyroidotomy is placement of a catheter through the cricothyroid membrane to establish an airway. This surgical airway may be used as a temporizing airway when oral and nasal intubation is not possible. This is done by first identifying the anatomy. The cricothyroid membrane is located between the thyroid cartilage and the cricoid cartilage. The first landmark to find is the thyroid cartilage (Adam's apple), then move inferiorly to the groove below the thyroid cartilage. The cricothyroid membrane is in the space between the thyroid cartilage and the crycoid cartilage located as the next hard ring of tissue inferior to the thyroid cartilage. If time permits the neck should be prepped with alcohol or povidone-iodine and the skin anesthetized locally before the first incision is made. The initial incision is made vertically thought the skin (3–4 cm) over the cricothyroid membrane. The next step is to identify the cricothyroid membrane immediately inferior to the thyroid cartilage. Once it is identified, a 1–2-cm horizontal incision is made. Insert a tracheostomy tube or a 5–6-mm endotracheal tube (3 mm for a child) and secure the tube with tape.
- If there is not enough time to perform the surgical procedure a needle cricothyroidotomy may be performed by locating the cricothyroid membrane as above and inserting a 12–16 gauge over the needle catheter that is attached to a syringe can be utilized. This allows the syringe to be connected to a pressurized oxygen source or a 3.0 endotracheal tube for ventilation while transport is taking place. There are prepackaged cricothyroidotomy kits available commercially. These kits will

TABLE 29-1   Sideline Cricothyroidotomy Kit

Alcohol pads	Povidone-iodine pads or swabs
# 11 Scalpel	3- or 5-cc syringe
25-gauge needle	1% or 2% lidocaine with or without epinephrine
4-in. hemostat	5- to 6-mm endotracheal tube or tracheostomy tube
3-mm endotracheal tube	12–16 guage catheter over needle

TABLE 29-2   Risks and Contraindications for Surgical Airway

RISKS	CONTRAINDICATIONS	
	ABSOLUTE	RELATIVE
Hemorrhage	Ability to place	Coagulopathy
Laceration to	another type	Overlying tumor
surrounding structures	of airway	Hematoma
Subcutaneous emphysema		Age less than 10 years
Hypoxia		Indistinct landmarks
Aspiration		Previous intubation
Infection		longer than 3 days
Tracheal stenosis		
Vocal cord damage		

come prepackaged for either the blind percutaneous method or the insertion through the skin incision. The contents for a sideline cricothyroidotomy kit are outlined in Table 29-1. The complications to this procedure should be weighed against the risk of death in the athlete prior to availability of definitive care. The complications as well as the contraindications are listed in Table 29-2 (Blanda and Gallo, 2003; Norris and Peterson, 2001*a*; 2001*b*; Roberts, 2000).

CONCLUSION

- Ear, nose, and throat injuries are among the most common injuries seen on the sidelines and can be quite serious in nature. The team physician must have a thorough knowledge of the anatomy in order to provide adequate care to the injured athlete. These injuries can range from cosmetic (wrestler's ear), to the severely life threatening (laryngeal fracture). Essential equipment and training for the team physician can mean the difference between life and death.

REFERENCES

Blanda M, Gallo UE: Emergency airway management. *Emerg Med Clin North Am* 21:1, 2003.

Douglass AB, Douglass JM: Common dental emergencies. *Am Fam Phys* 67(3):511, 2003.

Hart LE: Full facial protection reduces injuries in elite young hockey players. *Clin J Sport Med* 12(6):406, 2002.

Luke A, Micheli L: Sports injuries: Emergency assessment and field side care. *Pediatr Rev* 20(9):291, 1999.

Norris RL, Peterson J: Airway management for the sports physician part 1: Basic techniques. *Phys Sportsmed* 29(10), 2001*a*.

Norris RL, Peterson J: Airway management for the sports physician part 2: Advanced techniques. *Phys Sportsmed* 29(11), 2001*b*.

Roberts WO: Sideline airway access. *Phys Sportsmed* 28(4), 2000.

Shaikh ZS, Worrall SF: Epidemiology of facial trauma in a sample of patients aged 1–18 years. *Int J Care Injured* 33:669, 2002.

Swinson B, Lloyd T: Management of maxillofacial injuries. *Hosp Med* 64(2):72, 2003.

Truman B, Gooch B, Sulemana I, et al: Reviews of evidence on interventions to prevent dental caries, oral and pharyngeal cancers, and sports-related craniofacial injuries. *Am J Prev Med* 23(1 supp):21, 2002.

BIBLIOGRAPHY

Lane SE, Rhame GL, Wroble RL: A silicone splint for auricular hematoma. *Phys Sportsmed* 26(9), 1998.

Mahmood S, Lowe T: Management of epistaxis in the oral and maxillofacial surgery setting: An update on current practice. *Oral surg Oral Med Oral Pathol Oral Radiol Endod* 95:23, 2003.

Sander, R: Otitis extera: A practical guide to treatment and prevention. *Am Fam Phys* 63(5):927, 2001.

Stackhouse T: On-site management of nasal injuries. Phys Sportsmed 26(8), 1998.

30 DENTAL

Elizabeth M O'Connor, DDS

INTRODUCTION

- There are many benefits to participating in athletic activities, such as enhanced physical fitness and the enjoyment from competition. Sport, however, also increases the risk of sustaining an injury, especially injuries to the teeth and mouth.
- Sports medicine physicians are in an ideal position to facilitate early intervention to preserve dental health, and promote proper preventative strategies.

EPIDEMIOLOGY

- An oral injury can be defined as dental avulsions, dental fractures, dental luxations, lacerations or contusions to the gum, cheeks, tongue, lips and jaw injuries (fracture, locked open or closed, temporomandibular joint pain, and chewing difficulty). A concussion from a blow under the chin can also be included (Kvittern et al, 1998).

- Contact sports, such as basketball, hockey, and football have a great risk of orofacial related injuries. According to a study by Soporowski, based on 159 injuries reported by pediatric dentists during a 1-year period, the sports receiving the most orofacial injuries were baseball and biking followed by hockey and basketball (Tesini and Soporowski, 2000).
- Noncontact sports such as golf, billiards, and bowling have a much lower incidence of orofacial injury. Although not a contact sport, biking, as previously noted, has a great risk of orofacial injury (Tesini and Soporowski, 2000).
- The literature suggests that more boys than girls (3:1) are involved in orofacial sports related injuries. Parents additionally seem more inclined to have their sons wear mouth-guards as opposed to their daughters (Tesini and Soporowski, 2000).
- Studies have also shown that by the time a student graduates from secondary school, one out of three boys and one out of four girls will have suffered from a traumatic dental injury (Tesini and Soporowski, 2000).
- Injury rates appear to be highest from about 7 to 14 years of age (Douglas and Douglas, 2003).

ANATOMY

- The tooth is composed of three layers: enamel, dentin, and the pulp chamber (see Fig. 30-1).
- The enamel is the most external layer of the three. Enamel protects the crown of the tooth because of its hardness and structure.

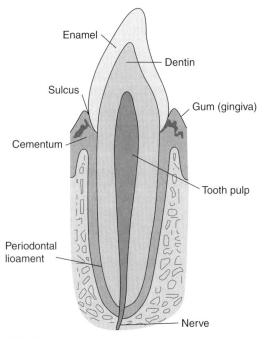

FIG 30-1   Anatomy of the tooth.

- The next layer is called the dentin. The dentin is softer than the enamel and has dentinal tubules that contain neurovascular structures. When dentin is exposed it is very prone to decay.
- The internal structure of a tooth is the pulp. The pulp contains the blood vessels and nerves that supply the tooth from the jaw.
- The *periodontal ligament* (PDL) connects the alveolar bone to the root and anchors the tooth in the socket.

FIELD SIDE ASSESSMENT

- It is important not to overlook dental injuries as part of the side line evaluation (Roberts, 2000; Cohen et al, 2002).
- Initial examination should be external beginning with checking for lacerations of the head or injury to the neck injury. The *tempormandibular joint* (TMJ) can be externally palpated while the patient opens and closes. The opening pattern should be closely evaluated to check for deviation which could indicate a unilateral mandibular fracture. Palpation of the zygomatic arch, angle, and lower border of the mandible should be checked for tenderness, swelling, and bruising to rule out bone fracture.
- Intraoral examination of the lips, tongue, cheek, palate, and floor of the mouth to check for laceration. Tenderness, swelling, and bruising of the facial and lingual gingival need to be checked. The anterior border of the ramus can be palpated intraorally.
- If there is a laceration to the lip or tongue it must be palpated and if need be radiographed to rule out embedded foreign bodies.

SPECIFIC INJURIES

TRAUMA

- Maxillomandibular relationships can increase risk for orofacial injury. Many studies have shown that the orthodontic status increases the rate of incisal trauma. A class-ll molar relationship (a malocclusion where the upper teeth protrudes past the lower teeth, also called an *overbite* or *buck teeth*), having an overjet greater than 4 mm, having a short upper lip, incompetent lips or a mouth breather will increase chance of dental injury. A referral to an orthodontist to evaluate for orthodontic correction to reduce such risks is very important (Roberts, 2000).
- A tooth fracture can be classified as a root fracture, crown fracture, or a chipped tooth. The most serious complication of the tooth fracture would involve injury to the pulp. Pulpal involvement can be seen by examining the fractured area and looking for a bleeding spot or a red dot. This type of involvement can be painful so care should be taken not to expose the tooth to air, saliva, and temperature changes. A patient with such a tooth fracture involving injury to the pulp should see their dentist for an examination and treatment on an emergent basis. A patient with dentin involvement should also not return to play, and seek immediate dental attention. A patient with enamel only involvement does not need immediate referral and can return to normal play with a protective mouth guard but must see a dentist for follow-up within 24 h.
- A tooth with a minor chip and without displacement does not need immediate dental attention but should be evaluated at a near future date, preferably within 24 to 48 h (Kenny and Barrett, 2001). Any tooth fragments that can be saved should be given to the patient to bring to the dental examination.
- Intrusion is the most complicated and controversial types of luxation injuries. If the intrusion is (>6 mm) then the prognosis is extremely poor. The eventual outcome of an intrusive injury depends on the severity of the injury, concurrent crown fracture, and treatment methods. The permanent tooth loss of severe intrusions is quite possible. This type of injury needs an immediate referral to a dentist. The tooth should not be attempted to be put back in correct position (Roberts, 2000).
- A tooth that has had an extrusion injury will interfere with normal occlusion—the patient seems to contact prematurely on the injured tooth. The displaced tooth will be in front of or behind the normal tooth row. These teeth will be quite painful to return to normal position, therefore these patients need immediate dental evaluation, treatment, and follow-up. An extruded tooth may be gently attempted to be repositioned in the field if not too painful (Roberts, 2000; Trope, 2002).
- An avulsed tooth is a tooth that has completely come out of the socket. The tooth has been separated from the socket and often there are vital PDL cells on the root surface. The prognosis is much higher for successful reimplantation if the tooth is not given a chance to dry out. The tooth must first be located; it may be in the patient's mouth, on their clothing, or near the injury site. The avulsed tooth should be handled very carefully-only by the crown/enamel therefore not causing further damage to the root surface. The tooth should be implanted within the first 20 min of injury to increase success of reimplantation. Immediate reimplantation onsite gives the best prognosis but requires onsite knowledge of emergency treatment (Kenny and Barrett, 2001). The tooth should be gently cleansed with saline and repositioned in the socket, if the patient

is alert. The tooth will click into place, but make sure the tooth is properly positioned. After reimplantation onsite temporary splinting can be done with aluminum foil, silly putty, or chewing gum to the surrounding teeth (Kenny and Barrett, 2001). The athlete should then follow up with a dentist immediately for definitive diagnosis and management.

- If reimplantation is not able to be done onsite then a proper medium for tooth transport is critical. The most suitable transport medium is *Hank's balanced salt solution* (HBSS) because of its pH-preserving fluid and trauma-reducing suspension. Save-a-Tooth (Biologic Rescue Products, Conshohacken, PA) is one HBSS-type product. HBSS should be readily available at schools, emergency rooms, athletic coach trainer kit, and at private medical offices.
- If HBSS is not available then milk, saliva, and physiologic saline are good alternatives. Tap water is not a good alternative because it can cause periodontal cell death within minutes (Kenny and Barrett, 2001). Cool milk has been shown to work as a better medium than warm milk. Also, getting the tooth into a medium within the first 15 min increases cell survival and reimplantation success (Trope, 2002).
- An avulsed tooth needs immediate attention and referral to a dentist because speed of treatment affects prognosis. A tooth that has been out of the mouth greater than 30 min decreases chance of survival. If the tooth is reimplanted within 15–30 min there is a 90% chance the tooth will be retained for life (Douglas and Douglas, 2003).
- Primary avulsed teeth should not be reimplanted because this could injure the permanent tooth follicle (Douglas and Douglas, 2003).

INFECTION

- Pulpitis is when an inflamed pulp will become necrotic causing inflammation around the apex of the tooth. The tooth will then have localized pain and swelling and sensitivity to percussion. Referral to dentist for either a root canal or extraction is needed. Pain medication may be given but antibiotics are not necessary (Douglas and Douglas, 2003).
- An apical abscess is localized, but if not treated a cellulitis may follow. Cellulitis is a diffuse painful swelling. This infection may spread into the fascial spaces of the head and neck possibly causing airway problems. The infection may spread to the periorbital area with complications such as loss of vision, cavernous sinus thrombosis, and *central nervous system* (CNS) involvement. A patient with cellulitis should be placed on antibiotics and incision and drainage

performed whether cellulitis is indurated or fluctuant to allow for a pathway of drainage.

- Patients with severe swelling in the head/neck with possible airway compromise often need hospitalization. These patients will need surgical drainage and IV broad spectrum antibiotics immediately.
- Periodontal disease is an inflammatory destructive process resulting in loss of attachment of tooth and bone. The PDL and alveolar bone are destroyed by bacterial plaque. Athletes with evidence of periodontal disease should be referred to the care of a periodontist.
- Dental decay or caries is caused by oral bacterial demineralizing tooth enamel and dentin. The acid production from the fermentation of dietary carbohydrates by oral bacteria demineralizes the tooth. Dental caries begins with no symptoms but can be seen as opaque areas on the enamel that progress to brownish cavities (Padilla, 2003).

PREVENTION

- A properly fitted mouth guard should be protective, comfortable, resilient, tear resistant, odorless, tasteless, not bulky, cause minimal interference to speaking and breathing, and have excellent retention, fit, and sufficient thickness in critical areas. Mouth guards are worn in football and it has been reported to have 0.07% orofacial injuries. On the contrary in basketball where mouth guards are not routinely worn oral facial injuries are 34% (Dorn, 2002). The American Dental Association (ADA) estimates mouth guards have prevented 200,000 injuries per year. A properly fitting mouth guard will protect the teeth and may reduce the incidence of concussion from a blow to the jaw (Padilla, 2003).
- There are four types of mouth guards: stock, boil and bite, vacuum custom, and pressure laminated custom.
- Stock mouth guards are available at most sporting good stores and are the least expensive and least protective. They are ready to use out of the package but considered bulky and have little retention.
- Boil and bite mouth guards are the most common on the market. The mouth guard is immersed in boiling water and formed in the mouth by fingers, tongue, and biting pressure. This mouth guard does not cover all the posterior teeth decreasing the protective qualities and increasing concussion chance.
- Custom mouth guards are made by a dentist after a complete dental examination and proper questioning. An impression is taken of the athlete's mouth allowing the dentist to make a stone cast of the mouth. A single layer thermoplastic mouth guard material is adapted over the cast. A vacuum custom mouth guard can be made in the office.

- Increased evidence has shown that a multilayer guard or laboratory pressure laminated may be preferred to a single layer. These can either be made by the dentist in office if proper materials are available or need to be sent to a qualified laboratory.
- When properly worn helmets and facemasks will increase safety and decrease morbidity. They protect the skin and bones of the head/face.
- The ADA recommends mouth guard use for these sports: acrobatics, basketball, boxing, field hockey, football, gymnastics, handball, ice hockey, lacrosse, martial arts, racquetball, roller hockey, rugby, shot putting, skateboarding, skiing, skydiving, soccer, squash, surfing, volleyball, water polo, weightlifting, and wrestling (Kvittern et al, 1998).
- Injury rates in football rates have gone from 50% to less than 1% since the onset of mouth guard and face mask use (Kvittern et al, 1998).
- In athletes who are undergoing orthodontic treatment (braces are a greater risk for orofacial injuries) a custom mouth guard is indicated (Kvittern et al, 1998).
- Compliance can be a problem with mouth guard use—coaches, parents, and athletic trainers are encouraged to explain to the athletes the benefit of mouth guard use (Ranalli, 2002).

DENTAL MAINTENANCE

- It is important for athletes as well as the general public to have regular dental checkups. An initial comprehensive dental examination should be performed, including chief complaint, health history, intraoral and extraoral examination, and radiographs where applicable; then the dentist will recommend a recall schedule as needed dictated by the evaluation.
- Oral jewelry has become a recent fad with the youth of this country. Dental professionals are advised to give these patients information about the problems that can occur with the jewelry. Tongue piercing can cause teeth fractures and also gingival stripping. Dental professionals should also inform patients that the jewelry should be removed prior to any contact sporting participation.
- Dentists can also screen patients who are using smokeless (spit) tobacco and inform them it is not a safe substitute for smoking.
- Anorexia and bulimia nervosa can also be picked up during routine dental checkup. The clinical signs are erosion of the lingual enamel of the teeth, bilateral swelling of the theparotid gland and floating amalgam because of quicker erosion of enamel versus metal.
- It is important for patients to follow through with any recommended dental treatment thereby preventing any future problems.

REFERENCES

Cohen S., Burns RC., et al: Traumatic injuries, in Cohen S, Burns RC (eds.): *Pathways of the Pulp*, 8th ed. St. Louis, MO, Mosby, 2002, p 605.
Dorn SO: Sports dentistry for Endodontist. *J Endod* 28:9, 2002.
Douglas AB Douglas JM: Common dental emergencies. *Am Fam Phys* 67:3, 2003.
Kenny DJ Barrett EJ: Recent developments in dental traumatology. *Am Acad Pediatr Dent* 23:6, 2001.
Kvittern B, Hardie NA, Roettger M, et al: Incidence of orofacial injuries in high school sports. *J Public Health Dent* 58:289, 1998.
Lee JL, Vann WF, Sigurdsson A: Management of avulsed permanent incisors: A decision analysis based on hanging concepts. *Pediatr Dent* 23:3, 2001.
Padilla RR: Sports dentistry online. www.sportsdentistry.com, 10 Jan. 2003.
Ranalli DN: Sports dentistry and dental traumatology. *Dental Traumatol* 18:231–236, 2002.
Roberts WO: Field Care of the injured tooth. *Phys Sportsmed* 28:1, 2000.
Tesini D Soporowski N: Epidemiology of orofacial sports-related injuries, in Holland, Kerry (eds.): *The Dental Clinic of North America Advances in Sports Dentistry*. Philadelphia, PA, Saunders. Jan. 2000. p 8.
Trope M: Clinical management of the avulsed tooth: Present strategies and future directions. *Dental Traumatol* 18:1–11, 2002.

31 INFECTIOUS DISEASE AND THE ATHLETE

John P Metz, MD

INTRODUCTION

- Among 170 surveyed marathoners, 90% definitely or mostly agreed they "rarely got sick" (Nieman, 1995). Ninety percent of nonelite athletes who engaged in regular, moderate exercise reported they rarely got sick (Pedersen and Bruunsgaard, 1995; Eichner, 1993; Nieman, 1999). In a 1989 *Runner's World* survey, 60.7% of subscribers reported catching fewer colds since starting running, while 4.9% reported catching more (Nieman, 1994).
- Elite athletes feel that intense training lowers their immunity and increases their vulnerability to illness (Eichner, 1993; Nieman, 1999).

- Regarding infectious diseases, the team physician should have the ultimate authority in return to play issues (Boschert, 2002).

IMMUNOLOGY AND EXERCISE

- The immune system has two parts, the innate and the acquired. The innate, composed of barrier and non-barrier elements, is nonspecific regarding host defense. The acquired protects the body against specific infectious agents.
- The body's first lines of defense are physical barriers, such as the skin and mucous membranes that can be impaired by temperature, wind, sun, humidity, and trauma (Simon, 1987).
- Airflow patterns, mechanical barriers, ciliary action, and mucosal immunoglobulin-A (IgA) activity affect airborne respiratory pathogens (Nieman, 1999).
  1. During nasal breathing at rest, viruses are suspended until they reach the bronchi and bronchioles where the mucous barrier, rich in IgA, impedes further invasion (Shephard and Shek, 1999).
  2. During mouth breathing with exercise, there is increased deposition of harmful particles in the lower respiratory tract, and increased cooling and drying of the respiratory mucosa, slowing ciliary movement and increasing mucous viscosity (Shephard and Shek, 1999).
  3. Depressed IgA levels have been noted in cross-country skiers, cyclists, and swimmers (Eichner, 1993; Nieman, 1999; Brenner, 1984).
  4. There is thus a decreased clearance of infectious particles and a theoretically increased infection risk (Nieman, 1999; Shephard and Shek, 1999).
- The nonbarrier components to the innate immune system include *natural killer* (NK) cells, phagocytes, cytokines, and neutrophils.
  1. NK counts (Woods, 1999) and *natural killer cell activity* (NKCA) (Nieman, 1999) increase immediately after high intensity exercise lasting less than 1 h, but fall soon after to below preexercise levels (Woods et al, 1999). NKCA is elevated chronically in elite versus untrained athletes (Nieman, 2000), but not with moderate exercise (Woods et al, 1999).
  2. Acute exercise increases macrophage count and function. Chronic exercise attenuates this response, but macrophage function is greater than in nonathletes (Woods et al, 1999).
  3. Cytokines mediate communication between immune and nonimmune cells. Proinflammatory cytokines, like *tumor necrosis factor-alpha* (TNF-alpha), *interleukin-1* (IL-1), and *interleukin-6* (IL-6), and anti-inflammatory cytokines, like interleukin-10 and IL-1 receptor antagonist, increase with acute exercise (Moldoveanu, Shephard, and Shek, 2001).
  4. Neutrophil counts increase with acute intense exercise, and several hours later. Long-term moderate exercise seems to elicit an increase in neutrophil activity, but chronic intense exercise seems to suppress it (Woods et al, 1999; Pyne, 1991).
- The acquired immune system, mainly T- and B-lymphocytes and plasma cell-secreted antibodies, attacks specific foreign particles that invade the body (Goodman, 1991). Overall lymphocyte counts increase with any type of acute exercise. Lymphocyte counts and B-cell function are decreased after intense exercise but not after moderate exercise (Pedersen and Toft, 2000).
- Antibody production, notably IgA, is affected by exercise. Cross-country skiers and cyclists have low baseline salivary IgA levels that drop after racing (Eichner, 1993; Nieman, 1999; Brenner, 1984; Pedersen et al, 1996). Longitudinal studies of salivary IgA in elite swimmers, however, have reported increases (Bruunsgaard et al, 1997), decreases (Gleeson et al, 1999), and no change with training (MacKinnon and Hooper, 1994).
- Among T-lymphocytes are CD4 (T-helper) and CD8 (T-suppressor) cells. A CD4/CD8 ratio of >1.5 is considered necessary for proper immune function. Intense exercise decreases CD4 and increases CD8 counts, decreasing the CD4/CD8 ratio. In one study (Bruunsgaard et al, 1997), male triathletes showed diminished skin test measures of cellular immunity 48 h after a half-ironman triathlon compared to noncompeting triathletes and recreational athletes.
- The brief period of immunosuppression after acute, intense physical activity when ciliary action, IgA levels, NK count, NKCA, T-lymphocyte count, and CD4/CD8 ratio are decreased has been described as the immunologic "open window" when infectious organisms are theoretically more likely to invade the host and cause an infection (Nieman, 1999; Shephard and Shek, 1999; Brenner, 1984; Pedersen et al, 1996).

INFECTIONS AND EXERCISE

- Marathon runners have a higher incidence of self-reported *upper respiratory tract infections* (URI's) after competition (Peters and Bateman, 1983; Nieman et al, 1990*a*). URI incidence was higher with increased training volume. Danish elite orienteers have increased incidence of URI compared to controls (Linde, 1987).
- Studies of moderate physical activity, however, have had variable results.

1. High levels of self-reported exercise, occupational, and leisure time activities were associated with a 20–30% decrease in the annual incidence of URI in healthy, nonathletic, and middle-aged adults (Matthews et al, 2002).

2. A similar study of healthy, elderly people noted an inverse relationship between the amount of energy expended in daily moderate activities and URI incidence (Kostka, 2000).

3. Runners in short races (5K, 10K, half-marathon) had no increased incidence of infection after the race compared to before. Training more than 15 mi a week showed a nonsignificant trend towards fewer infections (Nieman, Johanssen and Lee, 1989). Another study (Heath et al, 1991), however, found running 16–26 mi a week increased the risk of having ≥1 URI compared to running <9 mi a week. Running 9–16 mi or >26 mi a week conferred intermediate risk.

EXERCISE, IMMUNOLOGY, AND INFECTION

- In premenopausal women, no exercise or a 15-week walking program made no difference in NK cell counts. NKCA was significantly increased in the training group at 6 weeks, but was elevated equally in both groups at 15 weeks. The training group reported 50% fewer days with URI symptoms, but the same number of separate URIs compared to controls. NKCA at 6 weeks was negatively correlated with URI symptom days (Nieman et al, 1990b).

- A similar study (Nieman et al, 1993) of sedentary, elderly women found no significant difference in lymphocyte counts, T-cell counts, and NKCA. The exercise group, however, had significantly fewer URIs than the control group (3/14 vs. 8/16). A comparison group of elite elderly athletes had significantly higher NKCA and lymphocyte activity and even fewer URIs (1/12).

- NK counts (Gleeson et al, 2000) and resting neutrophil oxidative burst capacity (a measure of neutrophil activity) (Pyne et al, 1995) decreased in 22 elite swimmers during a 12-week training cycle but were not correlated with the risk of URI.

- A study (Nieman et al, 2000) of elite female rowers and sedentary controls found no difference in baseline measures of granulocyte/monocyte phagocytosis, neutrophil oxidative burst capacity, and concentrations of IL-6, TNF-alpha, and IL-1ra. NKCA and lymphocyte proliferative response were significantly higher in the rowers. Days of self-reported URI symptoms, however, were similar in both groups and did not correlate with immunologic changes.

- Gleeson (Gleeson et al, 1999) found an inverse correlation between pretraining salivary IgA levels and risk of infection in elite swimmers and controls, and predicted an additional infection for each 10% drop in IgA. Swimmers and controls had equal incidence of infections, however. A follow-up study (Gleeson et al, 2000) showed no correlation between salivary IgA levels and infection risk.

- Three 30-s Wingate leg cycling tests over 9 min decreased salivary IgA an average of 27.8% in healthy adult females, but without an increased incidence of URI (Fahlman et al, 2001).

- Klentrou et al (Klentrou et al, 2002) studied 19 sedentary men and women randomized to no exercise or exercise for 12 weeks. There was a negative correlation between salivary IgA levels and number of days of illness and flu symptoms, but not days of cold symptoms.

- Studies of immune marker changes with exercise have failed to show consistent correlation with risk of infection (Nieman, 2002).

- A popular theory regarding exercise intensity and infection risk is the "J-curve" proposed by Nieman (Fig. 31-1). Moderate exercise lowers infection risk to below that of being sedentary, while strenuous exercise imposes the highest risk of all (Nieman, 2002).

- More evidence is needed, however, as the link between moderate exercise and infection is less clear (Shephard and Shek, 1999). Most studies of infection and exercise are relatively small and rely on patient recall and self-reporting for diagnosis. Also, other factors such as pathogen exposure, stress, sleep, nutrition, and environment may play a confounding role (Shephard and Shek, 1999).

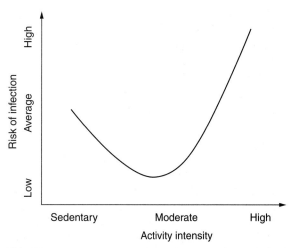

FIG. 31-1 "J" curve of exercise and susceptibility to infection.

INFECTION AND TRAINING

FEVER

- Fever impairs concentric muscle strength, mental cognition, and pulmonary perfusion; and increases overall caloric and oxygen demand and insensible fluid loss resulting in decreased exercise capacity and increased risk of injury (Brenner et al, 1984).
- Options to treat fever include acetaminophen (650–1000 mg q 4–6 h) and *nonsteroidal anti-inflammatory drugs* (NSAIDs) like ibuprofen (800 mg TID) (Kauffman, 1999).
- When an athlete is dehydrated, using NSAIDs during exercise may reduce renal blood flow and precipitate acute renal failure (McDonald, 1997).

RHINORRHEA AND NASAL CONGESTION

- The most common complaints related to infections in athletes are rhinorrhea and nasal congestion, most commonly seen with URIs and acute sinusitis.
- Typical URI symptoms include rhinorrhea, congestion, sneezing, sore throat, cough, hoarseness, malaise, and headache. Typical findings include nasal mucosa edema and erythema, rhinorrhea, oropharyngeal erythema, and cervical lymphadenopathy. Temperature greater than 100°F (37.7°C) is unusual (Levy and Kelly, 1999).
- URI treatment is aimed at symptom relief with rest and good hydration being paramount.
  1. Oral or nasal decongestants can help relieve congestion, but side effects can include nervousness, insomnia, tachycardia, and increased blood pressure.
  2. Sedating antihistamines are good choices for sneezing and rhinorrhea as their anticholinergic action dries the nasal mucosa and increases mucous viscosity. Side effects can include sedation, dry mouth, urinary retention, blurry vision, and constipation (Levy and Kelly, 1999). Athletes in warm climates should use them with caution since they impair sweating and increase the risk of heat exhaustion or heat stroke (Lillegard, Butcher, and Rucker 1999).
  3. Nasal ipratropium can provide the anticholinergic effect of the nonsedating antihistamines without the systemic side effects. (Hayden et al, 1996).
- Diagnosis of acute sinusitis relies on combining a constellation of signs and symptoms. Common indicators are unilateral sinus pain and tenderness, purulent rhinorrhea, lack of response to standard URI therapy, sinus pain with leaning forward, maxillary toothache, and "double sickening." "Double sickening" is when a patient has a URI that starts to improve, but

then gets acutely worse. Fever and other constitutional symptoms may be present. Transillumination and radiographs of the sinuses are generally not useful (Fagnan, 1998).
- Treatment of acute sinusitis is as follows:
  1. Analgesics and decongestants in doses discussed above.
  2. Nasal saline rinses, $1/4$ tsp of table salt in 8 oz of warm water, can give short-term relief and help remove mucous. Placing a warm washcloth over the affected sinus and its corresponding nostril may also help.
  3. Sedating antihistamines are not recommended because they increase mucous viscosity and may impede sinus drainage.
  4. Antibiotics should cover the most common causative pathogens, *Streptococcus pneumoniae, Haemophilus influenza,* and *Moraxella catarrhalis.* Appropriate first-line choices include 10–14 day regimens of amoxicillin (500 mg TID), and trimethoprim-sulfamethoxazole DS (one pill bid). Second-line choices include cefuroxime (250–500 mg bid), amoxicillin-clavulanate (875 mg bid), doxycycline (100 mg bid), and clarithromycin (500 mg bid) (Fagnan, 1998).

COUGH

- Most commonly seen with URIs, sinusitis, bronchitis, and pneumonia (Williamson, 1999).
- Focusing treatment on the underlying infection, cessation of smoking, and adequate hydration may provide significant relief (Simon, 1995).
- If the cough is especially irritating, however, cough medicines may be tried.
  1. The most effective cough suppressant is a narcotic such as codeine (10–30 mg q 3–4 h). It will suppress cough as well as provide sedation to help the patient sleep.
  2. Nonnarcotic options include dextromethorphan (10–20 mg q4h), benzonatate (100 mg TID), and guaifenesin (600–1200 mg bid) (Simon, 1995).
- Symptoms of acute bronchitis may include URI symptoms, but cough, productive or nonproductive, is typically the most predominant feature (Levy and Kelly, 1999).
- Most cases of acute bronchitis, in the absence of underlying lung disease, are viral. Atypical bacteria such as *Mycoplasma pneumonia* and *Chlamydia trachomatis* may also cause bronchitis in a small percentage of cases (Williamson, 1999). *Bordetella pertussis* should also be suspected, even in adults immunized as children (Birkebaek et al, 1999).

- Pulmonary findings are variable and can range from normal to diffuse rhonchi, and/or wheezing. Chest X-rays are usually normal but may be useful to exclude other diseases (Williamson, 1999).
- As in URIs and acute sinusitis, rest and hydration are key. Bronchodilators such as albuterol (1–2 puffs q 4–6 h) may be useful, especially in patients with wheezing or cough that increases with activity.
- Antibiotics are often not indicated in the first 2 weeks since most cases are viral.
- The decision to prescribe antibiotics may involve non-medical factors such as upcoming competitions and risk of deconditioning while monitoring the course of illness.
- Antibiotic treatment should primarily target *Bordetella* species (Gilbert, Moellering and Sande, 2002). The first line choice is erythromycin estolate (500 mg qid for 14 days). Second line choices include trimethoprim-sulfamethoxazole-DS (1 bid for 14 days) or clarithromycin (500 mg bid for 7 days).
- During recovery, the healing bronchi are more sensitive to changes with exercise such as increased minute ventilation, increased inhalation of antigens and irritants, and drying and cooling of inspired air. These can trigger bronchospasm and impede training. The clinician must provide considerable reassurance as complete symptom resolution may take 4–5 weeks (Williamson, 1999). Management relies on avoiding irritant stimuli and using bronchodilators such as albuterol (1–2 puffs q 4–6 h). Inhaled corticosteroids such as fluticasone (88–440 mcg bid), beclomethasone (2–4 puffs qid), flunisolide (2–4 puffs bid), or triamcinolone (2–4 puffs bid-qid) may be useful too (McDonald, 1997).
- Acute cough with a history of fever, sputum production, myalgias, pleuritic chest pain, and shortness of breath, and physical findings such as hypoxia, tachypnea, and localized pulmonary rales or rhonchi, suggest the diagnosis of community-acquired pneumonia (Masters and Weitekemp, 1998).
- Chest X-rays often show localized or diffuse infiltrates, but may not early in the course of disease. Sputum gram stain and culture may provide clues to the causative organism (Masters and Weitekemp, 1998).
- Healthy subjects can usually be treated as outpatients (Levy and Kelly, 1999). Proper rest, hydration, and nutrition are critical, as well as antibiotics to cover the common bacterial pathogens (*Streptococcus pneumoniae, Mycoplasma pneumoniae, Legionella pneumoniae, Chlamydia pneumoniae, Haemophilus influenzae*). First line therapy includes azithromycin (500 mg for one day then 250 mg a day for 4 days), or clarithromycin (500 mg bid for 7–14 days). One may also consider a flouroquinolone with increased *S. pneumoniae* activity such as levafloxacin (500 mg qd for 7–14 days), an oral second-generation cephalosporin such as cefuroxime (250–500 mg bid for 7–14 days), amoxicillin/clavulanate (875 mg bid for 7–14 days), or doxycycline (100 mg bid for 7–14 days) (Gilbert, Moellering, and Sande, 2002).
- Pneumonia patients, by virtue of their damaged pulmonary parenchyma, will require more time to recover and return to full training. Absolute rest while the patient is symptomatic is critical to avoid prolonged illness, pulmonary abscess, and empyema (McDonald, 1997).

SORE THROAT

- Common infectious causes of acute pharyngitis include viral URIs, *group A beta-hemolytic strep* (GABHS), *infectious mononucleosis* (IM), and enterovirus infections, like coxsackievirus, which have been linked to infectious myocarditis (Perkins, 1997; Francis, 1995).
- History should cover time of onset, ill contacts, presence of cough and/or fever, difficulty swallowing, and difficulty speaking.
- On examination look for tonsillar erythema and exudates, asymmetric tonsillar swelling, ulcerations, palatal petichiae, fever, cervical adenopathy, and splenomegaly.
- The most common etiology is viral (Perkins, 1997). Symptomatic treatment with warm salt water gargles, humidified air, throat lozenges, and analgesics is often all that is needed.
- A rapid strep test gives a quick diagnosis of GABHS pharyngitis. If negative, then a throat culture should be done and the patient treated if positive (Perkins, 1997).
- The combination of sore throat, fever, cervical adenopathy, tonsillar exudates, and absence of cough suggests a greater than 50% likelihood of strep throat and warrants empiric treatment (Perkins, 1997).
- Penicillin (500 mg bid for 10 days) remains the drug of choice for GABHS. Second line choices include azithromycin (500 mg qd for 1 day and then 250 mg a day for 4 days) or erythromycin (250 mg qid for 10 days) (Perkins, 1997). Antibiotics hasten recovery, render the patient noninfectious after 24 h, and protect against rheumatic fever (McDonald, 1997).
- IM, caused by *Ebstein-Barr virus* (EBV), occurs most commonly between ages 15 and 24 and affects 1–3% of college students each year (Maki and Reich, 1982).
- Typical symptoms include a 3–5-day prodrome of headache, anorexia, and malaise, followed by sore throat, fever, lymphadenopathy, and fatigue lasting typically 2 weeks. Anorexia, nausea, fatigue, and malaise are often present for longer, and can lengthen an athlete's return to preillness training levels by up to 3 months (Maki and Reich, 1982).

- Physical findings include fever, diffuse posterior lymphadenopathy, and tonsillar erythema and exudates. A morbiliform rash may occur in patients prescribed amoxicillin to treat a presumed strep throat, a finding that can aid in diagnosis.
- Diagnostic studies include a lymphocytosis of >50%, >10% atypical lymphocytes on a peripheral smear, and a positive heterophil antibody (monospot) test. Ten percent of IM sufferers will have a negative monospot (Bailey, 1994) in which case EBV serology should be ordered. Approximately 25% of affected individuals will also have GABHS pharyngitis (Bailey, 1994).
- Rest, hydration, saline gargles, and analgesics are all that are generally needed. Antiviral treatment is not indicated (Bailey, 1994).

- Severe tonsillar swelling responds well to prednisone (40–60 mg qd for 5–10 days) (Bailey, 1994).
- Splenic rupture occurs in 0.1–0.2% of all cases, and almost always occurs between illness days 4 and 21 in patients with splenomegaly. There is no correlation between the severity of the illness and the susceptibility to splenic rupture. Left upper quadrant pain that radiates to the left shoulder (Kehr's sign) suggests splenic rupture and demands immediate medical attention (McDonald, 1997). Splenic rupture can occur in the absence of significant physical exertion, trauma, or strain and may be the presenting clinical feature (Maki and Reich, 1982).
- The guidelines in Fig. 31-2 will help guide return to play decisions (Maki and Reich, 1982).

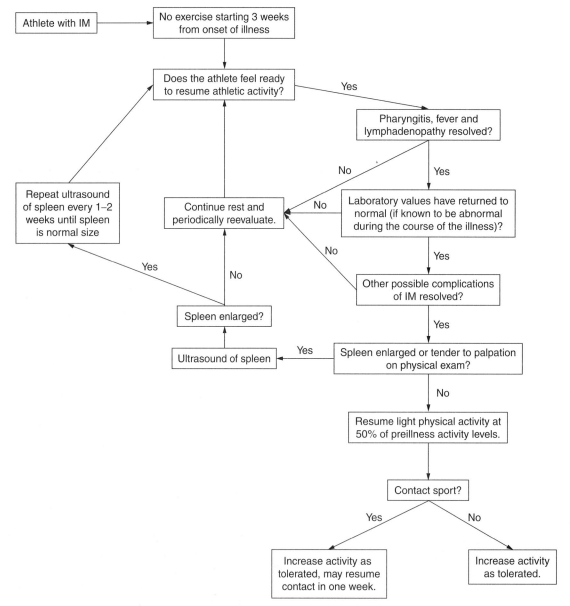

FIG. 31-2   Algorithm for return to play guidelines for athletes with infectious mononucleosis.

- If indicated by the algorithm in Fig. 31-2, ultrasound measurement of the spleen to left kidney ratio (Loftus and Metreweli, 1998) every two weeks can be useful, especially in athletes at the extremes of body habitus. A ratio of less than 1.25 is normal.

ACUTE DIARRHEA

- Diarrhea is >3 loose stools a day for up to 7 days (Mayer and Wanke, 1999) and is most often caused by a viral infection. Other causes to consider include hyperthyroidism, inflammatory bowel disease, bacterial colitis, and antibiotic-induced colitis.
- The history should focus on travel, hobbies, animal contacts, antibiotic usage, dietary habits, and ill contacts. The review of systems should cover stool appearance (mucous, bloody, or watery), fever, weight loss (acute and chronic), and abdominal pain (Mayer and Wanke, 1999).
- Stool examination for fecal leukocytes, ova and parasites, and occult blood and *C. difficile* toxin (if indicated), are helpful in identifying the cause. Five or more fecal leukocytes per high-powered field suggests bacterial colitis (Mayer and Wanke, 1999).
- Most cases can be treated with oral rehydration, but severe cases may require intravenous hydration (Mayer and Wanke, 1999).
- Antidiarrheal agents may be used, and include loperamide (4 mg × 1, then 2 mg after each loose stool, maximum 16 mg a day), and bismuth subsalicylate (262 mg, 2 qid prn). Loperamide should be avoided in patients who are toxic, febrile, or are having bloody diarrhea. Lomotil contains atropine and causes anticholinergic side effects (Fenton, 2000).
- The decision to use antibiotics empirically remains in the hands of the provider. Bacterial colitis (*Salmonella, Shigella, E. coli, Campylobacter*) can be treated with ciprofloxacin (500 mg bid) or trimethoprim-sulfamethoxazole DS (1 bid) for 3–5 days. *Salmonella* should not be treated unless the illness is severe or the patient is immunocompromised as antibiotic treatment may prolong the carrier state. *C. difficile* is treated with metronidazole (500 mg tid) or vancomycin (125 mg orally qid) for 10–14 days (Gilbert, Moellering, and Sande, 2002).

HIV INFECTION

- In HIV+ patients, moderate and high intensity aerobic exercise programs do not change leukocyte, lymphocyte, CD4, and CD8 counts or the CD4:CD8 ratio (Terry, Sprinz and Ribeiro, 1999). Progressive resistance training increases lean body mass and physical functioning in patients with HIV-associated wasting (Roubenoff and Wilson, 2001). Regular exercise is associated with slower progression to AIDS and decreased short-term mortality (Mustafa, 1999).
- Patients with a CD4 count <200 or an AIDS defining-infection, however, should be limited to moderate exercise (Stringer, 1999).
- Documented sports transmission of HIV is exceedingly rare. The risk of HIV transmission in professional football is estimated at one in 85 million game contacts (Feller and Flanigan, 1997).
- In 1995, the American Medical Society for Sports Medicine (AMSSM) and the American Academy of Sports Medicine (AASM) stated that mandatory HIV testing should not be a requirement for competitive sports participation, though they strongly encourage counseling and voluntary testing in individuals at high risk (AMSSM and AASM, 1995).
- The National Collegiate Athletic Association (NCAA) mandates removal of bloody uniforms and covering open wounds prior to returning to competition. Universal precautions are the norm in dealing with any blood or body fluid (Feller and Flanigan, 1997).

RETURN TO PLAY

- Experimental rhinovirus infection does not decrease pulmonary function tests, VO_{2max}, or submaximal exercise testing (Weidner et al, 1997). Exercise during such an infection does not alter its length or severity (Weidner et al, 1998). Other respiratory viruses, such as influenza virus (Blair et al, 1976; O'Connor et al, 1979), however, have been shown to impair pulmonary function.
- The "neck check" (Eichner, 1993; Primos, 1996) helps guide return to play decisions. If symptoms are above the neck (i.e., runny nose, nasal congestion, sore throat, or sneezing) and not associated with below the neck symptoms (i.e., fever, myalgias, arthralgias, severe cough, GI symptoms), then the athlete may train at half intensity for 10 min. If symptoms do not worsen, then the workout may continue as tolerated. If symptoms worsen, the workout should end and the athlete should rest until symptoms improve. Exercise should be delayed until below the neck symptoms have resolved (Eichner, 1993).
- When resuming training after recovering from an illness, the athlete should start at a 50% intensity and gradually increase to preillness training levels over 1–2 days for every training day missed (Primos, 1996).
- Training delay serves three purposes. First, training with below the neck symptoms hampers the workout and limits desired training effects. Second, without a medical evaluation athletes may not realize the severity

of their illness (Eichner, 1993). Third, no training may prevent the spread of disease to other athletes (Primos, 1996) as demonstrated by the documented transmission of Norwalk virus during a college football game (Becker, 2000).

CONCLUSION

- Moderate exercise seems to be an immune stimulant while intense exercise causes immune suppression. There are no reliable immune markers, however, that can help the physician make return to play decisions.
- When athletes become ill proper care and advice can minimize lost training time and maximize recovery.
- Athletes with HIV can safely exercise without fear of affecting their own illness or increasing the risk of transmission to other athletes during competition.
- Slowing or suspending training according to the "neck check" protocol is critical to facilitating return to full training.

REFERENCES

AMSSM, AASM: Human immunodeficiency virus and other blood-borne pathogens in sports: The American Medical Society for Sports Medicine (AMSSM) and the American Academy of Sports Medicine (AASM) joint position statement. *Clin J Sports Med* 5:199, 1995.

Bailey R: Diagnosis and treatment of infectious mononucleosis. *Am Fam Phys* 49(4):879–885, 1994.

Becker KM et al: Transmission of Norwalk virus during a football game. *N Engl J Med* 343:1223, 2000.

Birkebaek NH et al: *Bordetella pertussis* and chronic cough in adults. *Clin Infect Dis* 29:1239, 1999.

Blair HS et al: Effects of rhinovirus infection on pulmonary function of healthy human volunteers. *Am Rev Respir Dis* 114:95, 1976.

Boschert S: Team physician should control 'Return to Play'. *Fam Pract News* 32(16):36, 2002.

Brenner I et al: Infection in athletes. *Sports Med* 17:86, 1984.

Bruunsgaard H et al: In vivo cell-mediated immunity and vaccination response following prolonged, intense exercise. *Med Sci Sports Exerc* 29(9):1176, 1997.

Eichner R: Infection, immunity, and exercise: What to tell patients. *Phys Sportsmed* 21:125, 1993.

Fagnan LL: Acute sinusitis: A cost-effective approach to diagnosis and treatment. *Am Fam Phys* 58(8):1795, 1998.

Fahlman MM et al: Mucosal IgA response to repeated Wingate tests in females. *Int J Sports Med* 22:127, 2001.

Feller A, Flanigan TP: HIV-infected competitive athletes: What are the risks? What precautions should be taken? *J Gen Inter Med* 12:243, 1997.

Fenton BW: Infectious diarrhea, in Rakel RE (ed.): *Saunders Manual of Medical Practice*, 2nd (ed.): Philadelphia, PA, Saunders, 2000, p 1123.

Francis G: Viral myocarditis detection and management. *Phys Sportsmed* 23:63, 1995.

Gilbert DN, Moellering RC, Sande MA: *The Sanford Guide to Antimicrobial Therapy*, 32nd ed. Hyde Park, VT, Antimicrobial Therapy Inc, 2002.

Gleeson M et al: Immune status and respiratory illness for elite swimmers during a 12-week training cycle. *Int J Sports Med* 21:302, 2000.

Gleeson M et al: Salivary IgA levels and infection risk in elite swimmers. *Med Sci Sports Exerc* 31(1):67, 1999.

Goodman J: The immune response, in Stites D Terr A (eds.): *Basic Clinical Immunology*, 7th ed. Norwalk, CT, Appleton & Lange, 1991, p 34.

Hayden FG et al: Effectiveness and safety of intranasal ipratropium bromide in common colds. *Ann Int Med* 125:89, 1996.

Heath GW et al: Exercise and the incidence of upper respiratory infections. *Med Sci Sports Exerc* 23(2):152, 1991.

Kauffman R: Fever, in Rakel RE (ed.): *Conn's Current Therapy*, 51st ed. Philadelphia, PA, Saunders, 1999, p 23.

Klentrou P et al: Effect of moderate exercise on salivary immunoglobulin A and infection risk in humans. *Eur J Appl Physiol* 87:153, 2002.

Kostka T et al: The symptomatology of upper respiratory tract infections and exercise in elderly people. *Med Sci Sports Exerc* 32(1):46, 2000.

Levy BT, Kelly MW: Common cold, in *Griffith's 5 Minute Clinical Consult*. Baltimore, MD, Lippincott, Williams, and Wilkins, 1999, p 246.

Lillegard WA, Butcher JD, Rucker KS: *Handbook of Sports Medicine: A Symptoms Oriented Approach*, 2nd ed. Boston, MA, Butterworth & Heinemann, 353, 1999.

Linde F: Running and upper respiratory tract infections. *Scand J Sports Sci* 9(1):21, 1987.

Loftus W. Metreweli C: Ultrasound assessment of mild splenomegaly: Spleen/kidney ratio. *Pediatr Radiol* 28:98, 1998.

MacKinnon LT, Hooper S: Mucosal (secretory) immune system responses to exercise of varying intensity and during overtraining. *Int J Sports Med* 15:S179, 1994.

F RM: Infectious mononucleosis in the athlete: Diagnosis, domplications, and management. *Am J Sports Med* 10(3):162, 1982.

Masters PA, Weitekemp MR: Community-acquired pneumonia, in *Pulmonary and Critical Care Medicine*, St. Louis, MO, Mosby-Year Book, 1998, p J1-1.

Matthews DE et al: Moderate to vigorous physical activity and risk of upper-respiratory tract infection. *Med Sci Sports Exerc* 34(8):1242, 2002.

Mayer M, Wanke C: Acute infectious diarrhea, in Rakel RE (ed.): *Conn's Current Therapy*, 51st ed. Philadelphia, PA, Sanders 1999, p 13.

McDonald W: Upper Respiratory Tract Infections, in Fields and Fricker (eds.): *Medical Problems in Athletes*, Malden, MA, Blackwell Science 1997, p 9.

Moldoveanu AI, Shephard RJ, Shek PN: The cytokine response to physical activity and training. *Sports Med* 13(2):115, 2001.

Mustafa T, et al: Association between exercise and HIV disease progression in a cohort of homosexual men. *Ann Epidemiol* 9:127, 1999.

Nieman DC: Is infection risk linked to exercise workload? *Med Sci Sports Exerc* 32(7):S406, 2002.

Nieman DC, Johanssen LM, Lee JW: Infectious episodes in runners before and after a roadrace. *J Sports Med* 29:289, 1989.

Nieman DC et al: Infectious episodes in runners before and after the Los Angeles marathon. *J Sports Med Phys Fitness* 30:316, 1990a.

Nieman DC et al: The effects of moderate exercise training on natural killer cells and acute upper respiratory tract infections. *Int J Sports Med* 11(6):467, 1990b.

Nieman DC et al: Physical activity and immune function in elderly women. *Med Sci Sports Exerc* 25(7):823, 1993.

Nieman DC: Exercise, upper respiratory tract infection, and the immune system. *Med Sci Sports Exerc* 26(2):128, 1994.

Nieman DC et al: Immune function in marathon runners versus sedentary controls. *Med Sc Sports Exerc* 27(7): 986, 1995.

Nieman DC: Nutrition, exercise, and immune system function. *Clin Sports Med* 18(3), 537, 1999.

Nieman DC et al: Immune function in female elite rowers and non-athletes. *Br J Sports Med* 34:181, 2000.

O'Connor S et al: Changes in pulmonary function after naturally acquired respiratory infection in normal persons. *Am Rev Respir Dis* 120:1087, 1979.

Pedersen B, Bruunsgaard H: How exercise influences the establishment of infections. *Sports Med* 19:393–400, 1995.

Pedersen BK, Toft AD: Effects of exercise on lymphocytes and cytokines. *Br J Sports Med* 34:246–251, 2000.

Pedersen B et al: Immunity in athletes. *J Sports Med Phys Fitness* 36:36, 1996.

Perkins A: An approach to diagnosing the acute sore throat. *Am Fam Phys* 55:131, 1997.

Peters EM, Bateman ED: Ultramarathon running and upper respiratory tract infections: an epidemiological survey. *S Afr Med J* 64:582, 1983.

Primos WA: Sports and exercise during acute illness: Recommending the right course for patients. *Phys Sports Med* 24(2):44, 1996.

Pyne DB: Regulation of neutrophil function during exercise. *Sports Med* 17(4):245, 1991.

Pyne DB et al: Effects of an intensive 12-wk training program by elite swimmers on neutrophil oxidative activity. *Med Sci Sports Exerc* 27(4):536, 1995.

Roubenoff R, Wilson IB: Effect of resistance training on self-reported physical functioning in HIV infection. *Med Sci Sports Exerc* 33(11):1811, 2001.

Shephard R, Shek P: Exercise, immunity, and susceptibility to infection: A j-shaped relationship?, *Phys Sports Med*, 27(6):47–66, 1999.

Simon H: Exercise and infection. *Phys Sports Med* 15:135, 1987.

Simon HB: Management of the common cold, in *Primary Care Medicine*, 3rd ed. Philadelphia, PA, Lippincott-Raven, 1995, p 277.

Stringer W: HIV and aerobic exercise: Current recommendations. *Sports Med* 28(6):389, 1999.

Terry L, Sprinz E, Ribeiro JP: Moderate and high intensity exercise training in HIV-1 seropositive individuals: A randomized trial. *Int J Sports Med* 20:142, 1999.

Weidner TG et al: Effect of rhinovirus-caused upper respiratory illness on pulmonary function test and exercise responses. *Med Sci Sports Exerc* 29(5):604, 1997.

Weidner TG et al: The effect of exercise training on the severity and duration of viral upper respiratory illness. *Med Sci Sports Exerc* 30(11):1578, 1998.

Williamson HA: Acute bronchitis, in Rakel RE (ed.): *Conn's Current Therapy,* 51st ed. Philadelphia, PA, Saunders, 1999, p 210.

Woods J et al: Exercise and cellular innate immune function. *Med Sci Sports Exerc* 31(1):57, 1999.

32 ENDOCRINE CONSIDERATIONS

William Dexter, MD
Shireen Rahman, MD

INTRODUCTION

ENDOCRINE OVERVIEW

- Endocrine and nervous system work together to regulate homeostasis.
- Endocrine glands secrete hormones directly into the blood.
- Hormones alter activity of effector sites which have receptors for specific hormone binding.
- Plasma hormone concentration is the major determinant of the effect of the hormone.

CLASSES OF HORMONES

- Amino acid derivatives are most common.
- Steroidal derivatives of cholesterol

HORMONE–RECEPTOR INTERACTIONS

- Specificity of hormone to target tissue
- Hormone effect dependent on the following:
  a. Hormone concentration
  b. Target tissue receptor site availability
  c. Affinity
- Blood hormone concentration
  a. Rate of production/secretion and clearance
  b. Plasma volume
  c. Levels of releasing or inhibiting hormones
- Receptor number
  a. Desensitization to hormone
  b. Specificity

ENDOCRINE GLANDS

- Anterior/posterior pituitary
- Adrenal (cortex, medulla)
- Thyroid
- Pancreas
- Parathyroid
- Gonadal

ANTERIOR PITUITARY HORMONES AND EXERCISE (TABLE 32-1)

A. Growth Hormone

- **Endurance exercise:** Magnitude of increased secretion related to both duration and intensity of exercise (Felsing et al, 1992)
  - Exercise must be at least 10 min in duration.
  - Many studies suggest exercise must be above lactate threshold for greatest *growth hormone* (GH) stimulus (Godfrey et al, 2003; Vanhelder et al, 1984).
  - Suggests a linear relationship between acute GH release and exercise intensity.

- Following a single bout of exercise, GH release transiently decreases; 24 h GH is not elevated by single bout.
- Possible mechanisms for increased secretion include the following:
  1. Increased sympathetic outflow (Weltman et al, 2000)
  2. Hypoxia (Vanhelder et al, 1984)
  3. Exercise-released endorphin has inhibitory effect on somatostatin (Borer et al, 1986).
- **Resistance exercise:** Increased GH secretion may be related to load, frequency, and rest intervals (Godfrey et al, 2003).
  1. Kraemer et al (1991) reported significant increases in GH when utilizing a 10-*repetition maximum* (10-RM), 1-min rest interval versus 5-RM with a 3-min rest protocol.
  2. Higher volumes of resistance training (single set vs. multiple set) results in a significant increase in GH levels during recovery phase.
- Greater demands on anaerobic glycolysis appear to have more profound effect on GH release (Kraemer et al, 1993).

TABLE 32-1   Anterior Pituitary Hormones

GLAND	HORMONE	CONTROL	ACTION	ENDURANCE	RESISTANCE	CHRONIC
Anterior pituitary	Growth (GH)	**Hypothalamus;** stimulated by GHRH; inhibited by somatostatin; Plasma levels of FFA and glucose; feedback loops; pulsatile release	Promotes growth; glucose sparing through (+) lipolysis, amino acid uptake, (−) glucose uptake	*Increased* Glucose sparing aids in endurance activities; dependent on intensity	*Increased* Anabolic effects; recovery through protein synthesis	*Remains controversial*
	Thyrotropin (TSH)	**Hypothalamus** TRH **Anterior Pituitary** TSH Negative feedback loops via thyroid gland	Secretion of T3, T4; increases metabolism, lipolytic, (+) protein synthesis; increase HR, contractility of heart	*Conflicting*	*Decreased* Reserve energy	*Unknown*
	Corticotropin (ACTH)	Hypothalamus ACTH releasing hormone (CRH) in response to stress; negative feedback via cortisol; diurnal	(+) production and release of adrenal hormones (cortisol, aldosterone, sex steroids and the like); lipolytic	*Increased* Glucose-sparing Increased	*Increased;* during and throughout recovery; dependent on intensity	*Conflicting*
	Follicular Stimulating Hormone (FSH), Lutenizing Hormone (LH)	**Hypothalamus** FSH, LH releasing hormone **Female** Estrogen, Progesterone **Male** Testosterone; Pulsaltile	(+) production of estrogen, progesterone, and testosterone	*Conflicting*	*No effect*	*Conflicting;* Trained Females may have lower resting values dependent on menstrual stage; Men's values remain unchanged
	Prolactin (PRL)	**Hypothalamus** PRL releasing hormone; PRL inhibiting hormone	(+) milk secretion from mammary glands in females; (−) testosterone; lipolytic	*Increased;* higher intensity	*Unknown*	*May lower resting values*
	Endorphins	Stress	(−) pain; "exercise high"	*Increased;* duration Dependent		*Lower levels needed; Increase ex. tolerance*

- Effects of resistance training are difficult to study because of pulsatile release requiring frequent sampling.
- **Chronic exercise:** Conflicting data require further investigation; adaptation and mechanisms remain unknown.
- Godfrey et al (2003) report decreased resting GH values and blunted exercise-induced GH release with chronic endurance training.
- Wideman et al (2002) report aerobically trained females training at intensities greater than the lactate threshold experience a twofold increase in 24-h GH release.
  - GH release was not significant in those who trained at or below the lactate threshold (Weltman et al, 1992)
- Short-term GH release appears to be blunted with exercise training
  - GH was reduced within 3 weeks of exercise training, decreasing further at 6 week measurement (Weltman et al, 1997).
  - Decline may be due to increased tissue sensitivity and/or enhanced clearance.
- As a result of difficulty in measurement, the impact of chronic resistance training remains relatively unknown.

B. Thyroid Stimulating Hormone
- **Endurance exercise/resistance exercise:** Six rowers underwent 3 weeks of high intensity resistance training followed by 3 weeks of endurance training.
  1. Each 3 weeks was separated by a week of rest.
  2. Investigators found a significant decline in *thyroid stimulating hormone* (TSH) which continued to decrease during the rest period.
  3. At the start of the endurance training, TSH increased.
  4. Values returned to baseline during the subsequent rest period (Simsch et al, 2002).
- Following 6 weeks of endurance training, TSH remained unchanged in recreational athletes (Lehmann et al, 1993).

C. Adrenocorticotropic Hormone
- **Endurance exercise:** Repetitive bouts (2) of aerobic exercise at 75% Vo_{2max} demonstrate a significant increase in *adrenocorticotropic hormone* (ACTH) during and after the second bout; each bout was followed by 3-h rest (Ronsen et al, 2001).
- Aerobic exercise to exhaustion revealed a significant acute increase in ACTH when compared to resting values (de Diego et al, 2001).
- Postmenopausal women undergoing exhaustive bicycle exercise experienced a pronounced ACTH increase immediately following the exercise session (Pompe van der et al, 2001).
- **Resistance exercise:** High intensity (load 100%) showed a significantly greater increase in ACTH when compared to moderate intensity (70% load) (Raastad et al, 2000).

- Heavy resistance training significantly increased ACTH in young and older men.
  - The levels in younger men remained elevated throughout 30 min of recovery (Kraemer et al, 1998).
- **Exercise training:** Prolonged endurance training in recreational athletes (6 weeks) revealed a significant increase in ACTH after training period (Lehmann et al, 1993).
- Endurance trained individuals had comparable resting ACTH values as their sedentary counterparts (Duclos et al, 2001).

D. Luteinizing Hormone/Follicle-Stimulating Hormone
- **Endurance exercise:** Four successive days of low intensity, long duration (8 h) walking revealed the following:
  1. Decreased *luteinizing hormone* (LH) during the 1st and 2nd days by 31%.
  2. *Follicle-stimulating hormone* (FSH) suppression occurred each day after day 2 (19%) when compared to resting values.
  3. LH returned to baseline following the 4-day exercise protocol, whereas FSH maintained its exercise value (Vaananen et al, 2002).
- **Resistance exercise:** LH and FSH showed no response to high or moderate intensity strength exercise (Raastad et al, 2000).
- **Chronic exercise:** Six weeks of endurance training in male recreational athletes had no influence on baseline or exercise serum LH or FSH.
  - After training period, FSH synthesis–secretion capacity was increased whereas LH synthesis–secretion capacity was decreased (Lehmann et al, 1993).
- Vasankari et al (1993) showed increased FSH in endurance trained male athletes with years of physical training.
- Baseline and post race LH and FSH were not significantly different when comparing two elite cycling teams, one of which had more racing days than the other (Fernandez-Garcia et al, 2002).

E. Prolactin
- **Endurance exercise:** Plasma *prolactin* (PRL) was significantly increased following an acute graded, maximal treadmill test (Dohi et al, 2003).
- Cyclists involved in a 3-week stage competition showed a significant increase in PRL between week 1 and week 2 (Fernandez-Garcia et al, 2002).
- Postmenopausal women performing exhaustive aerobic exercise experienced a 114% increase (peak) in PRL 15 min postexercise (Pompe van der et al, 2001).
- **Resistance exercise:** Relatively unknown

TABLE 32-2 Posterior Pituitary Hormones

GLAND	HORMONE	CONTROL	ACTION	ENDURANCE	RESISTANCE	CHRONIC
Posterior pituitary	Oxytocin	Hypothalamic neurons	Stimulate uterine muscles and breasts	*Conflicting;* no change, controls for ex-induced tachycardia; may effect other hormone secretions	*Unknown*	*Unknown*
	Vasopress in (ADH)	Hypothalamic neurons	Controls water excretion; blood volume; blood osmolality; attenuates the inhibitory effect of glucoorticoidson CRH release of ACTH	*Increased effect;* increased water reabsorption by kidney as a result of result of sweating; conserves fluids; BP and HR control; intensity related; circadian influence	*Unknown*	*Possibly blunted during exercise itself;* training results in increased plasma volume

- **Chronic exercise:** Repeated exercise-induced release of PRL may result in menstrual cycle alterations (McCardle, Katch, and Katch, 1991).

POSTERIOR PITUITARY HORMONES AND EXERCISE

A. Oxytocin
- **Endurance exercise/chronic exercise:** Graded exercise to exhaustion in professional cyclists did not result in any response to plasma oxytocin levels (Chicharro et al, 2001).
- Pathways of oxytocin from the hypothalamus to the brain stem restrain the tachycardic response in trained individuals without compromising cardiac output or circulatory demand during exercise (Michelini, 2001).
- Six weeks of high intensity exercise decreased oxytocin levels in rats; this may be a result of overtraining (Peijie et al, 2003).

B. Vasopressin
- **Endurance exercise/chronic exercise:** Following a 1-h continuous cycling session at both 5 a.m. and 5 p.m., vasopressin levels were significantly higher with both exercise sessions.
  1. Levels were significantly greater with the a.m. session versus the p.m. session.
  2. This difference between sessions persisted through 1-h recovery period (Zhao et al, 2003; abstract).
- Ninety minutes of exercise at 60% peak VO_2 in untrained individuals significantly increased plasma vasopressin.
  - When plasma volume was expanded as with endurance training, this increase in vasopressin was blunted during exercise (Roy et al, 2001).
- Two female ultradistance triathletes who experienced hyponatremia and increases in plasma volume failed to show any change in vasopressin levels from pre- to postevent (Speedy et al, 2000).
- Takmata and coworkers (2000) found that exercise increases vasopressin.

- Correlated with increased osmolality.
- Dynamic running in rats increased vasopressin levels in the ventral and dorsal portions of the brain stem.
  - Contributes to *heart rate's* (HR's) response to increased circulatory demand with exercise (Michelini and Morris, 1999).
- Following two treadmill tests (100% VO_{2max} and 90% VO_{2max}), plasma vasopressin significantly increased in an intensity-dependent manner.
  - Higher values were found in women versus men (Deuster et al, 1998).

ADRENAL CORTEX HORMONES AND EXERCISE

A. Cortisol
- **Endurance exercise:** Cortisol levels increase acutely in middle-aged, postmenopausal women following exhaustive exercise.
  - Those who reported "low vigour" had lower cortisol responses than those who did not (Pompe van der et al, 2001).
- High intensity exercise of short duration (<15 min) results in peak cortisol levels immediately after activity (Consitt et al, 2002).
- Acute cortisol increases with endurance activity returns to baseline levels within hours of activity cessation.
- Viro et al (2001) revealed variable results in regard to cortisol levels following a 2-h exercise session.
  - High responders increased their performance in a 1 min anaerobic test.
  - Low responders decreased their performance in the anaerobic test.
- **Resistance exercise:** Following 8 weeks of heavy resistance training (3 sets of 6–12 RM with 2-min rest; 2 days/week), cortisol significantly increases above preexercise values (Kraemer et al, 1997).
  1. Men experienced increased values at weeks 1, 6, and 8.
  2. Women experienced increased values at weeks 6 and 8.

TABLE 32-3   Adrenal Cortex Hormones

GLAND	HORMONE	CONTROL	ACTION	ENDURANCE	RESISTANCE	CHRONIC
Adrenal cortex	Cortisol *Glucocorticoid*	Stress, diurnal rhythm, hypothalamic CRH, ACTH	Glucose sparing; promotes use of fatty acids and protein; insulin antagonist; anti-inflammatory effects	*Increased;* increased intensity and/or increased duration; glucose sparing	*Increased acutely*	*Decreased with resistance training;* decreases protein degradation leading to fiber hypertrophy; volume related
	Aldosterone *Mineralcorticoid*	Angiotensin, renin, potassium levels; ACTH (stress at the hypothalamus)	Balance Na$^+$ and K$^+$ levels; kidney fluid maintenance	*Increase;* intensity and duration dependent; because of constriction of blood flow to kidney	*Unknown*	*Unknown*

3. There was no significant difference between men and women.
4. Cortisol levels were significantly reduced at rest (8 weeks).
- Cortisol levels acutely increase with heavy resistance protocols in men and women (Hakkinen and Pakarinen, 1995; Kraemer et al, 1990; 1998).
- Cortisol levels increase in women immediately after resistance training.
  - Higher levels were seen with a multiple set protocol when compared to a single set protocol (Consitt et al, 2002).
- **Chronic exercise:** Increased levels of cortisol have been reported in overtraining (Consitt et al, 2002).
- Elite endurance female athletes had significantly greater cortisol levels than their sedentary counterparts.
- Chronic resistance exercise results in decreased resting levels of cortisol (anabolic effect).
  1. Kraemer et al (1998) found decreased values after 8 weeks of heavy resistance training.
  2. Marx et al (1998) showed a decline in resting cortisol in female athletes who completed a high-volume protocol versus low-volume protocol.

B. Aldosterone
- **Endurance exercise:** Aldosterone increases to help decrease the sweat loss of sodium chloride following acclimatization to a hot environment (Brooks, Fahey, and White, 1995).

- Prolonged exercise (90 min at 60% VO$_{2max}$) significantly increased aldosterone levels in untrained men.

ADRENAL MEDULLA HORMONES AND EXERCISE

Epinephrine/Norepinephrine (Catecholamines)
- **Endurance exercise:** Ninety minutes at 60% VO$_{2max}$ significantly increased catecholamine levels in previously untrained men (Roy et al, 2001).
- Intensity less than 50% VO$_{2max}$ had no effect on catecholamine levels; intensity above 50% VO$_{2max}$ increased catecholamine release.
- Norepinephrine increased more than epinephrine (Brooks, Fahey, and White, 1995).
- Untrained men exercising for 60 min at 50% VO$_{2max}$ increased catecholamine levels during the exercise session (Marion-Latard et al, 2003).
- A significant increase in epinephrine/norepinephrine resulted with 2 bouts of exercise (75 min, 75% VO$_{2max}$)
  1. Bouts were followed by a 3-h rest period or 6 h of rest.
  2. Increased levels were more profound than after 2 bouts of exercise with 6 h of rest.
  3. The 2nd bout exhibited greater increase in catecholamine levels (Ronsen et al, 2002).
- Catecholamine levels increased two- to fourfold with moderate exercise (<80% VO$_{2max}$)
  1. Intense exercise (>80% VO$_2$) resulted in a fourteen- to eighteenfold increase of epinephrine/norepinephrine.

TABLE 32-4   Adrenal Medulla Hormones

GLAND	HORMONE	CONTROL	ACTION	ENDURANCE	RESISTANCE	CHRONIC
Adrenal medulla	Epinephrine Norepinephrine nerves	Hypothalamic sympathetic	Augment SNS; glycogen catabolism; FA release; increases cardiac output; flight or fight response	*Increases;* intensity and duration dependent; blood flow distribution, cardiac contractility, glycogenolysis and lipolysis		*Intensity dependent;* response decreased during submaximal exercise; with maximal exercise response > or = to untrained

2. Catecholamines are the prime regulator of glucose production (Kriesman et al, 2001; 2002).
- **Resistance exercise:** On completion of 5 sets of 10 knee extensions at 40% RM load followed by 2 sets to exhaustion:
  1. Norepinephrine increased in women, men, and in pubescent boys postsubmax exercise and at max exercise.
  2. Epinephrine increased significantly post submax exercise in woman, and significantly in all groups after maximal exercise.
  3. Woman and boys had twice the values when compared to preexercise levels (Pullinen et al, 2002).
- **Chronic exercise:** Training dampened catecholamine response in mild to moderate exercise (lower sympathetic stimulation).
  1. During hard to maximal exercise trained individuals experienced increased catecholamines when compared to untrained individuals.
  2. Exercise at 60% VO_{2max} caused only slight increases; whereas, exercise at 100% VO_{2max} resulted in exaggerated epinephrine/norepinephrine levels.
  3. Hundred and ten percent VO_{2max} sprint caused further increases (Kjaer et al, 1986).
- Training 6 days a week (7 weeks) progressively decreased catecholamines in men over the training period.
  1. The most rapid decrease was found early in the training (Winder et al, 1968).
  2. When comparing endurance trained with untrained, the trained subjects have higher epinephrine secretion capacity at identical intensities: "sports adrenal medulla" (Kjaer, M., 1998).

THYROID HORMONE AND EXERCISE

- **Endurance exercise:** Twenty weeks of endurance training resulted decreased free T3 levels versus baseline by the 5th week (6.2%) and 10th week (7.9%).
  1. Values returned toward baseline levels as they approached 20th week.
  2. TSH levels followed the same pattern.
  3. Decreased TSH may indicate reduced hypothalamic drive (Baylor and Hackney, 2002).

- Six months of intensive training (rowing), resulted in a decrease in thyroid volume which was correlated with a decrease in LBM (Wesche et al, 2001).
- **Resistance exercise:** In eight trained weight lifters performing three sets of six exercises to exhaustion:
  1. T3 levels were unchanged immediately after exercise and during nocturnal measurements.
  2. T4 levels were increased for the 1st 20-min period postexercise but lowered at the nocturnal measurement when compared to the control (no exercise) period may suggest nocturnal muscle anabolism (McMurray et al, 1995).
- Twelve hours after an anaerobic exercise session there was a decrease in T4:T3; free T4, free T3 did not change with aerobic, anaerobic immediate post measurements (Umschied, 1998).
- **Chronic exercise:** Highly trained rowers performed 3 weeks of high intensity resistance training followed by 3 weeks of endurance training with 1 week of recovery in between each.
  - Resistance training resulted in a significant decrease in TSH and free T3 (free T4 unchanged).
  - Endurance training resulted in a significant increase in TSH and patterns of increasing values in free T3 and T4 (nonsignificant).
  - Changes were independent of body fat suggesting that high intensity exercise may decrease the hypothalamic-thyroid-axis (Simsch et al, 2001).
- Physically active men had significantly higher T3 levels than sedentary men; whereas, TSH values were significantly lower than their sedentary counterparts (Ravaglia et al, 2001).

PANCREATIC HORMONES AND EXERCISE

A. Insulin
- **Endurance exercise:** Blood glucose levels will likely decrease as activity continues.
  - Insulin is, in part, suppressed by epinephrine thus increasing hepatic glucose release.
- Intense exercise (80% VO_{2max}) resulted in an approximate eightfold increase in glucose production and only a fourfold increase in uptake.
  - Insulin did not change significantly and glucagon increased less than twofold (Kreisman et al, 2003).

TABLE 32-5 Thyroid Hormones

GLAND	HORMONE	CONTROL	ACTION	ENDURANCE	RESISTANCE	CHRONIC
Thyroid	Thyroxine (T4) Triiodothyronine (T3)	Hypothalamus; TRH; TSH	Stimulate metabolic rate; calorigenic, fuel metabolism, sympathomimetic	*Increased;* intensity dependent	*Conflicting*	*Decrease total T3; increased free T3 at rest; increased turnover without hyperthyroidism*

TABLE 32-6 Pancreatic Hormones

GLAND	HORMONE	CONTROL	ACTION	ENDURANCE	RESISTANCE	CHRONIC
Pancreas	Insulin	Glucose levels	(+) glucose, fatty acid, and amino acid transport into cell; regulate glucose metabolism with the exception of brain; anabolic hormone	*Decreased;* dependent on increasing intensity and duration; glucose levels also drop with similar exercise because of catecholamine release; induces more energy from FFA and hepatic glucose	*Improves insulin sensitivity;* moderate to intense (50–100% 1RM)	*Increased insulin sensitivity;* normal drop in insulin during an acute bout of ex. is significantly less; maintained close to resting values
	Glucagon	Glucose levels	(+) glycogenolysis and gluconeogenesis; insulin antagonist	*Increased with increasing exercise*		*Blunted response similar to resting values*

- With intense exercise (>80% VO_{2max}) it appears that catecholamines, *not insulin*, become the major regulators of glucose homeostasis during and immediately after a single bout.
  - Insulin regains control during recovery and insulin levels rise (Marliss et al 2002).
- During moderate exercise, glucagon and insulin appear to be the main regulators of glucose production.
  - Prolonged (>2 h) increases the role of catecholamines in glucose production (Richter et al 1995).
  - Increased glucagon and decreased insulin result in hepatic glycogenolysis and gluconeogenesis.
- High levels of catecholamines (high intense exercise) can prevent glucose stimulation of insulin release (Marliss et al, 2000).
- Insulin levels will increase during recovery because of immediate decrease in catecholamines aiding in the replacement of muscle glycogen.
- **Resistance exercise:** Progressive resistance training has been shown to improve insulin sensitivity and glucose tolerance (Willey and Singh, 2003).
- An acute single resistance bout decreased total insulin response to an oral glucose tolerance test.
- In nine subjects with type 2 diabetes, insulin sensitivity improved by 48% after 4–6 weeks of moderate intensity resistance training.
- Resistance trained rats performed three sets of 10 repetitions at 75% 1-RM, 3 days/week for 1–12 weeks:
  1. Increased rates of glucose transport were found in exercise specific muscles.
  2. Resistance exercise may improve insulin's effect on glucose uptake and transport in muscles recruited for exercise (Yaspelkis et al, 2002).
- **Chronic exercise:** In trained individuals, insulin did not fall as much as their untrained counterparts.
  - Blunted decrease may be a result of increased sensitivity to insulin or normoglycemia in trained individuals, increased dependence on *free fatty acids* (FFA) (Gyntelberg et al, 1977).

- An increased number of insulin receptors are found in trained individuals when compared to untrained counterparts; increased insulin sensitivity continues up to 24 h following exercise (Landry and Allen, 1992).

B. Glucagon
- **Endurance exercise:** Unchanged or increased glucagon levels and decreased insulin increased glucose production with moderate exercise (Wasserman et al, 1989).
- Glucagon: Insulin is the main regulator in glucose production with moderate exercise.
- As exercise increases in duration, glucagon secretion increases hepatic glucose production.
- **Resistance exercise:** College men participated in a 10-week progressive resistance training program:
  - No significant change in glucagon was found in a 3-h oral glucose tolerance test following the intervention.
- **Chronic exercise:** Blunted response may result with training.

PARATHYROID HORMONE AND EXERCISE

A. Parathyroid
- **Endurance exercise:** When examining the effect of a recovery period between (40 min) two periods of exercise (2×21 min at 70–85% VO_{2max}) versus two successive exercise sessions with no recovery:
  1. *Parathyroid hormone* (PTH) levels increased significantly with both protocols.
  2. PTH levels remained high 24 h into recovery with "no recovery" protocol.
  3. "No recovery" caused higher PTH levels when compared to "recovery."
  4. Ca^{2+} levels returned to resting after recovery (Bouassida et al, 2003).
- Male marathon runners were examined during training, during a 3-week training hiatus, and within 2 weeks of retraining:

TABLE 32-7 Parathyroid Hormone

GLAND	HORMONE	CONTROL	ACTION	ENDURANCE	RESISTANCE	CHRONIC
Parathyroid	Parathormone	Plasma Ca^{2+}	*Calcium homeostasis; stimulates bone growth;* increase plasma Ca^{2+}; *Phosphate regulation;* lowers Phosphate levels; bone resorption by stimulating osteoclasts and inhibiting osteoblasts; activation of Vit-D	*Increased;* compensate for decrease in plasma Ca^{2+}	*Increased*	*Increased over time*

1. Oxygen capacity decreased with haitus and increased with retraining.
2. Ca^{2+} levels decreased with retraining as PTH levels increased throughout the break and retraining periods (Klausen et al, 1993).
- One acute bout of prolonged endurance exercise to exhaustion in well trained individuals increased PTH levels thus inhibiting bone formation and stimulating bone resorption (Brahm and Ljunghall, 1996).
- Five hours of endurance exercise at 50% maximum capacity resulted in increased PTH levels after the first hour and throughout the remainder of the exercise (5–7% preexercise levels).
  - Ca^{2+} in plasma tended to be low during exercise (Ljunghall et al, 1986).
- **Resistance exercise:** Strength training consisting of 85% of 3-RM leg press significantly increased PTH levels (Rong et al, 1997).
- **Chronic exercise:** Well-trained individuals performed one single bout of long-term exhaustive exercise had increased PTH levels thus stimulating bone resorption and Ca^{2+} efflux to plasma (Brahm and Ljunghall, 1996).
  - Increased PTH levels following a maximal exercise test were significantly higher in endurance trained elderly men versus untrained elderly men (Zerath et al, 1997).

OVARIAN HORMONES AND EXERCISE
- **Endurance exercise:** Progesterone and estradiol levels taken during graded exercise showed only small increases in both the follicular and luteal phase.

1. Greatest increase with increasing intensities
2. LH and FSH did not change; the effects on progesterone/estradiol may only be because of increases in plasma volume (Jurowski, 1978).
- At similar intensities, increases in estradiol are greater during the luteal phase when compared to follicular phase (Consitt et al, 2002).
- When comparing three varying intensities: light (20 min at 30–45%), heavy (20 min at 60–66%), and exhaustive (20 min at 85–95%) exercise.
  1. The luteal phase showed a significant increase in estradiol with heavy and exhaustive exercise.
  2. The follicular phase showed a significant increase with exhaustive exercise (Consitt et al, 2002).
- A significant decrease in metabolic clearance rate of estradiol decreased after a short bout (10 min) of exercise (Keizer et al, 70).
- Following 2 h of exercise, an increase in metabolic clearance rate resulted in decreased estradiol levels.
- **Resistance exercise:** Untrained women had increased estradiol levels with three sets of four exercises at 10 RM, in both luteal and follicular phase; increased levels were similar to those found with endurance exercise (Consitt et al, 2002).
- **Chronic exercise:** Several studies report decreased levels of estradiol following only 8 weeks of intense endurance training (Consitt et al, 2002).

A. Testosterone
- **Endurance exercise:** Various studies have shown a short-term increase (returning to resting values within hours of recovery) in testosterone after short bouts of endurance exercise in women (Consitt et al, 2002).

TABLE 32-8 Ovarian Hormones

GLAND	HORMONE	CONTROL	ACTION	ENDURANCE	RESISTANCE	CHRONIC
Ovary	Estradiol/Progesterone	FSH, LH	Menstrual cycle; female sex characteristics; inhibition of glucose uptake; fat deposition, maintain bone density	*Increase/decrease with acute exercise;* may be influenced by menstrual phase and intensity; metabolic clearance rate may influence change	*Understudied*	*Decreased;* intensity and training volume dependent

TABLE 32-9 Hormones of the Testes

GLAND	HORMONE	CONTROL	ACTION	ENDURANCE	RESISTANCE	CHRONIC
Testes	Testosterone	LH, FSH	Anabolic; protein synthesis; androgenic	*Increased;* intensity and duration related; may be influence by decrease in metabolic clearance rate (decreased hepatic blood flow)	*Increased; conflicting findings in women*	*Resting levels may be lower in endurance trained*

- Various studies have shown that short-term maximal exercise results in increased testosterone levels in men (Hackney AC, 2001).
- Consitt et al (2001) showed increased levels of testosterone in woman who performed 40 min of cycling at 75% *maximum heart rate* (MHR) when compared to resting controls:
  - Testosterone did not change with three sets of eight exercises at 10 RM.
- Exercise that consists of moderate to hard exercise to exhaustion (>2 h) resulted in lowered testosterone levels in men (Hackney AC, 2001).
- **Resistance exercise:** Most research investigating the relationship between testosterone and short-term resistance training in women have found no significant changes even with measurable muscle gains (Consitt et al, 2002).
- Effects of acute resistance exercise and 8 weeks of resistance training were measured at pre-ex, immediate postexercise:
  - During the 1st week, 6 weeks, and 8 weeks, testosterone was significantly higher in men at all measurement points (Kraemer et al, 1998).
- **Chronic exercise:** Decreased testosterone levels were found in women after 3 months of endurance training.
  - This finding was only apparent in the luteal phase (Keizer et al 110).
- Many studies have shown that testosterone levels of endurance-trained men were 60–85% the levels (lower) of untrained counterparts (Hackney and Dolny, 1988; Hackney and Fahrner, 1997; Gulledge et al, 1996).
- Baseline testosterone levels and testosterone production rates were significantly lower in endurance trained men when compared to sedentary counterparts.
  - Blunted values may help the endurance athlete avoid excessive muscle mass which could overwhelm oxygen delivery during prolonged exercise (Hackney et al, 2002).

Type 1 Diabetes and Exercise

- Physiologic adaptations result within the exercising muscle, energy needs, and regulatory hormones.
- Increased dependence on hepatic glycogenolysis, FFAs, blood-borne glucose.

- Catecholamines become primary regulators of glucose as insulin levels decrease with exercise.
- Insulin may be needed to regulate ketone production; without insulin, exercise-induced increases in glucagon/catecholamines will result in increased ketone production.
- **Normoglycemic athletes:** During exercise, use of oxygen, muscle and liver glycogen, triglycerides, and FFAs increase in exercising muscles. This increased mobilization of substrates results from enhanced epinephrine, glucagon, cortisol, and growth hormone action. In addition, the counterregulatory function of insulin allows for stable blood glucose regulation (Drazin and Patel, 1998).
- Plasma insulin decrease with exercise.
- Glucagon/catecholamines promote increased hepatic glucose production to match the level of glucose usage.
- Increased insulin sensitivity postexercise, muscle, and hepatic glycogen restoration.
- **Athletes with type 1 diabetes:** Plasma insulin levels may not decrease during exercise.
- Insulin-stimulated glucose uptake may be blunted.
- Dependent on injection site, insulin could increase with exercise.
- Relies more on gluconeogenesis than hepatic glycogenolysis to maintain blood glucose levels.
- Glucose production > glucose clearance; less glucose oxidation
- Increased lipolysis can result in ketogenesis.
- Increased risk of hypoglycemia hours after exercise, increased insulin sensitivity, decreased levels of glycogen stores, and injection site.
- Hyperglycemia can result from poor control; insulin deficiency can lead to decreased glucose uptake, increased lipolysis, and therefore ketogenesis; and insulin coma.
- **Benefits of regular exercise**
  1. Cardiorespiratory and muscular fitness
  2. Improved insulin sensitivity
  3. Improved vascular endothelial function
  4. Improved lipid profiles, blood pressure (BP), and body fat percentage
  5. Enhanced quality of life: social, self-confidence, and the like.

TABLE 32-10   Clinical Implications

GLAND/HORMONE	HYPERSECRETION	HYPOSECRETION
Anterior Pituitary Hormones 1) GH 2) TSH 3) ACTH 4) FSH/LH 5) PRL 6) Endorphins	1) Insulin resistance; peripheral neuropathy 2) Increased BMR; weight loss; arrhythmia 3) Hyperglycemia; muscle wasting; bone protein loss; water and salt retention; hypertension 4) Unknown 5) Menses cessation in females; impotence in males 6) Unknown	1) Increased insulin sensitivity; decreased muscle strength, decreased bone density 2) Decreased BMR; weight gain; dry skin; fatigue 3) Rare 4) Decline in sexual maturation; menstrual disorder 5) Decreased milk production in women 6) Endorphins
Posterior Pituitary Hormones 1) Oxytocin 2) Vasopressin	1) Unknown 2) Hyponatremia; low plasma osmolality; poor fluid control	1) Unknown 2) Increased urine production; poor fluid control
Adrenal Cortex Hormones 1) Cortisol 2) Aldosterone	1) Hypertension; hypokalemia; protein depletion; muscle weakness; osteoporosis; decreased Ca absorption and increased excretion of Ca; suppressed immune function; impaired CHO metabolism 2) Sodium and water retention; hypokalemia; hypertension	1) Abnormal CHO, fat, and protein metabolism; muscle weakness; loss of appetite; weight loss; decreased sodium; increased potassium; hypotension; dehydration 2) Loss of sodium; hyperkalemia; hypotension; dehydration
Adrenal Medulla Hormones 1) Epinephrine/Norepinephrine	1) Hypertension; increased BMR	1) Rare
Thyroid Hormones 1) T4/T3	1) Elevated BMR; heat intolerance; excessive perspiration; weight loss; muscle weakness; tachycardia; arrhythmias; hypertension; increased metabolism of CHO, fat, protein; decreased ovarian function	1) Reduced BMR, cold intolerance; dry skin; fatigue; slow reflexes, muscle cramping; weight gain; CNS affects (poor memory, slow mentation); bradycardia; decreased contractility of heart; hypotension; increased cholesterol levels; decreased ovarian function
Pancreatic Hormones 1) Insulin 2) Glucagon	1) Hypoglycemia; anxiety, overall weakness 2) Hyperglycemia	1) Diabetes mellitus; hyperglycemia; altered CHO, fat, protein metabolism; increased ketogenesis; glucosuria; hypotension, dehydration; weight loss; fatigue 2) Hypoglycemia; decreased plasma protein levels
Parathyroid Hormones 1) PTH	1) Loss of Ca from bone; hypercalcemia; weakening of bone; muscle weakness; neurologic symptoms; kidney stones	1) Hypocalcemia; uncontrolled muscle spasm
Ovarian Hormones 1) Estrogen/Progesterone	1) Progesterone may enhance masculinization	1) Menstrual disorders; decreased bone growth; decreased BMR;
Testes 1) Testosterone	1) Masculization; liver disorders; lipid alterations; muscle hypertrophy	1) Feminization; muscle atrophy

• **Preparticipation examination**
1. Stable control
   (1) Glycosylated hemoglobin
   (2) Self-monitoring around activity
   (3) Urine ketone measurement if warranted
   (4) Insulin regimen, peak action time, and injection sites
   (5) Meal planning

2. Assess level of self-care
   (1) Recognition of hypo/hyperglycemia
   (2) Treatment strategies for hypo/hyperglycemia, ketoacidosis, and sick day regimen
   (3) Changes in insulin types, dosage, and injection site
   (4) Medical identification
   (5) Monitoring regimen

(6) Skin care

(7) Meal planning and CHO counting

3. Complications present

   (1) BP, neurology, mobility, opthalmology, blood lipids, nephropathy, microalbuminuria, PVD, proliferative retinopathy, autonomic neuropathy, thermoregulation

   (2) Graded exercise test recommended if >35 yoa or >25 yoa with diagnosed type-1 diabetes for >15-year duration.

4. Consider sports participation

   (1) Heavy-weight training should be avoided to avoid high ocular pressures.

   (2) Practice and game times, duration and intensity levels

   (3) Travel time

   (4) Meal planning

   (5) Do coaches, athletic trainers, and others have adequate knowledge of needs?

   (6) Is support-staff prepared for emergency situation?

   (7) Consider *high-risk* sports; mountain climbing, scuba diving and the like.

   (8) Consider complications, i.e., athletes with peripheral neuropathy should avoid weight bearing exercise.

   (9) Consider environment (hot or cold)–may experience problems with thermoregulation.

PARTICIPATION GUIDELINES

Before Exercise

- Estimate intensity, duration, and kilocalories of event.
- Eat 1–3 h prior to event.
- Inject insulin more than 1 h before exercise.
- Inject away from an exercising muscle.
- Decrease insulin dosage that may peak within activity.
- If blood glucose <100 mg/dL, ingest CHO snack.
- If blood glucose >250 mg/dL, postpone exercise, ketone measurement, and add insulin.
- Delay exercise until stable control is established.

During Exercise

- Supplement caloric expenditure with CHO supplementation—30 g per 30 min of exercise.

   1. <130 mg/dL, two CHO exchanges (120 kcal) per 35 min with exercise <60% VO_{2max}, three exchanges (180 kcal) with >70% VO_{2max} (heavy ex)

   2. 130–180 mg/dL, 1 CHO (60 kcal) per 30 min of light, and two CHO exchanges with heavy exercise

   3. 180–240 mg/dL, no food before exercise; if prolonged, intense exercise retake glucose levels during exercise

   4. >250, postpone exercise; ketone measurements; may need increased insulin

- Replace fluids.
- Monitor glucose levels with prolonged exercise.

Post-exercise

- Monitor blood glucose, delayed hypoglycemia is common.
- Increase caloric intake for 12–24 h after activity, CHO ingestion immediately after.
- Reduce insulin if necessary.
- Proper foot care.
- Proper rehydration.

REFERENCES

American Diabetes Association: Physical activity and diabetes mellitus. *Diabetes Care* 26 (suppl 1): S73–S77, 2003.

Baylor L, Hackney A: Resting thyroid and leptin hormone changes in women following intense, prolonged exercise training. *Eur J Appl Physiol* 88(4): 480–484, 2003.

Borer, KT, Nicoski DR, Owens V: Alteration of pulsatile growth hormone secretion by growth-inducing exercise: involvement of endogenous opiates and somatostatin. *Endocrinology* 118(2): 844–850, 1986.

Bouassida A, Zalleg D, Ajina M, Gharbi N, Duclos M, Richalet JP, Tabka Z: Parathyroid hormone concentrations during and after two periods of high intensity exercise with and without an intervening recovery period. *Eur J Appl Physiol* 88: 339–344, 2003.

Brahm H, Piehl-Aulin K, Ljunghall S: Bone Metabolism During Exercise and Recovery: The influence of plasma volume and physical fitness. *Calcif Tissue Int.* 61(3): 192–198, 1997.

Brooks GA, Fahey TD, White TP: *Exercise Physiology: Human Bioenergetics and its Applications*; Mayfield: Toronto, 1996.

Chicharro JL, Hoyos H, Bandres G, Gomez G, Perez M, Lucia A: Plasma oxytocin during intense exercise in professional cyclists. *Hormone Research* 55(3): 155–159, 2001.

Consitt LA, Copeland JL, Tremblay MS: Endogenous anabolic hormone responses to endurance versus resistance exercise in women. *Sports Med* 32(1): 1–22, 2002.

Consitt, LA, Copeland JL, Tremblay MS: Hormone responses to resistance vs. endurance exercise in premenopausal females. *Can J Appl Physiol* 26(6): 574–587, 2001.

Deuster PA, Petrides JS, Singh A, Lucci EB, Chrousos GP, Gold PW: High intensity exercise promotes escape of adrenocorticotropin and cortisol from suppression by dexamethasone: sexually dimorphic responses. *J Clin Endo Metab* 83(9): 3332–3338, 1998.

Dohi, K, Kraemer WJ, Mastro AM: Exercise increases prolactin-receptor expression on human lymphocytes. *J Appl Physio* 94(2): 518–24, 2003.

Duclos M, Corcuff J, Pehourcq F, Tabarin A: Decreased pituitary sensitivity to glucocorticoids in endurance-trained men. *Eur J Endocr* 144(4): 363–368, 2001.

Felsing NE, Brasel JA, Cooper DM: Effect of low and high intensity exercise on cirulating growth hormone in men. *J Clin Endocrinol Metab* 75(1): 157–162, 1992.

Fernandez-Garcia B, Lucia A, Hoyos J, Chicharro JL, Rodriguez-Alonso M, Bandres F, Terrados N: The response of sexual and stress hormones of male pro-cyclists during continuous intense competition. *Int J Sports Med* 23(8) 555–560, 2002.

Godfrey R, Madgwick Z, Whyte G: The exercise-induced growth hormone response in athletes. *Sports Med* 33(8): 599–613, 2003.

Gotshalk L, Loebel C, Nindl B, Putukian N, Sebatianelli W, Newton R, Hakkinen K, Kraemer W: Hormonal responses of multiset versus single-set heavy resistance exercise protocols. *Can J Appl Physiol* 22(3): 244–255, 1997.

Gulledge TP and Hackney, AC: Reproducibility of low testosterone concentrations in endurance trained men. *Eur J Appl Physiol* 73:582–583, 1996.

Hackney A.C. Endurance exercise training and reproductive endocrine dysfunction in men: alterations in the hypothalamic-pituitary-testicular axis. *Curr Pharm Des* 7:261–273, 2001.

Hackney AC, Dolny DG, Ness RJ: *Biology of Sport* 4:200, 1988.

Hackney AC, Fahrner CL: Reproductive hormonal responses to maximal exercise in endurance-trained men with low resting testosterone levels. *Exp Clin Endocrinol Diabetes* 105(5): 291–295, 1997.

Hackney AC, Sinning WE, Bruot BC: Reproductive hormonal profiles of endurance trained and untrained men. *Med Sci Exerc Sport* 20: 60–65, 1998.

Hough D: Diabetes mellitus in sports. *Sports Medicine* 78(2): 423–436, 1994.

Kanaley J, Hartman M: Cortisol and growth hormone responses to exercise. *Endocrinologist* 12(5): 421–432, 2002.

Kjaer M: Adrenal medulla and exercise training. *Eur J Appl Physiol* 77:195–199, 1998.

Kjaer M, Farrell PA, Christensen NJ, Galbo H: Increased epinephrine response and inaccurate glucoregulation in exercising athletes. *J Appl Physiol* 61:1693–1700, 1986.

Klausen T, Breum L, Sorensen HA, Schifter S, Sonne B: Plasma levels of parathyroid hormone, vitamin D, calcitonin, and calcium in association with endurance exercise. *Calcif Tissue Int* 52(3): 205–208, 1993.

Kraemer W, Hakkinen K, Newton R, et al: Acute hormonal responses to heavy resistance exercise in younger and older men. *Eur J Appl Phyiol* 77: 206–211, 1998.

Kraemer W, Volek J, Bush J, Putukian M, Sebastianelli W: Hormonal responses to consecutive days of heavy-resistance exercise with or without nutritional supplementation. *J Appl Physiol* 85: 1544–1555, 1998.

Kreaemer WJ, Volek JS, Clark KL, et al: Physiological adaptations to a weight-loss regimen and exercise programs in women. *J Appl Physiol* 83(1): 270–279, 1997.

Kreisman SH, Halter JB, Vranic M, Marliss EB: Combined infusion of epinephrine and norepinephrine during moderate exercise reproduces the glucoregulatory response to intense exercise. *Diabetes* 52(6): 1347–1354, 2003.

Kreisman, SH, Ah Mew N, Halter JB, Vranic M, Marliss EB: Norepinephrine infusion during moderate intensity exercise increases glucose production and uptake. *J Clin Endocrinol Metab* 86: 2118–2124, 2001.

Landry GL and Allen DB: Diabetes mellitus and exercise. *Clin Sports Med* 11(2): 403–418, 1992.

Lehmann M, Foster C, Keul J: Overtraining in endurance athletes: a brief review. *Med Sci Sports Exerc* 25(7): 854–862, 1993.

Lucia A, Hoyos J, Perez M, Chicharro J: Thyroid hormones may influence the slow component of V_{02} in professional cyclists. *Jap J Physio* 51(2): 239–242, 2001.

Marion-Latard F, Crampes F, Zakaroff-Girard A, et al: Post-exercise increase of lipid oxidation after a moderate exercise bout in untrained healthy obese men. *Horm Metab Res* 35(2): 97–103, 2003.

Marliss EB and Vranic M: Intense exercise has unique effects on both insulin release and Its role in glucoregulation: implications for diabetes. *Diabetes* 51(suppll):S271–S283, 2002.

Marliss EB, Kreisman SH, Manzon A, Halter JB, Vranic M, Nessim SJ: Gender differences in glucoregulatory responses to intense exercise. *J Appl Physiol* 88(2): 457–466, 2000.

McArdle WD, Katch F, Katch C: *Exercise Physiology: Energy, Nutrition, and Human Performance*; Williams and Wilkins; Maryland, 1996.

McMurray R, Eubank T, Hackney A: Nocturnal hormonal responses to resistance exercise. *Eur J Appl Physio and Occup Physio* 72(1/2): 121–126, 1995.

Michelini LC: Oxytocin in the NTS. A new modulator of cardiovascular control during exercise. *Ann NY Acad Sci* 940: 206–220, 2001.

Michelini LC and Morris M: Endogenous vasopressin modulates the cardiovascular response to exercise. *Ann NY Acad Sci* 897: 198–211, 1999.

Morris F, Payne W, Wark JD: Prospective decrease in progesterone concentrations in female lightweight rowers during the competition season compared with the off season: a controlled study examining weight loss and intensive exercise. *Br J Sports Med* 33: 417–422, 1999.

Peijie C, Hongwu L, Fengpeng X, Jie R, Jie Z: Heavy load exercise induced dysfunction of immunity and neuroendocrine responses in rats. *Life Sci* 72(20): 2255–2267, 2003.

Pompe van der G, Bernards N, Kavelaars A, Heijnen C: An exploratory study into the effect of exhausting bicycle exercise on endocrine and immune responses in post-menopausal women: relationships between vigour and plasma cortisol concentrations and lymphocyte proliferation following exercise. *Inter J Sports Med* 22(6): 447–453, 2001.

Pullinen T, Mero A, Huttunen P, Pakarinen A, Komi PV: Hormonal responses to a resistance exercise performed under the influence of delayed onset muscle soreness. *J Strength Cond Res* 16(3): 383–389, 2002.

Raastad T, Bjoro T, Hallen J: Hormonal response to high and moderate intensity exercise. *Eur J Appl Physiol* 82(1–2): 121–128, 2000.

Ravaglia G, Forti P, Maioli F et al: Regular moderate intensity physical activity and blood concentrations of endogenous anabolic hormones and thyroid hormones in aging men. *Mech Ageing Dev* 122(2): 191–203, 2001.

Rong, H, Berg U, Torring O, Sundberg CJ, Granberg B, Bucht E: Effect of acute endurance and strength exercise on circulating calcium-regulating hormones and bone markers in young healthy males. *Scand J Med Sci Sports* 7(3): 152–159, 1997.

Ronsen O, Haug E, Pedersen B, Bahr R: Increased neuroendocrine responses to a repeated bout of endurance exercise. *Med Sci Sports Ex* 33(4): 568–575, 2001.

Ronsen O, Kjeldsen-Kragh J, Haug E, Bahr R, Pedersen BK: Recovery time affects immunoendocrine responses to a second bout of endurance exercise. *Am J Physio* 283(6): 161–120, 2002.

Roy B, Green H, Grant S, Tarnopolsky M: Acute plasma volume expansion in the untrained alters the hormonal response to prolonged moderate-intensity exercise. *Horm Metab Res* 33(4): 238–245, 2001.

Salvesen, H, Johansson AG, Foxdal P, Wide L, Piehl-Aulin K, Ljunghall S: Intact serum parathyroid hormone levels increase during running exercise in well-trained men. *Calcif tissue Int* 54(4): 256–261, 1994.

Schmidt W, Hyner G, Lyle R, Corrigan D, Bottoms G, Melby C: The effects of aerobic and anaerobic exercise conditioning on resting metabolic rate and the thermic effect of a meal. *Inter J Sports Nutr* 4(4): 335–346, 1994.

Simsch C, Lormes W, Petersen K, et al: Training intensity influences leptin and thyroid hormones in highly trained rowers. *Int J Sports Med* 23(6): 422–427, 2002.

Speedy DB, Noakes TD, Rogers IR, et al: A prospective study of exercise-associated hyponatremia in two ultradistance triathletes. *Clin J Sports Med* 10(2): 136–141, 2000.

Takamata A, Nose H, Hirose M, Itoh T, Morimoto T: Effect of acute hypoxia on vasopressin release and intravascular fluid during dynamic exercise. *Am J Physio* 279(1): R 161–168, 2000.

Umsheid JM. *The Influence of Aerobic vs Anaerobic Exercise on Thyroid Hormone Concentrations.* Microform Publications, U of Oregon, 1998.

Vaananen I, Vasankari T, Mantysaari M, Vihko V: Hormonal responses to daily strenuous walking during 4 successive days. *Eur J Appl Phyisol* 88(1–2): 122–127, 2002.

Vanhelder WP, Radomski MW, Goode RC: Growth hormone responses during intermittent weight lifting exercise in men. *Eur J Appl Occup Physiol* 53(1): 31–34, 1984.

Vanhelder, WP, Goode RC, Radomski MW: Effect of anaerobic and aerobic exercise of equal duration and work expenditure on plasma growth hormone levels. *Eur J Appl Occup Physiol* 52(3): 255–257, 1984.

Viru A, Hackney A, Valja E, Karelson K, Janson T, Viru M: Influence of prolonged continuous exercise on hormone responses to subsequent exercise in humans. *Eur J Appl Physiol* 85(6): 578–585, 2001.

Wasserman DH, Spalding JA, Lacy DB, Colburn CA, Goldstein RE, Cherrington AD: Glucagon is a primary controller of hepatic glycogenolysis and gluconeogenesis during muscular Work. *Am J Physiol Endocrinol Metab* 257: E108–E117, 1989.

Weltman A, Weltman J, Womack C, Davis S, Blumer J, Gaesser G, Hartman M: Exercise training decreases the growth hormone response to acute constant-load exercise. *Med Sci Sports Ex* 29(5): 669–676, 1997.

Wesche M, Wiersinga W: Relation between lean body mass and thyroid volume in competition rowers before and during intensive physical training. *Horm Metab Res* 33: 423–427, 2001.

Wideman L, Weltman J, Hartman M, Veldhuis J, Weltman A: Growth hormone release during acute and chronic aerobic and resistance exercise: recent findings. *Sports Medicine* 32(15): 987–1004, 2002.

Willey K, Singh, M: Battling insulin resistance in elderly obese patients with type 2 diabetes; bring on the heavy weights. *Diabetes Care* 26(5): 1580–1588, 2003.

Zerath E, Holy X, Douce P, Guessenne CY, Chatard JC: Effect of endurance training on postexercise parathyroid hormone levels in elderly men. *Med Sci Sports Exerc* 29(9): 1139–1145, 1997.

33 HEMATOLOGY IN THE ATHLETE
William B Adams, MD

INTRODUCTION

- Athletes as a group tend to be healthier; however, they are still susceptible to the same hematologic diseases as nonathletes. Symptoms from hematologic disturbances, though, may present earlier and at lower severity, often manifesting as impaired physical performance (Fields, 1997; Eichner and Scott, 1998).
- Maximal or prolonged exertion efforts typically cause transient changes in several hematologic indices. Regular endurance and altitude training generally result in more sustained alterations of hematologic parameters (Selby and Eichner, 1994). Dietary inadequacies, not uncommon in athletes, may cause hematologic problems because of a deficit of calories or critical nutrients (Harris, 1995).

ANEMIA

- Anemia is the reduction of total *red blood cell* (RBC) volume (i.e., *hematocrit* (Hct)) or *hemoglobin* (Hgb) concentration below normal values. Symptoms and physical manifestations depend on decrements in RBC volume and oxygen delivery to tissues, the rate at which these changes occur and the cardiopulmonary compensatory capacity (Lee, 1999*b*; 1999*c*).
  a. Prevalence in US males: 6/1000 below age 45 to 18.5/1000 males age 75 and above (Little, 1999).
  b. Prevalence in US women of all ages is 30/1000 (Little, 1999).
  c. By reason of either excessive loss or inadequate production of RBCs, or a combination of both (Lee, 1999*b*; 1999*c*).
  d. Athletes trying to restrict weight or follow special diets that are deficient in iron, vitamins, or calories may have a higher prevalence of anemia (Selby and Eichner, 1994; Cook, 1994).

ATHLETIC PSEUDOANEMIA

- Regular consistent aerobic or endurance level training causes an increase in both red cell production and plasma volume; however, plasma volume expansion typically exceeds the increase in red cell mass causing a slight reduction in Hgb and Hct in the resting state. This condition, common in athletes, is not a true anemia but rather a physiologic adaptation that promotes increased cardiac output, enhanced oxygen delivery to tissues, and protects against hyperviscosity (Selby and Eichner, 1994; Eichner, 1992; 1997).

- Plasma volume can decrease 5 to 20% with endurance exercise (sweat losses and intravascular fluid shifts) (Selby and Eichner, 1994).
- Conditioned endurance athletes tend to have greater reductions as a result of greater sweat losses.
- Hgb values typically run 0.5 g/dL lower for athletes regularly pursuing moderate intensity training and 1.0 g/dL lower for elite level athletes (Eichner, 1997).
- Diagnosis may be confirmed by
  1. Testing the athlete after several days rest from training as the hemodilution of conditioning reverses within days of terminating endurance level training (Selby and Eichner, 1994).
  2. Inferred from laboratory testing yielding:
     a. Normal RBC indices and *red cell distribution width* (RDW) on *complete blood count* (CBC).
     b. Normal reticulocyte count.
     c. Normal serum ferritin level (normal ferritin levels in athletes may be as low as 12 µg/L, particularly with high intensity training) (Cook, 1994).

IRON DEFICIENCY ANEMIA

- Deficiency of iron in the body is the most common cause of *true* anemia in the athlete as in the nonathlete (Eichner, 1992; 1997). It may arise from inadequate dietary intake, excess losses through blood loss, or a combination of the both.
  a. Occurs more often in female athletes mostly because of menstrual losses coupled with inadequate consumption of meat or other sources of iron (Cook, 1994; Eichner, 1992).
  b. Laboratory testing reveals a low Hgb and Hct with low *mean corpuscular volume* (MCV) and *mean corpuscular hemoglobin* (MCH).
  c. RDW is increased, unless iron deficiency is chronic.
  d. Peripheral smear reveals hypochromic microcytic cells with a low to normal reticulocyte count.
  e. Serum ferritin levels are low (<12 µg/L) and better reflect total body iron content as serum iron levels are inconsistent.
  f. *Total iron binding capacity* (TIBC) tends to be elevated.

g. Transferrin saturation (Serum iron × 100/TIBC) tends to be low (particularly <16%) (Lee, 1999b; 1999c).

- In evaluation of iron deficiency anemia, it is imperative to determine the cause of the deficiency in order to best effect therapy and avoid overlooking potentially serious conditions. Iron replacement should continue until 6 to 12 months after anemia has resolved (Selby, 1991).

ANEMIA FROM BLOOD LOSS

- Acute bleeding as well as significant hemolysis and cumulative insidious blood loss may cause anemia. Acute hemorrhage is typically obvious from history or examination findings of gross blood, melena, or hypovolemia. Bleeding contained within tissues or body cavity may be less obvious, particularly in the retroperitoneal space. Characteristics of rapid blood loss:
  a. Hgb and Hct (both concentration values) are *initially* normal in the absence of any fluid administration (Lee, 1999a; 1999b).
  b. Platelet counts *initially* drop with hemorrhage but become elevated within 1 h if no hemorrhage stops (Lee, 1999a; 1999b).
  c. Hgb and Hct values decline over the ensuing days with plasma expansion from endogenous reservoirs (Lee, 1999a; 1999b).
  d. RBC indices are initially normal. After 3 to 5 days MCV and RDW increase because of reticulocyte response (Lee, 1999a; 1999b).
  e. Bilirubin levels are normal unless bleeding is internal. Similar to hemolysis, internal bleeding causes a rise in unconjugated bilirubin and *lactate dehydrogenase* (LDH), but without evidence of hemolysis on peripheral smear (Lee, 1999a; 1999b).
- If blood loss is slow and insidious as in *gastrointestinal* (GI) bleeding or menstrual blood loss in women, anemia may not manifest until iron stores are depleted. This situation may be revealed by a reticulocytosis with concomitant increase in RDW well before iron stores are depleted and MCV becomes low.
- **Gastrointestinal blood loss:** GI bleeding is a very common and often serious cause of anemia. It may arise from peptic ulcer disease, vascular anomalies, inflammatory bowel diseases, ischemic syndromes, infection, diverticuli, or tumors. Thus a stool occult blood test is indicated in any anemia evaluation (Little, 1999). Athletes often manifest GI bleeding in marathons and similar endurance events.
- Features of exercise associated GI Bleeding:
  1. Occurs exclusively with prolonged endurance events and is low grade (Selby and Eichner, 1994; Cook, 1994; Selby, 1991).

2. Source of this bleeding is seldom detectable; it is theorized to arise form acute transient ischemia or mechanical contusion (e.g., cecal slap syndrome) (Selby and Eichner, 1994; Harris, 1995; Cook, 1994; Selby, 1991).
3. In the absence of this or other pathology, bleeding is seldom significant enough to cause anemia (Fields, 1997).

• Note use of *nonsteroidal anti-inflammatory drugs* (NSAID) is common among athletes and may cause enough cumulative blood loss to impact RBC mass (Selby and Eichner, 1994; Eichner, 1997; Selby, 1991). All GI bleeding warrants thorough investigation to rule out serious conditions.

• **Menstrual blood loss:** Menstrual blood and iron losses often coupled with inadequate iron replacement are common causes of anemia in women. Menstrual flow and adequacy of iron replacement for chronic menstrual losses should be considered when evaluating all women athletes with anemia. Treatment is focused on reduction of menstrual flow if excessive and iron replacement. Indications of significant menstrual losses:

1. Heavy and/or frequent menses
2. Twelve or more soaked pads throughout menses (Lee, 1999c)
3. Passage of clots beyond the first day (Lee, 1999c)
4. Flow greater than seven days (Lee, 1999c)
5. More than one episode of menstrual flow per month
6. Diet is inadequate to compensate for cumulative menstrual losses (e.g., low intake of dietary iron sources) (Harris, 1995).

• **Exertional hemolysis (e.g., Footstrike hemolysis):** Intravascular destruction of RBCs may occur in association with various exertional activities. Originally described as "march hemoglobinuria" in foot soldiers in the late 1800s, it was thought arise from the footstrike causing compression of capillaries and rupturing RBCs; however, it is also seen in swimmers, rowers, and weight lifters, though usually to a much lesser degree (Selby and Eichner, 1994; Eichner, 1992; Selby, 1991). It is now hypothesized that intravascular turbulence, acidosis, and elevated temperature in muscle tissues may be causative factors as well (Eichner, 1997).

1. Typically hemolysis is not significant enough to affect CBC parameters (Selby and Eichner, 1994; Eichner, 1992; 1997).
2. Reticulocyte count, RDW, and MCV may be elevated (Selby and Eichner, 1994; Eichner, 1992; 1997).
3. Haptoglobin levels may be reduced if there is enough cumulative hemolysis (Selby and Eichner, 1994; Eichner, 1992; 1997).

4. Transient hemoglobinuria may occur if hemolysis exceeds binding capacity of serum haptoglobin (approximately 20 cc of blood) (Selby and Eichner, 1994; Eichner, 1992; 1997).

• Generally no treatment is necessary; reducing impact forces to the feet (e.g., improved shoe cushioning, softer running terrain) may benefit some, particularly elite level runners (Eichner, 1997).

SICKLE CELL TRAIT

• *Sickle cell trait* (SCT), the heterozygous state where Hgb S is present with Hgb A in RBCs is a common condition. It typically does not cause anemia and has little impairment of athletic performance (Fields, 1997; Eichner, 1993).

1. Present in 8% of Blacks in the United States (Eichner, 1993; Kark and Ward, 1994).
2. May confer heightened risk of complications with exercise at altitude: sickling may be provoked in hypoxic environments, particularly altitudes above 10,000 ft and cause a clinical picture similar to sickle cell anemia. Vigorous exertion at altitudes of 5000 ft or more may produce enough hypoxic and metabolic stress to induce sickling and its sequelae (Eichner, 1993; Kark and Ward, 1994).
3. Epidemiologically associated with increased risk of sudden death in heat stress environments and settings of rapid accelerated conditioning and sustained maximal exertion efforts (Kark and Ward, 1994).
4. May manifest mild microscopic hematuria independent of physical exertion which is rarely significant (Eichner, 1993).
5. May confer higher risk of exertion related rhabdomyolysis particularly in heat stress conditions (Eichner, 1993).

ERYTHROCYTHEMIA (POLYCYTHEMIA)

• Red blood cell mass may be increased as a physiologic response to hypoxic stress, disease processes or induced by drug use. Smoking, carbon monoxide exposure (e.g., ice rinks), and training at altitude may also increase RBC mass in athletes. A spurious erythrocytosis may also arise from transient plasma volume contraction (e.g., exercise, dehydrated status) (Means, 1999). True polycythemia arises from conditions of excess RBC production, either as part of a hyperplastic marrow response (polycythemia vera) or secondary response to excess erythropoietin production (secondary polycythemia).

ETIOLOGIES OF ERYTHROCYTOSIS

- **Pseudoerythrocytosis:** Phlebotomy when patient in a dehydrated state.
- **Polycythemia vera:** A myeloproliferative disorder involving trilineage marrow hyperplasia. RBC mass increase associated with leukocytosis and thrombocytosis. Erythropoeitin levels are low with markedly elevated Hct. These patients require regular phlebotomy to prevent a hyperviscosity state (Levine, 1999).
- **Secondary erythrocytosis:** results from intrinsic elevated erythropoietin or excess erythrocyte production (Means, 1999).
  1. Hypoxic stress
  2. Endogenous conditions of excessive erythropoietin production
  3. Endogenous conditions of isolated excess erythrocyte production
- **Blood doping**
  1. Transfusion (Simon, 1994)
  2. Exogenous erythropoietin (e.g., rEPO)-characterized by elevated RBC and erythropoietin levels with normal WBC and platelet counts (Means, 1999; Simon, 1994).

WBC LINE ABNORMALITIES

- Strenuous or prolonged vigorous exercise may produce acute profound perturbations of WBC populations. This effect, however, resolves with rest and is not typically associated with persistent abnormalities of white cell lines. Various drugs may either elevate or depress WBC production, as may infection. Persistent leukopenia may be indicative of human immunodeficiency virus infection or marrow disorders. Some populations (e.g., Black males) may manifest a mild neutropenia that is nonpathologic (Jandl, 1996).
- If blood work indicates a pathologic alteration of the WBC population, examination should include a thorough assessment of lymphatic and hematologic systems with investigation for infectious, toxic, or oncologic causes.
- Readily treatable etiologies such as infection are addressed as indicated. Referral to a hematologist for bone marrow assessment may be necessary, particularly if there is profound leukopenia, leukocytosis, or disturbances of other cell lines suggestive of malignancy (Tenglin, 1999).

ABNORMALITIES OF PLATELETS AND COAGULATION

- The effects of exercise, particularly endurance activities, seem to have a net neutral effect on platelets and coagulation. Athletes manifesting petechiae, unusual bruising or bleeding problems should undergo prompt investigation for causes of these. Long-standing history of mild bleeding or bruising problems may indicate Von Willebrand's disease or mild factor VIII or IX deficiency. Certain drugs, toxins, autoimmune disorders, infections, malignancies, and other conditions that trigger *disseminated intravascular coagulation* (DIC) may produce thrombocytopenia ranging from mild to severe (Tenglin, 1999). Diets deficient in green vegetables may manifest coagulopathy because of impairment of vitamin K dependent factors (Tenglin, 1999).
- Evaluation of platelet and coagulation disorders focuses on identification of causative conditions as listed above. Laboratory assessment should start with a CBC with peripheral smear looking for abnormalities in all hematologic cell lines. Coagulation studies (*prothrombin time*, PT; *partial thromboplastin time*, PTT; and *international normalized ratio*, INR) should be conducted as well. If the clinical picture suggests DIC (low platelets, fragmented RBCs, and prolonged coagulation times) confirmatory testing to include fibrinogen, fibrin split products, and D-dimer should be added (Tenglin, 1999).
- Thrombocytosis is often a transient condition, typically a manifestation of an acute response to physiologic stress. Transient isolated thrombocytosis is rarely of significance. Persistent thrombocytosis should prompt investigation for infection, inflammatory disorders, malignancies, or other hyperproliferative disorders (e.g., polycythemia vera, myeloproliferative diseases) (Levine, 1999).

OTHER DISORDERS CAUSING ANEMIA/CELL LINE ABNORMALITIES

- Anemia and other cell line abnormalities may result from several other conditions or as a consequence various disease processes. These may manifest in the form of accelerated cell destruction or hemolysis, or through impaired erythropoiesis. Details regarding diagnosis and evaluation of these conditions may be found in hematology reference books (Abramson and Aramson, 1999; Lee, 1999*d*).

SPECIAL CONSIDERATIONS— EXERTIONAL RHABOMYOLYSIS AND MYOGLOBINURIA

EXERTIONAL RHABDOMYOLYSIS

- Rhabdomyolysis is a condition of skeletal muscle breakdown with release of myocyte contents into the circulation. *Exertional rhabdomyolysis* is the term applied to rhabdomyolysis precipitated by exercise or exertion. It is most frequently seen in running or prolonged exertion activity, particularly in settings of accelerated physical training. Often it occurs with exertional heat illness (Kark and Ward, 1994; Baggaley; Saad, 1997; Gardner and Kark, 2002). Biochemically, muscle injury causes a release of myoglobin and muscle enzymes—*creatine phosphokinase* (CPK), LDH, transaminases. Severe states with a large volume of muscle damage typically cause electrolytes disturbances (potassium, phosphate, and calcium) plus extracellular fluid shifts into injured tissues (Baggaley; Saad, 1997; Vivweswaran and Guntupalli, 1999). Various extrinsic and intrinsic factors may enhance susceptibility to rhabdomyolysis (Baggaley; Saad, 1997; Gardner and Kark, 2002; Vivweswaran and Guntupalli, 1999). These include the following:

a. Drug or toxin exposure (e.g., stimulants, antihistamines, alcohol, ephedra, and statin drugs)
b. Infection
c. Heat stroke
d. Dehydration
e. Excessive muscle overload activities (especially eccentric loading)
f. Genetic-muscle diseases/enzyme deficiencies
g. Metabolic diseases or disorders (diabetes, thyroid disease, chronic electrolyte disorders or acidosis)
h. Sickle cell trait
i. Autoimmune disorders (e.g., polymyositis)
j. Deconditioned state (especially with rapidly accelerated physical training)

• Exertional rhabdomyolysis is a spectrum condition. Manifestations range from mild muscle injury with negligible symptoms or systemic effects, to fulminate cases with large muscle mass injury, severe metabolic derangements, *disseminated intravascular coagulation* (DIC), and death (Kark and Ward, 1994; Baggaley; Saad, 1997; Gardner and Kark, 2002; Vivweswaran and Guntupalli, 1999). Myoglobin release may cause nephrotoxicity, but may not directly correlate with muscle enzyme levels or metabolic disturbance. Severity of rhabdomyolysis is gauged initially by magnitude of symptoms and early perturbations of blood chemistries. Collapse short of a finish line, severe pain with inability to walk and early sustained acidosis are ominous indicators; however, symptoms may start off relatively mild but progress in intensity in subsequent hours or days. Also muscle enzyme levels may be deceptively low early on and typically peak 1 to 2 days after the injury.

• Management thus focuses on early recognition, initiating interventions appropriate to degree of injury and monitoring for progression. Initial laboratory studies should include basic electrolyte panel including *creatinine* (Cr), CPK, transaminases, LDH, uric acid,

CBC, and urinalysis with microscopy. In more severe cases, calcium, phosphate, PT, PTT, fibrinogen, and fibrin split products should be added (Gardner and Kark, 2000).
• Positive Hgb with no RBCs on urinalysis are used as indicators of myoglobinuria as myoglobin studies are not quickly available in most settings (Baggaley; Gardner and Kark, 2000). Muddy casts indicate heavy myoglobin load and likely renal toxicity (Vivweswaran and Guntupalli, 1999).

MILD RHABDOMYOLYSIS

• Mild muscle soreness that typically resolves within 1–2 days, otherwise no complaints.
• On examination has mild soreness to palpation, minimal to no soreness with passive muscle stretch.
• Laboratory studies reveal isolated CPK elevation (generally ≤3000 but may be up to 5000); transaminases may peak slightly above normal in 1–2 days (generally ≤2 × normal values).
• Treat with oral hydration and avoidance of strenuous exertion for 1–2 days.
• Monitor for escalation or recurrence of symptoms; educate regarding concerning preventive measures.
• May return to activity the next day if these individuals remain asymptomatic and laboratory studies improved.

MODERATE RHABDOMYOLYSIS

• Symptoms of moderate muscle soreness or stiffness.
• On examination has moderate muscle soreness to palpation and toward extremes of passive stretch.
• Moderate elevation of CPK in first few hours with mild increase in Cr (1.5–2 mg/dL) LDH, AST, and ALT rise (≥3 × normal) several hours to 1 day post injury with CPK peak typically <30,000 mg/dL; uric acid and electrolyte studies remain normal.
• Initial treatment is 2 L isotonic fluids and assess response (symptoms and studies):
1. Symptoms and laboratory studies improved: oral hydration and reevaluate in 12–24 h.
2. Symptoms improved, laboratory studies little changed: assess need for further *intravenous* (IV) hydration; reassess every 4–6 h until laboratory studies improving or refer for hospitalization if not improving.
3. Symptoms not improving, laboratory studies rising: refer to hospital for continued IV hydration and monitoring (watch for developing severe or fulminant state).

SEVERE RHABDOMYOLYSIS

- Severe rhabdomyolysis has marked muscle soreness and pain with any muscle activity.
- Examination reveals tight muscles that are painful to palpation and limited passive stretch.
- Laboratory studies reveal transient acidosis, elevated uric acid, and minor electrolyte alterations that resolve with hydration; Cr is elevated typically >2 mg/dL and CPK progressively rises well above 30,000; LDH, AST, and ALT progressively rise peaking above three times normal at 2–3 days after insult.
- Treatment is IV fluids (2L bolus) and arrange for continued IV fluid therapy and laboratory monitoring After several hours IV fluid therapy:
  1. Symptoms and laboratory studies improved: oral hydration and evaluate response over next 12–24 h.
  2. Symptoms improved, laboratory studies little changed: assess adequacy of hydration and need for additional measures (e.g., compartment pressure testing); reassess every 4–6 h.
  3. Symptoms not improving, laboratory studies rising: transfer to *intensive care unit* (ICU) addressing comorbid issues of electrolyte disturbances, myoglobinuria, and compartment syndrome.
- In subacute setting (days after injury) if stable to improving symptoms and labs may manage as moderate rhabdomyolysis with particular focus on renal injury and exclusion of myoglobinuria.

FULMINANT RHABDOMYOLYSIS

- Patient often presents with collapse and obtundation. Extreme muscle tightness and pain with weakness and extreme difficulty moving involved muscle(s).
- Often associated with findings typical of heat stroke, shock, and dehydration (Gardner and Kark, 2000).
- May manifest as progressively escalating symptoms refractory to less aggressive interventions.
- On examination, involved muscles are tense, very tender, and extremely painful to any passive stretch.
- Laboratory studies at time of collapse may manifest only acidosis, hypokalemia, hypocalcemia, elevated uric acid ± decreased phosphate. Studies in subsequent hours manifest shift to hyperkalemia, hypercalcemia, and hyperphosphatemia with rapidly rising CPK, LDH, AST, and ALT (Vivweswaran and Guntupalli, 1999).
- Treatment necessitates cardiac monitoring for dysrhythmias with advance life support materials, aggressive IV fluids hydration, and transfer to ICU for management of the metabolic derangements (Kark and Ward, 1994; Baggaley).

- Consult orthopedic surgeon for fasciotomy evaluation. Mild to moderate increased compartment pressures perpetuates muscle necrosis and condition improves with early fasciotomy of involved muscle areas (Wise and Fortin, 1997; Kuklo et al, 2000).

RHABDOMYOLYSIS OF AN ISOLATED MUSCLE OR MUSCLE GROUP

- Typically occurs with excessive overload in weight lifting.
- CPK levels may become elevated into the tens of thousands.
- Typically this is self limited, rarely manifesting systemic effects beyond the involved muscle.

RHABDOMYOLYSIS FOLLOW UP

- Healthy individuals with uncomplicated mild to moderate rhabdomyolysis may return to activity immediately after all enzymes have returned to normal. It may be prudent though, to resume exercise in a graduated manner. Recurrent bouts of rhabdomyolysis and any severe or fulminant episodes warrant investigation for an underlying disease process (Kark and Ward, 1994; Gardner and Kark, 2000; 2002).

CONCLUSION

- With the exception of athletic pseudoanemia, it is uncommon to encounter significant persistent hematologic alterations from running. While high intensity and prolonged endurance training may result in alterations of several hematologic parameters, and occasionally lysis of RBCs, rarely are these of pathologic significance; however, signs and symptoms of hematologic disease may manifest at an earlier state in the athlete because of physiologic demands that require maximal hematologic system performance.
- The condition of exertional rhabdomyolysis may occasionally manifest in athletes advancing training too rapidly, but may also appear in a conditioned athlete in association with underlying disease states or as a consequence of severe over-exertion or exertional heat illness. Identification and early treatment of those with myoglobin release or severe myocyte injury is crucial to preclude serious complications.

REFERENCES

Abramson SD, Aramson N: "Common" uncommon anemias. *Am Fam Phys* 59(4):851–861, 1999.

Baggaley PA: Rhabdomyolysis. http://members.tripod.com/~baggas/rhabdo.html#pathogenesis

Cook JD: The effect of endurance training on iron metabolism. *Semin Hematol* 31(3):146–154, 1994.

Eichner ER: Sports anemia, iron supplements and blood doping. *Med Sci Sports Exerc* 24(9) suppliment:315–318, 1992.

Eichner ER: Sickle cell trait, heroic exercise and fatal collapse. *Phys Sportsmed* 21(7):51–64, 1993.

Eichner ER: Anemia and blood doping, in Sallis RE, Massimino F (eds.): *Essentials of Sports Medicine.* Mosby, 1997, pp 35–38 (Chpt 6).

Eichner ER, Scott, WA: Exercise as Disease Detector. *Phys Sportsmed* 26(3):41–52, 1998.

Fields KB: The Athlete with Anemia, in Fields KB and Fricker PA (eds.): *Medical Problems in Athletes.* Malden MA, Blackwell Science, 1997, pp 259–265.

Gardner JW, Kark JA: Heat-Associated Illness, in Srickland GT (ed.): *Hunter's Tropical Medicine*, 8th ed., Philadelphia, PA, Saunders, 2000, pp 140–147.

Gardner JW, Kark JA: Clinical diagnosis, management, and surveillance of exertional heat illness: *Textbooks of Military Medicine, Medical Aspects of Harsh Environments,* Vol 1. Government Printing Office, 2002, pp 231–181.

Harris SS: Helping active women avoid anemia. *Phys Sportsmed* 23(5):35–48, 1995.

Jandl JH: Blood cell formation, in Jandl JH (ed.): *Blood Textbook of Hematology*, New York, NY, Little Brown, 1996, pp 53–55.

Kark JA, Ward FT: Exercise and hemaglobin S. *Semin Hematol* 31(3):181–225, 1994.

Kuklo TR et al: Fatal rhabdomyolysis with bilateral gluteal, thigh, and leg compartment syndrome after the army physical fitness test. *Am J Sports Med* 28(1):112–116, 2000.

Lee GR: Acute posthemorrhagic anemia, in *Wintrobe's Clinical Hematology*, 10th ed. Baltimore, MD, Lippincott, Williams & Wilkins, 1999a, pp 1485–1488.

Lee GR: Anemia: A diagnositc strategy, in *Wintrobe's Clinical Hematology*, 10th ed. Baltimore, MD, Lippincott, Williams & Wilkins, 1999b, pp 908–940.

Lee GR: Anemia: General aspects, in *Wintrobe's Clinical Hematology*, 10th ed. Baltimore, MD, Lippincott, Williams & Wilkins, 1999c, pp 897–907.

Lee GR: Hemolytic disorders: General considerations, in *Wintrobe's Clinical Hematology*, 10th ed. Baltimore, MD, Lippincott, Williams & Wilkins, 1999d, pp 1109–1131.

Levine SP: Thrombocytosis, in *Wintrobe's Clinical Hematology*, 10th ed. Baltimore, MD, Lippencott, Williams & Wilkins, 1999, pp 897–940, 1109–1131, 1485–1488, 1648–1660.

Little, DR: Ambulatory management of common forms of anemia. *Am Fam Phys* 59:1598–1604, 1999.

Means RT: Polycythemia: Erythrocytosis, in *Wintrobe's Clinical Hematology*, 10th ed. Baltimore, MD, Lippincott, Williams & Wilkins, 1999, pp 1538–1554.

Saad EB (1997): Rhabdomyolysis and Myoglobinuria. http://www.medstudents.com.br/terin/terin3.htm

Selby G: When does an athlete need iron? *Phys Sportsmed* 19(4):96–102, 1991.

Selby GB, Eichner ER: Hematocrit and performance: The effect of endurance training on blood volume. *Semin Hematol* 31(2):122–127, 1994.

Simon TL: Induced erythrocythmia and athletic performance. *Semin Hematol* 31(2):128–133, 1994.

Tenglin R: Hematologic abnormalitites, in Lillegard WA, Butcher JD, Rucker, KS (eds.): *Handbook of Sports Medicine: A Symptom-Oriented Approach*, 2nd ed. Boston, MA, Butterworth-Heinemann, 1999, pp 331–335 (Chap. 23).

Vivweswaran P, Guntupalli J: Environmental emergencies: Rhabdomyolysis. *Crit Care Clin* 15(2):415–428, 1999.

Wise JJ, Fortin PT: Bilateral exercise induced thigh compartment syndrome diagnosed as exertional rhabdomyolysis. A case report and review of the literature. *Am J Sports Med* 25(1):126–129, 1997.

34 NEUROLOGY

Jay Erickson, MD

INTRODUCTION

- With chronic headache affecting over 40 million Americans (Mauskop and Leybel, 1998) and considering that posttraumatic headache affects millions of athletes annually, the appropriate evaluation and treatment methodology can be critical to a positive outcome.
- *Mild traumatic brain injury* (MTBI), or concussion, is a common consequence of collisions, falls, and other forms of contact in sports. The rapid yet accurate determination of which athletes require immediate emergency room evaluation may be critical to an athlete's survival.
- The lack of participation in exercise and team sports by athletes with epilepsy is based largely on unfounded fears and misconceptions. For students with epilepsy, restriction from sports activity can contribute to isolation and stigma.

HEADACHE

CLASSIFICATION

- The *International Headache Society* (IHS) provides an extensive classification system for headaches

TABLE 34-1 International Headache Society Classification of Headache

1. Migraine
2. Tension-type headache
3. Cluster headache and chronic paroxysmal hemicrania
4. Miscellaneous headaches unassociated with structural lesion
5. Headache associated with head trauma
6. Headache associated with vascular disorders
7. Headache associated with nonvascular intracranial disorder
8. Headache associated with substances or their withdrawal
9. Headache associated with noncephalic infection
10. Headache associated with metabolic disorder
11. Headache or facial pain associated with disorder of cranium, neck, eyes, ears, nose, sinuses, teeth, mouth, or other facial or cranial structures
12. Cranial neuralgias, nerve trunk pain, and deafferentation pain
13. Headache not classifiable

(Table 34-1). While academically accurate, the provider on site is better served by a decision analysis tool that quickly distinguishes between those headaches that require minimal medical involvement and those that might require rapid evaluation and treatment.

- **Serious headache:** Requires immediate evaluation and treatment. Occurs with or without trauma and is associated with other neurologic symptoms to include mental status changes, nausea, vomiting, increased neck stiffness, or focal neurologic findings on examination.
- **Concerning headache:** Requires evaluation and treatment but not immediately. Patient meets criteria for concussion (confusion, amnesia, incoordination, slurred speech, emotional lability, or delayed motor or verbal response) but has none of the serious headache signs or symptoms.
- **Benign headache:** No further evaluation or treatment required. Best described as a tension-type headache that occurs as a result of exertion or effort. Should only be used as a diagnosis of exclusion once an evaluation has ruled out both concerning and serious headaches.
- Clues to the correct diagnosis and effective treatment of an athlete with headache lie in a detailed history. Four key aspects of any headache include the following:
  1. Precipitating factors
  2. Character of headache pain
  3. Location of headache
  4. Preceding and accompanying symptoms
- These factors allow the clinician to properly categorize the patient with headache symptoms, thereby ensuring the appropriate and timely diagnostic testing and treatment.
- One small study of benign exertional headache found organic brain lesions as the headache source in nearly 10% of its patients (Rooke, 1968).
- Benign exertional headache is typically precipitated by even minimal physical activity and is best described as dull and throbbing in nature and can be located unilaterally, bilaterally, or occipitally and may last for several hours.
- Effort migraine is a vascular headache brought on by extremely intense exercise. It is commonly unilateral and throbbing in nature and is generally preceded by scotomata or visual aura as seen in other forms of migraine headaches.
- Weightlifter's headache is typically a posterior headache occurring in athletes straining to lift heavy weights. Symptoms may last for days to weeks and resolve relatively slowly when compared to other benign headaches. Of note, several forms of underlying pathology can present as a strain type headache including Arnold Chiari malformations.
- Trauma-induced migraine is seen in athletes competing in contact sports and is typically preceded by minor head trauma without loss of consciousness followed within minutes by visual, motor, and sensory aura including scotomata, paresthesias, and even hemiplegic symptoms. The headache is usually unilateral, throbbing, and retro-orbital. It may be accompanied by photophobia, nausea, and vomiting and may last for hours to days in duration.

TREATMENT

- Treatment of benign exertional headaches includes the use of nonsteroidal anti-inflammatory medications either acutely or prophylactically (see Table 34-2).
- For athletes with effort migraine whose symptoms resolve abruptly, treatment is not indicated. For those athletes with prolonged debilitating symptoms, the use of classic migraine medications may allow for a faster return to activities (see Table 34-2). Instead of prophylactic medications, symptoms can be prevented by the use of longer warm-up periods.
- While treatment for weightlifter's headache may include rest, ice, and nonsteroidal anti-inflammatories, recurrent strain type headaches warrant further neurologic evaluation to include *computed tomography* (CT) and/or *Magnetic resonance imaging* (MRI) to rule out any underlying pathology as the headache source.
- Although the initial trauma-induced migraine must be fully evaluated via complete neurologic evaluation including neuroimaging studies because of its confounding presentation, subsequent similar headaches can be treated as classic migraines including the use of acute migraine medications. Prophylactic migraine medications are generally not recommended because of the unpredictable timing of these headaches.

TABLE 34-2 Headache Medications for Athletes

CATEGORY/AGENT	TRADE NAME	ROUTE	DOSING
Analgesics			
Acetaminophen	Tylenol	Oral	325–1000 mg every 4–6 h as needed
Nonsteroidal Anti-Inflammatories			
Aspirin	Ecotrin	Oral	325–650 mg every 4–6 h as needed
Ibuprofen	Motrin, Advil	Oral	400–800 mg every 8 h as needed
Naproxen	Naprosyn, Anaprox, Alleve	Oral	220–500 mg every 12 h as needed
Muscle Relaxants (Potential Sedating Effect)			
Cyclobenzaprine	Flexeril	Oral	10 mg every 12 h as needed
Methocarbamol	Robaxin	Oral	500–1500 mg every 6 h as needed
Migraine Sedatives (Potential Sedating Effect)			
Butalbital, Acetaminophen, Caffeine	Fioricet	Oral	One every 6 h as needed
Butalbital, Aspirin, Caffeine	Fiorinal	Oral	One every 6 hours as needed
Isometheptine, Dichloralphenazone, Acetaminophen	Midrin	Oral	Two at onset, then one per hour until headache relieved.
Ergotamines			
Ergotamine tartrate, Caffeine	Cafergot	Oral	Two at onset, then one per hour until headache relieved.
Dihydroergotamine mesylate, caffeine	Migranol Nasal	Nasal	One spray in each nostril, repeat in 15 min if needed.
Triptans			
Sumatriptan	Imitrex	Oral	One at onset, repeat every 2 h as needed to max of 200 mg.
	Imitrex	Nasal	One spray in each nostril, repeat may repeat once in two hours.
	Imitrex	Subcutaneous	One injection at onset, may repeat once after 1 h.

CONCUSSION

- Mild traumatic brain injury, or concussion, is a common consequence of collisions, falls, and other forms of contact in sports. The rapid yet accurate determination of which athletes require immediate emergency room evaluation may be critical to an athlete's survival.
- The severity of an injury may not correlate with loss of consciousness in traumatic brain injury (Kushner, 2001).
- Second impact syndrome is typically seen in football players, hockey players, and boxers in whom a relatively minor blow to the head is followed within one week by a second concussive trauma incident. In the worst case scenario, the athlete undergoes rapid neurologic demise and death within hours of the second head injury.
- While various theories account for the cause of death in second-impact syndrome, it appears that the initial trauma causes a loss of vasomotor tone allowing for an increase in intracranial volume. Receiving a second minor head impact during this brief period of decreased intracranial compliance may cause diffuse and uncontrollable cerebral edema and subsequent death.

- Most guidelines for concussion classification and return to lay criterion classify concussions as Grade I, II, or III and require an athlete to be completely asymptomatic for some period of time prior to returning to competition (Tables 34-3, 34-4, 34-5).
- The *standardized assessment of concussion* (SAC) is a simple, reproducible, and fast method of providing a gross measurement of mental status. The SAC evaluates orientation, immediate memory, concentration, and delayed memory recall (Johnston et al, 2001).

POSTCONCUSSIVE SYNDROME

- The most common symptoms of postconcussive syndrome include headaches, dizziness, tinnitus, diplopia, blurred vision, irritability, anxiety, depression, fatigue, sleep disturbance, poor appetite, poor memory, impaired concentration, and slowed reaction times.
- Because the symptoms are so wide ranging and neurologic examination is usually normal, neuropsychologic testing and treatment is indicated in any

TABLE 34-3 Guidelines for Return to Sports After Cerebral Concussion

GRADE	FEATURES	MANAGEMENT	RETURN TO PLAY
1 (mild)	No loss of consciousness	Remove from contest	May return if asymptomatic at rest and with exertion (no headache, dizziness, or impaired concentration plus full recall of the events occurring before injury)
	Posttraumatic amnesia less than 30 min	Observe on the sidelines	Second grade 1 concussion: May return in 2 weeks if asymptomatic at that time for 1 week
			Third grade 1 concussion: terminate season, may return next year if asymptomatic
2 (moderate)	Loss of consciousness less than 5 min or posttraumatic amnesia longer than 30 min	Remove from contest and disallow return that day	Return after asymptomatic for 1 week
		Athlete should be evaluated by a neurologist at a medical facility	Second grade 2 concussion: wait at least 1 month, may return then if asymptomatic for 1 week, consider terminating season
		Cervical spine precautions as indicated	Third grade 2 concussion: terminate season, may return next year if asymptomatic
3 (severe)	Loss of consciousness longer than 5 min or posttraumatic amnesia longer than 24 h	Transport athlete to nearest hospital with neurosurgical facilities with head and neck immobilization	Wait at least 1 month, may return then if asymptomatic for 1 week
		Admit to hospital to check for intracranial bleeding	Second grade 3 concussion: terminate season, may return next season if asymptomatic

SOURCE: Cantu R: Guidelines for return to contact sports after a cerebral concussion. *Phys Sportsmed* 14:75–76, 79, 83, 1986. (With permission)

posttraumatic head injury athlete who is suspected of having neuropsychologic symptoms.
• Testing and treatment of postconcussive athletes includes standard neuroimaging along with more specific evaluations to include audiologic testing, electronystagmography, posturography, and a battery of tests to evaluate everything from orientation and attention to visual scanning and motor coordination.
• Treatment of postconcussive syndrome is symptom related and can include analgesics, nonsteroidal anti-inflammatories, antidepressants, and muscle relaxants. Education and reassurance that most patients with postconcussive syndrome have complete

TABLE 34-4 Guidelines for Management of Concussion in Sports

GRADE	FEATURES	MANAGEMENT	RETURN TO PLAY
1	Confusion without amnesia	Remove from contest	May return if asymptomatic at rest and with exertion for at least 20 min
	No loss of consciousness	Examine immediately and at 5-minute intervals for development of mental status abnormalities or postconcussive symptoms at rest with exertion	Second grade-1 concussion in same contest: disqualify athlete for that day
			Third grade-1 concussion: terminate season
2	Confusion with amnesia	Remove from contest and disallow return that day	May return after 1 full asymptomatic week at rest and with exertion
	No loss of consciousness	Examine on site frequently for signs of evolving intracranial pathology	Second grade-2 concussion: return to play after 1 month symptom free at rest and with exertion, consider termination of season
		CT scan or MR imaging if symptoms worsen or persist for longer than 1 week	Third grade-2 concussion: terminate season
3	Any loss of consciousness	Transport athlete to nearest emergency department by ambulance with cervical spine precautions, if necessary	May return after 1 month if asymptomatic at rest and with exertion for at least 2 weeks
			Second grade-3 concussion: terminate season, return to any contact sport seriously discouraged

SOURCE: Colorado Medical Society Sports Medicine Committee: *Guidelines for the Management of Concussion in Sports.* Denver, CO, Colorado Medical Society, 1991. (With permission)

TABLE 34-5 Guidelines for the Management of Concussion in Sports

GRADE	FEATURES	MANAGEMENT	RETURN TO PLAY
1	Transient confusion No loss of consciousness Concussion symptoms resolve in less than 15 min	Remove from contest Examine immediately and at 5-min intervals for development of mental status abnormalities or postconcussive symptoms at rest and with exertion	Return if clear within 15 min Second grade-1 in same contest: disqualify athlete, return in 1 week if asymptomatic at rest and with exercise
2	Transient confusion No loss of consciousness Concussion symptoms last more than 15 min	Remove from contest and disallow return that day Examine on site frequently for signs of evolving intracranial pathology CT scan or MR imaging if symptoms worsen or persist for longer than 1 week	May return after 1 full asymptomatic week with exertion Second grade-2 concussion: return to play after 2 weeks symptom free at rest and with exertion
3	Any loss of consciousness, either brief (seconds) or prolonged (minutes)	Transport athlete to nearest emergency department by ambulance with cervical spine precautions, if necessary	Brief (seconds) grade 3 concussion: withhold from play until asymptomatic for 2 weeks at rest and with exertion Second grade-3 concussion withhold from play for a minimum of 1 asymptomatic month

SOURCE: Kelly JP, Rosenburg JH: Practice parameter: The management of concussion in sports. *Neurology* 48:575–580, 1997. (With permission)

resolution of symptoms within 3–6 months is a vital component of any therapeutic regimen.

EPILEPSY

- Epileptic syndromes are typically classified into one of three categories:
  1. Generalized epileptic syndromes that are often idiopathic, have a genetic predisposition, have bilateral electrical discharges on *electroencephalogram* (EEG), and have a good prognosis.
  2. Localization-related epileptic syndromes that are further divided into three subcategories: (*a*) idiopathic; (*b*) age-related onset; and (*c*) symptomatic.
  3. The *idiopathic* subtype is usually hereditary and is notable for negative diagnostic studies. The most common age-related subtype is benign rolandic epilepsy. It is a self-limited childhood condition that is hereditary and typically outgrown before puberty. The symptomatic category comprises epileptic syndromes caused by focal brain abnormalities, such as cortical malformations and those secondary to trauma or tumors. The seizures of this category tend to have a poorer prognosis for either complete control or cure. Resective epileptic surgery can be the only treatment option and may reduce the seizure burden.
- Unfortunately, because of misconceptions by parents, school administrators, coaches, physicians, and many youth are never allowed to participate in sports,

thereby isolating them from their peers and increasing their risk of comorbid behavior. The most current and standard recommendations are from the International League Against Epilepsy and restrict only scuba diving and sky diving (Commission of Pediatrics of the International League Against Epilepsy, 1997).

- By age 20, approximately 1% of the U.S. population will have developed some form of epilepsy. Of those affected, 75% experience their first seizure before their third decade of life (Daniel, 2002). The chance of a recurrent seizure after a first seizure is 30–40%. Once a child has experienced a second seizure, the chance of recurrence approaches 90%.
- Although team sports involving collision or contact must be pursued cautiously, many athletes with epilepsy can complete successfully in these sports. Additionally, the reports of epilepsy developing after participation in contact sports including boxing, football, and hockey are extremely rare. The decision regarding participation by any athlete with epilepsy must be made only after a careful risk/benefit analysis.
- In a patient-by-patient approach, all aspects of an athlete's seizure history must be considered. This includes type, frequency, loss of consciousness, prodromes, duration, and postictal symptoms. Also, any medications used and their physiologic and psychologic effects must be fully evaluated during the preparticipation examination.
- The preparticipation evaluation of an athlete with epilepsy or other seizure history can be considered a *fear* evaluation:

a. Frequency of seizures and adequacy of control
b. Effects of medications that might impact performance of safety
c. Activity or sport being considered for participation
d. Readiness or desire by athlete to participate in a specific sport or activity

- Athletes with epileptic triggers should understand that participation in activities that might initiate seizures should be avoided. Specific instances would include hyperventilation brought on by running or fatigue caused by prolonged athletic activities.
- While participation in water sports would appear to be a danger to any athlete with epilepsy, the fact that most competitive swimming competitions are observed by not only parents but coaches and trainers significantly reduces the inherent risk.
- Contraindications for swimming are *small*:
  a. Seizures have occurred recently or are poorly controlled.
  b. Medications have recently been changed or the patient is noncompliant.
  c. *Antiepileptic drug* (AED) blood levels are unstable.
  d. Lack of one-on-one supervision during the event.
  e. Lake or murky water events, including all prolonged underwater events.
- Scuba diving and underwater swimming would include a restricted ability to observe any seizure activity and the increased risk would need to be factored in to any decision regarding participation.
- Gymnastic events requiring a significant amount of swinging or separation from equipment at any height would pose an increased risk of falls and subsequent trauma. The presence of coaches and observers would provide little protection from injury because of an inability to be within reach of a falling athlete. The use of safety harnesses and direct contact observers for those athletes with epilepsy may be required for participation.
- If a seizure does occur during a sporting event, further participation should be restricted because of potential post-ictal effects. Special consideration could be made for the athlete who experiences an absence type event with minimal residual effects.
- The appropriate categorization of the seizure type and epileptic syndrome is the most important criterion in deciding on medical treatment.

MEDICAL TREATMENT OF EPILEPSY

- The medical treatment of epilepsy is a difficult task for the physician working with athletes. While the older antiepileptic medications are conveniently formulated for once or twice daily regimens, thereby improving compliance, they also have more significant side effects that may impact on an athlete's performance capability.
- While each medication has specific side effects, only those that would be considered to have a negative impact on athletic performance or function will be discussed.
- Phenytoin has been reported to depress cognitive function, slow overall performance, and produce sedation (Aubry et al, 2001).
- The toxic side effects of carbamazepine include dizziness, diplopia, sedation, ataxia, and nausea. Also, the concurrent use of erythromycin may increase carbamazepine levels.
- The most common side effects of valproate include weight gain secondary to increased appetite and mild tremors. In rare cases it can even cause an encephalopathy with sedation and cognitive impairment.
- Gabapentin is generally well tolerated with minimal side effects and has no significant drug interactions. Since it is not metabolized by the liver, it does not induce the P-450 enzyme system.
- Allergic skin rash is the most common side effect of lamotrigine, but additional side effects include dizziness, headaches, diplopia, sedation, and movement disorders.

REFERENCES

Aubry M, Cantu R, Dvorak J, et al: *Concussion in Sport Group.* Summary and agreement of the first International Symposium on Concussion in Sport, Vienna 2001. *Clin J Sports Med* 12: 6–11, 2002.

Bergman AI et al: *Heads Up: Brain Injury in Your Practice.* National Center for Injury Prevention and Control, Centers for Disease Control and Prevention, 2002.

Commission of Pediatrics of the International League Against Epilepsy: Restrictions for children with epilepsy. *Epilepsia* 38(9):1054–1056, 1997.

Daniel JC: The implementation and use of the standardized assessment of concussion at the U.S. Naval Academy. *Mil Med* 167, 873, 2002.

Johnston KM, McCrory P, Mohtaddi NG, et al: Evidence-based review of sport-related concussion: clinical science. *Clin J Sports Med* 11: 155–159, 2001.

Kushner DS: Concussion in sports: minimizing the risk for complications. *Am Fam Phys* 64, 1007, 2001.

Mauskop A, Leybel B: Headache in sports, in Jordan BD (ed.): *Sports Neurology,* 2nd ed. Philadelphia, PA, Lippincott-Raven, 1998, chap. 18.

Rooke ED: Benign exertional headache. *Med Clin North Am* 52, 801–809, 1968.

35 GASTROENTEROLOGY

David L Brown, MD
Chris G Pappas, MD

INTRODUCTION AND EPIDEMIOLOGY

- From a *gastrointestinal* (GI) perspective, long distance runners have been the most scrutinized group, but recent studies have looked at the GI symptoms of long distance walkers, cyclists, triathletes, and weight lifters. Upper and lower GI tract symptoms occur with equal prevalence in cyclists. Lower GI symptoms predominate nearly two to one over upper GI symptoms in endurance runners. Whether running or riding, these same patterns also hold true in triathletes (Peters, 1999*a*). In low-intensity long-distance walking, the overall occurrence of GI symptoms is much lower than in other sports studied. The most common symptoms are flatulence and nausea each of which occurs in only 5% of walkers (Peters, 1999*b*).
- Symptomatic gastroesophageal reflux is extremely common in athletes. Cyclists have the lowest esophageal acid exposure, followed closely by runners. Weight lifters have the highest rates of reflux. All groups have increased reflux when exercising postprandially. Cyclists have a modest increase in reflux after eating, while weight lifters nearly double and runners triple their reflux (Collings et al, 2003).
- *Peptic ulcer disease* (PUD) is associated with the primary risk factors of *Helicobacter pylori* infection and *nonsteroidal anti-inflammatory drugs* (NSAID) use.

H. pylori is associated with 65–95% of gastric ulcers and 75% of duodenal ulcers. The estimated risk of a clinically significant NSAID-induced event, including bleeding and perforation, is 1 to 4% per year for nonselective NSAID. Either of these factors alone increases ulcer risk twentyfold. When both risk factors are present, an individual is 61 times more likely to develop ulcer disease (Tytgat et al, 1985).
- The primary lower GI condition of athletes is runner's diarrhea, affecting up to 26% of marathon runners (Keefe et al, 1984). Runner's diarrhea is not typically associated with bleeding; however, studies in marathon runners showed that 20% of runners completing a marathon had occult blood in their stools, another 6% had bloody diarrhea, and 17% had frank hematochezia while in training (McCabe et al, 1986).

UPPER GI DISEASES

GASTROESOPHAGEAL REFLUX DISEASE

- The most common presenting complaints for *gastroesophageal reflux disease* (GERD) are heartburn and acid regurgitation. The classic presentation is retrosternal burning, exacerbated by meals, intense workouts, and recumbency with resolution on antacids. Atypical symptoms include nausea, excessive salivation (water brash), bloating, and belching (Richter, 1996). Extraintestinal complaints include sore throat, exertional dyspnea, cough, or wheezing (Table 35-1).
- GERD pathophysiology involves retrograde movement of gastric acid and the proteolytic enzyme pepsin, which causes irritation of the esophageal epithelium. Reflux alone is insufficient to explain why individuals become symptomatic because affected patients have

TABLE 35-1   GERD Symptom Patterns

CLASSIC SYMPTOMS	ATYPICAL SYMPTOMS/SIGNS	RED FLAG SYMPTOMS
Heartburn	**Pulmonary**	Chronic untreated symptoms
Acid regurgitation	Asthma	Dysphagia
	Chronic cough	Weight loss
Nonspecific Symptoms		Hemetemesis
	ENT	Melena
Nausea		Odynophagia
Dyspepsia	Dental erosions	Vomiting
Bloating	Halitosis	Early satiety
Belching	Lingual sensitivity	
Indigestion	Chronic pharyngitis	
Hypersalivation/water brash	Hoarseness	
	Rhinitis/Sinusitis	
	Globus	
	Cardiac	
	Atypical chest pain	

reflux rates similar to healthy individuals (Hirschowitz, 1991). The critical factor in symptom development appears to be that the contact time between refluxed material and the epithelium is so excessive that the normal gastric contents overwhelm the epithelial protective mechanisms. Alternatively, symptoms may develop when normal contact time occurs in the face of insufficient protective mechanisms.

• Symptomatic reflux episodes during exercise are likely multifactorial, but correlate best with *transient lower esophageal sphincter relaxations* (TLESR's). This vagally-mediated reflex facilitates *lower esophageal sphincter* (LES) relaxation and gas venting in response to gaseous stomach distention. The decrease in LES tone and reflux associated with TLESRs last longer and are not accompanied by a swallow-induced peristaltic sweep, leading to prolonged acid exposure. Supine or forward-flexed posture during particular

modes of exercise increases intra-abdominal pressure overcoming the mechanical protection of the LES and negating bolus acid clearance achieved by gravity. Increasing exercise intensity is associated with increased reflux episodes and duration of acid exposure (Soffer et al, 1993). As exercise intensity increases, the frequency, duration, and amplitude of esophageal contractions progressively decrease. High intensity exercise also reduces splanchnic blood flow, which may inhibit restoration of acid base balance and deprive the epithelium of the oxygen and nutrients needed for damage repair.

• If the history and physical raise red flags, symptoms are particularly severe, or the diagnosis is unclear, the athlete should be referred for gastroenterology evaluation (Fig. 35-1). In patients with extraintestinal manifestations or atypical GERD symptoms, providers can consider an initial therapeutic trial. If empiric

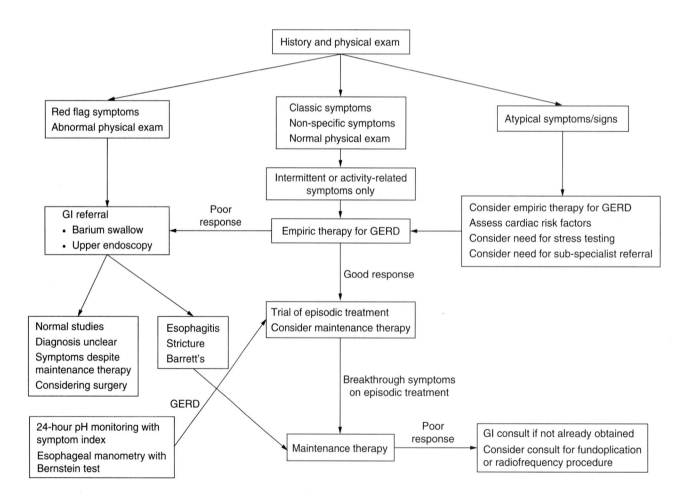

Adapted from O'Connor, FG. "Gastrointestinal Problems in Runners" in *Textbook of Running Medicine*. McGraw-Hill, 2001. With permission.

FIG. 35-1 Evaluation of GERD.

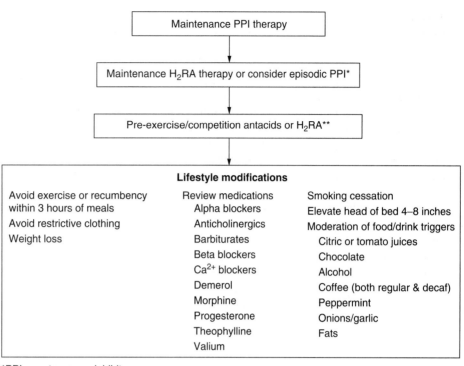

FIG. 35-2 Therapeutic Pyramid for Exercise-Related Gastroeso-phageal Reflux Disease.

*PPI = proton pump inhibitor
**H₂RA = histamine 2 receptor antagonist

Adapted from O'Connor, FG. "Gastrointestinal Problems in Runners" in *Textbook of Running Medicine*. McGraw-Hill, 2001. With permission.

therapy fails, it is important not only to consult gastroenterology, but also the specialty that would evaluate for extraintestinal complications. In the face of a classic history and normal physical examination, it is reasonable to institute empiric therapy in a stepwise fashion (Fig. 35-2).

• Persistent symptoms despite behavioral interventions warrant medical therapy. Episodic complaints are treated with *over-the-counter* (OTC) antacids or an *H-2 receptor antagonist* (H2RA) as needed. This can be advanced to prescription-strength H2RA therapy if control is insufficient. Should symptoms continue after 6 weeks of H2RA therapy, neither continuing therapy nor increasing the dose are likely to achieve control (Kahrilas, Fenerty, and Joelsson, 1999). At this point, it was previously common practice to consider add-on therapy with a prokinetic agent to improve LES tone, gastric emptying, and peristalsis. These agents all have side effects that make them undesirable for use in athletes. Bethanechol has generalized cholinergic effects. Metoclopramide has a high incidence of fatigue, restlessness, tremor, and tardive dyskinesia, making it a poor choice for anything more than sporadic use. Cisapride, formerly the prokinetic agent of choice, was found to be associated

with arrhythmia development, especially with concomitant use of macrolides, imidazoles, or protease inhibitors (Wysowski and Bacsanyi, 1996). This discovery led to severe prescribing restrictions in the United States.

• In individuals who fail to respond to H2RAs, standard-dose *proton pump inhibitors* (PPI) are the treatment of choice. PPIs provide more rapid relief of symptoms (Bardhan et al, 1999) and are more likely than H2RAs to heal and prevent recurrence of erosive esophagitis (Chilba et al, 1997). The agents in this class are equally efficacious in controlling heartburn and have similar healing and relapse rates (Caro, Salas, and Ward, 2001). Because reported differences in initial bioavailability and antisecretory potency are not clinically significant with long-standing use, one PPI cannot be recommended over another (Williams et al, 1998). If the response to episodic treatment is generally favorable but symptoms are occurring on a more chronic basis, maintenance therapy is beneficial. Because their efficacy is dose-dependent, PPI therapy can be stepped-up to control symptoms. Failure to respond to high dose PPI therapy requires gastroenterologist evaluation to rule out complications of GERD. In the absence of findings consistent with reflux disease, further GI testing will be necessary to confirm GERD and assess for other esophageal disorders.

- More invasive treatments are available for patients with an established diagnosis of GERD who respond poorly to PPIs, who are intolerant of medical therapy, or who desire a permanent solution to potentially eliminate their need for medication. Laparoscopic antireflux surgery has been shown to provide a 96% improvement in primary symptoms and 96% long-term satisfaction rate; however, 2% of patients were worse after surgery and 14% still required medication (Bammer et al, 2001). Other endoscopic therapies, including suturing, radiofrequency ablation, injection therapy, and bulking therapy are currently being investigated.

PEPTIC ULCER DISEASE

- Epigastric pain is the hallmark of PUD. Both gastric and duodenal ulcers typically present with deep burning or gnawing pain, sometimes with radiation to the back. Duodenal ulcer symptoms usually develop 2 to 3 h after meals and are relieved with food or antacids. Gastric ulcer symptoms develop sooner after meals but are less consistently relieved with food or antacids. Food ingestion can actually precipitate gastric ulcer pain in some individuals. Most PUD patients have associated anorexia and weight loss. Some patients, particularly with duodenal ulcers, experience hyperphagia and weight gain, presumably because of the mitigating effects of food. Not uncommonly, the initial presentation of PUD can be life-threatening upper GI hemorrhage or perforation (Spechler, 2002).
- Peptic ulcers are erosions in the surface of the stomach or duodenum that extend down to the muscularis mucosa. *H. pylori* induces ulcers by both direct and indirect mechanisms. Bacterial phospholipases weaken the protective mucus barrier, allowing the toxic compounds created from its breakdown of urea to directly damage the epithelium. The same urease enzyme that promotes this direct cell damage acts as a potent antigenic stimulator of immune cells. By inciting an exuberant host inflammatory response, *H. pylori* produces indirect epithelial damage as well (Nilius and Malfertheiner, 1996).
- NSAID inhibition of prostaglandins affects multiple layers of the GI tract's protective barrier. With increasing concentration, they diminish mucosal blood flow and penetrate the epithelial cells, eventually leading to mitochondrial oxidative uncoupling and cell death (Lichtenstein, Syngal, and Wofe, 1995). There are no studies directly relating NSAID use to

upper GI symptoms or bleeding specifically in athletes. Nevertheless, the increased mucosal permeability and decreased splanchnic blood flow that occurs with prolonged exercise may magnify the effects of *H. pylori* and the NSAIDs.

- Athletes should be questioned regarding any relationship of symptom onset with NSAID use. Laboratory analysis should assess for occult GI bleeding and anemia. If any alarm signs or symptoms are present, an individual has new onset dyspepsia after the age of 45, or has a family history of gastric cancer, early gastroenterology referral is recommended.
- If NSAID use is discovered, it should be discontinued if possible. If analgesic therapy is crucial, replacing a nonselective NSAID with acetaminophen or a COX-2 inhibitor would be prudent. Upper GI safety and tolerability studies have shown that COX-2 inhibitors have a 46% lower rate of medication withdrawal for adverse events, a 71% lower risk of ulcers on endoscopy, and a 39% lower incidence of symptoms because of ulcers, perforations, bleeding, or obstruction compared to nonselective NSAIDs (Deeks, Smith, and Bradley, 2002).
- If symptoms are not predominantly GERD-related, there are no markers for severe disease, and medication-induced disease is eliminated, consensus recommendations support a "test and treat" approach in adults under the age of 45 with persistent dyspepsia. These patients should have a noninvasive test for *H. pylori* infection. Urea breath analysis is the favored test with the stool antigen assay as an alternative. Those who are *H. pylori* negative, should receive short term H2RA or PPI therapy (4–6 weeks). If they fail empiric antisecretory therapy or symptoms recur upon cessation of treatment, they should have endoscopy. Symptomatic individuals who test positive for *H. pylori* require eradication therapy. PPI or ranitidine bismuth citrate along with clarithromycin and amoxicillin are to be used as first line therapy. Metronidazole can be substituted for amoxicillin in penicillin allergic patients. Subsequent second-line therapy should be with a PPI, bismuth, tetracycline, and metronidazole (Table 35-2). All patients should be retested for evidence of a cure no sooner than 4 weeks after therapy. The athlete should be off any antisecretory medication, especially PPIs, for a minimum of 1 week prior to retesting. Urea breath analysis is the posttreatment diagnostic test of choice. Stool antigen testing can be used if urea breath testing is unavailable. Individuals who fail second-line therapy and those with persistent dyspepsia should be referred to gastroenterology for further evaluation (Malfertheiner et al, 2002).

TABLE 35-2 Regimens for Treatment of *Helicobacter pylori* Infection

REGIMEN	ERADICATION RATE*
PPI bid	
Amoxicillin 1000 mg bid Clarithromycin 500 mg bid	96.4%
PPI bid	
Bismuth subsalicylate 525 mg qid Tetracycline 500 mg qid Metronidazole 250 mg qid	85–90%
PPI bid	
Metronidazole 500 mg bid Clarithromycin 500 mg bid	89.8%
PPI bid	
Amoxicillin 1000 mg bid Metronidazole 500 mg bid	79.0%

SOURCE: O'Connor FG: Gastrointestinal problems in runners, in *Textbook of Running Medicine,* 1st ed. New York, NY, McGraw-Hill. 2001. (With permission)
*All eradication are rates based on a 7-day regimen. Though European data suggest 7 days are adequate, this has not been confirmed by U.S. studies. Thus, a full 14-day treatment course is recommended.

LOWER GI DISEASES

RUNNER'S DIARRHEA

- Runner's diarrhea is a spectrum of exertional or immediately postexertional lower GI symptoms. Complaints range from abdominal cramping and fecal urgency to diarrhea and frank incontinence. Often runner's diarrhea occurs in association with increases in training mileage or with particularly strenuous training sessions and competitions. An individual may be able to endure an episode by transiently reducing their pace. When symptoms are more severe, it may be necessary to suspend their workout and quickly seek relief.
- While the true etiology of runner's diarrhea remains unknown, several physiologic mechanisms have been proposed. One theory is that it is related to the autonomic nervous system. Increased parasympathetic output during moderate exercise may intensify peristalsis leading to cramping and rapid bowel transit. Heightened sympathetic tone during more intense exercise, could lead to increased bowel activity by increasing the release of hormones such as gastrin and motilin (Cammack et al, 1982). Alternatively, strenuous exercise may lead to rapid shifts in intestinal fluid and electrolytes, causing colonic irritability (Rehrer et al, 1989). Another hypothesis is that the 70–80% reduction in splanchnic blood flow with vigorous exercise may lead to an ischemic enteropathy. Poor tissue perfusion maintained over the length of the

exercise session could cause mucosal ischemia leading to fluid shifts and diarrhea. This theory could also explain the high prevalence of GI bleeding in marathon runners (Bounous and Mcardle, 1990).
- In addition to the basics, the history should document any recent travel, unusual food ingestion, or exposure to sick contacts to determine a potential infectious etiology. Diarrhea not associated with training should prompt a more intensive investigation. A focused lab assessment includes fecal occult blood testing and a complete blood count to look for anemia. In the presence of severe diarrhea, serum electrolytes should be drawn. Liver enzymes and pancreatic enzymes can be considered. If the history is suggestive of an infectious process, the stool should be examined for leukocytes, ova, parasites, and stool cultures.
- Treatment starts with a temporary reduction in training intensity and duration for 1 to 2 weeks. In most cases this alone is enough to abolish symptoms (Fogoros, 1980). During this time, cross training with low or non-impact activities can be used to maintain the athlete's aerobic capacity. Any dietary or fluid replacement triggers should be eliminated. If a specific trigger is not identified, individuals with ongoing symptoms may benefit from dietary manipulation. A diet low in fiber can be helpful (Brouns, Saris, and Reher, 1987). While not an adequate regimen for the control of chronic symptoms, some individuals may benefit from a complete liquid diet on the day prior to competition or scheduled intense exercise session. Once the diarrhea is under control, a full return to high intensity exercise can be achieved by gradually increasing training as symptoms tolerate. Antidiarrheal medication should be used sparingly and with great caution. Anstispasmodics such as loperamide, are generally safe; however, anticholinergic medications such as diphenoxylate with atropine (Lomotil) are to be avoided because of the increased heat injury risk secondary to their effect on sweating. Consult GI for unresolved symptoms despite conservative therapy or for red flag symptoms.

ABDOMINAL PAIN—"SIDE STITCH"

- In the young, active population, abdominal pain with exertion is common. The conditions previously discussed notwithstanding, the "side stitch" is the most common cause of this in athletes. Typically seen in runners, it presents as a somewhat pleuritic aching sensation, usually in the right upper abdominal quadrant. It is often seen in deconditioned individuals starting an exercise program, but can also be observed in athletes intensifying their training. Exercise in the postprandial period is a frequent exacerbating factor. Side stitches usually stop immediately on ceasing exercise. As an individual gains aerobic fitness, the frequency and severity of attacks tend to subside.

- While their true etiology remains elusive, they are most likely caused by hypoxia-induced diaphragmatic muscle spasm (Pate, 1988). Other potential etiologies include pleural irritation, hepatic capsule irritation, symptomatic abdominal adhesions, and right colonic gas pain (Lauder and Moses, 1995).
- The management involves using the history to rule out not only the other GI diseases discussed in this chapter, but also other exertional pain syndromes, especially angina. Fortunately, other serious causes of abdominal pain with exercise such as mesenteric ischemia, bowel infarction, omental infarction, and hepatic vein thrombosis are rare; however, in the setting of unremitting pain, especially with signs of systemic illness or shock, these conditions need to be considered in the differential and patients referred for potential surgical evaluation.
- Athletes with the typical features of a side stitch should be reassured that this is a benign process and will get better as their conditioning improves. They should be advised against exercise immediately after eating. If an episode of pain does occur, temporarily stopping exercise, stretching the right arm over their head and exhaling through pursed lips can help abort it quickly (Stamford, 1985).

ELEVATED LIVER ENZYMES

- Liver enzyme elevations observed in otherwise asymptomatic long distance runners and other athletes are usually incidental findings. The suspected etiology is an ischemic insult secondary to reduced splanchnic blood flow and oxygen tension during vigorous exercise (Lijnen et al, 1988). Observed increases in *alanine aminotransferase* (ALT), *aspartate aminotransferase* (AST), alkaline phosphatase, creatinine phosphatase, and lactate dehydrogenase are confounded by the fact that these enzymes can be elevated in response to musculoskeletal injury. Hepatocellular injury can be confirmed by measuring glutamate dehydrogenase and *gamma-glutamyl-transferase* (GGT), enzymes more specific to the liver. (www.mamc.amedd.army.mil/referral/guidelines, 1999).
- Since these asymptomatic enzyme abnormalities are often discovered in the convalescent setting, the history and physical should focus on recent training sessions and environmental exposure, evaluating for evidence of a missed heat injury or episode of exertional rhabdomyolysis. The athlete should be

questioned regarding any history of chronic liver disease or alcohol dependence and their medication list reviewed for any potentially hepatotoxic agents. With the nearly ubiquitous use of nutritional supplements, it is crucial to investigate this often-overlooked area.

- The majority of athletes can be reassured that this is a benign process and the enzyme abnormalities usually revert to normal within just 1 week after abstaining from exercise. The first step in the laboratory evaluation is to obtain a repeat liver enzyme panel after abstaining from NSAIDs, alcohol, and exercise for 1 week. If the liver enzymes are elevated at that time, they can be rechecked in 1 month. If the liver enzyme abnormalities persist on serial examinations, further evaluation should start with an iron panel, TIBC, and hepatitis serologies. Second tier tests include ANA titer, antismooth muscle antibody, ceruloplasmin, alpha-1-antitrypsin and serum protein electrophoresis. A right upper quadrant ultrasound is useful to evaluate for fatty liver, cholelithiasis or other obstruction. GI referral should occur for abnormal lab testing, mildly elevated liver enzymes for over 6 months despite a negative evaluation, significantly elevated (AST or ALT >150) without improvement for 2 months, or signs of evolving hepatic insufficiency (www.mamc.amedd.army.mil/referral/ guidelines, 1999).

REFERENCES

Bammer T et al: Five-to eight-year outcome of the first laparoscopic Nissen fundoplications. *J Gastrointest Surg* 16, 2001.

Bardhan KD, et al: Symptomatic gastro-oesophageal reflux disease: Double-blind controlled study of intermittent treatment with omeprazole or ranitidine. *BMJ* 318, 1999.

Bunch T: Blood test abnormalities in runners. *Mayo Clin Proc* 55, 1980.

Cammack J, Read N, et al: Effect of prolonged exercise on the passage of a solid meal through the stomach and small intestine. *Gut* 23, 1982.

Caro JJ, Salas M. Ward A: Healing and relapse rates in gastroesophageal reflux disease treated with the newer proton-pump inhibitors lansoprazole, rabeprazole, and pantoprazole compared with omeprazole, ranitidine, and placebo: evidence from randomized clinical trials. *Clin Therapeutics* 23(7), 2001.

Chilba N et al: Speed of healing and symptom relief in grade II to IV gastroesophageal reflux disease: a meta-analysis. *Gastroenterol* 112, 1997.

Collings KL et al: Esophageal reflux in conditioned runners, cyclists, and weightlifters. *Med Sci Sports Exerc* 35(5), 2003.

Deeks JJ, Smith LA, Bradley, MD: Efficacy, tolerability, and upper gastrointestinal safety of celecoxib for treatment of osteoarthritis and rheumatoid arthritis: Systematic review of randomized controlled trials. *BMJ* 325, 21 Sep 2002.

Fogoros R: Runner's trots. *JAMA* 243, 1980.

Hirschowitz BI: A critical analysis, with appropriate controls of gastric acid and pepsin secretion in clinical esophagitis. *Gastroenterol* 101, 1991.

Kahrilas PJ, Fenerty MB, Joelsson B: High-versus standard-dose ranitidine for control of heartburn in poorly responsive acid reflux disease: A prospective, controlled trial. *Am J Gastroenterol* 94, 1999.

Keefe EB et al: Gastrointestinal symptoms of marathon runners. *West J Med* 41, 1984.

Lauder TD, Moses FM: Recurrent abdominal pain from abdominal adhesions in an endurance triathlete. *Med Sci Sports Exerc* 27(5), 1995.

Lichtenstein DR, Syngal S, Wofe MM: Nonsteroidal anti-inflammatory drugs and the gastrointestinal tract. *Arthritis Rheum* 38(5), 1995.

Lijnen P et al: Indicators of cell breakdown in plasma in men during and after a marathon race. *Int J Sports Med* 9(2), 1988.

Liver enzyme elevation referral guideline. www.mamc.amedd.army.mil/referral/guidelines, 30 September 1999.

Malfertheiner P et al: Current concepts in the management of *Helicobacter pylori* infection—the Maastrict 2-2000 consensus report. *Aliment Pharmacol Ther* 16(2), 2002.

McCabe, ME 3d, et al: Gastrointestinal blood loss associated with running a marathon. *Dig Dis Sci* 31, 1986.

Nilius M, Malfertheiner P: *Helicobacter pylori* enzymes. *Aliment Pharmacol Ther* 10 (Suppl 1), 1996.

Pate R: Principles of training, in Kulund D (ed.): *The injured athlete*. Philadelphia, PA, JB Lippincott, 1988.

Peters HP et al: Gastrointestinal symptoms in long-distance runners, cyclists, and triathletes: Prevalence, medication, and etiology. *Am J Gastroenterol* 94(6), 1999a.

Peters HP et al: Gastrointestinal symptoms during long-distance walking. *Med Sci Sports Exerc* 31, 1999b.

Rehrer N et al: Fluid intake and gastrointestinal problems in runners competing in a 25-km marathon. *Int J Sports Med* 10, 1989.

Richter JE:. Typical and atypical presentations of gastroesophageal reflux disease. *Gastroenterol Clin* 25(1), 1996.

Soffer EE et al: Effect of graded exercise on esophageal motility and gastroesophageal reflux in trained athletes. *Dig Dis Sci* 38, 1993.

Spechler JS: Peptic ulcer disease and its complications, in Feldman M, Friedman LS, Sleisinger MH (eds.): *Sleisenger and Fordtran's Gastrointestinal and Liver Disease*, 7th ed. Philadelphia, PA, Saunders, 2002.

Stamford B: A "stitch" in the side. *Phys Sportsmed* 13, 1985.

Tytgat G et al: Campylobacter-like organism (CLO) in the human stomach. *Gastroenterology* 88, 1985.

Williams MP et al: A placebo-controlled trial to assess the effects of 8 days of dosing with rabeprazole versus omeprazole on 24-hour intragastric acidity and plasma gastrin concentrations in young healthy male subjects. *Aliment Pharmacol Ther* 12, 1998.

Wysowski KD, Bacsanyi J: Cisapride and fatal arrhythmia. [letter] *N Engl J Med* 335, 1996.

36 PULMONARY

Carrie A Jaworski, MD

INTRODUCTION

- Patients with pulmonary disorders can benefit greatly from exercise when their disease process is under proper control.
- Awareness of when and when not to participate as well as the ability to use pharmacologic agents and environmental controls greatly enhances one's ability to participate safely.

ASTHMA

- Asthma is a pulmonary disorder characterized by chronic inflammation of the airways leading to bronchial hyperreactivity. While in the past, asthmatics were discouraged from exercise, today it is recognized that regular exercise can reduce airway reactivity and decrease medication use (Disabella and Sherman, 1998).
- Approximately 17 million adults and 5 million children in the United States have chronic asthma (NIH, 1997).
- The National Heart, Lung, and Blood Institute (NHLBI) has set forth guidelines on the diagnosis and management of asthma in an effort known as the National Asthma Education and Prevention Program (NAEPP). This program is evidence-based and routinely updates its recommendations based on the newest research. See NHLBI website for most recent recommendations @www.NHLBI.org.

DIAGNOSIS OF ASTHMA

- History or presence of episodic symptoms of airflow obstruction such as wheezing, chest tightness, shortness of breath, or cough. Absence of symptoms at time of examination does not exclude diagnosis.
- Airflow obstruction needs to be at least partially reversible demonstrated through the use of spirometry. First establish airflow obstruction: FEV_1 <80% predicted and FEV_1/FVC <65% or below the lower limit of normal. Then establish reversibility by an FEV_1 increase of ≥12% and at least 200 mL after using a short-acting inhaled beta2-agonist. (FEV_1 = Forced expiratory volume in 1 s; FVC = Forced vital capacity) (NIH, 1997).

TABLE 36-1 Stepwise Approach for Managing Asthma in Adults and Children Older Than 5 Years of Age

Goals of Asthma Treatment

- Prevent chronic and troublesome symptoms (e.g., coughing or breathlessness in the night, in the early morning, or after exertion)
- Maintain (near) normal pulmonary function
- Maintain normal activity levels (including exercise and other physical activity)
- Prevent recurrent exacerbations of asthma and minimize the need for emergency department visits or hospitalizations
- Provide optimal pharmacotherapy with minimal or no adverse effects
- Meet patients and families expectations of and satisfaction with asthma care

Classify Severity of Asthma

Clinical Features Before Treatment*

	Symptoms**	Nighttime Symptoms	Lung Function
Step 4 Severe persistent	• Continual symptoms • Limited physical activity • Frequent exacerbations	Frequent	• FEV_1 or PEF ≤60% predicted • PEF variability >30%
Step 3 Moderate persistent	• Daily symptoms • Daily use of inhaled short-acting beta$_2$-agonist • Exacerbations affect activity • Exacerbations ≥2 times a week; may last days	>1 time a week	• FEV_1 or PEF >60%–≤80% predicted • PEF variability >30%
Step 2 Mild persistent	• Symptoms >2 times a week but <1 time a day • Exacerbations may affect activity	>2 times a month	• FEV_1 or PEF ≥80% predicted • PEF variability 20–30%
Step 1 Mild Intermittent	• Symptoms ≤2 times a week • Asymptomatic and normal PEF between exacerbations • Exacerbations brief (from a few hours to a few days); intensity may vary	≤2 times a month	• FEV_1 or PEF ≥80% predicted • PEF variability <20%

*The presence of one of the features of severity is sufficient to place a patient in that category. An individual should be assigned to the most severe grade in which any feature occurs. The characteristics noted in this figure are general and may overlap because asthma is highly variable. Furthermore, an individual s classification may change over time.

**Patients at any level of severity can have mild, moderate, or severe exacerbations. Some patients with intermittent asthma experience severe and life-threatening exacerbations separated by long periods of normal lung function and no symptoms.

- Must exclude other diagnoses such as vocal cord dysfunction, vascular rings, and reflux disease, if spirometry is normal.
- Classification of asthma severity is based on history and spirometry (see Table 36-1)
- Management should focus on patient education, environmental control, and objective monitoring.
- **Patient education:** Patients and their families should understand signs and symptoms of an asthma exacerbation, the chronicity of the disease, and potential triggers of an attack. A written plan should be reviewed and instruction on proper use of inhaled medications and peak flow monitoring should be provided.
- **Environmental control:** Avoidance of exposure to precipitating factors is paramount. Potential triggers include, pollen, mold, ozone, exercise, and cold air. Athletes should exercise indoors on bad weather days, or use measures such as masks to decrease chance of attack. Indoor swimming is considered an excellent option secondary to the warm, moist environment at the pool.
- **Monitoring:** Athletes need to be monitoring their peak flows on a daily basis to recognize decline in function as well as response to treatment. Formal spirometry is recommended for initial diagnosis, after treatment and peak flows have stabilized, and then every 1 to 2 years when asthma is stable, more often when unstable (Consensus Guideline, Expert opinion NHLBI).
- Pharmacologic therapy should be instituted to control inflammation and treat episodes of bronchoconstriction. Use a stepwise approach to treatment as outlined in Table 36-2.

MEDICATION CLASSES

ANTI-INFLAMMATORIES

- Inhaled glucocorticoids are the mainstay of treatment in moderate to severe asthma. Must be taken on a regular basis, therefore not useful as a rescue medication. Side effects can include local irritation, dysphonia, and oral candidiasis. Systemic forms may be needed in asthma flares and cases recalcitrant to inhaled glucocorticoids.

- Khellin derivatives, cromolyn sodium (Intal), and nedocromil sodium (Tilade) act to stabilize mast cells thus preventing the release of inflammatory mediators. Both are inhaled medications and are for preventive use. Cromolyn has no significant side effects, and is approved for children of age 5 and up. It may take 3 to 4 weeks for full clinical benefit (Smith and MacKnight, 1998). Nedocromil becomes effective in 3 to 4 days, but can cause headache, cough, and bitter taste. It is approved in children over age 6.

TABLE 36-2   Stepwise Approach for Managing Asthma in Adults and Children Older Than 5 Years of Age: Treatment

	Long-Term Control	Quick Relief	Education
Step 4 Severe persistent	Daily medications: • Anti-inflammatory: inhaled corticosteroid (high dose) And • Long-acting bronchodilator: either long-acting inhaled beta$_2$-agonist, sustained-release theophylline, or long-acting beta$_2$-agonist tablets And • Corticosteroid tablets or syrup long term (make repeat attempts to reduce systemic steroids and maintain control with high dose inhaled steroids)	• Short-acting bronchodilator: inhaled beta$_2$-agonists as needed for symptoms. • Intensity of treatment will depend on severity of exacerbation; see component 3-Managing Exacerbations. • Use of short-acting inhaled beta$_2$-agonists on a daily basis, or increasing use, indicates the need for additional long-term-control therapy.	Steps 2 and 3 actions plus: • Refer to individual education/counseling
Step 3 Moderate persistent	Daily medication: Either • Anti-inflammatory: inhaled corticosteroid (medium dose) Or • Inhaled corticosteroid (low-medium dose) and add a long-acting bronchodilator, especially for nighttime symptoms; either long-acting inhaled beta$_2$-agonist, sustained-release thephylline, or long-acting beta$_2$-agonist tablets. If needed • Anti-inflammatory: inhaled corticosteroids (medium-high dose) And • Long-acting bronchodilator, especially for nighttime symptoms; either long-acting inhaled beta$_2$-agonist, sustained-release theophylline, or long-acting beta$_2$-agonist tablets.	• Short-acting bronchodilator: inhaled beta$_2$-agonists as needed for symptoms. • Intensity of treatment will depend on severity of exacerbation; see component 3-Managing Exacerbations. • Use of short-acting inhaled beta$_2$-agonists on a daily basis, or increasing use, indicates the need for additional long-term-control therapy.	Step 1 actions plus: • Teach self-monitoring • Refer to group education if available • Review and update self-management plan

(Continued)

TABLE 36-2   (*Continued*)

	Long-Term Control	Quick Relief	Education
Step 2 Mild persistent	One daily medication: • Anti-inflammatory: either inhaled corticosteroid (low doses) or cromolyn or nedocromil (children usually begin with a trial of cromolyn or nedocromil). • Sustained-release theophylline to serum concentration of 5–15 mcg/mL is an alternative, but not preferred, therapy. Zafirlukast of zileuton may also be considered for patients ≥12 years of age, although their position in therapy is not fully established.	• Short-acting bronchodilator: inhaled beta$_2$-agonists as needed for symptoms. • Intensity of treatment will depend on severity of exacerbation; see component 3-Managing Exacerbations. • Use of short-acting inhaled beta$_2$-agonists on a daily basis, or increasing use, indicates the need for additional long-term-control therapy.	Step 1 actions plus: • Teach self-monitoring • Refer to group education if available • Review and update self-management plan
Step 1 Mild intermittent	• No daily medication needed.	• Short-acting bronchodilator: inhaled beta$_2$-agonists as needed for symptoms. • Intensity of treatment will depend on severity of exacerbation; see component 3-Managing Exacerbations. • Use of short-acting inhaled beta$_2$-agonists more than 2 times a week may indicate the need to initiate long-term-control therapy.	• Teach basic facts about asthma • Teach inhaler/spacer/holding chamber technique • Discuss roles of medications • Develop self-management plan • Develop action plan for when and how to take rescue actions, especially for patients with a history of severe exacerbations • Discuss appropriate environmental control measures to avoid exposure to known allergens and irritants (see component 4)

Step down	**Step up**
Review treatment every 1 to 6 months; a gradual stepwise reduction in treatment may be possible.	If control is not maintained, consider step up. First, review patient medication technique, adherence, and environmental control (avoidance of allergens or other factors that contribute to asthma severity).

Note:
• The stepwise approach presents general guidelines to assist clinical decisionmaking; it is not intended to be a specific prescription. Asthma is highly variable; clinicians should tailor specific medication plans to the needs and circumstances of individual patients.
• Gain control as quickly as possible; then decrease treatment to the least medication necessary to maintain control. Gaining control may be accomplished by either starting treatment at the step most appropriate to the initial severity of the condition or starting at a higher level of therapy (e.g., a course of systemic corticosteroids or higher dose of inhaled corticosteroids).
• A rescue course of systemic corticosteroids may be needed at any time and at any step.
• Some patients with intermittent asthma experience severe and life-threatening exacerbations separated by long periods of normal lung function and no symptoms.
• This may be especially common with exacerbations provoked by respiratory infections. A short course of systemic corticosteroids is recommended.
• At each step, patients should control their environment to avoid or control factors that make their asthma worse (e.g., allergens, irritants); this requires specific diagnosis and education.
• Referral to an asthma specialist for consultation of comanagement is *recommended* if there are difficulties achieving or maintaining control of asthma or if the patient requires step 4 care. Referral may be *considered* if the patient requires step 3 care (see also component 1-Initial Assessment and Diagnosis).

ANTILEUKOTRIENES
• Leukotrienes are potent bronchoconstrictors and inflammatory mediators. Antileukotrienes block this effect in one of two ways. Zileuton (Zyflo) blocks the synthesis of leukotrienes, while zafirlukast (Accolate) and montelukast (Singulair) are leukotriene-receptor antagonists that block the effects of leukotrienes after they are formed. All three medications decrease airway inflammation and offer a more rapid onset of action than other anti-inflammatory medications.

Montelukast and zafirlukast are approved in children, have a favorable safety profile, and are taken orally qd or bid. Zileuton is not approved in children <12-year old, requires qid dosing and monitoring of hepatic function (Nathan and Spector, 1999).

MEDICATIONS

BRONCHODILATORS

- **Short-Acting B2-agonists:** Inhaled albuterol is the main rescue medication for acute bronchoconstriction. Inhaled forms have a good safety profile with primarily mild *central nervous system* (CNS) side effects. Medication has an immediate effect, and is, therefore, subject to overuse. Overuse can also lead to decreases in efficacy and increased bronchial hyperreactivity (Bhagat, Kalra, and Swystun, 1995). Oral forms are not approved for use by the Olympics or National Collegiate Athletic Association (NCAA).
- **Long-Acting B2-agonists:** Salmeterol (Serevent) has a duration of action of 12 h and is useful in assisting with long-term control. Not intended to be used as a rescue medication.
- **Anticholinergics:** Ipratropium bromide (Atrovent) is a bronchodilator used more often in patients with *chronic obstructive pulmonary disease* (COPD). It can be an adjunct for patients who have an inadequate response to β2-agonists. The duration of action is 3 to 4 h with an onset of 30 to 90 min.
- Use caution when prescribing medications to collegiate, professional, and elite athletes. Always check with the sport's governing body in regards to banned substances. U. S. Olympic Committee has an up-to-date list available through their website @www.usantidoping.org or call their drug control hotline 1-800-233-0393.
- Once asthma is well controlled, exercise should be encouraged. Studies have demonstrated decreased numbers of exacerbations, less medication use, and fewer missed days of work/school in asthmatics who exercised (Cochrane and Clark, 1990; Szentagothai et al, 1987).
- Normal ranges of ventilation, work capacity, blood pressure, and maximal heart rate are exhibited in asthmatics that are well conditioned and have their disease under control (Bundgaard, 1985).
- The exercise presciption should include a preexercise assessment to document control. FEV_1 should be ≥80% of expected levels (Disabella and Sherman, 1998). The exercise goal should be consistent with the American College of Sports Medicine's recommendation to exercise on most days of the week for 20 to 30 min (American College of Sports Medicine, 1998). The type of exercise can be anything that the patient enjoys, but should provide aerobic benefit as well as strength and flexibility conditioning.

- Advise caution on risky activities such as exercising outside on a cold day, when wheezing or when peak flows suggest a decline in lung function, as exercise can trigger symptoms of bronchoconstriction. (See exercise-induced bronchospasm section below.)

EXERCISE-INDUCED BRONCHOSPASM

- *Exercise-induced bronchospasm* (EIB) is defined as the transitory increase in airway resistance that typically occurs following vigorous exercise. EIB will usually resolve spontaneously.
- EIB is found in 12–15% of the general population (Randolph, Randolph, and Fraser, 1991; Rupp, Guill, and Brudno, 1992). Ninety percent of patients with chronic asthma and 40% of patients with allergic rhinitis or atopic dermatitis will have EIB (Feinstein et al, 1996).
- The prevalence of EIB in athletes varies by sport with ranges between 12 and 55% (Langdeau and Boulet, 2001) and occurs in amateur to elite level athletes. Higher risk sports include those with high minute ventilation such as basketball, track, and soccer as well as those in cool, dry air such as cross-country skiing, ice skating, and hockey.
- The pathophysiology of EIB remains debatable. Two main theories exist:
- The *water loss theory* attributes EIB to the loss of water through the bronchial mucosa as the body tries to warm rapidly inhaled air during exercise. This dries the mucosa and causes local changes in pH, osmolarity, and the temperature of the airway, which may trigger bronchoconstriction (Storms, 1999).
- The *thermal expenditure theory* holds that EIB is the result of respiratory heat loss that occurs during exercise. The increased ventilation of exercise causes a cooling of the airways. Once exercise ceases, the blood vessels dilate and engorge to rewarm the epithelium, which may lead to rebound hyperemia and bronchoconstriction (Storms, 1999).

PRESENTATION

- Clinical symptoms may include coughing, wheezing, chest tightness, or shortness of breath during or after intense exercise. Atypical symptoms can include stomach cramps, chest pain, nausea, headache, or feeling out of shape. Examination during an attack may demonstrate increased respiratory rate, prolonged expiration, decreased breath sounds, and wheezing. Some athletes may describe a late-response 6 to 8 h after the onset of exercise. This occurs in ~30% of patients with EIB, and is more frequently seen in children (Lacroix, 1999).

DIAGNOSIS

- The diagnosis of EIB is often based on history and self-reported symptoms. Numerous studies have demonstrated that this approach is unreliable (Tikkanen and Peltonen, 1999; Rice et al, 1985; Thole et al, 2001). Tikkanen *et al* found that only 61% of athletes with a positive field exercise challenge had reported symptoms, while 45% of athletes with a negative field test did report symptoms (Rice et al, 1985). More reliable diagnosis is based on pulmonary function testing after a thorough history and physical examination has ruled out any other explanation of the symptoms.
- Office spirometry should be done at rest to rule out underlying chronic asthma in anyone suspected of having EIB. A normal resting test with suspicion of EIB warrants a bronchoprovocation test. Many physicians will give a trial of a prophylactic bronchodilator if classic history and mild symptoms exist.
- Options for confirming EIB include direct and indirect challenge tests.
- Direct challenge testing involves administration of increasing doses of a pharmacologic agent, such as methacholine, to cause bronchoconstriction. These tests are highly sensitive, but have a poor specificity for EIB (Anderson, 1997).

INDIRECT CHALLENGE TESTS

EXERCISE CHALLENGE TEST
- Performed either in a laboratory or in the field, this test seeks to simulate the athlete's sport in order to provoke EIB. Formal pulmonary function tests are done with FEV_1 being the index most often measured in the lab versus *peak expiratory flow rate* (PEFR) in the field. Solitary EIB will have a preexercise baseline FEV_1 or PEFR between 80 and 100% of normal predicted values. The exercise is most commonly free or treadmill running for 5 to 8 min at a high intensity ($\geq$85–90% maximum predicted heart rate). FEV_1 or PEFR is measured at 1-, 3-, 5-, 10-, and 15-min intervals. Positive test = a fall in FEV_1 or PEFR of 15%. Mild EIB = 15 to 25% drop, moderate EIB = 25 to 40% drop, and severe EIB = more than a 40% drop (Smith and MacKnight, 1998).
- Field testing offers the advantage of more closely mimicking actual sport, but can be difficult to control environmental factors as well as hard to control/monitor rate of exertion (Eliasson et al, 1992).
- Laboratory testing is more costly and eliminates possible contributing environmental triggers. Offers advantage of controlled cardiovascular workload and ability to monitor pulmonary and cardiovascular function during exercise (Rundell et al, 2000).
- Other indirect challenge tests include the *eucapnic voluntary hyperventilation* (EVH) challenge test, the hyperosmolar saline challenge test, and the mannitol challenge test. These tests offer promise in difficult to diagnose and elite athletes, but are not readily available other than at research centers (Holzer, Brukner, Douglass, 2002).
- **Pharmacologic treatments** (Also see asthma section above): A variety of agents are available to treat EIB. Treatment should be tailored to the individual athlete and his or her sport.

BETA-AGONISTS
- First-line therapy is usually with an inhaled short-acting beta-agonist, such as albuterol, 2–4 puffs taken 15 to 30 min prior to activity. Albuterol's onset of action is $\leq$5 min and duration of effect is ~2–6 h. It is 90% effective (Lemanske and Henke, 1989). All athletes with EIB should carry a short-acting beta-agonist inhaler with them during exercise to relieve acute exacerbations that occur despite prophylaxis. The long acting beta-agonist, salmeterol, lasts 12 h and should be considered in athletes involved in endurance/all day events as well as in children where activity is unpredictable. It needs to be taken at least 1 h before exercise, but preferably more than 4 h before activity (Tan and Spector, 1998). Usual duration of action is 12 h, but with regular bid use, effect can wane after 9 h (Nelson et al, 1998). This effect can be counteracted if combined with an inhaled steroid.

MAST-CELL STABILIZERS
- Cromolyn sodium blocks late phase EIB while nedocromil sodium blocks immediate and late phase EIB. Both should be administered as 2–4 puffs 20 min prior to exercise. The duration of action is ~2 h. They are ~70–85% effective (Smith and LaBotz, 1998). Not to be used to treat acute symptoms, but useful for repeated bouts of exercise as they have minimal/no side effects. Combining with beta-agonists does not appear to be better than beta-agonist alone (Smith and LaBotz, 1998).
- **Inhaled corticosteroids:** Steroids are not effective when used as prophylaxis prior to exercise. Studies show decreased airway responsiveness to exercise after 4 weeks of inhaled corticosteroids (Henriksen and Dahl, 1983; Waalkans et al, 1993). Based on the potential for side effects, corticosteroids should be reserved for those patients refractory to beta-agonists or mast-cell stabilizers. This lack of response should also prompt reevaluation for chronic asthma.

ANTILEUKOTRIENES

- This class offers the advantage of oral administration and long duration of action. Both montelukast and zafirlukast have demonstrated an immediate protective effect against EIB (Leff et al, 1998). Montelukast is 10 mg daily in adults and 5 mg in 6–14-year old children. It has a 3–4-h onset of action and duration of 24 h. Zafirlukast is 20 mg bid in adults and 10 mg bid in children 5–11-year old. It has an onset of action of 30 min and duration of 12 h. Zileuton is 600 mg qid in adults and children ≥12. It has an onset of 30 min to 2 h and duration of 5–8 h.

IPRATROPIUM

- This drug has limited usefulness in preventing EIB.
- **Nonpharmacologic treatments:** The use of masks or scarves to decrease the amount of heat and water lost with exercise in cold weather may diminish EIB.
- Aerobic conditioning may reduce severity of EIB by improving rate of ventilation during exercise, but no proof it prevents EIB (Cochrane and Clark, 1990; Holzer, Brukner, and Douglass, 2002).
- Appropriate cool downs help decrease EIB. Cooling down helps by allowing gradual rewarming of the airways which decreases vascular dilation and edema.
- **Refractory period:** Defined as the time after spontaneous recovery from an episode of EIB where >50% of athletes will not experience another episode of bronchoconstriction with exercise. Effect is usually 1 to 2 h in duration. Can benefit athletes who experience this effect in that they can induce a refractory period prior to their actual competition to lessen the severity of EIB during their event. Various methods exist to induce the effect, including 20 to 30 min of low-intensity exercise or seven 30-s sprints separated by short intervals (Disabella and Sherman, 1998; Holzer, Brukner, and Douglass, 2002). Recent studies demonstrate that a continuous low-intensity warm-up is more beneficial than interval training to decrease risk of EIB (McKenzie, McLuckie, and Stirling, 1994). Studies also demonstrate that this effect is inhibited with use of nonsteroidal anti-inflammatories (O'Byrne and Jones, 1986; Margolskee, Bigby, and Boushey, 1988; Wilson, Bar-Or, and O'Byrne, 1994). Athletes should be counseled to still use their prescribed EIB medications, as effect is partial for most people (Storms and Joyner, 1997).

CHRONIC OBSTRUCTIVE PULMONARY DISEASE

- Chronic obstructive pulmonary disease is a progressive disease that primarily refers to emphysema and chronic bronchitis. It is a condition of slowly deteriorating pulmonary function whereby expiratory airflow obstruction leads to dyspnea and deconditioning. While exercise cannot reverse the process, it can provide improvements in quality of life and decreased disability (Mink, 1997).
- Approximately 15–25 million Americans are afflicted with COPD. It is responsible for 200,000 deaths annually and is a major cause of disability (Shayevutz and Shayevitz, 1986).
- The primary cause is chronic tobacco use, but other etiologies such as alpha1-antitrypsin deficiency and environmental exposures do play a role.
- The pathophysiology of COPD is multifactorial. Airway hyperreactivity and/or increased respiratory secretions lead to chronic obstruction. This results in air trapping and respiratory muscle dysfunction, which, over time, causes generalized deconditioning. Additionally, the emphysematous component causes destruction of alveolar capillary membranes, which leads to hypoxemia. Chronic hypoxemia results in pulmonary hypertension and right ventricular failure (Smith and MacKnight, 1998).
- Severe limitations in respiratory function and chronic hypoxemia cause great fear and anxiety in COPD patients. This can result in fear of exercise and further deconditioning (Casaburi, 1993).
- Our role as sports medicine physicians is to enable COPD patients to exercise comfortably and safely. The most dramatic improvements in function are often the most severely compromised (Mink, 1997).
- **Evaluation:** Prior to providing an exercise prescription, patients must have an assessment of their current status through a physical examination and pulmonary function testing. One can expect reductions in FEV_1 and increased ventilatory muscle effort.
- A careful assessment of cardiac risk and exercise capacity including exercise testing is recommended for all patients (Mink, 1997). Many protocols exist for both treadmill and stationary cycle testing. Exercise testing can help to determine safe levels of exercise to prevent arrhythmias and hypoxemia, the amount of supplemental oxygen needed during exercise and any need for bronchodilators.
- **Management:** The care of the COPD patient is aimed at maintaining, or improving, the functional capacity through a multidisciplinary approach.
- **Exercise:** Studies demonstrate that exercise improves dyspnea, provides an aerobic training response, reduces ventilation, and improves overall exercise tolerance (Casaburi et al, 1991; O'Donnel, Webb, and McGuire, 1993; Reardon et al, 1994). No evidence exists that exercise lengthens life expectancy in the COPD patient, but it provides immense physical and psychologic benefits.

- Supervised exercise through a rehabilitation program is warranted if patient has significant disease. Most can graduate to independent exercise within 6 weeks (Mink, 1997).
- Independent exercise goal should be to exercise 3 days a week at 60 to 80% of maximal heart rate for 20 to 30 min. Type of exercise will vary based on patient's ability and comorbidities. Stationary cycling is useful initially as many patients are unsteady on their feet and arm ergometry can be used for those with lower extremity limitations. These goals may take months to reach, if at all. Start with several minutes of exercise and progress at a rate appropriate for the individual (Mink, 1997).
- Exercise aids can include supplemental oxygen and medications. Bronchodilators and anticholinergics are the mainstay of pharmacologic therapy in COPD and should be used aggressively. Mucolytics can assist with excessive secretions. Inhaled corticosteroids can also assist in decreasing airway inflammation. Oral corticosteroids are reserved for more severe cases, and theophylline remains a controversial therapy.
- Bronchopulmonary toilet and pursed lip breathing are two other mechanical techniques that can aid COPD patients in achieving activity goals.
- Careful attention to preventive health care such as influenza and polyvalent pneumococcal immunizations can help COPD patients avoid setbacks in their exercise programs and enhance overall well-being.

CYSTIC FIBROSIS

- *Cystic fibrosis* (CF) is an autosomal recessive disorder that affects multiple organ systems, including the pulmonary, gastrointestinal, reproductive, and skeletal systems as well as the sweat glands. Chronic pulmonary disease is the leading cause of morbidity and mortality as the thick mucus found with CF leads to infection as well as inhibits pulmonary function. Aerobic exercise has been shown to aid in the clearance of secretions and improve quality of life in patients with CF.
- Diagnosis of CF is made by an abnormal sweat chloride test. Prenatal screening is now available and should be offered to couples at higher risk, particularly those of Northern European descent. Pulmonary function tests are similar to an asthmatic, but also demonstrate a decreased *forced vital capacity* (FVC).
- Management of CF is dependent on the extent of disease. A goal of preventing recurrent respiratory infections is attempted through chest physiotherapy, bronchodilators, and antibiotics. Corticosteroids,

oxygen, recombinant deoxyribonuclease I, and possibly lung transplantation in advanced cases may also be warranted.
- Exercise can augment mobilization of secretions when combined with chest physiotherapy (Thomas, Cook, and Brooks, 1995). A study also demonstrated less loss of FVC compared to controls (Schneiderman-Walker et al, 2000). In mild forms of CF, athletes should be allowed to participate as their pulmonary function allows. Moderate to severe cases of CF benefit from more formal rehabilitation programs where the need for supplemental oxygen can be tracked.
- All athletes with CF need to be counseled on safe exercise in the heat, as they are subject to increased sodium and chloride losses in their sweat when compared to those without CF.

RESPIRATORY INFECTIONS

- Respiratory tract infections are one of the most common medical problems encountered in the care of athletes (Hanley, 1976). *Upper respiratory tract infections* (URIs) comprise the majority of these infections.
- Immune function affects avoidance and occurrence of URIs. Studies demonstrate moderate exercise can protect against URIs, while intense exercise can decrease immunity and increase the risk of URIs (Smith and MacKnight, 1998; Nieman, 1994).
- Prevention of URIs can be augmented through avoidance of overtraining, adequate sleep, proper nutrition, and limiting stress. Influenza vaccination of athletes in winter sports should be considered.
- Treatment of URIs is primarily symptomatic. Nasal ipratropium bromide and oral/topical decongestants can be helpful short-term. Caution must be exercised with antihistamines in athletes as they can impair temperature regulation and cause sedation. Inhaled beta-agonists can help with URI-associated coughs. Antibiotics are only indicated if progression to a secondary bacterial infection occurs. Zinc and vitamin C may reduce the duration of URI symptoms (Hemila, 1994; Mossad et al, 1996).
- Athletes with a common cold can continue to participate to a lesser degree provided no fever is present. Care should be taken to increase hydration and cease activity if constitutional symptoms occur, such as fever, myalgias, productive cough, vomiting, or diarrhea.
- Progression to diseases such as pneumonia and complicated bronchitis warrant up to 10–14 days of rest before resuming full activity.

REFERENCES

American College of Sports Medicine: ACSM's Position stand on the recommended quantity and quality of exercise for developing and maintaining cardiorespiratory and muscular fitness, and flexibility in healthy adults. *Med Sci Sports Exerc*–30(6): 975–991, 1998.

Anderson SD: Exercise-induced asthma, in Kay AB (ed.): *Allergy and Allergic Diseases*. Boston, MA, Blackwell Scientific, 1997, pp 692–711.

Bhagat R, Kalra S, Swystun A: Rapid onset of tolerance to the bronchoprotective effect of salmeterol. *Chest* 108:1235–1239, 1995.

Bundgaard A: Exercise and the asthmatic. *Sport Med* 2(4):254–266, 1985.

Casaburi R: Exercise training in chronic obstructive lung disease, in Casaburi R, Petty TL (eds.): *Principles and Practice of Pulmonary Rehabilitation*. Philadelphia, PA, Saunders, pp 204–224.

Casaburi R, Patessio A, Ioli F, et al: Reductions in exercise lactic acidosis and ventilation as a result of exercise training in patients with obstructive lung disease. *Am Rev Respir Dis* 143(1):9–18, 1991.

Cochrane LM, Clark CJ: Benefits and problems of a physical training programme for asthmatic patients. *Thorax* 45(5):345–351, 1990.

Disabella V, Sherman C: Exercise for asthma patients: little risk, big rewards. *Phys Sportsmed* 26(6):75–85, 1998.

Eliasson AH, Phillips YY, Rajagopal KR, et al: Sensitivity and specificity of bronchial provocation testing. An evaluation of four techniques in exercise-induced bronchospasm. *Chest* 102:347–355, 1992.

Feinstein RA, LaRussa J, Wang-Dohlman A, et al: Screening adolescent athletes for exercise-induced asthma. *Clin J Sport Med* 6(2):119–123, 1996.

Hanley DF: Medical care of the US Olympic team. *JAMA* 236(2): 147–148, 1976.

Hemila H: Does vitamin C alleviate the symptoms of the common cold? A review of current evidence. *Scand J Infect Dis* 26(1): 1–6, 1994.

Henriksen JM, Dahl R: Effects of inhaled budesonide alone and in combination with a low dose terbutaline in children with execise-induced asthma. *Am Rev Respir Dis* 128:993–997, 1983.

Holzer K, Brukner P, Douglass J: Evidence-based management of exercise-induced asthma. *Curr Sports Med Rep* 1:86–92, 2002.

Lacroix VJ: Exercise-induced asthma. *Phys Sportmed* 27(12), 1999.

Langdeau JB, Boulet LP: Prevalence and mechanism of development of asthma and airway hyperresponsiveness in athletes. *Sports Med* 31:601–616, 2001.

Leff JA, Busse WW, Pearlman D, et al: Montelukast, a leukotriene antagonist for the treatment of mild asthma and exercise-induced bronchoconstriction. *N Engl J Med* 339:147–152, 1998.

Lemanske RF, Jr, Henke KG: Exercise-induced asthma, in Gisolfi C, Lamb DR (eds.): *Youth, Exercise and Sport: Perspectives in Exercise Science and Sports Medicine*, vol. 2. Indianapolis, Benchmark Press, 1989, pp 465–511.

Margolskee DJ, Bigby BG, Boushey HA: Indomethacin blocks airway tolerance to repetitive exercise but not to eucapnic hyperpnoea in asthmatic subjects. *Am Rev Respir Dis* 137:842–846, 1988.

McKenzie DC, McLuckie SL, Stirling DR: The protective effects of continuous and interval exercise in athletes with exercise-induced asthma. *Med Sci Sports Exerc* 26:951–956, 1994.

Mink, BD: Exercise and chronic obstructive pulmonary disease: Modest fitness gains pay big dividends. *Phys Sportsmed* 25(11), 1997.

Mossad SB, Macknin ML, Medendorp SV, et al: Zinc gluconate lozenges for treating the common cold. *Ann Intern Med* 125(2):81–88, 1996.

Nathan RA, Spector SL (eds.): Asthma 2000: The role of antileukotrienes in clinical practice. Asthma 2000 Monograph Series, Western Region Monograph, Deerfield, IL, Discovery International, 1999, pp 1–52.

Nelson JA, Strauss L, Skowronski M, et al: Effect of long-term salmeterol treatment on exercise-induced asthma. *N Engl J Med* 339(3):141–146, 1998.

Nieman DC: Exercise, upper respiratory infection, and the immune system. *Med Sci Sport Exerc* 26(2):128–139, 1994.

NIH: Highlights of the expert panel report 2: Guidelines for the diagnosis and management of asthma, *National Institutes of Health publication No. 97–4051A*. Bethesda, MD, National Institutes of Health, National Heart, Lung, and Blood Institute, May 1997.

O'Byrne PM, Jones GL: The effect of indomethacin on exercise-induced bronchoconstriction and refractoriness after exercise. *Am Rev Respir Dis* 134:69–72, 1986.

O'Donnel DE, Webb KA, McGuire MA: Older patients with COPD: benefits of exercise training. *Geriatrics* 48(1):59–66, 1993.

Randolph C, Randolph M, Fraser B: Exercise-induced asthma in school children. *J Allergy Clin Immunol* 87:341, 1991.

Reardon J, Awad E, Normandin E, et al: The effect of comprehensive outpatient pulmonary rehabilitation on dyspnea. *Chest* 105(4)1046–1052, 1994.

Rice SG, Bierman CW, Shapiro GG, et al: Identification of exercise-induced asthma among intercollegiate athletes. *Ann Allergy* 55:790–793, 1985.

Rundell KW, Wilber RL, Szmedra L, et al: Exercise-induced asthma screening of elite athletes: fileds versus laboratory exercise challenge. *Med Sci Sports Exerc* 32(2):309–316, 2000.

Rupp NT, Guill MF, Brudno DS: Unrecognized exercise-induced bronchospasm in adolescent athletes. *Am J Dis Child* 146:941–944, 1992.

Schneiderman-Walker J, Pollock SL, Corey M, et al: A randomized controlled trial of a 3-year home exercise program in cystic fibrosis. *J Pediatr* 136:304, 2000.

Shayevutz MB, Shayevitz BR: Athletic training in chronic obstructive pulmonary disease. *Clin Sports Med* 5 (3):471–491, 1986.

Smith BW, LaBotz M: Pharmacologic treatment of exercise-induced asthma. *Clin Sports Med* 17(2):343–363, 1998.

Smith BW, MacKnight JM: Pulmonary, in Safran MR, McKeag DB, VanCamp SP (eds.): *Manual of Sports Medicine.* Philadelphia, PA, Lippincott-Raven, 1998, pp 244–254.

Storms WW: Exercise-induced asthma: diagnosis and treatment for the recreational or elite athlete. *Med Sci Sports Exerc* 31(suppl 1):S33–S38, 1999.

Storms WW, Joyner DM: Update on exercise-induced asthma: A report of the Olympic Exercise Asthma Summit Conference. *Phys Sportsmed* 25(3):45–55, 1997.

Szentagothai K, Gyene I, Szocska M, et al: Physical exercise program for children with bronchial asthma. *Pediatr Pulmonol* 3(3):166–172, 1987.

Tan RA, Spector SL: Exercise-induced asthma. *Sport Med* 25(1):1–6, 1998.

Thole RT, Sallis RE, Rubin AL, et al: Exercise-induced bronchospasm prevalence in collegiate cross-country runners. *Med Sci Sports Exerc* 33(10):1641–1646.

Thomas J, Cook DJ, Brooks D: Chest physical therapy management of patients with cystic fibrosis: A meta-analysis. *Am J Respir Crit Care Med* 151:846, 1995.

Tikkanen HO, Peltonen JE: Asthma-cross-country skiing. *Med Sci Sports Exerc* 31(5) (suppl): S99, 1999.

Waalkans HJ, van-essen-Zandvliet EEM, Gerritsen J, et al, and the Dutch CNSLD Study Group: The effect of an inhaled corticosteroid (budesonide) on exercise-induced asthma in children. *Eur Resp J* 6:523–526, 1993.

Wilson BA, Bar-Or O, O'Byrne PM: The effects of indomethacin on refractoriness following exercise both with and without bronchoconstriction. *Eur Respir J* 12:2174–2178, 1994.

37 ALLERGIC DISEASES IN ATHLETES

David L Brown, MD
David D Haight, MD
Linda L Brown, MD

INTRODUCTION

- Allergic rhinitis alone affects over 40 million Americans (American Academy of Allergy, Asthma and Immunology, 2003). It is the fifth most common chronic disease and the most prevalent in patients under 18 years of age (Public Health Service, 1997).
- Urticaria and angioedema affect 20–30% of the population during their lifetime (Kaplan, 2002).
- Approximately 20,000–50,000 patients with anaphylaxis present for medical care in the United States each year, resulting in 400–1000 deaths (Neugut, Ghalak, and Miller, 2001).

ALLERGIC RHINITIS

- Allergic rhinitis occurs when an individual develops IgE sensitization to aeroallergens. Inhalation of the aeroallergens leads to mast cell activation and release of histamine and other chemical mediators of inflammation.
- Common symptoms include—rhinorrhea, post-nasal drip, congestion, sneezing, cough, and pruritus of the nasal and soft palate. Patients may complain of generalized irritability and fatigue. Eye pruritus, injection, irritation, and watery discharge may indicate coexisting allergic conjunctivitis.
- Symptoms recur on exposure to any aeroallergen to which a patient is sensitized.
- Spring and early summer exacerbations occur with tree and grass pollination. Late summer and fall symptoms are usually because of weeds and mold. Indoor flares suggest sensitivity to cockroach, dust mites, pet dander, or molds. Perennial symptoms may be sensitivity to a combination of these allergens or indicate nonallergic rhinitis.

NONALLERGIC RHINITIS

- The etiology of nonallergic rhinitis is unknown.
- The prominent complaint is nasal congestion. Nasal, eye, and soft palate pruritus are usually absent. Symptoms are often perennial and triggered by strong odors or smoke. Seasonal air temperature, humidity, and barometric pressure changes may lead to exacerbations, making it difficult to distinguish from allergic rhinitis.

EVALUATION

- The history should focus on isolating an allergen exposure. A personal or family history of asthma, allergies, and eczema leads to a higher suspicion for allergic rhinitis.
- Physical examination will not distinguish allergic and nonallergic rhinitis.
  1. The nasal mucosa in allergic rhinitis is classically pale or bluish, but can be red, edematous, or appear normal. Postnasal drip of any etiology causes posterior pharyngeal cobblestoning. "Allergic shiners" from infraorbital venous congestion are also nonspecific.
  2. Findings suggestive of allergic rhinitis include accentuated transverse nasal crease seen in children who repeatedly rub their nose because of pruritus and atopic stigmata, such as eczema and wheezing on auscultation.

MANAGEMENT

- Allergen avoidance is essential in managing allergic rhinitis.
  1. Avoidance of animal dander is always best. Exclusion of the pet from the bedroom and hepa filter use may provide some benefit.
  2. For dust mite allergy, use occlusive covers on the pillows, mattress, and box springs. Frequent washing of bed linens and blankets in hot water is helpful. Dehumidifiers and removing carpet may help. Hepa filters are ineffective because dust mite products are not airborne for an extended period of time.
  3. Mold allergen can be difficult to control, but dehumidifiers and scrupulous cleaning can be beneficial.

MEDICAL THERAPY

- Medical therapy is initiated in a stepwise fashion (see Fig. 37-1). Available medications include: decongestants, oral and topical antihistamines, cromolyn, corticosteroids, leukotriene receptor blockers, and topical ipratropium bromide.

- Oral decongestants relieve congestion in allergic and nonallergic rhinitis. In allergic rhinitis, they are most effective combined with an oral antihistamine (Sussman et al, 1999). Side effects include insomnia, irritability, tachycardia, and palpations. Because they decrease heat dissipation via peripheral vasoconstriction, they should be avoided during training or competition in the heat.
- Topical nasal decongestants are for short-term control of severe congestion. Their use should not exceed 3 days. If used more than 5–7 days they can cause severe rebound congestion and rhinorrhea.
- Antihistamines relieve sneezing, itching, and rhinorrhea in allergic rhinitis. Their efficacy is roughly equivalent to nasal cromolyn but less than nasal steroids. They provide little relief of nasal obstruction and are generally ineffective in the treatment of nonallergic rhinitis. First generation antihistamines can cause significant sedation, decreased alertness, and performance impairment—making them undesirable for most competitive athletes. These effects can exist without an individual's awareness and can be present even with nighttime-only dosing. Second generation antihistamines are at least as effective as first generation antihistamines and possess much lower rates of

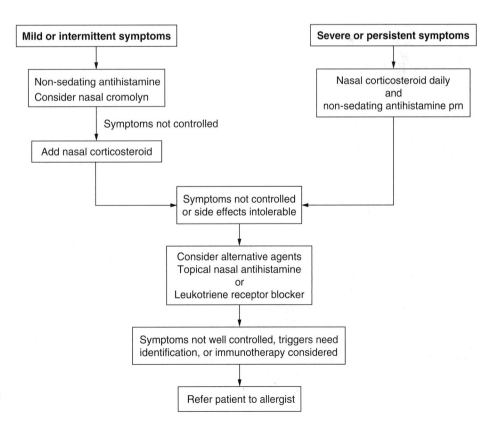

FIG. 37-1 Suggested Therapeutic Strategy for Allergic Rhinitis in Athletes.

TABLE 37-1   Second Generation Oral Antihistamines

2ND GENERATION ORAL ANTIHISTAMINE	DOSE	SEDATION
Fexofenadine (Allegra)	Age ≥12: 180 mg qd or 60 mg bid Age 6–11: 30 mg bid	No different than placebo
Cetirizine (Zyrtec)	Age ≥6: 5–10 mg qd Age 2–5: 2.5–5 mg qd (syrup)	Slightly higher than placebo, but less than 1st generation
Loratadine (Claritin)	Age >6: 10 mg qd Age 2–6: 5 mg qd	No different that placebo at 10 mg, sedating at higher doses
Desloratadine (Clarinex)	Age ≥12: 5 mg qd	No different than placebo*

*7% of population may have sedation because of decreased metabolism of the drug.

sedation (see Table 37-1). Antihistamines can decrease heat dissipation by their anticholinergic effects on sweat glands and should be used with caution in athletes.

• Topical nasal antihistamines can be beneficial in both allergic and nonallergic rhinitis. Side effects include drowsiness and an unpleasant aftertaste. While intranasal steroids provide greater relief of nasal symptoms, nasal antihistamines can be considered as an alternative when the response to an oral antihistamine and a nasal steroid is inadequate (Yanez and Rodrigo, 2002).

• Cromolyn, a topical mast cell stabilizer, provides modest improvement in the sneezing, itching, and rhinorrhea associated with allergic rhinitis and has a low potential for toxicity. It is useful when given prior to allergen exposure, but often requires dosing up to 4 to 6 times daily to be effective.

• Nasal steroids are the most effective therapy for persistent or severe symptoms (Pullerits et al, 2002). Several days of treatment are usually necessary for maximal effectiveness. They can be used periodically for an athlete's allergy season, but once initiated, the steroid needs regular administration for efficacy (see Table 37-2). Side effects are low and include irritation, burning, sneezing, and bloody nasal discharge.

• Chronic nasal steroids, when used properly, are not associated with significant adrenal suppression, nasal

TABLE 37-2   Topical Nasal Corticosteroids

TOPICAL NASAL CORTICOSTEROID	DOSE: SPRAYS PER NOSTRIL
Flonase (fluticasone)	Age ≥12: 1 bid or 2 qd; Age 4–11: same but start at 1 qd
Nasonex (mometasone furoate)	Age ≥12: 2 qd; Age 3–11: 1 qd
Rhinocort Aqua (budesonide)	Age ≥12: 1–4 qd; Age 6–11: 1–2 qd
Nasarel (flunisolide)	Age >14: 2 bid to qid; Age 6–14: 1 tid
Nasacort AQ (triamcinolone)	Age ≥12: 2 qd; Age 6–11: 1–2 qd
Beconase AQ (beclomethasone)	Age ≥12: 1–2 bid; Age 6–11: 1 bid
Vancenase AQ DS (beclomethasone)	Age ≥6: 1–2 qd

or pharyngeal candidiasis, cataracts, or glaucoma (Boner; Krahnke and Skoner, 2002). Studies using the newer agents mometasone furoate and fluticasone in children showed no difference in growth compared to placebo (Skoner et al, 2000; Schenkel et al, 2000; Allen et al, 2002).

• *Leukotriene receptor antagonists* (LRAs) provide mild improvement in allergic rhinitis with efficacy similar to second-generation antihistamines (Nathan, 2003). Their side effect profile is no different than placebo. They should be considered when nasal steroids and/or antihistamines fail or have intolerable side effects and when concomitant asthma may benefit from LRA therapy.

• Ipratropium bromide 0.03% nasal spray is effective for treating rhinorrhea, particularly vasomotor-induced rhinorrhea triggered by cold air or exercise. It has no effect on pruritus or congestion. Side effects include occasional epistaxis and nasal dryness, but no systemic anticholinergic or rebound effects. It is effective when dosed 30 min prior to exercise or exposure.

• When treatments fail, consider medication inadequacy and noncompliance, as well as the possibility of other diagnoses such as anatomical or physical obstruction and/or chronic sinusitis.

ATHLETE-SPECIFIC MEDICATION ISSUES

• As restrictions on over-the-counter and prescription medications can change, an athlete should discuss a medication's status with the governing body for their particular sport or level of competition prior to its use. This would include the National Collegiate Athletic Association (NCAA) and U. S. Olympic Committee (USOC).

• The NCAA has no restrictions on any allergy-related products with the exception that any products containing ephedrine are banned.

TABLE 37-3 Allergic Conjunctivitis Topical Medications

TOPICAL AGENT	MECHANISM OF ACTION	DOSE
Patanol (Olopatadine)	Mast cell blocker/antihistamine	1 drop bid; age >3
Zaditor (Ketotifen)	Mast cell blocker/antihistamine	1 drop bid to tid
Alomide (Lodoxamide)	Mast cell blocker	1–2 drops qid
Alamast (Pemirolast)	Mast cell blocker	2 drops qid
Alocril (Nedocromil)	Inhibits activation and mediator release from inflammatory cells	1–2 drops bid
Livostin (Levocabastine)	Antihistamine	1–2 drops qid
Emadine (Emadastine)	Antihistamine	1 drop qid
Optivar (Azelastine)	Antihistamine	1 drop bid
Crolom (Cromolyn):	Mast cell blocker	1–2 drops 4–6 times/day
Naphcon A, Opcon A, Vasocon A, Visine A	Antihistamine/Decongestants	Up to qid

- The USOC is much more stringent. All sympathomimetic-containing medications are banned. Antihistamines are allowed in all but the shooting sports in which they are completely banned. While the USOC does not restrict cromolyn or leukotriene receptor blockers, written permission should be obtained for nasal or inhaled steroid use (Fuentes and Rosenberg, 1999).

ALLERGY TESTING

- In patients with a history suggestive of allergic rhinitis, indications for referral for skin testing include targeting allergens for avoidance as well as institution of immunotherapy when medical therapy is failing. Allergy consultation is recommended prior to drastic environmental interventions such as pet elimination, taking up carpets, or purchasing new mattresses, bedding, dust mite covers, and the like.
- Antihistamines should be stopped 1 week prior to testing so as not to blunt the cutaneous response to skin testing.
- Allergy testing is contraindicated in the setting of severe lung disease or poorly controlled asthma with a FEV1 (*forced expiratory volume in 1 s*) less than 70%.
- Skin testing is preferred over in vitro *radioallergosorbent testing* (RAST) because it is more sensitive. In vitro RAST is helpful for validating the diagnosis and supporting environmental controls. It is a reasonable alternative when skin testing cannot be performed.

ALLERGEN IMMUNOTHERAPY

- *Allergen immunotherapy* (AIT) is effective for allergic rhinitis and allergic asthma. Advantages include long lasting symptom remission and reducing the risk of developing new allergies and asthma in children (Ledford, 2000). Notable symptom relief usually takes several months of treatment. Three to five years of AIT is required to sustain symptom remission. Any

individual who cannot fully commit to treatment, has poorly controlled asthma, or is on a beta-blocker should not receive AIT. It should be prescribed and administered by a board certified allergist to ensure a thorough discussion of the benefits and potential risks of therapy and to provide ongoing follow-up.

ALLERGIC CONJUNCTIVITIS

- Etiology is the same as for allergic rhinitis. Symptoms occur on inoculation of the allergen onto the mucosa of the eyes.
- Symptom control can be achieved with the same measures as discussed with allergic rhinitis. Persistent eye symptoms may require targeted ocular medications (see Table 37-3). Combination mast cell blocker and antihistamine topical therapy is very effective. Other options include topical mast cell blockers or antihistamine alone, topical decongestants, and topical mast cell stabilizers. Topical corticosteroids are associated with significant complications and should only be used after consultation with an ophthalmologist.

URTICARIA AND ANGIOEDEMA

PATHOPHYSIOLOGY

- Urticaria is caused by mast cell degranulation in the superficial dermis and is characterized by pruritic, erythematous, cutaneous elevations that blanch with pressure. Hives may appear anywhere on the body, but occur primarily on the trunk and extremities. Mast cell mediators involved include: histamine, prostaglandins, leukotrienes, platelet activating factor, anaphylatoxins, bradykinin, and hageman factor. All cause blood vessel dilation and tissue edema.
- Angioedema is similar to urticaria but occurs in the deeper dermis and subcutaneous tissues. It is more painful and burning than pruritic and often involves the face.

TABLE 37-4 Common Triggers for Urticaria

Medications

Antibiotics
  Beta-lactams
  Sulfa compounds
NSAIDs
Progesterone
Local Anesthetics
Opioid analgesics

Physical Contacts

Latex
Nickel
Plants and plant resins
Fruits/vegetables
Raw fish
Animal saliva

Insect Stings

Foods and food additives
  Milk
  Egg
  Peanut
  Nuts
  Soy
  Wheat
  Fish/shellfish
  Sulfites

Infections

Coxsackie A and B
Hepatitis A, B, C
HIV
Ebstein-Barr virus
Herpes simplex
Intestinal parasites
Dermatophyte infections

- Acute urticaria is defined as new onset symptoms of less than 6 weeks in duration. If symptoms persist more than 6 weeks, it is considered chronic urticaria.
- In chronic urticaria, 75% have symptoms over 1 year, 50% have symptoms over 5 years, and 20% have symptoms for decades. Urticaria occurs at any age, but is most common in children and young adults. Approximately 50% of patients at presentation have both urticaria and angioedema, 40% have urticaria only and 10% have angioedema only (Tharp, 1996).
- Most cases are idiopathic but potential triggers are medications, insect stings, infections, and foods and food additives. Table 37-4 lists the most common known triggers.
- Physical stimuli can also cause urticaria. Physical urticarias are important to consider in athletes because they are triggered by conditions occurring during practice and competition. See Table 37-5 for their evaluation and management (Casale et al, 1988).
  1. Cholinergic urticaria, from elevation in core body temperature, is precipitated by exercise or use of hot tubs. Classically, patients develop small, punctate wheals with prominent erythematous flare. Symptom usually occur within 2 to 30 min of exposure and last up to 90 min.
  2. Cold urticaria is precipitated by rewarming following contact with a cold object. Within 2–5 min, the exposed area develops swelling and pruritus. Symptoms generally worsen as the area is warmed and last up to 2 h. Patients with cold urticaria should avoid swimming and diving because this condition carries a risk of anaphylaxis if patients have a significant drop in core body temperature.
  3. Aquagenic urticaria is caused by contact with water. For athletes in water sports, this condition could be confused with cholinergic or cold urticaria. Unlike cholinergic urticaria, aquagenic urticaria occurs even when the water temperature is cool and even when the patient is not exercising in the water. Unlike cold urticaria, aquagenic urticaria will not be precipitated by application of a cold object that is not water-based.

TABLE 37-5 Physical Urticarias

TYPE	PRECIPITANT	EVALUATION	TREATMENT
Cholinergic urticaria	Elevation in core temperature; Exercise, hot tubs, and the like.	History and classic "pencil eraser-sized" punctate wheals	Premedicate with nonsedating antihistamine prior to exercise
Cold urticaria	Rewarming after contact with cold object	Place cold object on skin for 15 min and look for urticaria on rewarming	Nonsedating antihistamines as needed; Avoidance of swimming and diving sports because of risk of anaphylaxis
Aquagenic urticaria	Water contact	History; Expose skin to water and look for changes	Nonsedating antihistamines
Solar urticaria	UV light exposure	Expose small, unprotected patch of skin to sunlight	Limit sun exposure; Protective clothing and sunscreen use
Pressure urticaria/ angioedema	Direct pressure on skin. Running, prolonged sitting, clapping and the like.	Place 15 lb weight on patient for 20 min—look for skin changes; Test for fever and leukocytosis 3–12 h later	Avoidance of precipitants; Nonsedating antihistamines and NSAIDs; Consider steroid burst/taper if symptoms severe
Symptomatic Dermatographism	Stroking or rubbing skin; Areas where clothing or equipment abrades skin	Look for linear, pruritic wheal 2–5 min after rubbing the skin	Loose fitting clothing; Treatment usually not necessary. Nonsedating antihistamines only for severe symptoms

4. Solar urticaria occurs with exposure to ultraviolet light. Anaphylaxis could occur if large body areas are exposed.
5. Pressure urticaria (angioedema) is precipitated by direct pressure on the skin. Skin pressure is followed 3–12 h later by localized hives, fever, malaise, and leukocytosis. It can be precipitated by running, clapping, sitting, or using hand equipment. Symptoms can last up to 24 h.
6. Symptomatic dermatographism is another type of physical urticaria. Patients develop linear, pruritic wheals 2–5 min after an area of skin is stroked.

EVALUATION

- In the acute setting, providers should assess for symptoms indicating anaphylaxis rather than isolated urticaria or angioedema. (See Anaphylaxis and Anaphylactoid Reactions.)
- While in most cases the precipitant remains unknown, a detailed history may isolate the cause. Searching for a trigger is more beneficial in acute urticaria as compared to chronic urticaria where the cause is found in less than 10% of cases. For known causes, drug hypersensitivity is most common. Individuals should be asked about any recent prescription, over-the-counter medications, or supplement use. Food and food additives rarely cause isolated urticaria, but the relationship to food inhalation, contact, and consumption should be documented. It is important to document physical triggers, occupational exposures, insect envenomations, and any recent illnesses. A thorough review of systems will help rule out any disease associations, such as an acute bacterial or viral illness, parasitic infection, autoimmune/collagen vascular disease, serum sickness, endocrine disease, or malignancy (Stafford, 1990).
- The physical examination is especially helpful in the acute setting when skin manifestations are present. It can help document whether urticaria and angioedema are occurring together or in isolation and whether there are any signs of anaphylaxis. The examination should also look for evidence of other diseases that are rarely associated with urticaria and angioedema.
- The use of laboratory and imaging studies should be targeted by the history and physical. Consider the following tests: Monospot or Epstein-Barr virus antibody titers if acute mononucleosis is suspected; Hepatitis A, B, and C panel; and HIV testing given the right clinical setting. The association of urticaria with other viral infections remains unclear and routine testing for other viral pathogens is not recommended.

- If a significant travel history is discovered and the complete blood count shows eosinophilia, stool studies should be obtained looking for intestinal parasites. Progressive weight loss and/or the presence of lympadenopathy or hepatosplenomegaly on examination would warrant an evaluation for an underlying lymphoreticular malignancy.
- If enlargement or nodularity of the thyroid is present, a thyroid function panel, thyroid autoantibodies, thyroid ultrasound, and nuclear medicine thyroid studies should be considered.
- Testing for C1 esterase inhibitor deficiency should be considered for any athlete presenting with recurrent isolated angioedema.
- A skin biopsy for vasculitis is indicated when individual urticarial lesions last longer than 24 h or are associated with purpura, pain, hyperpigmentation, or systemic symptoms (Kaplan, 1993).
- If the history and physical examination are unrevealing, a limited laboratory evaluation consisting of a complete blood count with differential, urinalysis, erythrocyte sedimentation rate and liver panel is reasonable to screen for occult conditions.

MANAGEMENT

- After the initial evaluation, the management of urticaria and angioedema becomes primarily symptomatic. Known triggers should be avoided if possible. Mild symptoms can be controlled with a low sedating antihistamine (see Table 37-1). Athletes with exercise-induced symptoms only, such as cholinergic urticaria, can take the antihistamine 1–2 h prior to exercise. Those who exercise regularly and those with chronic symptoms often require daily medication to prevent exacerbations. For moderate or poorly controlled symptoms, the antihistamine dose should be maximized prior to considering add-on therapy. Additive therapies include leukotriene antagonists, H-2 blockers and nighttime doxepin. For periods of moderate to severe symptoms prednisone therapy can be helpful.
- Because food and food additives are a rare cause of chronic urticaria and angioedema, elimination diets are unnecessary unless the history pinpoints a specific food.
- Referral to an allergist is recommended when there is suspicion of an allergic component precipitating symptoms, when symptoms are not well controlled with the therapies listed above, when there is a history of respiratory distress or hypotension suggesting anaphylaxis, or when there is severe angioedema. The athlete should be referred to dermatology for skin biopsy if urticarial vasculitis is suspected.

ANAPHYLACTIC AND ANAPHYLACTOID REACTIONS

PATHOPHYSIOLOGY

- Anaphylaxis is an acute, life-threatening, systemic reaction mediated through IgE antibodies and their receptors. It requires previous sensitization and subsequent reexposure to an allergen.
- Anaphylactoid reactions are clinically indistinguishable from true anaphylaxis. Both are caused by massive release of potent chemical mediators from mast cells and basophils. The differences are: anaphylactoid reactions are not mediated by IgE antibodies, they do not require prior sensitization, and they are less commonly associated with severe hypotension and cardiovascular collapse. Both are managed with the same treatment measures discussed here.
- Anaphylaxis includes cutaneous signs or symptoms accompanied by obstructive respiratory symptoms and/or hemodynamic changes. Additional features include gastrointestinal complaints and experiencing a "sense of impending doom" (see Table 37-6).

TABLE 37-6   Symptoms and Signs of Anaphylaxis

Psychologic

"Sense of impending doom"

Cutaneous

Tingling/Pruritus
Generalized erythema
Urticaria
Angioedema

Upper Airway

Nasal Congestion
Rhinorrhea
Sneezing
Globus sensation
Throat tightness
Dysphonia
Dysphagia

Lower Airway

Dyspnea
Wheezing
Cough

Cardiovascular

Lightheadedness
Syncope
Palpitations
Shock

Gastrointestinal

Abdominal cramps
Bloating
Nausea/Vomiting

The onset of symptoms typically begins seconds to minutes after the inciting cause. More rarely, symptoms may be delayed for up to 2 h.

- Approximately half of cases have a uniphasic course with abrupt, severe onset, and death within minutes despite treatment. Up to 20% of cases have a biphasic presentation. After the acute stage and a 1–8 h asymptomatic period, a late phase reaction ensues with recurrence of severe symptoms. The late phase symptoms can be protracted, persisting for several hours in 28% of individuals (Kemp, 2001).

EVALUATION

- The diagnosis of anaphylaxis is affected by variability in the standard case definition. Obtaining as much information from the affected athlete and any witnesses will define the time course, severity of the reaction, and the potential cause.
- Anaphylaxis triggers include: food, medications, and insect stings (see Table 37-7). Any food exposure prior to the onset of symptoms should be documented. Of special concern would be exposure to the most common food allergens, which include eggs, peanut, cow's milk, nuts, fish, soy, shellfish, and wheat. Several medications have been known to cause anaphylaxis with the most common being beta-lactam antibiotics. Documenting exposure to prescription medications as well as over-the-counter medications and supplements is important. Bee-sting sensitivity

TABLE 37-7   Causes of Anaphylaxis

Idiopathic
Medications
   Antibiotics
   IV and local anesthetics
   Aspirin/NSAIDs
   Chemotherapeutic agents
   Opiates
   Vaccines
   Allergy immunotherapy sera
Radiographic contrast media
Blood products
Latex
Hymenoptera envenomation
Foods
   Eggs
   Peanut
   Cow's milk
   Nuts
   Seafood
   Soy
   Wheat
Exercise

should be suspected in any athlete with a reaction that occurs outdoors, even if the patient does not recall being stung.

- Exercise-induced anaphylaxis is a rare condition associated with exercising within 2–4 h after food ingestion. It is characterized by the usual manifestations of anaphylaxis beginning within 5 to 30 min of exercise and lasting up to 3 h. The medical history should explore the relationship of symptom onset to physical exercise to assess for this rare trigger.

- The physical manifestations of anaphylaxis involve multiple sites including the skin, upper airway, lower airway, and cardiovascular system. The physical examination should start by evaluating upper airway patency by listening for inspiratory stridor and looking for oral or pharyngeal edema. The respiratory status can be assessed by observing work of breathing and accessory muscle use. Auscultation may reveal wheezing indicating acute bronchospasm. A set of vital signs is critical to patient management, looking for any evidence of cardiovascular or respiratory compromise. Once the ABCs are assessed and secured, the skin can be examined for the presence of generalized erythema, urticaria, and angioedema.

ACUTE MANAGEMENT

- Initial management of anaphylaxis should always start with epinephrine 0.2–0.5 cc *intramuscular* (IM) or *subcutaneous* (SQ) of 1:1000, even if symptoms are mild. The IM route is preferred, especially in children, as SQ injection may delay absorption. Doses may be repeated every 10–15 min if symptoms persist. *Intravenous* (IV) epinephrine at 1 mcg/min of 1:10,000 (10 mcg/mL) can be considered for symptoms resistant to repeated SQ or IM administration. The IV dosage can be increased to 2–10 mcg/min for severe reactions. Patients on beta-blockers may not respond to epinephrine. In these cases Glucagon 2–5 mg IM/SQ is beneficial. Supportive therapy includes: oxygen for hypoxemia, recumbent positioning and IV fluids for hypotension, and inhaled beta-agonists or racemic epinephrine for bronchospasm. Antihistamines (diphenhydramine 1–2 mg/kg or 25–50 mg IV/po) may provide additional benefit. Corticosteroids, (prednisone 0.5–2.0 mg/kg up 125 mg) should also be considered to prevent late phase reactions. Neither antihistamines nor steroids should be used as substitutes for epinephrine. Their onset of action

is much slower and they are insufficient to prevent or treat more severe anaphylaxis with respiratory or cardiovascular involvement.

- Mild anaphylaxis cases should be observed a minimum of 3 h after symptoms have resolved. Severe reactions should be observed at least 6 h and hospitalization should be strongly considered to monitor for late phase reactions.

LONG-TERM MANAGEMENT

- All patients with anaphylaxis need an action plan to include allergen identification, symptom recognition, and appropriate treatment. A provider knowledgeable in allergic disease should provide education on allergen avoidance, hidden allergens, and cross-reacting substances. All individuals should have an epinephrine autoinjector with them at all times and be educated on the indications and proper technique for its use. The trainer and coach should be familiar with anaphylaxis recognition and epinephrine use as well. The athlete should wear a medical alert bracelet at all times, indicating their condition and allergy if known.

- Because there are no measures proven to prevent exercise-induced anaphylaxis, affected athletes should never exercise alone. Pretreatment with antihistamines is not effective. The primary preventative strategy is to avoid eating for 4 h prior to exercise. Other measures that may limit attacks are to avoid NSAIDs and aspirin prior to exercise and to avoid outdoor exercise during periods of high humidity, temperature extremes, and the individual's allergy season (Shadick, 1999). Occasionally skin testing can identify a specific food that the patient can avoid, but often the results are inconclusive. Athletes should carry an epinephrine autoinjector on their person when they don't have immediate access to their gear bag. They should discontinue exercise at the first sign of symptoms and self-administer epinephrine.

- Indications for allergy referral include: when further testing is necessary for an unclear diagnosis or an unknown inciting agent, when reactions are recurrent and difficult to control, or when desensitization is required such as for stinging insects or antibiotic administration. Allergists also serve as an important resource for athletes, parents, and coaches needing education on allergen avoidance as well as institution or reinforcement of an individual's action plan.

REFERENCES

Allen DB et al: No growth suppression in children treated with the maximum recommended dose of fluticasone propionate aqueous nasal spray for one year. *Allergy Asthma Proc* 23(2), Nov–Dec 2002.

American Academy of Allergy, Asthma and Immunology: *The Allergy Report.* http://www.aaaai.org/. Accessed: April 13, 2003.

Boner AL: Effects of intranasal corticosteroids on the hypothalamic-pituitary-adrenal axis in children. *J Allergy Clin Immunol* 108(1), 2001.

Casale TB, Sampson HA et al: Guide to physical urticarias. *J Allergy Clin Immunol* 82, 1988.

Fuentes RJ, Rosenberg JM: *Athletic Drug Reference '99.* Durham, NC, Clean Data, 1999.

Joint task force on practice parameters: diagnosis and management of rhinitis. *Ann Allergy Asthma Immunol* 81, 1998.

Kaplan AP: Urticaria and angioedema, in Middleton E, Jr, Reed CE, Ellis EF, et al (eds.): *Allergy: Principles and Practice.* St. Louis, MO, Mosby, 1993, pp 1553–1580.

Kaplan AP: Clinical practice. Chronic urticaria and angioedema. *N Engl J Med* 346:175, 2002.

Kemp SF: Currents concepts in the pathophysiology, diagnosis, and management of anaphylaxis. *Allergy Immunol Clin N Am* Nov 21(4), 2001.

Krahnke J, Skoner D: Benefit and risk management for steroid treatment in upper airway diseases. *Curr Allergy Asthma Rep* 2(6), Nov. 2002.

Ledford DK: Efficacy of Immunotherapy. *Immunol Allergy Clin N Am* August 20(3), Aug. 2000.

Nathan, RA: Pharmacotherapy for allergic rhinitis: a critical review of leukotriene receptor antagonists compared with other treatments. *Ann Allergy Asthma Immunol* 90(2), Feb. 2003.

Neugut AI, Ghalak AT, Miller RL: Anaphylaxis in the United States: An investigation into its epidemiology. *Arch Intern Med* 161(17), 2001.

Public Health Service: US Dept of Health and Human Services publication (PHS) 93-1522, Jan. 1997.

Pullerits T et al: Comparison of a nasal glucocorticoid antileukotriene, and a combination of antileukotriene and antihistamine in the treatment of seasonal allergic rhinitis. *J Allergy Clin Immunol* 109, 2002.

Schenkel EJ et al: Absence of growth retardation in children with perennial allergic rhinitis after one year of treatment with mometasone furoate aqueous nasal spray. *Pediatrics* 105:E22, 2000.

Shadick NA: The natural history of exercise-induced anaphylaxis: survey results from a 10-year follow-up study. *J Allergy Clin Immunol* July 104(1), 1999.

Skoner DP et al: Detection of growth suppression in children during treatment with intranasal beclomethasone dipropionate. *Pediatrics* 105(2), 2000.

Stafford CT: Urticaria as a sign of systemic disease. *Ann of Allergy* 64, 1990.

Sussman GL et al: The efficacy and safety of fexofenadine HCL and pseudoephedrine alone and in combination in seasonal allergic rhinitis. *J Allergy Clin Immunol* 104, 1999.

Tharp MD: Chronic urticaria: Pathophysiology and treatment approaches. *J Allergy Clin Immunol* 98, 1996.

Yanez A, Rodrigo GJ: Intranasal corticosteroids versus topical H1 receptor antagonists for the treatment of allergic rhinitis: A systematic review with meta-analysis. *Ann Allergy Asthma Immunol* 89(5), Nov. 2002.

38 OVERTRAINING SYNDROME/ CHRONIC FATIGUE

Thomas M Howard, MD

INTRODUCTION

- Overtraining has been described and has been well known to athletes and trainers for decades. In 1923 Dr Parmenter described overtraining as "a condition difficult to detect and still more difficult to describe. Evaluation should focus on training load, nutrition, sleep, rest, competition stress, and psychological state" (Parmenter, 1923).
- It has only been in the last 10 years that there has been a surge in the literature to further define the condition, the pathophysiology and identify markers for treatment and prevention.
- Overtraining, if left unrecognized or untreated, results in injury and poor performance during key competitions and early retirement.

TERMS

- **Training:** A series of stimuli or displacement of homeostasis to provide stimulation for adaptation. A progressive overload in an effort to improve performance.
- **Adaptation:** A physiologic response to stress which results in an adjustment in function.
- **Recovery:** Period of time following a training stimulus when adaptation occurs resulting in supercompensation to allow better performance in the future, i.e., the training effect. Recovery includes hydration, nutritional replenishment, sleep/rest, stretching, relaxation, and emotional recovery.
- **Periodization:** Planned sequencing of increased training loads and recovery periods within a training program.
- **Overreaching/Overwork:** Acute phase where training load (intensity or volume) is significantly increased resulting in a short-term decrement in performance (generally thought to be <2 weeks). Physiologic Fatigue (Derman et al, 1997).

- **Overtraining:** Maladaptive response to training from extended overload with inadequate recovery resulting in decrements of performance generally lasting >2 weeks. It is manifested by increased fatigability, pronounce vegetative somatic complaints, sleep disorder, altered psychic excitability, overuse injuries, immune dysfunction, and some blood chemistry changes. Pathologic Fatigue (Derman et al, 1997)

PHYSIOLOGIC CHANGES WITH TRAINING

IMMUNOLOGIC

- Decreased salivary *immunoglobulin A* (IgA)
- Increased *white blood cells* (WBC), lymphocytes, natural killer cells, and *poly morphonuclear cells* (PMN) activity
- Transient decrease in the *T helper/T suppressor* (Th/Ts) ratio
- Decreased serum glutamine

ENDOCRINE

- Increased testosterone proportional to exercise intensity and muscle mass stimulating glycogen regeneration and protein synthesis (Anabolism).
- Transient increased cortisol relative to the duration and intensity of exercise. The stress response (Catabolism).
- The ratio of *free testosterone to cortisol* (FTCR) represents the balance of catabolism and anabolism. A 30% decrease in this ratio may suggest inadequate recovery or overreaching (Fry and Kraemer, 1997).
- Norepinephrine increase preexercise (anticipation) and early in exercise, stimulating lypolysis.
- Epinephrine increase proportional to exercise intensity.
- *Sex hormone binding globulin* (SHBG) decreased production with intense exercise.
- Suppression of pulsatile secretion of *gonadotropin releasing factor* (GnRH); probably affected by stress and poor nutrition.
- Growth hormone peak secretion at night and with exercise ~50% VO_{2max}; blunted response with intense exercise.

EPIDEMIOLOGY

- Overtraining affects 5–15% of elite athletes at any one time and as much as two-thirds of runners during and athletic career.
- It may be higher in amateur athletes.

- Seen more commonly in endurance events like swimming, cycling, or running. Overtraining in power lifters is probably different.
- Susceptible athletes include highly motivated, goal-oriented individuals, exercise programs designed by the athletes themselves, those athletes that tend to be focused, conventional, and conservative.

HYPOTHESES

- **Chronic glycogen depletion:** A chronic nutritional deficiency leading to chronic glycogen depletion with peripheral muscle fatigue. Central fatigue is interrelated to changes in branched-chain amino acids, see central fatigue hypothesis (Snyder, 1998).
- **Autonomic imbalance:** An increase in sympathetic activity form stress and overloaded target organs and increased catabolism leading to decreased sympathetic intrinsic activity. Chronically increased catecholamine levels causes a receptor down regulation and fatigue (Lehmann et al, 1998).
- **Central fatigue hypothesis:** Peripheral fatigue and nutrient depletion leading to the consumption of *branched-chain amino acids* (BCAAs) with subsequent change in the BCAA to *free Tryptophan ratio* (fTry) in the plasma. This change favors increased transport of Try into the central nervous system. Try is a precursor for serotonin *5-hydroxytryptamine* (5HT) which causes central fatigue (Gastman and Lehmann, 1997; Davis and Bailey, 1996).
- **Glutamine hypothesis (immune dysfunction):** Overload training leads to depressed glutamine production from stressed muscle tissue. Glutamine deficiency as well as acute exercise stress on the immune system creates immunologic open windows leading to repeated minor infections and systemic stress (Walsh et al, 1998).
- **Cytokine hypothesis:** Incomplete recovery of locally damage tissues with overload causing a local inflammatory response that becomes systemic with elevated proinflammatory cytokines IL-1β, TNF-α, and IL-6. These cytokines cause CNS fatigue (Smith, 2000).

CATEGORIES OF OVERTRAINING

- **Sympathetic overtraining:** Probably represents early overtraining. It is manifested by increased resting *heart rate* (HR) and blood pressure, loss of appetite, loss of *lean body mass* (LBM), irritability, sleep disturbance, and fatigue (Fry and Kraemer, 1997).
- **Parasympathetic overtraining:** Probably represents more chronic, prolonged overtraining. It is manifested by low resting HR and blood pressure, sleep disturbance, depressed mood, and fatigue. (Fry and Kraemer, 1997).

PHYSICAL FINDINGS

- Elevated resting HR (usually >10 bpm over baseline); decreased LBM; depressed mood on various evaluation tools; otherwise essentially normal examination.

DIFFERENTIAL DIAGNOSIS (HAWLEY AND SCHOENE, 2003)

COMMON CAUSES
- Caffeine withdrawal, environmental allergies, exercise-induced asthma, infectious mononucleosis, insufficient sleep, iron deficiency with or without anemia, overtraining, performance anxiety, mood disorder (anxiety, depression, adjustment reaction), psychosocial stress, and upper respiratory infection.

LESS COMMON CAUSES
- Dehydration, diabetes mellitus, eating disorder, hepatitis (A, B, or C), hypothyroidism, inadequate carbohydrate or protein intake, lower respiratory infection, medication side effect (antidepressants, antihistamines, anxiolytics, beta-blockers), post concussive syndrome, pregnancy, and substance abuse.

RELATIVELY RARE, BUT IMPORTANT
- Adrenocortical insufficiency or excess, congenital or acquired heart disease, arrhythmia, bacterial endocarditis, congestive heart failure, coronary heart disease, hypertrophic cardiomyopathy, myocarditis/pericarditis, HIV, malabsorbtion, lung disease, Lyme disease, malaria, malignancy, neuromuscular disorder, renal disease, and syphilis.

EVALUATION (FIG. 38-1)

FIRST VISIT
- A thorough history focusing on chief complaint, training program, diet, medications, nutrition, illness, review of systems, and an assessment of the goals of the athletes training program.
- Initial lab studies to consider include *complete blood count* (CBC), *erythrocyte sedimentation rate* (ESR), metabolic panel, *thyroid-stimulating hormone* (TSH),

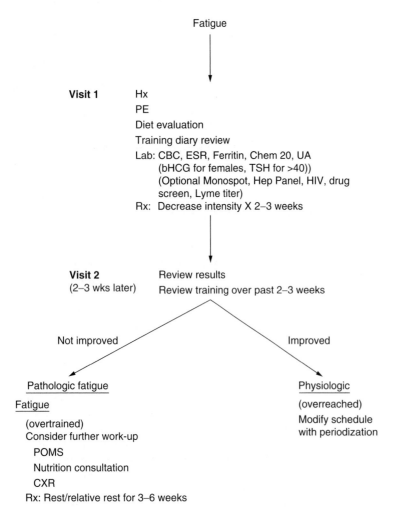

FIG. 38-1 Evaluation of fatigue in an athlete.

Ferritin, serum β-*human chorionic gonadotropin* (β-HCG), Monospot, and other specifically indicated tests based on history, review of systems (ROS), and examination.

• Prescribe decrease in intensity or even absolute rest for 2 weeks. During that time consider cross training for enjoyment and evaluation of other confounding stressors.

SECOND VISIT

• Review lab results, training over the past 2 weeks, and symptoms.
• If improved consider the diagnosis of physiologic fatigue (overreached) and focus on adjustments to the training schedule with periodization, cross training, and addressing other stressors identified.
• If not improved consider the diagnosis of pathologic fatigue or overtraining. They will require prolonged relative rest from intense training and further work up. Consider consultation with a sports psychologist, dietician, and further evaluation to work through the differential diagnosis.

MONITORING

• Poor markers for overtraining include body mass, hemoglobin, ferritin, CPK.
• Indicators of inadequate recovery, but not necessarily overtraining include FTCR ratio decrease >30%, a decrease in SHBG, and a glutamine to glutamate level <3.58 (Smith and Norris, 2000; Halson et al, 2003).
• Psychiatric indicators generally change before biologic markers.
• **Good markers for monitoring:** Athletes, trainers and coaches often use baseline HR. A rise of >10 beats is considered abnormal. This rise represents an imbalance between sympathetic and parasympathetic systems with heightened sympathetic tone (Dressendorfer, Hansen, and Timmis, 2000). In the past this was not considered to be a great monitoring tool because of multiple confounding factors.
• HR variability is another research tool that also monitors the balance of parasympathetic and sympathetic activity. Increase in HR variability indicates inadequate recovery (Pichot et al, 2002).
• Performance in time trials and standard exercise challenges.
• Foster recently described a "session RPE," or relative perceived exertion, as the athlete's self-described intensity of the training session multiplied by the duration of the session. Daily mean load and *standard deviation* (SD) can calculated to quantitative monotony (daily mean/SD) and strain (weekly load * monotony) (Foster, 1998).
• **Psychologic tools:** Profile of Mood State-a 65-item questionnaire assessing five negative (tension, depression,

TABLE 38-1   TQR Action

RATING OF PERCEIVED EXERTION (RPE)	TOTAL QUALITY RECOVER (TQR)
6	6
7 Very, very light	7 Very, very poor recovery
8	8
9 very light	9 very poor recovery
10	10
11 Faintly light	11 Poor recovery
12	12
13 Somewhat hard	13 Reasonable recovery
14	14
15 Hard	15 Good recovery
16	16
17 Very hard	17 Very good recovery
18	18
19 Very, very hard	19 Very, very good recovery
20	20

SOURCE: (Foster, 1998).

anger, fatigue, and confusion) and one positive mood state (vigor) (McNair, Lorr, and Dropplemann, 1992).
• *Total quality recovery* (TQR) action and perceived scales (Kentta and Hassmen, 1998)
  a. Action: A total score in four major areas of recovery
    (a) Nutrition/Hydration   10 pts
    (b) Sleep/Rest   4 pts
    (c) Relaxation/emotional support 3 pts
    (d) Stretching/Active rest   3 pts
  b. Perceived: A reverse Borg RPE scale of perceived recovery (Table 38-1)
• Recovery-stress-questionnaire for athletes (RESTQ-Sport) (Kellman and Günther, 2000).
  a. Ninety nine question survey tool answered on a Likert-type scale to assess training stress and recovery.

PREVENTION

• Individualized and variable training programs
• Coaching and supervised training
• Periods of "time out"
• Cross training
• Reasonable goal setting (short and long term)
• Relaxation and visualization techniques or use of a sports psychologist

REFERENCES

Davis MJ, Bailey SP: Possible mechanism of central nervous system fatigue during exercise. *Med Sci Sports Exerc* 29(1):45, 1996.

Derman W et al: The worn-out athlete: A clinical approach to chronic fatigue in athletes. *J Sports Sci* 15(3):341, 1997.

Dressendorfer RH, Hansen AM, Timmis GC: Reversal of runners bradycardia with training overstress. *Clin J Sport Med* 10:279, 2000.

Foster C: Monitoring training in athletes with reference to overtraining syndrome. *Med Sci Sports Exerc* 30(7):1164, 1998.

Fry A, Kraemer WJ: Resistance exercise overtraining and overreaching. *Sports Med* 23(2):106, 1997.

Gastman UA, Lehmann MJ: Overtraining and the BCAA hypothesis. *Med Sci Sports Exerc* 30(7):1173, 1997.

Halson SL et al: Immunological responses to overreaching in cyclists. *Med Sci Sports Exerc* 35(5):854, 2003.

Hawley CJ, Schoene RB: Overtraining Syndrome a guide to diagnosis, treatment and prevention. *Phys Sport Med* 31(6):25, 2003.

Kellman M, Günther K-D: Changes in stress and recovery in elite rowers during preparation for the Olympic Games. *Med Sci Sports Exerc* 32(3):676, 2000.

Kentta G, Hassmen P: Overtraining and recovery. A conceptual model. *Sports Med* 26(1):1, 1998.

Lehmann MC et al: Autonomic imbalance hypothesis and overtraining syndrome. *Med Sci Sports Exerc* 30(7):1140, 1998.

McNair D, Lorr M, Dropplemann CF: *POMS Manual: Profile of Mood States.* San Diego, CA, Education and Industrial Testing Sevice, 1992.

Parmenter DC: Some medical aspects of the training of college athletes., *Med Surg J* 189:45, 1923.

Pichot V et al: Autonomic adaptations to intensive and overload training periods: A laboratory study. *Med Sci Sports Exerc* 34(10):1660, 2002.

Smith LL: Cytokine hypothesis of overtraining: A physiological adaptation to excessive stress. *Med Sci Sports Exerc* 32(2):317, 2000.

Smith DJ, Norris SR: Changes in glutamine and glutamate concentrations for tracking training tolerance. *Med Sci Sports Exerc* 32(3):684, 2000.

Snyder AC: Overtraining and glycogen depletion hypothesis. *Med Sci Sports Exerc* 30(7):1146, 1998.

Walsh NP et al: Glutamine, exercise, and immune function. *Sports Med* 26(3):177, 1998.

39 ENVIRONMENTAL INJURIES
Brian V Reamy, MD

HYPOTHERMIA

DEFINITION

- Hypothermia occurs when the body's core temperature drops below 35°C (95°F).

EPIDEMIOLOGY

- Individuals younger than 2 years of age and older than 75 years of age are most at risk.

- Increasing homelessness and sports activities in inclement environments have contributed to an increased incidence of hypothermia in the past decade.
- Risk factors include the use of intoxicants, psychiatric illness, medical illnesses, sleep deprivation, dehydration, malnutrition, and trauma. Impaired judgement resulting from psychiatric illness or the use of ethanol is the most common predisposing factor (Danzl and Pozos, 1994b).

PATHOPHYSIOLOGY

- The body combats the fall in core temperature through shivering thermogenesis and increased gluconeogenesis. When the core temperature drops below 35°C the victim becomes poikilothermic and cools to the ambient temperature.
- *Central nervous system* (CNS) function is directly depressed by the cold. The *electroencephalogram* (EEG) becomes abnormal below a temperature of 33.5°C (92.5°F) and silent at 19°C (66°F).
- Initial reflex tachypnea continues until core temperature falls below 30°C (86°F). Failure of brainstem control of respiratory drive and the freezing of the thoracic musculature eventually lead to a cessation of breathing.
- Cold triggers peripheral vasoconstriction and tachycardia. Below 34°C (93°F), bradycardia, hypotension, decreased cardiac output, and a lengthening of cardiac electrical conduction ensue. A J-wave (Osborn hypothermic hump) may be noted at the QRS–ST junction. The myocardium becomes increasingly irritable, and spontaneous atrial and ventricular dysrhythmias can occur (Graham, McNaughton, and Wyatt, 2001).
- Below 28°C (82°F) ventricular fibrillation can develop with minor stimuli such as removing a patient's wet clothing or ambulance transport.

CLINICAL FEATURES

- Nonspecific symptoms and signs predominate and mimic the effects of mild dementia or ethanol intoxication. The CNS effects of cold lead to impaired memory, judgement, slurred speech, and decreased alertness. Paradoxic bradycardia and hypoventilation occur despite hypotension. Multiple cardiac dysrhythmias develop as the core temperature falls. A cold-induced ileus, abdominal spasm and rigidity can mimic an acute abdomen.

DIAGNOSIS

- An accurate core temperature is crucial and is ideally obtained with a rectal thermistor probe. At a minimum, a rectal temperature obtained with a thermometer scaled for hypothermia is required. Oral and ear temperatures are grossly inaccurate. A core temperature above 35°C can rapidly exclude hypothermia.

- Common laboratory findings include a falsely elevated hematocrit caused by dehydration, a low leukocyte count caused by sequestration, hyperamylasemia resulting from pancreatic injury, an aberrant coagulation profile, hypokalemia and hypoglycemia caused by glycogen depletion. Below 30°C insulin is rendered inactive and a paradoxic hyperglycemia can ensue (Danzl, 2001).

TREATMENT

- Field treatment should focus on *gentle handling* of the victim so as to not cause cardiac dysrhythmias. Wet clothing should be removed and dry clothing or a blanket applied. Massage of cold-injured limbs should be avoided; it can damage fragile, frozen parts and trigger dysrhythmias. Traumatic injuries to the spine or limbs should be stabilized. An airway should be maintained and cardiac monitoring begun if available. If the skin is frozen, needle electrodes should be used or fashioned by passing a 20-gauge needle through an electrode pad into the frozen skin. If the patient is alert—warm, non-caffeinated beverages can be provided.
- Fluid resuscitation with IV D5NS should be started. Lactated Ringers should be avoided because of problems with the metabolism of lactate by a cold-injured liver (level of evidence B/C, nonrandomized clinical trials and expert opinion). (Danzl, 2001; ECC Guidelines of the American Heart Association, 2000).
- Emergency room treatment should focus on rewarming of the patient. Defibrillation is limited to three countershocks until the core temperature is raised above 30°C (86°F) (level of evidence B, nonrandomized clinical trials). (ECC Guidelines of the American Heart Association, 2000).
- *Passive external rewarming* (PER) by covering the victim with a blanket or wrap is ideal in an alert patient whose core temperature is greater than 32°C (90°F).
- Below 90°F, rewarming should proceed with *active core rewarming* (ACR) (level of evidence B, systematic reviews, uncontrolled trials) (Lazar, 1997; Danzl et al, 1987; Danzl and Pozos, 1994*a*). This can be accomplished with IV D5NS warmed to 40–42°C (104–108°F), or the inhalation of humidified oxygen warmed to 104–108°F. More invasive techniques include peritoneal lavage with dialysate warmed to 104–108°F, thoracic lavage with normal saline at 104–108°F or warming of the gastrointestinal tract with gastric/colonic lavage.

TABLE 39-1 Hypothermia Severity and Treatment

TEMPERATURE	CLINICAL FEATURES	TREATMENT
35°C/95°F	Maximum shivering	Passive external rewarming
33°C/91°F	Ataxia, apathy, tachypnea	Passive external warming
32°C/90°F	Stupor, shivering stops	Active core rewarming (± active external rewarming)
28°C/82°F	Decreased v-fibrillation threshold, hypoventilation	Active core rewarming
14°C/57°F	Lowest adult accidental hypothermia survival	Active core rewarming
9°C/48°F	Lowest therapeutic survival	Active core rewarming

- *Active external rewarming* (AER), (fires, hot water bottles, and heating pads) should be employed only when ACR has already begun to avoid the life-threatening risk of core temperature afterdrop. This devastating process occurs when sudden exposure of vasoconstricted cool extremities to AER, causes peripheral vasodilatation, a drop in central blood pressure, and a sudden influx of cool blood from the periphery to the core that can trigger dysrhythmias and shock (Danzl, 2001). Table 39-1 provides an overview of hypothermia severity and ideal treatment modalities (Danzl, 2001).

PREVENTION

- Good conditioning, proper nutrition, experienced leadership in backcountry environments, normal hydration, avoidance of ethanol or tobacco, habituation to the cold environment (both physiologic and behavioral), and the use of proper clothing help prevent hypothermia.
- Clothing choice centers on the 3 Ls: layered, loose, and lightweight. A waterproof outer layer is key. If exercise is occurring in a temperature of <0°F three-layered hand and footwear are optimal for the prevention of frostbite.

FROSTBITE

DEFINITIONS

- Frostbite is freezing of tissues leading to damage. Frostnip is the formation of superficial ice crystals and causes *no tissue damage*. Chilblains is an *autoimmune* lymphocytic vasculitis, common in women, that leads to localized nodules or ulcers on the extremities 12 h after cold exposure.

TABLE 39–2   Risk Factors for Frostbite

PREDISPOSING FACTORS	
BEHAVIORAL	ORGANIC
Ethanol use	Prior cold injury
Psychiatric illness	Wound infection
Motor vehicle problems	Atherosclerosis
Homelessness	Diabetes mellitus
Smoking	Fatigue
Improper Clothing	
High-risk outdoor activities (back-country skiing/mountaineering)	

EPIDEMIOLOGY

- Frostbite is most common in active individuals from 30–49 years of age. High-risk outdoor activities in inclement environments account for a large percentage of injuries.
- Risk factors for frostbite are shown in Table 39-2. Ethanol and psychiatric problems underlie up to 70% of most cases of frostbite. The need for amputation correlates with the *duration* of cold exposure rather than the *lowness* of the temperature. This explains why the impaired judgement resulting from ethanol use and psychiatric illness account for such a large percentage of injuries (Reamy, 1998).
- Anatomic sites of injury are in order: feet and hands (90% of all frostbite), ears, nose, cheeks, and the penis (a particular concern for runners).

PATHOPHYSIOLOGY

- There are three synchronous pathways that lead to tissue damage in frostbite: tissue freezing, hypoxia, and the release of inflammatory mediators. Each pathway multiplies and catalyses the damage caused by the other pathways. Freezing leads to denaturation of the membrane lipid-protein matrix and cellular disruption. Hypoxia occurs from cold-induced vasoconstriction that triggers acidosis, increased viscosity, microthrombosis, and vessel endothelial damage. Inflammatory mediators, (PGF2α, Thromboxane A2) are released from damaged endothelium which triggers more vasoconstriction, platelet aggregation, thrombosis, hypoxia, and cell death. The same prostaglandins are found in the blister fluid of heat and frostbite damaged skin (Reamy, 1998).
- The release of these prostaglandins peaks during rewarming, *therefore cycles of recurrent freezing and rewarming must be avoided to lessen the extent of injury* (level of evidence B, nonrandomized clinical trials and systematic review) (Heggers et al, 1987; McCauley et al, 1983).

CLINICAL FEATURES

- Symptoms include numbness, clumsiness, tingling, and throbbing pain after rewarming.
- The signs of frostbite were classically divided into first through fourth degrees. This scheme is not prognostically useful. It is better to distinguish between two types of injury: superficial and deep frostbite. Superficial injury is characterized by normal skin color, large blisters filled with clear or milky fluid, intact pinprick sensation, and skin that will indent with pressure. Deep frostbite shows small blood-filled dark blisters, nonblanching cyanosis, skin that is wooden to the touch and will not indent with pressure.

DIAGNOSIS

- Tissue viability is not ultimately determined until 22–45 days post injury. The primary utility of diagnostic tests is to help define tissue viability at an earlier time.
- Doppler flow studies and angiography can determine tissue viability and predict the need for surgical intervention as early as 7 days postinjury. Technitium 99 m scintigraphy can be employed as soon as 72 h from injury to assess tissue viability with a *positive predictive value* (ppv) of 0.84. A scan on day 7 raises the ppv to 0.92 (level of evidence A, randomized clinical trial). (Cauchy et al, 2000)
- *Magnetic resonance imaging/magnetic resonance angiography* (MRI/MRA) may emerge as the optimal modality for early tissue assessment.

TREATMENT

- Field warming should not be instituted until refreezing can be prevented. The injured part should be protected with a loose bulky splint during transport for definitive care. Hypothermia should be treated, and smoking, ethanol, and massage of the frozen part should be avoided.
- Definitive emergency department care is outlined in Table 39-3. It is based on the work of Heggars and McCauley (Murphy et al, 2000). Adjuvant therapies with heparin, warfarin, steroids, dextran, vitamin C, and hyperbaric oxygen have not been proven to be helpful. Studies using TPA are still preliminary. Pentoxifylline (Trental) has been shown to be useful in pedal frostbite (Hayes et al, 2000).

TABLE 39-3   Stepwise Treatment of Frostbite

Treat hypothermia and any concomitant injuries.
Rapidly rewarm the affected parts in water at 40–42°C (104–108°F) until thawing is complete and the skin is pliable in texture. (Typically 15–30 min of rewarming).
Debride blisters filled with clear or milky fluid. Apply Aloe Vera (at least 70%; Dermaide Aloe). Cover with a bulky dressing. Leave hemorrhagic blisters intact.
Splint and elevate the extremity.
Administer ibuprofen orally at standard doses. (Avoid aspirin or steroids, but consider use of pentoxyfylline 400 mg po tid).
Give tetanus toxoid and tetanus immune globulin if >10 years since last booster.
Administer IV penicillin 500,000 units q. 6 hours for 72 hours. (Clindamycin is the recommended alternative for penicillin allergic patients)
Treat pain with parenteral narcotics as needed.
Begin daily hydrotherapy with hexachlorophene at 40°C for 30–60 min daily.
No smoking.

HEAT ILLNESS

DEFINITIONS

- Heat illness is best thought of as a continuum of disease that progresses along a spectrum from the mild (heat cramps), through the moderate (heat exhaustion), to the life-threatening (heatstroke). Heat cramps are involuntary, painful contractions of skeletal muscle typically occurring during or after prolonged exercise. Heat exhaustion is a sign of systemic vascular strain in the body's attempt to maintain normothermia—*untreated it will progress to heatstroke*. Heatstroke occurs when heat generation exceeds heat loss leading to a rise in core temperature and thermoregulatory failure. Classical heatstroke is confined to individuals without access to cool environments or debilitated by medical illness. Exertional heatstroke is the form most common in athletes.

EPIDEMIOLOGY

- Frequency correlates with the *wet bulb globe temperature* (WBGT). WBGT = (wet bulb temp × 0.7) + (dry bulb × 0.1) + (black globe × 0.2) where the wet bulb represents the humidity, the dry bulb the air temperature, and the black globe the radiant heat.
- Risk factors for exertional heatstroke include obesity, dehydration, fatigue, recent episode of heat illness, concomitant febrile illness, wear of impermeable garments, lack of acclimatization, sustained exercise, use of medicines, or supplements that decrease sweating and increase thermogenesis (antihistamines, ephedra, caffeine, diuretics) (Haller and Benowitz, 2000).

PATHOPHYSIOLOGY

- The cause of heat cramps is unclear. Heat illness occurs when heat storage outpaces heat loss that leads to deleterious changes at the cellular level. Core temperature >41°C leads to a release of many inflammatory mediators to include *interleuken 1* (IL-1), *interleuken 6* (IL-6), and *tumor necrosis factor* (TNF). These cytokines amplify cellular and endothelial damage that triggers systemic vascular collapse and multiorgan failure (Khosla and Guntupalli, 1999).

CLINICAL FEATURES

- Symptoms of heat exhaustion and heatstroke overlap. The diagnosis of heatstroke rests not on absolute temperature criteria—rather it is due to the presence of an altered mental status and the progression of disease despite first line treatments. Initial symptoms include headache, dizziness, fatigue, irritability, anxiety, chills, nausea, vomiting, and heat cramps. Seizures and disordered thoughts are evidence of heatstroke.
- Signs include a core temperature greater than 39.4°C, tachycardia, hyperventilation, hypotension, and syncope. Temperature elevations greater than 41°C (106°F), a lack of spontaneous cooling with cessation of exertion, and profuse sweating that *ceases* despite an elevated core temperature are all ominous signs that point toward heatstroke.

DIAGNOSIS

- The diagnosis hinges on an elevated core temperature *combined* with the presence of the symptoms and signs noted above. Ideally this temperature should be rectal. Any collapse during exertion should include heat illness in the differential and early core temperature measurement is crucial. Of note, healthy athletes can raise their core temperature to 39°C simply from exertion alone and be asymptomatic.
- Laboratory tests are normal until heatstroke is present. Lab alterations such as increased liver function tests, disordered coagulation profile, leukocytosis, electrolyte disturbances, and evidence of acute renal failure are nonspecific and similar to other shock states.

TREATMENT

- The key is to not delay treatment while trying to determine where on the continuum of heat illness a

TABLE 39-4 Treatment of Heatstroke

Immediate cooling. If available, ice water immersion is best. If not, fanning after misting the patient should be undertaken. Cool until rectal temp reaches 39°C (102.2°F).

Avoid antipyretics. The hypothalamic set point is normal! They can aggravate hepatic or renal injury.

Avoid alcohol baths. Vasodilated skin can lead to systemic absorption.

Monitor core temperature until it is <38°C (100.5°F).

Consider diazepam (5 mg) or lorazepam (2 mg) to control shivering and as prophylaxis against seizures.

Monitor renal function closely. Early dialysis is indicated.

Correct *persistent* electrolyte abnormalities.

Check coagulation profile at admission and serially until 72 h have passed. Use fresh frozen plasma (FFP) and/or platelets as needed.

Rehydrate vigorously–monitor for fluid overload and hyponatremia.

particular patient is located. Immediate treatment increases the likelihood of the body's return to normal thermoregulation and prevents progression to heatstroke.

- Field treatment should involve cessation of activity, removal to a shaded, cool environment, fluid replacement beverages, and fanning after spraying the patient with a cool mist. Heat cramps can be treated with passive stretching of the affected muscles.
- In case of altered mental status, seizures, or a core temperature greater than 104°F, heatstroke should be presumed, and the patient should be evacuated for definitive emergency care. If the patient responds to field treatment they should avoid exertion for at least 24–48 h to avoid a transient, but increased risk of recurrent heat illness.
- Heatstroke treatment involves the nine steps shown in Table 39-4 (Moran and Gaffan, 2001). Concerns that ice water immersion would increase seizures or trigger shivering thermogenesis have been allayed by recent studies (level of evidence B, nonrandomized clinical trials) (Costrini, 1990; Gaffin, Gardner, and Flinn, 2000; Weiner and Khogali, 1980).

FIVE KEYS TO PREVENTION

- *Acclimatization* to high heat and humidity for 10–14 days prior to competition is ideal. The first 4 to 5 days are when two key physiologic changes occur: changes in sweat composition and an increase in the ability of the body to rapidly dissipate heat.
- *Clothing* should be light colored, lightweight, and offer sun-protection.
- *Medications* that impair heat loss should be stopped or changed, e.g., change antihistamines to nasal steroids to treat allergic rhinitis and stop ephedra compounds.
- *Activity planning or reduction* should be based on the WGBT scale: <65 low risk for heat illness, 65–75

moderate risk, 75–85 high risk individuals should not exercise, 85–90 unacclimated athletes should stop, >90 all activities should stop (Armstrong et al, 1996).
- *Prehydration and hydration per ACSM* recommendations. These can be summarized for patients as follows: drink 16 oz of water or sports beverage 2 h before exercise—if no urination, repeat 15 min before exercise. During exercise drink 20–40 oz every hour divided in 5–10 oz amounts every 20 min. After exercise, replace each pound of weight lost with 32 oz of fluid (Armstrong et al, 1996).

ALTITUDE ILLNESS

DEFINITIONS AND CLINICAL SYNDROMES

- Rapid ascent past 8000 ft leads to the onset of the physiologic effects of decreased oxygen concentration at altitude. These effects are most pronounced for those attempting exercise at altitude. Several clinical syndromes exist:
- *High altitude headache* (HAH) is the first symptom of altitude exposure. It may or may not progress to acute mountain sickness.
- *Acute mountain sickness* (AMS) is a syndrome that includes HAH and at least one of four symptoms: nausea/vomiting, fatigue/lassitude, dizziness, or insomnia.
- *High altitude cerebral edema* (HACE) is the clinical progression of AMS so that severe CNS symptoms develop, such as ataxia, altered consciousness, confusion, drowsiness, stupor, or coma.
- *High altitude pulmonary edema* (HAPE) is the most common cause of altitude related death. It is characterized by classic signs of pulmonary edema: wet cough, dyspnea at rest, weakness, and orthopnea.

EPIDEMIOLOGY

- Altitude illness is most common in the unacclimatized, regardless of fitness level, who ascend rapidly past 8000 ft. The severity is linked to the rate of ascent, altitude attained, sleeping altitude, length of altitude exposure, level of exertion, and an individual's inherent physiologic susceptibility that remains static despite reexposure.

PATHOPHYSIOLOGY

- A rapid rate of ascent, an inappropriately slowed hypoxic ventilatory response to ambient hypoxia and hypercarbia, fluid retention, and vasogenic edema are the initial pathologic changes. Days later, cerebral edema, pulmonary hypertension, and alveolar leakage lead to death if untreated.

- *Maximal oxygen uptake* (VO_{2max}) falls 10% for each 3281 ft of altitude gained over 5000 ft (Hackett and Roach, 2001*a*). VO_{2max} at sea level is *not* predictive of performance at altitude. Many of the world's elite mountaineers have average sea level VO_{2max} values (Hackett and Roach, 2001*b*). Past performance and personal problems with altitude illness are the best predictors of future performance and the need for aggressive preventive interventions.

DIFFERENTIAL DIAGNOSIS

- Any of the symptoms of AMS on ascent past 8000 ft should trigger suspicion for altitude illness. Key differential diagnostic considerations include dehydration, hypothermia and a viral infection. Dehydration can be differentiated by response to a fluid challenge. Hypothermia can be distinguished by a low core temperature and improvement with exertion/increased body temperature. Altitude illness worsens with exertion. Although viral syndromes have similar symptoms, they are typically accompanied by fever, myalgia, or diarrhea and are more subacute in onset than AMS. Dyspnea at rest, worsening of symptoms after sleeping, and gait disturbance point toward altitude illness. Abnormal tandem gait is a sensitive examination finding for severe AMS progressing to HACE. Improvement with descent confirms the diagnosis.

TREATMENT

- Initial field treatment involves stopping the ascent and rest. A lack of improvement in 12 h should lead to a descent in altitude. Typically, descending 1000–3000 ft is sufficient. Acetazolamide (125 to 250 mg bid) should be given. If available, low flow oxygen, and portable hyperbaric bags are helpful. Additional useful medications are ibuprofen or aspirin for headache and promethazine (25–50 mg) or prochlorperazine (5–10 mg) for nausea and vomiting.
- Treatment of HACE or HAPE should include *immediate* descent and evacuation. Dexamethasone (4 mg po/IM q 6 h) for HACE and nifedipine (10 mg po once followed by 30 mg of the extended release tablet bid) should be instituted for HAPE (level of evidence B, nonrandomized clinical trial) (Bartsch et al, 1991).
- Hospital treatment will also include high flow oxygen or hyperbaric oxygen, and loop diuretics for pulmonary edema. Mechanical ventilation is only required in cases of coma.

TABLE 39-5   Prevention of Altitude Illness

1. Begin exertion below 8,000 ft. Spend two to three nights sleeping between 8000 and 10,000 ft before ascending above 10,000 ft.
2. Sleep no more than 1500 ft higher each day above 10,000 ft.
3. Avoid alcohol or sedatives.
4. Avoid dehydration or hypothermia.
5. Consider acetazolamide 250 mg po bid beginning the day before ascent: for any individual with a prior history of AMS, when climbing above 11,400 ft., or when acclimatization is not possible. (Continue until after 48 h at maximum altitude.)
6. In the face of symptoms of AMS—do not go higher. Descend if symptoms do not improve in 12 h.
7. Reserve dexamethasone for the treatment of severe AMS or HACE.

PREVENTION

- Altitude illness can be prevented by proper acclimatization. Physiologic changes of hyperventilation, tachycardia, erythropoesis, and a variety of cellular changes take from minutes to months to reach their peak. Recommendations for the prevention of altitude illness are provided in Table 39-5 (Hackett and Roach, 2001*b*).

REFERENCES

Armstrong LE, Epstein Y, Greenleaf JE, et al: American college of sports medicine position stand. Heat and cold illnesses during distance running. *Med Sci Sports Exerc* 28(12):I–X, 1996.

Bartsch P et al: Prevention of high-altitude pulmonary edema by Nifedipine. *N Engl J Med* 325:1284, 1991.

Cauchy E, Marsigny B, Allamel G, et al: The value of technetium 99 scintigraphy in the Prognosis of Amputation in severe frostbite injuries of the extremities. *J Hand Surg* 25(5):969–978, 2000.

Costrini AM: Emergency treatment of exertional heatstroke and comparison of whole body cooling techniques. *Med Sci Sports Exerc* 22:15, 1990.

Danzl DF: Accidental hypothermia, in Auerbach PS (ed.): *Wild-erness Medicine*; 4th ed. St Louis, MO, Mosby, 2001, pp 135–177.

Danzl DF, Pozos RS: Accidental hypothermia. *N Engl J Med* 331:1756, 1994*a*.

Danzl DF, Pozos RS: Accidental hypothermia. *N Engl J Med* 331:1756–1760, 1994*b*.

Danzl DF et al: Multicenter hypothermia survey. *Ann Emerg Med* 16:1042, 1987.

ECC Guidelines of the American Heart Association: Advanced challenges in resuscitation. *Circulation* 102:I229–I259, 2000.

Gaffin SL, Gardner J, Flinn S: Current cooling method for exertional heatstroke. *Ann Intern Med* 132:678, 2000.

Graham CA, McNaughton GW, Wyatt JP: *Wilderness Environ Med* 12(4):232–235, 2001.

Hackett PH, Roach RC: High-altitude illness. *New Engl J Med* 345:107–114, 2001*a*.

Hackett PH, Roach RC: High-altitude medicine, in Auerbach PS (ed.): *Wilderness Medicine,* 4th ed. St Louis, MO, Mosby, 2001*b,* pp 2–43.

Haller CA, Benowitz NL: Adverse cardiovascular and central nervous system events associated with dietary supplements containing ephedra alkaloids 343:1833–1838, 2000.

Heggers JP et al: Experimental and clinical observations on frostbite. *Ann Emerg Med* 16:1056, 1987.

Hayes DW, Mandracchia VJ, Considine C, et al: Pentoxifylline adjunctive therapy in the treatment of pedal frostbite. *Clin Podiatr Med Surg* 17(4):715–722, 2000.

Khosla R, Guntupalli KK: Heat-related illnesses. *Crit Care Clin* 15:251–263, 1999.

Lazar HL: The treatment of hypothermia. *N Engl J Med* 337: 1545, 1997.

McCauley RL et al: Frostbite injuries: A rational approach based on pathophysiology. *J Trauma* 23:143, 1983.

Moran DS, Gaffan SL: Clinical management of heat-related illnesses, in Auerbach PS (ed.): *Wilderness Medicine,* 4th ed. St Louis, MO, Mosby, 2001, pp 290–316.

Murphy JV, Banwell PE, Roberts AHN, et al: Frostbite: Pathogenesis and treatment. *J Trauma* 48:171–181, 2000.

Reamy BV: Frostbite: Review and current concepts. *J Am Board Fam Pract* 11:34–40, 1998.

Weiner JS, Khogali M: A physiological body-cooling unit for treatment of heatstroke. *Lancet* 1:507, 1980.

Section 4
MUSCULOSKELETAL PROBLEMS IN THE ATHLETE

40 HEAD INJURIES

Robert C Cantu, MD, FACS, FACSM

- If we define a direct fatality as one occurring directly from participation in the skills of a sport, as opposed to an indirect fatality which is one caused by systemic failure as a result of exertion while participating in a sport, head injury is the most frequent direct cause of death in sport (Mueller and Blyth, 1985).
- Injury to the head takes on a singular importance when we realize the brain is neither capable of regeneration nor, unlike many other body parts and organs, of transplantation.
- Every effort must be made to protect the athlete's head as injury can lead to dementia, epilepsy, paralysis, and death.
- Starting with President Theodore Roosevelt's threat to ban American football in 1904, injuries from this sport have received more media attention and reports in the medical literature than any other organized sport because none has contributed more fatalities (Kraus and Conroy, 1984).
- Brain injuries have been the most common direct cause of death among American football players since the annual recording of football-related deaths began in 1931 (Cantu and Mueller, 2003).
- Brain injury-related fatalities accounted for 69% of all football fatalities from 1945 through 1999 (Cantu and Mueller, 2003).
- Most brain injury-related fatalities involved a subdural hematoma sustained by high school football players while either tackling or being tackled in a game (Cantu and Mueller, 2003).

- Fatalities in American football from 1973 to 1983 exceeded deaths in all other competitive sports combined (Kraus and Conroy, 1984).
- Yet per 100,000 participants American football is not as likely to result in a fatal head injury as horseback riding (Barclay, 1978; Barber, 1973), sky diving (Krel, 1965; Petras and Hoffman, 1983), or car or motorcycle racing.
- Football has about the same risk of a fatal head injury as gymnastics and ice hockey (Goldberg, 1980; Fekete, 1968).
- Other sports historically shown to have a high rate of head injury including boxing (Hillman, 1980; Van, 1983; Lundberg, 1983), the martial arts (McLarchie, Davies, and Caulley, 1980), and rugby football (McCoy et al, 1984), although a fatal head injury in rugby is rare (Gibbs, 1994; Ryan and McQuillen, 1992).
- A cerebral concussion is the most common athletic head injury (Cantu, 1991).
- More than 90% of all cerebral concussions fall into this most mild category where there has not been a loss of consciousness but rather only a brief period of posttraumatic amnesia or loss of mental alertness (Cantu, 1991).

CEREBRAL CONCUSSION

- Concussion is derived from the Latin *concussus* which means "to shake violently." Initially it was thought to produce only a temporary disturbance of brain function due to neuronal, chemical, or neuroelectrical changes without gross structural damage. We now know that structural damage with loss of brain cells does occur with some concussions.
- The rates of concussion in some popular sports are listed in Tables 40-1 and 40-2.

TABLE 40-1   Sports with Helmets

Ice hockey	0.27
Football	0.25
Men's lacrosse	0.19
Woman's softball	0.11

SOURCE: (Dick, 1994)
Rate of concussions per 1000 athlete exposures.

TABLE 40-2   Sports without Helmets

Men's soccer	0.25
Women's soccer	0.24
Field hockey	0.20
Wrestling	0.20

SOURCE: (Dick, 1994)
Rate of concussions per 1000 athlete exposures.

TABLE 40-3   AAN Practice Parameter (Kelly and Rosenberg) Grading System for Concussion

Grade 1	Transient confusion; no loss of consciousness; concussion symptoms or mental status abnormalities on examination resolve in less than 15 min
Grade 2	Transient confusion; no loss of consciousness; concussion symptoms or mental status abnormalities on examination last more than 15 min
Grade 3	Any loss of consciousness, either brief (seconds) or prolonged (minutes)

TABLE 40-4   Data Driven Cantu Grading System for Concussion

Grade 1	(Mild)	No LOC, PTA, PCSS <30 min
Grade 2	(Moderate)	LOC < 1 minute or PTA >30 min <24 h PCSS >30 min <7 days
Grade 3	(Severe)	LOC ≥1 min or PTA ≥24 h, PCSS >7 days

SOURCE: Cantu RC: Post traumatic (retrograde/anterograde) amnesia; pathophysiology and implications in grading and safe return to play. *J Athl Train* 36(3):244–248, 2001.
ABBREVIATIONS: LOC = Loss of consciousness; PTA = post-traumatic amnesia; PCSS = postconcussive signs/symptoms other than amnesia.

TABLE 40-5   Post Concussion Signs/Symptoms Checklist

Bell rung	Nausea
Depression	Nervousness
Dinged	Numbness/tingling
Dizziness	Poor balance
Drowsiness	Poor concentration
Excessive sleep	Ringing in the ears
Fatigue	Sadness
Feeling "in a fog"	Sensitivity to light
Feeling "slowed down"	Sensitivity to noise
Headache	Trouble falling asleep
Irritability	Vacant stare/glassy eyed
Loss of consciousness	Vomiting
Memory problems	

- The risk of sustaining a concussion in football is four (Gerberuch et al, 1983) to six (Zemper, 1994) times greater for the player who has sustained a previous concussion. It can occur with direct head trauma in collisions or falls, or may occur without a direct blow to the head when sufficient force is applied to the brain, as in a whiplash injury (Lindberg and Freytag, 1970).
- While earlier estimates of concussion in football were as high as 20% (Gerberuch et al, 1983), current estimates place the incidence at 5–10%.
- It must be realized that universal agreement on the definition and grading of concussion does not exist. This renders the evaluation of epidemiological data extremely difficult.
- Tables 40-3 and 40-4 are the most widely cited guidelines.
- Table 40-3 guidelines are at odds with subsequent studies of Lovell et al (2003), Collins et al (2002), and Erlanger et al (2002) that found on the field memory problems/amnesia best correlated with the number and severity of postconcussion symptoms and postconcussion neuropsyche scores at 48 h. Brief *loss of consciousness* (LOC) did not.
- In the clinical evaluation of concussion—*postconcussion signs and symptoms* (PCSS) checklist (see below) should be employed, and all of the signs and symptoms noted in Table 40-5 should be sought.
- Today it is recognized that after concussion the ability to process information may be reduced (Gronwell and Wrightson, 1974), and the functional impairment may be greater with repeated concussions (Gronwell and Wrightson, 1974; Symonds, 1962).
- The late effects of repeated head trauma of concussive or even subconcussive force leads to anatomical patterns of chronic brain injury with correlating signs and symptoms.

POSTCONCUSSION SYMPTOMS

- A second late effect of concussion is the postconcussion syndrome. This syndrome consisting of headache (especially with exertion), dizziness, fatigue, irritability, and especially impaired memory and concentration has been reported in football players, but its true incidence is not known.
- The persistence of these symptoms reflects altered neurotransmitter function and usually correlates with the duration of posttraumatic amnesia (Guthkelch, 1980).
- When these symptoms persist, the athlete should be evaluated with a *computed tomography* (CT) scan and neuropsychiatric tests. Return to competition should

be deferred until all symptoms have abated and the diagnostic studies are normal.

INTRACRANIAL HEMORRHAGE

- The leading cause of death from athletic head injury is intracranial hemorrhage. There are four types of hemorrhage: epidural, subdural, subarachnoid, and intracerebral, to which the examining trainer or physician must be alert in every instance of head injury.
- Because all four types of intracranial hemorrhage may be fatal, a rapid and accurate initial assessment, as well as an appropriate follow up, is mandatory after an athletic head injury.

POSTTRAUMATIC SEIZURE

- If a seizure occurs in an athlete with a head injury, it is important to log-roll the patient onto his side. By this maneuver, any blood or saliva will roll out of the mouth or nose and the tongue cannot fall back and obstruct the airway.
- Usually such a traumatic seizure will last only for a minute or two. The athlete will then relax, and transportation to the nearest medical facility can be effected.

MALIGNANT BRAIN EDEMA

- This condition is found in athletes in the pediatric age range and consists of rapid neurological deterioration from an alert conscious state to coma and sometimes death minutes to several hours after head trauma (Pickles, 1950; Schnitker, 1949).
- Pathology studies show diffuse brain swelling with little or no brain injury (Schnitker, 1949). Rather than true cerebral edema, Langfitt and colleagues have shown that the diffuse cerebral swelling is the result of a true hyperemia or vascular engorgement (Langfitt and Kassell, 1978; Langfitt, Tannenbaum, and Kassell, 1966).
- Prompt recognition is extremely important because there is little initial brain injury and the seriousness of fatal neurological outcome is secondary to raised intracranial pressure with herniation.
- Prompt treatment with intubation, hyperventilation, and osmotic agents has helped to reduce the mortality (Bowers and Marchall, 1980; Bruce et al, 1978).

SECOND IMPACT SYNDROME

- The syndrome occurs when an athlete who sustains a head injury—often a concussion or worse injury, such as a cerebral contusion—sustains a second head injury before symptoms associated with the first have cleared (Cantu, 1992; Cantu and Voy, 1995; Saunders and Harbaugh, 1984).
- The second blow may be remarkably minor, perhaps only involving a blow to the chest that jerks the athlete's head and indirectly imparts accelerative forces to the brain.
- Usually within seconds to minutes of the second impact, the athlete—conscious yet stunned—quite precipitously collapses to the ground, semicomatose with rapidly dilating pupils, loss of eye movement, and evidence of respiratory failure.
- The pathophysiology of second impact syndrome is thought to involve a loss of autoregulation of the brain's blood supply. This loss of autoregulation leads to vascular engorgement within the cranium, which in turn markedly increases intracranial pressure and leads to herniation either of the medial surface (uncus) of the temporal lobe or lobes below the tentorium or of the cerebellar tonsils through the foramen magnum.

INCIDENCE

- Second impact syndrome is not confined to American football players. Head injury reports of athletes in other sports almost certainly represent the syndrome but do not label it as such (Fekete, 1968; Cantu, 1992; Cantu and Voy, 1995; Saunders and Harbaugh, 1984; McQuillen, McQuillen, and Morrow, 1988; Kelly et al, 1991).
- Physicians who cover athletic events, especially those in which head trauma is likely, must understand the second impact syndrome and be prepared to initiate emergency treatment.
- For a catastrophic condition that has a mortality rate approaching 50% and a morbidity rate nearing 100%, prevention takes on the utmost importance.
- An athlete who is symptomatic from a head injury *must not* participate in contact or collision sports until all cerebral symptoms have subsided, and preferably not for at least 1 week after.

DIFFUSE AXONAL INJURY

- This condition results when severe shearing forces are imparted to the brain and axonal connections are literally severed, in the absence of intracranial hematoma.

TABLE 40-6   Guidelines for Return to Sports After Concussion

	FIRST CONCUSSION	SECOND CONCUSSION	THIRD CONCUSSION
GRADE I (Mild)	May return to play if asymptomatic for 1 week	Return to play in 2 weeks if asymptomatic at that time for 1 week	Terminate season; may return to play next season if asymptomatic
GRADE II (Moderate)	Return to play after asymptomatic 1 week	Minimum of 1 month; may return to play then if asymptomatic for 1 week; consider terminating season	Terminate season; may return to play next season if asymptomatic
GRADE III (Severe)	Minimum of 1 month; may return to play if asymptomatic	Terminate season; may return to play next season	

- The patient is usually deeply comatose with a low Glasgow coma scale, a negative head CT, and immediate neurologic triage for treatment of increased intracranial pressure is indicated.

MANAGEMENT GUIDELINES

- **Immediate treatment:** With a head injury the ABCs of first aid must be followed. Before a neurological examination is undertaken, the treating physician must determine if the airway is adequate, and that circulation is being maintained. Thereafter attention may be directed to the neurological examination.
- **Definitive treatment:** Definitive treatment of Grade II and Grade III concussions as well as of the second impact syndrome and intracranial hematoma should take place at a medical facility where neurosurgical and neuroradiological capabilities are present.
- **What tests to order and when:** After a Grade I concussion, observation alone may be all that is indicated. In instances of Grade II and Grade III concussion, however, a CT scan or MRI of the brain is recommended.
- **When to refer:** Head injuries other than a Grade I concussion should be referred for neurological or neurosurgical evaluation following removal of the athlete from the contest.
- **Appropriate time course for resolution:** Table 40-6 provides guidelines for return to competition after a cerebral concussion whether Grade I, Grade II, or Grade III, and whether this was a first, second, or third concussion sustained in a given season.

CONCLUSION

- Although fatalities and catastrophic head injury will never be totally eliminated from athletics, their occurrence, especially in American football, is now low compared to previous decades.

REFERENCES

Barber HM: Horse-play: Survey of accidents with horses. *BMJ* iii:532, 1973.

Barclay WR: Equestrian sports. *JAMA* 240:1892–1893, 1978.

Bowers SA, Marchall LF: Outcome in 200 consecutive cases of severe head injury treated in San Diego County: A prospective analysis. *Neurosurgery* 6:237, 1980.

Bruce DA et al: Outcome following severe head injuries in children. *J Neurosurg* 48:679, 1978.

Cantu RC: Minor head injuries in sports, iN Dyment PG (ed.): *Adolescent Medicine: State of the Art Reviews.* Philadelphia, PA, Hanley & Belfus, 1991.

Cantu RC: Second impact syndrome: immediate management. *Phys Sportsmed* 20:55–66, 1992.

Cantu RC, Mueller FO: Brain fatalities in American football 1945–1999. *Neurosurgery* 52:847–853, 2003.

Cantu RC, Voy R: Second impact syndrome a risk in any contact sport. *Phys Sportsmed* 23:27–34, 1995.

Collins M, Lovell M, Iverson G, et al: Cumulative effects of concussion in high school athletes. *Neurosurgery* 51:1175–1179, 2002.

Dick RW: A summary of head and neck injuries in collegiate athletes using the NCAA injury surveillance system, in Hoerner E (ed.): *Head and Neck Injuries in Sports.* Philadelphia, PA, American Society for Testing and Materials, 1994.

Erlanger D, Cantu R, Barth J, et al: Loss of consciousness, anterograde memory dysfunction, and history of concussion: Implications of return-to-play decision making. *JAMA* 2002. (submitted)

Fekete JF: Severe brain injury and death following rigid hockey accidents. The effectiveness of the "safety helmets" of amateur hockey players. *Can Med Assoc J* 99:1234, 1968.

Gerberuch SG, Priest JD, Boen JR, et al: Concussion incidences and severity in secondary school varsity football players. *Am J Public Health* 73:1370–1375, 1983.

Gibbs N: Common rugby league injuries. Recommendation for treatment and preventative measures. *Sports Med* 18:438–450, 1994.

Goldberg MJ: Gymnastic injuries. *Orthop Clin North Am* 11:717, 1980.

Gronwell D, Wrightson P: Delayed recovery of intellectual function after minor head injury. *Lancet* ii:605, 1974.

Guthkelch AN: Post-traumatic amnesia, post concussional symptoms and accident neurosis. *Eur Neurol* 19:91, 1980.

Hillman H: Boxing. *Resuscitation* 8:211, 1980.

Kelly JP et al: Concussion in sports: guidelines for the prevention of catastrophic outcome. *JAMA* 266:2867–2869, 1991.

Kraus JF, Conroy C: Mortality and morbidity from injuries in sports and recreation. *Annu Rev Public Health* 5:163, 1984.

Krel FW: Parachuting for sport—study of 100 deaths. *JAMA* 194:264, 1965.

Langfitt TW, Kassell NF: Cerebral vasodilations produced by brainstem stimulation. Neurogenic control vs autoregulation. *Am J Physiol* 215:90, 1978.

Langfitt TW, Tannenbaum HM, Kassell NF: The etiology of acute brain swelling following experimental head injury. *J Neurosurg* 24:47, 1966.

Lindberg R, Freytag E: Brainstem lesions characteristics of traumatic hyperextension of the head. *Arch Pathol* 90:509–515, 1970.

Lovell M, Collins M, Iverson G, et al: Recovery from concussion in high school athletes. *J Neurosurgery* 98:293–301, 2003.

Lundberg GD: Boxing should be banned in civilized countries. *JAMA* 249:250, 1983.

McCoy GF et al: Injuries of the cervical spine in schoolboy rugby football. *J Bone Joint Surg Br* 66:500, 1984.

McLarchie GR, Davies JE, Caulley JH: Injuries in karate: a case for medical control. *J Trauma* 2:956, 1980.

McQuillen JB, McQuillen EN, Morrow P: Trauma, sports and malignant cerebral edema. *Am J Forensic Med Path* 9:12–15, 1988.

Mueller FO, Blyth CS: Survey of catastrophic football injuries: 1977–1983. *Phys Sportsmed* 13:75, 1985.

Petras AF, Hoffman EP: Roentgenographic skeletal injury patterns in parachute jumping. *Am J Sports Med* 11:325, 1983.

Pickles W: Acute general edema of the brain in children with head injuries. *N Eng J Med* 242:607, 1950.

Ryan JM, McQuillen R: A survey of rugby injuries attending an accident and emergency department. *Irish Med J* 82:72–73, 1992.

Saunders RL, Harbaugh RE: Second impact in catastrophic contact-sports head trauma. *JAMA* 252:538–539, 1984.

Schnitker MT: A syndrome of cerebral concussion in children. *J Pediatr* 35:557, 1949.

Symonds C: Concussion and its sequelae. *Lancet* i:1, 1962.

Van Allen MW: The deadly, degrading sport. *JAMA* 249:250, 1983.

Zemper E: Analysis of cerebral concussion frequency with the most common models of football helmets. *J Athl Train* 29:44–50, 1994.

41 CERVICAL SPINE

Gerard A Malanga, MD
Garrett S Hyman, MD, MPH
Jay E Bowen, DO

BACKGROUND

- Sports-related cervical spine injuries, while relatively uncommon, can be season-ending, career-ending, life-altering, or even life-ending.
- The majority of neck injuries are ligament sprains, muscle strains, or contusions (Cantu, 2000).
- The Sports Medicine physician can take steps to help prevent catastrophic neck injuries in athletes. The training of physicians who wish to care for athletes, therefore, should impart an understanding of the mechanisms and management of cervical spine injuries.
- The majority of athletic cervical spine injuries in the United States occur in football players, partly related to the large numbers of participants in the sport. As a result, most of the sports literature has examined the epidemiology and pathomechanics of cervical spine injuries in football players. Regardless of the sport, the principles for management of athletic cervical spine injuries remain constant.

EPIDEMIOLOGY

- Athletes sustain 10% of the 10,000 cervical spinal cord injuries that occur each year.
- Sports with a greater risk of cervical spine injuries include diving, football, rugby, surfing, skiing, boxing, ice hockey, wrestling, and gymnastics (Vaccaro et al, 2001).
- While the prevalence of sports-related cervical spine injuries has not been adequately researched, it is estimated that 10–15% of football players may experience a soft-tissue or neurologic injury of the cervical spine that results in time loss from sport (Meyer et al, 1994).

- In football, those most at risk play defensive positions, i.e., defensive backs, linemen, and linebackers (Cantu and Mueller, 2000; Castro et al, 1997).
- The prevalence of the stinger or burner (i.e., neurapraxic injury to the nerve root or brachial plexus) is reported to be ≥50% in football players (Levitz, Reilly, and Torg, 1997).
- Helmets have decreased fatalities but may have increased the risk of nonfatal cervical spine injury due to the emergence of spear-tackling and by imparting a sense of invincibility to the athlete in his "armor."

FUNCTIONAL ANATOMY

- There are seven cervical vertebrae and eight exiting nerve roots.
- The cranium articulates with C1 at the atlantooccipital joint, where approximately 50% of all flexion and extension occur (the "yes" joint). The first and second cervical vertebrae form the atlantoaxial joint and are uniquely designed to allow for 50% of all cervical rotatory motion (the "no" joint).
- Lateral bending occurs coupled with rotation via motion from C3 to C7.
- Intervertebral discs between C2 and C7 serve to dissipate and transmit compressive or axial loads.
- The discs are thicker anteriorly and this design contributes to the normal cervical lordosis.
- Normal sagittal diameter of the cervical spinal canal between C3 and C7 is ≥15 mm, and spinal stenosis is present below 13 mm. Functional spinal stenosis refers to the loss of protective cushioning from cerebrospinal fluid around the spinal cord as documented on MRI, CT, or myelography (Cantu, Bailes, and Wilberger, 1998).
- Each nerve root occupies between 25 and 33% of the neural foramen, which is bordered by the uncovertebral joints anteromedially, the intervertebral disc medially, the zygapophyseal or facet joints posterolaterally, and superiorly/inferiorly by the pedicles of adjoining vertebrae. Degenerative arthritic changes of any of the structures that form or border the foramina may contribute to nerve root compression.
- From C2 to C7, the nerve roots exit above their corresponding numbered vertebral body, while C1 exits between the occiput and atlas, and C8 exits between the C7 and T1 vertebrae (Malanga, 1997).
- The cervical spine depends on both static (i.e., osseocartilaginous and ligamentous) and dynamic (i.e., musculotendinous) stabilizing factors to absorb and/or dissipate forces.
- Pain in the cervical spine is mediated by free nerve endings in the outer 1/3 of the annulus fibrosus of each intervertebral disk, in the zygapophyseal (facet) joints, in the ligaments (i.e., posterior longitudinal ligament, ligamentum flavum, interspinous, and supraspinous ligaments), and the supporting musculature.

SPORT-SPECIFIC BIOMECHANICS

- The cervical spine is normally able to absorb significant multidirectional external forces by virtue of several supportive mechanisms.
- The cervical lordosis aids in dissipating axial loads through the intervertebral disks, facet joints, interspinous ligaments, and paraspinal muscles. Tucking the chin during a tackle or before an impact can lead to reversal of the normal lordosis and impairs the mechanism for dissipating axial loads.
- Axial loading has been shown to be the mechanism of catastrophic cervical spine injury in all National Football League cases that were documented well enough to allow detailed analysis (Torg, Guille, and Jaffe, 2002).
- Hyperflexion or hyperextension of the cervical spine in an athlete with a congenitally or developmentally narrowed canal may cause neurologic injury by a *pincer* mechanism (Penning, 1962).
- External forces that cause a combination of lateral bending and extension may lead to neuroforaminal compression and the neurologic injury commonly called a stinger or burner.
- A second proposed mechanism for the stinger or burner is flexion or extension combined with lateral bending and ipsilateral shoulder depression resulting in a traction injury to the cervical nerve roots.
- Acceleration/deceleration forces, such as those that occur in whiplash injuries, occur commonly in contact/collision sports, and commonly cause injury to the muscular or ligamentous supports (cervical strain/sprain) or the cervical facet joints.

CLINICAL FEATURES

DIFFERENTIAL DIAGNOSIS OF NECK PAIN IN THE ATHLETE

- Cervical muscle strain or ligament sprain
- Herniated nucleus pulposus
- Burner/stinger (i.e., cervical nerve root, brachial plexus, or peripheral nerve neuropraxia)
- Cervical radiculopathy
- Brachial plexopathy
- Fracture or dislocation
- Facet arthropathy

- Medical causes of neck pain, such as cardiovascular (MI), endocrine (thyroid), pulmonary (pneumomediastinum), infection (osteomyelitis or diskitis)

HISTORY

- Sideline physicians at an athletic event should keep in mind that most cervical spine injuries in athletes are cervical sprains or strains, followed by the stinger or burner. Fortunately, fracture-dislocation injuries are rare (Torg, Vesgo, and Sennett, 1985).
- That said, the sports medicine physician must err on the side of caution. Neck pain in any downed athlete is treated as an unstable cervical spine injury until proven otherwise.
- The stinger or burner (cervical nerve root, brachial plexus, or peripheral nerve neurapraxia) typically involves the C5 and C6 innervated muscles (i.e., deltoid, biceps, and rotator cuff), and so the athlete may complain of an inability to raise the arm (Feinberg, 2000).
- Head injuries frequently occur concomitantly with spinal injuries. An athlete with both a suspected concussion and neck pain should be considered to have a cervical spine injury until proven otherwise.
- Immobilize the spine-injured athlete immediately to prevent further neurologic deterioration. Manipulating an individual with an unstable cervical spine injury may worsen the neurologic outcome (McAlindon, 2002).
- The examiner should always inquire about the following:
  a. Neck, shoulder, arm, and leg pain
  b. Arm or leg numbness, tingling, or weakness
- Rule of thumb:
  a. Symptoms in one arm → peripheral nerve injury
  b. Symptoms in two arms, or in one or both legs → spinal cord injury
  c. Signs of head injury such as headache, blurred vision, dizziness, and disorientation
  d. Previous head or neck injuries
  e. Bowel or bladder dysfunction
  f. Prior treatments and functional status (if not seen acutely)
- Athletes with Down's syndrome (Trisomy 21) may be at increased risk for rupture of the transverse and/or alar ligaments and atlantoaxial instability. Minor trauma in such persons may cause complete atlantoaxial dissociation.

PHYSICAL EXAMINATION

- Inspection for the normal spinal curvature, ecchymosis, laceration, and obvious deformity
- Palpation for deformity or step-off, bony or soft-tissue tenderness
- Range of motion, including flexion, extension, lateral bending, and rotation
- Strength examination via manual muscle testing
- Sensation testing in all cervical dermatomes
- Reflex assessment of the C5 (biceps), C6 (brachioradialis), C6/7 (pronator), and C7 (triceps), as well as the L4 (patellar), L5 (medial hamstring), and S1 (Achilles) myotomes
- Pathologic reflex testing (Hoffman's and Babinski)
- Special tests such as the Spurling's and Lhermitte's signs

ON-SITE ACUTE MANAGEMENT

- A physician and/or certified athletic trainer with skills in the acute management of cervical spine injuries should always be on-site at collision sporting events. The aim of acute care is to prevent further neurologic deterioration, immobilize the spine, and safely transport the athlete to a trauma center for definitive evaluation and treatment. An emergency care plan should be in place and rehearsed *before* the opportunity arises to put it into action.

DIAGNOSTIC STUDIES

IMAGING

- Plain radiographs are appropriate if osseoligamentous disruption is a concern or in cases of recurrent stingers or burners or cervical cord neurapraxia. AP, lateral, and open-mouth views should always be obtained. Flexion and extension views may be indicated to rule out abnormal segmental motion.
- Studies of intact cadaver cervical spine segments have shown that horizontal movement of one vertebra on the next does not normally exceed 3.5 mm, and the angular displacement of one vertebral body on another is always ≤11° These measurements may be made with lateral neutral or flexion/extension radiographs. One caveat, however, is that younger athletes are more likely to demonstrate ligamentous laxity, and these criteria may not always be applicable (Cantu, 2000; White et al, 1975; Albright et al, 1976).
- The Torg–Pavlov ratio compares the diameter of the spinal canal to that of the vertebral body. A ratio of less than 0.8 is used to predict cervical stenosis, and has been found commonly in persons with an episode of transient cervical cord neurapraxia. The ratio has been found, however, to have low positive predictive

value for determining future injury. It is not, therefore, a recommended screening tool.

- A diagnosis of "spear tackler's spine" constitutes an absolute contraindication to participation in collision sports. It is identified as follows:
  1. Developmental cervical canal stenosis
  2. Reversal of the normal cervical lordosis on lateral radiographs
  3. Preexisting posttraumatic radiographic abnormalities of the cervical spine
  4. Documentation of the athlete having used spear tackling techniques
- Advanced imaging such as a CT scan is recommended to investigate a clinically suspected fracture when plain radiographs are unrevealing or equivocal. CT scan with myelography is a sensitive measure of spinal stenosis.
- MRI is used to evaluate soft tissues for ligamentous disruption or herniated nucleus pulposus, and can also demonstrate spinal cord contusions. T2-weighted images may be used to determine the extent of *functional reserve*, the protective cushioning of cerebrospinal fluid around the spinal cord.

ELECTRODIAGNOSTICS

- *Electromyography and nerve conduction* (EMG/NCS) studies may be useful in evaluating an athlete after neurologic insult with persistent motor or sensory abnormalities. Such testing can help delineate whether the lesion is at the level of the nerve root, brachial plexus, or peripheral nerve.

TREATMENT

- Sideline management of any athlete with neck pain or tenderness and neurologic symptoms, excluding those with a clear diagnosis of a stinger or burner, mandates immobilizing the athlete on a spine-board and emergent transport to a trauma center for evaluation by a spine specialist. The helmet should *not* be removed. Trainers and physicians should be trained in equipment to remove the athlete's facemask.
- Fractures should be referred to an orthopedic spine specialist for definitive treatment.
- Cervical sprains or strains are generally self-limited injuries managed with relative rest, icing, and nonsteroidal anti-inflammatory medications for pain and inflammation, and early mobilization and strengthening in a pain free range of motion.
- There is no benefit to using a soft cervical collar for cervical sprains or strains other than perhaps providing

a sense of security and local warmth. In fact, the use of a collar can delay recovery by causing a decrease in cervical spine range of motion.

- Stingers or burners are generally self-limited, with symptom resolution in minutes to hours. Once an athlete's neurologic examination has normalized, a tailored rehabilitation program should be instituted to prevent recurrence.
- Unresolved neurologic symptoms should be observed closely for progression.

REHABILITATION

- Rehabilitation is the cornerstone of ensuring prompt return of an athlete to competition and for preventing recurrent injury. Alternative methods of conditioning should be used while the athlete is kept out of play.
- The sports rehabilitation paradigm is as follows:
  1. Decrease pain and inflammation.
  2. Restore pain-free, full cervical spine range of motion.
  3. Optimize head and neck posture.
  4. Strengthen the cervical spine musculature (dynamic stabilizers), scapular stabilizers, upper extremities, and trunk.
  5. Maintain cardiovascular endurance according to the demands of the sport.
  6. Direct sport-specific training.
  7. Review and refine specific techniques such as tackling skills. Determine, if possible, the issues surrounding the initial injury.
  8. Optimize use of well-fitted protective gear, e.g., pads, collars, and the like.

RETURN-TO-PLAY GUIDELINES

- Several authors have published guidelines to assist clinicians in determining when an athlete should be allowed to return to collision sports following a cervical spine injury (Cantu 2000; Torg and Ramsey-Emrhein, 1997; Morganti et al, 2001). All of these guidelines are based on expert opinion (Table 41-1).
- In general, return-to-play may be contemplated when the athlete:
  1. Demonstrates full and pain-free range of motion
  2. Displays a normal neurologic examination including strength, sensation, and reflexes
  3. Does not have an osseous or unstable ligamentous injury
  4. Controversy exists over returning an athlete to sport after sustaining an episode of cervical cord neuropraxia (transient quadriparesis).

TABLE 41-1 Torg & Ramsey-Emrhein Collision Sport Participation Guidelines

NO CONTRAINDICATION

Congenital

Spina bifida occulta
Type II Klippel-Feil at C3 and below

Developmental

Torg-Pavlov ratio <0.8
Nondisplaced stable healed fracture at compression or endplate, no
 posterior involvement; or clay shoveler fracture
Healed herniated nucleus pulposus
One-level fusion

RELATIVE CONTRAINDICATION

Developmental

Pavlov ratio <0.8, with motor and/or sensory neurapraxia
Previous episodes of neurapraxia
Two- or three-level fusions
Healed but displaced stable fracture C3-C7 at posterior ring or
 compression fracture
Healed, nondisplaced stable fracture C1-C2
Instability <3.5 mm or 11°
Healed herniated nucleus pulposus with residual facet instability

ABSOLUTE CONTRAINDICATION

Congenital

Odontoid (C2) abnormalities such as odontoid agenesis, odontoid
 hypoplasia, or os odontoidium
Atlantooccipital fusion
C1-C2 anomaly or fusion
Klippel-Feil anomaly with congenital fusion of one or more vertebral
 segments and a loss of segmental motion or instability

Developmental

Spear tackler's spine
Residual pain or limited range of motion
Acute fracture or central herniated nucleus pulposus
Recurrent cervical cord neurapraxia
Fracture or ligamentous laxity at C1-C2
Acute or chronic hard disk
C1-C2 fusion
Instability >3.5mm or 11°
Body fracture with sagittal compression, arch fracture, ligament
 injury, fragmentation at canal
Lateral mass fracture with facet incongruity
>Three level fusion

SOURCE: (Malanga, 1997; Torg, Guille, and Jaffe, 2002)

PREVENTION

- Reductions in the numbers of cervical spine injuries in sport can be made by the following:
  1. Rule changes: In the National Football League, for instance, rule changes in 1976 eliminated the head as an initial contact area for blocking and tackling. Coaches are encouraged to instruct players to block and tackle with their head up. Spearing with the head has been banned.

  2. Conditioning exercises to strengthen the neck and sports-specific training.
  3. Prohibiting spearing or tackling using the head as a battering ram or grabbing the facemask.
  4. Strict enforcement of the rules by officials and intolerance of illegal play.
  5. Understand that football players playing defensive positions are more likely to sustain a catastrophic injury, so safe blocking and tackling techniques should be reinforced and stressed.
  6. Ensure that equipment properly fits.
  7. Expert on-site medical care. A certified athletic trainer, and if possible, a sports medicine physician should be available at the playing field. A plan for managing a catastrophic neck injury must be rehearsed and be in place.
  8. Any athlete with a suspected head or neck injury should be managed as if they have an unstable cervical spine fracture until proven otherwise. The player should be instructed not to move, the head and neck should be immobilized, and trained professionals should coordinate safe transfer onto a spine board and referral to a trauma center.
  9. When possible identifying congenital anomalies of the spine through a thorough preparticipation history and physical examination.

REFERENCES

Albright JP, Moses JM, Feldich HG, et al: Non-fatal cervical spine injuries in interscholastic football. *JAMA* 236:1243–1245, 1976.

Cantu RC: Cervical spine injuries in the athlete. *Semin Neurol* 20(2):173–178, 2000.

Cantu RC, Bailes JE, Wilberger JE: Guidelines for return to contact or collision sport after a cervical spine injury. *Clin Sports Med* 17(1):137–146, 1998.

Cantu RC, Mueller FO: Catastrophic football injuries: 1977–1998. *Neurosurg* 47(3): 673–677, 2000.

Castro FP, Ricciardi J, Brunet ME, et al: Stingers, the Torg ratio, and the cervical spine. *Am J Sports Med* 25(5):603–608, 1997.

Feinberg JH: Burners and stingers. *Phys Med Rehabil Clin N Am* 11(4):771–784, 2000.

Levitz CL, Reilly PH, Torg JS: The pathomechanics of chronic, recurrent cervical nerve root neurapraxia—the chronic burner syndrome. *Am J Sports Med* 25(1):73–76, 1997.

Malanga GA: The diagnosis and treatment of cervical radiculopathy. *Med Sci Sports Exerc* 29(7 Suppl):S236–S245, 1997.

McAlindon RJ: On field evaluation and management of head and neck injured athletes. *Clin Sports Med* 21(1):1–14, 2002.

Meyer SA, Schulte KR, Callaghan JJ, et al: Cervical spinal stenosis and stingers in collegiate football players. *Am J Sports Med* 22(2):158–166, 1994.

Morganti C, Sweeney CA, Albanese SA, et al: Return to play after cervical spine injury. *Spine* 26(10):1131–1136, 2001.

Penning L: Some aspects of plain radiography of the cervical spine in chronic myelopathy. *Neurology* 12:513–519, 1962.

Torg JS, Guille JT, Jaffe S: Current concepts review—Injuries to the cervical spine in American football players. *J Bone Joint Surg* 84–A(1):112–122, 2002.

Torg JS, Ramsey-Emrhein JA: Management guidelines for participation in collision activities with congenital, developmental, or post-injury lesions involving the cervical spine. *Clin J Sports Med* 7(4):273–291, 1997.

Torg JS, Vesgo JJ, Sennett B: The National Football Head and Neck Injury Registry: 14 year report on cervical quadriplegia, 1971–1985. *JAMA* 254:3439–3443, 1985.

Vaccaro AR, Watkins B, Albert TJ, et al: Cervical spine injuries in athletes: current return-to-play criteria. *Orthopedics* 24(7): 699–703, 2001.

White AA, Johnson RM, Pangabi MM, et al: Biomechanical analysis of clinical stability in the cervical spine. *Clin Orthop* 109:85–89, 1975.

42 THORACIC AND LUMBAR SPINE

Scott F Nadler, DO
Michele C Miller, DO

INTRODUCTION AND EPIDEMIOLOGY

- Back pain is a frequent complaint and source of morbidity among athletes in all sports, with low back pain accounting for 5–8% of injuries (Stanish, 1987).
- Fortunately, most episodes are self-limiting and respond to conservative treatment.
- By age 20, 50% of the general population has experienced low back pain (Sinaki and Mokri, 2000).
- Low back pain is second only to the common cold for reasons to visit a physician (Agency for Health Care Policy and Research, 1994).
- Low back pain is second only to headache as a cause of pain (Agency for Health Care Policy and Research, 1994).
- In contrast to the general population, the mechanism of injury in athletes may be more likely secondary to a sprain or strain, contusion or fracture from a direct blow to the spine (including a compression fracture, comminuted fracture, fracture of the growth plate at the vertebral end plate, lumbar transverse process fracture, and fracture of the spinous process), facet syndrome, spondylolysis, and spondylolisthesis related to repeated and forceful hyperextension maneuvers, and disc herniations (Harvey and Tanner, 1991).

- Female athletes have demonstrated to be more likely to suffer from its occurrence than males for unknown reasons (NCAA, 1998).
- Risk factors for back pain in the general population may include—history of low back pain, obesity, increasing age, lack of fitness, poor health, smoking, drug or alcohol abuse, postural factors and scoliosis, occupational hazards, and psychosocial issues.
- Risk factors in athletes usually have more to do with strength and flexibility imbalances, and functional deficits (Nadler et al, 1998; 2002b).
- Additional risk factors in young athletes may include growth spurts, an abrupt increase in the intensity or duration of training, improper technique, poor equipment, and leg length discrepancies (Harvey and Tanner, 1991).
- Hip extensor imbalance has been found to play a significant role in the past history and in the future occurrences of low back pain in female college athletes (Nadler et al, 2000; 2001).

ANATOMY

ANTERIOR ELEMENTS

VERTEBRAL BODY
- The vertebral body functions as the weight bearer of the spine.
- They are mainly trabecular bone surrounded by a thin layer of cortical bone.
- The cortical layer can proliferate with age at the sites of ligamentous attachment and result in osteophyte formation.
- The vertebral bodies are weakest anteriorly, a potential site for collapse, and often seen with compression fractures.
- There are 12 thoracic vertebral bodies.
- The vertebrae in T1–T3 diminish in size and then increase progressively in size until T12.
- The thoracic vertebral bodies are unique in that they have facets for the ribs as do the transverse processes.
- The anterior height of the vertebral body is shorter by approximately 1.5–2 cm than the posterior height and this results in the normal thoracic kyphosis.
- Conditions in which there is prominence of the thoracic kyphosis include the following:
  1. Gibbus (or humpback), caused by a localized sharp, posterior angulation often resulting from a wedging of the body of one or two vertebrae
  2. Dowager's hump caused by postmenopausal osteoporosis
  3. Postural round back resulting from decreased pelvic inclination (20°, normal 30°) with a thoracolumbar or thoracic kyphosis (Bogduk, 1997).

- There are five lumbar vertebral bodies.
- Being the largest vertebrae in the spine, they constitute 25% of the height of the entire vertebral column.

INTERVERTEBRAL DISC

- The function of the disc is for weight bearing and load transfer.
- The outer portion of the disc is the annulus fibrosis, composed of concentric rings of fibrocartilaginous tissue.
- The anterior portion is thicker than the posterior.
- The outer one-third of the disc is innervated by the vertebral and sinuvertebral nerve.
- The inner portion of the disc is the nucleus pulposus and is a gelatinous material of loose, nonoriented, collagen embedded in a matrix of glucosaminoglycans, water, and salt.
- With age, the amount of water within the disc decreases and therefore the height of the disc decreases.
- The vertebral endplate is composed of two layers of cartilage that cover the top and the bottom of each disc.
- The blood supply to the disc is obliterated within the first three decades of life, and therefore nutritional support is disrupted.
- The discs must then rely on diffusion from the endplate and the annulus for its nutrients.
- The thoracic disc is thinner, but has a stronger annulus than the cervical and lumbar discs.

COSTOVERTEBRAL JOINTS OF THE THORACIC SPINE

- These joints are synovial joints located between the vertebral bodies and the ribs.
- There are four articulations/joints (two pairs) on each vertebral body, with the exception of T1 and T10–T12 which have only one pair each.
- This joint is strengthened by the radiate ligament.

COSTOTRANSVERSE JOINTS OF THE THORACIC SPINE

- These joints are also synovial joints located between ribs 1 and 10, and the transverse processes of the vertebra of the same level.
- The ribs for T11 and T12 do not articulate with the transverse processes and therefore this joint does not exist there.
- This joint is strengthened by the costotransverse ligament.

PEDICLES

- The pedicle channels forces between the zygopophyseal joint, the transverse process and the spinous process.

POSTERIOR ELEMENTS

- The posterior elements are composed of the lamina, transverse processes, zygopophyseal/facet joint (superior and inferior), and a spinal process.
- The lamina channels forces from the spinous and inferior processes.
- The zygapophyseal joint resists sliding and twisting of the vertebral bodies.
- The superior facet of the inferior vertebral body articulates with the inferior facet of the superior vertebral body.
- This joint is a synovial joint and is subject to inflammation.
- With respect to the facets from T2 to T11 the superior facets face up, back, and slightly laterally, while the inferior facets face down, forward, and slightly medially.
- The positioning of these facets allows for the slight rotation that occurs in the thoracic spine.
- The facets for T1 and T12 are considered transitional since they are situated similar to that of the cervical and lumbar spine facets respectively.
- With respect to the lumbar spine facets, L1–L4 are oriented in a sagittal plane which is conducive to flexion and extension.
- L4–L5 and L5–S1 facets are oriented in the coronal plane which is conducive to lateral bending and rotation.
- The pars interarticularis is a portion of the lamina that intervenes between the superior and inferior zygopophyseal joints.
- The spinous processes of the thoracic spine face obliquely downward.
- The area of greatest angulation is at T7.
- T1–T3 spinous processes project posteriorly and are on the same plane as their transverse process of the same vertebrae.
- T4–T6 spinous processes project slightly downward and therefore they are on the plane halfway between their own transverse process and that of the vertebral body below.
- T7–T9 spinous processes project downward and therefore the tip is at the level of the transverse process of the vertebrae below.
- T10 spinous process is at the level of the transverse process of the vertebra below, like that of T9.
- T11 spinous process is halfway between the two transverse processes, like that of T6.
- T12 spinous process is on the same plane as its transverse process of the same vertebrae, like that of T3.
- This spinous process arrangement of the thoracic spine is sometimes referred to as the rule of 3s (Greenman, 1996).

INTERVERTEBRAL FORAMEN
- The foramen lies between the pedicles of adjacent vertebra.
- The AP diameter is larger superiorly.
- Nerve roots emerge in the upper portion and the intervertebral disc occupies the lower portion.
- This is clinically relevant because with respect to disc herniations, posterolateral herniations frequently will spare the nerve in the foramen because of this arrangement and will impinge on the roots that emerge from the lower intervertebral foramen.

LIGAMENTS
- The anterior longitudinal ligament traverses the axis to the upper sacrum and prevents hyperextension.
- It is twice as strong as the posterior longitudinal ligament.
- The posterior longitudinal ligament helps prevent hyperflexion.
- It is broader in the cervical region than in the lumbar region.
- Because of this narrowing, the lumbar region tends to be more susceptible to disc herniations as there is an inherent weakness in the posterolateral aspect of the intervertebral disc.
- Ossification of this ligament can contribute to spinal stenosis.
- The ligamentum flavum attaches lamina to lamina.
- It is continuous with the anterior capsule of the zygopophyseal joint and helps to resist flexion.
- This ligament can buckle and impinge on the spinal canal when there is intervertebral disc degeneration.
- The supraspinous and interspinous ligaments lie between the spinous processes and resist flexion and are generally weaker ligaments.

SPINAL MUSCULATURE
- There are multiple vertebral column muscles and when describing them, they are often divided into layers.
- The most superficial layer can be divided into the trapezius, latissimus dorsi, and lumbodorsal fascia.
- The next layer can be divided into the levator scapulae, and the major and minor rhomboids.
- Below that layer is the erector spinae muscle group consisting of the spinalis, semispinalis, longissimus, and iliocostalis.
- The deepest layer can be divided into the multifidi, rotatores, and intertransversarii (Greenman, 1996).

NERVES
- The anterior primary ramus forms the lumbosacral plexus innervating the lower extremity musculature.
- The posterior primary ramus forms the cutaneous and muscular innervation to the back, erector spinae, fascia, ligaments, and facet joints.
- The sinuvertebral nerve supplies the posterior and anterior longitudinal ligament, dural sac, posterior annulus fibrosis, and posterior vertebral body.

DIAGNOSTIC ASSESSMENT
- An assessment of an injured athlete or patient with low back pain should be comprehensive and determine whether the injury is attributable to a traumatic or overuse mechanism.
- Please refer to Table 42-1 for *history* and *physical examination*.
- Evaluation of the entire lower extremity kinetic chain is a key component of the physical examination as distal involvement may result in future low back injury and residual functional deficits (Nadler et al, 1998; 2002c).
- It has been determined that athletes with lower extremity acquired ligamentous laxity or overuse may be at risk for development of noncontact low back pain during athletic competition (Nadler et al, 1998).
- Effective diagnosis and management of athletes with low back pain must include an understanding of which injuries are often associated with particular sports and with the relative age of the athlete (Keene, 1985).

X-RAYS
- X-rays can help to rule out fractures, dislocations, degenerative joint disease, spondylolisthesis, narrowed intervertebral disc joint space, bony disease, and tumors.
- An oblique view may be helpful for evaluating the neural foramina.
- Flexion and extension views are useful for evaluating subluxation and stability.

CT SCAN
- CT scan is useful for evaluating spondylolysis, herniated nucleus pulposus, neoplasm, facet arthrosis, spinal stenosis, and osteoporosis.
- Overall, it is better for bony evaluation than a *magnetic resonance imaging* (MRI).

MRI
- MRI is useful to evaluate a herniated nucleus pulposus, neoplasm, spinal stenosis, and spinal infection.
- Overall, it is better for soft-tissue evaluation than a *computed tomography imaging* (CT scan).

TABLE 42-1   Historical Information to Obtain When Evaluating a Patient with Back Pain Complaints

Age and sport or occupation of patient	Onset- acute vs. insidious
Course (progressive, improving, fluctuating, episodic)	Mechanism of injury
Character of pain (sharp, dull, achy, numbing, etc.)	History of injury
Frequency of pain (constant vs. intermittent)	Location/radiation of pain
Paresthesias or abnormal sensory complaints	Weakness
Aggravating vs alleviating factors (sitting, standing, walking, supine, medication)	
Pain with inspiration, expiration or both and any difficulty breathing	
Pain with coughing, sneezing or straining (valsalva maneuver)	
Any skin lesions that might be present	Digestive complaints
History of surgery	Medical history
Social history (tobacco, alcohol, drug abuse)	
Relation to work, automobile, or other related injury	Nighttime pain and sleep history
Time of day pain occurs or is worst	

Any treatment that has been previously tried including medication, therapy, modalities, manipulation, injection

RED FLAGS bowel or bladder dysfunction, history of cancer, fever, unexplained weight loss, significant trauma, age >50, failure to improve with appropriate treatment, alcohol, or drug abuse
Generalized disorders such as HIV/AIDS, drug use, Paget's disease, osteoporosis, or end stage renal disease warrants additional laboratory or imaging studies.

Physical Examination

General appearance
Gait evaluation including heel and toe walking, tandem walking, one foot stand, and squat and return to upright positioning
Inspection including posture
Palpation
Range of motion
Strength
Sensation to light touch/pinprick in the dermatomal and peripheral nerve distribution
Muscle stretch reflexes/deep tendon reflexes and cutaneous reflexes
Upper motor neuron signs such as Babinski response, ankle clonus and spasticity
Provocative maneuvers of the thoracic spine such as a sitting slump test, passive scapular approximation, and first thoracic nerve root stretch
Provocative maneuvers of the lumbar spine such as the modified Schober test, sitting slump test, straight leg raise, crossed straight leg raise, bowstring test, reverse straight leg raise, Patrick's/Faber's, Gaenslen's test, measurement for leg length discrepancy

- Gymnasts, in particular, demonstrate disc degenerative changes and other abnormalities of the thoracolumbar spine seen on MRI.
- There appears to be a significant correlation between back pain and the decreased signal intensity and abnormalities on MRI seen in gymnasts (Basmajian and DeLuca, 1985).

BONE SCAN

- A bone scan is useful to evaluate spondylolysis, neoplasm, infection, inflammatory arthritis, and pseudoarthrosis.

ELECTRODIAGNOSTICS

- Electrodiagnostics provide an objective picture of a pathologic process and provide physiologic information.
- It may be used at the onset of nerve injury for evaluation of the H reflex and motor unit recruitment.
- It may also be used to determine recovery/chronicity.

LABORATORY

- A comprehensive evaluation may also include a *complete blood count* (CBC) with differential, erythrocyte sedimentation rate, and urinalysis, as well as other specific tests as indicated.
- Utilizing laboratory diagnostics is often appropriate to determine if an infection or malignancy may be the possible source of the back pain.

BIOMECHANICS

- Thoracic spine mobility is limited by the rib cage.
- Rotation and sidebending are the primary motions of the thoracic spine.
- There is progressively increasing flexion and extension from T1 to T12, and progressively decreasing rotation from T1 to T12.
- Flexion occurs as the inferior articular process of the superior vertebrae glides anterior and superior, and is limited by the posterior longitudinal ligament, interspinous ligament and the ligamentum flavum.
- Extension, which is the most restricted motion of the thoracic spine, occurs as the inferior articular process of the superior vertebrae glides posteriorly and inferiorly stretching the anterior longitudinal ligament and the costal cage.
- The lumbar spine region is capable of axial compression, forward flexion, extension, lateral flexion, and rotation.
- When the lumbar spine is in extreme flexion, there is spontaneous electrical silence of the musculature.
- With initial flexion there is increasing activity of the erector spinae muscles.
- Progressing to mid flexion activates the gluteus maximus until late flexion which activates the hamstrings.
- With lateral flexion of the lumbar spine, there is electrical silence of the obliques, contralateral greater than ipsilateral.

- Synergistic activity of the right external oblique and the left internal oblique, along with the transversospinalis is demonstrated during rotation to the left (Sward et al, 1991).

DIFFERENTIAL OF BACK PAIN

- Muscle strains and sprains are common and can occur at any age and with any sport.
- Gymnasts and divers may experience interspinous process bursitis or stress fractures of the pars interarticularis (Keene, 1985).
- Swimmers, in particular those who swim the butterfly stroke, and weightlifters with upper thoracic or lumbar pain, may be diagnosed with a Scheuermann's kyphosis (Keene, 1985).
- Spondylolysis—caused typically by repeated hyperextension with wrestlers, ballet dancers, gymnasts, divers, and polevaulters—has also been found to be a cause of low back pain in swimmers (Nyska et al, 2000; Gainor, Hagen, and Allen, 1983).
- Skiers, especially young elite alpine skiers and ski jumpers, demonstrate significantly higher rates of end plate lesions and this may be attributable to excessive loading and repetitive trauma of the immature spine under high velocity situations and performed in a forward bent position (Rachbauer, Sterzinger, and Eibl, 2001).
- There have been case reports of football and rugby players with thoracic spine fractures, and rugby players with acute disc prolapse (Bartlett and Robertson, 1994; Davies and Kaar, 1993; Elattrache, Fadale, and Fu, 1993; Geffen, Gibbs, and Geggen, 1997).
- It has been reported that with respect to athletes with disabilities the most commonly injured area is the thorax and spine, generally secondary to a sprain type mechanism of injury (Ferrara et al, 2000).
- Lastly, athletes of all ages and sports, with persistent midline lumbar pain, may have a disc injury or chronic instability secondary to a fracture of the vertebral body or posterior elements (Keene, 1985).
- Please refer to Table 42-2 for differential diagnosis.

TABLE 42-2   Differential Diagnosis

Myofascial pain	Sacroiliac dysfunction	Herniated nucleus pulposus
Facet pain	Spondylosis/Spinal stenosis	Spondylolysis/Spondylolisthesis
Osteoporosis	Neoplasm	Paget's disease
Radiculopathy	Congenital vs. Developmental	Medical (other)

GENERAL TREATMENT CONSIDERATIONS

- With respect to modalities, more recently benefits have been found with the use of a continuous low-level heat wrap (Nadler et al, 2003).
- Core conditioning has recently come into prominence with focus on the stabilization of the abdominal, paraspinal, and gluteal musculature in order to improve the stability and control during sports participation.
- The theory behind core conditioning is based on past studies that have demonstrated the importance of pelvic stabilization in training (Pollock et al, 1989; Jeng, 1999).
- At this time core conditioning has not yet been correlated to decrease the incidence of low back pain in the athlete; however, larger studies are required (Nadler et al, 2002a).
- Overall, aggressive rehabilitation using nonoperative intervention and education should be the focus (Spencer and Jackson, 1983).
- Surgical intervention is rarely necessary and should be reserved strictly for problems that are refractory to nonsurgical measures (Stanish, 1987).
- The goals of treatment for athletes are also different from the general population.
- The primary goal in athletes who have experienced an acute episode of low back pain is pain modulation and return to play and with episodes of chronic low back pain, return to play and the prevention of recurrence are the primary concerns (George and Dellitto, 2002).
- Return to play can be gradual and steady, and previous performance levels can usually be obtained (Spencer and Jackson, 1983).

CLINICAL SYNDROMES OF THE THORACIC SPINE

THORACIC DISC HERNIATIONS

- Thoracic disc herniations are often difficult to diagnose and to treat.
- The thoracic spine anatomy is predisposed to impingement of the spinal cord secondary to its small ratio of thoracic canal area to spinal cord area.
- The incidence of clinically significant thoracic disc herniations is estimated at less than 1% of all disc ruptures (Errico, Stecker, and Kostuik, 1997).
- The number of asymptomatic thoracic disc herniations may have a prevalence of 11–13.3% (Errico, Stecker, and Kostuik, 1997).

- There is generally no typical presentation on history or physical examination.
- Herniations typically occur from the fourth to sixth decades of life, they may also be found in children (Errico, Stecker, and Kostuik, 1997).
- The majority of herniations occur in the lower thoracic segments with 75% below T8 with 28% located at T11–T12 (Errico, Stecker, and Kostuik, 1997).
- Pain when present, can vary in character and location, possibly occurring in the thoracic or lumbar region, and possibly radiating to the trunk anteriorly, the groin, and the lower extremities.
- Neurologic findings as described in the history and physical examination section may be present.
- Diagnosis is often made by a high clinical suspicion based on examination and correlating this with diagnositic studies.
- MRI is the most sensitive method for diagnosis of a thoracic disc herniation.
- CT with myelography may also be used to provide information on bony structure, and in particular, if it is anticipated that the patient will require surgical intervention.
- In situations where disc herniation is associated with radicular pain only, conservative treatment may be most appropriate.
- Conservative treatment may include relative rest, anti-inflammatory medications, and therapies (Errico, Stecker, and Kostuik, 1997).
- Surgical intervention for thoracic disc herniations is indicated when signs of myelopathy are present.
- Once the disc is removed, fusion is often recommended secondary to cases of kyphotic deformity resulting from the surgery.

THORACIC DISCOGENIC PAIN

- As with other thoracic pain generators, thoracic discogenic pain is often poorly recognized.
- Patients who experience disc pain without radicular symptoms and without true evidence of a disc herniation or a significant herniation can often be refractory to conservative treatment.
- Discography may be useful for determining the diagnosis; however, it does remain controversial as previously described.
- With discography typically three or four levels are examined.
- When conservative treatment fails, which may include therapies for general conditioning and strengthening, surgery utilizing discectomy and fusion may be a consideration.

THORACIC SPINAL STENOSIS

- Spinal stenosis may affect the central canal or lateral recess or both, and may affect one or more spinal levels.
- Stenosis may be secondary to congenital, developmental or acquired mechanisms.
- As with the other areas of the spine although much less common than the cervical or lumbar spine, thoracic spinal stenosis is generally the result of degenerative changes that cause narrowing of the canal thereby generating pain and neurologic symptoms (Errico, Stecker, and Kostuik, 1997).
- The most common cause of stenosis is degenerative joint disease and this can be a result of any or all the following: spur formation, disc disease, narrowing intervertebral space, ligament or facet hypertrophy, and subluxation.
- There has been little published data on the treatment of thoracic spinal stenosis.
- In the lumbar spine, the L4–L5 level is most commonly affected followed by L3–L4, L2–L3, L5–S1, and T12–L1.
- Clinically, stenosis can lead to the syndrome of neurogenic claudication (pseudoclaudication).
- Patients may complain of unilateral or bilateral pain that radiates, paresthesias or weakness, pain that is generally worse with standing or walking, and improves with sitting, lying down, or with forward flexion at the waist (the classically described shopping cart syndrome).
- By forward flexing at the waist the patient can increase the anterior–posterior diameter of the spinal canal and often find relief.
- Extension will usually exacerbate the pain.
- Patients will often describe walking uphill as easier than downhill, and find comfort in a fetal position.
- The diagnosis can often be confirmed with radiographs, CT myelography, CT scan, MRI, and electrodiagnostics.
- Treatment when there is progressive neurologic deficit requires surgical intervention.
- Otherwise conservative treatment utilizing *nonsteroidal anti-inflammatory drugs* (NSAIDs), and therapy emphasizing strengthening the abdominal and spinal musculature and flexion based exercise is most appropriate.

SCHEURMANN'S DISEASE

- Scheurmann's disease may be a cause of back pain in adolescents, most commonly affecting males.

- It is believed to be a result of a herniation of a disk through the endplate into the vertebral body (Sinaki and Mokri, 2000).
- Five percent of the population demonstrates radiographic evidence of this disease without symptoms.
- Radiographic evidence comprises (*1*) anterior wedging, (*2*) endplate irregularity, (*3*) Schmorl's nodes, and (*4*) apophyseal ring fracture (Sinaki and Mokri, 2000).
- Conservative management is directed at correction of postural issues, strengthening core musculature with occasional use of a spinal orthosis in those refractory to conservative management.

FACET JOINT SYNDROME

- With facet joint syndrome, pain is generally localized to the spine, with only occasional radicular features.
- The pain is typically exacerbated by extension, and improves with activity.
- Isolated facet arthropathy is a rare finding (Errico, Stecker, and Kostuik, 1997).
- Manipulative therapy should be the initial treatment for this condition in conjunction with a comprehensive exercise program with attention toward postural biomechanics.
- Additional treatment may include relative rest, weight control, analgesics/NSAIDs, flexion-based exercise therapies, lumbosacral support, facet injections, and radiofrequency neurotomy in refractory episodes.

COSTOVERTEBRAL JOINT PAIN

- Costovertebral joint pain is a result of osteoarthritic changes and most commonly involves the ribs that are single articulations with the vertebral bodies (ribs 1, 11, and 12) and the ribs that are the longest (ribs 6–8).
- Pain is often unilateral, and may be described as achy, burning, or radiating.
- Palpation of the costovertebral junction may reproduce pain as can manipulation of the rib.
- The diagnosis may be confirmed with an injection of a local anesthetic.
- Treatment may include a corticosteroid injection or surgical excision of the affected joint in refractory cases.

THORACIC COMPRESSION FRACTURES

- Compression fractures are usually the result of a compressive flexion movement or trauma.
- The fractures are generally seen with osteoporosis, trauma (usually associated with a burst fracture),

metastatic disease, multiple myeloma or hyperparathyroid disease (Sinaki and Mokri, 2000).
- The most common areas prone to fractures are the mid and lower thoracic, and upper lumbar vertebral bodies.
- On physical examination there is often tenderness when the affected vertebral body is percussed.
- The diagnosis can be established by radiographs, MRI, CT scan, and/or bone scan.
- Treatment may include relative rest, pain medications, therapy utilizing an extension-based program, a brace with a three-point contact system.
- In the young female athlete with a compression fracture, evidence for the female athlete triad of amenorrhea, osteoporosis, and anorexia needs to be a part of the evaluation.

NEOPLASM

- Neoplasms in the thoracic spine may be categorized as primary and metastatic.
- Primary neoplasms are rare compared to metastasis.
- Common sources for the metastasis may include breast, lung, kidney, thyroid, prostate, malignant melanoma, myeloma, lymphoma, colon, and bladder (Errico, Stecker, and Kostuik, 1997).
- The hallmark of this disease process is considered to be complaints of localized back pain, particularly nocturnal pain that can disrupt sleep.
- Early there may be sensory changes and loss of bowel and bladder function along with other myelopathic symptoms.
- Often there may be a mixed picture of radiculopathy, myelopathy, and long tract signs.
- The diagnosis can often be established through the use of MRI.
- Radiation may be the treatment of choice, and at times high dose dexamethasone may be necessary when there is cord compression present (Sinaki and Mokri, 2000).
- Chemotherapy, hormonal therapy and surgical decompression and/or corpectomy may be considered when appropriate.
- Additional treatment with appropriate pain medication management and spinal support or bracing should also be addressed.

DIFFUSE IDIOPATHIC SKELETAL HYPEROSTOSIS

- *Diffuse idiopathic skeletal hyperostosis* (DISH) is a nondeforming ossification process that can involve any level of the spine, but most commonly affects the thoracic spine.

- There is ossification of the anterior and lateral spinal ligaments without disk narrowing.
- It typically affects middle aged to elderly individuals, and generally males more than females.
- Patients may be asymptomatic or may find associated pain, stiffness, and decreased range of motion.
- Treatment is generally conservative and includes NSAIDs therapeutic modalities and range of motion/flexibility exercises.

COSTOCHONDRITIS (TIETZE'S SYNDROME)

- Costochondritis involves a painful inflammatory process of the costal cartilage.
- The second rib is most commonly affected (Errico, Stecker, and Kostuik, 1997).
- Palpation of the chest wall often reproduces the pain and is important in distinguishing this syndrome from a cardiac source of pain.
- Bone scan may help confirm the diagnosis and the extent of involvement.
- Treatment often consists of anti-inflammatory medications or in refractory cases, a corticosteroid injection.

RIB-TIP SYNDROME

- This syndrome involves pain that radiates, generally from the lower four ribs, anteriorly to posteriorly.
- It is often reproducible with palpation.
- Treatment may include a steroid injection or in extremely rare cases, excision of a rib has been performed (Errico, Stecker, Kostuik, 1997).

CLINICAL SYNDROMES OF THE LUMBAR SPINE

MECHANICAL LOW BACK PAIN

- Mechanical low back pain is often a term used to describe nondiscogenic pain that is often provoked by physical activity and relieved by rest (Sinaki and Mokri, 2000).
- There is often an associated stress or strain type mechanism of injury to the spinal musculature, tendons, or ligaments.
- The symptoms are typically described as dull, achy, varying in intensity, and are generally localized to the low back region with possible involvement of the buttocks.

- There are no neurologic deficits.
- Treatment should focus on therapies that emphasize postural training, abdominal and spine stabilization, and stretching and strengthening exercises.

FACET SYNDROME

- Please refer to this section in the clinical syndromes of the thoracic spine.

LUMBAR DISC HERNIATION AND RADICULOPATHY

- Disc herniation is a common cause of acute, chronic, or recurrent low back pain.
- The herniation may occur centrally or laterally and may cause unilateral or bilateral pain.
- The mechanism of injury is often a flexion-based movement with a component of rotation.
- Symptoms of pain may often be described as radiating to the buttocks, posterior thigh or to the level of the calf or foot.
- The most common level of herniation occurs at L5–S1, followed by L4–L5, L3–L4, and L2–L3.
- The diagnosis can often be made based on the history and physical alone, but is often confirmed by further diagnostic testing in the event of confusing objective findings or to help in prognostication.
- Conservative treatment is often most appropriate and may include activity modification, NSAIDs, a rapid steroid taper, McKenzie program, squat program, abdominal and spine strengthening, and possibly epidural steroids.
- Surgical intervention is indicated in refractory cases with progressive neurological deficit or persistent unrelieved pain.

SPONDYLOLYSIS AND SPONDYLOLISTHESIS

- Spondylolysis is a bony defect of the pars interarticularis.
- Studies suggest that spondylolysis is caused by repetitive microtrauma during growth (Morita et al, 1995).
- It is commonly seen with high-risk sports activities, such as a football block, military press, tennis serve, baseball pitch, gymnastic back walkover, and the butterfly swim stroke.
- Athletes who participate in these high-risk sports may be five times more likely to have an unfavorable outcome than those who participate in low risk sports (d'Hemecourt et al, 2002).

- Symptoms are more often noted in younger patients and include localized back pain.
- An acute onset of pain and tight hamstrings can be associated with a worse outcome (d'Hemecourt et al, 2002).
- When there is a bilateral spondylolysis there can be anterior slippage of the vertebral body on the adjacent vertebral body and this is known as spondylolisthesis.
- With respect to spondylolisthesis, this is more commonly seen in males and is located at the L5 vertebral body level, followed by L4, and then L3.
- Spondylolisthesis can result in compression of the nerve roots and present as radicular pain and/or with neurologic deficits.
- Meyerding's classification is useful for grading spondylolisthesis displacement: (*1*) less than 25%, (*2*) 25–50%, (*3*) 50–75%, and (*4*) greater than 75% displacement.
- On physical examination there is often an associated increase in the lumbar lordosis, decreased range of motion, and tight hamstrings.
- The diagnosis of spondylolysis is often confirmed with radiographs utilizing lateral and oblique views to demonstrate a break in the neck or collar of the "Scottie Dog."
- Bone scan with *spect* may be necessary to confirm a more difficult diagnosis.
- The diagnosis of spondylolisthesis may be confirmed with flexion and extension radiographs that will help to determine segmental instability.
- Treatment of these entities can be controversial, however, and may involve the use of a brace, corset, or custom molded body jacket, and therapy emphasizing abdominal strengthening and flexion based exercises.
- Athletes with symptomatic spondylolysis who are treated with an anti-lordotic brace may be able to expect improvement and possible return to sports participation in 4–6 weeks (d'Hemecourt et al, 2002).
- In particular, Morita found that when pars defects were found early, with conservative management, (rest and lumbosacral corset for 3–6 months) healing was produced in 73% of the patients versus 38.5% of progressive and 0% of terminal defects (Morita et al, 1995).
- Patients with neurologic symptoms as a result of their injury may require surgical intervention.

LUMBAR SPINAL STENOSIS

- Please refer to the section titled Thoracic Spinal Stenosis.

REFERENCES

Agency for Health Care Policy and Research: *Clinical Practice Guideline 14: Acute Low Back Pain in Adults.* Rockville, MD, U.S. Department of Health and Human Services Public Health Service, 1994.

Bartlett GR, Robertson PA: Acute thoracic disc prolapse with paraparesis following a rugby tackle: A care report. *N Z Med J* 107(973):86–7, 1994.

Basmajian JV, DeLuca CJ: *Muscles Alive: Their Functions Revealed by Electromyography,* 5th ed. Baltimore, MD, Williams & Wilkins, 1985: pp 1–561.

Bogduk N: *Clinical Anatomy of the Lumbar Spine and Sacrum,* 3rd ed. New York, NY, Churchill Livingstone, 1997.

Davies PR, Kaar G: High thoracic disc prolapse in a rugby player: The first reported case. *Br J Sports Med.* 27(3):177–8, 1993.

d'Hemecourt PA, Zurakowski D, Kriemler S, et al: Spondylolysis: returning the athlete to sports participation with brace treatment. *Orthopedics* 25(6):653–7, 2002.

Elattrache N, Fadale PD, Fu FH: Thoracic spine fracture in a football player. A case report. *Am J Sports Med* 21(1):157–160, 1993.

Errico TJ, Stecker S, Kostuik JP: Thoracic Pain Syndromes, in Frymoyer JW (ed.): *The Adult Spine: Principles and Practice,* 2nd ed. Philadelphia, PA, Lippincott-Raven, 1997, pp 1623–1637.

Ferrara MS, Palutsis GR, Snouse S, et al: A longitudinal study of injuries to athletes with disabilities. *Int J Sports Med.* 21(3):221–4, 2000.

Gainor BJ, Hagen RJ, Allen WC: Biomechanics of the spine in the polevaulter as related to spondylolyis. *Am J Sports Med* 11(2):53–57, 1983.

Geffen S, Gibbs N, Geggen L: Thoracic spinal fracture in a rugby league footballer. *Clin J Sport Med* 7(2):144–146, 1997.

George SZ, Dellitto A: Management of the athlete with low back pain. *Clin Sports Med* 21(1):105–120, 2002.

Greenman, PE: *Principles of Manual Medicine,* 2nd ed. Baltimore, MD, Williams & Wilkins, 1996.

Harvey J, Tanner S: Low back pain in young athletes. A practical approach. *Sports Med* 12(6):394–406, 1991.

Jeng S: Lumbar spine stabilization exercise. *Hong Kong J Sport Med Sports Sci* 8:59–64, 1999.

Keene JS: Mechanical back pain in the athlete. *Compr Ther* 11(1):7–14, 1985.

Morita T, Ikata T, Katoh S, et al: Lumbar spondylolysis in children and adolescents. *J Bone Joint Surg Br* 77(4):620–625, 1995.

Nadler SF, Wu KD, Galski T, et al: Low back pain in college athletes. A prospective study correlating lower extremity overuse or acquired ligamentous laxity with low back pain. *Spine* 23(7):828–833, 1998.

Nadler SF, Malanga GA, DePrince M, et al: The relationship between lower extremity injury, low back pain, and hip muscle strength in male and female collegiate athletes. *Clin J Sport Med* 10(2):89–97, 2000.

Nadler SF, Malanga GA, Feinberg JH, et al: Relationship between hip muscle imbalance and occurrence of low back pain in collegiate athletes: a prospective study. *Am J Phys Med Rehabil* 80(8):572–7, 2001.

Nadler SF, Malanga GA, Bartoli LA, et al: Hip muscle imbalance and low back pain in athletes: influence of core strengthening. *Med Sci Sports Exerc* 34(1):9–16, 2002*a*.

Nadler SF, Malanga GA, Feinberg JH, et al: Functional performance deficits in athletes with previous lower extremity injury. *Clin J Sport Med* 12(2):73–78, 2002*b*.

Nadler SF, Moley P, Malanga GA, et al: Functional deficits in athletes with a history of low back pain: a pilot study. *Arch Phys Med Rehabil* 83(12):1753–8, 2002*c*.

Nadler SF, Steiner DJ, Petty SR, et al: Continuous low-level heatwrap for treating acute nonspecific low back pain. *Arch Phys Med Rehabil* 84(3):329–334, 2003.

NCAA: *Injury Surveillance System (1997–1998).* Overland Park, KS, National Collegiate Athletic Association, 1998.

Nyska M, Constantini N, Cale-Benzoor M, et al: Spondylolysis as a cause of low back pain in swimmers. *Int J Sports Med* 21(5):375–379, 2000.

Pollock, ML, Leggett, SH, Graves JE, et al: Effect of resistance training on lumbar extension strength. *Am J Sports Med* 17:624–629, 1989.

Rachbauer F, Sterzinger W, Eibl G: Radiographic abnormalities in the thoracolumbar spine of young elite skiers. *Am J Sports Med* 29(4):446–449, 2001.

Sinaki M, Mokri B: Low back pain and disorders of the lumbar spine, in Braddom RL (ed.): *Physical Medicine and Rehabilitation,* 2nd ed. Philadelphia, PA, Saunders, 2000, pp 853–893.

Spencer CW, 3rd, Jackson DW: Back injuries in the athlete. *Clin Sports Med* 2(1):191–215, 1983.

Stanish W: Low back pain in athletes: An overuse syndrome. *Clin Sports Med* 6(2):321–344, 1987.

Sward L, Hellstrom M, Jacobsson B, et al: Disc degeneration and associated abnormalities of the spine in elite gymnasts. A magnetic resonance imaging study. *Spine* 16(4):437–443, 1991.

43 MAGNETIC RESONANCE IMAGING: TECHNICAL CONSIDERATIONS AND UPPER EXTREMITY

Carolyn M Sofka, MD

TECHNICAL CONSIDERATIONS

- Nuclei with an inherent magnetic dipole moment (i.e., odd number of protons or neutrons) are suitable for *magnetic resonance* (MR) imaging (Hendrick, 1994). In clinical medical imaging, most often, this is hydrogen (H^+).

- When an external magnetic field (B_0) is applied to living tissues the hydrogen nuclei align either with or against the external magnetic field, producing a local magnetization force (Hendrick, 1994).

- Precession (ω_0) is the continuous change in the direction of this regional tissue magnetization and is determined by both the strength of the external magnetic field, B_0, as well as the gyromagnetic ratio of the nucleus (H^+) being used in the MR experiment, γ, (the Larmor frequency) $\omega_0 = \gamma B_0$ (Hendrick, 1994).

- Longitudinal magnetization is the amount of tissue magnetization in the direction of the main magnetic field B_0 (Hendrick, 1994).

- T_1 (relaxation time) is the time required for longitudinal magnetization to recover 63% of its value before a second 90° *radiofrequency* (RF) pulse is applied (Hendrick, 1994).

- T_2^* is the time for transverse magnetization to decay 37% of its original value. Both the inevitable effects of dephasing as well as the strength of the external magnetic field determine T_2^* (Hendrick, 1994).

- A basic spin echo pulse sequence resulting from applying a 90° RF pulse, waiting a certain time interval (TE/2), applying an additional 180° RF pulse, and then measuring the signal (spin echo) (Hendrick, 1994). *Repetition time* (TR) is the time between 90° pulses and *Echo time* (TE) is the time from 90° pulse to the center of the spin echo (Hendrick, 1994).

- Tissues with short T_1 values (e.g., fat) are bright on a T_1-weighted sequence and those with long T_1 times (water) are dark on T_1-weighted images. A T_1-weighted image has a short TR and a short TE.

- The TR value of a sequence determines the ultimate T_1-weighting of an image and the TE determines the amount of T_2-weighting (Plewes, 1994).

- In fast spin echo sequencing, raw data is collected simultaneously using multiple 180° refocusing pulses, resulting in multiple spin echoes being acquired during one sequence (Plewes, 1994). This results in an overall shortened imaging time.

- Other MR pulse sequences such as gradient echo imaging, fat suppression or inversion recovery techniques, and contrast-enhanced imaging are often performed in musculoskeletal imaging.

- Fat suppression and inversion recovery sequences are water-sensitive pulse sequences; these are used to evaluate for bone marrow edema, intramuscular edema, joint effusions, and tendon sheath effusions.

- Contrast-enhanced imaging uses a T_1-shortening agent (gadolinium), injected either intravenously or intra-articularly. As gadolinium is a T_1-shortening agent, areas of enhancement will be bright on T_1-weighted sequences; the conspicuity of contrast-enhancement is increased if fat suppression technique is used in addition the T_1-weighting; areas of contrast enhancement will be bright against an overall low signal intensity background. Contrast-enhanced imaging is often used in tumor imaging as well to evaluate for osteomyelitis.

- MR arthrography is a technique whereby gadolinium is injected intra-articularly. The theory of MR arthrography is to create a conspicuous (bright) joint effusion, that can help outline areas of potential pathology (Zlatkin, 1999; Beltran et al, 1997; Helgason, Chandnani, and Yu, 1997).

- Patients with orthopaedic hardware (joint prostheses, fracture plates, and screws) can be imaged with MR. Techniques to reduce regional magnetic susceptibility should be performed to improve image quality, such as using fast spin echo imaging as opposed to routine spin echo and fast inversion recovery as opposed to frequency selective fat suppression as a water sensitive pulse sequence (Tartaglino et al, 1994; Potter et al, 1996; White et al, 2000; Sofka et al, 2003) as the latter is more sensitive to magnetic field inhomogeneities (i.e., in the presence of metal).

SHOULDER

- High sensitivity and specificity of MR of the shoulder for diagnosing rotator cuff pathology has been repeatedly demonstrated (Zlatkin et al, 1989; Burk et al, 1989; Iannotti et al, 1991). The utility of fast spin echo imaging with resultant decreased examination time for diagnosing rotator cuff tears has also been validated (Carrino et al, 1997).

- Normal tendons are seen as linear hypointense (dark) bands of tissue with no internal signal on all pulse sequences.

- Tendinosis is diagnosed by observing a change in the morphology of the tendons, to include thickening, and increased signal intensity within the substance of the tendon.

- Tendon tears, including those of the rotator cuff, are diagnosed by visualizing a discrete, focal area of tendinous discontinuity, often with a fluid-filled gap.

- The degree of tendon slip retraction, if any, should be noted as well as any possible muscle atrophy in cases of full thickness tears.

- Secondary signs of rotator cuff tears include fluid distention of the subacromial-subdeltoid bursa and muscle atrophy, often seen in the setting of chronic full thickness tears.

- Muscle atrophy is diagnosed on MR as fatty infiltration of the muscle (areas of high signal intensity on T_1-weighted images) as well as thinning of the muscle and decreased muscle bulk (Bredella et al, 1999).

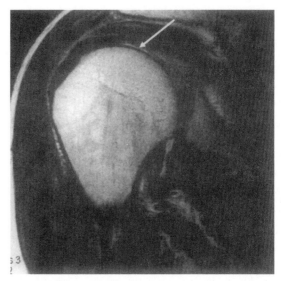

FIG 43-1(a)   Oblique coronal fast spin echo image of the shoulder demonstrating focal chondral shearing injury at the superior aspect of the humeral head (arrow).

- Care should be taken in interpreting areas of abnormal signal intensity in tendons that are recently post repair, as areas of abnormal signal or frank tendon defects can persist for some time (Zanetti et al, 2000).

- One of the most common indications for MR imaging of the shoulder is for cartilage evaluation, whether this be the articular cartilage or the fibrocartilaginous labrum.

- Some authors have demonstrated good success with diagnosing labral tears with MR arthrography (Jee et al, 2001); however, with appropriate pulse sequences, unenhanced fast spin echo imaging is highly reliable and accurate in diagnosing labral pathology (Gusmer et al, 1996; Connell et al, 1999).

- MR imaging with appropriate imaging parameters and surface coils can produce high resolution images of articular cartilage. Areas of minimal fibrillation, softening, or even focal cartilage defects can be evaluated, without the use of intra-articular contrast (Figs. 43-1(*a*), 43-1(*b*)).

- In the setting of the unstable shoulder, MR imaging can provide information as to the integrity of the glenohumeral ligaments, the joint capsule as well as any possible osseous pathology.

- After an anterior dislocation, MR can demonstrate acute osseous abnormalities (Hill Sachs fractures) as well as soft tissue injuries such as an anteroinferior labral tear (Bankart lesion) (Fig. 43-2).

- Paralabral cysts can occur in the setting of a labral tear or a degenerated labrum. MR arthrography is of limited use in diagnosing a paralabral cyst as the intra-articular contrast does not often extend into or

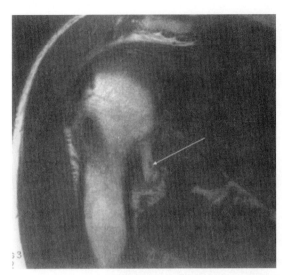

FIG 43-1(b) Oblique coronal fast spin echo image of the same shoulder at a slightly more posterior level demonstrates a linear chondral fragment in the axillary recess (arrow).

communicate with the cyst (Tung et al, 2000). Unenhanced fast spin echo imaging can clearly not only demonstrate paralabral cysts but also their communication with the labrum (Fig. 43-3).

• The fibrocartilaginous glenoid labrum helps to deepen the glenoid and maintain glenohumeral joint stability. The glenoid labrum is normally seen as a smooth uniform triangular hypointense focus adherent to the osseous glenoid on all pulse sequences. Tears of the

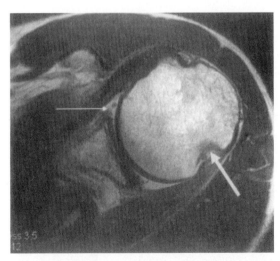

FIG 43-2 Axial fast spin echo image of the shoulder demonstrates the sequela of an anterior dislocation. Focal contour abnormality at the posterior aspect of the humeral head is a Hill Sachs impaction fracture (thick white arrow). There is, in addition, a Bankart lesion (anteroinferior labral tear) (thin white arrow).

glenoid labrum can be diagnosed as abnormal irregular high signal coursing through the substance of the labrum, with associated abnormal labral morphology. Detached fragments of the glenoid can also be seen.

• In addition to the glenoid labrum and capsule, three glenohumeral ligaments help to maintain stability of the shoulder. These are the superior, middle, and inferior glenohumeral ligaments.

• The diagnosis of adhesive capsulitis, usually diagnosed clinically and often confirmed with conventional arthrography, can be suggested at MR imaging, with thickening and occasionally hyperintensity of the joint capsule, preferential fluid distention of the biceps tendon sheath, absence of conspicuous fluid in the glenohumeral joint and scarring in the rotator interval.

• The rotator interval is the anatomic space bordered by the subscapularis and supraspinatus tendons containing the coracohumeral and superior glenohumeral ligaments (Ho, 1999; Potter, 2000). Rotator interval injuries and lesions can be associated with glenohumeral joint instability (Ferrari, 1990; Harryman et al, 1992).

• Various named labral injury patterns exist. These include the *superior labrum anterior and posterior* (SLAP) lesion (Snyder et al, 1990), the *anterior labral ligamentous periosteal sleeve avulsion* (ALPSA) lesion (Neviaser, 1993), and the *humeral avulsion of the glenohumeral ligament* (HAGL) lesion (Bui-Mansfield et al, 2002).

• SLAP lesions are generally classified into four types, all of which can be diagnosed on high-resolution noncontrast MR imaging; however, some authors have found the use of intra-articular gadolinium helpful (Jee et al, 2001).
  • Type I: Fraying and degeneration of the superior labrum (inhomogeneous and hyperintense on MR without detachment)
  • Type II: Stripping of the superior labrum and biceps anchor from the glenoid
  • Type III: A bucket-handle type tear of the superior labrum with an intact biceps
  • Type IV: Bucket handle type tear of the superior labrum with involvement of the biceps anchor (Snyder et al, 1990)

• The glenohumeral joint is the most prone to dislocate all the joints in the body. Types of glenohumeral joint dislocations include subcoracoid, subglenoid, subclavicular, and intrathoracic.

• Injuries to the *acromioclavicular* (AC) joint can be evaluated with MR imaging, with detailed depiction of the AC joint capsule and well as the supporting ligamentous structures, such as the coracoclavicular ligament.

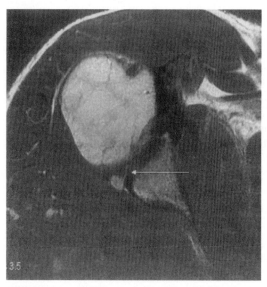 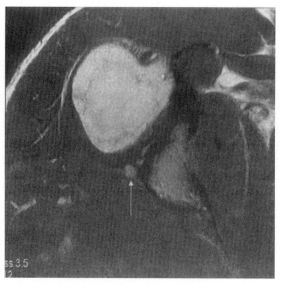

FIG 43-3 Axial fast spin echo image of the shoulder at the level of the mid glenohumeral joint demonstrates a small cyst arising from a tear in the posterior labrum (thin white arrow). Axial image at a slightly more inferior level (left) demonstrates the multilobulated paralabral cyst (arrow).

- AC joint sprains are generally classified into three types:
  - Type I: Partial disruption of the AC joint (capsular hyperintensity on fat suppressed MR sequences)
  - Type II: Partial injury to the AC joint capsule and coracoclavicular ligament. The coracoclavicular ligament is generally seen to best advantage on oblique sagittal or oblique coronal MR images.
  - Type III: Complete disruption of the AC joint capsule and coracoclavicular ligament

ELBOW

- One of the more common indications for MR imaging of the elbow is for epicondylitis. While the diagnosis of epicondylitis can be made clinically, the advantage of MR is that it can provide detailed morphologic information about the status of the tendons, including possible tendon tears, as well as reactive edema in the epicondyle. MR can also exclude other possible causes of elbow pain mimicking lateral epicondylitis, for example, such as compression of the posterior interosseous nerve.
- Epicondylitis is actually a misnomer; there is no active inflammatory component involved (Potter et al, 1995). At histology, there is primarily neovascularization and mucoid degeneration of the tendon (Potter et al, 1995).
- Degeneration of either the extensor or flexor tendons about the elbow is demonstrated by thickening, hyperintensity, and fraying of the tendon fibers (Fig. 43-4). In the case of lateral epicondylitis, the extensor carpi radialis brevis tendon, with or without involvement of

the more laterally located extensor carpi radialis longus is the primary tendon affected.
- The elbow can be imaged either with the arm at the side or with the hand over the head. Pulse sequences

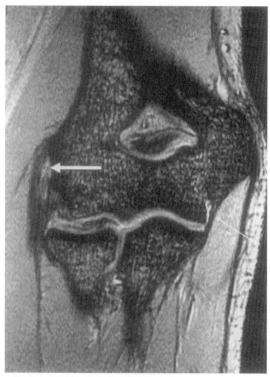

FIG 43-4 Coronal gradient echo image of the elbow demonstrates moderate tendinosis of the extensor tendons at the humerus (thick white arrow). Note the normal appearance of the medial collateral ligament (thin white arrow).

for imaging the elbow vary, but most authors agree on a volumetric gradient echo coronal sequence to evaluate the major ligamentous stabilizers and tendons about the elbow (Decker and Potter, 1998; Steinbach et al, 1997; Fritz et al, 1997).

- Medial elbow pain, typically encountered in throwing athletes from repetitive valgus stress, is often as a result of injury to the medial collateral ligament, which can be seen to best advantage on high resolution three dimensional volumetrically acquired gradient echo sequences (Gaary, Potter, and Altchek, 1997) (Fig. 43-4).
- Posteromedial impingement, with osteophyte formation about the humeral-ulnar joint, also often encountered with chronic repetitive valgus stress and overuse throwing injuries, can be imaged with MR (Gaary, Potter, and Altchek, 1997), often demonstrating subtle proliferative change and cartilage wear before any findings are apparent on conventional radiographs.
- Posterolateral rotatory instability, resulting from laxity of the ulnar band of the lateral collateral ligament, with an intact annular ligament (O'Driscoll, Bell, and Morrey, 1991) can be diagnosed prospectively with high resolution MR images (Potter et al, 1997).
- MR is especially useful in diagnosing osteochondral injuries of the elbow (osteochondritis dissecans) and localizing potential intraarticular cartilage fragments. MR provides more information as to the behavior of the osteochondral lesion than conventional radiographs or *computed tomography* (CT). In addition to identifying the abnormality as well as possible intraarticular fragments, identification of high signal (fluid) tracking about an osteochondral lesion suggests an unstable fragment.

WRIST AND HAND

- Common indications for MR imaging of the hand and wrist are for evaluating triangular fibrocartilage complex (TFCC) lesions, intercarpal ligamentous injuries, and possible ganglion cysts.
- Both the extrinsic as well as the intrinsic ligaments of the wrist can be evaluated with high resolution MR imaging (Rominger et al, 1993).
- The TFCC is composed of multiple structures, including the articular disk, the ulnar collateral ligament, the volar and dorsal radioulnar ligaments, the extensor carpi ulnaris tendon sheath, and the ulnolunate and ulnotriquetral ligaments (Palmer and Werner, 1981).
- High resolution MR imaging can be used not only to identify TFCC tears but can further classify abnormalities as radial or ulnar sided avulsions, central tears, degenerative tears as well as degenerative changes, thus appropriately directing treatment, possibly to

include arthroscopy (Potter et al, 1997). The articular disk and supporting ligamentous structures are low signal intensity on all pulse sequences.

- The interosseous scapholunate ligament has a variable appearance at MR imaging depending on the level of the wrist one is imaging. It has been demonstrated that the more volar portion of the scapholunate ligament is somewhat more patulous and hyperintense than the dorsal aspect, suspected to be due to the higher concentration of loose connective tissue in the palmar aspect of the ligament; the higher concentration of collagen in the more dorsal fibers result in a more uniform low signal intensity appearance (Totterman and Miller, 1996).
- Carpal bone fractures, often nonvisualized on conventional radiographs, can be clearly seen with a water-sensitive pulse sequence, such as inversion recovery MR imaging.
- Cartilage-sensitive pulse sequences can evaluate the articular cartilage in the radiocarpal, intercarpal, and carpometacarpal joint spaces, identifying abnormalities before secondary changes of joint space narrowing and subchondral sclerosis appear on conventional radiographs.
- The carpal tunnel can be evaluated with dedicated MR of the wrist. The median nerve is seen as a tubular intermediate signal intensity structure with fine internal linear fascicles amidst the hypointense flexor tendons. Mass lesion such as a ganglion cyst in the carpal tunnel causing compression of the median nerve can be visualized.
- The contents of the carpal tunnel, clearly seen on axial images through the wrist, include the eight superficial and deep flexor tendons, the median nerve and the flexor pollicus longus tendon.
- Repetitive overuse injuries in the adolescent can result in abnormalities of the physes about the wrist (especially in gymnasts) such as early closure (Shih et al, 1995; Liebling et al, 1995). A dedicated MR physeal pulse sequence can provide exquisite anatomic information about the status of the physis compared with conventional radiographs or CT.
- Ulnar impaction syndrome is a clinical entity with positive ulnar variance and degenerative changes along the ulnar side of the wrist, primarily involving the lunate, triquetrum and distal ulna (Escobedo, Bergman, and Hunter, 1995; Cerezal et al, 2002). Edema, subchondral cystic change and sclerosis can be seen, resulting from altered load-bearing across the ulnar side of the wrist. MR imaging can demonstrate findings in the early stages, observing signs of lunate chondromalacia, and thus can direct treatment (potential ulnar shortening).
- In the finger, high resolution, small dedicated surface coils are needed to achieve adequate resolution.

- In addition to osseous and articular injuries, MR imaging of the finger can be used to evaluate the integrity of the extensor and flexor tendons.
- In the fingers, disruption of any of the flexor pulleys can result in bowstringing of the tendon (Parellada et al, 1996). Detailed MR imaging can demonstrate the individual flexor pulleys (Hauger et al, 2000) with the A2 pulley (level of the proximal phalanx) most commonly injured, often in rock climbers.
- Gamekeeper's thumb, generally seen in skiers, is injury to the ulnar collateral ligament, with an avulsion fracture at the base of the proximal phalanx, ulnarly (Campbell, 1955). These injuries are seen to best advantage on small field of view high-resolution gradient echo MR images, centered over the *metacarpal-phalangeal* (MCP) joint. Associated Stener lesions, which is retracted ulnar collateral ligament fibers superficial to the adductor pollicis aponeurosis (Stener, 1962), can also be seen with MR imaging as a globular retracted mass of tissue superficial to the aponeurosis.

REFERENCES

Beltran J, Bencardino J, Mellado J, et al: MR arthrography of the shoulder: Variants and pitfalls. *Radiographics* 1403–1412, 1997.

Bredella MA, Tirman PF, Fritz RC, et al: Denervation syndromes of the shoulder girdle: MR imaging with electrophysiologic correlation. *Skeletal Radiol* 28(10):567–572, 1999.

Bui–Mansfield LT, Taylor DC, Uhorchak JM, et al: Humeral avulsions of the glenohumeral ligament: imaging features and a review of the literature. *Am J Roentgen* 179:649–655, 2002.

Burk, Jr DL, Karasick D, Kurtz AB, et al: Rotator cuff tears: Prospective comparison of MR imaging with arthrography, sonography, and surgery. *Am J Roentgen* 153(1):87–92, 1989.

Campbell CS: Gamekeeper's thumb. *J Bone Joint Surg Br* 37: 148–152, 1955.

Carrino JA, McCauley TR, Katz LD, et al: Rotator cuff: Evaluation with fast spin–echo versus conventional spin–echo MR imaging. *Radiology* 202:533–539, 1997.

Cerezal L, del Pinal F, Abascal F, et al: Imaging findings in ulnar–sided wrist impaction syndromes. *Radiographics* 22:105–121, 2002.

Connell DA, Potter HG, Wickiewicz TL, et al: Noncontrast magnetic resonance imaging of superior labral lesions: 102 cases confirmed at arthroscopic surgery. *Am J Sports Med* 27(2):208–213, 1999.

Decker MJ, Potter HG: Current concepts in MR imaging of the elbow and wrist. *Applied Radiol* 27–35, April 1998.

Escobedo EM, Bergman AG, Hunter JC: MR imaging of ulnar impaction. *Skeletal Radiol* 24:85–90, 1995.

Ferrari DA: Capsular ligaments of the shoulder: anatomical and functional study of the anterior superior capsule. *Am J Sports Med* 18:20–24, 1990.

Fritz RC, Steinbach LS, Tirman PFJ, et al: MR imaging of the elbow. *Radiol Clin NA* 35(1):117–144, 1997.

Gaary EA, Potter HG, Altchek DW: Medial elbow pain in the throwing athlete: MR imaging evaluation. *Am J Roentgen* 168:795–800, 1997.

Gusmer PB, Potter HG, Schatz JA, et al: Labral injuries: Accuracy of detection with unenhanced MR imaging of the shoulder. *Radiology* 200:519–524, 1996.

Harryman DT, Sidles JA, Harris SL, et al: The role of the rotator interval capsule in passive motion and stability of the shoulder. *J Bone Joint Surg Am* 74:53–66, 1992.

Hauger O, Chung CB, Lektrakul N, et al: Pulley system in the fingers: Normal anatomy and simulated lesions in cadavers at MR imaging, CT and ultrasound with and without contrast material distention of the tendon sheath. *Radiology* 217: 201–212, 2000.

Helgason JW, Chandnani VP, Yu JS: MR arthrography: A review of current technique and applications. *Am J Roentgen* 168:1473–1480, 1997.

Hendrick RE: Basic physics of MR imaging: An introduction. *Radiographics* 14:829–846, 1994.

Ho CP: MR imaging of rotator interval, long biceps, and associated injuries in the overhead–throwing athlete. *Magn Reson Imaging Clin N Am* 7(1):23–37, 1999.

Iannotti JP, Zlatkin MB, Esterhai JL, et al: Magnetic resonance imaging of the shoulder: Sensitivity, specificity, and predictive value. *J Bone Joint Surg Am* 73(1):17–29, 1991.

Jee WH, McCauley TR, Katz LD, et al: Superior labral anterior posterior (SLAP) lesions of the glenoid labrum: reliability and accuracy of MR arthrography for diagnosis. *Radiology* 218:127–132, 2001.

Liebling MS, Berdon WE, Ruzal–Shapiro C, et al: Gymnast's wrist (pseudorickets growth plate abnormality) in adolescent athletes: Findings on plain films and MR imaging. *Am J Roentgen* 164:157–159.

Neviaser TJ: The anterior labroligamentous periosteal sleeve avulsion lesion: A cause of anterior instability of the shoulder. *Arthroscopy* 9:17–21, 1993.

O'Driscoll SW, Bell DF, Morrey BF: Posterolateral rotatory instability of the elbow. *J Bone Joint Surg Am* 73(3): 440–446, 1991.

Palmer AK, Werner FW: The triangular fibrocartilage complex: of the wrist: Anatomy and function. *J Hand Surg* 6:153–162, 1981.

Parellada JA, Balkissoon ARA, Hayes CW, et al: Bowstring Injury of the flexor tendon pulley system: MR imaging. *Am J Roentgen* 167:347–349, 1996.

Plewes DB: Contrast mechanisms in spin–echo MR imaging. *Radiographics* 14:1389–1404, 1994.

Potter HG: Magnetic resonance imaging of the unstable shoulder. *Tech Shldr and Elbow Surg* 1(1):25–38, 2000.

Potter HG, Asnis–Ernberg L, Weiland AJ, et al: The utility of high–resolution magnetic resonance imaging in the evaluation of the triangular fibrocartilage complex of the wrist. *J Bone Joint Surg* 79–A(11):1675–1684, 1997.

Potter HG, Hannafin JA, Morwessel RM, et al: Lateral epicondylitis: Correlation of MR imaging, surgical and histopathologic findings. *Radiology* 196:43–46, 1995.

Potter HG, Rodeo SA, Wickiewicz TL, et al: MR imaging of meniscal allografts: Correlation with clinical and arthroscopic outcomes. *Radiology* 198(2):509–514, 1996.

Potter HG, Weiland AJ, Schatz JA, et al: Posterolateral rotatory instability of the elbow: Usefulness of MR imaging in diagnosis. *Radiology* 204:185–189, 1997.

Rominger MB, Bernreuter WK, Kenney PJ, et al: MR Imaging of anatomy and tears of wrist ligaments. *Radiographics* 13:1233–1246, 1993.

Shih C, Chang CY, Penn IW, et al: Chronically stressed wrists in adolescent gymnasts: MR imaging appearance. *Radiology* 195:855–859, 1995.

Snyder SJ, Karzel RP, del Pizzo W, et al: SLAP lesions of the shoulder. *Arthroscopy* 6(4):274–279, 1990.

Sofka CM, Potter HG, Figgie M, et al: Magnetic resonance imaging of total knee arthroplasty. *Clin Orthop* 406:129–135, 2003.

Steinbach LS, Fritz RC, Tirman PFJ, et al: Magnetic resonance imaging of the elbow. *Eur J Radiol* 25:223–241, 1997.

Stener B: Displacement of the ruptured ulnar collateral ligament of the metacarpophalangeal joint of the thumb: A clinical and anatomical study. *J Bone Joint Surg Br* 44:869, 1962.

Tartaglino LM, Flanders AE, Vinitski S, et al: Metallic artifacts on MR images of the postoperative spine: Reduction with fast spin–echo techniques. *Radiology* 190:565–569, 1994.

Totterman SMS, Miller RJ: Scapholunate ligament: Normal MR Appearance on three–dimensional gradient–recalled–echo images. *Radiology* 200:237–241, 1996.

Tung GA, Entzian D, Stern JB, et al: MR imaging and MR arthrography of paraglenoid labral cysts. *Am J Roentgen* 174:1707–1715, 2000.

White LM, Kim JK, Mehta M, et al: Complications of total hip arthroplasty: MR imaging—initial experience. *Radiology* 215:254–262, 2000.

Zanetti M, Jost B, Hodler J, et al: MR imaging after rotator cuff repair: Full–thickness defects and bursitis–like subacromial abnormalities in asymptomatic subjects. *Skeletal Radiol* 29:314–319, 2000.

Zlatkin MB: Techniques for MR imaging of joints in sports medicine. *Magn Reson Imaging Clin N Am* 7(1):1–21, 1999.

Zlatkin MB, Iannotti JP, Roberts MC, et al: Rotator cuff tears: Diagnostic performance of MR imaging. *Radiology* 172 (1):223–229, 1989.

44 SHOULDER INSTABILITY

Robert A Arciero

CLASSIFICATION

- Instability of the shoulder is a common problem. There is no report of incidence because of the large range in variability of presentation. There are three basic categories of instability. Instability should be considered as a spectrum of pathology: unidirectional traumatic instability on one end of the spectrum, acquired instability and atraumatic multidirectional instability at the other end. (Thomas and Matsen, 1989)

A. TRAUMATIC

- Anterior: Fall with the arm in an abducted and externally rotated position or an anterior force with the arm in abduction and external rotation (arm tackling in football, falling while snow skiing).
- Posterior: Posterior directed force with the arm forward elevated and adducted (MVA or pass blocking in football). Grand mal seizure or electrical shock can also produce a traumatic posterior dislocation.

B. ACQUIRED

- Microinstability: Subtle instability associated with pain in a throwing athlete or associated with rotator cuff tendinosis/dysfunction. This instability can occur from repetitive stretching of shoulder ligaments from activity or sports requirements.

C. ATRAUMATIC

- Multidirectional: These patients have symptomatic glenohumeral subluxation or dislocations in more than one direction. Many patients will present with severe pain as an initial complaint and not overt instability. For treatment purposes it is important to differentiate by patient history and physical examination the primary direction of instability.
  1. Primary Anterior: Pain associated with the arm in an abducted, externally rotated position
  2. Primary Posterior: Pain with pushing open a heavy door
  3. Primary Inferior: Pain associated with carrying heavy objects at the side
- Shoulder instability can be further classified:
  1. Degree of Instability: Dislocation, subluxation, apprehension
  2. Chronology of Instability: Congenital, acute, chronic, recurrent
  3. Direction of Instability: Anterior, posterior, inferior, superior
  4. Laxity is not Instability: Laxity refers to translation of the humerus within the glenoid fossa. Many individuals are extremely lax but are asymptomatic. Instability refers to the symptomatic complaint of instability and dysfunction.

PATHOLOGY OF INSTABILITY

- The primary pathologic entity for traumatic instability is disruption of the anterior inferior labrum combined with damage to the capsule. The primary pathology for multidirectional instability is a loose, redundant capsule.

DYNAMIC RESTRAINTS

- This is a term that refers to the stability provided by contraction of the rotator cuff (supraspinatus, infraspinatus, subscapularis, and teres minor) and scapular stabilizers (serratus anterior, trapezius, and levator scapulae). The long head of the biceps can stabilize when contracting as well as the acromial arch (coracoacromial ligament and conjoined tendon)

STATIC RESTRAINTS

- These restraints comprise bony, ligamentous, and labral anatomy that restrain translation statically and is independent of muscle contraction. It is important to recognize that the shoulder capsule only stabilizes at the end ranges of motion.
  1. Labrum: Labrum provides stability to the humeral head like a chock block for a tire. Fibrocartilagenous structure attached to both the capsule as well as the glenoid. Surrounds the entire glenoid and is generally tightly attached in the anterior inferior quadrant, has a variable attachment in the superior quadrant, and is generally less prominent posteriorly.
  2. Ligaments: The glenohumeral ligaments represent thickenings of the shoulder capsule. These are checkreins for stability. They are visualized arthroscopically on the inside of the shoulder but are difficult to distinguish on the outside.
  3. Physical pressure adhesions/cohesions
  4. Finite joint volume
  5. Joint conformity

CONGENITAL FACTORS

- Individual collagen laxity
- Bone configuration (small glenoid, retroverted glenoid)
- Age

CLINICAL PRESENTATION (PHYSICAL EXAMINATION)

- **Examination:** A careful and complete vascular and neurologic examination is essential. (The frequency of axillary nerve injuries increases with age, incidence 5–35%) (Blom and Dahlback, 1970)

A. TRAUMATIC
- **Anterior:** This patient is in acute distress. Arm held in slight abduction and internal rotation. There is a loss of deltoid contour and there will be a prominence of the acromion. (Arciero, 1999)
- **Posterior:** Associated either with a high energy event with a posterior directed force or a subluxation. Arm held in significant internal rotation. An anterior dimple can be appreciated. A hallmark physical examination feature is inability to externally rotate the arm.

B. ATRAUMATIC MULTIDIRECTIONAL
- These patients present with complaints of pain and multiple subluxation events. A hallmark physical examination feature is generalized ligamentous laxity and a sulcus sign. They may or may not have global joint laxity and due to pain and spasm sometimes do not have significant glenohumeral translation. (Neer and Foster, 1980)

RADIOGRAPHIC EXAMINATION

- It is essential to obtain three views of the shoulder to determine direction of dislocation but also to ascertain the involvement of other bony pathology.
- **AP:** The arm is held in slight internal rotation. This view will assist in identification of greater tuberosity fractures. The glenoid in profile or an AP with the beam angled perpendicular to the glenohumeral joint will allow more accurate identification of glenoid rim fractures.
- **West point:** This is a special view taken with the patient prone and the beam directed inferiorly. It is a view which allows visualization of the anterior glenoid with no other overlying bone involvement. A traditional axillary view is also very useful for evaluating direction of dislocation and fractures of the glenoid.
- **Supraspinatus outlet view, scapular lateral view, or Y view:** This is a lateral view of the shoulder which can provide information on direction of dislocation as well as angulation of proximal humerus fractures.
- **Stryker notch:** This is a view taken to evaluate the humeral head. A Hill Sachs lesion is an impression fracture of the humeral head and if large enough can impact on clinical outcome. The patient is supine with the shoulder and elbow flexed and the beam directed through the axilla.

IMAGING

- Various imaging technology is used to quantify the amount of capsular labral damage as well as evaluate the articular surface, rotator cuff, and bony architecture.

- **Computed tomography arthography:** This study allows axial cuts to evaluate glenoid morphology (amount of excess retroversion or anteversion) with size and shape of glenoid fracture fragment
- **Magnetic resonance imaging:** The MRI allows visualization of the articular cartilage and rotator cuff. It also allows visualization of the glenolabral structures, capsule, and if there is a *humeral avulsion of the glenohumeral ligaments* (HAGL) which would predicate a much different operative course.

METHODS OF REDUCTION

- After a complete history, physical examination and radiographic evaluation reduction should be completed as quickly as possible.
- **Rockwood method:** An assistant provides countertraction with a sheet draped around the torso stabilizing the chest. The caregiver then applies counter traction of the dislocated extremity distally. Slight internal and external rotation may be used to "free" up the engaged humeral head. (Neer and Rockwood, 1996)
- **Stimpson method:** The patient is placed in a prone position with the thorax supported by the table. Five to 10 lb of weight are applied to the wrist with the arm straight. In time the muscle will relax and the shoulder will be reduced. (Matsen, Thomas, and Rockwood, Jr, 1998)
- **Westin method:** Stockinette placed around the proximal forearm flexed at 90° and the patient sitting. A foot is placed in the loop created by the stockinette and a gentle force applied with internal and external rotation. (Westin et al, 1995)
- **Scapula manipulation technique:** The patient is placed prone with the arm flexed, hanging over the gurney or table and 5 to 15 lb of traction placed at the elbow. The scapula is rotated medially by pushing medially on the inferior tip and rotating the superior aspect of the scapula outward.
- **Milch Technique:** The patient is supine and the arm is elevated slowly to 90°. It is the abducted with external rotation and thumb pressure is used to gently reduce the shoulder. (Milch, 1938)
- **Kocher Technique:** The arm is flexed to 90° and traction applied in the line of the humerus. The arm is then fully externally rotated and then adducted across the chest. The arm is then internally rotated until the hand is placed on the opposite shoulder. This has been associated with proximal humerus fractures in the elderly. (Neer and Rockwood, 1996)

POST REDUCTION CARE

- It is paramount to examine and document neurovascular status after reduction. A sling can be provided for comfort and pendulum exercises should be taught to the patient. Follow up evaluation should be in 10–14 days when spasm and pain have subsided. Rehabilitation can then be employed to establish full strength and range of motion. (Arciero, 1999)
- **Rotator cuff injury:** In patients over 40 years, tears of the rotator cuff can occur with an incidence of 15% (Neviaser, Neviaser, and Neviaser, 1988). In patients over 50, there is a 63% incidence of rotator cuff pathology or proximal humerus fractures (Ribbans, Mitchell, and Taylor, 1990).
- **Axillary nerve injury:** This complication has been reported to be between 1 and 7%. At 4 weeks postreduction if active abduction cannot be established an *electromyogram* (EMG) may be necessary to diagnose and follow an axillary nerve injury. Full functional and EMG recovery is typically documented 3 to 6 months after this complication (Arciero, 1999).
- **Proximal humerus fractures:** Fractures of the greater tuberosity have been observed in up to 40% of patients over the age of 50. Displacement of 1 cm may require surgical treatment.
- *Note:* associated injuries involving the rotator cuff, proximal humerus fractures, and axillary nerve injuries increase with age at time of dislocation.

NATURAL HISTORY AND NONOPERATIVE TREATMENT

- **Traumatic anterior:** Recurrence rates after primary dislocation
- 65–95% in patients less than 20 years depending on the author
- 60% in patients 20–40 years old
- 10% in patients older than 40
- Both investigators demonstrated that immobilization had little effect on outcome (Hovelius et al, 1996; McLaughlin and MacLellan, 1967; Rowe, 1956). There are new, recent data that arm position with immobilization may play a role in nonoperative treatment. Immobilization of the arm in 35° of external rotation better approximates the labrum to the glenoid than the traditional position of internal rotation (Itoi et al, 2001).
- **Posterior:** Posterior subluxation patients responded better to nonoperative treatment than anterior subluxation patients (Burkhead and Rockwood, Jr, 1992).
- **Multidirectional Instability (MDI):** The natural history of MDI patients involves a much larger spectrum

of pathology. Eighty percent of MDI diagnosed patients respond favorably to nonoperative treatment (Burkhead and Rockwood, Jr, 1992).

REHABILITATION

- Rehabilitation for instability involves activation of the dynamic stabilizers of the shoulder to aide in the overall stabilization. There are three main components—*range of motion* (ROM), strengthening, and brace wear.
- **ROM:** Full external, internal, abduction, and forward elevation should be established. This is obtained by passive, active assisted, and finally active range of motion. A trained therapist is critical for accuracy of movement, safety, and motivation.
- **Strengthening:** This begins with isometric contractions within a range of motion that is comfortable for the patient. Once this is established, theraband exercises can begin. Finally isokinetic and isotonic strengthening with a complete arc of motion complete the program. Strengthening of the rotator cuff and scapular stabilizers is critical.
- **Brace:** Braces are used to limit the "at risk" position for return to sports.
  - SSI brace: (Boston Brace International) Limits motion and protects against blows.
  - The SAWA Shoulder Orthosis: Brace International provides anterior support and ads a check rein.
  - The Duke–wire harness–Lace up corset
  - The SSI brace was the most effective in limiting anterior shoulder subluxation while the SAWA was considered to be the most comfortable (DeCarlo et al, 1996).

OPERATIVE TREATMENT OPTIONS

- **Recurrent traumatic anterior**: Recurrence rates in the young athletic population after nonoperative treatment are unpredictable (65–95%). Surgical stabilization should be considered in a young athlete who desires return to sport. Arthroscopic surgery has the advantage of creating less morbidity and allowing a more detailed examination of the shoulder. Although controversial acute stabilization arthroscopically in the high demand patient has been very successful and should be considered in the correct setting (Arciero et al, 1994; Kirkley, Griffin, and Richards, 1999).
  1. **Arthroscopic results:** Arthroscopic techniques have evolved over the last 35 years. The literature is replete with methods involving staples, transglenoid sutures, cannulated implants, and suture anchors. In the last 3–5 years arthroscopic techniques have

evolved to the level where they mimic the open technique. This involves plication of redundant inferior capsule, reattachment of the anterior inferior labrum directly to bone with suture anchors and closure of the rotator interval. Recent reports place the recurrent dislocation event after surgery at 5 to 15% (Bacilla, Field, and Savoie, 1997). In high demand patients a recurrent subluxation event was 15% (2/13 patients) with one requiring surgery (Mazzocca et al, 2004).
  2. **Open results:** Historically many procedures have been described for glenohumeral instability. Many of these did not repair the labral lesion and high rates of instability were still found.
     a. Magnuson-stack-muscle transposition of the subscapularis
     b. Putti-Platt-shortening of the subscapularis and capsule
     c. Bristow-transfer of the coracoid process
     d. Weber-osteotomy of the proximal humerus
     e. Meyer-Burgdorff-osteotomy of glenoid
     f. Gallie-reconstruction with fascia lata
     g. Nicola-biceps tendon through humeral head
     h. Du Toit-staple repair of labrum
     i. Bankart-suture repair of labrum
- Bankart lesions (tears of the anterior inferior labrum) were found in 84% of patients with continued instability after surgery. Stability was restored in 92% with repair of labrum. Uncorrected capsular redundancy was also a reason for failure in over 80% of patients (Rowe, Zarins, and Ciullo, 1984).
  3. **Bone reconstruction:** There are instances where the anterior inferior glenoid has a large fracture or is deficient secondary to impaction or chronic instability. In these instances soft tissue procedures are not adequate and bone graft may be required.
     a. **Glenoid deficiency:** A 21% glenoid defect caused instability and limited range of motion after Bankart repair (Itoi et al, 2000). For large defects two procedures exist:
        1. **Laterjet/Bristow:** Coracoid bone graft placed to the glenoid (Burkhart and De Beer, 2000).
        2. **Extracapsular iliac crest:** Iliac crest autograft placed extracapsular with 3.5 mm screws 20/21 excellent results after chronic instability (Churchill et al, 2001).
     b. **Hill sachs lesion:** If the humeral head lesion is large (greater than 33%) or engages the glenoid in a functional range of motion then various procedures can be considered (Burkhart and De Beer, 2000).
        1. Humeral head allograft
        2. Open capsular shift

3. Lesser tuberosity transfer with subscap tendon

4. Rotational osteotomy of the humerus

- **Recurrent traumatic posterior:** This is a less frequent multifactorial condition with several modes of presentation.

  1. Open capsular posterior shift: Associated with a posterior Bankart lesion and good success. Posterior capsule is shifted superiorly and laterally through a posterior approach (Bigliani et al, 1995).

  2. Arthroscopic: Suture anchor or bioabsorbable tack fixation arthroscopically of the posterior Bankart lesion, associated with an 8% re–operation rate for failure (Williams et al, 2003).

- **Acquired microinstability:** This is a condition that exists in the throwing or overhead athlete. Subtle anterior instability may lead to an impingement of the articular supraspinatus/infraspinatus tendons against the posterior superior labrum termed internal impingement.

- **Multidirectional:** Open inferior shift: This procedure first reported by Neer and Foster has been successful. Reports of 2–8% failure rates in multidirectional instability patients (Neer and Foster, 1980; Cooper and Brems, 1992).

REFERENCES

Anderson D, Zvirbulis, Ciullo J: Scapular manipulation for reduction of anterior shoulder dislocation. *Clin Orthop* 164:181–183, 1982.

Arciero RA: Acute Anterior Dislocations, in Warren RF, Craig EV, Altchek DW (eds.): *The Unstable Shoulder.* Philadelphia, PA, Lippincott–Raven, 1999, pp 159–175.

Arciero RA, Wheeler JH, Ryan JB, et al: Arthroscopic Bankart repair versus nonoperative treatment for acute, initial anterior shoulder dislocations. *Am J Sports Med* 22(5):589–594, 1994.

Bacilla P, Field L, Savoie F: Arthroscopic Bankart repair in a high demand patient population. *Arthroscopy* 13(1):51–60, 1997.

Bigliani L, Pollock G, McIlveen S, et al: Shift of the posterior inferior aspect of the capsule for recurrent posterior glenohumeral instability. *J Bone Joint Surg* 77–A:1011–1020, 1995.

Blom S, Dahlback LO: Nerve injuries in Dislocations of the Shoulder Joint and Fractures of the Neck of the Humerus: A clinical and Electromyographical Study. *Acta Chir Scand* 136:461–466, 1970.

Burkhart S, De Beer J: Traumatic Glenohumeral bone defects and their relationship to failure of arthroscopic Bankart repairs: Significance of the inverted–pear glenoid and the humeral engaging Hill Sachs lesion. *Arthroscopy* 19(7):677–694, 2000.

Burkhead WZ, Rockwood CA, Jr: Treatment of instability of the shoulder treated with an exercise program. *J Bone Joint Surg* 74A:890– 896, 1992.

Churchill R, Moskal M, Lippitt S, et al: Extracapsular anatomically contoured anterior glenoid bone grafting for complex glenohumeral instability. *Tech Shldr and Elbow Surg* 2(3):210–218, 2001.

Cooper RA, Brems JJ: The inferior capsular shift procedure for multidirectional instability of the shoulder. *J Bone Joint Surg* 74A:1516– 1521, 1992.

DeCarlo M, Malone K, Geric B, et al: Evaluation of Shoulder Instability Braces. *J Sports Rehab* 1996;5:143–150.

Hovelius L, Augustine BG, Fredin H, et al: Primary anterior dislocation of the shoulder in young patients. A ten–year prospective study. *J Bone Joint Surg* 78(11):1677–1684, 1996.

Itoi E, Lee S, Berglund L, et al: The effect of a glenoid defect on anteroinferior stability of the shoulder after Bankart repair: a cadaveric study. *J Bone Joint Surg* 82–A(1):35–46, 2000.

Itoi E, Sashi R, Minigawa H, et al: Position of immobilization after dislocation of the glenohumeral joint. A study with use of magnetic resonance imaging. *J Bone Joint Surg* 84–A(5):661–667, 2001.

Kirkley A, Griffin S, Richards C: Prospective randomized clinical trial comparing the effectiveness of immediate arthroscopic stabilization versus immobilization and rehabilitation in first traumatic anterior dislocations of the shoulder. *Arthroscopy* 155:507–514, 1999.

Matsen FA, Thomas SC, Rockwood CA, Jr: Anterior glenohumeral instability, in Rockwood CA, Jr, Matsen FA (eds.): *The Shoulder,* vol. 2, 2nd ed. Philadelphia, PA, Saunders, 1998, pp 669–672.

McLaughlin HL, MacLellan DI: Recurrent anterior dislocation of the shoulder. *J Trauma* 7:191–201, 1967.

Mazzocca AD, Brown FM, Carriera DS, et al: Arthroscopic Stabilization of Collision Athletes. *AJS* 2003. (in press)

Milch H: Treatment of Dislocation of the Shoulder. *Surgery* 3:732–740.

Neer CS, II, Foster CR: Inferior Capsular Shift for Inferior and Multidirectional Instability of the Shoulder: A Preliminary Report. *J Bone Joint Surg A* 62:879–908, 1980.

Neer CS, Rockwood CA, Jr: Fractures and Dislocations of the Shoulder, in Rockwood CA, Jr. Green DP (eds.): *Fractures in Adults,* vol. 1, 4th ed. Philadelphia, PA, JB Lippincott, 1996.

Neviaser RJ, Neviaser TJ, Neviaser JS: Concurrent rupture of the rotator cuff and anterior dislocation of the shoulder in the older patient. *J Bone Joint Surg* 70A:1308–1311, 1988.

Ribbans WJ, Mitchell R, Taylor GJ: Computerized arthrotomography of primary anterior dislocation of the shoulder. *J Bone Joint Surg* 72B:181–185, 1990.

Rowe CR: Prognosis in dislocation of the shoulder. *J Bone Joint Surg* 38A:957–977, 1956.

Rowe CR, Zarins B, Ciullo JV: Recurrent anterior dislocation of the shoulder after surgical repair. *J Bone Joint Surg* 66A:159, 1984.

Thomas SC, Matsen FA, III: An approach to the repair of avulsion of the glenohumeral ligaments in the management of traumatic anterior glenohumeral instability. *J Bone Joint Surg* 71A:506–513, 1989.

Westin CD, Gill EA, Noyes ME, et al: Anterior shoulder dislocation. A simple and rapid method for reduction. *AJS* 23:369–371, 1995.

Williams R, Strickland S, Cohen M, et al. Arthroscopic repair for traumatic posterior shoulder instability. *AJS* 31(2):203–209, 2003.

45 ROTATOR CUFF PATHOLOGY

Patrick St Pierre, MD

HISTORY

- John Gregory Smith published the first detailed series of rotator cuff ruptures, describing seven cases obtained by grave robbing, in a letter to the editor of the London Medical Gazette in 1834. Muller and Perthes were the first to perform repairs in the late 1800s. Codman and later McLaughlin were pioneers in the early 1900s, describing their approach to the shoulder and detailing rotator cuff repair techniques that have been followed until today (Burkhead and Habermeyer, 1996).
- In 1972, Charles Neer II (Neer, 1972) first proposed the phrase "Impingement Syndrome" for pain involving the subacromial bursa and superior rotator cuff. He described the clinical presentation of the painful shoulder and proposed a mechanism for how the pathology developed. He noted that many of these patients had a hooked acromion and his hypothesis was that the bursa and rotator cuff were impinged between the humeral head and acromion with elevation of the arm. This would usually start as mild inflammation of the tendon, would progress to fibrosis and tendonitis, and eventually could lead to full thickness rotator cuff tear.

IMPINGEMENT OR ROTATOR CUFF SYNDROME (NEER, 1972;1983)

- Stage I, as described by Neer, included edema and hemorrhage in the tendon. Tendinosis of the supraspinatus and less frequently, the infraspinatus or subscapularis is involved.
- Stage II, consisted of fibrosis and tendonitis in the subacromial space. This is a secondary process resulting from the underlying etiology.
- Stage III, resulted in the development of spurs and eventually tendon rupture.
- The long head of the biceps tendon may also be involved with pathology ranging from inflammation to rupture (Crenshaw and Kilgore, 1966). Dislocation of the biceps tendon from the bicipital groove is pathognomonic for a tear of the upper border of the subscapularis muscle from its humeral insertion (Gerber, Hersche, and Farron, 1996; Gerber and Krushell, 1991).

- Pain will often occur along the anterior–lateral acromion, in the infraspinatus fossa, or distally at the deltoid insertion on the humerus. This pain is likely to be referred pain from the inflamed bursa, which irritates the deep deltoid. Pain referring proximally to the neck usually originates from the *acromioclavicular* (AC) joint (Chen, Rokito, and Zuckerman, 2003; Valadie et al, 2000; Warner et al, 2001; Yocum, 1983).
- There have been several other etiologies proposed for shoulder pain emanating from the subacromial space following Dr. Neer's initial description (Jobe and Jobe, 1983; Jobe, Kvitne, and Giangarra, 1989; Walch et al, 1992). These different etiologies may or may not lead to actual impingement of the cuff by the acromion. Because multiple pathologies are often factors in this condition, including tendinosis and bursitis, the best global term to describe this condition is Rotator Cuff Syndrome, reserving Impingement Syndrome for cases of true external impingement caused by AC arthritis or from the development of a *coracoacromial* (CA) ligament spur. Specific etiologies, as discussed later, may also be used.

PATHOPHYSIOLOGY

- **Rotator cuff syndrome**
  - Historically, patients will occasionally remember a direct blow or some other form of trauma. There may be history of a traction injury or a fall directly on a patient's shoulder.
  - Overuse injury is also a frequent cause of this syndrome. Patients will often not recall a specific injury, but may have carried luggage all weekend, cleaned out their attic, or worked on their car. Often the patient will be a weekend athlete who plays a full day of tennis, softball or other activity that they are not sufficiently trained for.
  - These conditions occur primarily because of injury to the rotator cuff causing tendinosis and rotator cuff dysfunction. The subacromial impingement occurs chronically with the development of subacromial spurs and superior humeral head migration due to lower rotator cuff inhibition or fatigue.
- **Secondary impingement:** Subtle shoulder instability can lead to rotator cuff dysfunction and thus to rotator cuff syndrome. Jobe described this as secondary or internal impingement syndrome (Jobe and Jobe, 1983; Jobe, Kvitne, and Giangarra, 1989). This condition was originally noted in overhead throwing athletes, but should be suspected in all younger athletes who complain of impingement type pain. Treatment of this condition must address the underlying instability and not just the secondary pathology in the subacromial space.

- **Posterosuperior glenoid impingement:** This condition, as described by Walch (Walch et al, 1992), has also been proposed as an etiology in occurring in patients who play repetitive overhead sports such as baseball, tennis, and swimming. Walch did not find the anterior instability described by Jobe in his patients, but rather noted an impingement of the supraspinatus and infraspinatus tendons between the posterosuperior glenoid labrum and the humeral head.
- These internal impingement syndromes are characterized by partial tears of the articular surface of the rotator cuff, in distinction to the external compression described by Neer (McFarland et al, 1999).
- Whatever the etiology, weakness of the rotator cuff results, especially the lower cuff, and superior humeral head migration occurs. The humeral head then compresses the bursa and tendon into the acromion, leading to impingement. This causes more bursitis, more tendinosis, and eventually more weakness. Often with chronic injury, shoulder mechanics will change leading to abnormal scapulothoracic motion. Physical therapy will need to include rehabilitation of the scapular stabilizing musculature as well as the lower rotator cuff muscles (Jobe and Moynes, 1982).
- Any subacromial changes, such as lateral hooking, CA ligament calcification, or AC joint arthritis (inferior spurs), will cause the condition to get worse and will more likely need operative intervention than when the acromion is flat.
- **Calcific tendinitis:** The etiology of calcific tendinitis remains unknown. Degenerative changes and relative hypoxia has been suggested as possible explanations. Conservative treatment similar to that for rotator cuff syndrome is reported as successful in 60–90% of patients (DePalma and Kruper, 1961; Harmon, 1958; Moseley, 1963). Repetitive needling and injection of local anesthetic has also been successful in relieving symptoms and often disappearance of the calcified mass. Infrequently, the patient's symptoms will persist and they will require operative intervention. The mass is localized within the substance of the tendon while viewing in the subacromial space. The calcified substance is then evacuated and debrided. Some argue that a repair of the tendon is not necessary, but the surgeon should evaluate the cuff after debridement in each case to determine if repair is necessary.

EXAMINATION (YAMAGUCHI ET AL, 2001)

- Inspection should focus on normal alignment of chest wall, shoulders, and clavicle. Have the patient perform active *range of motion* (ROM) in forward flexion,

abduction, adduction, external rotation, and internal rotation. Look from the back and front for asymmetric motion or atrophy. Often patients will have a painful arc of motion over 120° of elevation.
- Palpation of the AC and *sternoclavicular* (SC) joints, the anterior and lateral acromion edges and the infraspinatus fossa. Tenderness at the AC joint should lead you to further evaluation and treatment of AC joint arthrosis. Cross-arm adduction is often painful with AC arthrosis; however, this test is not very specific and is often positive with rotator cuff syndrome.
- Palpation of the long head of the biceps tendon within the bicipital groove is helpful to determine biceps involvement.
- Strength testing should involve the deltoid muscles, biceps muscles, and triceps muscles. Although there is no way to totally isolate each of the rotator cuff muscles, the tests that have shown to be most specific are as follows (Kelly et al, 1996):
  1. Supraspinatus: Active elevation against resistance with the elbow in extension and the arm elevated to 90° and externally rotated to 45°. The hand should be supinated to neutral as if holding a full can of soda.
  2. Infraspinatus/teres minor: Active external rotation with arm at the side and elbow flexed to 90°.
  3. Subscapularis: Active internal rotation with elbow flexed to 90° and hand placed behind the back. This is often referred to as the Gerber lift-off test (Gerber, Hersche, and Farron, 1996; Gerber and Krushell, 1991; Greis et al, 1996). In patients who are unable to internally rotate their hand behind their back, a belly press test or "Napoleon's test" is performed. Patient place their hands on their belly and press hard into their abdomen while bringing their elbow forward in the sagittal plane. Subscapularis tear or dysfunction is indicated if they are unable to do this maneuver and the elbow stays close to the side (Warner, Allen, and Gerber, 1994).
- Lag tests are also often used to detect rotator cuff tears. The Hornblower's sign, ER lag and IR lag tests were described by Gerber and Hertel and are helpful to determine subtle weakness (Gerber and Krushell, 1991; Hertel et al, 1996).
- Special tests include the Neer impingement sign and test and Hawkins' sign.
  1. Neer's impingement sign is similar to the supraspinatus testing described above, except the arm is held in maximal internal rotation as if pouring out a can of soda. This rotates the greater tuberosity under the acromion to elicit a painful response if the bursa or tendons are injured. A positive Neer's test is when a subacromial injection of local anesthetic relieves the pain elicited prior to the injection (Neer, 1972; 1983).

2. Hawkins' test forward flexes the arm to 90° and applies maximum internal rotation to the flexed elbow. If one supplies downward pressure at the elbow while the patient resists, the sensitivity of the exam increases (Hawkins and Kennedy, 1980; Valadie et al, 2000).

RADIOGRAPHIC EXAMINATION

- Standard radiographs include an *anteroposteior* (AP), axillary, and supraspinatus outlet view. These views will allow you to determine if there is degenerative joint disease in the AC or glenohumeral joints, spurring from the acromion or calcification within the tendon (calcific tendonitis). Chronic rotator cuff tears will often result in superior humeral head migration secondary to atrophy of the lower rotator cuff. A true scapular AP view will allow better examination of the glenoid and internal and external rotation view will allow better assessment of the humeral head for defects or impression fractures.
- Special radiographs are indicated in certain conditions. A supraspinatus outlet view is often obtained to evaluate the morphology of the acromion in rotator cuff or impingement syndrome. A West Point view is helpful in evaluating the anterior glenoid for bony deficiency in cases of instability.
- MRI is an excellent tool for determining rotator cuff pathology, but is often overused and/or obtained too soon.
- Certain signal characteristics are indicative of full tears versus partial tears versus AC arthritis. A *magnetic resonance imaging* (MRI) can determine labral pathology (Bankart lesions, or SLAP tears), bursitis, acromial morphology, and articular cartilage condition. More details about MRI for upper extremity injuries can be found in chapter 43.
- An MRI does not need to be obtained immediately if the patient has full ROM and only complains of pain and weakness. These patients can be started on the nonoperative treatment described below and the vast majority will improve. An MRI can be obtained after the next visit if the patient's symptoms have not resolved with therapy.

NONOPERATIVE TREATMENT

- Rotator cuff strengthening is essential for recovery and many patients improve after surgical intervention because they finally commit themselves to the rehabilitation.

- The focus of rehabilitation should be to reduce inflammation (usually bursal), restore motion, and strengthen muscles to help stabilize the scapula and humerus. Therapists will start with anti-inflammatory modalities, work on ROM and begin periscapular strengthening to stabilize the scapula (Jobe and Moynes, 1982; Wilk and Arrigo, 1993).
- Nonsteroidal anti-inflammatory drugs (NSAIDs) are usually helpful to help decrease the bursitis and reduce the pain. They are not curative in themselves, but decrease pain so the patient can do therapy. In rare instances, the pain is severe enough for a short course of narcotics.
- A subacromial injection can be performed as a diagnostic test or as part of the treatment plan. When the Neer sign is positive, an injection is made into the subacromial space using a local anesthetic. The patient is retested after 3–5 min and the Neer test is positive if the pain is relieved. Many physicians who are certain of their diagnosis will proceed with a therapeutic injection of 2–3 cc of an injectable corticosteroid at the same time. Others will inject a second time if the initial injection relieves the patient's symptoms.
- If there is a diagnostic dilemma between whether the AC joint is the cause of pain or the bursa, injections can be performed in one location and then the second to determine the source. The subacromial injection should be done first because with AC pathology—the capsule is often disrupted and an AC injection is likely to go into the bursa as well. The reader is referred to chapter 72 on injections for more information.
- Once the pain is reduced and the ROM restored, more aggressive strengthening exercises are instituted. Internal and external rotation exercises using rubber tubing or resistance bands are very useful, and the patient progresses to heavier tubing, as they get stronger. Supine or lateral decubitus exercises with small weights are also started at this time.
- Core strengthening exercises to help stabilize the scapula are also instituted. These exercises are very important and often neglected. Simple exercises such as squeezing the shoulder blades together or scapular rows are often effective. Progress is monitored by observing normal scapulothoracic motion with elevation. If scapular winging is severe or fails to improve with treatment, further workup for other etiologies such as trapezius or long thoracic nerve palsy should occur.
- Deltoid strengthening, to include isolated training of all three parts of the deltoid.
- Strengthening of the supraspinatus is not instituted immediately because it will aggravate symptoms. Supraspinatus strengthening should be started when

ROM is restored and lower cuff strength is sufficient to allow overhead motion without pain.

- Most patients' symptoms resolve with this program. Injections are usually limited to three, but each patient treatment is individualized. Many practitioners are concerned about the effects of corticosteroids on the damaged tendon and either forego this step or limit the number of injections. Patients who have developed subacromial spurs and AC arthritis are less likely to improve due to fixed impingement and may require surgery. On the other hand, a younger patient with normal radiographs may get more injections and physical therapy prior to surgical intervention.

SURGICAL INTERVENTION

- **Subacromial decompression**
  - Originally described by Neer as an open operation to remove anterior and lateral spurs on the acromion, remove the inflamed bursa, and resection or release of the CA ligament (Neer, 1972).
  - Nirschl has proposed that the development of spurs is a secondary process and is not causative in nature as once thought by Neer (Nirschl, 1989). The spurs are usually anterior and medial and due to calcification of the CA ligament. He advocates inspection of the acromion and CA ligament, with the removal of bone only if abnormal ossification has occurred. He maintains that frequently an acromioplasty and CA ligament resection is not necessary. This is especially true for articular sided tears cause by intrinsic pathology.
  - Arthroscopy has led to a less invasive approach to decompression and the operative goal is usually to convert the acromion to a so-called type I acromion. A bursectomy and inspection of the cuff is included.
  - Pathology of the long head of the biceps tendon is often a part of this syndrome. A thorough inspection of the biceps tendon intra-articularly and into the bicipital groove is necessary. Treatment of these conditions is described in chapter 47.
- **AC joint surgery (Also discussed in chapter 46)**
  - Originally described as an open operation by Mumford (Blevins et al, 1996), 1.5–2.0 cm of the distal clavicle is removal for treatment of AC joint arthritis (Chen, Rokito, and Zuckerman, 2003).
  - This surgery relies on the coracoclavicular ligaments providing stabilization of the clavicle. The acromioclavicular ligaments are repaired at closure.
  - Arthroscopic surgeons have found that resection of 8–10 mm is all that is necessary for adequate decompression and pain relief.

- Often neglected is medial spurring on the acromion at the AC joint. This should also be resected with either an open or arthroscopic procedure.
- **Rotator cuff repair**
  - The indications and necessity of rotator cuff repair remains controversial. The fact that many patients—with a full thickness rotator cuff tear—are asymptomatic indicates that the mere presence of a hole in the supraspinatus tendon does not necessitate surgical repair. Many patients also do well with a simple lower rotator cuff rehabilitation program to strengthen and balance the anterior and posterior forces providing humeral head depression (Burkhart, Esch, and Jolson, 1993). Some surgeons advocate subacromial decompression alone without repair of the rotator cuff (Burkhart, 1993).
  - On the other hand, Yamaguchi has shown us that many tears will progress (Yamaguchi et al, 2001), leading to a dysfunctional shoulder. Once these tears are large, the muscles will atrophy and undergo fatty degeneration, making a functional repair impossible.
  - Therefore, most shoulder surgeons will repair rotator cuff tears whenever possible. Burkhart has shown us that balancing the forces of the infraspinatus and subscapularis, without necessarily a *water tight closure* is often sufficient for a successful repair (Burkhart, 1997; 2000; 2001; Burkhart et al, 1994); however, for large, massive tears, many advocate decompression alone or tendon transfers to restore some function of the lower rotator cuff (Gartsman, 1997). The use and technique of tendon transfer for rotator cuff deficiency is beyond the scope of this book.
  1. Open rotator cuff repair: Open repair of the rotator cuff to the tuberosities of the humerus has been the gold standard for many years (Cordasco and Bigliani, 1997; McLaughlin, 1944). This requires detachment of a portion of the deltoid off of the acromion. The risk of postoperative deltoid detachment leads some surgeons to take off a sliver of bone to enhance healing. The fear of deltoid failure or detachment has led surgeons to develop less invasive techniques.
  2. Mini-open repair (Blevins et al, 1996): Development of shoulder arthroscopy methods has allowed surgeons to perform subacromial decompression by burscoscopy. This allows visualization of the rotator cuff, and the ability to address subacromial bursitis, AC joint pathology, and acromial changes such as the development of spurs or ossification of the CA ligament. The mini-open repair takes advantage of this preparation and utilizes a deltoid split to access the rotator cuff tear and perform an open repair (Blevins et al, 1996). The advantage is that the deltoid is preserved

(barring over retraction and iatrogenic deltoid detachment); however, large tears are difficult to address with this approach.

3. Arthroscopic rotator cuff repair: Further development of arthroscopic suture management, arthroscopic knot tying, and use of arthroscopically delivered suture anchors has led to the ability to perform rotator cuff repairs arthroscopically. The ability to preserve cortical bone enhances the strength of fixation while maintaining the ability of the tendon to heal to bone (St Pierre et al, 1995). These techniques require a significant amount of practice and skill at arthroscopic techniques. Newer techniques and instruments are being developed and this procedure now can be done as effectively as open repair (Ellman, Kay, and Wirth, 1993; Gartsman, Khan, and Hammerman, 1998; Murray, Jr, et al, 2002; Tauro, 1998; Wilson, Hinov, and Adams, 2002).

• **Postoperative rehabilitation**
  • Following surgery, a good rehabilitation program should be instituted to ensure optimal recovery (Wilk and Arrigo, 1993).
  • The rehabilitation is tailored to the operative treatment. Following arthroscopic subacromial decompression, a sling is used for a few days for comfort, and active motion may be resumed immediately. Once motion is achieved, strengthening exercises are started.
  • Strengthening should focus on lower rotator cuff strength and scapular stabilization.
  • Pool therapy is often very effective for shoulder rehabilitation for regaining proper motion and allowing protected use of the shoulder muscles in the recovery period.
  • Following rotator cuff repair, the recovery is slower to allow the cuff to heal to the tuberosities.
  • The surgeon will direct postoperative range of motion based on the size of the tear and the stability of the repair at the time of surgery.
  • Passive internal and external rotation can be started early, with active motion being delayed if the corresponding tendon was repaired.
  • Forward elevation may be delayed if the motion will cause stress on the repair.
  • More aggressive range-of-motion exercises are instituted after 4–6 weeks.
  • Return to sports is recommended when full painless motion is recovered following surgery. This will differ for each patient; however, 6–8 weeks is usually sufficient for decompression alone, and 4–6 months for rotator cuff repair.
• Rotator cuff pathology is a frequent cause of pain in active patients in all stages of life. From younger

patients participating in throwing sports, to the weekend athlete developing overuse injuries, to the elderly patient throwing a baseball with his grandson, the proper diagnosis and treatment of this condition can lead to resolution of symptoms and return the patient to a more functional and usually normal use of their arm.

REFERENCES

Blevins FT, Warren RF, Cavo C, et al: Arthroscopic assisted rotator cuff repair: Results using a mini–open deltoid splitting approach. *Arthroscopy* 12(1):50–59, 1996.

Burkhart SS: Arthroscopic debridement and decompression for selected rotator cuff tears: Clinical results, pathomechanics, and patient selection based on biomechanical parameters. *Orthop Clin North Am* 24:111–123,1993.

Burkhart SS: Partial repair of massive rotator cuff tears: The evolution of a concept. *Orthop Clin North Am* 28:125–132, 1997.

Burkhart SS: Arthroscopic repair of massive rotator cuff tears: Concept of margin convergence. *Tech Shldr Elbow Surg* 1:232–239, 2000.

Burkhart SS: Arthroscopic treatment of massive rotator cuff tears. *Clin Orthop* 390:107–118, 2001.

Burkhart SS, Esch JC, Jolson RS: The rotator crescent and rotator cable: An anatomic description of the shoulder's "suspension bridge." *Arthroscopy* 9:611–616, 1993.

Burkhart SS, Nottage WM, Ogilvie–Harris DJ, et al: Partial repair of irreparable rotator cuff tears. *Arthroscopy* 10:363–370, 1994.

Burkhead WZ, Habermeyer P: The rotator cuff: A historical review of our understanding, in Burkhead WZ (ed.): *Rotator Cuff Disorders*. Baltimore, MD, Williams & Wilkins, 1996, pp 3–18.

Chen AL, Rokito AS, Zuckerman JD: The role of the acromioclavicular joint in impingement syndrome. *Clin Sports Med* 22:343–357, 2003.

Cordasco FA, Bigliani LU: The rotator cuff: Large and massive tears. Techniques of open repair. *Orthop Clin North Am* 28:179–193, 1997.

Crenshaw AH, Kilgore WE: Surgical treatment of bicipital tenosynovitis. *J Bone Joint Surg* 48A:1496–1502, 1966.

DePalma AF, Kruper JS: Long term study of shoulder joints afflicted with and treated for calcific tendinitis. *Clin Orthop* 20:49–60, 1961.

Ellman H, Kay SP, Wirth M: Arthroscopic treatment of full-thickness rotator cuff tears: 2- to 7-year follow-up study. *Arthroscopy* 9:195–200, 1993.

Gartsman GM: Massive, irreparable tears of the rotator cuff. Results of operative debridement and subacromial decompression. *J Bone Joint Surg* 79A:715–721,1997.

Gartsman GM, Khan M, Hammerman SM: Arthroscopic repair of full-thickness tears of the rotator cuff. *J Bone Joint Surg* 80A:832–840, 1998.

Gerber C, Hersche O, Farron A: Isolated rupture of the subscapularis tendon. Results of operative repair. *J Bone Joint Surg* 78A:1015–1023, 1996.

Gerber C, Krushell RJ: Isolated rupture of the tendon of the sub-scapularis muscle. Clinical features in 16 cases. *J Bone Joint Surg* 73B:389–394, 1991.

Greis PE, Kuhn JE, Schultheis J, et al: Validation of the lift-off test and analysis of subscapularis activity during maximal internal rotation. *Am J Sports Med* 24:589–593,1996.

Harmon HP: Methods and results in the treatment of 2580 painful shoulders. With special reference to calcific tendinitis and the frozen shoulder. *Am J Surg* 95:527–544, 1958.

Hertel R, Ballmer FT, Lombert SM, et al: Lag signs in the diagnosis of rotator cuff rupture. *J Shoulder Elbow Surg* 5:307–313,1996.

Hawkins RJ, Kennedy JC: Impingement syndrome in athletes. *Am J Sports Med* 8:151–158, 1980.

Jobe FW, Jobe CM: Painful athletic injuries of the shoulder. *Clin Orthop* 173:117–124, 1983.

Jobe FW, Kvitne RS, Giangarra CE: Shoulder pain in the over-hand or throwing athlete: The relationship of anterior stability and rotator cuff impingement. *Orthop Rev* 18:963–975, 1989.

Jobe FW, Moynes DR: Delineation of diagnostic criteria and a rehabilitation program for rotator cuff injuries. *Am J Sports Med* 10:336–339, 1982.

Kelly BT, Kadrmas WR, Kirkendall DT, et al: Optimal normalization tests for shoulder muscle activation: An electromyographic study. *J Orthop Res* 14:647–53, 1996.

MacDonald PB, Clark P, Sutherland K: An analysis of the diagnostic accuracy of the Hawkins and Neer subacromial impingement signs. *J Shoulder Elbow Surg* 9:299–301, 2000.

McFarland EG, Hsu CY, Neira C, et al: Internal impingement of the shoulder: A clinical and arthroscopic analysis. *J Shoulder Elbow Surg* 8:458–460,1999.

McLaughlin HL: Lesions of the musculotendinous cuff of the shoulder. Part I. The exposure and treatment of tears with retraction. *J Bone Joint Surg* 26A:31–51, 1944.

Moseley HF: The results of nonoperative and operative treatment of calcified deposits. *Surg Clin North Am* 43:1505–1506, 1963.

Murray TF, Jr, Lajtai G, Mileski RM, et al: Arthroscopic repair of medium to large full-thickness rotator cuff tears: Outcome at 2- to 6-year follow-up. *J Shoulder Elbow Surg* 11:19–24, 2002.

Neer CS, II: Anterior acromioplasty for the chronic impingement syndrome in the shoulder: A preliminary report. *J Bone Joint Surg* 54A:41–50, 1972.

Neer CS, II: Impingement lesions. *Clin Orthop* 173:70–77, 1983.

Nirschl RP: Rotator cuff tendinitis: Basic concepts of pathoetiology. *Instr Course Lect* 439–445, 1989.

St Pierre P, Olson EJ, Elliott JJ, et al: Tendon-healing to cortical bone compared with healing to a cancellous trough. A biomechanical and histological evaluation in goats. *J Bone Joint Surg* 77A:1858–66, 1995.

Tauro JC: Arthroscopic rotator cuff repair: Analysis of technique and results at 2- and 3-year follow-up. *Arthroscopy* 14:45–51, 1998.

Valadie AL, III, Jobe CM, Pink MM, et al: Anatomy of provocative tests for impingement syndrome of the shoulder. *J Shoulder Elbow Surg* 9:36–46, 2000.

Walch G, Bioleau P, Noel E: Impingement of the deep surface of the supraspinatus on the posterosuperior glenoid rim: An arthroscopic study. *J Shoulder Elbow Surg* 1:238–245, 1992.

Warner JJP, Allen AA, Gerber C: Diagnosis and management of subscapularis tendon tears. *Tech Orthop* 9:116–125, 1994.

Warner JJ, Higgins L, Parsons IM, IV, et al: Diagnosis and treatment of anterosuperior rotator cuff tears. *J Shoulder Elbow Surg* 10:37–46, 2001.

Wilk KE, Arrigo C: Current concepts in the rehabilitation of the athletic shoulder. *J Orthop Sports Phys Ther* 18:365–378, 1993.

Wilson F, Hinov V, Adams G: Arthroscopic repair of full-thickness tears of the rotator cuff: 2- to 14-year follow-up. *Arthroscopy* 18:136–144, 2002.

Yamaguchi K, Tetro AM, Blam O, et al: Natural history of asymptomatic rotator cuff tears: A longitudinal analysis of asymptomatic tears detected sonographically. *J Shoulder Elbow Surg* 10:199–203, 2001.

Yocum LA: Assessing the shoulder. History, physical examination, differential diagnosis, and special tests used. *Clin Sports Med* 2:281–289, 1983.

46 STERNOCLAVICULAR, CLAVICULAR, AND ACROMIOCLAVICULAR INJURIES

Carl J Basamania, MD, FACS

INTRODUCTION

- Few animals other than primates, birds, humans and, surprisingly, marsupials have a functional clavicle.
- Injuries to the clavicle and its articulations are very common.
- High energy injuries have been seen in increasing frequency as more people participate in higher risk sports such as mountain biking and rollerblading.
- Since man is an upper extremity dependent animal, these injuries can lead to significant disabilities and limitations.

STERNOCLAVICULAR JOINT

- The sternoclavicular joint is the only true articulation between the upper extremity and the rest of the axial skeleton.
- Although the sternoclavicular joint has the least amount of osseous stability of any major joint, it is seldom injured in comparison to other joints.

STERNOCLAVICULAR ANATOMY

- The medial physis of the clavicle is the last to form and the last to stop growing. The medial physis of the clavicle does not close until around 24 years of age.
- Many injuries seen in young patients are actually physeal injuries rather than true dislocations.
- The sternoclavicular joint is a saddle joint that articulates with the clavicular notch of the sternum (Rockwood and Young, 1990). Less than half of the medial clavicle actually articulates with the sternum.
- The sternoclavicular joint capsule and the intra-articular disk, in addition to the very strong costoclavicular and interclavicular ligaments, stabilize the sternoclavicular joint. The two parts of the costoclavicular ligament cross in a V-type fashion and provide stability during rotation and elevation.

STERNOCLAVICULAR JOINT FUNCTION

- The sternoclavicular joint acts as the stabilizing base of the clavicle and, therefore, the upper extremity.
- Studies have shown that there is quite a bit of motion at the *sternoclavicular* (SC) joint, especially compared to the *acromioclavicular* (AC) joint. In a study by Rockwood, he found that there approximately 40° of rotation between the clavicle and the sternum as compared to 6° of rotation between the clavicle and the acromion (Rowe, 1968).

STERNOCLAVICULAR PATHOLOGIC CONDITIONS

- The three primary pathologic conditions of the SC joint are dislocations, instabilities, and degenerative arthritis. The SC joint can also become septic.
- It takes a considerable amount of force, applied either directly or indirectly to the shoulder and clavicle to disrupt the SC joint.
- The most common mechanism of injury to the SC joint is indirect force, typically an axial load from falling directly on the lateral aspect of the shoulder. The direction of the force and the position of the shoulder, either flexed or extended, determine if the dislocation is anterior or posterior.
- The SC joint is often disrupted by a direct force to the clavicle, which results in a posterior dislocation of the joint. This is seen in motor vehicle accidents where the patient is driven forward against a shoulder harness or a direct blow from the steering wheel against the clavicle.

- SC joint dislocations are typically the result of a single traumatic event. Instability can result either from a single event or from repeated microtrauma, much like the glenohumeral joint. Instabilities are often seen in individuals with ligamentous laxity and can be seen in skeletally immature individuals.
- Degenerative arthritis can be seen in patients who had previously experienced a traumatic injury to the shoulder with one notable exception: postmenopausal women can develop spontaneous arthritis of the sternoclavicular joint, particularly on the right side. This is often seen in the 6th and 7th decade.

STERNOCLAVICULAR JOINT PATHOLOGY DIAGNOSIS

- Since it usually takes a significant force to injure the SC joint, the mechanism of injury is usually traumatic, but often missed. This is due to the soft tissue swelling over the region and the fact that patients often have other life-threatening injuries. SC injuries should be suspected in any high-energy injury such as a high impact motor vehicle accident. They can also be seen after a hard fall on to the lateral aspect of the shoulder such as that seen with a football tackle.
- Anterior dislocations are typically associated with significant pain and swelling at the SC joint. Almost any arm motion will exacerbate the discomfort. There is a firm palpable mass from the prominence of the medial clavicle.
- Posterior dislocations can often be mistaken clinically for an anterior dislocation because of the soft tissue swelling in the region. Patients may also complain of difficulty swallowing and breathing and shortness of breath. Occasionally, there may also be venous distention of the affected arm due to compression of the underlying vessels.
- Plain radiographs, including *anteroposteior* (AP) and lateral views of the chest, may be of limited usefulness in the acute setting. The most helpful plain radiograph of the SC joint is the serendipity view described by Rockwood, which is a 40–45° cephalic tilt AP of the chest centered on the SC joint (Rockwood and Young, 1990). An anterior dislocation will appear to be higher on the affected side; whereas, a posterior dislocation will appear lower. *Computed tomography* (CT) scan is the ideal imaging technique in both acute and chronic conditions. *Magnetic resonance imaging* (MRI) can be useful in evaluation of the soft tissues. More specialized tests, such as a CT arteriogram, are dictated by the situation, e.g., to rule out compression of the great vessels in a chronic posterior dislocation.

STERNOCLAVICULAR JOINT TREATMENT

- Anterior and posterior dislocations are best reduced within the first 7 days of the injury.
- Unfortunately, anterior dislocations typically are not well maintained after a closed reduction. They are best treated postreduction with a figure of eight harness as a standard sling can put a medially directed load on the SC joint.
- Posterior dislocations must be treated as soon as possible. Failure to do so can result in compromise of the trachea and mediastinal structures. A very thorough physical examination and prereduction radiographic evaluation is mandatory. Assuming there is no involvement of the underlying structures, they can be managed with a closed reduction, if seen within the first 7 days postinjury, followed by immobilization for 6–10 weeks. If an adequate closed reduction is not obtained, an open reduction and stabilization must be performed.
- Chronic anterior dislocations should be treated with activity modification and support treatment for 6–12 months as most of these become less symptomatic with time. If still symptomatic, they can be treated with a resectional arthroplasty and stabilization.
- Chronic posterior dislocations also require a very thorough radiographic evaluation to determine compromise of the underlying soft tissues. If it has been longer than 7–10 days since the original injury, an open reduction and resectional arthroplasty of the medial clavicle is usually required.
- As the medial physis does not close till 23–25 years of age, anterior and posterior dislocations under that age are typically physeal injuries and are best managed with observation as the deformity can remodel.
- Degenerative arthritis of the SC joint can typically be managed with supportive measures such as activity modification and anti-inflammatory drugs. If the patient continues to have symptoms for more than 6–12 months, and the symptoms can be alleviated with an injection in the SC joint, they can be considered for a resectional arthroplasty and stabilization (Rockwood and Young, 1990).
- Under no circumstances should hardware, especially smooth pins, be used to stabilize the medial clavicle as numerous cases of hardware migration have been reported in which some resulted in death.

RETURN TO PLAY CRITERIA

- For a mild sprain of the SC joint, the patient can be treated with ice, rest, and a sling for 4–5 days. Activity can then be advanced as tolerated.
- For a more severe sprain or subluxation, that is not a true dislocation, ice and rest should be used; however, the involved extremity should be immobilized in a sling or figure of eight harness for 6–8 weeks before resuming activity. The patient should have full, pain-free motion before returning to sports, particularly overhead sports. This may take up to 3 months.
- In the case of a true dislocation, a closed reduction maneuver should be made and the extremity immobilized in a sling or figure of eight harness for 6–8 weeks. That extremity should be protected for an additional 2 weeks before resumption of strenuous activity and then only advanced as tolerated. Again, the return to play criteria is full, pain-free range of motion.

CLAVICLE FACTS

- The clavicle is the first bone to ossify and the last to finish growing. The physes of the clavicle do not close till approximately 23–25 years of age. Prior to this time, most injuries actually represent physeal injuries. The clavicle grows through intramembranous ossification much like the flat bones of the body such as the pelvis and skull and the medial physis accounts for approximately 80% of the growth.
- The middle third of the clavicle has poor muscle coverage much like the mid-tibia, which may contribute to healing problems.
- There does not appear to be an intraosseous blood supply to the clavicle, unlike most bones. All of its blood is supplied through the periosteum.

CLAVICLE FRACTURES

- Clavicle fractures are very common, accounting for 5–15% of all fractures and nearly half of all shoulder fractures.
- Middle third fractures are by far the most common, accounting for 80% of all clavicle fractures with lateral third fractures accounting for about 10–15% and medial third fractures accounting for about 5%.
- Although commonly thought to be a result of a direct blow, the clavicle is typically fractured by a fall on to the lateral aspect of the shoulder; however, it can also be fractured by a direct blow as seen in seat belt fractures or in sports such as lacrosse. There are reported cases of stress fractures of the clavicle, typically in overhead athletes (Taft, Wilson, and Oglesby, 1987).
- Midshaft clavicle fractures tend to occur in younger individuals while lateral third fractures tend to occur in older individuals.

- Earlier literature suggested that the rate of healing with nonoperative treatment was quite high—approximately 99% were reported to heal without complication (Neer, 1960; Stanley, Trowbridge, and Norris, 1988); however, recent studies have not been able to reproduce these results. In fact, most recent studies have shown a nonunion rate of 15–25% (Eskola et al, 1986; Harris et al, 2000; Nowak, 2002). More importantly, when looking at patient satisfaction, 30–50% of patients who had sustained a clavicle fracture, even as long as 10 years previously, felt that they had not fully recovered and were dissatisfied with the result (Nowak, 2002).
- Most clavicle fractures are multiplanar injuries, that is, the fracture displacement occurs in multiple planes: angulation, shortening, and medial rotation. This is due to the weight of the arm and the pull of the various muscles about the shoulder, particularly the anterior muscles such as the pectoralis (Basamania, Craig, and Rockwood, 2003).

FRACTURE CLASSIFICATION

- There are numerous classification systems for clavicle fractures; however, it is really only important to describe them as displaced or nondisplaced and comminuted or simple. Lateral third fractures are usually referred to as type II or III fractures; however, in this case, it is important only to recognize whether or not the stabilizing *coracoclavicular* (CC) ligaments are involved. If the ligaments are involved, as would typically be the case in a fracture in the region of the coracoid, the fracture is inherently unstable, whereas fractures occurring in the lateral most aspect of the clavicle or medial to the CC ligaments are inherently stable.

CLINICAL EVALUATION

- Clavicle fractures typically do not present as a diagnostic dilemma because the injury is rather obvious in most cases. There is usually a clear history of some form of either direct or indirect injury to the shoulder. There is usually tenting of the skin over the fracture site; however, open fractures of the clavicle are quite rare.
- It is of utmost importance to assess for other associated injuries due to the trauma. A careful neurovascular exam should be documented in all clavicle fractures. The obvious nature of the clavicle fracture should not detract from detecting other bony injuries such as those to the scapula and underlying ribs.

RADIOGRAPHIC EVALUATION

- Many physicians accept a single AP radiographic view to assess injuries to the clavicle; however, it is impossible to assess fracture displacement on a single radiograph. Unfortunately, it is not possible to obtain orthogonal views (views at right angles to each other) of the clavicle. The next best technique is to obtain an AP and 45° cephalic tilt AP radiograph. The contour and displacement can best be seen on the 45° cephalic tilt view (Basamania, Craig, and Rockwood, 2003).
- Lateral third clavicle fractures must include an axillary radiograph to assess posterior displacement of the medial fragment relative to the lateral fragment.
- It is not possible to assess accurately shortening of a clavicle fracture on plain radiographs. This is because the shortening occurs obliquely to the plane of the radiograph. In fact, short of *three-dimensional* (3D) CT reconstructions with side-to-side comparisons, shortening can only be measured clinically.

TREATMENT

- The statement that "all clavicle fractures heal well" is probably one of the greatest fallacies in all orthopedics (Eskola et al, 1986; Jupiter, 2000; Nowak, 2002). Many clavicle fractures can be treated nonoperatively; however, as more and more studies have suggested a poorer outcome with nonoperative treatment, it is important to recognize those that may require operative intervention.
- For those fractures that are nondisplaced or are minimally displaced (100% or less displacement and less than 15–20 mm of shortening), patients can be treated in a sling or a figure of eight harness. Studies have suggested that there is no difference in these two treatment modalities; however, both have significant limitations. First, the figure of eight harness tends to be very awkward to put on and maintain. It should be adjusted frequently to keep proper tension on the brace. Second, the figure of eight harness itself usually lies directly over the fracture and can actually exacerbate the discomfort rather than alleviate it. The advantage of the figure of eight harness is that it frees up both upper extremities for day-to-day activities. The primary problem with the sling is that it is typically worn with the arm internally rotated and this can exacerbate the shortening and rotation of the fracture. If used, the sling is better if the arm is held in a neutral position, i.e., with the forearm pointing straight ahead.
- An attempt at closed reduction of clavicle fractures is not only painful but also futile. At best, patients will

remain in the position they present with on first evaluation. Repeat examinations and radiographs are justified to make sure a minimally or nondisplaced fracture remains so.

- There are certain cases where operative intervention is indicated:
  1. Neurovascular injury or compromise that is progressive or that fails to reverse with closed reduction of the fracture
  2. Severe displacement caused by comminution with resultant angulation and tenting of the skin severe enough to threaten its integrity and that fails to respond to a closed reduction
  3. An open fracture that will require operative debridement
  4. Multiple trauma, when mobility of the patient is desirable and closed methods of immobilization are impractical or impossible
  5. A *floating* shoulder resulting from a displaced clavicular fracture, an unstable scapular fracture, and compromise of the acromioclavicular and coracoacromial ligaments
  6. Factors that render the patient unable to tolerate closed immobilization, such as the neurological problems of Parkinsonism, seizure disorders, or other neurovascular disorders
  7. The very rare patient for whom the cosmetic lump over the healed clavicle would be intolerable

- A relative indication for operative intervention is displacement of the fracture fragments more than 100% (the width of the clavicle) and shortening more than 20 mm. Most poor outcomes after nonoperative treatment of clavicle fractures occur in patients who have more this much displacement. In addition, patients who have a butterfly fragment that is flipped 90° on the 45° cephalic tilt radiograph tend to have poorer outcomes and should be considered for operative intervention (Basamania, Craig, and Rockwood, 2003).

OPERATIVE TREATMENT

- There are two primary forms of operative treatment of midshaft clavicle fractures: plate and screw fixation and intramedullary fixation. Due to the significant forces placed on the clavicle, most other types of fixation, such as circlage wires, are inadequate, and should not be considered.
- One type of fixation that is contraindicated in clavicle fractures is smooth wire fixation. Smooth wires have a significant tendency to migrate and the literature is replete with cases of smooth wires migrating from the shoulder to locations such as the lung, abdomen, and spine (Lyons and Rockwood, 1990; Mazet, 1943).

- Both intramedullary fixation and plate fixation have good outcomes in treating clavicle fractures. The choice is usually due to the experience and comfort level of the surgeon in regard to operating in this area. The primary advantage of plate and screw fixation is that most orthopedic surgeons are comfortable with using this technique. The primary disadvantage is that this type of surgery is performed through a rather large, noncosmetic incision with the risk of compromise of the bone's blood supply due to soft tissue stripping. Removal of the plate and screws requires a second major procedure that can leave the clavicle with multiple stress rises and can place the patient at risk for later refracture (Bostman, Manninen, and Pihlajamaki, 1997; Poigenfurst, Rappold, and Fischer, 1992). The primary advantage of intramedullary fixation is that it can be accomplished through a small, cosmetic incision and the hardware can later be removed under local anesthesia. The primary disadvantage of this type of fixation is that most surgeons are unfamiliar with this technique and that fact that there is less rotational control of the fragments with the intramedullary fixation (Basamania, Craig, and Rockwood, 2003).
- Lateral third clavicle fractures represent a special dilemma: most occur in older patients from standing height falls; however, the nonunion rate from nonoperative treatment is rather high. Some surgeons suggest that many of these nonunions are relatively asymptomatic; however, most surgeons feel that operative intervention is indicated due to the high nonunion rate (Eskola et al, 1987; Kona et al, 1990; Nordqvist, Petersson, and Redlund-Johnell, 1993).
- Fixation of lateral third fractures can be difficult due to the location of the fracture and the difficulty in getting enough adequate purchase with the fixation devices. Plate and screw fixation is very difficult to achieve unless the plate extends out on to the acromion. Newer plates that hook under the acromion are being devised. Most surgeons prefer suture circlage or coracoclavicular screw fixation. With suture fixation, sutures are passed around the coracoid or through the medial clavicle fragment to achieve and hold the reduction. Although relatively easy to do, there is a risk of the sutures sawing through the clavicle or coracoid if nonabsorbable sutures are used (Martell, 1992). Absorbable sutures can be used; however, these may weaken and fail before adequate healing has taken place. With coracoclavicular screw fixation, a screw is passed through the medial fragment into the coracoid. This is a very strong form of fixation when properly placed; however, it is technically more difficult and the screw should be removed once healing is achieved, necessitating a second operative procedure (Harris et al, 2000).

- Late treatment of lateral third nonunions usually comprises excision of the distal fragment. The medial fragment must be stabilized with a ligament transfer caused by the earlier injury to the CC ligaments. Failure to do so will result in significant instability of the clavicle.
- Intra-articular distal clavicle fractures are treated with rest until there is evidence of radiographic and clinical healing. If the patient has later symptoms, they can be treated with a simple distal clavicle resection. Stability of the remaining clavicle should be assessed at the time of surgery.

RETURN TO PLAY CRITERIA

- **Nonoperative treatment:** The involved extremity should be held immobilized in a sling or figure of eight harness with no forward elevation of the arm more than 45° for 4–6 weeks or until there is evidence of radiographic and clinical healing (fracture site nontender). The immobilization can then be discontinued and range of motion increased as tolerated. For adults, return to full activities, particularly contact sports, cannot occur till there is evidence of complete radiographic healing and no tenderness at the fracture site. This may take 3–6 months.
- **Operative treatment:** A sling is not necessary and simple midline activities of daily living can be resumed as tolerated with the exception that the patient should avoid elevation of the involved hand higher than should level for 4–6 weeks to avoid excessive torque on the fracture site. Once radiographic and clinical healing is obtained, usually 4–6 weeks, activities including full shoulder range of motion, can be started. Return to full activity should not take place until the patient has full, pain-free range of motion and radiographic union of the fracture.
  - In the case of intramedullary fixation, the device can be removed at about 12 weeks post-op if there is clinical and radiographic healing. Full range of motion and noncontact sports can be resumed as soon as the sutures are removed and contact sports can be resumed 6 weeks after removal of the device.

ACROMIOCLAVICULAR JOINT FACTS

- The acromioclavicular joint, or AC joint, and the SC joint represent the only true joints that link the entire upper extremity to the rest of the axial skeleton.
- There is approximately 5–10° of differential motion between the clavicle and the acromion as compared to 40° of differential motion between the clavicle and the sternum.
- The acromioclavicular joint is stabilized by a very strong ligamentous complex consisting of the conoid, trapezoid, and acromioclavicular ligaments. The acromioclavicular ligaments, particularly the posterior band, are the primary restraints to superior and posterior translation of the clavicle relative to the acromion. The trapezoid ligament is the primary constraint to axial translation of the acromion in a compression mode while the conoid ligament acts as a restraint to superior translation and rotation of the clavicle. The load to failure strength of this complex is about 1000 N (Fukuda et al, 1986; Harris et al, 2000).

INJURIES TO THE ACROMIOCLAVICULAR JOINT

- In addition to wear and tear due to strenuous activity, the AC joint is commonly injured though falls on to the lateral aspect of the shoulder. In fact, the AC joint is second most commonly dislocated major joint, with the glenohumeral joint being first.
- It is the most commonly injured joint in martial arts and hockey.
- With a fall on to the lateral aspect of the shoulder, a load is placed on the AC joint ligament complex. If the tensile strength of the ligaments is exceeded, the ligaments can then rupture, probably in a sequential pattern, with the acromioclavicular ligaments failing first, followed by the trapezoid and conoid ligaments (Basamania, 2000).
- If the entire ligament complex is damaged, the patient can be left with significant inability of the AC joint and disability, particularly with overhead work and lifting.

CLINICAL EVALUATION

- Most patients present with the complaint of pain and actively splint the injured shoulder with the uninjured arm. There may be ecchymosis or abrasions over the later aspect of the shoulder, particularly the posterolateral aspect of the acromion.
- Due to swelling about the AC joint and splinting of the injured side, there may or may not be obvious deformity of the AC joint itself.
- There is typically exquisite tenderness on palpation of the AC joint.
- Patients should be reexamined after a few days because once the initial pain has subsided, many patients who

initially appeared to have minor injuries will have much more obvious deformity and instability.

ACROMIOCLAVICULAR INJURY CLASSIFICATION

- The two most commonly used classification system for injuries to the AC joint were described by Allman-Tossey and Rockwood.
- The Allman-Tossey classification is broken down into three grades:
  1. A type I injury involves a strain of the acromio-clavicular ligaments. There is usually some widening of the AC joint on plain radiographs but no increase in the coracoclavicular interval.
  2. A type II injury involves tearing of the acromio-clavicular ligaments and strain of the coracoclavic-ular ligaments.
  3. A type III injury is characterized by complete rupture of the acromioclavicular and coracoclavicular ligaments.
- Rockwood felt that not all type III injuries were equivalent and further broke this type into type IV, V, and VI.
  1. A type IV injury involves complete rupture of the AC and CC ligaments; however, the clavicle is displaced posteriorly into or through the trapezius muscle.
  2. A type V injury represents a severe type III injury with significant displacement of the clavicle relative to the acromion. Radiographically this is seen as a 100–300% increase in the distance between the clavicle and the coracoid.
  3. A type VI injury is a very rare event where the CC and AC ligaments are completely ruptured and the clavicle is displaced inferior to the coracoid. Only handfuls have ever been reported in the literature (Rowe, 1968).
- One of the most significant problems with these two classification systems is that they are often used interchangeably and there tends to be little interobserver reliability.

RADIOGRAPHIC EVALUATION

- It is difficult to obtain radiographs that adequately reflect the extent of the injury in the early postinjury period. This is due to pain and the splinting of the shoulder girdle muscles. The most accurate radiographs are obtained a few weeks after the injury; however, if operative intervention is indicated, it is best performed within the first 2 weeks after injury.
- Standard radiographs should include an AP and axillary view of the shoulder. If there is posterior displacement of the clavicle relative to the scapular, it can be seen best on the axillary view.
- Stress radiographs, although commonly obtained in urgent care settings, are of questionable value because if the patient is actively guarding due to the pain of the injury, the results will not show the full extent of the injury.
- A very useful view is the cross-body adduction radiograph. The radiograph is taken similar to a standard AP radiograph except that the patient is instructed to pull the elbow of the affected shoulder across their chest to the midline. Since the patients cannot splint or actively restrain motion of the shoulder in this position, subtle instability patterns can be detected in the early postinjury period. In the case of complete rupture of the AC and CC ligaments, the scapula will rotate anteriorly and medially relative the distal clavicle and, on this view, the acromion will appear to go medial and under the distal clavicle. If either of the CC ligaments is intact, this will not happen. This obvious radiographic finding can easily differentiate severe injuries that may need operative intervention from lesser ones that can be treated nonoperatively (Basamania, 2000).
- In the case of high demand athletes with questionable injuries, MRI studies can be used to detect injuries to the AC and CC ligaments.

TREATMENT

- Few injuries have had as much controversy over treatment as acromioclavicular joint injuries. Although there is a consensus on the treatment of type I, II, IV, V, and VI injuries, there is little, if any agreement, on the treatment of type III injuries. Most studies support nonoperative treatment of all type I and II injuries while most studies support operative intervention in type IV through VI injuries. To add further confusion, many studies do not distinguish whether they are referring to an Allman-Tossey type III injury or a Rockwood type III injury, potentially including Rockwood type IV–VI injuries in the former. An equal number of studies showing good results from both operative and nonoperative treatment of type III injuries are found in the literature (Bergfeld, Andrish, and Clancy, 1978; Bjerneld, Hovelius, and Thorling, 1983; Eskola et al, 1991; Galpin, Hawkins, and Grainger, 1985).
- One particular exception to the treatment régime is the contact athlete. In those athletes who are high risk for a recurrent injury, such as a hockey player, it makes little sense to put them through an operative treatment program when they will probably go on to have another injury. It is better to wait until the end of their

playing career when the injury can be treated operatively if the former player is still symptomatic.

- **Type I and II injuries**
  1. These are treated with ice, rest, and immobilization for 7–14 days. Gradual resumption of full activities can then progress as the patient tolerates.
  2. Heavy lifting and contact sports is avoided for 8–12 weeks, especially in the case of type II injuries.
- **Type III injuries**
  1. There is little, if any, agreement as to the best treatment of these injuries. A prospective, randomized study was performed accessing operative versus nonoperative treatment revealed no difference between the two groups; however, this study combined two types of operative fixation: coracoclavicular lag screw fixation and transacromial pin fixation. There were a significant number of failures in the transacromial fixation group; whereas, there were no failures in the lag screw fixation group. Taken together, the average failure was the same as nonoperatively treated patient; however, this would seem to support lag screw fixation as being superior to nonoperative treatment of these injuries.
  2. This author has found the cross-body adduction radiograph to be the most helpful in differentiating these patients: if there is no evidence of medial instability, most of these patients do fine with nonoperative treatment. If there is medial instability, this represents a more severe injury and these patients typically will do better with operative intervention.
- **Type IV, V, and VI injuries:** Most authors agree that due to the severity of these injuries, operative intervention is indicated (Rowe, 1968).
- Operative intervention can be broken down into three types:
  1. Transacromial fixation: Pins are passed through the acromion into the distal clavicle to hold it reduced. The primary limitation with this procedure is that it can be difficult to pass pins accurately through the acromion, especially in a patient with a thin acromion. Furthermore, the joint surfaces of the distal clavicle and acromion are disrupted by the pins and, as noted earlier, smooth pins can migrate.
  2. Coracoclavicular lag screw fixation: a screw is passed through the distal clavicle into the base of the coracoid to hold the joint reduced. This is by far the strongest fixation; however, the technique can be rather demanding for an inexperienced surgeon, as the exact placement of the screw into the coracoid can be difficult to obtain. Furthermore, the screw needs to be removed because of the risk of hardware breakage and reabsorption of

the bone around the screw (Weaver and Dunn, 1972).
  3. Coracoclavicular cerclage fixation: Sutures are passed around the clavicle and coracoid to hold the AC joint reduced. This is probably the easiest to perform and does not require fluoroscopy in the operating room; however, permanent sutures can saw through the clavicle or coracoid while absorbable sutures may not last long enough to achieve adequate healing (Martell, 1992). Furthermore, if weaved sutures are used, the fixation is less stable due to the *bungee cord* nature of the sutures and this can interfere with ligament healing.
  4. These procedures and be combined with or without distal clavicle resection and with or without ligament transfer, typically the acromioclavicular ligament.

RETURN TO PLAY CRITERIA

- **Type I injuries:** Activities can be advanced after 7 days of rest and ice. Return to full, unrestricted activity can occur when the player has full, pain-free range of motion. This usually occurs after 2 weeks.
- **Type II injuries:** Ice, rest, and immobilization for 7–14 days or until symptoms subside. Activities of daily living can then be started and activities are gradually progressed as tolerated; however, due to the risk of exacerbation of the injury, most contact sports should be avoided for 8 to 12 weeks.
- **Type III injuries:** Nonoperative treatment—same as type II injuries.
- **Type III (operative) and Type IV–VI injuries:** Sling for 4–6 weeks followed by 6 weeks of simple activities of daily living. The fixation can be removed after 8–12 weeks and then activities slowly progress over the following 6 weeks to allow the repaired ligament to strengthen. Once they have full, painless range of motion and strength, they can return to sports.

REFERENCES

Basamania CJ: Medial instability of the shoulder: A new concept of the pathomechanics of acromioclavicular separations. Presented at American Orthopaedic Society for Sports Medicine Specialty Day Meeting, Orlando, FL, 2000.

Basamania CJ, Craig EV, Rockwood CA, Jr: Fractures of the clavicle, in Rockwood CA, Jr, Matsen FA, III (eds.): *The Shoulder*. Philadelphia, PA, Saunders, 2003.

Bergfeld JA Andrish JT, Clancy WG: Evaluation of the acromioclavicular joint following first- and second-degree sprains. *Am J Sports Med* 6:153–159, 1978.

Bjerneld H, Hovelius L, Thorling J: Acromio-clavicular separations treated conservatively: A 5-year follow-up study. *Acta Orthop Scand* 54:743–745, 1983.

Bostman O, Manninen M, Pihlajamaki H: Complications of plate fixation in fresh displaced midclavicular fractures. *J Trauma* 43:778–783, 1997.

Eskola A, Vainionpaa S, Myllynen P, et al: Outcome of clavicular fracture in 89 patients. *Arch Orthop Trauma Surg* 105:337–338, 1986.

Eskola A, Vainionpaa S, Patiala H, et al: Outcome of operative treatment in fresh lateral clavicle fracture. *Ann Chir Gynaecol* 76:167–168, 1987.

Eskola A, Vainionpaa O, Korkala S, et al: Four year outcome of operative treatment of acute acromioclavicular dislocation. *J Orthop Trauma* 5:9–13, 1991.

Fukuda K, Craig EV, An KN, et al: Biomechanical study of the ligamentous system of the acromioclavicular joint. *J Bone Joint Surg* 68A:434–440, 1986.

Galpin RD, Hawkins RJ, Grainger RW: A comparative analysis of operative vs. nonoperative treatment of grade III acromioclavicular separations. *Clin Orthop* 193:150–155, 1985.

Harris RI, Wallace AL, Harper GD, et al: Structural properties of the intact and the reconstructed coracoclavicular ligament complex. *Am J Sports Med* 28:103–108, 2000.

Jupiter JB: *American Shoulder and Elbow Surgeons,* 1st Open Meeting, Miami, FL 2000.

Kona J, Bosse NJ, Staeheli JW, et al: Type II distal clavicle fractures: A retrospective review of surgical treatment. *J Orthop Trauma* 4:115–120, 1990.

Lyons FA, Rockwood CA, Jr: Migration of pins used in operations on the shoulder. *J Bone Joint Surg* 72A:1262–1267, 1990.

Martell JR: Clavicular nonunion: Complication with the use of Mersilene tape. *Am J Sports Med* 20:360–362, 1992.

Mazet R: Migration of a Kirschner wire from the shoulder region into the lung: Report of two cases. *J Bone Joint Surg* 25:477–483, 1943.

Neer CS, II: Nonunion of the clavicle. *JAMA* 172:1006–1011, 1960.

Nordqvist A, Petersson C, Redlund-Johnell I: The natural course of lateral clavicle fracture. *Acta Orthop Scand* 64:87–91, 1993.

Nowak J: *Clavicular Fractures: Epidemiology, Union, Malunion, Nonunion.* Uppsala, Sweden, Acta Universitatis Upsalaiensis, 2002.

Poigenfurst J, Rappold G, Fischer W: Plating of fresh clavicular fractures: Results of 122 operations. *Injury* 23:237–241, 1992.

Rockwood CA, Young DC: Disorders of the acromioclavicular joint, in Rockwood CA, Jr, Matsen FAA, III: *The Shoulder.* Philadelphia, PA, Saunders, 1990, pp 413–476.

Rowe CR: An atlas of anatomy and treatment of mid-clavicular fractures. *Clin Orthop* 58:29–42, 1968.

Stanley D, Trowbridge EA, Norris SH: The mechanism of clavicular fracture. *J Bone Joint Surg* 70B:461–464, 1988.

Taft TN, Wilson FC, Oglesby JW: Dislocation of the acromioclavicular joint: An end-result study. *J Bone Joint Surg* 69A:1045–1051, 1987.

Weaver JK, Dunn HK: Treatment of acromioclavicular injuries, especially acromioclavicular separation. *J Bone Joint Surg* 54A:1187–1198, 1972.

BIBLIOGRAPHY

Abbot AE, Hannafin JA: Stress fracture of the clavicle in a female lightweight rower. A case report and review of the literature. *Am J Sports Med* 29:370–372, 2001.

Allman FL: Fractures and ligamentous injuries of the clavicle and its articulation. *J Bone Joint Surg* 49A:774–784, 1967.

Egol KA, Connor PM, Karunakar MA, et al, F: The floating shoulder: Clinical and functional results. *J Bone Joint Surg Am* 83-A:1188–1194, 2001.

Fallon KE, Fricker PA: Stress fracture of the clavicle in a young female gymnast. *Br J Sports Med* 35:448–449, 2001.

Hill JM, McGuire MH, Crosby LA: Closed treatment of displaced middle-third fractures of the clavicle gives poor results. *J Bone Joint Surg Br* 79:537–539, 1997.

Rockwood CA: Fractures of the outer clavicle in children and adults. *J Bone Joint Surg* 64B:642, 1982.

Tossy JD, Mead NC, Sigmond HM: Acromioclavicular separations: Useful and practical classification for treatment. *Clin Orthop* 28:111–119, 1963.

Tsou PN: Percutaneous cannulated screw coracoclavicular fixation for acute acromioclavicular dislocations. *Clin Orthop* 243:112–121, 1989.

47 SHOULDER SUPERIOR LABRUM BICEPS AND PEC TEARS

Jeffrey S Abrams, MD

INTRODUCTION

- Shoulder injuries that were felt to be rare and uncommon are being diagnosed more frequently with clinical examination, magnetic resonance imaging, and arthroscopic surgery.
- Increased participants in overhead athletics and weight training have precipitated many of these injuries.
- Eccentric muscle contraction can place excessive loads on muscle tendon units, placing the superior labrum, biceps, and pectoralis major structures at risk.

SUPERIOR LABRUM

- The superior labrum is the superior part of the cartilaginous ring that surrounds the glenoid. The labrum contributes to depth of the shallow glenoid, increasing humeral head contact and stability.

- Superior labral tears have been described, as shoulder arthroscopy experience has increased. Open surgery with the arthrotomy placed deep to the subscapularis does not demonstrate this anatomy, and therefore little has been mentioned in the literature (Snyder et al, 1990).
- There can be anatomic variants and gradual developmental changes with age and use, overuse leading to tissue failure, and traumatic instability events. *Superior labrum anterior to posterior* (SLAP) tears may be an isolated etiology for shoulder pain or combined with rotator cuff pathology.
- Overhead sports as in baseball pitching may place additional stresses on the superior labrum. As sports participation and injury recognition increases, so does the experience in treatment of injuries to the superior labrum (Andrews, Carson, Jr, and McLeod, 1985; Abrams, 1991).

SUPERIOR LABRUM ANATOMY

- The labrum is a cartilaginous ring around the shallow glenoid, contributing to depth and humeral head contact (Howell and Galinat, 1989). Superior labrum lesions can occur alone or combined with anterior or posterior labral avulsions.
- The superior labrum consists of dense fibrocartilage and elastin that connects the superior and middle capsular ligaments and long head of the biceps to the glenoid.
- Common normal variants include a fovea, a Buford complex, and a peel-back labrum. The fovea is an incomplete anterior superior labral attachment to the glenoid with a hole or thin fibrous tissue between the labrum and the glenoid (Cooper et al, 1992). A Buford complex is a thickened middle glenohumeral ligament band that inserts at the biceps labral junction with an absent anterior superior labrum (William, Snyder, and Buford, 1994). A large fovea or superior labral absence may mistakenly resemble an avulsion injury. The posterior superior labrum may be attached to the glenoid neck rather than to the articular surface. Variations of labral attachment can be normal embryonic variants or repetitive activity adaptations.
- Normal variants may predispose shoulders to additional injuries. Buford complexes do not have anterosuperior labrum. Visualizing below the biceps and labrum often demonstrates abnormal wear suggesting instability of the biceps anchor.
- Superior labral tears (SLAP tears) have been classified by Snyder as type I degenerative, type II avulsion, type III bucket-handle tears, and type IV combined labral tear and biceps insertion split (Snyder, Banas,

and Karzel, 1995). Expanded classification includes extension of Bankart lesions (Maffet, Gartsman, and Moseby, 1995), associated rotator cuff articular-side pathology, continuations of ganglion cysts.
- The anatomy can be arthroscopically visualized in a static and dynamic exam. The peel-back labrum can be seen arthroscopically as loss of posterior superior, glenoid contact when the shoulder is placed in abduction and external rotation (Burkhart and Morgan, 1998). An otherwise normal finding may increase with repetitive stresses leading to a painful condition.

SUPERIOR LABRUM FUNCTION

- Superior labrum contributes to superior, anteroinferior, and posterior glenohumeral stability. Superior humeral head translation can be reduced with secure attachment of the superior labrum and its biceps and capsular attachments. Investigators have increased anteroinferior translation after creating superior labral tears (Rodosky, Harner, and Fu, 1994; Pagnani et al, 1995). In addition, arthroscopists have noted SLAP tears associated with some cases of posterior instability, multidirectional shoulder instability (Abrams, 2003).
- The rotator cuff interval plays a role in stabilizing the adducted shoulder (Harryman et al, 1992). This interval consists of the superior labrum, superior glenohumeral ligament, middle glenohumeral ligament, and coracohumeral ligament. Reduction of an enlarged interval has decreased inferior translation or sulcus, reduced anterior translation, and external rotation augmenting anterior repairs, and reduced posterior translation augmenting posterior repairs.
- Superior translation of the humeral head can be limited with an intact superior labrum and biceps anchor with the humerus in external rotation (Abrams, 1991). The long head of the biceps attaches to the superior labrum and glenoid tubercle. When the shoulder is in the cocked throwing position (abduction, external rotation, and extension), the head is translated posteriorly (Howell et al, 1988). Capsular changes and tears in the superior labrum may alter these relationships.
- The superior labrum may contribute to articular lesions on the undersurface of the rotator cuff. Internal impingement is a common pathologic finding in overhead throwers with shoulder pain. Excessive contact of the posterosuperior labrum with the supraspinatus during early acceleration can create partial-thickness rotator cuff tears. Subscapularis tears can abrade on the anterosuperior labrum with flexion and interval rotation.

SUPERIOR LABRAL PATHOLOGIC CONDITIONS

- SLAP tears can be a source of pain and disability either in isolation or coexistent with other shoulder pathology (Kim et al, 2003; Morgan et al, 1998). SLAP tears have been associated with instability, rotator cuff pathology, and ganglion cyst origination.
- SLAP tears can result from a single traumatic event. A fall on an outstretched arm or elbow can create a superior humeral translation that can avulse or tear the superior labrum. Shoulder hyperextension, as in an arm tackle or seat-belt restraint injury, can place traction on the biceps and capsular attachments avulsing the superior labrum. Large Bankart avulsions can include the superior labrum and biceps anchor. SLAP avulsion can increase inferior translation of the shoulder contributing to shoulder instability.
- SLAP tears often coexist with other shoulder pathology as a result of overuse and developmental conditions. Baseball pitchers develop upper extremity velocity by placing the arm in maximum extension as they externally rotate and abduct. Torso forward projection places additional contact forces on the undersurface of the rotator cuff against the superior labrum. Internal impingement occurs when excessive compressive forces occur and may be associated with rotator cuff tears, superior labral tears, posterior capsular changes, and scapular dyskinesia.
- Juxta-articular ganglions adjacent to the glenohumeral joint have been diagnosed with increasing frequency, as magnetic resonance imaging of the shoulder has been utilized. Ganglions often originate from the joint space and communicate with the ganglion with a defect or tear in the superior or posterosuperior labrum. Ganglions may be asymptomatic or cause neurologic dysfunction due to peripheral pressure on the suprascapular nerve prior to the supraspinatus innervation at the scapular notch or adjacent to the scapular spine prior to the infraspinatus innervation.

SUPERIOR LABRAL DIAGNOSIS

- Patients most often complain of pain in provocative positions. A painful click may occasionally be reproducible, especially when associated with instability.
- The mechanism of injury can be traumatic and overuse. Traumatic events include a fall on an outstretched arm, hyperextension injury, and seat-belt injury. The body torso projects forward as the shoulder and arm are restrained. Overuse injuries as in baseball pitching accentuates internal impingement contact forces. Forced inferior translation may create superior labral avulsions due to traction on the biceps and capsular attachments.

- Degenerative changes are commonly found in the superior labrum, and their significance has not been established.
- Physical examination has had variable results (Kim et al, 2003; Morgan et al, 1998; McFarland, Kim, and Savino, 2002). Examination of the biceps with provocative testing has been helpful in anterior tears (Speed's, Yergason) Translation test (load and shift, jerk tests), provocative position (relocation test, O'Brien) testing can reproduce pain, but is often associated with common complaints exterior to the shoulder, i.e., the acromioclavicular joint. Most SLAP lesions are not diagnosed preoperatively, but rather at the time of arthroscopic surgery.
- Imaging tests can be helpful. *Magnetic resonance imaging* (MRI) without contrast can identify ganglion cysts adjacent to the shoulder. MRI with articular contrast may illustrate superior labral tear. Anatomic variants may contribute to abnormal imaging findings.

SUPERIOR LABRAL TREATMENT

- Most common treatment for intersubstance tears of the superior labrum is debridement (type I and III).
- Tears in young active individuals associated with shoulder instability, advanced rotator cuff pathology, ganglion origin, and as isolated source of pain are considered for repair. These repairs may be done in combination with capsulorrhaphies, cuff repairs, ganglion decompression, and subacromial decompressions.
- Superior labral repairs are most commonly performed with suture anchors. An anchor is inserted along the articular margin of an abraded glenoid neck. Sutures are advanced under the labrum and through the capsule and tied. Anterior labral repairs include the biceps anchor. Posterosuperior SLAP repairs may need accessory portals to properly place anchors along the glenoid to secure the labrum (Morgan et al, 1998).
- Postoperative management should include immobilization and regulated movement, followed by strengthening. Return to demanding activities take 3 to 6 months.

BICEPS (SHOULDER)

- The biceps is susceptible to injury in multiple locations in the shoulder region. The long head of the biceps has a twisted pathway before attaching to the superior labrum and glenoid. As the shoulder is positioned in abduction and external rotation, additional stresses are placed on these attachments (Burkhart and Morgan, 1998).

- The articular portion of the tendon as it exits the shoulder and enters the intertuberal groove may develop tendinosis due to repetitive humeral movements, friction below the subacromial arch, and compromised blood supply.
- Instability of the long head of the biceps may occur when capsular ligaments or rotator cuff tendons are disrupted. Clicking as the humerus is rotated may reproduce these findings in a painful shoulder.
- Tendonopathies and instability of the biceps are most often associated with additional injuries of the shoulder. Rotator cuff pathology and impingement syndromes are common coexistent pathologies.

BICEPS ANATOMY

- The biceps has two proximal origins and inserts below the elbow on the tubercle of the proximal radius. It traverses both the shoulder and the elbow and plays a role in shoulder flexion, elbow flexion, and forearm supination. From a shoulder perspective, the long head of the biceps is the most susceptible to injury. The short head originates from the coracoid process and is rarely injured.
- The musculocutaneous nerve (C5, C6, C7) innervates the biceps. The nerve can be seen to enter the short head inferior to the coracoid. The second portion is innervated more distally, prior to this nerve becoming a cutaneous nerve along the anterolateral aspect of the forearm. Injury to this nerve can result from anterior shoulder instability and surgical retractors.
- The long head of the biceps originates from the glenoid tubercle and superior labrum (Habermeyer and Walch, 1996). This tendon changes direction as it exits the shoulder. Capsular ligaments act as a pulley as the tendon exits the articular space and traverses under the transverse ligament (Paavolainen, Slatis, and Aalto, 1984). Extra-articularly, it runs within a groove between the greater and lesser tuberosities. The muscle tendon junction is adjacent to the inferior border of the pectoralis major tendon. Anatomic variations including attachments to the rotator cuff and absence of glenoid attachment may be rarely found without consequence.
- Biceps pathology involving the elbow will be discussed in the appropriate section.

BICEPS FUNCTION

- The biceps functions during arm elevation, flexes and supinates the elbow. Shoulder function includes assist in arm elevation, stabilizing or depressing the humeral

head, while the arm is externally rotated (Burkhead, Jr et al, 1998).
- Due to two proximal attachment sites, the long head may rupture and not severely impact these functions if the rotator cuff or short head attachments can compensate for this tear (Mariani, Cofield, and Askew, 1988).
- During the throwing motion, the biceps is positioned with the arm in abduction, extended and externally rotated. A complex change in pull occurs as the shoulder changes from cocking to acceleration (Glousman et al, 1988). In addition to shoulder stresses, elbow extension occurs simultaneously placing additional eccentric tension on the proximal anatomy (Andrews, Carson, Jr, and McLeod, 1985; Abrams, 1991).

BICEPS PATHOLOGIC CONDITIONS

- Shoulder biceps tears can be located adjacent to the superior labrum, along the articular portion, beneath the transverse ligament, within the groove, or at the muscle tendon junction.
- Biceps tendinosis is most commonly located adjacent to the location where the tendon has a directional change as it exits the shoulder. Since the shoulder abducts and adducts, these tears extend proximally and can be seen arthroscopically during the articular exam (Curtis and Snyder, 1993).
- Biceps tendon subluxation can occur when the supporting capsular ligaments are disrupted. This can occur when the superior portion of the subscapularis is detached from the lesser tuberosity (Peterson, 1986). Capsular and coracohumeral ligament injury can allow medial subluxation without significant tendon tear (Paavolainen, Slatis, and Aalto, 1984; Walch et al, 1998).
- Tears at the muscle tendon junction can result from traumatic events. Abrupt eccentric contraction may create a tear (Garrett, Jr et al, 1987). Exclusion of a pectoralis major tear is important since there is overlap in the clinical exam.
- Biceps long head tendinosis can be coexistent with rotator cuff pathology in the impingement syndrome (Neer, Bigliani, and Hawkins, 1977). The tendon is aligned along the leading edge of the supraspinatus. During forward flexion, these structures can contact the anterior acromion and the coracoacromial ligament.

BICEPS COMPLAINTS AND FINDINGS

- The most common complaint is pain along the anteromedial aspect of the shoulder. Some patients can demonstrate a click with rotation of the humerus.

- The impingement test is not specific, but can be sensitive to biceps pathology. Localized tenderness along the groove can help distinguish this from supraspinatus tendinosis.
- Á Speed's test is performed by an examiner applying resistance to arm flexion while the arm is supinated. A Yergason sign reproduces pain while palpating the tendon while applying resistance against supinating a flexed forearm. Pain and weakness caused by pain can be reproduced with these maneuvers (Burkhead et al, 1998; Curtis and Snyder, 1993).
- Muscular biceps examination is done with elbow flexion and the arm in neutral and supination. Additional testing can be performed with resistive elbow flexion or supination while the shoulder is in the overhead throwing position (Bell and Noble, 1996).
- Disruptions of the long head of the biceps may produce a "biceps Popeye muscle" if the tendon retracts distally beyond the transverse ligament. A tear at the muscle tendon junction can create a similar deformity. This appears as a bulging muscle located distal to the contralateral side. There is often ecchymosis initially and it is commonly associated with a rotator cuff tear (Neer, Bigliani, and Hawkins, 1977).
- Biceps imaging can be best accomplished with MRI without enhancement. The sagittal views can demonstrate the articular portion, and the transverse cuts demonstrate the extra-articular portions. Rotator cuff tears in the coronal view may raise suspicion of associated pathology. Transverse cuts may demonstrate the biceps medial to the bicipital groove. An important coexistent pathology is disruption of the subscapularis insertion.

BICEPS TENDON TEARS TREATMENT

- Biceps pathology is often coexistent with rotator cuff problems. Tendinosis and impingement can coexist with supraspinatus tears. Biceps instability following trauma can be associated with a subscapularis tear. Rotator cuff deficiency is important in determining treatment options.
- Traditionally treatment has been divided into biceps tears involving 50% of tendon or greater (Curtis and Snyder, 1993). More mild tears are debrided and larger tears are considered for tenotomy or tenodesis. This concept is controversial, and sports physicians have individualized treatment rather than degree of tendon involvement (Gill et al, 2001).
- Biceps tendon debridement can be done arthroscopically or through an open approach. The articular part of the tendon can be easily debrided arthroscopically. To visualize the extra-articular portion, the tendon needs to be drawn into the articular viewing area or has to be visualized on the bursal side after the supporting capsule has been divided.
- Current controversy exists between cutting the damaged biceps tendon (tenotomy) (Gill et al, 2001) versus reattachment of the biceps tendon in a different location (tenodesis) (Curtis and Snyder, 1993). Generally, older individuals who are less active are comfortable with tenotomy supported by a minimal postoperative recovery. Younger and high-demand individuals may wish to avoid a possible biceps muscle deformity that may be created by completing the tear of the biceps and prefer a tenodesis. Functional deficits from a long head rupture or iatrogenic division of the long head of the biceps are usually temporary (Mariani, Cofield, and Askew, 1988). Patients' concerns and options should be discussed preoperatively.
- Biceps tenodesis can be performed after completing the tear adjacent to the superior labrum. The stump can be fastened to the proximal humerus or to adjacent soft tissue. Bone repairs can be performed with suture anchors, bone tunnels, or interference screw fixation. Soft tissue repairs can be maintained with sutures, tendon to tendon, or tendon to ligament.
- Patients can be categorized as rotator cuff intact with biceps tear or coexistent cuff and biceps tears. In the latter, the arthroscopic or open suture anchor repair can be used to create a secure tendon-to-bone repair of both the cuff and the biceps. Patients with an intact cuff may have tenodesis performed, but will need postoperative activity restriction during the initial healing period to protect the biceps attachment. Resistive exercises are generally started at 8 weeks postoperatively.
- Subpectoral open tenodesis repairs have been popularized when extensive tendon involvement includes the extra-articular portion. This allows for excision of the diseased portion prior to tendon-to-humerus reattachment. The muscle tendon junction is aligned along the inferior border of the pectoralis major tendon.

PECTORALIS MAJOR

- The pectoralis major is a large muscle responsible for arm flexion, internal rotation, and adduction.
- Pectoralis tears were considered uncommon but have been recognized with increasing frequency due to weight lifting, contact sports, anabolic steroids, and MRI diagnosis (Noble and Bell, 1996).
- Chest strengthening has always placed a large emphasis on the pectoralis. Supine and seated *flys* and bench

press emphasize pectoralis contraction. As the shoulders extend posterior to the chest wall, significant eccentric stresses are placed on the muscle tendon junction and the tendon insertion. Anabolic steroids may place this structure at additional risk of injury.

PECTORALIS MAJOR ANATOMY

- The pectoralis major comprises two muscular portions originating on the clavicle and sternocostal (ribs 1 through 5). There are additional inferior attachments along the external oblique fascia. The tendon has a trilaminar insertion along the humerus, lateral to the biceps groove (McEntire, Hess, and Coleman, 1972).
- Muscular portions have independent neural innervation from branches of the lateral pectoral nerve (C5, C6, C7) and medial pectoral nerve (C8, T1). Vascular supply is from the pectoral major branch of the coracoacromial artery.
- There are independent tendon insertions along the proximal humerus. The clavicular head is more superficial, and the sternal costal head is deep and more superior. There are muscular attachments more distally extending the insertion.
- There is intimate contact along the anterior edge of the deltoid. Pectoralis injuries may appear as deltoid injuries if detachment or atrophy is detected. The cephalic vein travels along the superficial portion of this interval.

PECTORALIS TEARS

- The most common mechanism of injury is forced adduction against resistance. Direct injury can create tears at the muscle and muscle tendon junction. Indirect injuries via muscular eccentric contraction including bench press, breaking a fall, and wrestling are more commonly humeral avulsion injuries (Noble and Bell, 1996).
- Tears can be classified as sprain, partial tear (most common), or complete tear. Location of tear can be humerus avulsion, muscle tendon junction, tendinous ruptures, and muscular tears.
- Clinical presentation of a tear is hematoma, weakness of shoulder adduction and internal rotation, deformity of the anterior axillary fold, prominent deltoid, asymmetric pectoralis muscular bulge, and arm swelling.
- Provocative testing can be performed on seated patients with their hands on their hips. Asking them to apply an adduction force recreates pain and visual asymmetry of the pectoralis compared to the uninjured extremity.

- On a supine patient with the arm abducted, palpation along the humerus insertion and the muscular tendon junction may be helpful in identifying the location of the tear. Slight forward flexion and neutral rotation allows for deeper examination.
- Magnetic resonance imaging can identify tear and hematoma. Location of the tear is important to prognosis and treatment options. Tears within the muscle or at the muscle tendon junction have poorer surgical outcomes than tendon avulsion injuries.

PECTORALIS TEARS TREATMENT

- Early surgical repair is recommended for patients who participate in athletics and strenuous activities (Zeman, Rosenfeld, and Lipscomb, 1979). Reduction in adduction strength can be 50% or greater if treated nonoperatively (Wolfe, Wickiewicz, and Cavanaugh, 1992).
- Complete tears and avulsions should be repaired early with anticipated satisfactory results. Delayed repairs 2–3 months may require a graft due to adhesions and muscular atrophy.
- Surgical repair of tendon avulsions are best achieved with suture anchors or bone tunnels. Anchors should be located along the lateral aspect of the biceps groove. Superior reinforcement can be added including deltoid pectoralis interval closure.
- Muscular repairs have increased risk of failure (Noble and Bell, 1996). Tissue augmentation as in xenograft or allografts may increase successful repairs when compromised tissue is detected at surgery.
- Postoperative management includes a sling for 4 to 6 weeks. Early pendulum exercises with restricted flexion to the face, external rotation to 30°, and avoidance of extension for 6 weeks. Strengthening can begin at 10–12 weeks. Restrictions for maximal resistance are commonly greater than 4 months.
- Conservative treatment to partial and muscular tears includes stretching at 2 weeks, terminal stretching at 4–6 weeks, and strengthening at 12 weeks. Muscular compensation can occur with subscapularis, deltoid, latissimus dorsi, and teres major.

REFERENCES

Abrams JS: Special shoulder problems in the throwing athlete: Pathology, diagnosis and nongenerative management. *Clinic Sports Med* 10(4):839–861, 1991.

Abrams JS: Arthroscopic treatment of posterior instability, in Tibone JE, Savoie FH III, Shaffer BS (eds.): *Shoulder Arthroscopy*. New York, NY, Springer-Verlag, 2003, pp 97–103.

Andrews JR, Carson WG, Jr, McLeod WD: Glenoid labrum tears related to the long head of the biceps. *Am J Sports Med* 13:337–341, 1985.

Bell RH, Noble JS: Biceps disorders, in Hawkins RJ, Misamore GW (eds.): *Shoulder Injuries in the Athlete*. New York, NY, Churchill Livingstone, 1996, pp 267–282.

Burkhart SS, Morgan CD: The peel-back mechanism: Its role in producing and extending posterior type II SLAP lesions and its effect on SLAP repair rehabilitation. *Arthroscopy* 14:637–640, 1998.

Burkhead WZ, Jr, Arcand MA, Zeman C, et al : The biceps tendon, in Rockwood CA, Jr, Matsen FA (eds.): *The Shoulder*, 2nd ed. Philadelphia, PA, Saunders, 1998, pp 1009–1063.

Cooper DE, Arnoczky SP, O'Brien SJ, et al: Anatomy, histology, and vascularity of the glenoid labrum: An anatomical study. *J Bone Joint Surg* 47A:46–52, 1992.

Curtis AS, Snyder SJ: Evaluation and treatment of biceps tendon pathology. *Orthop Clin North Am* 24(1):33–43, 1993.

Garrett WE, Jr, Safran MR, Seaber AV, et al: Biomechanical comparison of stimulated and nonstimulated skeletal muscle pulled to failure. *Am J Sports Med* 15:448–454, 1987.

Gill TJ, McIrvin E, Mair SD, et al: Results of biceps tenotomy for treatment of pathology of the long head of the biceps brachii. *J Shoulder Elbow Surg* 10:247–249, 2001.

Glousman R, Jobe F, Tibone J, et al: Dynamic electromyographic analysis of the throwing shoulder with glenohumeral instability. *J Bone Joint Surg* 70:220–226, 1988.

Habermeyer P, Walch G: The biceps tendon and rotator cuff disease, in Burkhead WZ, Jr, (ed.): *Rotator Cuff Disorders*. Baltimore, MD, Williams & Wilkins, 142–159, 1996.

Harryman DT, Sidles JA, Harris SL, et al: The role of the rotator interval capsule in passive motion and stability of the shoulder. *J Bone Joint Surg* 74A:53–66, 1992.

Howell SM, Galinat BJ: The glenoid labral socket: a constrained articular surface. *Clin Orthop* 243:122–125, 1989.

Howell SM, Galinat BJ, Penz AJ, et al: Normal and abnormal mechanics of the glenohumeral joint in the horizontal plane. *J Bone Joint Surg* 70:227–232, 1988.

Kim TK, Quele WS, Cosgarea AJ, et al: Clinical features of different types of SLAP lesions. *J Bone Joint Surg* 85A:66–71, 2003.

Maffet MW, Gartsman GM, Moseby B: Superior labrum biceps tendon complex lesions of the shoulder. *Am J Sports Med* 23:93–98, 1995.

Mariani EM, Cofield RH, Askew LJ: Rupture of the tendon of the long head of the biceps brachii: Surgical versus nonsurgical treatment. *Clin Orthop* 228:233–239, 1988.

McEntire JE, Hess WE, Coleman SS: Rupture of the pectoralis major muscle. *J Bone Joint Surg* 54A:1040–1046, 1972.

McFarland EG, Kim TK, Savino RM: Clinical assessment of three common tests for superior labral anterior-posterior lesions. *Am J Sports Med* 30(6):810–815, 2002.

Morgan CD, Burkhart SS, Palmieri M, et al: Type II SLAP lesions: Three subtypes and their relationships to superior instability and rotator cuff tears. *Arthroscopy* 14:553–565, 1998.

Neer CS, III, Bigliani LU, Hawkins RJ: Rupture of the long head of the biceps related to subacromial impingement. *Orthop Trans* 1:114, 1977.

Noble JS, Bell RH: Pectoralis ruptures in shoulder injuries in the athlete, in Hawkins RJ, Misamore GW (eds.): *Churchhill Livingstone*. New York, NY, 1996, pp 283–290.

Paavolainen P, Slatis P, Aalto R: Surgical pathology in chronic shoulder pain, in Bateman JE, Welsh R (eds.): *Surgery of the Shoudler*. Philadelphia, PA, BC Decker 1984, pp 313–318.

Pagnani MJ, Deng XH, Warren RF, et al: Effects of lesions of the superior portion of the glenoid labrum on glenohumeral translation. *J Bone Joint Surg* 77A:1003–1010, 1995.

Peterson CJ: Spontaneous medial dislocation of the tendon of the long biceps brachii. *Clin Orthop* 211:224–227, 1986.

Rodosky MW, Harner CD, Fu FH: The role of the long head of the biceps muscle and superior glenoid labrum in anterior stability of the shoulder. *Am J Sports Med* 22:121–130, 1994.

Snyder SJ, Banas MP, Karzel RP: An analysis of 140 injuries to the superior glenoid labrum. *J Shoulder Elbow Surg* 4:243–248, 1995.

Snyder SJ, Karzel RP, DelPizzo W, et al: SLAP lesions of the shoulder. *Arthroscopy* 6:274–279, 1990.

Walch G, Nove-Josserand L, Boileau P, et al: Subluxations and dislocations of the tendon of the long head of the biceps. *J Shoulder Elbow Surg* 7:100–108, 1998.

William MM, Snyder SJ, Buford D: The Buford complex—the cord-like middle glenohumeral ligament and absent anterosuperior labrum complex: A normal anatomic capsulolabral variant. *Arthroscopy* 10:241–247, 1994.

Wolfe SW, Wickiewicz TL, Cavanaugh JT: Rupture of the pectoralis major muscle: an anatomic and clinical analysis. *Am J Sports Med* 20:587–593, 1992.

Zeman SC, Rosenfeld RT, Lipscomb PR: Tears of the pectoralis major muscle. *Am J Sports Med* 7:343–347, 1979.

48 THE THROWING SHOULDER
Carlos A Guanche, MD

INTRODUCTION

THROWING MOTION

- Throwing in baseball has been analyzed extensively, with the specific maneuvers being broken down into six phases (Gowan et al, 1987). While the analysis of the baseball throw is the best understood and most studied, other throwing, racquet and overhand sports have also been evaluated. The mechanics of a baseball throw are transferable, for the most part, to other sports with some modifications depending on the size of the ball or the maneuver being analyzed. The baseball throw, by virtue of its speed and frequency, however, is the most traumatic to the shoulder.

- The phases of throwing are summarized as follows:
  - Wind-up
    a. Readying phase
    b. Minimal shoulder stress
  - Early cocking
  - Late cocking
    a. Scapular retraction for stable throwing base
    b. Maximal external rotation
    c. Posterior translation of the humeral head as a result of abduction/external rotation
    d. Shear force across anterior shoulder of 400 N
    e. Compressive force of 650 N generated by cuff
  - Acceleration
    a. Transition from eccentric to concentric forces anteriorly (vice-versa posteriorly)
    b. Rotation occurs at 7000°–9000°/s
    c. Only 1/3 of the kinetic energy leaves with the ball (the remainder is dissipated through the extremity)
  - Deceleration
    a. Most violent phase (responsible for dissipation of energy not imparted to ball)
    b. Largest joint loads
      1. Posterior shear force of 400 N
      2. Inferior shear forces of greater than 300 N
      3. Compressive forces of greater than 1000 N
      4. Adduction torque >80 N-m; horizontal abduction torque 100 N-m
  - Follow-through
    a. Rebalancing phase
    b. Compressive forces 400 N
    c. Inferior shear of 200 N
- The entire motion takes less than 2 s with most of the time (1.5 s) taken up by the early phases (wind-up and cocking)
- Two critical points in the motion
  a. Cocking: Full external rotation maximizes anterior shear forces and applies the highest torque to the shoulder.
  b. Acceleration: The body falls ahead of the shoulder while the internal rotators are maximally contracting and the angular velocity exceeds 7000°/s.

PATHOPHYSIOLOGY

ROTATOR CUFF

- Supraspinatus, infraspinatus, and teres minor fire in late cocking to move to maximal external rotation, followed by eccentric firing in deceleration.
- Tensile stress developed in tissues that may speed normal degeneration. Factors of stressful loading, distraction, excessive internal, and external rotation can cause acute inflammatory responses early (leading to impingement) or tendon failure in the later stages (rotator cuff tears).

LABRAL TEARS (*SUPERIOR LABRUM ANTERIOR TO POSTERIOR* (SLAP))

TRACTION MECHANISM
- During deceleration, biceps muscle contraction is strong as both elbow extension and glenohumeral distractions occur. The biceps muscle has been shown to be essential to limiting torsional forces to the shoulder in the abducted, externally rotated position (Rodosky, Harner, and Fu, 1994). By this mechanism, the effect on the superior labrum would be one of failure either by tension or direct compression.

PEEL BACK MECHANISM
- Tension overload develops in the abducted/externally rotated extremity (Morgan et al, 1998) based on three observations:
  1. A type II SLAP (posterosuperior) lesion can cause anterior pseudolaxity.
  2. *Abduction/External Rotation* (ABER) causes peel-back of posterosuperior labrum.
  3. Posterior inferior capsule tightens in overhand throwers. Axis of rotation of humeral head is shifted posterosuperiorly and increases internal impingement.

CAPSULAR

EXTERNAL ROTATION EXCESS
- Excessive external rotation leading to soft tissue adaptive changes and subsequent instability (Kvitne and Jobe, 1993).
- With failure of ligamentous restraints, coracoacromial arch impingement may result (secondary impingement).
- Secondary posterior capsular tightness also occurs.

INTERNAL IMPINGEMENT
- Rotator cuff impinges on the posterosuperior rim of the glenoid in ABER (Jobe and Sidles, 1992).
- Causes pain in ABER position and correlates with positive apprehension and relocation maneuvers (Walch et al, 1992).
- Etiology: Two theories
  1. Physiologic phenomenon causing labral and cuff tearing with repetitive activity
  2. Secondary internal impingement as a result of excessive external rotation developing with repetitive throwing

- Analysis of rotator cuff contact in throwing and non-throwing extremities, however, has revealed contact in both arms when in ABER position, lending credence to the theory of physiologic impingement which develops problems as a result of repetitive trauma (Halbrecht, Tirman, and Atkin, 1999).

BONY CHANGES

- Bennett's lesion: Bony reactive changes at the posterior glenoid margin (Bennett, 1959)
  - Symptom complex includes pain in posterior deltoid in follow-through phase
    1. Exostosis typically at the posterior, inferior glenoid margin.
    2. Size of lesion not correlated with symptoms.
    3. Symptoms may occur gradually or acutely.
  - Not always clinically symptomatic.
  - Symptomatic exostoses usually respond to rest and occasional steroid injections.
  - Excision is performed through either an arthroscopic or posterior open approach (Lombardo et al, 1977; Meister et al, 1999).

MANAGEMENT OF SPECIFIC INJURIES

SLAP LESIONS

- Variable amounts of detachment encountered. The established classification system defines the clinically unstable lesions as those that involve the biceps anchor (Snyder et al, 1990).
- Conservative management in an established SLAP lesion does not fare well.
- Attempts at rehabilitation center around increasing rotator cuff strength and management of secondary scapulothoracic dyskinesia.
- Surgical management is arthroscopic stabilization with the use of suture anchors. The use of solid, arthroscopically delivered tacks is contraindicated in throwing athletes and is reserved for less active patients (Morgan et al, 1998).

CAPSULAR LAXITY (MICROINSTABILITY)

- Most commonly present with impingement (secondary).
- Initial treatment is focused on decreasing pain and inflammation, followed by a cuff strengthening program emphasizing flexibility, strength, power, and endurance of the rotator cuff.

- Surgery is indicated with failure to progress within 3 to 6 months.
- Surgical intervention has been shown to be successful with either open (capsulolabral reconstruction) (Rubenstein et al, 1992) or arthroscopic capsular imbrication.
- Thermal capsulorrhaphy alone may be indicated in those cases where labral pathology is nonexistent and the patient has excessive external rotation with a total arc of motion greater than 30° as compared to the contralateral side (D'Alessandro et al, 1998).
- Surgical intervention with the goal of limiting motion, especially external rotation, should be undertaken following a thorough rehabilitation course and careful discussion with the patient.
  - All of these procedures, to some extent, limit motion.
  - Rate of return is not always 100%.

INTERNAL IMPINGEMENT

- Overlap with laxity has made treatment difficult.
- In cases where no obvious instability is present, debridement may be an option with approximately 65% return to prior activity level (Walch et al, 1992).
- Capsular imbrication:
  - May be performed with any method available, including open capsulolabral reconstruction, arthroscopic plication or heat capsulorrhaphy (Levitz, Andrews, and Dugas, 2000).
  - Variable results with no long-term series are available.
- Derotation:
  - This is a highly invasive surgical procedure.
  - This may be used in extreme cases following failure of debridement and/or capsulorrhaphy with a desire to return to high level throwing.

ROTATOR CUFF TEARS

- Partial thickness tearing is most common. Partial tears result from the excessive tension developed within fibers.
  - Intra-articular partial tears are most common.
  - Diagnosis is done via MRI with intra-articular gadolinium.
    a. Assess arm in ABER position
    b. Highly suspicious of diagnosis in high level throwers
  - Surgical indications
    a. Arthroscopic evaluation of joint is important as a result of high incidence of labral lesions and partial cuff tears.

    b. Repair is considered in those lesions greater than 50% of tendon thickness (normal 12–16 mm).

    c. Debridement is in lower grade lesions and in those with normal preoperative strength.

    d. Consider acromioplasty and/or coracoacromial ligament release.

IMPINGEMENT

PRIMARY

- Rare as an isolated entity.
- High incidence of intra-articular pathology.
- Arthroscopy indicated in all patients to assess for additional pathology.
- Conservative resection.
  a. Do not resect type I acromion.
  b. Release of coracoacromial ligament (no resection).

SECONDARY

- Most often missed and inappropriately treated as primary problem:
  - Requires treatment of the primary problem either with rehabilitation or surgical intervention.
- Arthroscopy helps assess for primary intra-articular pathology.
- The employment of subacromial decompression in isolation has been shown to be unpredictable with respect to return to prior activity level.
  a. In one study, only 43% of patients with surgical decompression returned to preinjury level of competition (Tibone et al, 1985).
  b. Return is perhaps more indicative of improvement in their muscular imbalance through thoughtful rehabilitation than as a result of the surgical procedure.

REHABILITATION ISSUES

SCAPULOTHORACIC ARTICULATION

- Often the cause of secondary impingement.
- Scapula has five specific functions that have implications in throwers (Kibler, 1998).
  a. Stable part of the glenohumeral articulation, where rotation of the glenohumeral joint allows maximal concavity and compression.
  b. The scapula retracts and protracts the shoulder complex along the thoracic wall.
  c. Acromial elevation to avoid impingement with arm elevation.
  d. Base for muscular attachments.
  e. Energy transfer from the legs, back, and trunk.

SCAPULOTHORACIC DYSKINESIA

- Abnormal set of motions and positions affecting the relative position of the scapula and the proximal humerus.
  a. Etiologies include nerve or muscle injury, muscle inhibition, and glenohumeral stiffness or laxity.
  b. Mechanical dysfunction may result in impingement as well as insufficient translation of energy from the lower body.
    1. Excessive stress results in overuse injuries.
    2. Clinical picture is confusing as a result of secondary impingement and capsular changes that may occur as a result of the adaptations to scapular malalignment.

PROPRIOCEPTION (LEPHART AND HENRY, 2000)

- Excessive joint laxity associated with capsuloligamentous injury and resulting microtrauma cause damage to the neural receptors and lead to deafferentation.
- Neuromuscular deficits impair reflexive muscular stabilization, predisposing shoulder to episodes of functional instability.
  a. Diminished joint position sense, kinesthetic awareness, and abnormal humeroscapular firing patterns (Lephart et al, 1996).
  b. Abnormal firing patterns documented on EMG studies in throwers with glenohumeral instability (Glousman et al, 1988).
  c. Following surgical reconstruction, joint position sense, and reproduction of passive positioning improve to baseline levels (Lephart et al, 1996).
- Restoration of functional stability.
  a. Traditional strengthening exercises do not address neuromuscular deficits.
  b. Four elements necessary to restore functional stability (Lephart et al, 1996):
    1. Peripheral somatosensory, including visual and vestibular
    2. Spinal reflexes:
      - Sudden alteration in joint position that requires reflex muscular stabilization.
    3. Cognitive programming:
      - Appreciation of joint position.
    4. Brain stem.
  c. All four elements need to be addressed in order to fulfill the objective of stimulating all subsystems:
    1. Dynamic stabilization:
      a. Promotes coactivation of force couples
      b. Centers humeral head
    2. Joint position sensibility:
      - Restore through conscious and unconscious pathways.

3. Reactive neuromuscular control:
   a. Reflexive muscular stabilization induced by sudden alterations in joint position.
   b. Eccentric activities useful.
4. Functional motor patterns:
   a. Progression to the actual throwing activity.
   b. Analyze direction of force, amount of loading, and resultant muscle action to incorporate functional progression.

REFERENCES

Bennett GE: Elbow and shoulder lesions of baseball players. *Am J Surg* 98:484–492, 1959.

D'Alessandro DF, Bradley JP, Fleischli JF, et al: Prospective evaluation of electrothermal arthroscopic capsulorrhaphy (ETAC) for shoulder instability: Indications, technique and preliminary results. *Annual Closed Meeting of American Shoulder and Elbow Surgeon*, New York, NY, 1998.

Glousman R, Jobe FW, Tibone, et al: Dynamic electromyographic analysis of the throwing shoulder with glenohumeral instability. *J Bone Joint Surg* 70:220–226, 1988.

Gowan ID, Jobe FW, Tibone JE, Moynes DR: A comparative electromyographic analysis of the shoulder during pitching. Professional versus amateur pitchers. *Am J Sports Med* 15:586–590, 1987.

Halbrecht JL, Tirman P, Atkin D: Internal impingement of the shoulder: Comparison of findings between throwing and nonthrowing shoulders of college baseball players. *Arthroscopy* 15:253–258, 1999.

Jobe CM, Sidles J: Evidence for a superior glenoid impingement upon the rotator cuff: Anatomic, kinesiologic, MRI and arthroscopic findings (Abstract). *5th International Conference on Surgery of the Shoulder*. Paris, France, July 1992.

Kibler WB: The role of the scapula in athletic shoulder function. *Am J Sports Med* 26:325–337, 1998.

Kvitne RS, Jobe FW: The diagnosis and treatment of anterior instability in the throwing athlete. *Clin Orthop* 291:107–123, 1993.

Lephart SM, Henry TJ: Restoration of proprioception and neuromuscular control of the unstable shoulder, in Lephart SM and Fu FH (eds.): *Proprioception and Neuromuscular Control in Joint Stability*. New York, NY, Human Kinetics, 2000, pp 405–413.

Lephart SM, Kocher MS, Fu FH, et al: The physiological basis for open and closed kinetic chain rehabilitation for the upper extremity. *J Sport Rehab* 5:71–87, 1996.

Levitz CL, Andrews JR, Dugas J: The use of thermal capsular shrinkage in the management of labral detachments in elite throwing athletes. *Annual Meeting American Academy of Orthopaedic Surgeons*. Orlando, FL, 2000.

Lombardo SJ, Kerlan RK, Jobe FW, et al: Posterior shoulder lesions in throwing athletes. *Am J Sports Med* 5:106–110, 1977.

Meister K, Andrew JR, Batts J, et al: Symptomatic thrower's exostosis. Arthroscopic evaluation and treatment. *Am J Sports Med* 27:133–136, 1999.

Morgan CD, Burkhart SS, Palmeri M, et al: Type II SLAP lesions: Three subtypes and their relationships to superior instability and rotator cuff tears. *Arthroscopy* 14:553–565, 1998.

Rodosky MW, Harner CD, Fu FH: The role of the long head of the biceps muscle and superior glenoid labrum in anterior stability of the shoulder. *Am J Sports Med* 22:121–130, 1994.

Rubenstein DL, Jobe FW, Glousman RE, et al: Anterior capsulolabral reconstruction of the shoulder in athletes. *J Shoulder Elbow Surg* 1:229–237, 1992.

Snyder SJ, Karzel RP, Delpizzo W, et al: SLAP lesions of the shoulder. *Arthroscopy* 6:274–279, 1990.

Tibone JE, Jobe FW, Kerlan RK, et al: Shoulder impingement syndrome in athletes treated by anterior acromioplasty. *Clin Orthop* 198:134–140, 1985.

Walch G, Boileau P, Noel E, et al: Impingement of the deep surface of the supraspinatus tendon on the posterior glenoid rim: An arthroscopic study. *J Shoulder Elbow Surg* 1:238–245, 1992.

49 ELBOW INSTABILITY

Derek H Ochiai, MD
Robert P Nirschl, MD, MS

INTRODUCTION

- The elbow is a highly congruent, complex hinge joint.
- Although constrained by bony architecture and the stabilizing ligaments, it accounts for 20% of all dislocations (Josefsson, Johnell, and Gentz, 1984).
- Most instabilites result from either a single trauma (straight posterior or *posterolateral rotatory instability,* [PLRI]) or chronic overuse in the overhead athlete (valgus instability). A congenitally shallow ulnohumeral joint may contribute to single trauma instabilities.

FUNCTIONAL ANATOMY

- The elbow joint comprises the humeroradial, humeroulnar, and proximal radioulnar joints.
- The lateral portion of the distal humerus, the capitulum, articulates with the radial head. The medial portion of the humerus, the trochlea, articulates with the trochlear notch of the ulna. The radial notch of

the ulna articulates with the radial head (Netter, 1987).

- The ulnohumeral joint affords flexion and extension of the elbow, while the proximal radioulnar joint affords pronation and supination. The humeroradial joint moves in both rotation and flexion/extension.
- The primary restraints of the elbow are the congruous ulnohumeral articulation, the anterior band of the *medial collateral ligament* (MCL) and the *lateral ulnar collateral ligament* (LUCL) (O'Driscoll et al, 2000).
- The MCL, the main constraint to valgus instability, originates on the anteroinferior medial epicondyle and inserts onto the body of the coronoid process. The injury pattern is usually midsubstance to proximal failure.
- The LUCL, the main constraint to PLRI, originates from the lateral epicondyle and inserts into the annular ligament and on the supinator crest of the ulna. The injury pattern is usually an avulsion of the humeral origin.

HISTORY (MCL)

- MCL injuries are most common in overhead throwing athletes (Conway, Jobe, and Glousman, 1992).
- The most common complaint is pain typically felt during late cocking and early deceleration of the throwing motion. Throwing velocity may also be diminished.
- In elite pitchers, valgus forces in excess of 120 N-m have been documented (Williams and Altchek, 1999).
- Athletes usually *do not* have complaints of pain during activities of daily living or symptoms of elbow instability, such as popping, locking, or clicking; however, associated abnormalities such as synovitis, plica, or loose bodies may present with these symptoms.
- Patients may also have neuritis of the ulnar nerve, with numbness and tingling in the ulnar digits as well as loss of strength in the finger intrinsic.

HISTORY (LUCL)

- Injury to the LUCL is usually the result of trauma causing a dislocation, such as a fall on an outstretched hand. An occasional iatrogenic cause may occur secondary to previous lateral tennis elbow surgery, especially if a full release was performed, instead of a partial resection.
- The main complaints of athletes are instability symptoms of popping and clicking of the elbow and a sensation of giving way. Push-ups or lifting can be painful (Hotchkiss and Yamaguchi, 2002).

PHYSICAL EXAMINATION (MCL)

- Athlete may be tender to palpation over the MCL. This is more easily appreciated when palpation is done concurrently with valgus stress.
- Possible Tinel's sign may be present over the ulnar nerve in the cubital tunnel.
- Valgus stability is tested with the elbow flexed beyond 25° to minimize the bony restraints, and a valgus stress is applied while the examiner supports the elbow (Williams and Altchek, 1999).

PHYSICAL EXAMINATION (LUCL)

- The lateral pivot shift test is used for diagnosis. As originally described by O'Driscoll (Jobe, Stark, and Lonbardo, 1986), the patient is supine with the shoulder at 90° of flexion with the elbow flexed 90° overhead. The examiner gently supinates the forearm, and a valgus moment is applied. The arm is brought from near extension to flexion. The athlete should have apprehension during the beginning of the test, with further flexion causing a reduction of subluxation and diminution of the apprehension. We prefer a modification of this test, first bringing the elbow from flexion to extension, causing the apprehension or pain. As the elbow is brought back into a flexed position, the feeling of apprehension or pain is diminished. Frank palpable subluxation and reduction is rare, unless the patient is under general anesthesia or has had intra-articular local anesthetic.

IMAGING STUDIES

- Plain radiographs may reveal associated intra-articular loose bodies, osteophytes, or calcification of the MCL (O'Driscoll, Bell, and Morrey, 1991). A shallow ulnohumeral joint may be evident on the lateral view.
- Stress views with a valgus force can show a side to side difference, confirming MCL insufficiency.
- Fluoroscopy can be useful for demonstrating PLRI.
- MRI can show damage to ligaments on either side, and can be useful when the diagnosis is in doubt or for preoperative planning. Injection of gadolinium dye may enhance the MRI.

TREATMENT (NONOPERATIVE)

- Immediate treatment is reduction of any dislocation and splinting in 90° of flexion, with X-rays to look for intra-articular pathology as well as associated fractures.

- Immobilization in a cast or splint for an unstable elbow is contraindicated for more than 10 days, because prolonged immobilization of the elbow can lead to intractable stiffness.
- Treatment is dictated by the athlete's symptoms and desire to return to play.
- For MCL injuries, a trial of nonoperative treatment with modalities to reduce swelling and medial sided flexor-pronator strengthening as well as rotator cuff strengthening may be sufficient.
- For LUCL injuries, physical therapy is usually ineffective for athletics as well as pain and dysfunction with daily living. A hinged brace may be tried for low demand people, but this is rarely tolerated.

TREATMENT (OPERATIVE)

- For MCL injuries, the indications for surgery are a failure of a quality rehabilitation regimen and the athlete's desire to return to previous level of activity. The surgical treatment consists of a tendon graft approximating the attachments of the MCL (Morrey, 1996). Graft choices are palmaris longus or plantaris tendons. The reconstruction described by Jobe (Jobe, Stark, Lonbardo, 1986) is technically demanding, requiring five tunnels with a tendon weave. Newer techniques such as the docking procedure (Rohrbough et al, 2002) or use of interference screws are promising (Ahmad, Lee, and ElAttrache, 2003). Results of primary repair of the MCL (without reconstruction with a graft) have been disappointing, and are usually reserved for patients with a bony avulsion at the MCL origin or insertion (Williams and Altchek, 1999).
- For LUCL injuries, the indications are pain and dysfunction, either in activities of daily living or with athletics. Surgical treatment consists of either repair of the LUCL, or surgical reconstruction of the LUCL with a tendon graft (O'Driscoll, Bell, and Morrey, 1991).

REFERENCES

Ahmad CS, Lee TQ, ElAttrache NS: Biomechanical evaluation of a new ulnar collateral ligament reconstruction technique with interference screw fixation. *Am J Sports Med* 31:332–337, 2003.
Conway JE, Jobe FW, Glousman RE: Medial instability of the elbow in throwing athletes: Treatment by repair or reconstruction of the ulnar collateral ligament. *J Bone Joint Surg Am* 74:67–83, 1992.
Hotchkiss RN, Yamaguchi K: Elbow reconstruction. *Ortho Knowledge Update: Sports Medicine 7;* 31:317–327, 2002.
Jobe FW, Stark H, Lonbardo SJ: Reconstruction of the ulnar collateral ligament in athletes. *J Bone Joint Surg Am* 68:1158–1163, 1986.
Josefsson PO, Johnell O, Gentz CF: Long-term sequelae of simple dislocation of the elbow. *J Bone Joint Surg Am* 66:927–930, 1984.
Morrey BF: Acute and chronic instability of the elbow. *J Am Acad Orthop Surg* 4:117–128, 1996.
Netter FH: *The CIBA Collection of Medical Illustrations:* vol. 8. Summitt, NJ, CIBA-GEIGY, 1987, pp 42–43.
O'Driscoll SW, Bell DF, Morrey BF: Posterolateral rotatory instability of the elbow. *J Bone Joint Surg Am* 73:440–446, 1991.
O'Driscoll SW, Jupiter JB, King GJW, et al: The unstable elbow. *J Bone Joint Surg Am* 82:724–728, 2000.
Rohrbough JT, Altchek DW, Hyman J, et al: Medial collateral ligament reconstruction of the elbow using the docking technique. *Am J Sports Med* 30L:541–548, 2002.
Williams RJ, Altchek DW: Atraumatic injuries of the elbow. *Ortho Knowledge Update: Sports Medicine 2;* 23:229–236, 1999.

50 ELBOW ARTICULAR LESIONS AND FRACTURES
Edward S Ashman, MD

INTRODUCTION

- Elbow articular lesions and fractures are not uncommon in the athlete. Seven percent of all fractures occur in the elbow (Regan, 1994). It is important for the sports physician to become familiar with patterns of injury and treatment options for athletic injuries of the elbow.
- The elbow's high degree of bony congruity, soft tissue aspects, and high potential for stiffness make the elbow uniquely challenging to treat after athletic injury. A common theme of elbow injury is that early motion is important to minimize stiffness and to nourish the joint. *Range of motion* (ROM) required for activities of daily living is defined as 30–130° of flexion and 50° of supination and pronation (Scheling, 2002). Athletic activities may require far more motion than this.
- Pediatric and adult elbow fractures differ considerably and will be discussed separately.

PEDIATRIC FRACTURES

RADIOGRAPHIC EVALUATION

- Physicians evaluating pediatric elbow fractures must be familiar with normal developmental anatomy as well as secondary ossification centers about the elbow.
- It may be helpful to obtain contralateral comparison view for comparison because of the confusion between ossification centers and fractures.
- The proximal radius should point to the capitellum in all views. The long axis of the ulna should line up with or be slightly medial to the long axis of the humerus on a true *anteroposteior* (AP) view. The anterior humeral line should bisect the capitellum on the lateral view. The humeral-capitellar (Baumann's) angle should be within the range of 9–26° of valgus (Vitale and Skaggs, 2002).
- A posterior fat pad sign is always considered to be an abnormal radiographic finding, and represents an elbow fracture 76% of the time as per a recent prospective study (n = 45) (Skaggs and Mirzayan, 1999).
- An anterior fat pad sign represents a superficial part of anterior fat pad and should be in front of coronoid fossa. In normal elbow the anterior fat pad should be barely visualized.
- Look for small radiolucent area between bony rim and moderate opaque shadows of brachialis.
- With joint effusion, there will be anterior and superior displacement of anterior fat pad (Skaggs and Mirzayan, 1999).

OSSIFICATION CENTERS OF THE ELBOW

- Capetellum (appears age 1–2)
- Radial Head (appears age 2–4)
- Medial epicondyle (appears age 4–6)
- Trochlea (appears age 8–11)
- Olecranon (9–11 years)
- Lateral epicondyle (appears age 10–11) (Vitale and Skaggs, 2002)
- A well known, but ribald, mnemonic exists to remember this order, but will not be repeated here. (So sue me; just remember: you *Can't Resist My Team Of Lawyers*.)

SUPRACONDYLAR FRACTURES

- Extra-articular supracondylar fractures are extremely common in the pediatric population, and represent 10% of all pediatric fractures. Occur due to fall on hand or elbow. Extension pattern is far more common (98%) (Vitale and Skaggs, 2002).
- Performance of a careful neurovascular examination is crucial. Any of the neurovascular structures crossing the elbow joint may be at risk. Radiographs are mandatory. The pulseless, poorly perfused hand is a true emergency. It is important to rule out vascular injury. Vascular injuries are more commonly associated with posterolateral displacement, and higher grade injuries. The medial spike may tether the brachial artery. One must perform frequent rechecks of the radial pulse to document its presence as well as its quality. An intimal arterial injury may not be initially apparent, but may develop over hours. Compartment syndromes must be treated emergently, and must be carefully watched for (Shaw et al, 1990).
- The *anterior interosseus* (AI) nerve is most frequently injured nerve, most recover spontaneously within 6 months. The AI nerve can be checked by having the patient make an "OK" sign. With posteromedial displacement, the lateral spike of proximal fragment may tether the radial nerve (Ippolito, Caterini, and Scola, 1986).
- Clinical signs include the "dimple sign" that occurs when the fracture ends are caught in the brachialis and subcutaneous soft tissues. The olecranon and the two epicondyles should form a straight line in the extended position, and a triangle when the elbow is flexed to 90°. This relationship is unchanged in a supracondylar fracture, but is altered by an elbow dislocation (Harris, 1992).
- Treatment is defined by stability of fracture pattern as defined by Gartland classification. Type I is nondisplaced, type II exhibits anterior gapping, limited rotational malalignment, and an intact posterior hinge. Type III fractures have no cortical continuity and are totally unstable. Minimally displaced may be treated with splinting, types II and III require reduction most require operative intervention to maintain stability while in a 90° position of flexion (Harris, 1992).
- Following reduction, it is crucial to perform a repeat neurovascular examination and again check radiographs.
- Long term sequelae of the supracondylar fracture are extremely important and include the following (Ippolito, Caterini, and Scola, 1986):
  1. Cubitus varus is the most common complication following supracondylar humerus fracture. It is primarily a cosmetic deformity, and does not usually create a loss of function. Previously, cubitus varus was thought to be created by growth disturbamce, but it is now believed to be due to imperfect fracture reduction. It is extremely important to have perfect fracture rotation.

2. Volkmann's contracture can be caused by brachial artery injury leading to a severe compartment syndrome, muscle necrosis and degeneration. This was often a result of maintaining the arm in severe flexion in order to maintain a reduction. A closed reduction should be maintained with the arm in 90° of flexion. If more flexion is needed to maintain the reduction, percutaneous pinning should be considered. Treatment options are focused on restoring vascular flow and reducing compartment pressure. It is usually too late to avoid severe morbidity. It is imperative to avoid this complication with proper fracture care and neurovascular monitoring.

3. Arterial injury occurs in approximately 5% of children with supracondylar fractures. Arteriography is indicated if the pulse is decreased following reduction. If no pulse is present before and after reduction, emergent surgery is required, and a delay for arteriography is contraindicated.

4. Nerve injuries are usually anterior interosseus or radial nerve and can be quite common (up to 50% AI injury with type III fractures). Most nerve palsies resulting from supracondylar fractures are neuropraxias, and will resolve spontaneously within 3 to 6 months.

LATERAL EPICONDYLE FRACTURE

- Exceedingly rare in adults (as is the medial epicondyle fracture), essentially a pediatric fracture. Intra-articular fractures must be considered potentially unstable. May need MRI to see intra-articular component of fracture. Even benign appearing injuries may have high complication rates. Potential complications include nonunion, delayed union, and tarda ulnar nerve palsy secondary to progressive cubital valgus (Wilson et al, 1988).
- With less than 2 mm of displacement the fracture may be treated with cast immobilization, but must be followed closely with serial radiographs. Any displacement greater than 2 mm must be surgically reduced and fixed (Wilson et al, 1988).

MEDIAL EPICONDYLE FRACTURE

- More common in young throwing athletes (i.e., pitchers) that subject their elbows to high valgus stress. If chronic, the condition is termed "Little Leaguer's Elbow."
- Must perform careful neurologic examination, as ulnar nerve may be involved (Wilson et al, 1988).

- Must test for stability, as it is possible that elbow dislocated and spontaneously reduced, as youths have less inherent stability than adults (Fowles, Slimane, and Kassab, 1990). Valgus instability should be assessed at 25° of flexion. Also gravity stress test may be used. The patient lies supine, externally rotate and abduct the shoulder to 90°, flex the elbow to 20°, and observe for pain and laxity. Stress X-ray views may also be performed (Vitale and Skaggs, 2002).
- Even minimally displaced fractures may be well tolerated in the nonathlete (Wilson et al, 1988). In the young athlete that is expected to have valgus stress on the elbow (throwers), however, operative intervention more likely necessary. Surgical indications include the following (Wilson et al, 1988):
  1. Displacement greater than 10 mm may cause loss strength of the flexor mass and should be fixed.
  2. Ulnar neuropathy with displaced fracture
  3. Valgus instability as determined above
  4. Displaced fracture that blocks joint motion

OLECRANON FRACTURE

- Occur with other elbow fractures 20% of time.
- Displacement of 5 mm or articular step off of 2 mm are operative indications. Hardware used depends on stability of fracture pattern, with plates used for less stable injury.
- Treat nonoperatively in 20° of flexion to minimize triceps pull (Vitale and Skaggs, 2002).

PROXIMAL RADIUS FRACTURE

- Radial neck fractures are more common in 8–12-year olds. Treatment determined by angulation. Less than 30° angulation of neck is accepted. Greater than 30° requires reduction, and greater than 60° may require the use of a wire to "joystick" the fracture into position (Vitale and Skaggs, 2002).

ADULT ELBOW TRAUMA

DISTAL HUMERUS FRACTURES

- Rare in the athlete. Requires high energy to cause this injury in young adult population. In the general population, represent one-third of elbow fractures, or 2% of all fractures (Scheling, 2002). Have a high propensity for stiffness. It is important to maintain a functional range of motion for activities of daily living.

- Operative treatment for displaced articular fractures aims for anatomic reduction and early motion to minimize stiffness. Intra-articular distal humerus fractures tend to be extremely complicated to treat operatively.

CAPITELLAR FRACTURE

- Rare! <1% of all elbow fractures (Scheling, 2002). Often associated with radial head fractures. Diagnosis may be difficult, and the lateral plain film must be carefully checked. A *computed tomography* (CT) scan may be necessary to better delineate the fracture type. Nonoperative treatment for nondisplaced fractures.
- There are three basic types of capitellar fractures: Hahn-Steinthal fracture includes a large portion of bone with the capitellar articular surface, and usually is able to be primarily reduced, and fixed operatively. The Kocher-Lorenz fragment involves a small amount of articular surface of the capitellum only, and must often be excised. A third type of fracture is comminuted and is also difficult to fix.
- Early motion is mandatory after these injuries.

RADIAL HEAD FRACTURES

- Common: 20–30% of elbow fractures (Scheling, 2002). Adults tend to sustain radial head as opposed to neck fractures. May be isolated or associated with elbow dislocation, ulnar shaft fractures, distal radial joint injury (Essex-Lopresti lesion), or carpal fractures, as well as additional fracture patterns.
- Must rule out associated *medial collateral ligament* (MCL) injury, interosseus membrane, *distal radioulnar joint* (DRUJ) injury.
- Operative indications include displacement greater than 2 mm, mechanical block to motion (pain may be ruled out as cause with intra-articular lidocaine injection), greater than 20–30% articular depression, or open fracture (Scheling, 2002). Surgical options depend on fracture type as well as associated lesions and include excision, ORIF or hemiarthroplasty. Radial head should never be excised if interosseus ligament or MCL injury.

OLECRANON FRACTURE

- Nondisplaced fractures <2 mm are treated nonoperatively with long arm casting. Care must be taken to avoid prolonged immobilization and stiffness (Scheling, 2002).

- Displaced fracture required ORIF, with technique dependent upon fracture pattern stability. Although excision of up to 50% of olecranon has been described (Scheling, 2002), this should only be used in very low demand patients, and not in the athletic population.

CORONOID FRACTURES

- Caused by humeral hyperextension. Associated with dislocation of elbow 10–33% of time. Coronoid-trochlear articulation provides up to 50% of elbow stability (Scheling, 2002).
- Treatment depends on fracture stability pattern, which is defined by amount of coronoid involved in fracture. Greater than 50% involvement requires ORIF, less than 50% fracture may be treated nonoperatively if it is stable.
- As with most elbow fractures, basic treatment plan is to obtain stability so as to allow early motion.

OSTEOCHONDRITIS DESSICANS

- *Osteochondritis dessicans* (OCD) of the capitellum occurs in adolescent and young adult athletes who are involved in repetitive upper extremity exercises.
- Throwers, gymnasts, and weight lifters are particularly susceptible.
- Etiology involves microtrauma, but exact cause is uncertain.
- AP and lateral radiographs are usually sufficient for diagnosis, but MRI or CT may be helpful to further delineate extent of lesion. There may be a localized area in capitellum without rarefaction and crater formation.
- Osteochondrosis of the capitellum or Panner's disease occurs in children age 4–8 years and involves *entire* ossific nucleus self-limiting with conservative treatment (Schenck, Jr and Goodnight, 1996).
- OCD of the capitellum occurs in individuals 10 years old or greater and involves a *portion* of the capitellum. It is believed to be due to valgus high stress forces caused during the acceleration phase of throwing, when the capitellum becomes loaded. Symptoms include poorly defined lateral elbow pain, with later stages of disease showing catching and locking. Laxity of the MCL may be present. Permanent deformity may result. Strict restriction from throwing for 8–12 weeks or until full, pain-free motion is restored for nondisplaced lesion with intact articular cartilage (Schenk and Goodnight, 1996).
- Indications for surgery include partially or completely detached fragment. Treatment options are dependent on lesion type and chronicity and include removal,

reattachment, bone grafting, drilling, and debridement. Operative techniques continue to evolve (Vitale and Skaggs, 2002).

REFERENCES

Fowles JV, Slimane N, Kassab MT: Elbow dislocation with avulsion of the medial humeral epicondyle. *J Bone Joint Surg Br* 72(1):102–104, Jan. 1990.

Harris IE: Supracondylar fractures of the humerus in children. *Orthopedics-pcm* [JC:pcm] 15(7):811–817, Jul. 1992.

Ippolito-E, Caterini-R, Scola-E: Supracondylar fractures of the humerus in children: Analysis at maturity of fifty-three patients treated conservatively. *J Bone Joint Surg Am* 68(3): 333–344, Mar. 1986.

Regan WD: Acute traumatic injuries of the elbow in the athlete, in Griffin LY (ed.): *OKU Sports Medicine*. Rosemont, PA, AAOS, 1994, pp 191–204.

Scheling GJ: Elbow and forearm: Adult trauma, in Koval KJ (ed.): *OKU 7*. Rosemont, PA, AAOS, 2002, pp 307–316.

Schenck RC, Jr, Goodnight JM: Osteochondritis dissecans. *J Bone Joint Surg Am* 79(3):439–456, 1996.

Shaw BA, Kasser JR, Emans JB, et al: Management of vascular injuries in displaced supracondylar humerus fractures without arteriography: *J Orthop Trauma* [JC:jh4] 4(1):25–29, 1990.

Skaggs DL, Mirzayan R: The posterior fat pad sign in association with occult fracture of the elbow in children. *J Bone Joint Surg Am* 81-A:1429–1433, 1999.

Vitale MG, Skaggs DL: Elbow: Pediatric aspects, in Koval KJ (ed.): *OKU 7* Rosemont, PA, AAOS, 2002, pp 299–306.

Wilson NI, Ingram R, Rymaszewski L, et al: Treatment of fractures of the medial epicondyle of the humerus: *Injury; Br J Accid Surg* 19(5):342–344, Sep. 1988.

51 ELBOW TENDINOSIS

Robert P Nirschl, MD, MS
Derek H Ochiai, MD

INTRODUCTION

- Elbow tendinosis is a result of tendon overuse and a failure of tendon healing.
- Elbow tendinosis can affect the lateral side (extensor carpi radialis brevis, extensor digitorum communis), the medial side (pronator teres, flexor carpi radialis), or the posterior side (triceps) (Nirschl, 1992)

SYMPTOMS/SIGNS

- Initial symptoms are activity related pain followed by pain at rest as the condition becomes more chronic.
- Some loss of extension common in medial elbow tendinosis
- Tenderness over lateral or medial tendon origins or posterior insertion of triceps
- Pain with provocative procedures (resisted wrist/finger extension for lateral tendinosis, wrist flexion/pronation for medial tendinosis, and elbow extension for posterior tendinosis)
- Since medial and lateral affected tendon units cross the elbow joint, pain is more severe with provocative testing with the elbow in extension. Therefore, pain with provocative testing with the elbow flexed indicates more severe involvement.
- Functional strength loss is common.

HISTOPATHOLOGY

- Histology of surgically resected tissue fails to reveal inflammatory cells. Thus, the term *tendinosis* is preferable to *tendonitis*.
- The epicondyle (bone) itself is not affected in the disease process. Therefore, epicondylitis is a misnomer; however, bony exostosis may be noted as a companion problem in 20% of lateral elbow tendinosis cases.
- Pathological tendinosis tendon shows disruption of normal collagen matrix by the characteristic invasion of fibroblasts and vascular granulation tissue termed *angiofibroblastic proliferation* (Nirschl and Pettrone, 1979).

DIFFERENTIAL DIAGNOSIS/ ASSOCIATED LESIONS

- Lateral tendinosis can be confused with the rare entity of *posterior interosseous nerve* (PIN) entrapment that would have diffuse pain along the radial nerve in the extensor mass of the proximal forearm, painful resisted supination, and *electromyogram* (EMG) changes of distal muscle groups (Lubahn and Cermak, 1998).
- Lateral tendinosis can be seen in combination or association with intra-articular abnormalities such as synovitis, plica, chondromalacia, and *osteochondritis dessicans* (OCD).
- Medial elbow associated abnormalities may include degeneration/rupture of medial collateral ligament, entrapment of the ulnar nerve, and congenital subluxation of the ulnar nerve.

- Posterior elbow associated abnormalities may include extra-articular olecrenon bursitis and intra-articular olecrenon fossa issues (synovitis, chondromalacia, and loose fragments).
- The mesenchymal syndrome, coined by Nirschl, has been used to describe a subset of patients with apparent decreased tissue durability who present with multiple affected areas that are often bilateral, including rotator cuffs, medial and lateral elbow tendinosis, carpal tunnel syndrome, trigger finger, deQuervain's disease, plantar neuromaplantar fasciosis, Achilles' insertional tendinosis, and hip trochanteric bursitis (Nirschl, 1992).

TREATMENT CONCEPTS

- Anti-inflammatory medications can be helpful in controlling pain and can be first line therapy allowing patients to comfortably proceed with curative rehabilitative exercises.
- Cortisone injections, when done correctly under the origin of the *extensor carpi radialis brevis* (ECRB) or flexor pronator mass can also be effective in relieving pain; however, cortisone injections are not without risks including fat atrophy, skin pigmentation changes, and infection, especially if injected superficially. Recently, injection of autologous blood has shown promising results (Edwards and Calandruccio, 2003).
- Physical modalities such as high voltage electrical stimulation, ultrasound, heat/cold, and dexamethasone iontophoresis (Nirschl et al, 2003) also are useful in relieving pain.
- Promotion of a tendon healing response (neovascularization, fibroblastic infiltration with collagen deposition and maturation) can be accomplished by the following:
  1. Rehabilitative exercise
  2. High-voltage electrical stimulation
  3. General/aerobic conditioning that provides increased regional blood perfusion and minimization of loss of strength of adjacent tissue
  4. Rest from inciting trauma
- Control of force loads
  1. Counter-force strap bracing to constrain key muscle groups while maintaining muscle balance
  2. Improved sports technique, such as improved backhand stroke in tennis (lateral tendinosis) and less trailing arm activity in the golf swing (medial tendinosis)
  3. Equipment changes in sports, such as low string tension on tennis racquets and perimeter weighting in golf clubs

INDICATIONS FOR SURGERY

- Chronic symptoms usually exceeding one year duration
- Failure of response to a good quality rehabilitation program
- Failed permanent response to cortisone injections (up to three)
- Unacceptable quality of life as determined by the patient

SURGICAL PRINCIPLES

- Historically, elbow tendinosis was treated by the total release of the origin of the combined tendon groups from the epicondyle.
- Currently, surgical treatment is directed at resecting only the pathologic tissue, protecting all normal tissues and attachments, followed by quality postoperative rehabilitation.
- Surgical goals can be accomplished through a small incision (3 cm or less).
- Associated lesions, when present, such as OCD, loose bodies, and synovitis can be addressed with a miniarthrotomy at the time of the tendinosis resection (Kraushaar, Nirschl, and Cox, 1999).
- Recently, interest has risen in arthroscopic treatment of lateral elbow tendinosis with encouraging early results (Owens, Murphy, and Kuklo, 2001); however, at this time we feel the arthroscopic approach does not afford the visualization necessary to resect all the pathologic tissue.
- Ulnar nerve entrapment can be addressed along with medial tendinosis resection through the same incision.

TREATMENT RESULTS

- The vast majority of patients with elbow tendinosis respond to nonoperative intervention.
- Of those that do require surgery, 97% will experience significant or total pain relief and return of strength with minimal complications (Nirschl and Ashman).

REFERENCES

Edwards SG, Calandruccio JH: Autologous blood injections for refractory lateral epicondylitis. *J Hand Surg Am* 28:272–278, 2003.

Kraushaar BS, Nirschl RP, Cox W: A modified lateral approach for release of posttaumatic elbow flexion contracture. *J Shoulder Elbow Surg* 8:476–480, 1999.

Lubahn JD, Cermak MB: Uncommon nerve compression syndromes of the upper extremity. *J Am Acad Ortho Surg* 6:378–386, 1998.

Nirschl RP: Elbow tendinosis/tennis elbow. *Clin Sports Med* 11(4):851–870, 1992.

Nirschl RP, Ashman EA: Elbow tendinopathy: tennis elbow. *Clin Sports Med* 22:813–836, 2003.

Nirschl RP, Pettrone FA: Tennis elbow. The surgical treatment of lateral epicondylitis. *J Bone Joint Surg Am* 61:832–839, 1979.

Nirschl RP, Rodin DM, Ochiai DH, et al: Iontophoretic administration of dexamethasone sodium phosphate for acute epicondylitis: A randomized, double-blinded, placebo-controlled study. *Am J Sports Med* 31:189–195, 2003.

Owens BS, Murphy KP, Kuklo TR: Arthroscopic release for lateral epicondylitis. *Arthroscopy* 17:582–587, 2001.

52 SOFT TISSUE INJURIES OF THE WRIST IN ATHLETES

Steven B Cohen, MD
Michael E Pannunzio, MD

INTRODUCTION

• Injuries to the wrist are common in sports. In the past, these injuries were frequently designated as sprains. More recently, however, the waste basket term *wrist sprain* has given way to a specific diagnosis and a defined treatment plan. An understanding of wrist anatomy, biomechanics, and function allows the physician to pinpoint specific pathology and treatment, thus allowing quicker return to sport for the athlete with a wrist injury.

EPIDEMIOLOGY

• The incidence of injuries to the wrist varies according to sport. Hand and wrist injuries occur more frequently in younger athletes than adults. A study performed at the Cleveland Clinic found that 9% of all athletic participants under the age of 16 sustained injuries involving the wrist (Bergfeld et al, 1982). In another study, 35% of all injuries in adolescent football players involved the wrist (Roser and Clawson, 1970). Ligamentous laxity is often seen in athletes. This joint hypermobility can lead to partial or complete ligament tears following a loading of the wrist or

may predispose to cumulative injury after repetitive stress (Taleisnik, 1992). Overuse syndromes of the wrist are also common in athletes as a result of tension failure or shear stresses (Pitner, 1990).

DORSAL WRIST SYNDROMES

• Chronic wrist pain on the dorsal aspect of the wrist can be a result of occult dorsal ganglion or dorsal impaction/dorsal impingement syndromes. Ganglions account for the most frequent soft-tissue tumors of the wrist. Of these, 60% to 70% originate from the dorsal scapholunate ligament and are extra-articular manifestations of a connection to the scapholunate joint. A history of wrist trauma is found in 15% of patients with a dorsal ganglion (Angelides and Wallace, 1976). An occult dorsal ganglion is difficult to detect on clinical examination and may only be palpable with extreme flexion (Angelides and Wallace, 1976). Symptoms are generally inversely related to the size of the ganglion, as smaller, tense ganglions produce more pain than larger, soft cysts. Patients often complain of localized tenderness, limitation of motion, and/or weakness of grip. Ultrasound or *magnetic resonance imaging* (MRI) can be more useful than plain radiographs. Often the diagnosis is made by exclusion. Initial treatment should include steroid injection of the dorsal capsule followed by immobilization (Sanders, 1985). When conservative treatment has failed to relieve the symptoms, excision of the capsule and ganglion from the scapholunate ligament are performed. Results are generally favorable with ultimate full return to competition in the majority of cases.

• Dorsal impaction syndromes occur as a result of repetitive loading of the wrist in maximum extension and happen most frequently to gymnasts. The shear forces created by this action may lead to localized synovitis or even osteocartilaginous fractures (Linscheid and Dobyns, 1985). The athlete will often complain of pain and point tenderness on the mid-dorsal aspect of the wrist, at the projection of the lunocapitate joint (Halikis and Taleisnik, 1996). Progression of the problem may lead to radiographic changes including a hypertrophic ridge of the dorsal rim of the scaphoid, or the dorsal border of the lunate as a result of impingement with the capitate during hyperextension. Successful treatment usually results from restriction of wrist hyperextension, strengthening of the wrist flexors, and local steroid injection. Failure of relief of symptoms should be followed by immobilization and cessation from sport for 4 to 6 weeks. If symptoms should continue to persist, either abandonment from the activity or surgical treatment consists of limited synovectomy and cheilectomy of hypertrophic margins that impinge during hyperextension. Return to sport may not be possible in all cases, but relief of pain generally occurs following treatment.

CARPAL INSTABILITY

• Carpal instability can be seen in any athlete in a contact sport following a collision injury, but may also be a result of chronic repetitive loading in noncontact sports. Carpal instability can be seen as a spectrum of injuries ranging in symptoms and functional deficit. Initial injury may present as something as innocuous as an occult dorsal or intracapsular ganglion (mentioned above) and progress to dynamic instability, then static instability, and ultimately to *scapholunate advanced collapse* (SLAC). The dynamic instability is not apparent on routine radiographs, but is reproduced by manipulation and seen on stress radiographs (pronated clenched fist views (Dobyns et al, 1975)). Static instability can be seen on routine radiograph as abnormal carpal alignment (Taleisnik, 1980). Carpal collapse is seen following complete disruption initially of ligaments between the scaphoid and lunate, and progressing to disruption between the lunate and triquetrum and finally to the midcarpal joints.

SCAPHOLUNATE DISSOCIATION

• Scapholunate instability occurs as the ligamentous support of the proximal pole of the scaphoid is disrupted, and the scaphoid rotates into palmarflexion. This can be reproduced clinically during physical examination by performing the Watson maneuver (Watson and Dhillon, 1993). Radiographically, this is shown by widening of the scapholunate space (compared to the uninjured wrist), an increase in the scapholunate angle (>70°, normal 30° to 60°), and a cortical *ring* sign in which the distal pole of the perpendicular scaphoid is seen end-on on the anteroposterior view of the wrist.
• Successful treatment may consist of closed reduction and percutaneous pinning if initiated within the first 3 to 4 weeks after injury. This may also be performed under arthroscopic guidance. In most cases, open reduction, ligamentous repair, and internal fixation with Kirschner wires is the most reliable treatment in the management of scapholunate ligament injuries in athletes. For chronic scapholunate dissociation without advanced arthritic changes, a dorsal capsulodesis and ligament reconstruction as described by Blatt (Blatt, 1987) or when ligament reconstruction is not possible,

a scaphotrapezial-trapezoidal fusion as described by Watson (Watson and Hempton, 1980) may be performed. Postoperatively, the wrist is immobilized in slight palmar flexion and pronation. Return to contact sports is limited after treatment for carpal instability.

LUNOTRIQUETRAL INSTABILITY

• Injuries to the lunotriquetral ligaments may range from sprain to partial tear to complete tear with or without carpal malalignment. The carpal instability associated with this injury is a *volar intercalated segment instability* (VISI) deformity. This complete injury occurs rarely in athletes. Symptoms consist of pain on the dorsoulnar side of the carpus with a positive lunotriquetral ballotment test as described by Reagan et al (Reagan, Linscheid, and Dobyns, 1984). Injection of local anesthetic to the lunotriquetral joint usually relieves symptoms and restores grip strength. Routine radiographic evaluation is able to detect static instability as evident by volarflexion of the lunate in neutral deviation. Midcarpal arthrography and MRI may demonstrate incomplete or complete tears of the lunotriquetral ligaments or radiocarpal arthrography may detect a simultaneous injury to the triangular fibrocartilage particularly in an ulna positive patient. Ulnar variance has been shown to be associated with the location of injury. An ulnar minus variance is related with radial axis injury, while an ulnar neutral or plus variance has been linked to ulnar axis injury.
• Treatment of acute or untreated chronic injuries with no evidence of a tear consists of injection of a corticosteroid preparation followed by immobilization. Surgical treatment is considered when disabling pain continues and cessation from sport is not an alternative, and consists of lunotriquetral ligament repair when possible. Arthroscopy may be valuable in staging and determining treatment, and may be used to assist in reduction and pinning in both acute and chronic ligament tears without advanced collapse (Weiss et al, 2000). In patients with an ulna plus variance, ulna shortening is the treatment of choice. Lunotriquetral arthrodesis has been performed, but without uniform success (Taleisnik, 1992) and is rarely performed in athletes (Weiss et al, 2000).

ULNAR TRANSLOCATION

• Ulnar translocation is an extremely rare injury in athletes, which is usually a result of a severe violent impact, such as in motor sports. In order for complete translocation to occur, complete disruption of both the volar and dorsal radiocarpal ligaments must take place. As a result, the carpus is allowed to slide along the incline of the radius in the ulnar direction. Physical examination includes severe swelling, loss of motion, and deformity. Radiographic evaluation will demonstrate translation of the carpus, as well as rotation of the proximal carpal row into palmarflexion, and scapholunate disastasis due to ulnar displacement of the lunate.

- There is no role for nonoperative treatment in this injury. Surgical exploration reveals extensive capsular tears, frequently including the scapholunate ligament. Taleisnik believes that capsular reattachment commonly results in recurrence and if stability is achieved, it is usually at the expense of loss of motion (Taleisnik, 1980). As a result, he recommends radiolunate arthrodesis to maintain reduction that results in a stable, pain-free wrist with satisfactory preservation of motion. This may allow an athlete to return to strenuous activity when full range of motion is not mandatory.

TRIANGULAR FIBROCARTILAGE COMPLEX INJURY

- The *triangular fibrocartilage complex* (TFCC) is made up of the *triangular fibrocartilage* (TFC) a cartilaginous disc, which lies on the ulnar head, and several supporting ligaments, and acts as a stabilizer of the *distal radioulnar joint* (DRUJ). Injury to this structure may result in two forms, perforation of the disk (traumatic or degenerative), or avulsion (traumatic) of the disk with or without avulsion of the supporting ligaments. Avulsion of the TFCC occurs following acute dislocation or subluxation of the distal ulna relative to the radius. Degenerative tears usually occur after the third decade (Mikic, 1978). Ulnar variance may play a role in degenerative changes of the TFC. Palmer found the center of the TFC to be thinner in ulna plus wrists (Palmer, Glisson, and Werner, 1984). Lunotriquetral tears may occur following degenerative perforation of the TFC leading to carpal instability. Young athletes with ulna plus variants, who participate in repetitive loading of the wrist, may be susceptible to degenerative changes of the TFC similar to older patients (Halikis and Taleisnik, 1996).
- Patients with injury to the TFC frequently complain of ulnar sided wrist pain, exacerbated by forearm rotation. It is important to discern injury to TFC from injury to the DRUJ. Injury to the TFC is suspected when tenderness and crepitus are palpated between the ulna and triquetrum. Relief of pain during manual stabilization of the DRUJ during forearm rotation may be an indicator of DRUJ instability. Diagnostic evaluation may include plain radiographs, MRI, arthrography, and/or arthroscopy. Demonstration of ulna plus variance on plain radiographs adds to suspicion of TFC injury. Arthrography may exhibit a communication between the radiocarpal and distal radioulnar joints. MRI and arthroscopy have been helpful in determining the size and location of lesion of the TFC.

- Treatment of acute injury of the TFC includes immobilization of the wrist in neutral rotation for up to 4 to 6 weeks. Gradual progression of activities may then begin with the use of supportive splinting. An injection into the ulnocarpal space with steroid may also be helpful and diagnostic prior to immobilization. If the athlete is unable to return to sport and symptoms persist, then surgical debridement of the perforation and/or decompression of the ulnocarpal space should be performed. Decompression can be obtained through ulnar shortening (Linscheid, 1987), DRUJ excisional hemiarthroplasty (Bowers, 1985), or the Kapanji procedure (Goncalves, 1974). If a peripheral tear is found in the outer 15 to 20% of the TFC, a repair may be considered in conjunction with ulnar recession (Taleisnik, 1992). For patients with ulna plus variance and a degenerative tear of the TFC, ulnar shortening is the treatment of choice, while excision of the TFC and Darrach procedure should be avoided. For patients with ulna minus variant, debridement of the TFC defect may relieve pain and will not increase load transmission providing only the central third is removed. For acute avulsions causing DRUJ instability, above elbow immobilization with the DRUJ reduced, usually is successful. If instability persists, reattachment of the TFC is performed, usually at the fovea of the ulnar styloid using suture and drill holes (Hermansdorfer and Kleinman, 1991).

COMPRESSION NEUROPATHIES

- Compression neuropathies in athletes may be subtle and often overlooked. Nerve injuries can result from a single violent injury, or from repetitive stress. Compression may also result from anatomic structures (e.g., muscles, vessels, fibrous bands), or pathologic structures (e.g., ganglia, aneurysms, inflammation). Nerve injuries are often classified as described by Seddon (1943) in order of severity as neurapraxia, axonotmesis, or neurotmesis.

MEDIAN NERVE

- Compression of the median nerve at the carpal tunnel is the most common compressive neuropathy in the general population, but is not regularly seen in athletes.

Carpal tunnel syndrome (CTS) can be caused by direct trauma, repetitive use, or anatomic anomalies. It is commonly seen in the dominant upper extremity of athletes who participate in repetitive flexion and extension of the wrist such as lacrosse and gymnastics, and in grip-intensive activities such as cycling, racquet sports, and archery (Plancher, Peterson, and Steichen, 1996). Hypertrophy of the lumbrical muscles as seen in weightlifters can also cause CTS. Athletes have similar classic complaints as other patients with CTS such as pain and paresthesias in the radial three and one-half digits, especially at night. They may also complain of clumsiness and weakness with grip related activities. Phalen's and Tinel's tests are variably positive. Electrodiagnostic study results fluctuate, but commonly exhibit delays across the wrist.

- Treatment consists of rest, anti-inflammatory medication, nighttime splinting, and activity modification. Corticosteroid injection into the carpal tunnel may be diagnostic and therapeutic, but often relief is only temporary. Surgical decompression with release of the transverse carpal ligament is the treatment of choice when symptoms persist. Patients returning to sports using a racquet, club, or bat should use a specially padded glove to protect the hand from shock and vibratory trauma until pillar pain resolves (Rettig, 2001).

ULNAR NERVE

- Ulnar tunnel syndrome is compression of the ulnar nerve at the level of the wrist as it enters Guyon's canal or as the deep branch curves around the hook of the hamate and traverses the palm. Compression may occur due to ganglias, lipomas, anatomic anomalies, carpal fractures (e.g., hook of hamate), local inflammation, or ulnar artery thrombosis (Plancher, Peterson, and Steichen, 1996; Sicuranza and McCue, III, 1992). The most common mechanism of injury in sports occurs in cyclists, owing to the term cyclist's or handlebar palsy. It can also be seen in baseball players, golfers, hockey players, and racquet sports as well as a result of performing numerous push-ups (push-up palsy (Walker and Troost, 1988)). Compression of the nerve may cause motor, sensory, or mixed symptoms. A fixed motor deficit results in a claw hand appearance and is rare. Sensory complaints involve usually the ulnar one and one-half digits. EMG is performed on both ulnar and median nerves, as coincident involvement is frequent (Plancher, Peterson, and Steichen, 1996). Treatment consists of rest, anti-inflammatory medication, and activity modification including changing hand position on the handlebars or padding of affecting object. If symptoms persist, surgical decompression of

the ulnar nerve in Guyon's canal should be performed and provides excellent relief from symptoms with return to activity in 4 to 8 weeks.

RADIAL NERVE

DISTAL POSTERIOR INTEROSSEOUS NERVE SYNDROME

- Compression and/or irritation of the terminal sensory branch of the radial nerve is called distal posterior interosseous nerve syndrome. The terminal branch crosses over the dorsal aspect of the distal radius and enters the wrist capsule and is susceptible to injury from repetitive and forceful wrist dorsiflexion such as in gymnastics (Linscheid and Dobyns, 1985). Symptoms include a deep, dull ache in the wrist, pain with forceful wrist extension, and tenderness with deep palpation during wrist hyperflexion. This is a diagnosis of exclusion and should only be made after other conditions such as occult fracture, carpal instability, ganglions, and dorsal impaction syndrome have been ruled out. Radiographs should be taken to rule out other causes. A local injection of anesthetic may be diagnostic and provide short-term relief. If conservative therapy fails, surgical excision of the nerve as it exits under the extensor digitorum communis on the floor of the fourth extensor compartment is indicated (Dellon, 1985).

SUPERFICIAL RADIAL NERVE COMPRESSION

- Compression of the superficial radial nerve is also called Cheiralgia paresthetica, or Wartenberg syndrome. The nerve is subcutaneous and is susceptible to injury as it pierces the deep fascia between the tendons of the *extensor carpi radialis longus* (ECRL) and brachioradialis. Constriction of the nerve may occur during sports that include pronation and supination, such as batting, throwing, and rowing (Dellon and Mackinnon, 1986). It also may occur from external compression from tight wristbands, tape, watches, archery guards, gloves, or straps from a racquetball racquet (Plancher, Peterson, and Steichen, 1996; Sicuranza and McCue, III, 1992). Direct trauma may also cause nerve irritation from contact sports, e.g., hockey, football, and lacrosse.
- The athlete complains of numbness or paresthesias over the dorsoradial aspect of the wrist, hand, dorsal thumb, and index finger. There may also be associated dorsoradial pain with thumb flexion and wrist ulnar deviation, similar to that in de Quervain's tenosynovitis; however, wrist pain is present when performing the Finklestein test regardless of thumb position in Cheiralgia paresthetica compared with thumb flexion

only in de Quervain's tenosynovitis (Eaton and Lister, 1992). A Tinel's sign is commonly positive. Wrist motion is full and pain free ruling out overuse conditions. Electrodiagnostic results are variable. Treatment consists of initial conservative treatment including rest, ice, anti-inflammatory medication, splinting, padding, and activity modification. Surgical treatment is considered if relief of symptoms has not occurred after 6 to 12 months. Decompression consists of extensive release of the deep fascia along the course of the superficial radial nerve with good to excellent results achieved in 86% following surgical decompression (Dellon and Mackinnon, 1986).

VASCULAR INJURY

HYPOTHENAR HAMMER SYNDROME

- Covered in chapter 53—Hand Injuries.

OVERUSE INJURIES

- The incidence of wrist problems in athletes is extremely high. Wrist syndromes account for the most common upper extremity overuse injuries (Rettig, 2001). Repetitive activities such as gymnastics, racquet sports, rowing, and throwing sports result in a high number of overuse injuries.

DE QUERVAIN'S TENOSYNOVITIS

- Stenosis of the first dorsal compartment (*abductor pollicis long* (APL) and *extensor pollicis brevis* (EPB)) is referred as *de Quervain's tenosynovitis*. It occurs in athletes who perform forceful grasp with repetitive use of the thumb and ulnar deviation (Kiefhaber and Stern, 1992). Sports that are more susceptible to this injury include racquet sports, golf (particularly the left thumb in right handed golfers (Rettig and Patel, 1995)), fly-fishing, javelin, and discus throwing. Athletes classically complain of pain over the radial styloid particularly with range of motion of the thumb and ulnar deviation of the wrist. Generally, there is tenderness over the first dorsal compartment along with swelling and occasional crepitus or triggering. The Finklestein test is frequently positive with wrist ulnar deviation while the thumb is adducted, and is pathognomonic for the diagnosis (Rettig, 2001). Initial treatment includes anti-inflammatory medication, thumb spica splinting, and corticosteroid injection into the first dorsal compartment. Poor response from injection

may be due to a longitudinal septum, which separates the APL and EPB in 20% to 30% of cases (Froimson, 1992), and may improve with a second more dorsal injection. If there is no improvement of symptoms, surgical treatment involves decompression of the first dorsal compartment with division of any septum when present. Complications of surgery include persistence of symptoms (possibly due to inadequate release), adhesions, injury to the superficial radial nerve, and volar tendon subluxation. Most athletes are able to return to full participation following surgical decompression in 6 to 9 weeks.

INTERSECTION SYNDROME

- Intersection syndrome is pain in the dorsoradial wrist where the first dorsal compartment crosses the second dorsal compartment (ECRL and *extensor carpi radialis brevis* (ECRB)). It occurs in athletes exposed to repetitive wrist motions such as rowers, racquet sports, weightlifters, and canoeists (Wood and Dobyns, 1986). It appears to be caused by tenosynovitis of the tendons in the second dorsal compartment. Athletes complain of dorsoradial pain and tenderness proximal to the wrist and may have swelling or crepitus 4 to 6 cm proximal to Lister's tubercle (Plancher, Peterson, and Steichen, 1996). Initial treatment consists of rest, splinting, anti-inflammatory medication, corticosteroid injection, and activity modification, and is successful 95% of the time (Plancher, Peterson, and Steichen, 1996). For the rare failure of conservative treatment, surgical management includes release of the second dorsal compartment, exploration and debridement of the intersection zone and bursal tissue, and release of the fascial sheaths of the tendons in the first dorsal compartment (Kiefhaber and Stern, 1992). Postoperatively, the wrist is splinted for 7 to 10 days followed by a stretching and strengthening program, and return to sport is allowed when the patient is symptom free.

EXTENSOR CARPI ULNARIS TENDINITIS/ SUBLUXATION

- *Extensor carpi ulnaris* (ECU) tendonitis is the second most common stenosis tenosynovitis of the hand after de Quervain's (Wood and Dobyns, 1986). It occurs in athletes involved in repetitive wrist motion such as racquet sports, baseball, golf, and rowing. It may also happen following traumatic ECU subluxation with rupture of the fibrous sheath overlying the ECU during forced supination, flexion, and ulnar deviation of the wrist (similar to that seen in a baseball swing)

(Kiefhaber and Stern, 1992). Athletes will typically complain of pain and swelling distal to the ulnar head, worsened by resisted wrist extension. A painful snap may be elicited as subluxation of the ECU occurs with supination and ulnar deviation of the wrist. Initial treatment includes rest, splinting, anti-inflammatory medication, corticosteroid injection, and activity modification. Patients who fail to respond to nonoperative treatment require surgical decompression of the sixth dorsal compartment with radial release of the fibroosseous tunnel and repair of the extensor retinaculum (to prevent postoperative subluxation) (Hajj and Wood, 1986). After surgery, the wrist is immobilized in 20° of extension for 3 weeks prior to starting activity (Rettig, 2001). Patients with acute ECU subluxation may be treated with long-arm casting with the wrist in full pronation and slight dorsiflexion (Wood and Dobyns, 1986). This frequently fails to respond to conservative treatment and often requires stabilization of the ECU with return to sport after a minimum of 8 to 10 weeks.

FLEXOR COMPARTMENT TENDINOPATHIES

- Inflammation of the flexor tendons most commonly occurs in the *flexor carpi radialis* (FCR) and *flexor carpi ulnaris* (FCU) as a result of repetitive wrist motions such as golf and racquet sports (Plancher, Peterson, and Steichen, 1996). FCR tendonitis usually presents with pain over the volar aspect of the wrist, proximal to the wrist crease over the FCR tendon. Pain may be elicited with abrupt wrist extension or resisted wrist flexion and radial deviation. Athletes with FCU tendonitis may complain of pain and swelling just distal to the pisiform. Pain may be exacerbated with passive wrist extension, or resisted wrist flexion and ulnar deviation. Initial treatment of both of these conditions includes rest, anti-inflammatory medication, splinting, corticosteroid injection, and activity modification. If symptoms persist, surgical decompression of the fibro-osseous tunnel containing the FCR is performed in the case of FCR tendonitis (Gabel, Bishop, and Wood, 1994). Surgical treatment of FCU tendonitis includes FCU lengthening with or without pisiform excision (Palmieri, 1982).

PEDIATRIC INJURY

GYMNAST'S WRIST

- The number of athletes competing in competitive gymnastics has been steadily increasing. As a result there has been a rise in the frequency of wrist pain in skeletally immature athletes. Mandelbaum et al found that 75% of all male and 50% of all female competitive gymnasts complained of some wrist pain (Mandelbaum et al, 1989). This is most likely due to repetitive axial loading across a hyperextended wrist (Le and Hentz, 2000). Injuries can result from either acute, high-energy trauma or chronic and repetitive stress. Physical examination of young gymnasts with wrist pain can be challenging due to difficulty in pinpointing the location of pain and fear of injury which would preclude competition. Female gymnasts more commonly complain of ulnar sided wrist pain, whereas males had similar frequency of radial and ulnar sided wrist pain (Mandelbaum et al, 1989).

- Initial radiographic evaluation includes plain X-rays that may reveal stress related changes of the distal radial epiphysis including widening of the growth plate, epiphyseal cystic changes with beaking of the distal epiphysis, and metaphyseal irregularity (Roy, Caine, and Singer, 1985). These changes may lead to premature physeal closure and ultimately a higher incidence of ulnar positive variance. As a result, following skeletal maturity, gymnasts may present with ulnar abutment syndrome, or Madelung-like deformity. MRI and technetium bone scanning may be useful in determining the presence or extent of physeal injury and assist determining return to sports participation, especially in the face of normal plain radiographs (Morgan and Slowman, 2001).

- It is rare that the treatment of wrist pain in a skeletally immature athlete is other than rest and withdrawal from the offending activity. Prevention may be the best form of treatment by using protective gear, spotters, proper warm up, and preclusion of sudden changes in activity intensity. If a physeal injury is suspected or found, the athlete generally is withdrawn from activity, treated symptomatically, and allowed to return to sport when symptoms have resolved. It may also be possible to remove the gymnast from the specific event causing symptoms and allow continued competition in other events that do not exacerbate symptoms.

REFERENCES

Angelides AC, Wallace PF: The dorsal ganglion of the wrist: Its pathogenesis, gross and microscopic anatomy, and surgical treatment. *J Hand Surg* 1:228–235, 1976.

Bergfeld JA, Weiker GG, Andrish JT, et al: Soft playing splint for protection of significant hand and wrist injuries in sports. *Am J Sports Med* 10:293–296, 1982.

Blatt G: Capsulodesis in reconstructive hand surgery: Dorsal capsulodesis for the unstable scaphoid and volar capsulodesis following excision of the distal ulna. *Hand Clin* 3:81–102, 1987.

Bowers WH: Distal radioulnar joint arthroplasty: The hemiresection-interposition technique. *J Hand Surg* 10:169–178, 1985.

Dellon AL: Partial dorsal wrist denervation : Resection of the distal posterior interosseous nerve. *J Hand Surg* 10:527–533, 1985.

Dellon AL, Mackinnon SE : Radial sensory nerve entrapment in the forearm. *J Hand Surg* 11:199–205, 1986.

Dobyns JH, Linscheid RL, Chao EYS, et al : Traumatic instability of the wrist. *Instr Course Lect* 24:182–198, 1975.

Eaton CJ, Lister GD: Radial nerve compression. *Hand Clin* 8:343–357, 1992.

Froimson A: Tenosynovitis and tennis elbow, in Green DP (ed.): *Operative Hand Surgery,* 3rd ed. New York, NY, Churchill Livingstone, 1992, pp 1989–2006.

Gabel G, Bishop AT, Wood MD: Flexor carpi radialis tendonitis: II results of operative treatment. *J Bone Joint Surg* 76A:1015–1018, 1994.

Goncalves D: Correction of disorders of the distal radioulnar joint by artificial pseudoarthrosis of the ulna. *J Bone Joint Surg* 56B:462–464, 1974.

Hajj AA, Wood MB: Stenosing tenosynovitis of the extensor carpi ulnaris. *J Hand Surg* 11:519–520, 1986.

Halikis MN, Taleisnik J: Soft tissue injuries of the wrist. *Clin Sports Med* 15:235–259, 1996.

Hermansdorfer JD, Kleinman WB: Management of chronic peripheral tears of the triangular fibrocartilage complex. *J Hand Surg* 16:340–346, 1991.

Kiefhaber TR, Stern PJ: Upper extremity tendonitis and overuse syndromes in the athlete. *Clin Sports Med* 11:39–55, 1992.

Le TB, Hentz VR : Hand and wrist injuries in young athletes. *Hand Clin* 16:597–607, 2000.

Linscheid RL: Ulnar lengthening and shortening. *Hand Clin* 3:69–79, 1987.

Linscheid RL, Dobyns JH: Athletic injuries of the wrist. *Clin Orthop* 198:141–151, 1985.

Mandelbaum BR, Bartolozzi AR, Davis CA, et al: Wrist pain syndrome in the gymnast: Pathogenetic, diagnostic, and therapeutic considerations. *Am J Sports Med* 17:305–317, 1989.

Mikic ZD: Age changes in the triangular fibrocartilage of the wrist join. *J Anat* 126:367–384, 1978.

Morgan WJ, Slowman LS: Acute hand and wrist injuries in athletes: Evaluation and management. *J Am Acad Orthop Surg* 9:389–400, 2001.

Palmer AK, Glisson RR, Werner FW: Relationship between ulnar variance and triangular fibrocartilage complex thickness. *J Hand Surg* 9:681–682, 1984.

Palmieri TJ: Pisiform area pain treatment by pisiform excision. *J Hand Surg* 7:477–480, 1982.

Pitner MA: Pathophysiology of overuse injuries in the hand and wrist. *Hand Clin* 6:355–364, 1990.

Plancher KD, Peterson RK, Steichen JB: Compressive neuropathies and tendinopathies in the athletic elbow and wrist. *Clin Sports Med* 15:331–371, 1996.

Reagan DS, Linscheid RL, Dobyns JH: Lunotriquetral sprains. *J Hand Surg* 9:502–514, 1984.

Rettig AC: Wrist and hand overuse syndromes. *Clin Sports Med* 20:591–611, 2001.

Rettig AC, Patel DV: Epidemiology of elbow, forearm, and wrist injuries in the athletes. *Clin Sports Med* 14:289–297, 1995.

Roser LA, Clawson DK : Football injuries in the very young athlete. *Clin Orthop* 69:219–223, 1970.

Roy S, Caine D, Singer K: Stress changes of the distal radial epiphysis in young gymnasts: A report of 21 cases and review of the literature. *Am J Sports Med* 13:301–308, 1985.

Sanders WE: The occult dorsal carpal ganglion. *J Hand Surg* 10B:257–260, 1985.

Seddon JH: Three types of nerve injury. *Brain* 66:237–281, 1943.

Sicuranza MJ, McCue FC III: Compressive neuropathies in the upper extremity of athletes. *Hand Clin* 8:263–273, 1992.

Taleisnik J: Post-traumatic carpal instability. *Clin Orthop* 149:73, 1980.

Taleisnik J: Soft tissue injuries of the wrist, in Strickland JW, Rettig AC (eds.): *Hand Injuries in Athletes*. Philadelphia, PA, Saunders, 1992, pp 107–127.

Walker FO, Troost BT: Push-up palmar palsy. *JAMA* 259:45–46, 1988.

Watson HK, Dhillon HS: Intercarpal arthrodesis, in Green DP (ed.): *Operative Hand Surgery:* vol. 1, 3rd ed. New York, NY, Churchill Livingstone, 1993, pp 113–168.

Watson HK, Hempton RF: Limited wrist arthrodesis: Part I. The triscaphoid joint. *J Hand Surg* 5A:320–327, 1980.

Weiss LE, Taras JS, Sweet S et al: Lunotriquetral injuries in the athletes. *Hand Clin* 16:433–438, 2000.

Wood MB, Dobyns JH: Sports related extra-articular wrist syndromes. *Clin Orthop* 202:93–102, 1986.

53 SOFT TISSUE INJURIES OF THE HAND IN ATHLETES

Todd C Battaglia, MD
David R Diduch, MD, MS

INTRODUCTION

• Hand injuries in athletes are common injuries that require a thorough knowledge of anatomy for accurate examination, diagnosis, and treatment. Most soft tissue injuries of the hand can be acutely treated by closed means, but many require definitive care by an orthopaedic or plastic hand surgeon. Missed or misdiagnosed injuries can result in permanent deformity and loss of function. Radiographs are indicated in nearly all cases to evaluate for fracture or the presence of foreign bodies in cases of fingertip injuries, and to evaluate for joint incongruity or avulsion fracture in cases of joint or tendon injury.

FINGERTIP INJURIES

SUBUNGUAL HEMATOMA

- Many crush injuries to the fingertips will damage the nail and underlying matrix, causing blood beneath the nail and throbbing pain. These injuries may also be associated with tuft fractures of the distal phalanx, which are typically open fractures because they communicate through the nail matrix disruption (Idler et al, 1990*b*).
- Hematoma involving less than 50% of the nail matrix may be drained using a heated paperclip, an 18-gauge needle, or a battery-operated cautery to create one or multiple holes in the nail. An anesthetic digital block may be necessary prior to drainage. Soaking the finger in sterile water with peroxide will facilitate drainage. A sterile dressing should then be applied, with a Stack splint in cases involving fracture (Idler et al, 1990*b*; Fassler, 1996).
- Hematoma involving more than 50% of the underlying nailbed is presumed to be associated with an open fracture. Radiographs, surgical removal of the nail, thorough irrigation and debridement of the wound, repair of the nail matrix, and replacement of the nail with splinting are recommended (Fassler, 1996).

NAIL AVULSION

- If nail avulsion occurs without damage to the underlying sterile matrix, the wound should be thoroughly cleansed and dressed with a nonadherent dressing. If the proximal portion of the nail has also been avulsed from the nail fold and germinal matrix, the patient's cleansed nail or a piece of sterile gauze or foil should be slid under the eponychial fold to prevent adherence (Fassler, 1996).
- If any part of the sterile or germinal matrix has been torn or lacerated, removal of any remaining nail fragments and repair of the nail bed injury are mandatory. Again, the eponychial fold should be splinted open (Fassler, 1996).

FINGERPAD INJURIES

- Simple lacerations may be cleansed and sutured using nonabsorbable monofilament in adults or absorbable suture in children. Grossly contaminated wounds may be cleansed and left open.
- Partial amputations with soft tissue loss measuring less than 1 cm² will heal by secondary intention and may be treated with cleansing and serial dressing changes. Even larger defects will heal well in children. Larger wounds involving exposed bone or tendon, nail bed injury, or more proximal amputation should be emergently treated by a hand surgeon (Idler et al, 1990*b*; Fassler, 1996).

JOINT INJURIES OF THE FINGERS

- Dislocations are usually clinically apparent; are characterized by pain, limited movement, and digit deformity; and should be radiographed prior to reduction to assess for associated fracture if there is any crepitus, bony point tenderness, or open injury.
- Other dislocations can be reduced, splinted, and a post-reduction radiograph obtained. Any irreducible dislocation or dislocation associated with an open wound requires emergent referral.
- Local or regional anesthesia may be necessary to obtain adequate pain relief and relaxation for reduction. Digital blocks are placed by injecting the ulnar and radial webspaces of a digit, anesthetizing the dorsal and volar digital nerves. The local anesthetic should not contain epinephrine, which could cause digital ischemia.

DISTAL INTERPHALANGEAL JOINT

- *Distal interphalangeal* (DIP) joint dislocations are uncommon, almost always dorsal, and often open. These injuries are frequently associated with extensor disruption (see section on Mallet Finger).
- If there is no open wound or tendon rupture and closed reduction is possible, extension splinting for 2–3 weeks is recommended.

PROXIMAL INTERPHALANGEAL JOINT

- *Proximal interphalangeal* (PIP) joint injuries are the most common joint injuries in sports, primarily occurring in athletes who participate in contact sports and ball-handling (Morgan and Slowman, 2001; Rettig, Coyle, and Hunt, 2002).

DORSAL DISLOCATIONS
- These injuries are frequently seen in football and basketball. Dorsal dislocations are most common and result from hyperextension with axial load. This causes distal volar plate rupture with or without bony avulsion. A true lateral x-ray should be obtained to rule out a fracture (Rettig, Coyle, and Hunt, 2002).

- Reduction is usually uncomplicated. Dynamic and static stability should be assessed after reduction, including collateral ligament stability (Kahler and McCue, 1992).
- If there is no associated fracture or ligament injury, splinting in 30° of flexion for 1–2 weeks, followed by buddy taping for sports for 4–6 weeks, is effective. Recurrent dislocation is rare. Swelling and tenderness can persist for several months. Motion exercises as soon as comfort permits can help to prevent stiffness (Rettig, Coyle, and Hunt, 2002).

Volar Dislocations

- Volar dislocations of the PIP joint are less common injuries, are more difficult to reduce, and are associated with more complications than are dorsal dislocations. They are caused by compression and rotation with PIP joint flexion. Pathology usually includes extensor tendon central slip avulsion, volar plate disruption, and collateral ligament tears (Rettig, Coyle, and Hunt, 2002; Kahler and McCue, 1992).
- If closed reduction is successful, the PIP joint should be splinted in full extension for 3–4 weeks to protect the central slip, allowing the DIP joint to remain free, followed by night splinting for an additional 3–4 weeks. If closed reduction is not possible, open reduction and pinning are necessary (Rettig, Coyle, and Hunt, 2002).
- Late development of boutonnière deformity is a potential complication.

Rotary PIP Subluxation

- This injury typically presents as an irreducible dislocation of the PIP joint. It involves buttonholing of one condyle of the proximal phalanx through a longitudinal rent in the extensor hood between the central slip and lateral band. A lateral profile of the proximal phalanx with an oblique profile of the middle phalanx is seen on lateral radiograph (Kahler and McCue, 1992).
- If closed reduction is successful, buddy taping with full active range of motion is usually sufficient. Open reduction is often necessary to disengage the proximal phalanx condyle from the central slip and lateral band.

Collateral Ligament Injuries

- Collateral ligament injuries occur as a result of radial or ulnar stress on the joint, most commonly in football, wrestling, and basketball. Disruption usually occurs at the proximal attachment, with radial collateral injury more common than ulnar collateral injury. The most commonly involved digit is the index finger (Rettig, Coyle, and Hunt, 2002).
- Tenderness and ecchymosis are usually present on examination. Radiographs should be obtained to rule out fracture. Examination and radiographs should be used to assess stability.
- Most collateral ligament injuries are treated with buddy taping to an adjacent finger, with continued participation in athletic activity. If the tear is associated with significant instability, the digit should be immobilized in a dorsal splint for 3–4 weeks. (Rettig, Coyle, and Hunt, 2002).

METACARPOPHALANGEAL JOINT

- *Metacarpophalangeal* (MCP) dislocations are relatively rare and usually involve dorsal dislocation of the proximal phalanx on the metacarpal. Most occur in the index or small finger.
- Simple dislocations may be reduced by closed reduction, and if stable following reduction, then consider buddy taping alone and allowing immediate active motion. Complex dislocations involve buttonholing of the metacarpal head between the flexor tendon and the lumbrical with volar plate interposition into the dislocated joint. These usually require formal open reduction.

JOINT INJURIES OF THE THUMB

INTERPHALANGEAL JOINT

- Thumb *interphalangeal* (IP) dislocations are uncommon injuries and are managed similarly to finger DIP dislocations.

METACARPOPHALANGEAL JOINT

- Dislocations of the thumb MCP joint are usually dorsal dislocations, resulting from hyperextension at the MCP joint with volar plate rupture. The metacarpal head may protrude through the volar plate, where it becomes buttonholed between the flexor pollicus longus and flexor pollicus brevis tendons (Kahler and McCue, 1992).
- The volar plate, flexor pollicus longus, or sesamoids may be interposed and prevent reduction, but closed reduction is usually possible, with splinting recommended for 3–4 weeks after reduction.

GAMEKEEPER'S THUMB

- Also known as *skier's thumb*, this refers to the acute rupture of the *ulnar collateral ligament* (UCL) of the thumb MCP joint. The mechanism of injury involves a fall on an outstretched thumb with hyperabduction at the MCP joint. Patients present with tenderness and swelling over the ulnar aspect of the thumb MCP joint with instability of the UCL on radial stress. Instability should be assessed with the MCP in 30° of flexion and at full extension. This can also be documented and quantified on stress radiographs (Morgan and Slowman, 2001; Abrahamson et al, 1990; Leddy, 1998; Rettig, 1992).

- The injury may be associated with the Stener lesion, in which the torn end of the UCL is displaced superficially to the aponeurosis of the adductor pollicus, preventing primary healing. Gross instability or a palpable lump suggests a Stener lesion, which can sometimes also be directly visualized with ultrasound or MRI. This lesion may be present in up to 70% of cases (Morgan and Slowman, 2001; Kahler and McCue, 1992).
- Many injuries will do well with immobilization for 4 weeks in a thumb spica cast, followed by 2–4 months of protected splinting during athletic competition.
- Surgical intervention with reattachment of the UCL is typically required for any injury with greater than 30–35° of instability in flexion, any instability in extension, a Stener lesion, or large bony avulsion (Morgan and Slowman, 2001; Kahler and McCue, 1992; Abrahamson et al, 1990; Leddy, 1998).

RADIAL COLLATERAL LIGAMENT INJURY

- Radial collateral ligament injury may involve proximal or distal ligament tears of the ligament.
- It is much less common than UCL injury but evaluated and treated in a similar manner. Injuries may be associated with volar subluxation of the joint and may require surgical stabilization (Rettig, Coyle, and Hunt, 2002; Kahler and McCue, 1992).

TENDON INJURIES

MALLET FINGER

- This injury is also known as *drop finger* or *baseball finger* and most commonly occurs in football receivers, baseball players, and basketball players. *Mallet finger* refers to a disruption of the extensor mechanism insertion into the distal phalanx, resulting from forced flexion of an actively extended DIP joint. A variably sized piece of bone may be avulsed with tendon (Rettig, Coyle, and Hunt, 2002; Leddy, 1998; Rettig, 1992).
- The patient will have a passively flexed DIP joint with full passive range of motion but inability to actively extend at the DIP joint (Idler et al, 1990*a*).

- Preferred treatment is continuous extension splinting of the DIP joint for at least 6 weeks while allowing PIP motion, then up to 4 weeks of nighttime splinting. If there is a large bony fragment avulsed, some recommend surgical fixation with reduction and pinning. Surgical treatment may be necessary for late, chronic cases (Rettig, Coyle, and Hunt, 2002; Leddy, 1998; Rettig, 1992; Aronowitz and Leddy, 1998).

BOUTONNIÈRE DEFORMITY

- This injury is also known as a *buttonhole* deformity and involves rupture or avulsion of the extensor mechanism central slip at the middle phalanx. The head of the phalanx may buttonhole through the defect. The lateral bands then contract, causing late extension deformity at the DIP joint (usually appearing 1–3 weeks later) (Rettig, Coyle, and Hunt, 2002; Leddy, 1998).
- This injury occurs with unrecognized palmer dislocation of the PIP joint, or more commonly, by forced flexion of the middle phalanx while the athlete is attempting to extend the joint. The patient will present with swelling and pain over the dorsal PIP joint, inability to extend the PIP, and possible hyperextension at the DIP joint (Rettig, 1992).
- Treatment consists of extension splinting of the PIP for 6 weeks, allowing DIP motion, followed by gradual PIP motion. Chronic cases usually respond to closed treatment as well. Cases associated with large bony fragments should be surgically addressed (Rettig, Coyle, and Hunt, 2002; Leddy, 1998; Rettig, 1992).

PSEUDOBOUTONNIÈRE DEFORMITY

- This injury has a similar clinical appearance to the Boutonnière deformity but a distinctly different mechanism and treatment. It is caused by a hyperextension injury to the DIP joint, disrupting the volar plate and either the radial or ulnar collateral ligament. Tissue contraction causes later development of progressive PIP flexion deformity. Differentiation from a Boutonnière deformity is possible by absence of tenderness over the PIP central slip and equivalent active and passive ranges of motion at the PIP joint in this injury (Kahler and McCue, 1992; Leddy, 1998).
- Treatment is difficult and often prolonged, with splinting recommended if PIP deformity is less than 45°. Surgical intervention with capsular release is often necessary for greater deformities (Leddy, 1998).

EXTENSOR TENDON SUBLUXATION AND DISLOCATION

- Extensor tendons usually subluxate or dislocate to the ulnar side of the metacarpophalangeal joint, usually resulting from a direct blow to the digit with forced flexion and ulnar deviation. Radial subluxation is rare. The middle finger is most commonly affected. Patients present with tenderness over the MCP joint, pain with resisted extension, inability to fully extend at the joint and often palpable tendon subluxation or dislocation (Rettig, Coyle, and Hunt, 2002; Rettig, 1992; Aronowitz and Leddy, 1998).
- Acute injuries (presenting within 4–6 weeks) may respond to extension splinting of the MCP joint. Chronic or recalcitrant cases often require surgical reconstruction with release of contractures and repair of the extensor hood and sagittal bands (Leddy, 1998; Rettig, 1992).

BOXER'S KNUCKLES

- This injury, also known as *soft knuckles*, is caused by repetitive trauma to the dorsal MCP joints, most commonly involving the index and long digits. The injury manifests as pain and swelling over involved joints, usually improving with rest but recurring with resumed training (Rettig, 1992).
- The anatomic basis of injury usually involves tears of the extensor hood, extensor tendon, or dorsal joint capsule. Rest or splinting is of little benefit; exploration with surgical repair of injured structures is often required (Leddy, 1998; Rettig, 1992; Hame and Melone, 2000).

JERSEY FINGER

- Jersey finger involves an avulsion of the *flexor digitorum profundus* (FDP) tendon from its insertion on the distal phalanx, commonly occurring in football and rugby players. Greater than 75% of cases involve the ring finger (Rettig, Coyle, and Hunt, 2002; Leddy, 1998; Leddy, 1985).
- Injury is caused by forced DIP extension during maximal FDP contraction, as in grabbing someone's jersey while attempting to tackle. Clinical findings include the inability to actively flex the DIP joint, with normal passive range of motion. Radiographs are usually negative unless a bony fragment is avulsed with the tendon (Rettig, 1992; Aronowitz and Leddy, 1998).
- Injuries are graded and treated according to severity that depends on the degree of tendon retraction.

In type I injuries, the tendon retracts into the palm. In type II injuries, the tendon retracts to the level of the PIP joint. In type III injuries, the tendon retracts only to the A4 pulley. These are nearly always associated with a large avulsed bony fragment (Leddy, 1998; Rettig, 1992; Aronowitz and Leddy, 1998; Leddy, 1985).
- All require surgical intervention, but the greater the degree of retraction, the more quickly surgical intervention is required. Type I injuries should be addressed within 7–10 days, whereas type III injuries are often successfully treated up to 2–3 months later (Rettig, Coyle, and Hunt, 2002; Leddy, 1998).

TRIGGER DIGITS

- Trigger digits involve inflammation of the flexor tendons as they pass through the digital flexor pulleys, especially the first annular (A1) pulley. Most occur secondary to chronic degenerative changes of the involved structures, but direct pressure from racquets, baseball bats, or golf clubs can also cause acute inflammation of the pulley and tendons (Rettig, 2001).
- The injury manifests as pain in the flexor area over the A1 pulley (metacarpal head) and may also produce catching or locking as swollen tendons attempt to pass through pulley.
- A large percentage of trigger digits will respond to steroid injection into the tendon sheath and pulley. Surgical release of the A1 pulley may be either a first-line treatment or reserved for cases unresponsive to injection (Rettig, 2001).

NERVE COMPRESSION INJURIES

HANDLEBAR PALSY

- This injury, also known as *cyclist's palsy,* is caused by compression of the ulnar nerve at the hand and wrist as the result of direct pressure from the grip on the handlebars and wrist hyperextension. Patients present with paresthesias and dysesthesias in the ulnar nerve distribution (ring and small digits), a positive Tinel's sign over Guyon's canal, and possible weakness of the intrinsic hand musculature (Rettig, 2001).
- Rest, stretching exercises, and anti-inflammatory medications usually help relieve the symptoms. Symptoms may take from several days to months to resolve. Surgical treatment is occasionally necessary. Applying less pressure or weight to the handlebars and avoiding hyperextension by altering handlebar

position and riding posture can help to prevent a recurrence.

BOWLER'S THUMB

- Bowler's thumb involves recurrent trauma to the ulnar digital nerve as a result of direct pressure from the edge of the bowling ball hole. This causes proliferation of the surrounding fibrous tissue and decreased nerve mobility. Findings include a positive Tinel's sign and possible decreased two-point discrimination in the nerve distribution (Rettig, 2001; Dobyns et al, 1972).
- Treatment consists of rest, anti-inflammatory medications, and redrilling of the bowling ball to remove pressure areas. Surgical decompression or nerve transfer is rarely indicated (Rettig, 2001).

VASCULAR INJURIES

CHRONIC DIGITAL ISCHEMIA

- Chronic compression or microtrauma to the hand and digital vasculature may cause distal ischemia. This is occasionally seen in baseball pitchers and catchers and handball players. Typical symptoms include cold intolerance, pallor, and pain in the involved digits (Rettig, 2001; Sugawara et al, 1986).
- Increased padding during causative activities, use of pharmacologic agents, or surgical decompression may be appropriate treatments.

FROSTBITE

- Ischemic cold injury depends on the duration and severity of exposure, as well as the presence of constrictive clothes, vasospasm, and wetness. Early symptoms include erythema, burning, and itching (the chilblains). The involved part later becomes numb as injury progresses. Vesicles and ulcers may also develop (Idler et al, 1990b; Murphy et al, 2000).
- First-degree frostbite is a superficial injury from which full recovery is expected. Second-degree injury involves partial-thickness dermal loss. In third-degree injury, full thickness dermal loss occurs, whereas involvement of deeper structures, including tendon and bone, indicates fourth degree injury (Idler et al, 1990b).
- Treatment involves gradual rewarming of involved digits in 40–42°C water. Advanced injuries and gangrenous areas will require surgical debridement, amputation, or skin grafting (Murphy et al, 2000).

HYPOTHENAR HAMMER SYNDROME

- This syndrome is caused by repetitive impact to the hypothenar region of the hand, with trauma to the ulnar nerve distal to Guyon's Canal resulting in arterial constriction, thickening, thrombosis, and possible aneurysm formation. It is most commonly seen in judo, karate, and lacrosse (Rettig, 2001).
- Symptoms are caused by distal ischemia and include cold intolerance, pain in the palm or ulnar digits, and an abnormal Allen's test. Ulnar nerve compression and the corresponding symptoms may occur secondary to aneurysm formation.
- Treatment includes rest from inciting activities, increased padding of the hypothenar area, vasolytic agents, or surgical intervention with excision of the thrombosed segment and artery ligation or reconstruction (Rettig, 2001).

REFERENCES

Abrahamson SO, Sollerman C, Lundborg G, et al: Diagnosis of displaced ulnar collateral ligament of the metacarpophalangeal joint of the thumb. *J Hand Surg (Am)* 15:457, 1990.
Aronowitz ER, Leddy JP: Closed tendon injuries of the hand and wrist in athletes. *Clin Sports Med* 17:449, 1998.
Dobyns JH, O'Brien ET, Linscheid RL, et al: Bowler's thumb diagnosis and treatment: Review of 17 cases. *J Bone Joint Surg (Am)* 54:751, 1972.
Fassler PR: Fingertip injuries. Evaluation and treatment. *J Am Acad Orthop Surg* 4:84, 1996.
Hame SL, Melone CP: Boxer's Knuckle. Traumatic disruption of the extensor hood. *Hand Clin* 16:345, 2000.
Idler RS, Manktelow RT, Lucas G, et al: *The Hand Examination and Diagnosis,* 3rd ed. New York, NY, Churchill Livingstone, 1990a.
Idler RS, Manktelow RT, Lucas G, et al: *The hand Primary care of common problems,* 2nd ed. New York, NY, Churchill Livingstone, 1990b.
Kahler DM, McCue FC: Metacarpophalangeal and proximal interphalangeal joint injuries of the hand, including the thumb. *Clin Sports Med* 11:57, 1992.
Leddy JP: Avulsions of the flexor digitorum profundus. *Hand Clin* 1:77, 1985.
Leddy JP: Soft-tissue injuries of the hand in athletes. *Am Acad Orthop Surg Instr Course Lect* 47:181, 1998.
Morgan WJ, Slowman LS: Acute hand and wrist injuries in athletes: Evaluation and management. *J Am Acad Orthop Surg* 9:389, 2001.
Murphy JV, Banwell PE, Roberts AH, et al: Frostbite: Pathogenesis and treatment. *J Trauma Injury Infect Crit Care* 48:171, 2000.
Rettig AC: Closed tendon injuries of the hand and wrist in athletes. *Clin Sports Med* 11:77, 1992.

Rettig AC: Wrist and hand overuse syndromes. *Clin Sports Med* 20:591, 2001.

Rettig AC, Coyle MP, Hunt TR: Hand and wrist problems in the athlete. *Am Orthop Soc Sports Med Instr Course* 108:AOSSM 28th Annual Meeting, Orlando, FL, 2002.

Sugawara M, Oginot T, Minami A, et al: Digital ischemia in baseball players. *Am J Sports Med* 14:329, 1986.

54 WRIST AND HAND FRACTURES

Baer G, MD
Chhabra AB, MD

EPIDEMIOLOGY

- Wrist and hand injuries account for 25% of athletic injuries (Amadio, 1990).
- Gymnasts have the highest level of wrist and hand injuries with up to 43% suffering chronic injuries. In one series 88% of elite male gymnasts complained of wrist pain and 58% required *nonsteroidal anti-inflammatory drugs* (NSAID) therapy to continue competing (Mandelbaum et al, 1989).

DISTAL RADIUS FRACTURES

- Distal radius fractures account for 10% of all bony injuries, up to 75% of all fractures to the forearm, and 16% of all fractures treated in the emergency room (Alffram and Bauer, 1962; Owen et al, 1982; Jupiter, 1991).
- Injury often occurs during running or contact sports when the hand is planted on the ground, the wrist hyperextends and the arm rotates. In addition to a fracture of the distal radius, injury to the *triangular fibrocartilage complex* (TFCC) and *distal radioulnar joint* (DRUJ) can result.
- On physical examination, examine for deformity (classic *silver fork* as described by Colles) (Colles, 1814), swelling, pain, and limited range of motion. Check the DRUJ for tenderness, dislocation or subluxation, and examine for any loss of pronation or supination.
- Carpal tunnel symptoms may be present in up to 15% of patients but controversy exists concerning acute versus delayed (48 to 72 h) release (Ford, 1986; Gelberman, Szabo, and Mortenson, 1984).
- Clinical symptoms of DRUJ disruption, including pain and instability, have been found in 5 to 15% of fractures (Lidstrom, 1959).

- The TFCC is the major stabilizer of the DRUJ. Disruption of the TFCC and other carpal ligaments including the scapholunate ligament has been identified at time of arthroscopy in 45 to 70% of cases (Mohanti and Kar, 1980; Geissler et al, 1996). Most TFCC tears are in the central or radial portion of the complex and are treated with debridement (Richards and Roth, 1995).
- Anatomic reduction of intra-articular distal radius fractures is required. Two millimeters of articular step-off increases the risk for subsequent degenerative arthritis (Knirk and Jupiter, 1986).

RADIOGRAPHIC EVALUATION

- True *posteroanterior* (PA) and lateral views required. Oblique and fossa lateral views, traction views as well as MRI, CAT scan, bone scan, and fluoroscopy may provide critical information regarding the nature of the fracture and associated injuries when planning for fracture management   (Batillas et al, 1981; Bindra et al, 1997; Breitenseher et al, 1997; Doczi et al, 1995).

MANAGEMENT OF DISTAL RADIUS FRACTURES

- Most stable fractures can be treated with closed reduction and casting while unstable fractures, suggested by (*1*) excessive fracture comminution, (*2*) fracture displacement, (*3*) radial articular surface angulation greater than 20°, (*4*) articular surface separation or step-off greater than 2 mm, and (*5*) comminution of both volar and dorsal cortices often require surgical intervention.
- **Extra-articular fractures:** Stable fracture treatment generally consists of closed reduction and placement of a well-fitted long-arm cast with a good 3-point mold and the forearm in neutral or supination to help stabilize the DRUJ and improve recovery of supination following fracture healing (Moir, Wardlaw, and Maffulli, 1999; Sarmiento, Zagorski, and Sinclair, 1980). Casting should be performed after acute swelling subsides. Close radiographic follow-up is required every 1 to 2 weeks to assure that loss of reduction and shortening does not occur. Unstable extra-articular fractures may require percutaneous pin fixation in conjunction with cast or external fixation for support.
- **Noncomminuted intra-articular fractures:** Barton's fractures are the result of shear forces across either the volar or dorsal lip of the distal radius resulting in two large fragments that extend into the joint (Barton, 1838). Closed reduction is usually obtained by reversal of the deformity but maintenance of reduction usually requires additional stabilization (Jupiter et al, 1996).

- **Comminuted or complex intra-articular fractures:** Highly comminuted articular fractures with dorsal comminution and subchondral bone defects frequently collapse and shorten thus requiring close radiographic observation and remanipulation if nonoperative management is chosen. Fractures with articular displacement greater than 2 mm often require external fixation with or without limited internal fixation. Accuracy of reduction may be assessed with either open or arthroscopic visualization of the articular surface to ensure anatomic restoration of the surface. Bone grafting is often required to fill bony defects especially in the subchondral region (Bass, Blair, and Hubbard, 1995; Trumble et al, 1998; Geissler and Freeland, 1996).

COMPLICATIONS

- Nonunion following distal radius fracture is a rare occurrence while malunion is a common complication (Harper and Jones, 1990; Cooney, Dobyns, and Linscheid, 1980). Correction of malunion should be undertaken when there is persistent pain and loss of the functional wrist arc of motion.

RETURN TO SPORTS

- Stable fractures treated with splint or cast immobilization should be maintained in a reduced position until fracture healing is evident (4 to 8 weeks). The athlete may then begin to rehabilitate the wrist using a removable thermoplastic splint for the next 4 to 6 weeks until full pain-free range of motion and strength has been achieved. Return to sports without protection is usually not allowed until 3 months from the time of injury. Fractures treated with rigid internal fixation can be protected by a thermoplastic splint with early range of motion exercises. Once radiographic evidence of healing is present, progressive strengthening exercises may be begun but full return to sport is not permitted before 3 months. Unstable intra-articular fractures are often immobilized for 6 to 12 weeks and full return to sports is discouraged until motion and strength have been restored (Morgan and Busconi, 1995; Christensen et al, 1995).

SCAPHOID FRACTURES

- Scaphoid fractures are the most common carpal bone fracture (1 in 100 college football players per year) and often the result of apparently minor trauma (Zemel and Stark, 1986).
- Fracture mechanism is forced hyperextension with ulnar deviation.

- Extraosseous vascular supply enters the scaphoid at the middle and distal poles while the proximal pole relies on retrograde flow. This results in a high rate of avascular necrosis and nonunion with proximal pole fractures.
- Patient presents with pain in the anatomic snuff box.
- Radiographs include PA, lateral, navicular, and closed fist views.
- Bone scan and MRI are useful in identifying nondisplaced fractures.
- Treatment—Nondisplaced fractures (less than 1 mm of displacement)
- Immobilize in long-arm thumb spica cast with the wrist in slight palmar flexion and radial deviation for 6 weeks followed by short-arm thumb spica cast until healing is evident on radiographs, usually within 3 months (Gellman et al, 1989).
- If there is no evidence of healing by 3 to 4 months then consider the use of bone grafting or electrical stimulation to enhance healing.
- Early operative intervention for nondisplaced fractures with percutaneous compression screw fixation is controversial but may allow the athlete an earlier return to sports and lower risk of fracture displacement and rehabilitation time (Koman, Mooney, and Poehling, 1990; Geissler, 2001).
- Athletes with snuffbox pain and negative radiographs should be immobilized in thumb spica cast and reassessed at 1–2-week intervals until the pain resolves or the diagnosis is made radiographically (Geissler, 2001).

TREATMENT—DISPLACED FRACTURES

- Most often requires open reduction and internal fixation to restore anatomic alignment and facilitate accurate reduction with compression screws.
- Compression screw fixation techniques have improved and permit minimal immobilization of 2 to 3 weeks followed by early restorative therapy and return to activities (Herbert and Fisher, 1984); however, with athletes susceptible to reinjury a 3- to 4-month period of healing and rehabilitation may allow a safer return to sports (Rettig et al, 1998).

RETURN TO SPORTS

- Athletes may participate in sport with immobilization; plastic, synthetic, and silastic casts have been used effectively in contact sports (Reister et al, 1985).
- Splint protection is continued for strenuous activities for an additional 2–3 months following radiographic healing until strength and motion approaches that of the contralateral side (McCue, Bruce, Jr, and Koman, 2003).

HAMATE FRACTURES

- Hook or body of the hamate fractures is present in 2 to 4% of carpal bone fractures (Rettig, Ryan, and Stone, 1992).

HOOK OF THE HAMATE FRACTURES
- Injury commonly occurs from direct force of bat, club, or racket.
- Diagnosis is often missed; chronic fractures are associated with flexor tendon rupture, and ulnar nerve neuropathy.
- Pain localized over the hamate in the hypothenar eminence.
- Carpal tunnel view and CT scans aid in diagnosis.
- Direct repair of the fracture results in high nonunion rates, therefore treatment usually requires removal of the hook through the fracture site with early return to sports (Parker et al, 1986; Bishop and Beckenbaugh, 1988).

BODY OF THE HAMATE FRACTURES
- Less common than hook fractures, often associated with dislocation of fourth and fifth metacarpals (Marck and Klasen, 1986).
- Oblique radiographs of the carpus and CT scans can assist in defining the fracture.
- Nondisplaced fractures treated with cast immobilization for 4 to 6 weeks.
- Displaced fractures are treated with open reduction, K-wire or screw fixation, and immobilization for 4 to 6 weeks.

RETURN TO SPORTS
- Athletes with fractures treated by conservative measures may return to sport immediately with protection until pain free (McCue, Bruce, and Koman, 2003).
- Athletes treated with excision of the hamate hook may return to sport as tolerated, they will often have hypothenar tenderness for several months and will require the use of well-padded gloves for return to sport (Geissler, 2001).
- Athletes with surgically treated fractures are restricted from sport until after healing is evident (4 to 6 weeks). Participation may resume with splint or cast protection until normal strength and range of motion return (McCue, Bruce, and Koman, 2003).

CAPITATE FRACTURES

- The capitate is centered within the carpus and is well protected from injury and accounts for only 1% to 2% of all carpal fractures (Geissler, 2001).
- Fractures often occur from either a direct blow to the dorsum of the wrist or from forced dorsi-flexion or volar-flexion. Capitate fractures are often associated with scaphoid fractures and perilunate dislocations (Rand, Linscheid, and Dobyns, 1982).
- Radiographic assessment with PA and lateral views, CT scan or MRI.
- Nondisplaced fractures are treated with immobilization in short-arm cast for 6 to 8 weeks.
- Capitate fractures are associated with poor outcomes because the fractures are inherently unstable and delayed union, nonunion and avascular necrosis are common complications (Rand, Linscheid, and Dobyns, 1982).
- Displaced fractures (2 mm of displacement) are treated with *open reduction, internal fixation* (ORIF) with K-wires or screw fixation and immobilized in short-arm cast for 6 weeks.

RETURN TO SPORTS
- Athletes with nonoperative fractures may return to sport immediately with protective casting (McCue, Bruce, and Koman, 2003). Close follow-up must be maintained to assure that fracture displacement does not occur obligating operative intervention.
- Athletes with surgically treated fractures are restricted from sport until after healing is evident (4 to 6 weeks). Participation may resume with splint or cast protection for an additional 3 months or until normal strength and range of motion return (McCue, Bruce, and Koman, 2003).

PISIFORM FRACTURES

- Pisiform fractures are rare and usually occur from direct blow to the palm and account for 1 to 3% of all carpal bone fractures (Geissler, 2001).
- Patients tend to have tenderness over the hypothenar region.
- Fractures are best visualized on 30° oblique AP view or carpal tunnel view.
- Acute nondisplaced fractures are managed by immobilization in a short-arm cast for 3 to 6 weeks.
- Comminuted fractures and symptomatic nonunions are managed by excision, with care to preserve the flexor carpi ulnaris tendon, with little or no functional impairment (Arner and Hagberg, 1984).

RETURN TO SPORTS
- Athletes return to sports as soon as acute pain subsides with taping, padded gloves, or casting as needed (McCue, Bruce, and Koman, 2003; Geissler, 2001; Rettig et al, 1998).

- Symptomatic nonunion may be excised following the season (McCue, Bruce, and Koman, 2003).

TRIQUETRUM FRACTURES

- Triquetrum fractures are common carpal bone fractures in sports accounting for 3 to 4% of all carpal bone injuries (Bryan and Dobyns, 1980).
- Fractures commonly consist of avulsion of the dorsal cortex following hyperextension injury causing impingement with the distal ulna.
- Treatment of this dorsal marginal fracture consists of immobilization in short-arm cast for 3 to 4 weeks (Geissler, 2001; Rettig et al, 1998).
- Isolated fractures through the body of the triquetrum are rare injuries and are often associated with scapholunate ligamentous disruption which must be clinically assessed (Geissler, 2001; Herzberg et al, 1993).

RETURN TO SPORTS
- Athletes may return to sport wearing a semi-rigid cast as soon as acute pain resolves or without immobilization when pain does not interfere with sporting activity (McCue, Bruce, and Koman, 2003; Hocker and Menshik, 1994).

LUNATE FRACTURES

- The lunate is enclosed in the radial fossa and fracture of the lunate is a rare entity.
- Athletes present with pain and swelling over the dorsum of the wrist.
- Lunate fractures occur through either a compressive force between the capitate and the distal radius fracturing through the body of the lunate or through traction from the ligamentous or capsular structures at the extremes of motion resulting in avulsion type fractures (Morgan and Reardon, 1995).
- CT scan is often needed for diagnosis as the bony architecture of the lunate is difficult to visualize on standard radiographs.
- Prompt diagnosis, immobilization, and protection from further injury until union is evident are critical as there is a possible association with fracture nonunion and the development of avascular necrosis of the lunate (Kienbock's disease) (Beckenbaugh et al, 1980).
- Nondisplaced fractures are immobilized in a short-arm cast, with the metacarpophalangeal joints flexed to reduce the compressive forces generated by gripping, for 6 weeks.
- Displaced fractures require open reduction and internal fixation versus percutaneous fixation to restore

radiocarpal and midcarpal stability as well as lunate vascularity with immobilization continuing until fracture healing is evident.

RETURN TO SPORTS
- Athletes may return to sport once fracture healing is evident. Protective splinting is recommended when athletes return to competition (Morgan and Reardon, 1995).
- Close observation for signs of avascular necrosis (dorsal wrist pain and swelling) are required following fracture healing, so it can be caught during the early stages when treatment options afford the best opportunity for return to competition (Geissler, 2001; Rettig et al, 1998).

TRAPEZIUM FRACTURES

- Fractures of the trapezium constitute 1 to 5% of all carpal fractures (Geissler, 2001; Botte and Gelberman, 1987).
- Trapezium fractures involve either the longitudinal ridge (the attachment site for the transverse carpal ligament) or the body.
- Ridge fractures are usually the result of direct trauma such as fall on outstretched hand or being struck by a ball.
- Body fractures are more common and result from falling on outstretched thumb with resultant splitting of the trapezium body and displacement of the thumb carpometacarpal joint (the mirror image of the Bennett's fracture-dislocation).
- Fractures of the body of the trapezium can often be seen on standard AP and lateral views. A pronated PA view can help visualize the articular surface and detect any displacement. The carpal tunnel view is useful to visualize trapezial ridge fractures. A CT scan may be useful in fractures difficult to visualize with plain radiographs.
- Nondisplaced fractures of the trapezium are treated with immobilization in a thumb spica cast for 4 to 6 weeks. Range of motion and strengthening are then initiated with continued use of a removable thumb spica splint for an additional 2 to 4 weeks (Morgan and Reardon, 1995).
- Body fractures are unstable and subject to displacement therefore close follow-up must be maintained until fracture union is evident (Geissler, 2001).
- Displaced body fractures are managed with open reduction and internal fixation with the use of compression screws, Kirschner wires, or a combination of both and repair of the capsular structures. Stable internal fixation allows early mobilization of the joint

(Rettig et al, 1998; Cordrey and Ferrer-Torells, 1974; Seitz, Jr, and Papandrea, 2001).

- Trapezial ridge fractures with minimal displacement have high rates of nonunion and surgical excision of the fragment allows for an uncomplicated recovery and early return to sport (Palmer, 1981).

RETURN TO SPORTS

- Nondisplaced fractures treated nonoperatively may return to sport with cast or splint immobilization once symptoms permit with protection continuing for up to 12 weeks or until strength and motion return (Morgan and Reardon, 1995).
- Trapezial body fractures treated operatively should be protected with cast or splint immobilization until complete healing and strength and motion has been restored.
- Trapezial ridge fractures treated with excision may return to sport once soft tissue healing allows; padded gloves are often required to minimize wound sensitivity that may last for several months (Geissler, 2001; Rettig et al, 1998).

TRAPEZOID FRACTURES

- The trapezoid is in a well-protected position anatomically and is the least commonly fractured carpal bone, involved in less than 1% of carpal fractures (Ruby, 1992).
- Fracture of the trapezoid is the result of high-energy axially directed trauma along the index metacarpal.
- Trapezoid fractures are usually visualized on standard AP, lateral, and oblique views.
- Treatment usually requires open reduction and internal fixation of the trapezoid with pinning of the index metacarpal in a reduced position. The Kirschner wires can be pulled at approximately 6 weeks followed by the initiation of hand therapy to restore motion and strength (Geissler, 2001).

RETURN TO SPORT

- Athletes may return to sport wearing a protective splint once the Kirschner wires are removed or when soft tissues allow (Geissler, 2001).

METACARPAL FRACTURES

- Metacarpal and phalangeal fractures are the most common fractures in the skeletal system, accounting for greater than 14% of all emergency room visits and greater than 36% of all hand fractures (Capo and Hastings, 1998; Packer and Shaheen, 1993).

- Often the result of a direct blow or crush type injury to the hand; can occur secondary to fall onto the hand.
- Typically presents with apex dorsal angulation secondary to deforming force of intrinsic muscles.
- Rotational deformity must be recognized and corrected in treating these fractures.
- Rotational alignment is best visualized with full flexion of the fingers.
- Fractures best visualized with standard AP, lateral, and oblique radiographs of the hand.
- Classified as transverse, oblique, spiral, and comminuted.

TRANSVERSE FRACTURES

- Apex dorsal fracture angulation is secondary to forces applied by intrinsic muscles. These forces are neutralized by *metacarpophalangeal* (MCP) joint flexion.
- Reduction is indicated for any angulation in the index and middle fingers, greater than 20° for ring finger, and greater than 30° for small finger (Capo and Hastings, 1998; Henry, 2001; Freeland, 2000).

TREATMENT

- Most stable fractures can be treated nonoperatively with cast immobilization for 2 weeks, followed by orthoplast splint immobilization of the affected digit and its neighbor for an additional 2 weeks, and buddy taping and initiation of active motion at 4 weeks post injury (Capo and Hastings, 1998).
- Rotational deformity is not acceptable—rotation is the most critical factor in evaluating metacarpal fractures.
- Treatment options for unstable fractures or fractures that fail closed treatment comprise closed reduction and percutaneous pinning, cross pinning to adjacent metacarpal, closed reduction and internal fixation, and open reduction and internal fixation (Capo and Hastings, 1998).
- Stable fixation requires no protection except for sport, with light active use being permitted within 5 days postoperatively (Capo and Hastings, 1998).

OBLIQUE AND SPIRAL FRACTURES

- Result of torsional forces to the metacarpal.
- Untreated fractures tend to shorten and rotate.
- Rotational deformity is unacceptable as 5° of malrotation can lead to 1.5 to 2 cm of digital overlap (Rolye, 1990).
- Five millimeters of shortening can be accepted without functional deficit (Bloem, 1971).

TREATMENT

- Isolated, minimally displaced fractures may be treated by closed methods similar to the treatment of transverse fractures.
- Fractures that cannot be maintained with closed methods require either percutaneous pinning or open reduction an internal fixation.
- Interfragmentary lag screw fixation may be used if fracture length is twice the bone diameter and provides the most biomechanically stable construct. For fractures with a shorter surface a lag screw and dorsal neutralization plate can provide stable fixation permitting early return to sport (Black et al, 1985).

COMMINUTED FRACTURES

- May be associated with soft tissue loss.
- Treatment often requires ORIF or external fixation to maintain length.
- May require delayed or primary bone grafting.

METACARPAL HEAD FRACTURES

- Rare fractures that occur from axial loading or direct trauma, must examine closely to assure that fracture is not the result of a fight bite.
- Nondisplaced fractures may be treated nonoperatively with initial splint immobilization followed by buddy taping and early range of motion (Palmer, 1998).
- Displaced fractures require open reduction and internal fixation to restore anatomic alignment and articular congruity with Kirschner wires, screws, minifragment plates or dynamic traction to allow for early motion; if early motion cannot be started then immobilization in the intrinsic plus position should be maintained until motion can be initiated (Palmer, 1998).
- Complications include limited motion and arthritis.

METACARPAL NECK FRACTURES

- Most commonly involves the ring or small finger (Boxer's fracture).
- Apex dorsal angulation and volar comminution can make it difficult to maintain reduction with cast immobilization.
- Angular deformity of 40° to 60° may be accepted at the ring and small fingers secondary to the mobility of the fourth and fifth carpometacarpal joints. More than 15° to 20° of angulation is unacceptable at the index or long metacarpals secondary to the lack of motion at

their carpometacarpal joints (Capo and Hastings, 1998; Henry, 2001).
- Treatment for the majority of fractures comprises closed reduction by the technique described by Jahss (1938) and immobilizing the fracture in a short-arm gutter splint with the fingers in the intrinsic plus position. Immobilization is continued for 2 weeks when buddy taping and motion are initiated (Capo and Hastings, 1998).
- Radiographs should be obtained weekly with index and long metacarpal fractures to assure that reduction is not lost.
- Surgical intervention is indicated for irreducible fractures or in fractures where reduction is lost. Operative intervention may include closed-reduction and percutaneous pinning, open reduction, and internal fixation with tension band or a laterally applied minicondylar plate (Capo and Hastings, 1998; Freeland, 2000).
- Bouquet pinning with the insertion of multiple small intramedullary Kirschner wires down the metacarpal shaft and across the fracture into the metacarpal head can provide stable fixation and early return of unrestricted hand function in fractures that would otherwise require lengthy immobilization (Capo and Hastings, 1998; Graham and Mullen, 2003).
- The hand is immobilized in a splint for 2 weeks after which motion is initiated with return to sports at preinjury level within 6 weeks.

METACARPAL BASE FRACTURES

- Metacarpal base fractures are rare fractures. They usually have a stable configuration secondary to set of four strong interosseous ligaments.
- Index and long CMC joints have limited motion while ring and small CMC joints have 15° and 30° of mobility respectively (Capo and Hastings, 1998).
- Nondisplaced or minimally displaced fractures are treated in a short-arm cast with the metacarpophalangeal joints flexed and the interphalangeal joints free.
- Immobilization is often maintained for 6 weeks followed by buddy taping for 2 to 3 weeks to maintain rotational control and allow initiation of motion (Palmer, 1998).
- Displaced fractures often require closed or open reduction followed by percutaneous fixation followed by splint immobilization and the gradual restoration of motion at 6 to 8 weeks post injury (Capo and Hastings, 1998; Henry, 2001; Freeland, 2000; Palmer, 1998).
- Fractures that proceed to malunion may cause weakness of grip or pain with evidence of arthritis and may

be treated with arthodesis without significantly compromising hand function (Palmer, 1998).

RETURN TO SPORTS FOLLOWING METACARPAL FRACTURES

- Most sports-related metacarpal fractures are stable and are treated initially with splint or cast immobilization. Return to sports with protection may be initiated within 1 to 2 weeks from injury depending upon the requirements of the specific sport. Protection is usually continued for 8 to 12 weeks depending upon the demands of the sport (Alexy and De Carlo, 1998).
- Fractures treated with rigid internal fixation may allow the athlete earlier return to play than nonoperative treatment. Athletes may begin early motion with return to sports with immobilization as early as 2 weeks and by 5 to 6 weeks buddy taping or a light splint may be all that is required to permit sport specific activities (Graham and Mullen, 2003; Alexy and De Carlo, 1998; Breen, 1995).

THUMB METACARPAL FRACTURES

- Thumb metacarpal fractures are unique from fractures of the other digits secondary to the thumb's critical role in hand function, especially grasp and power pinch.
- More than one fourth of all metacarpal fractures are to the thumb metacarpal base and result from axial loading across the partially flexed thumb (Gedda, 1954).
- Radiographic imaging requires views specifically of the thumb in AP and lateral projections.
- Joint anatomy comprises reciprocal saddle-shaped surfaces of the distal trapezium and proximal metacarpal.
- Intra-articular Bennett's (partial articular) and Rolando's (complete articular) fractures often have displacement dorsally and radially by pull of the abductor pollicis longus (Green and O'Brien, 1972; Langford, Whitaker, and Toby, 1998).
- Treatment is directed at minimizing posttraumatic arthritis by obtaining anatomic joint reduction.
- If less than 15 to 20% of the joint surface is involved then closed reduction and percutaneous pinning is successful (Freeland, 2000).
- Immobilization in a short-arm thumb spica cast for 4 to 6 weeks is recommended followed by removal of pins and initiation of motion (Palmer, 1998; Langford, Whitaker, and Toby, 1998).
- If greater than 25 to 30% of the joint surface is involved then open reduction and stable internal fixation with screws or pins is indicated (Green, 1993).
- Range of motion is initiated at 5 to 10 days postoperatively (Langford, Whitaker, and Toby, 1998).

- Severely comminuted intra-articular Rolando fractures often require external fixation followed by limited open reduction and internal fixation with bone grafting (Buchler, McCollam, and Oppikofer, 1991).
- Immobilization is continued for a minimum of 6 to 8 weeks followed by the initiation of hand based therapy to regain motion and strength.
- Extra-articular thumb metacarpal fractures usually occur toward the metacarpal base.
- Treatment often consists of closed reduction and immobilization in a thumb spica cast for 4 to 6 weeks followed by initiation of hand therapy.
- Twenty to thirty degrees of angulation is acceptable because of the multiple planes of thumb motion (Capo and Hastings, 1998).
- Unstable fractures may require operative intervention with either closed reduction and percutaneous pinning or internal fixation similar to the treatment for other metacarpal fractures (Capo and Hastings, 1998; Freeland, 2000).

RETURN TO SPORTS

- Athletes may return to sport with immobilization in thumb spica splint or cast as symptoms and sport specific activity permit.
- Protection should be maintained until fracture healing is evident on radiographs and strength, stability and motion are restored.
- Operative intervention with stable fixation may allow for earlier initiation of motion and return to sports (Langford, Whitaker, and Toby, 1998).

PHALANGEAL FRACTURES

PROXIMAL AND MIDDLE PHALANX FRACTURES

- Very common fractures in athletes participating in contact sports or sports requiring catching of a ball.
- Fracture displacement depends on mechanism of injury and deforming forces of muscles and tendons on bone.
- Proximal phalanx fractures typically have volar angulation with proximal segment flexed by the interossei and the distal segment extended by pull of the central slip portion of the extensor mechanism (Capo and Hastings, 1998; Henry, 2001).
- Middle phalanx fractures are deformed by both the central slip and by the flexor digitorum superficialis tendon resulting in either volar or dorsal angulation depending upon the location of the fracture (Capo and Hastings, 1998; Henry, 2001).
- Treatment depends upon the stability of the fracture, correction of rotational deformation, and no greater than 10° of angulation in any plane.

- Nondisplaced and stable fractures can be treated with buddy taping and early range of motion (Capo and Hastings, 1998). Careful clinical and radiographic follow-up is required to detect subsequent fracture displacement.
- Displaced fractures require closed reduction and immobilization with cast or splint and an outrigger with the affected finger held in the intrinsic-plus position including an adjacent digit to help maintain rotational alignment (Capo and Hastings, 1998).
- Fracture immobilization should be limited to 3 weeks prior to initiation of hand based therapy to facilitate maximal restoration of motion, protective splinting should be continued during sport specific activities until healing is evident (Capo and Hastings, 1998; Posner, 1995; Strickland et al, 1982).
- Intra-articular, unstable, or rotationally malaligned fractures may benefit from open or closed reduction and internal or percutaneous fixation to restore anatomic alignment and rotational control.
- If rigid fixation is obtained, mobilization to regain range of motion and edema control should begin within the first week after surgery, permitting earlier return to sport and a more predictable functional outcome (Capo and Hastings, 1998; Breen, 1995).
- Protective splinting should be maintained for 4 weeks or until fracture healing is evident. Simple buddy taping should be continued until range of motion and strength are restored.

DISTAL PHALANX FRACTURES

- Account for 50% of all hand fractures—especially thumb and middle finger (McNealy and Lichtenstein, 1940).
- Fibrous septa from skin minimize fracture displacement.
- Must examine for evidence of nail bed injury.
- Treatment is dictated by presence of soft tissue injury.
- If a nail bed injury is present, the nail bed must be repaired to prevent nail deformity (Simon and Wolgin, 1987).
- Immobilization is restricted to the distal interphalangeal joint for a period of 3 to 4 weeks after which motion is initiated (Capo and Hastings, 1998).
- Tenderness may persist for greater than 6 months requiring a program of desensitization to allow full return of function (DaCruz, Slade, and Malone, 1988).
- Mallet finger deformity can occur from loss of continuity of extensor mechanism through bony or tendinous disruption.
- Treatment is almost always nonoperative with continuous extension splinting of the *distal interphalangeal* (DIP) joint for at least 6 weeks followed by the removal of the splint several times a day for active

range of motion exercises for an additional 2 weeks (Henry, 2001; Posner, 1995).

RETURN TO SPORTS AFTER PHALANGEAL FRACTURES

- Athletes with stable fractures treated nonoperatively may return to sports with rigid cast immobilization, thermoplast splint protection, or buddy taping (as sport specific activities permit) as soon as symptoms allow often within the first week (Alexy and De Carlo, 1998).
- Close follow-up must be maintained to ensure that loss of reduction or malrotation do not occur.
- Protection should be maintained until radiographic evidence of complete healing is evident and functional recovery of range of motion and strength are complete (Posner, 1995).
- Athletes with surgically treated fractures may return to sports with protective splinting or casting once soft tissue healing allows.
- Edema control and active motion are typically initiated at 2 weeks and by 4 weeks 75% of motion should have been regained and strengthening can be initiated. Protective splinting should be maintained for sport specific activities until healing is evident (Capo and Hastings, 1998; Graham and Mullen, 2003; Alexy and De Carlo, 1998). Buddy taping should be maintained until strength and motion have been regained.

REFERENCES

Alexy C, De Carlo M: Rehabilitation and use of protective devices in hand and wrist injuries. *Clin Sports Med* 17:635–655, 1998.

Alffram PA, Bauer GC: Epidemiology of fractures of the forearm. A biomechanical investigation of bone strength. *J Bone Joint Surg [Am]* 44A:105–114, 1962.

Amadio PC: Epidemiology of hand and wrist injuries in sports. *Hand Clin* 6:379–381, 1990.

Arner M, Hagberg L: Wrist flexion strength after excision of the pisiform bone. *Scand J Plast Reconstr* 18:241–245, 1984.

Barton JR: Views and treatment of an important injury of the wrist. *Med Exam* 1:365, 1838.

Bass RL, Blair WF, Hubbard PP: Results of combined internal and external fixation for the treatment of severe AO-C3 fractures of the distal radius. *J Hand Surg* 20A:373–381, 1995.

Batillas J, Vasilas A, Pizzi WF, et al: Bone scanning in the detection of occult fractures. *J Trauma* 21:564–569, 1981.

Beckenbaugh RD, Shiver TC, Dobyns JH, et al: The natural history of Kienbock's disease and consideration of lunate fractures. *Clin Orthop* 149:98–106, 1980.

Bindra RR, Cole RJ, Yamaguchi K, et al: Quantification of the radial torsion angle with computerized tomography in cadaver specimens. *J Bone Joint Surg* 79A:833–837, 1997.

Bishop AT, Beckenbaugh RD: Fractures of the hamate hook. *J Hand Surg* 13A:135–139, 1988.

Black DM, Mann RJ, Constine RM, et al: Comparison of internal fixation techniques in metacarpal fracture. *J Hand Surg* 10A:466–472, 1985.

Bloem JJ: The treatment and prognosis of uncomplicated dislocated fractures of the metacarpals and phalanges. *Arch Chir Neer* 23:55–65, 1971.

Botte MJ, Gelberman RH: Fractures of the carpus excluding the scaphoid. *Hand Clin* 3:149–161, 1987.

Breen TF: Sport-related injuries of the hand, *in* Pappas AM (ed.): *Upper Extremity Injuries in the Athlete*. New York, NY, Churchill Livingstone, 1995, pp 451–491.

Breitenseher MD, Metz VM, Gilula LA, et al: Radiographically occult scaphoid fractures: Value of MR imaging in dectection. *Radiology* 203:245–250, 1997.

Bryan RS, Dobyns JH: Fractures of the carpal bones other than the lunate and navicular. *Clin Orthop* 14:107–111, 1980.

Buchler U, McCollam SM, Oppikofer C: Comminuted fractures of the basilar joint of the thumb: Combined treatment by external fixation, limited internal fixation, and bone grafting. *J Hand Surg* 16A:556–560, 1991.

Capo JT, Hastings H: Metacarpal and phalangeal fractures in athletes. *Clin Sports Med* 17:491–511, 1998.

Christensen OM, Christiansen TG, Krasheninnikoff M, et al: Length of immobilization after fractures of the distal radius. *Intern Orthop* 19:26–29, 1995.

Colles A: On the fracture of the carpal extremity of the radius. *Edinburgh Med Surg J* 10:182–186, 1814.

Cooney WP, Dobyns JH, Linscheid RL: Complications of Colles' fractures. *J Bone Joint Surg* 62A:613–619, 1980.

Cordrey LJ, Ferrer-Torells M: Management of fractures of the greater multangular: Report of five cases. *J Bone Joint Surg* 42A:1321–1322, 1974.

DaCruz DJ, Slade RJ, Malone W: Fractures of the distal phalanges. *J Hand Surg [Br]* 13B:350–352, 1988.

Doczi J, Springer G, Renner A, et al: Occult distal radial fractures. *J Hand Surg* 20B:614–617, 1995.

Ford DJ: Acute carpal tunnel syndrome: Complications of delayed decompression. *J Bone Joint Surg* 68B:758–759, 1986.

Freeland AE: Hand Fractures: Repair, Reconstruction, and Rehabilitation. Philadelphia, PA, Churchill Livingstone, 2000.

Gedda KO: Studies of Bennett's fractures: Anatomy, roentgenology, and therapy. *Acta Chir Scand Suppl* 5:193, 1954.

Geissler WB: Carpal fractures in athletes. *Clin Sports Med* 20:167–188, 2001.

Geissler WB, Freeland AE: Arthroscopically assisted reduction of intraarticular distal radial fractures. *Clin Orthop* 327:125–134, 1996.

Geissler WB, Freeland AE, Savoie FH, et al: Intracarpal soft-tissue lesions associated with an intra-articular fracture of the distal end of the radius. *J Bone Joint Surg* 78A:357–365, 1996.

Gelberman RH, Szabo RM, Mortenson WW: Carpal tunnel pressures and wrist position in patients with Colles' fractures. *J Trauma* 24:747–749, 1984.

Gellman H, caputo RJ, Carter V, et al: A comparison of short and long thumb-spica casts for nondisplaced fractures of the carpal scaphoid. *J Bone Joint Surg [Am]* 71:354–357, 1989.

Graham TJ, Mullen DJ: Athletic injuries of the adult hand, *in* DeLee JC, Dres D, Jr, Miller MD (eds.): *DeLee & Drez's Orthopaedic Sports Medicine; Principles and Practice*. Philadelphia, PA, Saunders, 2003, pp 1381–1431.

Green DP: *Operative Hand Surgery*. New York, NY, Churchill Livingstone, 1993.

Green DP, O'Brien ET: Fractures of the thumb metacarpal. *South Med J* 65:807–814, 1972.

Harper WM, Jones JM: Non-union of Colles' fracture: Report of two cases. *J Hand Surg* 15B:121–123, 1990.

Henry M: Fractures and dislocations of the hand, *in* Bucholz RW, Heckman JD (eds.): *Rockwood and Green's Fractures in Adults*. Philadelphia, PA, Lippincott Williams & Wilkins, 2001, pp 655–748.

Herbert TJ, Fisher WE: Management of the fractured scaphoid using a new bone screw. *J Bone Joint Surg [Br]* 66B:114–123, 1984.

Herzberg G, Comtet JJ, et al: Perilunate dislocations and fracture dislocations: A multicenter study. *J Hand Surg* 18A:768–779, 1993.

Hocker K, Menshik A: Chip fractures of the triquetrum: Mechanism, classification and results. *J Hand Surg* 19B:584–588, 1994.

Jahss S: Fractures of the metacapals: A new method of reduction and immobilization. *J Bone Joint Surg* 20:178–186, 1938.

Jupiter JB: Current concepts review: Fractures of the distal end of the radius. *J Bone Joint Surg [Am]* 73:461, 1991.

Jupiter JB, Fernandez DL, Toh CL, et al: Operative treatment of volar intra-articular fractures of the distal end of the radius. *J Bone Joint Surg* 78A:1817–1828, 1996.

Knirk JL, Jupiter JB: Intra-articular fractures of the distal end of the radius in young adults. *J Bone Joint Surg [Am]* 63A:647–659, 1986.

Koman LA, Mooney JF, Poehling GG: Fractures and ligamentous injuries of the wrist. *Hand Clin* 6:477–491, 1990.

Langford SA, Whitaker JH, Toby EB: Thumb injuries in the athlete. *Clin Sports Med* 17:553–566, 1998.

Lidstrom A: Fractures of the distal end of the radius: A clinical and statistical study of end results. *Acta Orthop Scand Suppl* 41:1–118, 1959.

Mandelbaum BR, Bartolozzi AR, Davis CA, et al. Wrist pain syndrome in the gymnasts. *Am J Sports Med* 17:305–317, 1989.

Marck KW, Klasen HJ: Fracture-dislocation of the hamato-metacarpal joint: A case report. *J Hand Surg* 11:128–130, 1986.

McCue FC, III, Bruce JF, Jr, Koman JD: The wrist in the adult, *in* DeLee JC, Dres D, Jr, Miller MD (eds.): *DeLee & Drez's Orthopaedic Sports Medicine; Principles and Practice*. Philadelphia, PA, Saunders, 2003, pp 1337–1364.

McNealy RW, Lichtenstein ME: Fractures of the bones of the hand. *Am J Surg* 50:563–570, 1940.

Mohanti RC, Kar N: Study of triangular fibrocartilage of the wrist joint in Colles' fracture. *Injury* 11:321–324, 1980.

Moir JS, Wardlaw D, Maffulli N: Functional bracing of Colles' fractures. *Hospital Joint Disease* 58:45–52, 1999.

Morgan WJ, Busconi BD: Injuries of the distal radius and distal radioulnar joint, in Pappas AM (ed.): *Upper Extremity Injuries in the Athlete.* New York, NY, Churchill Livingstone, 1995, pp 393–412.

Morgan WJ, Reardon TF: Carpal fractures of the wrist, *in* Pappas AM (ed.): *Upper Extremity Injuries in the Athlete.* New York, NY, Churchill Livingstone, 1995, pp 431–449.

Owen RA, Melton JJ, Johnson A, et al: Incidence of Colles' fracture in North American community. *Am J Public Health* 72:605, 1982.

Packer GJ, Shaheen MA: Patterns of hand fractures and dislocations in a district general hospital. *J Hand Surg* 18B:511–514, 1993.

Palmer AK: Trapezial ridge fractures. *J Hand Surg* 6:561–564, 1981.

Palmer RE: Joint injuries of the hand in athletes. *Clin Sports Med* 17:513–531, 1998.

Parker RD, Berkowitz MS, Brahms MA, et al: Hook of the hamate fractures in athletes. *Am J Sports Med* 14:517–523, 1986.

Posner MA: Hand injuries, *in* Nicholas JA, Hershman EB, and Posner MA (eds.): *The Upper Extremity in Sports Medicine.* St Louis, MO, Mosby 1995, pp 483–569.

Rand J, Linscheid RL, Dobyns JH: Capitate fractures: A long term follow-up. *Clin Orthop* 165:209–216, 1982.

Reister JN, Baker BE, Mosher JF, et al: A review of scaphoid fracture healing in competitive athletes. *Am J Sports Med* 13:159–161, 1985.

Rettig AC, Ryan RO, Stone JA: Epidemiology of hand injuries in sports, *in* Strickland JW, Rettig AC (eds.): *Hand Injuries in Athletes.* Philadelphia, PA, Saunders, 1992, pp 37–48.

Rettig ME, Dassa GL, Raskin KB, et al: Wrist fractures in the athlete–distal radius and carpal fractures. *Clin Sports Med* 17:469–489, 1998.

Richards RS, Roth JH: Common wrist injuries, *in* Chan KM (ed.): *The Hand and Upper Extremity: Sports Injuries of the Hand and Upper Extremity.* New York, NY, Churchill Livingstone, 1995, pp 213–226.

Rolye SG: Rotational deformity following metacarpal fracture. *J Hand Surg* 15B:124–125, 1990.

Ruby L: Fractures and dislocation of the carpus, *in* Brown BD, Jupiter JB, Levine AM, et al (eds.): *Skeletal Trauma.* Philadelphia, PA, Saunders, 1992, pp 1025–1062.

Sarmiento A, Zagorski JB, Sinclair WF: Functional bracing of Colles' fractures: A prospective study of immobilization in supination versus pronation. *Clin Orthop* 146:175–183, 1980.

Seitz WH, Jr, Papandrea RF: Fractures and dislocations of the wrist, *in* Bucholz RW, Heckman JD (eds.): *Rockwood and Green's Fractures in Adults.* Philadelphia, PA, Lippincott Williams & Wilkins, 2001, pp 749–813.

Simon RR, Wolgin M: Subungual hematoma: Association with occult laceration requiring repair. *Am J Emerg Med* 5:302–304, 1987.

Strickland JW, Steichen JB, Kleinman WB, et al: Phalangeal fractures, factors influencing digital performance. *Orthop Rev* 11:39–50, 1982.

Trumble TE, Wagner W, Hanel DP, et al: Intrafocal (Kapandji) pinning of distal radius fractures with and without external fixation. *J Hand Surg* 23A:381–394, 1998.

Zemel NP, Stark HH: Fractures and dislocations of the carpal bones. *Clin Sports Med* 5:709–724, 1986.

55 UPPER EXTREMITY NERVE ENTRAPMENT

Margarete Di Benedetto, MD
Robert Giering, MD

GENERAL PRINCIPLES OF UPPER EXTREMITY NERVE ENTRAPMENT

EPIDEMIOLOGY

- The most common nerve entrapment is that of the median nerve at the wrist, the *carpal tunnel syndrome* (CTS). Its occurrence is 3.46 cases per 1000 person-years. Female to male ratio for CTS is about 3:1 (Kimura, 2001). The next highest incidence is entrapment of the ulnar nerve at the elbow (Dumitru, Amato, and Zwarts, 2002). Krivickas and Wilbourn (2000) studied 180 athletes with sports injuries in his electrodiagnostic laboratory, of which 23% had median nerve injuries, 22% stingers, 10.5% radial nerve lesions, 10.5% ulnar nerve compression syndromes, 12% axillary nerve problems, and 7.8% entrapment of the suprascapular nerve only.

PATHOPHYSIOLOGY

- Nerve entrapment occurs when the nerve passes through a tight space, placing it at risk for mechanical compression as well as ischemia secondary to the pressure on the vasa nervorum. Persistent compression results in predictable, progressive degrees of nerve damage, as classified by Seddon: Neurapraxia, Axonotmesis, and Neurotmesis (Kimura, 2001).
1. *Neurapraxia* (conduction block) is reversible failure of conduction across the affected segment. Eventually demyelination results. Most vulnerable are large myelinated fibers. Duration of compression determines degree of damage. The presence of neurapraxia can vary from minutes to months.
2. *Axonotmesis* specifies axonal damage, with endoneurium and perineurium intact. Wallerian degeneration ensues (axonal breakdown distal to lesion). Preservation of endoneurial tubes provide a guide for regeneration of axons. Recovery is on the order of months.
3. *Neurotmesis* represents complete disruption of axons, endoneurium, and perineurium. Wallerian degeneration occurs. Poor functional outcome results, and surgical intervention is usually indicated.

RISK FACTORS AND ASSOCIATED MEDICAL CONDITIONS

- **Anatomy:** Narrowed space in bony and/or muscular/tendinous/fibrous canals/tunnels.
- **Examples:** Thoracic outlet, quadrilateral space, Struthers ligament, anomalous bone spurs, muscles or fibrous bands, cubital-, radial- and carpal tunnel, Guyon's canal, excessive callous formation after (especially malunited) fractures.
- **Functional/Injury:** Acute or chronic such as through repetitive motion, percussion, compression, stretch, excessive pressure from equipment.
- **Medical conditions:** Endocrine problems (pregnancy, hypothyroidism), compartment syndrome, *peripheral neuropathy* (PN), genetic PN with propensity to develop compression syndromes (*hereditary neuropathic peripheral polyneuropathy*).

CLINICAL FEATURES

- Symptoms and signs: Numbness, tingling, pain, and weakness in the distribution of the affected nerve. Feeling of coldness, heaviness, or burning (*paresthesias*).
- Common signs are sensory loss in the distribution of the affected nerve except in lesions of pure motor nerves, e.g., anterior, posterior interosseous, supracapular, and long thoracic nerves; weakness and/or atrophy of muscles supplied by the compressed nerve.
- Special tests include Tinel's, Phalen's, Spurling's, Adson's maneuver, pectoralis minor and costoclavicular maneuvers, and stress-abduction test that may or may not be positive.
- Persistent minor pain due to entrapment may cause a regional pain syndrome—*reflex sympathetic dystrophy* (RSD).

ELECTRODIAGNOSIS

- *Eletromyography* (EMG) and *nerve conduction studies* (NCS) are significant factors in establishing the correct diagnosis of entrapment syndromes. Typical findings include the following:
  1. Conduction delay across the site of the lesion. Amplitudes are reduced due to blocking or axonal loss (with normal duration), or secondary to demyelination (with increased duration).
  2. Electromyography shows decreased recruitment, increase in polyphasic waves, action potential durations and amplitudes, and in more severe cases fibrillations and positive sharp waves. *Complex repetitive discharges* (CRD) denote chronicity. EMG demonstrates the severity of the abnormality—especially if there is evidence of denervation—that has considerable impact on treatment decisions.
- In compression syndromes, major diagnoses to be ruled out with EMG and NCS are: radiculopathy, peripheral neuropathy, plexopathy including neuralgic amyotrophy (brachial plexitis), myopathy, and malingering.

SPECIFIC NERVE ENTRAPMENTS OF THE UPPER EXTREMITY

- **Radiculopathy:** Radiculopathy is caused by pressure on a spinal nerve as it exits the spine. It is the most significant differential diagnosis for upper extremity compression syndromes. Primary anterior compression (disk herniation) may selectively affect motor fibers. It may spare the dorsal ramus, sparing sensation. Posterior compression may selectively affect sensory fibers. Compression of the nerve root can occur from any direction within the intervertebral foramen, but most commonly occurs due to posterolateral disk herniation or facet degeneration.
- **Risk factors:** For cervical radiculopthy include patients with cervical spondylosis, cervical disk herniation, facet degeneration, space occupying lesions, and prior C-spine trauma or surgery. The most commonly affected level is C7 (31–81% of all cervical radiculopathy), followed by C6 (19–25%), C8 (4–12%), and C5 (2–14%) (Wilbourn and Aminoff, 1998).
- **Symptoms and signs:** Sensory complaints (findings are in root distribution), weakness, and reflex changes. Provocative maneuvers include Spurling's—pressure on laterally and posteriorly tilted head reproduces symptoms in the affected nerve root distribution.
- **Treatment:** Indications for immediate surgical referral are progressive neurologic deficit, bowel or bladder dysfunction, and severe pain refractory to other approaches. Surgery usually includes decompression of the nerve root, diskectomy if needed, and possibly cervical fusion.
  - Conservative treatment includes pain medications, *nonsteroidal anti-inflammatory drugs* (NSAIDs), antispasmodics, antiepileptics, and antidepressants. Physical therapy modalities include cervical traction, strengthening exercises, biomechanical mobilization (flexibility), and alignment techniques as indicated. Epidural steroid injections can help facilitate physical therapy when needed. *Transcutaneous electrical nerve stimulation* (TENS) units and biofeedback may help.

SPINAL ACCESSORY NERVE, CRANIAL NERVE XI

- **Anatomy:** The trapezius, the major muscle supplied by the spinal accessory nerve, is a significant scapular stabilizer and thereby critical for the maintenance of efficient shoulder function (Ewing and Martin, 1952). The spinal component of *cranial nerve* (CN) XI originates from the anterior horn cells of the cervical spinal cord (C1–C5). Fibers enter the skull through the foramen magnum and leave the skull through the jugular foramen. There is somatotopical arrangement with the fibers arising from C1 and C2 mainly innervating the sternocleidomastoid muscles while those arising from C3 and C4 constitute the nerve supply for the trapezius. In the neck, the spinal accessory nerve passes through the posterior triangle after giving off a branch to the sternocleidomastoid muscle. It then supplies the trapezius muscle.
- **Risk factors:** Intracranial—head injuries. Intraspinal cord—post traumatic syrinx.
  1. **Cervical:** Sports injuries involving percussion or compression in the posterior triangle of the neck, such as through ill fitting shoulder pads in football (stingers/burners) (Di Benedetto and Markey, 1984; Markey, Di Benedetto, and Curl, 1993), blows to the shoulder (e.g., with a hockey stick), compression with backpack straps, and shoulder dislocation.
  2. Traumatic penetrating injuries to the neck, atraumatic iatrogenic lesions, acute or delayed, mainly after radical neck dissections or lymph node biopsies, cannulation of the internal jugular vein or after carotid enterarterectomies (due to hemorrhages, hematomas, malpositioned suction drainage, infection, or scarring).
  3. Atraumatic weakness of trapezius must rule out neurologic or myopathic disease.
- **Symptoms and signs:** Shoulder syndrome (accessory nerve lesion) consists of shoulder drooping, acromion prominence, and limited lateral abduction, impaired forward shoulder flexion, aberrant scapular rotation, and abnormal scapulohumeral rhythm (Codman, 1934), pain and abnormal electromyographic findings. Significant pain and tenderness over trapezius, exacerbated by shoulder movement, and a feeling of heaviness in the affected arm may be present. Patients have difficulty with overhead activities, heavy lifting, prolonged writing, or driving. The patient may have impingement pain secondary to inability to rotate the scapula, thereby causing the greater tuberosity to abut the acromion (Bigliani et al, 1996). Late onset of pain is mostly due to adhesive capsulitis, a common sequela of spinal accessory nerve injury.

  1. Test trapezius strength by resistance to lateral abduction of the arm from about 100–180° with the arm internally rotated and hand pronated (Ewing and Martin, 1952) (check endurance). Isolation of trapezius must be assured since shoulder elevation can also be accomplished with the levator scapula and the rhomboids. Test strength of sternocleidomastoid muscles by resisting head turning, opposite to the side of the muscle tested. Also test tilting. Resistance to head flexion tests both sternocleidomostoid muscles at the same time. Lateral scapular winging is not as pronounced as with a long thoracic nerve lesion. The scapula is laterally translocated with medial rotation of the inferior angle.
- **Treatment:** Management includes *range of motion* (ROM) exercises to prevent contractures. Resistive exercises to restore strength to the shoulder girdle. If no improvement, surgery.
  - **Surgical intervention:** Eden-Lange dynamic muscle transfer is the procedure of choice. This consists of a lateral transfer of the insertions of the levator scapulae, rhomboids minor and rhomboids major muscles (Lange, 1951; Wiater and Bigliani, 1999).

BRACHIAL PLEXUS

- Brachial plexopathy secondary to sports or occupational injury mostly presents as compression, stretch, or the combination of the two.
- **Other risk factors:** Compression after prolonged anesthesia, postmedian sternotomy, coronary bypass surgery, jugular vein cannulation, and *Erb's* (birth) *palsy*. Nontraumatic causes for sudden onset of shoulder pain followed by weakness that has to be ruled out is brachial plexitis (neuralgic amyotrophy) (Krivickas and Wilbourne, 2000), which is believed to be a genetic disorder, or an inflammatory-immune response (Suarez et al, 1996). In addition the brachial plexus may be affected by space occupying lesions or radiation.

UPPER TRUNK PLEXOPATHY

- **Anatomy and origin:** C5–C6 cervical nerve roots/spinal nerves. In the upper trunk region the suprascapular nerve and the nerve to the subclavius originate. The fibers to the musculocutaneous, axillary, median, and radial nerve pass through.
- The best known brachial plexus injury is the *stinger* (*burner*) (Di Benedetto and Markey, 1984).
- **Risk factor:** At risk are football players (highest incidence in defensive backs), wrestlers and participants in

other collision sports. Some investigators believe that the lesion is more likely in the spinal nerves than the plexus, because of the lack of protective epi- and per- ineurium at that site (Weinstein, 1998); however, long thoracic nerve involvement with scapular winging is not a typical manifestation of most stinger injuries. Other risk factors include backpacking, especially car- rying heavy loads for a long time; foraminal stenosis (Castro, 2003; Kelly et al, 2000), especially during extension–compression injuries; poor technique, ill fit- ting equipment (shoulder pads) (Markey, Di Benedetto, and Curl, 1993). Risk factors for Erb's (birth) palsy include difficult childbirth, instrumentation (forceps).

- **Symptoms and signs:** Symptoms and signs of the stinger syndrome include burning pain and dysesthe- sia in the affected arm on impact lasting seconds to hours, followed by mostly transient weakness and no sensory symptoms. At times there is prolonged loss of strength (Di Benedetto and Markey, 1984). *Cervical cord neurapraxia* (CCN) has to be ruled out (Castro, 2003). Occasionally, the only objective change may be seen as postural abnormality (drooping of the shoulder, especially if the accessory nerve is also involved). Confirmation by objective tests is often dif- ficult. Findings include weakness in supra- and infra- spinatus, deltoid and biceps. Check for positive Tinel's sign at Erb's point and Spurling's sign to con- sider root involvement. More severe injuries may involve the middle and lower trunk and/or nerve roots.
- **Treatment:** There is no direct treatment for the stinger syndrome, other than prevention of recurrence. Shoulder pad and neck orthosis selection should be optimal to ensure best protection. Gradually increas- ing collision work and improved tackling techniques are recommended. Prolonged weakness will require a reconditioning program before returning to competi- tive contact sports (Cramer, 1999). Emphasis is placed on postural exercises with cervicothoracic stabiliza- tion training and resistive exercises to shoulder mus- cles (when no more evidence of denervation).
- The athlete may return to participation in contact sports on reestablishment of pain-free motion and full recovery of strength and functional status.
- Contraindication for return to play is two or more episodes of transient CCN, imaging confirmation of cervical myelopathy, evidence of neurological deficit, decreased ROM and/or neck pain (Weinberg, Rokito, and Silber, 2003).

LOWER TRUNK PLEXOPATHY

- **Anatomy and origin:** The 8th cervical and first tho- racic roots/spinal nerves. The lower trunk lies between

the clavicle and the first rib. It carries sensory and motor fibers of C8–T1 distribution (median and ulnar nerves). The closeness of median motor and ulnar sen- sory fibers at this level has diagnostic significance.

- The best known and most debated compression syn- drome here is the thoracic outlet syndrome (TOS).
- **Thoracic outlet syndromes:** Several are identified: *(1)* between the anterior and middle scalene muscles, *(2)* the scalenus anticus syndrome (nerve entrapment between the insertion of the scalenus anticus, the clav- icle and the first rib—more severe in the presence of a cervical rib), *(3)* the costoclavicular syndrome, and *(4)* the pectoralis minor syndrome.
- **Risk factors:** Risk factors include the presence of a cervical rib (with fibrous bands to the 1st rib) (Wilbourn, 1999), and slim asthenic females with long "swan" necks and droopy shoulders. Sternotomy places patients at risk for a pectoralis minor syn- drome, especially those with premorbid impaired shoulder motion. Space occupying lesions (e.g., Pancoast tumor) or bulky lymphadenopathy (of what- ever etiology), and radiculopathy. Entrapment may be of several types:
- **Vascular etiology:** Entrapment of subclavian or axil- lary artery or vein.
- **Neurogenic etiology:** Neurogenic etiology (much debated) specifically affects the lower trunk (Dumitru, Amato, and Zwarts, 2002). The incidence of true neu- rogenic TOS is thought to be near one in one million (Wilbourn, 1999).
- **Symptoms and signs:** With vascular etiology there is vague pain and fatigue (claudication), color change (pallor or cyanosis), distended veins of the arm and chest wall, and cool temperature of the upper limb. Confirmatory tests are arteriography or venography. Neurogenic etiology causes paresthesias along the medial aspect of the affected hand and forearm noted in conjunction with thenar wasting and weakness of the *abductor pollicis brevis* (APB). The ulnar hand intrin- sics may also be weak and atrophic. Characteristic EDX finding include reduced median motor and ulnar sensory response amplitudes.
- Provocative maneuvers include Adson's maneuver (decreasing the space between the clavicle and the first rib, by placing the shoulders in military position, head turned to the side and taking a deep breath, which elevates the ribcage). It is considered positive if the radial pulse can no longer be palpated, or if the neurologic symptoms increase. Unfortunately, there are many false positive and false negative results. Test for costo-clavicular compression with shoulders in military positions and then forcing clavicles down- ward posteriorly. The hyperabduction–extension test is used for pectoralis minor syndrome.

- **Treatment:** Most patients do very well with an intensive physical therapy program including biomechanical retraining, shoulder and ribcage elevation exercises that enlarge the entrapped space. Pain should be addressed adequately with specific agents for neuropathic pain (e.g., tricyclics, anticonvulsants). Surgical options include first rib removal, which may be indicated in cases of vascular etiology or the presence of a cervical rib and classic electrodiagnostic findings. Post surgical complications are of concern.

LONG THORACIC NERVE

- **Anatomy and origin:** The C5/C6 and occasionally also C7 anterior primary rami join to form the long thoracic nerve. It crosses the first rib, lies behind the brachial plexus and then runs down the lateral chest wall, giving off branches to the eight digitations of the serratus anterior.
- **Risk factors:** Compression/entrapment injuries are not common, but can occur after weightlifting exercises, in climbers, carrying heavy backpacks, in backstroke swimmers (Bateman, 1967), wrestlers, gymnasts, bowlers, golfers, soccer, volleyball, hockey, and football players (Gregg et al, 1979), motor vehicle accidents, and chiropractic manipulation. Depression of the shoulder girdle by a blow to the shoulder or downward traction of the arm may cause compression of the long thoracic nerve against the 2nd rib (Gozna and Harris, 1979). Differential diagnosis must include neuralgic amyotrophy. Scapular winging is not an unusual presentation for this disease (Suarez et al, 1996).
- **Symptoms and signs:** Scapular winging may be seen in the subject while standing with arms at the side; the inferior angle of the scapula is translocated medially. Pushing the hands/arms in forward flexion against a wall exaggerates the winging. No sensory changes are noted.
- Prognosis for spontaneous recovery is good, except in the case of root avulsion. Physical therapy includes resistive exercises and general shoulder muscle strengthening (in absence of denervation). A temporary shoulder sling support may avoid discomfort.

AXILLARY NERVE

- **Anatomy and origin:** Fifth and 6th nerve roots. Fibers travel through the upper trunk of the brachial plexus, then the posterior divisions and posterior cord. The first terminal branch is the axillary nerve. The nerve passes through the quadrilateral space (risk area

for compression). It then divides into a posterior trunk that supplies the teres minor muscle and the posterior deltoid, and terminates as the superior lateral brachial cutaneous nerve. The anterior trunk supplies the anterior and middle deltoid. Bounderies of the quadrilateral space are teres minor superior, teres major inferior, long head of the triceps medial, and the surgical neck of the humerus lateral. The axillary nerve and the posterior humeral circumflex artery traverse this space. The axillary nerve is the most common nerve effected in shoulder lesions.

- Compression injuries are observed as *quadrilateral space syndrome* (Cahill and Palmer, 1983). At risk are throwing athletes. Other sports placing participants at risk are football, crew, swimming, and backpacking. Lesions may also be due to a direct blow to the deltoid (percussion/contusion), after glenohumeral joint dislocation 12.3% (Toolanan et al, 1993) or humerus fracture or surgical procedures.
- **Symptoms and signs:** Isolated axillary nerve injury in contact sports may be unnoticed at first. In quadrilateral space syndrome there is posterior shoulder pain, and paresthesias over the lateral arm and weakness of the deltoid. Forward flexion and/or abduction and external rotation of the humerus aggravate the symptoms. Muscle hypertrophy and possibly fibrous bands are believed to be the cause (Cahill and Palmer, 1983). Subclavian arteriography may show compression of the posterior humeral circumflex artery with abduction and external rotation of the arm (Cahill and Palmer, 1983).
- Many, especially young subjects, recover full shoulder abduction even with continued denervation of the deltoid muscle by substituting the supraspinatus muscle for the deltoid. Throwing athletes experience difficulty. The deltoid provides 50% of the torque about the shoulder. With a direct blow to the deltoid prognosis is poorer than with lesions from other causes. Functional outcome, however, can still be adequate (Perlmutter, Leffert, and Zarins, 1997).
- **Treatment:** Rest in the acute phase and treatment of bony or other injuries as indicated. ROM, passive exercises to rotator cuff muscles, deltoid, and periscapular muscles, progressing to resistive exercises, after cessation of denervation. Shoulder contracture must be avoided. If there is no sign of reinnervation noted within 3–6 months after injury, surgical exploration of the axillary nerve may have to be considered. Neurolysis or nerve grafting (sural, neurotization with thoracodorsal, spinal accessory or intercostal nerves have been tried) can restore axillary nerve function (Perlmutter, Leffert, and Zarins, 1997).
- Surgery for quadrilateral space syndrome: Decompression by the release of fascia and fibrous

bands around the axillary nerve and posterior humeral circumflex vessels (Cahill and Palmer, 1983).

SUPRASCAPULAR NERVE

- **Anatomy and origin:** The C5–C6 nerve roots. Fibers travel through the upper trunk of the brachial plexus, pass through the supraclavicular fossa, and then through the scapular notch (incisura scapulae), covered by the transverse scapular ligament (the 1st site of possible entrapment). After innervating, and passing through the supraspinatus muscle, the suprascapular nerve bends around the spine of the scapula to innervate the infraspinatus (the 2nd site of potential entrapment, if enclosed by the spinoglenoid ligament, which is present in about 50% of people) (Pecina, 2001).
- **Risk factors:** Traumatic *risk factors* for compression of the suprascapular nerve include fracture of the scapula, rotator cuff tear, and shoulder arthrodesis. Nontraumatic risk factors include repetitive overhead loading activities, such as experienced in volleyball, tennis, weightlifting, boxing, basketball, baseball, and painting. Other sources of compression are backpack straps or ganglion cysts at the scapular notch.
- **Symptoms and signs:** Vague shoulder or *acromioclavicular* (AC) joint pain. Weakness and atrophy may be apparent in the supra- and infraspinatus muscles. Pain or a Tinel sign may be present upon palpation of the scapular notch. Overhead activities may worsen the symptoms. The crossed arm abduction test should exacerbate symptoms on the effected side. The differential diagnosis is cervical radiculopathy, diskogenic pain, shoulder or AC joint pathology, rotator cuff tear, or musculoskeletal pain syndromes.
- **Treatment:** Avoidance of exacerbating activities, e.g., overhead. Physical therapy should focus on maintaining ROM of the scapula, and on improving muscle strength. Dysfunction of scapulohumeral rhythm should be corrected as possible. Injection of local anesthetic into the scapular notch may assist in the diagnosis and the treatment. Most patients will respond to conservative measures; however, in some, surgical release may be necessary (release of the transverse scapular ligament with or without widening of the scapular foramen).

MUSCULOCUTANEOUS NERVE

- **Anatomy and origin:** The musculocutaneous nerve is the terminal nerve of the lateral cord of the brachial plexus (fibers from the C5–C7). It innervates the coracobrachialis, brachialis, and biceps brachii muscles. Its sensory terminal branch, the lateral antebrachial cutaneous nerve, innervates the volar and dorsal forearm along its radial aspect, but not the hand.
- **Risk factors:** Compression of the musculocutaneus nerve is uncommon. Shoulder dislocation is a risk factor. Nontraumatic lesions may occur during exercises, especially excessive resistive elbow extension, as in push-ups or arm presses (weightlifters) a hypertrophic coracobrachialis muscle may entrap the musculocutaneous nerve where it pierces the muscle. Entrapment of the sensory branch distal to the biceps aponeurosis, as the nerve enters the forearm is noted to occur in association with strongly resisted extension and pronation of the elbow.
- **Symptoms and signs:** Entrapment at the proximal site presents with elbow flexor weakness, lateral arm pain, and/or loss of sensation. A positive Tinel's sign and decreased biceps reflex may be observed. Entrapment at the distal location presents with lateral arm pain and numbness only. A positive Tinel's sign may also be elicited.
- **Treatment:** Rest, ROM exercises and gentle stretching, and anti-inflammatory medication and modalities. Entrapment of the lateral antebrachial cutaneous nerve near the cubital fossa mostly needs surgical decompression. Good long term outcome has been reported (Davidson, Nunley, and Bassett, 1998).

RADIAL NERVE

- **Anatomy and origin:** C5–C8 nerve roots. Fibers run between the medial and long heads of the triceps, through the spiral groove. There are four sites of potential entrapment. There is entrapment site 1 where the nerve gives off motor branches to the extensor carpi radialis longus muscle prior to and to the extensor carpi radialis brevis muscle after entering the cubital fossa. Just proximal to entering the supinator muscle, the radial nerve gives off the superficial radial nerve (sensory, which supplies sensation to the dorsum of the wrist, hand, and dorsum of the first three and one half digits). It then pierces the supinator at the Arcade of Frohse (entrapment site 3) and becomes the posterior interosseous nerve that is purely motor. It supplies the extensor forearm muscles. Cutaneous (sensory) nerve supply to the arm is by two branches to the posterior skin of the arm and one for the dorsal forearm, the posterior antebrachial cutaneous, which branches off the radial nerve in the proximal arm and runs with the main radial nerve through the spiral groove. It supplies a strip of skin over the dorsum of the forearm and wrist.

ENTRAPMENT SITE 1

- A common cause of radial nerve entrapment in this area is *humerus fracture*. The estimated incidence is 10–18% (Bodner et al, 2001). Most are neurapraxic, with return of function by 4–5 months (Kimura, 2001). *Saturday night/honeymooner's palsy,* the most common nontraumatic radial nerve lesion in the upper arm is also due to compression near the spiral groove. Deep sleep (mostly after excessive alcohol consumption) prevents awareness of discomfort and repositioning.
- **Symptoms and signs:** Frequently there is deformity of the humerus. Neurologic lesion presents with a wrist drop, slight weakness of elbow flexion caused by involvement of the brachioradialis. The triceps may be involved, but frequently is not. The triceps reflex may or may not be absent. There may be pain or numbness in the posterior antebrachial cutaneous and mostly in the superficial radial nerve distribution.
- **Treatment:** Bony stability is the first requirement in preventing further radial nerve injury after humerus fracture. Most radial nerve lesions are neurapraxic. Treatment can be conservative management, if nerve continuity can be demonstrated with stimulation study. If spontaneous recovery does not occur in several months surgical exploration is indicated.

ENTRAPMENT SITES 2 AND 3

- **Anatomy:** At the elbow the radial nerve passes through the radial tunnel (entrapment site 2), which is formed by the lateral intermuscular septum, the brachialis and brachioradialis muscles, until it reaches the supinator (the end of the radial tunnel). *Radial tunnel syndrome* is controversial. It usually refers to a treatment resistant chronic tennis-elbow. There is no definite neurologic deficit that can be demonstrated clinically or by electrodiagnosis.
- **Posterior interosseous nerve:** Syndrome is a compression at the Arcade of Frohse where the radial nerve pierces the supinator and becomes the *posterior interosseous nerve* (PIN), which is purely motor. *Risks* are mainly repetitive motion, scarring, lipomas, or other space occupying lesions. Imaging may help to demonstrate the cause. Surgery is frequently needed to free the nerve.
- **Symptoms and signs:** Partial wrist drop with radially deviated wrist extension present. No sensory deficits. Interossei appear weak secondary to loss of wrist stabilization.
- **Treatment:** Conservative management. If no improvement, consider surgical release.

ENTRAPMENT SITE 4—HANDCUFF NEUROPATHY

- *Handcuff neuropathy* occurs at the wrist and is mostly a purely sensory lesion, where the superficial radial nerve is compressed against the radius. *At risk* are prisoners—most common neurologic complaint of US prisoners returning from Operation Desert Storm (Cook, 1993). With more severe injury multiple nerves may be involved. Recovery is mostly complete within 6–8 weeks. Symptoms include sensory deficits in superficial sensory nerve distribution. Treatment is through conservative management.

MEDIAN NERVE

- The median nerve is one of the three nerves supplying all muscles of the forearm and hand.
- **Anatomy and origin:** C6–T1 nerve roots/spinal nerves. It traverses the upper, middle, and lower trunk, the anterior divisions, and the lateral and medial cord. It has five sites of potential entrapment.

ENTRAPMENT SITE 1—LIGAMENT OF STRUTHERS

- **Anatomy:** Some subjects have an anomalous supracondylar process on the humerus, from which a fibrous band arises and attaches to its medial epicondyle. This structure can entrap the median and/or the ulnar nerves and the brachial artery.
- **Risk factor:** At risk are the 2.7% of the population who have the anomaly.
- **Symptoms and signs:** Tingling, numbness, and weakness in all median innervated muscles. Sometimes the ulnar nerve may also be entrapped. Imaging studies may demonstrate the presence of the anomaly.
- **Treatment:** The reduction of aggravating activities and anti-inflammatory medications may help some, but surgery will usually be the treatment of choice.

ENTRAPMENT SITE 2—PRONATOR SYNDROME

- **Anatomy:** In the antecubital area the median nerve is located underneath the bicipital aponeurosis (lacertus fibrosus). Then it passes between the superficial and deep heads of the pronator teres, located underneath the flexor digitorum superficialis. Entrapment by these structures is known as pronator syndrome. An accessory head of the *flexor pollicis longus* (FPL) called Gantzer's muscle may also contribute to the pronator as well as the anterior interosseous nerve syndrome (site 3). An anomalous isolated brachialis muscle tendon may cause compression.
- **At risk:** At risk are pianists, fiddlers, harpists, baseball players, machine milkers, dentists.
- **Symptoms and signs:** Pain on active resistive forearm pronation. There may be cramping of fingers or *writer's cramp*. Provocative maneuvers include paresthesias in the hand after 30 s or less of manual compression of the

median nerve over the pronator teres muscle. Tinel's test may be positive, Phalen's test is negative.

- **Treatment:** Rest, splinting, anti-inflammatories, and/or steroid injections into the area of entrapment. If there is no improvement in 6 months, surgical exploration and release of offending structure leads to full recovery unless severe axonotmesis is present (Eversmann, 1992).

ENTRAPMENT SITE 3—ANTERIOR INTEROSSEOUS NERVE SYNDROME (KILOH-NEVIN SYNDROME)

- **Anatomy:** In the forearm, the median nerve gives off a large deep motor branch, the anterior interosseous nerve that supplies the flexor pollicis longus, the two lateral flexor digitorum profundus muscles and the pronator quadratus. Anterior interosseous nerve lesions are rare.
- **Risk factors:** Most discussions are case reports of complications with supracondylar humerus fracture (especially in children), or venipuncture. Anatomic variants also play a role. An important differential is neuralgic amyotrophy (brachial plexitis).
- **Symptoms and signs:** No sensory symptoms. A specific test is the "O" sign. Patients are unable to hold, and resist opening of an index to thumb tip to tip pinch. The two distal phalanges align flat against each other to hold the pinch. There is no sensory deficit.
- **Treatment:** Usually conservative management. Surgical exploration may become necessary.

ENTRAPMENT SITE 4—CARPAL TUNNEL SYNDROME

- **Anatomy:** At the wrist the median nerve (except for the sensory fibers supplying an area on the thenar eminence) passes through the carpal tunnel (entrapment site 4). It is formed by the arched carpal bones covered by the carpal ligament, which spans from the pisiform and hamate to the trapezium and scaphoid. It contains the median nerve, the tendons of the flexor digitorum superficialis, profundus, flexor pollicis longus, and flexor carpi radialis. In the hand, the median nerve supplies the lateral two lumbricals, and most of the thenar muscles, except for the deep head of the flexor pollicis brevis. Sensory fibers after traveling through the carpal tunnel supply the lateral $3^1/_2$ digits (entrapment site 5) and the lateral palm, except for a small area over the thenar eminence.
- CTS is the most common compression syndrome, even though not always symptomatic; most often bilateral, one being more involved than the other.
- **Risk factors:** Repetitive motion activities (jobs), low ratio of depth to width (<0.70) of the wrist (Gordon et al, 1988), hypothyroidism, pregnancy, and other causes of excessive soft tissue swelling, cycling,

wheelchair athletics, tennis, baseball, volleyball, violin, and piano playing.

- **Symptoms and signs:** Nocturnal numbness, tingling, and wrist pain. Symptoms increase with activities. Subjects are *dropping things*. There is sensory impairment in a median nerve distribution, and weak hand grip. When holding a pinch against resistance, the patient frequently will use the ulnar innervated deep flexor pollicis to oppose the index, instead of the APB.
- **Treatment:** Splinting, at night and during activities that provoke increased symptoms; avoidance of constant wearing of assistive device to prevent disuse atrophy; anti-inflammatories; Pyridoxine (deficiency often present); steroid injections surgical release.

ENTRAPMENT SITE 5—DIGITAL NERVE ENTRAPMENT

- **Anatomy:** Median nerve sensory nerve fibers are located on the medial and lateral side of digits 1–3 and on the lateral side of digit 4. They may become entrapped. *At risk* are baseball players, bowlers, flutists (lateral side of left index finger), violinists, cellists (right thumb), percussionists (left middle finger), and vibration exposure (vibration syndrome).
- **Treatment:** Anti-inflammatory drugs and splinting may reduce the acuteness of the syndrome. Steroid injections or surgical release are the treatments of choice.

ULNAR NERVE

- The ulnar nerve supplies only two muscles in the forearm and with the median nerve all intrinsic muscles of the hand. There are five distinct areas of potential entrapment.

ENTRAPMENT SITE 1—LIGAMENT OF STRUTHERS ENTRAPMENT

- **Anatomy:** The ulnar nerve (C8—T1) travels through the medial cord of the brachial plexus. It accompanies the brachial artery and the median nerve in a neurovascular bundle. The nerve then passes distally, between the coracobrachialis and triceps muscles. At the midpoint of the upper arm, the nerve enters the posterior compartment of the arm by piercing the intermuscular septum. The nerve runs along the medial head of the triceps in a tough investing fascia that comprises the *arcade of Struthers* (risk factor) (entrapment site 1).
- **Symptoms and signs:** Similar to those of median nerve compression at the same site.
- **Treatment:** Conservative management is usually not adequate. Surgery to release the constricting band is often favored.

ENTRAPMENT SITE 2—ULNAR SULCUS—TARDY ULNAR PALSY

- **Anatomy:** At the elbow the nerve leaves this fascia and passes posterior to the medial epicondyle of the humerus (ulnar sulcus—entrapment site 2). Compression at the elbow is the second most common nerve entrapment of the upper extremity. Common *risk factors* are leaning on elbows, tight casts after fracture, compressive trauma, wrestling without elbow pads, excessive flexion (as in prolonged driving), and extension have been implicated as causes of this problem. Anatomic predisposition to tardy ulnar palsy (Kimura, 2001) is also a risk factor.
- **Symptoms and signs:** Pain, paresthesia, and/or numbness in the volar aspect of the fifth and median fourth digits, and over the hypothenar eminence of the affected hand, increasing with elbow flexion. Motor weakness and/or atrophy often presents in the hand intrinsic muscles innervated by the ulnar nerve. Flexion contracture of the PIP, digit V or a claw hand may be present (partial flexion of the proximal and distal interphalangeal joints, with extension of the metacarpophalangeal joints). Grip strength may be diminished.
- **Treatment:** Conservative course of pain control, occupational therapy for muscle strengthening and maintaining the range of motion. Relative rest should include avoiding exacerbating activities. Padding and/or splinting around the elbow may be used. If neurologic symptoms are progressive, surgery may be required. Two primary surgical procedures used are simple *ulnar nerve release* (UNR) and *ulnar nerve transposition* (UNT). It should be recognized that the UNT is a relatively more involved procedure with a higher complication rate, including reentrapment.

ENTRAPMENT SITE 3—CUBITAL TUNNEL SYNDROME

- **Anatomy:** The ulnar nerve enters the cubital tunnel at the *humeroulnar aponeurotic arcade* (HUA). It lies on the ulnar collateral ligament between the two heads of the flexor carpi ulnaris. The nerve passes beneath the HUA, pierces the *flexor carpi ulnaris* FCU, and then exits at the distal end of the cubital tunnel through the *deep flexor pronator aponeurosis* (DFPA). The length of the cubital tunnel may be from 4–5 cm. Entrapment may occur at the entrance, midpoint, or exit of the tunnel.
- **Risk factors:** Lesions here are most often nontraumatic, repetitive motion injuries, and may have an anatomical predisposition.
- **Symptoms and signs:** Clinical presentation of the cubital tunnel syndrome will be similar to compression at the *retrocondylar* (RTC) groove, making these

diagnoses a challenge to distinguish from each other. A positive Tinel's sign over the cubital tunnel instead of over the RTC groove may be one of only a few differentiating clinical findings. Symptoms include Wartenberg's sign of weakness with fifth finger abduction, and Froment's sign (flexion of the thumb to activate the FPL). This may be observed by asking the patient to pinch a piece of paper between first and second metacarpals. In response to a strong pull on the paper, the patient contracts the FPL to substitute for the weak first dorsal interosseus and adductor pollicis muscles.
- **Treatment:** For cubital tunnel syndrome is initially conservative, as in the case of tardy ulnar palsy, mentioned above. Should symptoms progress with motor decline, surgery should be considered. The procedure of choice for nontraumatic cubital tunnel syndrome is a cubital tunnel release.

ENTRAPMENT SITES 4 AND 5

- **Anatomy:** These sites are at the wrist at Guyon's canal and/or in the palm. Borders are medially the pisiform bone, laterally the hook of the hamate, the roof is the tendon of the FCU and the floor the carpal ligament. In the canal the ulnar nerve divides into two branches. The deep branch accompanied by the ulnar artery winds around the hook of the hamate, supplies the interossei, the 3rd and 4th lumbricals, the adductor pollicis, the 1st dorsal interosseous and the deep head of the flexor pollicis brevis. The superficial branch supplies the palmaris brevis and terminates as sensory nerve to digits 4 and 5.
- **Risk factors:** Bicycle riding, push-ups, flute or violin playing, occupational trauma, scars, ganglion cysts, ulnar artery aneurysms, and lipomas. Compression after exit from Guyon's canal (palmar branch) results in weakness of ulnar innervated intrinsics, but no sensory deficit. Occasionally the abductor digiti minimi is spared. This syndrome is seen in bicyclists due to the pressure on the *horn handlebars* even after one ride, which formerly (using different handlebars) was only observed after prolonged multiple rides. Compression of superficial and deep branches within the canal affects motor and sensory branches. Compression of superficial branch in the canal causes sensory loss of the ulnar half of the 4th digit and the 5th digit.
- **Symptoms and signs:** Wrist pain, weakness especially in grasp, numbness, tingling in ulnar nerve distribution, worse at night. Physical examination may confirm the weakness in grasp and finger abduction. If sensory involvement is present, loss is in ulnar nerve distribution. Provocative maneuvers that may be positive are Tinel's, Phalen's, or reverse Phalen's (Wormer's test).

• **Treatment:** Conservative management—including activity modification, NSAIDs, padding, and steroid injections. If there is no improvement in 6 months, surgery is considered.

REFERENCES

Bateman JE: Nerve injuries about the shoulder in sports. *J Bone Joint Surg [Am]* 49:785–792, 1967.

Bigliani LU, Compito CA, Duralde XA, et al: Transfer of the levator scapulae, and rhomboid minor for paralysis of the trapezius. *J Bone Joint Surg* 78A:1534–1540, 1996.

Bodner G, Buchberger W, Schocke M, et al: Radial nerve palsy associated with humeral shaft fracture. *Radiology* 219(3): 811–816, 2001.

Cahill BR, Palmer RE: Quadrilateral space syndrome. *J Hand Surg* 8:65–69, 1983.

Castro FP: Stingers, cervical cord neurapraxia, and stenosis. *Clin Sports Med* 22:4893–92, 2003.

Codman EA: Rupture of the supraspinatus tendon and other lesions on or about the subacromial bursa. In Codman EA (ed.), *The Shoulder.* Boston, MA, Thomas Todd, 1934, pp 32–64.

Cook, AA: Handcuff neuropathy among prisoners of war from operation desert storm military medicine. *Mil Med* 158(4): 253–254, 1993 Apr.

Cramer CR: Reconditioning program to lower the recurrence rate of brachial plexus neurapraxia in collegiate football players. *J Athl Train* 34(4):390–396, 1999.

Davidson JJ, Nunley JA, Bassett FH: Musculocutaneous nerve entrapment revisited. *J Shoulder Elbow Surg* 7(3):250–255, 1998.

Di Benedetto M, Markey K: Electrodiagnostic localization of traumatic upper trunk brachial plexopathy. *Arch Phys Med Rehabil* 65(1):15–17, 1984.

Dumitru D, Amato AA, Zwarts MJ (eds.): *Electrodiagnostic Medicine,* 2nd ed. Philadelphia, PA, Hanley & Belfus, 2002.

Eversmann WW: Proximal median nerve compression. *Hand Clinics* 8(2):307–315, 1992.

Ewing MR, Martin H: Disability following radical neck dissection. *Cancer* 5:873–883, 1952.

Gordon C, Johnson EW, Gatens PF, et al: Wrist ratio correlation with carpal tunnel syndrome in industry. *Am J Phys Med Rehabil* 67(6):270–272, 1988.

Gozna ER, Harris WR: Traumatic winging of the scapula. *J Bone Joint Surg [Am]* 61(8):1230–1233, 1979.

Gregg JR, Labosky D, Harty M, et al: Serratus anterior paralysis in the young athlete. *J Bone Joint Surg [Am]* 63:825–832, 1979.

Kelly JD, Aliquo D, Sitler MR, et al: Association of burners with cervical canal and foraminal stenosis. *Am J Sports Med* 28(2): 214–217, 2000.

Kimura, J: *Electrodiagnosis in Diseases of Nerve and Muscle: Principles and Practice,* 3rd ed. New York, Oxford University Press, pp 717–718, 2001.

Krivickas LS, Wilbourne AJ: Peripheral nerve injuries in athletes: a case series of over 200 injuries. *Semin Neurol* 20(2):225–232, 2000.

Lange M: Die Behandlung der irreparablem Trapeziuslahmung: Langenbecks Arch. *Klin Chir* 270:437–439, 1951.

Markey K, Di Benedetto M, Curl WW: Upper trunk brachial plexopathy: The stinger syndrome. *Am J Sports Med* 21:650–656, 1993.

Pecina M: Who really first described and explained the suprascapular nerve entrapment syndrome? *J Bone Joint Surg [Am]* 83(8):1273–1274, 2001.

Perlmutter GS, Leffert RD, Zarins B: Direct injury to the axillary nerve in athletes playing contact sports. *Am J Sports Med* 25:65–68, 1997.

Suarez GA, Giannini C, Bosch EP, et al: Immune brachial plexus neuropathy suggestiveevidence for an inflammatory-immune pathogenesis. *Neurology* 46:559–561, 1996.

Toolanan G, Hildingsson C, Hedlund T, et al: Early complications after anterior dislocation of the shoulder in patients over 40 years. *Acta Orthop Scand* 64:549–552, 1993.

Weinberg J, Rokito S, Silber JS: Etiology, treatment and prevention of athletic "stingers." *Clin Sports Med* 21:493–500, 2003.

Weinstein SM: Assessment and Rehabilitation of the athlete with a "stinger." *Clin Sports Med* 17(1):127–135, 1998.

Wiater JM, Bigliani LU: Spinal accessory nerve injury. *Clin Orthop* 368:5–16, 1999.

Wilbourn AJ: Thoracic outlet syndromes. *Neurol Clin* 17(3): 477–497, 1999.

Wilbourn AJ, Aminoff MJ: AAEM minimonograph 32: the electrodiagnostic examination in patients with radiculopathies. *Muscle Nerve* 21(12):1612–1631, 1998.

56 MAGNETIC RESONANCE IMAGING: LOWER EXTREMITY

Carolyn M Sofka, MD

HIP

• Magnetic resonance (MR) imaging of the hip should be performed with dedicated surface coils and small field of view for high resolution imaging of the articular cartilage and acetabular labrum.

• MR arthrography of the hip is advocated by some to diagnose cartilage injuries in the hip (Schmid et al, 2002); however, noncontrast MR imaging of the hip can noninvasively diagnose osteochondral injuries (Weaver et al, 2002).

• Tears of the acetabular labrum are usually seen to best advantage on sagittal sequences (Fig. 56-1). A tear is diagnosed as a focal linear hyperintensity undermining

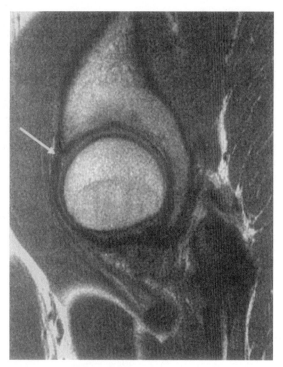

FIG. 56-1 Sagittal fast spin echo image of the hip demonstrating a tear of the anterior labrum (arrow).

the normally well-defined, hypointense, triangular acetabular labrum.
- Cartilage-sensitive pulse sequences are necessary to adequately evaluate for subtle areas of chondromalacia over the femoral head.
- A large field-of-view water sensitive pulse sequence (fast inversion recovery) should be performed to evaluate for other possible causes of hip pain: degenerative disc disease, sacroiliac joint pathology, possible sacral or pubic ramus insufficiency fracture, or bursitis.
- In addition to the hip joint proper, MR imaging of the hip can evaluate the regional muscles and tendons. With the adductor insertion avulsion syndrome ("thigh splints"), patients have mid thigh pain that is activity-related; MR imaging demonstrates hyperintensity and periosteal reaction along the mid femur. Findings are thought to be related to traction injury of the adductor longus and brevis tendons (Anderson, Kaplan, and Dussault, 2001).
- Subchondral insuffiency fractures, transient osteoporosis, and avascular necrosis of the femoral may all have similar clinical presentation. In the acute stage, MR findings may only include edema in the femoral head and neck; a discrete subchondral fracture line or a zone of demarcation in the setting of avascular necrosis may not be visible on large field-of-view images. Small field of view and dedicated surface

coils of the hip are necessary to visualize subtle fracture lines and early avascular necrosis.
- MR is of value in imaging the hip after a dislocation, to evaluate the soft tissue envelope as well as for evaluating for any osteochondral injuries and possible intra-articular chondral fragments.
- Tendinosis of the tendons about the hip is seen as thickening, hyperintensity, and ill-definition of the normally uniformly hypointense (dark) tendon.

KNEE

- In general three planes of imaging should be performed in addition to at least one fat suppression sequence to evaluate for bone marrow edema. High resolution imaging of the menisci is also suggested.
- Normal ligaments and tendons about the knee are uniformly hypointense (Fig. 56-2 and 56-3). In general, the sagittal sequence is best for evaluating the cruciate ligaments and the coronal sequence for evaluating the collateral ligamentous complexes. The cruciate ligaments, however, have an oblique course; and areas of potential signal abnormality should be confirmed in two planes, as some of the signal may be fictitious due to volume average with the ligament passing out of the plane of imaging.
- Cartilage sensitive pulse sequences are suggested for routine imaging of the knee. Cartilage should normally be intermediate signal intensity and of uniform thickness. Occasionally, the laminar microstructure of

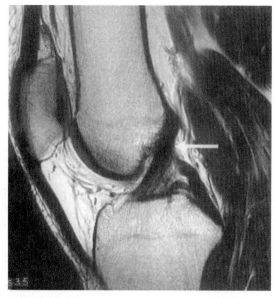

FIG. 56-2 Sagittal fast spin echo image demonstrating a normal hypointense anterior cruciate ligament (arrow).

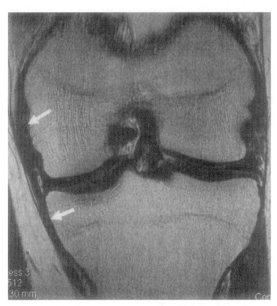

FIG. 56-3 Coronal fast spin echo image demonstrating a normal medial collateral ligament (arrows).

articular cartilage can be resolved (Waldschmidt et al, 1997) (Fig. 56-4).

- The high accuracy of MR imaging for diagnosing internal derangement of the knee has been demonstrated, with high reliability and accuracy in directing clinical treatment. A large series of 200 patients who had MR of the knee had arthroscopic correlation (Vincken et al, 2002). At the conclusion of the study, 179 of the 200 patients were felt to have had a need for

arthroscopic treatment based on the MR findings (MR sensitivity 93.2%, specificity 79.2%). Indications for arthroscopic surgery diagnosed on MR imaging included meniscal tears, cartilage lesions, cruciate ligament injuries, collateral ligament injuries, and synovial disorders.

- Magnetic resonance imaging, particularly of the knee and shoulder, are becoming some of the most requested diagnostic imaging tests (Helms, 2002).
- MR imaging has a high sensitivity for diagnosing bone marrow edema. Causes of bone marrow edema pattern are varied and include trauma, avascular necrosis, reactive edema due to altered weight-bearing and biomechanics or arthritic changes. In one study of 17 asymptomatic basketball players, 14 were found to have bone marrow edema (41%) suggesting that MR findings should be taken in concert with the clinical presentation (Major and Helms, 2002).
- Bone marrow contusion patterns seen on MR imaging often correlate with the mechanism of injury. For example, a valgus load applied to the knee, when the knee is in a degree of flexion, as in cases of clipping injuries in football or skiing injuries, result in tears of the anterior cruciate ligament (Sanders et al, 2000). The tibia anteriorly subluxes, and the posterolateral margin of the tibia impacts against the lateral femoral condyle (Fig. 56-5(*a*)). The bone marrow contusion

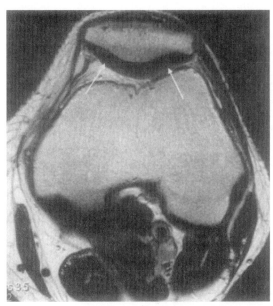

FIG. 56-4 Axial fast spin echo image demonstrating normal uniform thickness of articular cartilage over the patellar facets.

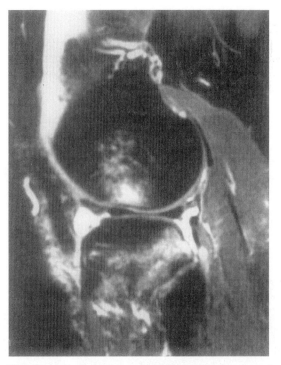

FIG. 56-5(a) Sagittal fat suppression image demonstrating bone marrow contusion pattern involving the anterior aspect of the lateral femoral condyle and the posterolateral aspect of the tibia.

pattern seen on MR imaging typically is one of edema in the posterior aspect of the tibia as well as the anterior margin of the lateral femoral condyle, just superior to the anterior horn of the lateral meniscus.

- There are many injury patterns and mechanisms encountered in sports injuries to the knee. These (and their resultant ligamentous injuries) include pure hyperextension (*posterior cruciate ligament* (PCL) and posterior capsule), hyperextension with varus (posterolateral corner, *anterior cruciate ligament* (ACL), popliteus tendon, posterior capsule), hyperextension with valgus (*medial collateral ligament* (MCL), posteromedial corner, posterior capsule, PCL), pure valgus (MCL, ACL ± PCL), pure varus (iliotibial band, *lateral collateral ligament* (LCL)), flexion valgus, external rotation (MCL, ACL), flexion varus, internal rotation (ACL, posterolateral corner), flexion with posterior tibial translation (isolated PCL, possible posterior dislocation), and a patellar dislocation (flexion and internal rotation of femur on fixed tibia) (medial patellar retinaculum, MCL, possible ACL) (Hayes et al, 2000).
- In view of anterior cruciate ligament injuries, determination of a full thickness tear is made by observing a focal discontinuity in the ligament fibers (Fig. 56-5(*b*)).
- Additional secondary signs of ACL injury may support the diagnosis at MR imaging. One of these is the Segond fracture, which is an avulsion fracture of the lateral tibial plateau, indicative of injury to the lateral capsule and often concomitant ACL injury (Goldman, Pavlov, and Rubenstein, 1988).
- Partial ACL tears are diagnosed by observing only a few fibers in discontinuity; these should be graded as high or low-grade injuries depending on the cross sectional area of ligament fibers that are affected. As

noted above, as the anterior cruciate ligament is an oblique structure and confirming the diagnosis of a partial ACL tear in another plane may be necessary; some authors have found the axial plane to be particularly helpful (Roychowdhury et al, 1997).

- Other MR findings in cases of ACL tears include a buckled posterior cruciate ligament with anterior translation of the tibia, an uncovered posterior horn of the lateral meniscus, visualizing the fibular collateral ligament in one coronal image due to anterior translation of the tibia and injury to the medial collateral ligament (Brandser et al, 1996).
- Postoperatively, the anterior cruciate ligament can be evaluated with MR imaging. Care should be taken in the postoperative setting to utilize fast spin echo sequences and fast inversion recovery as opposed to frequency selective fat suppression as a water-sensitive pulse sequence to evaluate for bone marrow edema as the latter is more susceptible to regional magnetic field inhomogeneities and will result in moderate to severe susceptibility artifact.
- As with the native ACL, tears of ACL grafts are diagnosed as focal areas of ligamentous discontinuity and partial tears as areas of partial ligamentous discontinuity (Horton et al, 2000).
- Normally, the postoperative anterior cruciate ligament graft should be parallel to the roof of the intercondylar notch as seen in the sagittal plane and should not demonstrate any areas of focal angulation or kinking (Schatz et al, 1997).
- After a complete knee dislocation, all of the supporting ligamentous structures of the knee can potentially be injured. These can all be evaluated with MR imaging. In the setting of a complete knee dislocation, magnetic resonance angiography can be performed to

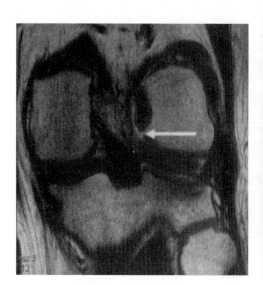 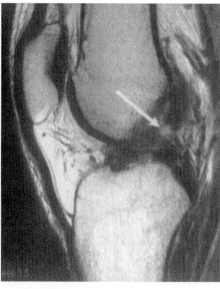

FIG. 56-5(b) Coronal (left) and sagittal (right) fast spin echo images of the knee demonstrating a complete tear of the anterior cruciate ligament (arrows).

evaluate the integrity of the popliteal artery and geniculate vessels (Potter et al, 2002).

- The *cyclops lesion*, a localized, often mass-like, form of arthrofibrosis seen postoperative ACL repair, has been demonstrated with high sensitivity and specificity on MR imaging (Bradley, Bergman, and Dillingham, 2000).

- Ganglion formation in ACL grafts, seen as thickening and hyperintensity of the graft without any other MR evidence for traumatic injury occurs not infrequently post-ACL reconstruction, especially noted with gracilis or semitendinosis autografts (Schatz et al, 1997).

- The meniscus is seen at MR imaging as a triangular hypointense focus of fibrocartilage on sagittal sequences. The posterior horn of the medial meniscus should be larger than the anterior horn on sagittal sequences. The lateral meniscus is less fixed to the tibia than the medial meniscus and therefore is less likely to be injured.

- The lateral meniscus is more circular in shape than the medial meniscus.

- Meniscal tears are diagnosed as abnormal linear hyperintense (fluid) signal reaching an articular surface as well as abnormal morphology. Wedge-shaped degenerative signal (sometimes classified as grade 2C signal) does not usually correlate with patient symptomatology (McCauley et al, 2002).

- When evaluating for meniscal tears, one should look for displaced meniscal fragments (Fig. 56-6). Bucket handle tears are a specific category of meniscal tears

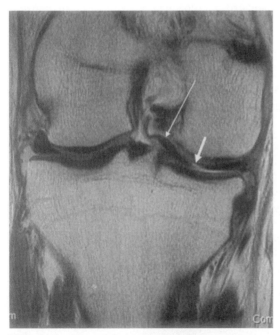

FIG. 56-6 Coronal fast spin echo MR image demonstrating a tear of the medial meniscus (short thick white arrow) with a displaced fragment of hypointense fibrocartilage into the intercondylar notch (long thin white arrow).

in which the meniscus is cleaved in an anteroposterior direction and the inner margin of the meniscus is displaced into the intercondylar notch; this often results in the "double PCL" sign whereby the paramidline sagittal sequence demonstrates an additional hypointense curvilinear density deep to and in addition to the posterior cruciate ligament.

- If a meniscal tear is found at MR imaging, the tear should be categorized as a horizontal, vertical, or radial split tear. In addition, the location of the tear with respect to the periphery in the anteroposterior dimension is important in determining repairability of the tear. The more in the periphery the tear is, the greater the vascular supply and therefore the greater likelihood of viability if the tear is repaired.

- Meniscal cysts, often encountered in cases of degenerative tears of the menisci, have been reported to occur with greater frequency in the medial compartment than laterally (Campbell, Sanders, and Morrison, 2001).

- Postoperatively, recurrent meniscal tears can be diagnosed with unenhanced MR imaging as well as MR arthrography. A slightly higher specificity for recurrent meniscal tears has been demonstrated with direct MR arthrography compared with unenhanced magnetic resonance imaging (78 vs. 67%); however, sensitivity is similar at 83 and 86% as well as positive predictive value of 90 versus 83%, respectively (White et al, 2002).

- There is a high accuracy of evaluating articular cartilage abnormalities with appropriate MR pulse sequences. A prospective study evaluating 616 articular surfaces in the knee with specific cartilage-sensitive pulse sequences found an accuracy of 92% of MR compared with arthroscopy (Potter et al, 1998).

- Surgical repair of articular cartilage defects can include microfracture, autologous chondrocyte implantation, fresh cadaver allografts, and mosaicplasty (Minas and Nehrer, 1997; Kish, Modis, and Hangody, 1999), all of which can be imaged with MR post operatively.

- Some authors have suggested a correlation between the presence of subchondral bone marrow edema and clinical outcome in cases of chondral injuries (Rubin, Harner, and Costello, 2000).

- Osteochondral injuries can occur on any articular surface. The classic *osteochondritis dissecans* lesion is located on the nonweight bearing aspect of the medial femoral condyle.

- Mosaicplasty is a procedure where multiple osteochondral plugs are harvested from a nonweightbearing portion of the knee, usually in the patellofemoral joint and used to fill an osteochondral defect (Kish, Modis, and Hangody, 1999; Hangody et al, 1998; Berlet, Mascia, and Miniaci, 1999).

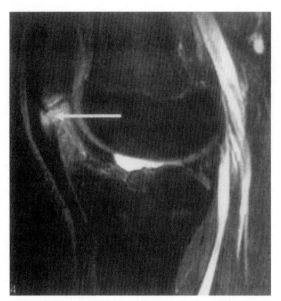

FIG. 56-7 Sagittal fat suppression MR image of the knee demonstrating moderate proximal patellar tendinosis (arrow) with hyperintensity and thickening of the proximal patellar tendon and reactive edema in the inferior pole of the patella.

- In the setting of a patellar dislocation and subsequent relocation, bone marrow edema pattern is typically localized in the anterolateral aspect of the femur and inferomedial aspect of the patella. MR imaging is recommended in cases of patellar dislocations to look for possible chondral or osteochondral fragments.
- Proximal patellar tendinosis is diagnosed on MR as focal thickening and hyperintensity of the proximal patellar tendon fibers (Fig. 56-7). Occasionally, reactive edema in the inferior pole of the patella or edema in the infrapatellar fat can also be seen.
- Tears of the extensor mechanism or patellar tendon are seen as focal areas of tendinous discontinuity, often replaced with heterogenous fluid, usually a hematoma (Fig. 56-8).
- Redundancy and laxity of the quadriceps mechanism and patella alta is often seen in cases of full thickness patellar tendon tears due to the unopposed pull of the quadriceps.

FOOT AND ANKLE

- At least one water sensitive pulse sequence should be used to evaluate for bone marrow edema in the ankle. Fast inversion recovery is suggested as opposed to fat suppression as the ankle is a peripheral joint and is more susceptible to regional field inhomogeneities.
- Stress fractures and insufficiency fractures can be seen earlier on MR than with conventional radiographs.
- Ankle sprains can result in a variety of osseous injuries than can often be overlooked on conventional radiographs. These include the fractures of the malleoli, the talus, the navicular, the anterior process of the calcaneus, and the base of the cuboid.
- MR is useful in evaluating chronic pain after an ankle sprain as causes of this pain are varied and can include osteochondral injuries, unrecognized fractures, and ligamentous injuries.
- Nondisplaced fractures can be overlooked on conventional radiographs, such as talar insufficiency fractures (Umans and Pavlov, 1995).

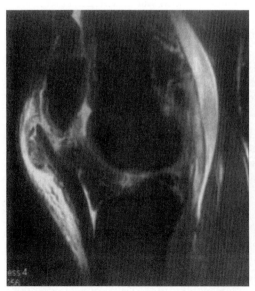 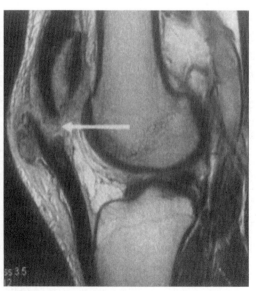

FIG. 56-8 Sagittal fat suppression (left) and fast spin echo (right) image of the knee demonstrating complete tear of the proximal patellar tendon (arrow).

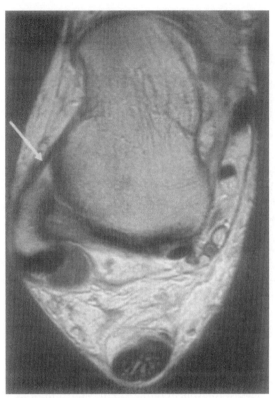

FIG. 56-9   Axial fast spin echo image of the ankle demonstrating an intact, normal anterior talofibular ligament (arrow).

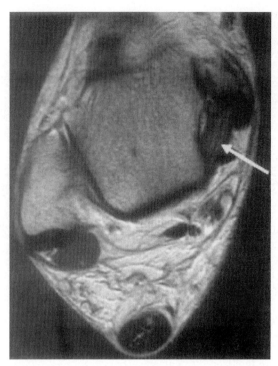

FIG. 56-10   Axial fast spin echo image demonstrating the deltoid ligament (arrow). Partial, nonacute injury to the deltoid ligament is suspected, with osseous remodeling involving the medial malleolus.

- Ligaments about the ankle are normally hypointense bands of tissue in continuity from bone to bone.
- The anterior talofibular ligament, one of the most commonly injured ligaments in an ankle sprain is seen to best advantage on axial images, with the ligament located at the very inferior tip of the lateral malleolus (Fig. 56-9).
- The deltoid ligament is a strong thick ligament located on the medial side of the ankle, connecting the medial malleolus to the talus (Fig. 56-10).
- The three main tendon compartments about the ankle should be evaluated on an MR examination of the ankle. As the tendons angle and curve around the ankle to enter the foot, care should be taken not to overestimate signal abnormalities seen on one plane, and confirmation of findings should be made in at least two planes.
- Osteochondral injuries of the tibiotalar joint are well evaluated with MR. These lesions can occur on the tibial side of the joint (Bui-Mansfield et al, 2000); however, they more commonly affect the talar dome (Hangody et al, 1997; Rosenberg, Beltran, and Bencardino, 2000) (Fig. 56-11).
- Identification and grading of posterior tibial tendon abnormalities is important in treatment planning. Posterior tibial tendon pathology is often associated with other abnormalities in the foot and ankle and so should be identified. These include abnormalities of

the spring ligament, the sinus tarsi, and plantar fascia, and often lead to flatfoot deformity (Balen and Helms, 2001; Pomeroy et al, 1999). Considering this, MR images of the ankle should extend plantarly enough to cover the plantar fascia, and be high resolution to identify and evaluate the spring ligament. Chronic posterior tibial tendon tears usually occur at the level of the medial malleolus as opposed to an acute more traumatic tear, which is usually at the insertion (Rosenberg, Beltran, and Bencardino, 2000).

- Tendon tears are diagnosed by focal high (fluid) signal within the tendon or identifying discrete tendinous discontinuity.
- The Achilles tendon is normally visualized as a thick hypointense band of tissue inserting onto the calcaneus. Tendinosis of the Achilles tendon is manifest as diffuse thickening and inhomogeneity of the tendon, often with intrasubstance signal (Fig. 56-12).
- The Achilles tendon usually tears approximately 2–6 cm proximal to the enthesis.
- If an Achilles tendon is seen on MR imaging, the signal abnormality should be traced cephalad to see if the injury extends to and involves the muscle tendon junction.
- The Achilles tendon can demonstrate dystrophic calcification and ossification in cases of chronic tendinosis (Schweitzer and Karasick, 2000).

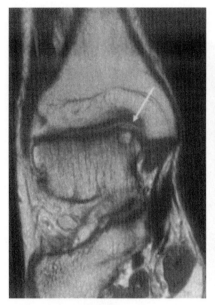
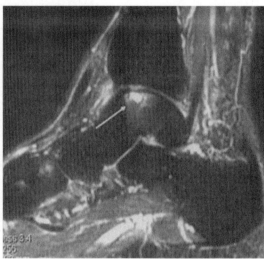

FIG. 56-11 Coronal fast spin echo (left) and sagittal inversion recovery (right) images of the ankle demonstrate an osteochondral impaction injury involving the medial aspect of the talar dome (arrows). Subchondral cystic change and edema are seen in the talar dome, as well as overlying hyperintense, frayed articular cartilage.

- Other findings in cases of chronic Achilles tendon injuries include reactive edema in the calcaneus and fluid in the deep retrocalcaneal bursa.
- The sinus tarsus is an anatomic region between the posterior subtalar joint and the talocalcaneonavicular joint (Klein and Spreitzer, 1993). Fat and blood vessels are normally seen in the sinus tarsi in addition to five ligaments: the medial, intermediate, and lateral roots of the inferior extensor retinaculum; the cervical ligament; and the ligament of the tarsal canal (Klein and Spreitzer, 1993). Patients with sinus tarsi syndrome may have a morphological abnormality in

the sinus tarsi, such as ligament tears or ganglion cysts.
- The location of the peroneal tendons with respect to the fibular groove should be evaluated; insufficiency of the superior peroneal retinaculum can result in peroneal tendon dislocation (Bencardino, Rosenberg, and Delfaut, 1999).
- Plantar fasciitis is diagnosed with MR as diffuse fascial thickening, usually at the calcaneal insertion with intrafascial hyperintensity (Narvaez et al, 2000). Occasionally, reactive edema in the calcaneus and edema in the heel fat pad can also be identified.
- The presence of osseous spurs at the anterior margin of the tibial plafond should be looked for, as these may be associated with anterior impingement.
- Posterior ankle impingement, classically described in ballet dancers, can be seen on fat suppressed MR images as abnormal intraosseous signal in the os trigonum or lateral talar tubercle (Bureau et al, 2000).

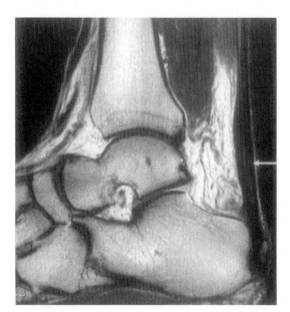

FIG. 56-12 Sagittal fast spin echo image demonstrating moderate Achilles tendinosis with thickening and mild intrasubstance hyperintensity in the Achilles tendon.

REFERENCES

Anderson MW, Kaplan PA, Dussault RG: Adductor insertion avulsion syndrome (thigh splints): spectrum of MR imaging features. *Am J Roentgen* 2001;177:673–675.

Balen PF, Helms CA: Association of posterior tibial tendon injury with spring ligament injury, sinus tarsi abnormality and plantar fasciitis on MR imaging. *Am J Roentgen* 2001;176:1137–1143.

Bencardino J, Rosenberg ZS, Delfaut E: MR imaging in sports injuries of the foot and ankle. *MRI Clinics of North America.* 1999;7(1):131–149.

Berlet GC, Mascia A, Miniaci A: Treatment of unstable osteochondritis dissecans lesions of the knee using autogenous osteochondral grafts (mosaicplasty). *Arthroscopy,* 1999;15(3): 312–316.

Bradley DM, Bergman AG, Dillingham MF: MR imaging of cyclops lesions. *Am J Roentgen* 2000;174:719–726.

Brandser EA, Riley MA, Berbaum KS, et al: MR imaging of anterior cruciate ligament injury: independent value of primary and secondary signs. *Am J Roentgen* 1996;167:121–126.

Bui-Mansfield LT, Kline M, Chew FS, et al: Osteochondritis dissecans of the tibial plafond: imaging characteristics and a review of the literature. *Am J Roentgen* 2000;175:1305–1308.

Bureau NJ, Cardinal E, Hobden R, et al: Posterior ankle impingement syndrome: MR imaging findings in seven patients. *Radiology* 2000;215:497–503.

Campbell SE, Sanders TG, Morrison WB: MR imaging of meniscal cysts: incidence, location, and clinical significance. *Am J Roentgen* 2001;177:409–413.

Goldman AB, Pavlov H, Rubenstein D: The Segond fracture of the proximal tibia: a small avulsion that reflects major ligamentous damage. *Am J Roentgen* 1988; 151:1163–1167.

Hangody L, Kish G, Karpati Z, et al: Treatment of osteochondritis dissecans of the talus: use of the mosaicplasty technique – a preliminary report. *Foot and Ankle International* 1997;18(10):628–634.

Hangody L, Kish G, Karpati Z, et al: Mosaicplasty for the treatment of articular cartilage defects: application in clinical practice. *Orthopaedics* 1998;21(7):751–756.

Hayes CW, Brigido MK, Jamadar DA, et al: Mechanism-based pattern approach to classification of complex injuries of the knee depicted at MR imaging. *Radiographics* 2000;20:S121–S134.

Helms CA: The impact of MR imaging in sports medicine. *Radiology* 2002;224:631–635.

Horton LK, Jacobson JA, Lin J, et al: MR imaging of anterior cruciate ligament reconstruction graft. *Am J Roentgen* 2000;175:1091–1097.

Kish G, Modis L, Hangody L: Osteochondral mosaicplasty for the treatment of focal chondral and osteochondral lesions of the knee and talus in the athlete. rationale, indications, techniques, and results. *Clinics in Sports Medicine* 1999;18 (1):45–65.

Klein MA, Spreitzer AM: MR imaging of the tarsal sinus and canal: normal anatomy, pathologic findings, and features of the sinus tarsi syndrome. *Radiology* 1993;186:233–240.

Major NM, Helms, CA: MR imaging of the knee: findings in asymptomatic collegiate basketball players. *Am J Roentgen* 2002;179:641–644.

McCauley TR, Jee WH, Galloway MT, et al: Grade 2C signal in the meniscus on MR imaging of the knee. *Am J Roentgen* 2002;179:645–648.

Minas T, Nehrer: Current concepts in the treatment of articular cartilage defects. *Orthopaedics.* 1997;20(6):525–538.

Narvaez JA, Narvaez J, Ortega R, et al: Painful heel: MR imaging findings. *Radiographics* 2000;20:333–352.

Pomeroy GC, Pike RH, Beals TC, et al: Acquired flatfoot in adults due to dysfunction of the posterior tibial tendon. *J Bone Joint Surg* 1999;81–A (8):1173–1182.

Potter HG, Linklater JM, Allen AA, et al: Magnetic resonance imaging of articular cartilage in the knee. *J Bone Joint Surg* 1998;80–A (9):1276–1284.

Potter HG, Weinstein M, Allen AA, et al: Magnetic resonance imaging of the multiple-ligament injured knee. *J Orthop Trauma* 2002;16(5):330–339.

Rosenberg ZS, Beltran J, Bencardino JT: MR imaging of the ankle and foot. *Radiographics* 2000;20:S153–S179.

Roychowdhury S, Fitzgerald SW, Sonin AH, et al: Using MR imaging to diagnose partial tears of the anterior cruciate ligament: value of axial images. *Am J Roentgen* 1997;168:1487–1491.

Rubin DA, Harner CD, Costello JM: Treatable chondral injuries in the knee: frequency of associated focal subchondral edema. *Am J Roentgen* 2000;174:1099–1106.

Sanders TG, Medynski MA, Feller JF, et al: Bone contusion patterns of the knee at MR imaging: footprint of the mechanism of injury. *Radiographics* 2000;20:S135–S151.

Schatz JA, Potter HG, Rodeo SA, et al: MR imaging of anterior cruciate ligament reconstruction. *Am J Roentgen* 1997; 169: 223–228.

Schmid MR, Notzli HP, Zanetti TF, et al: Cartilage lesions in the hip: diagnostic effectiveness of MR arthrography. *Radiology* 2002;226:382–386.

Schweitzer ME, Karasick D: MR imaging of disorders of the achilles tendon. *Am J Roentgen* 2000;175:613–625.

Umans H, Pavlov H: Insuffiency fractures of the talus: diagnosis with MR imaging. *Radiology.* 1995;197:439–442.

Vincken PWJ, ter Braak BPM, van Erkell AR, et al: Effectiveness of MR imaging in selection of patients for arthroscopy of the knee. *Radiology* 2002;223:739–746.

Waldschmidt JG, Rilling RJ, Kajdacsy-Balla AA, et al: In vitro and in vivo MR imaging of hyaline cartilage: zonal anatomy, imaging pitfalls, and pathologic conditions. *Radiographics* 1997;17:1387–1402.

Weaver CJ, Major NM, Garrett WE, et al: Femoral head osteochondral lesions in painful hips of athletes: MR imaging findings. *Am J Roentgen* 2002;178:973–977.

White LM, Schweitzer ME, Weishaupt D, et al: Diagnosis of recurrent meniscal tears: prospective evaluation of conventional MR imaging, indirect MR arthrography, and direct MR arthrography. *Radiology* 2002;222:421–429.

57 PELVIS, HIP, AND THIGH

Brett D Owens, MD
Brian D Busconi, MD

BONY INJURIES

AVULSION FRACTURES AND APOPHYSEAL INJURIES

- Avulsion fractures about the hip and pelvis are the result of failure of the bone at the tendonous insertion rather than the tendon itself. These injuries are more common in skeletally immature athletes with open apophyses that are more susceptible to failure than the tendonous insertion. These are usually the result of a sudden, forceful concentric or eccentric contracture or rapid, excessive passive lengthening. Common sites of these avulsions about the pelvis are the insertion of the sartorius into the anterior-superior iliac spine, the rectus femoris superior head insertion into the anterior-inferior iliac spine, and the insertion of the hamstrings into the ischial tuberosity. These injuries are also seen in the proximal femur with the insertion of the hip abductors into the greater trochanter and the insertion of the iliopsoas into the lesser trochanter.

TREATMENT

- Nonsurgical management has been the mainstay of treatment in most series with good to excellent results reported. In the case of severe displacement of the avulsed fragment (especially noted in avulsions of the ischial tuberosity or the greater trochanter) surgical intervention has been recommended; however, most authorities do not recommend surgery for these injuries. Metzmaker and Pappas defined a rehabilitation treatment protocol for these injuries including (*a*) rest, using proper positioning to unload the injured apophysis and ice/analgesics; (*b*) initiation of gentile active and passive range-of-motion excercises; (*c*) progressive resistance beginning when 75% of motion is achieved and ending when 50% of strength is returned; (*d*) integration of stretching and strengthening exercises with functional activity; and (*e*) return to competitive sport at 8 to 10 weeks (Metzmaker and Pappas, 1985).
- Skeletally immature patients are also susceptible to chronic traction injuries at these apophyses and this is referred to as apophysitis. Apophysitis is treated conservatively with rest followed by functional rehabilitation of the involved muscle group (Busconi and McCarthy, 1996).

STRESS FRACTURES

PELVIS

- Pelvic stress fractures should be suspected in athletes such as long-distance runners and military recruits. The most common site is the junction between the ischium and inferior pubic ramus. Tenderness to palpation directly over the fractured bone can be helpful in locating the lesion. A positive standing sign has been described in which a patient develops discomfort in the grain while standing unsupported on the ipsilateral leg.
- Plain radiographic signs, such as periosteal reaction or fracture line, can lag behind the clinical presentation

by as long as 3 weeks. Magnetic resonance imaging and bone scan can provide an earlier diagnosis. Tumors should at least be considered in the differential diagnosis. Treatment consists of rest with emphasis on protected weight-bearing, flexibility, and aerobic nonimpact exercises such as swimming or cycling. Return to sport can be delayed up to 6 months.

FEMORAL NECK

- While femoral neck stress fractures are not as common as pelvic stress fractures, if treated incorrectly, the results can be disastrous. Similar to pelvic stress fractures, these present with groin pain and an antalgic gait. Pain will be worsened by flexion and internal rotation of the hip. Again, radiographic evidence may lag behind by 3–4 weeks. Magnetic resonance imaging and bone scan may be helpful in earlier diagnosis. Two types of femoral neck stress fractures exist. The first type is a compression side femoral neck stress fracture. These occur in the inferior medial aspect of the neck and usually respond to restriction to nonweight-bearing status until radiographic evidence of healing has occurred. The more worrisome type is the tension side femoral neck stress fracture. This is a transverse fracture along the superior margin of the neck. Internal fixation is recommended for nondisplaced fractures. Immediate closed or open reduction and internal fixation is recommended for displaced fractures. Fracture displacement can lead to avascular necrosis of the femoral head (Boden and Osbahr, 2000).

OSTEITIS PUBIS

- Primary osteitis pubis is caused by repetitive microtrauma and is difficult to treat. Most cases of osteitis pubis are secondary, however. Retained sutures from hernia or urogynecological repair may cause osteitis pubis. Traumatic osteitis pubis is a fatigue fracture involving the bony origin of the gracilis muscle at the pubic symphysis. When the bony lesion is located at the lower margin of the symphysis, this may be referred to as gracilis syndrome. Endometriosis, pelvic inflammatory disease, and tumor must also be considered in the differential, often necessitating a biopsy.
- On physical examination, patients will have tenderness to palpation directly on the pubis. Although activity may aggravate the symptoms, patients with primary osteitis may get some relief. While the diagnosis is usually confirmed by *magnetic resonance imaging* (MRI) or bone scan, the distinction between

primary and secondary osteitis is usually made on physical examination. Initial treatment consists of rest, *range of motion* (ROM) exercises, oral *nonsteroidal anti-inflammatory drugs* (NSAIDs), and sometimes corticosteroid injection. Secondary osteitis will respond to treatment of the underlying condition. Surgical intervention can be required in recalcitrant cases, but has unpredictable results (Busconi, Wixted, and Owens, 2003).

FRACTURE AND DISLOCATION

- Pelvic and femoral diaphyseal fractures are rare in sports but can have devastating consequences. These injuries require great amounts of energy imparted in order to occur, although lower energy mechanisms can be seen in pathologic bone. The majority of pelvic fractures are stable injuries of the pelvic ring and requires symptomatic treatment with an initial course of protected weight bearing. The determination of pelvic ring stability should be confirmed by inlet/outlet radiographs, in addition to computed tomography. The standard of care for diaphyseal femur fractures is reduction followed by intramedullary nailing.
- Hip dislocation and fracture-dislocations can be seen more commonly, but are still rare injuries. Intertrochanteric hip fractures require surgical reduction and internal fixation. Femoral neck fractures in athletes are a true orthopedic emergency. Anatomic reduction and internal fixation are required in a timely fashion, as *avascular necrosis* (AVN) is associated with delays in treatment. Another injury that has the devastating risk of AVN is hip dislocation, which may also have associated femoral head or acetabular fractures. These require emergent closed (or open if necessary) reduction followed by *computed tomography* (CT) to assess a fracture if present or to rule out an osseous loose body. Even in the absence of fracture, the presence of chondral loose bodies and labral pathology can cause persistent symptoms. Hip arthroscopy has been useful in this scenario (Owens and Busconi, 2003).

SOFT TISSUE INJURIES

MUSCLE STRAINS

- Soft tissue injuries to the periarticular structures surrounding the hip and pelvis are the most common injuries seen in athletes. In general, the great majority of soft tissue injuries about the hip and pelvis are musculotendinous strains. The type of injury sustained is highly dependent on (*1*) skeletal age of the athlete, (*2*) physical condition, and (*3*) biomechanical forces involved in both the sport and nature of the trauma. The degree of injury can range from repetitive microinjury associated with each performance to a more significant single macroinjury caused by an abnormal biomechanical force. A certain degree of microtrauma occurs with every major exertional performance immediately manifested by swelling, sensitivity, and a recovery interval. If additional moderate or severe micro- or macroinjury occurs, there may not be a normal healing response that may lead to more significant changes in tissue structure and a negative effect on future athletic performance (Busconi, Wixted, and Owens, 2003).
- A strain is an injury to a musculotendinous structure caused by an indirectly applied force. The most common mechanism of injury is a result of eccentric contraction or stretching of an activated muscle. The site of injury is influenced by the rate of loading, mechanism of injury, and local anatomic factors. Low rates of loading will result in a failure at the tendon bone junction by bone avulsion or disruption at its insertion. High rates of loading result in intratendinous or myotendinous juncture injuries.
- These injuries can be graded on a three-scale clinical grading system. Grade 1 injuries involve a simple stretching of soft tissue fibers. Grade 2 strains involve partial tearing of the musculotendinous unit; and Grade 3, which are unusual, are secondary to extreme violent forces causing complete disruptions.

CONTUSIONS

- Among the most frequently experienced hip and pelvic injuries sustained by athletes are soft tissue contusions. Contusions usually result from direct blows to a specific soft tissue area usually overlying a bony prominence. Contusions are most common in contact sports, especially football, but are also seen other sports as well. In contact sports, the blow is usually caused by contact with another athlete. In noncontact sports, athletes usually sustain blows from contact with equipment (gymnastics), contact with high velocity projectiles (lacrosse ball), or contact from the playing surface.
- Contusions are often found over areas of bony prominences of the pelvis including the iliac crest (hip pointer), greater trochanter, ischial tuberosity, and pubic rami. Because of the varied anatomy of the pelvis, contusions can be superficial, especially when they overlie a relatively subcutaneous bone or lie deep within a large muscle mass. It is important to determine

possible presence and extent of muscular hemorrhage because an increase in muscular hemorrhage often results in more severe symptoms and longer time before returning to sport (Busconi, Wixted, and Owens, 2003).

HIP POINTER

- Pain and hemorrhage over the iliac crest has been referred to as a hip pointer. These injuries include contusions, avulsion of the iliac apophysis, periostitis, or avulsion of the muscles that insert onto the iliac crest. On physical examination, the patient will have superficial or muscular hemorrhage, which will be painful on palpation. It is important to note by touch a defect, which would indicate an avulsion injury. Patients will have difficulty with rotation and side bending of the trunk. Anterior-posterior and oblique X-rays of the pelvis will rule out an avulsion fracture, periostitis, or an acute fracture of the iliac wing.

THIGH CONTUSIONS

- Thigh contusions are common athletic injuries, most often encountered in football from direct trauma. These injuries can involve significant muscular damage, hematoma formation, and swelling. Therefore, the athlete can be extremely uncomfortable. Initial treatment is rest, ice, and compression to minimize hematoma formation. Immobilization in flexion and initiation of early flexion exercises have been recommended to decrease myositis ossificans formation and improve functional outcome (Ryan et al, 1991).

BURSITIS

- Bursitis about the hip is a common condition secondary to inflammation of one of the three major bursae about the hip: the trochanteric bursa, the iliopsoas bursa, and the ischiogluteal bursa. These bursae facilitate the gliding of musculotendinous or ligamentous structures. Bursitis may be secondary to direct injury, overuse of the adjacent musculotendinous structures, or degenerative changes in these structures. Because bursae are lined by true synovial tissue, bursitis also can occur with systemic disease, causing synovitis.
- The trochanteric bursa is a large bursa that lies between the greater trochanter and the overlying junction of the gluteus maximus and tensor fascia lata, as these merge to form the fascia lata and iliotibial tract. This is the most common bursitis in athletes and is common in runners.
- Ischiogluteal bursitis, inflammation of the bursa between the ischial tuberosity and the overlying gluteus

maximus, is usually associated with injury or with occupations requiring long periods of sitting. The patient complains of pain over the ischial tuberosity that is aggravated by sitting, and the pain may radiate into the posterior thigh.
- Iliopsoas bursitis is another relatively common bursitis in athletes. This bursa located between the iliopsoas muscle and the pelvis proximally and the hip capsule and psoas tendon distally. Communication between the hip joint and psoas bursa is common.
- Corticosteroid injections may provide temporary symptomatic relief. Use of local anesthetics can also provide diagnostic confirmation (Anderson, Strickland, and Warren, 2001).

PIRIFORMIS SYNDROME

- Yeoman in 1928 first described a syndrome involving compression of the sciatic nerve by the piriformis muscle. The compression of the nerve occurs as it exits deep to the piriformis muscle. Patients will complain of pain and symptoms in the sciatic nerve distribution. A history of past acute trauma to the buttock is often present. Patients will have difficulty sitting or participating in activities that cause hip flexion and internal rotation (ice skating). On physical examination, tenderness can be present over the piriformis tendon in the gluteal area. Pain is elicited by forced internal rotation on an extended thigh, or pain and weakness on resisted abduction and external rotation of the thigh (Pace's sign). Rectal or vaginal examination may produce pain in the piriformis area. An MRI can be helpful to demonstrate sciatic nerve inflammation in the area of the piriformis tendon (Meyers et al, 1999).

SNAPPING HIP SYNDROME

- Snapping hip syndrome is a collection of extra-articular and intra-articular pathologies that can be painful and disabling to the athlete. Extra-articular snapping of the hip joint can be caused by (*1*) the iliopsoas tendon as it passes over the iliopectineal eminence or the lesser trochanter of the femur; (*2*) the iliofemoral ligaments over the femoral head; (*3*) the long head of the biceps femoris over the ischial tuberosity; and (*4*) the iliotibial band over the greater trochanter of the femur. It can be very difficult to distinguish these entities from more disconcerting intra-articular lesions such as tears of the anterior labrum, synovitis, and loose bodies that can also create a snapping or clicking sensation in the hip; however, as CT, MRI, and hip arthroscopy become more refined we are able to better differentiate these entities (Meyers et al, 2000).

- The most common cause of snapping hip syndrome is irritation of the greater trochanter by the iliotibial band. The iliotibial band is a large flat tendinous structure that originates on the anterior superior portion of the iliac crest, crosses over the greater trochanter of the femur, and inserts onto the lateral condyle of the tibia. Iliotibial band syndrome is seen in athletes who undergo repetitive knee flexion, such as runners and cyclists. Athletes will have pain over the greater trochanter of the femur, the lateral thigh, or radiating pain down to the knee. Patients often report hip instability symptoms. If severe enough, the snapping sensation will occur during normal ambulation. Once this area becomes inflamed, running or rising from a seated position may hurt continuously.

HAMSTRING SYNDROME

- Hamstring syndrome, described in track athletes, involves severe pain in and around the ischial tuberosity which radiates down the posterior aspect of the thigh to the popliteal area. Any activity which puts the hamstring in stretch can create this radiating pain. Sprinting, hurdling, and even sitting for long periods will cause pain. Physical examination elicits exquisite tenderness at the ischial tuberosity and, at times, reproduction of sciatic pain with percussion of the nerve at the ischial tuberosity. Resisted leg extension will reproduce the pain. The sciatic nerve is thought to be entrapped between the semitendinosus and the biceps femoris by a fibrous band that constricts the two muscles (Busconi, Wixted, and Owens, 2003).

ATHLETIC PUBALGIA

- The term *athletic pubalgia* refers to a chronic inguinal or pubic area pain in athletes, which is noted with exertion. The pattern of symptoms in these patients, operative findings, and results of studies, all suggest that the lower abdominal/inguinal pain is not due to occult hernia. Only a small percentage of patients are found to have occult hernia at the time of surgery. When this does occur, the occult hernia is usually found on the side opposite the principal symptoms.
- The rectus tendon insertion on the pubis seems to be the primary site of pathology. Most patients describe a hyperextension injury in association with hyper abduction of the thigh. The location of pain suggests that the injury involves both the rectus abdominis and adductor longus muscles. Other tendinous insertion sites on the pubic bone may also be involved (Meyers et al, 2000).

DIAGNOSIS

- The athletes have lower abdominal pain with exertion. A minority of patients have pure adductor related pain that is disabling. Most of the patients remember a distinct injury during exertions. Usually, the abdominal pain involves the inguinal canal near the insertion of the rectus abdominis muscle on the pubis. The pain often causes a majority of patients to stop competing in sports.
- MRI findings in athletic pubalgia are often nonspecific. On the other hand 12% of patients have MRI findings that clearly indicate a problem at the rectus insertion site. The relatively small incidence of a specific diagnosis by imaging studies suggests that the problem may be an attenuation of the muscle or tendon due to repeated microtrauma. The finding in the MRI, of adductor longus inflammation, is consistent with athletic pubalgia.

TREATMENT

- Generally, the acute management of groin pain suspected to be athletic pubalgia consists of conservative management. This includes rest, ice, compression, anti-inflammatory medications, and massage. When the process continues over several months and the athlete cannot return to previously expected activity because of pain, an operation should be considered. Surgical treatment of athletic pubalgia requires a broad surgical reattachment at the inferolateral edge of the rectus muscle with its fascial investments to the pubis and adjacent anterior ligaments. Also performed is an anterior and lateral release of the epimysium of the adductor fascia in order to expand this compartment. The epimysium is the layer of connective tissue that encloses the entire muscle. This kind of fascial release is often very successful in relieving the adductor symptoms in athletic pubalgia.

REFERENCES

Anderson K, Strickland SM, Warren R: Hip and groin injuries in athletes. *Am J Sports Med* 29:521–533, 2001.

Boden BP, Osbahr DC: High-risk stress fractures: Evaluation and treatment. *J Am Acad Orthop Surg* 8:344–353, 2000.

Busconi B, McCarthy J: Hip and pelvic injuries in the skeletally immature athlete. *Sports Med Arthrosc Rev* 4:132–158, 1996.

Busconi BD, Wixted JJ, Owens BD: Differential diagnosis of the painful hip, in McCarthy JC (ed.): *Early Hip Disease: Advances in Detection and Minimally Invasive Treatment.* New York, NY, Springer-Verlag, 2003.

Metzmaker JN, Pappas AM: Avulsion fractures of the pelvis. *Am J Sports Med* 13:349–358, 1985.

Meyers WC, Ricciardi R, Busconi BD, et al: Groin pain in the athlete, in Arendt EA (ed.): *Orthopaedic Knowledge Update: Sports Medicine 2.* Rosemont, IL, American Academy of Orthopaedic Surgeons, 1999, pp 281–290.

Meyers WC, Ricciardi R, Busconi BD, et al: Athletic pubalgia and groin pain, in Garrett WE, Speer KP, Kirkendall DT (eds.): *Principles and Practice of Orthopaedic Sports Medicine.* Philadelphia, PA, Lippincott Williams & Wilkins, 2000, pp 223–230.

Owens BD, Busconi BD: Trauma, in McCarthy JC (ed.): *Early Hip Disease: Advances in Detection and Minimally Invasive Treatment.* New York, NY, Springer-Verlag, 2003.

Ryan JB, Wheeler JH, Hopkinson WJ, et al: Quadriceps contusions: West Point update. *Am J Sports Med* 19:299–304, 1991.

BIBLIOGRAPHY

Klingele KE, Sallay PI: Surgical repair of complete proximal hamstring tendon rupture. *Am J Sports Med* 30:742–747, 2002.

McCarthy JC, Day B, Busconi B: Hip arthroscopy: Applications and technique. *J Am Acad Orthop Surg* 3:115–122, 1995.

Melamed H, Hutchinson MR: Soft tissue problems of the hip in athletes. *Sports Med Arthrosc Rev* 10:168–175, 2002.

Scopp JM, Moorman CT: The assessment of athletic hip injury. *Clin Sports Med* 20:647–659, 2001.

58 KNEE MENISCAL INJURIES

John P Goldblatt, MD
John C Richmond, MD

INTRODUCTION

- The meniscus plays an important role in weight distribution, reduction in joint contact stresses, joint stabilization, and energy absorption (Greis et al, 2002(*a*); Fairbank, 1948; Arnoczky and McDevitt, 2000; Rath and Richmond, 2000; Lo et al, 2003). Injury to the meniscus can result in marked physical impairment.
- Once thought to be a vestigial organ, it is now recognized that meniscectomy often leads to a recognizable pattern of joint deterioration including, joint space narrowing, osteophyte formation, and squaring of the femoral condyles (Fairbank, 1948).

- Meniscal preservation is the goal of new surgical procedures.
- Arthroscopy facilitates optimal treatment of meniscal tears with minimally invasive techniques.

ANATOMY AND BASIC SCIENCE

- Each of the medial and lateral compartments of a knee has an intervening meniscus located between the femur and tibia.
- The menisci are peripherally thick and convex, and centrally taper to a thin free margin (Arnoczky and McDevitt, 2000).
- The meniscal surfaces conform to the femoral and tibial contours.
- Each meniscus has anterior and posterior bony attachment sites.

MEDIAL MENISCUS

- The medial meniscus is semicircular, crescent shaped, and measures approximately 3.5 cm in length.
- The medial meniscus covers 50–60% of the medial tibial plateau. The posterior horn is wider than the anterior horn in the *anteroposterior* (AP) dimension (Rath and Richmond, 2000; Lo et al, 2003).
- The attachment site for the anterior horn is variable, in the area of the intercondylar fossa in front of the *anterior cruciate ligament* (ACL), often to the anterior surface of the tibial plateau.
- The posterior fibers of the anterior horn merge with the transverse fibers of the intermeniscal ligament, which connects the anterior horns of the medial and lateral menisci. The intermeniscal ligament is located approximately 8 mm anterior to the ACL (Arnoczky and McDevitt, 2000).
- The posterior horn is firmly attached to the posterior intercondylar fossa of the tibia, anterior and medial to the PCL attachment site (Arnoczky and McDevitt, 2000).
- The periphery is attached to the capsule throughout its length, and the tibial portion of this attachment is called the coronary ligament. In addition, at its midpoint, the medial meniscus is firmly attached to the femur and tibia through a condensation of the joint capsule known as the deep medial collateral ligament (Rath and Richmond, 2000).

LATERAL MENISCUS

- The lateral meniscus is almost circular in gross morphology, and covers 70–80% of the lateral tibial

plateau (Arnoczky and McDevitt, 2000; Rath and Richmond, 2000).
- The lateral meniscus is nearly uniform in width from front to back.
- The bony attachments of the lateral meniscus are much closer to each other than those of the medial meniscus. The anterior horn inserts adjacent to the ACL, and the posterior horn inserts just posterior to the ACL, anterior to the posterior horn of the medial meniscus.
- There is a loose peripheral attachment of the lateral meniscus to the joint capsule that allows greater translation of the lateral meniscus, when compared to the medial (11.2 vs. 5.2 mm) (Arnoczky and McDevitt, 2000).
- The area of the lateral meniscus with no coronary ligament attachment, anterior to the popliteus tendon, is called the bare area of the lateral meniscus, or popliteal hiatus.

LATERAL MENISCUS ATTACHMENTS

- Motion of the lateral meniscus is guided by the capsular attachments, as well as additional ligamentous attachments. These ligaments include the meniscofemoral ligaments, and the anterior-inferior and posterior-superior popliteomeniscal fascicles from the popliteus muscle.
- The posterior horn has variably present attachments to the medial femoral condyle through the *meniscofemoral ligaments* (MFLs). The MFLs originate from the posterior horn of the lateral meniscus.
- The anterior MFL (of Humphrey) passes anterior to the *posterior cruciate ligament* (PCL) to insert on the femur between the distal margin of the femoral attachment of the PCL and the edge of the condylar articular cartilage.
- The posterior MFL (of Wrisberg) passes posterior to the PCL to insert at the proximal margin of the femoral attachment of the PCL.
- The overall incidence of at least one MFL is 91%. In the knees demonstrating at least one structure, the incidence of an anterior MFL is 48.2%, and posterior MFL is 70.4%. The incidence of both ligaments coexisting in one knee is 31.8% (Gupte et al, 2003).

MENISCAL VARIANTS

- Discoid variants occur with an estimated incidence of 3.5–5%, most commonly the incomplete type (Greis et al, 2002a).
- Discoid meniscus is almost universally located in the lateral compartment.
- Three types exist—incomplete, complete, and Wrisberg.
- Both the incomplete and complete types have firm posterior tibial attachments, and are considered stable.
- The Wrisberg variant occurs when the posterior horn bony attachment is absent, and the posterior meniscofemoral ligament of Wrisberg is the only stabilizing structure (Greis et al, 2002a).

MICROSCOPIC ANATOMY

- The menisci are fibrocartilagenous tissue comprised of cells interspersed in a matrix largely composed of collagen bundles, along with noncollagenous proteins including elastin, and proteoglycans.
- Two cell types are present—a more fusiform, fibroblastic cell, and a more rounded, chondrocytic cell.
- Water constitutes 72% of the extracellular matrix, and collagen makes up 75% of the dry weight (Lo et al, 2003).
- Elastin is estimated to be less than 0.6%, and noncollagenous proteins 8–13%, of the meniscus dry weight in humans (Lo et al, 2003).
- Type I collagen represents 90% of collagen present, and types II, III, V, and VI are present in varying quantities depending on location and age (Lo et al, 2003).
- The principle orientation of collagen fiber bundles is circumferential, with few radially directed "tie" fibers. Tie fibers provide structural rigidity to help resist forces that would split the circumferential fibers with compressive loading (Arnoczky and McDevitt, 2000; Lo et al, 2003).
- Fiber orientation changes with depth from the surface. Surface fibers are arranged as a network of irregularly oriented bundles. The deeper fibers are primarily circumferential (Lo et al, 2003).

NEUROVASCULAR ANATOMY

- Both medial and lateral menisci demonstrate an extensive microvascular network, arising from the respective superior and inferior geniculate arteries (Rath and Richmond, 2000; Klimkiewicz and Shaffer, 2002).
- The perimeniscal capillary plexus is oriented circumferentially, and branches extensively into smaller vessels to supply the peripheral border of the meniscus through its attachment to the capsule.
- The branches terminate after supplying the peripheral 10–30% of the meniscus, leaving the remainder avascular (Lo et al, 2003; Klimkiewicz and Shaffer, 2002).

- Free nerve endings and specialized end-receptors are present within the menisci. The most densely innervated regions are the anterior and posterior horns of both menisci (Lo et al, 2003).
- Nerve fibers originate in the perimeniscal tissues and radiate into the peripheral 30% of the meniscus.
- Three receptor types have been identified—Ruffini endings, Golgi tendon organs, and pacinian corpuscles.
- It is hypothesized that the nerves play a proprioceptive role in normal joint function. Meniscal derived signals generated during deformation and loading may be important to joint-position sense, and for protective neuromuscular reflex control of joint motion and loading (Lo et al, 2003).

NUTRITION OF THE MENISCI

- The bulk of meniscus nutrition is supplied by the synovial fluid, most notably to the avascular regions.
- Nutrients reach the tissue via passive diffusion and mechanical pumping with intermittent compression during loading (Lo et al, 2003).

BIOMECHANICS AND MENISCAL FUNCTION

- The menisci serve in load transmission, shock absorption, lubrication, prevention of synovial impingement, synovial fluid distribution, stability, and improved gliding motion (Rath and Richmond, 2000).
- Long term follow-up demonstrates that virtually all knees after total meniscectomy develop degenerative changes, and this is less frequent following partial meniscectomy (Fairbank, 1948; Andersson-Molina, Karlsson, and Rockborn, 2002).

MENISCUS MOTION

- With knee flexion from 0° to 120°, the menisci move posteriorly. In the midcondylar, parasagittal plane, the medial meniscus moves approximately 5.1 mm, and the lateral 11.2 mm (Arnoczky and McDevitt, 2000).
- The medial meniscus lacks the controlled mobility of the lateral meniscus.
- Posterior motion of the medial meniscus is guided by the deep MCL, and semimembranosus, while anterior translation is caused by the push of the anterior femoral condyle (Simon et al, 2000).
- The posterior oblique fibers of the deep MCL limit motion in rotation, and therefore the medial meniscus

is at increased risk of tear (Arnoczky and McDevitt, 2000; Klimkiewicz and Shaffer, 2002).
- The lateral meniscus is stabilized, and motion guided, by the popliteus tendon, popliteomeniscal ligaments, popliteofibular ligament, meniscofemoral ligaments, and lateral capsule.
- Meniscal motion allows continued load distribution during changes of position of the joint, during which the radius of curvature of the femoral condyles changes (Simon et al, 2000).

KNEE STABILITY

- The medial meniscus provides greater restraint to anterior translation than the lateral, by acting as a buttress (Levy, Torzilli, and Warren, 1982; Levy et al, 1989).
- ACL deficient knees demonstrate increased anterior translation when subjected to an anteriorly directed force, and this translation increases significantly with combined meniscectomy at all angles of flexion. This confirms the role of the ACL as a primary restraint to anterior translation, and demonstrates that the medial meniscus acts as a secondary stabilizer to resist anterior translation (Levy, Torzilli, and Warren, 1982).
- With sufficient anterior translation (in the ACL deficient knee), the posterior horn of the medial meniscus is wedged between the tibial plateau and the femoral condyle, and is the mechanism suggested for the resistance provided by the meniscus.
- In contrast, the soft tissue attachments of the lateral meniscus do not affix the lateral meniscus as firmly to the tibia. Combined lateral meniscectomy and ACL sectioning does not increase anterior translation significantly over ACL sectioning alone. This implies that the greater mobility of the lateral meniscus prevents it from contributing as efficiently as a posterior wedge to resist anterior translation of the tibia on the femur (Levy et al, 1989).

ADDITIONAL FUNCTIONAL ROLES OF THE MENISCI

- The menisci serve additional functional roles, including load bearing, and shock absorption (Rath and Richmond, 2000). The menisci transmit large loads across the joint, and their contact areas change with different degrees of knee flexion and rotation.
- Up to 50–70% of compressive load is transmitted through the menisci in extension, and 85% at 90° of flexion (Greis et al, 2002; Arnoczky and McDevitt, 2000; Rath and Richmond, 2000; Klimkiewicz and Shaffer, 2002).

- Removal of a portion of the meniscus results in a decreased contact area between the femur and tibia. Medial meniscectomy decreases the contact area by up to 70%.
- Resection of as little as 15–34% of the meniscus results in increased contact pressure by up to 350% (Simon et al, 2000).

EPIDEMIOLOGY

- The annual incidence of meniscal injury is 60–70 per 100,000 persons (Greis et al, 2002*a*).
- Meniscus injury is more common in males, with a male to female ratio between 2.5:1 and 4:1 (Greis et al, 2002*a*).
- Approximately one-third of all tears are associated with ACL injury, and approximately 80% of repairable meniscal tears occur during ACL injury (Klimkiewicz and Shaffer, 2002).
- Meniscal tears are also commonly associated with tibia plateau fractures, and femoral shaft fractures.
- Degenerative tears in men peak in the 4th through 6th decade, and in women remain relatively constant after the second decade (Greis et al, 2002*a*).
- Medial meniscus tears are more common than lateral, and tears are most frequently located in the midportion and posterior horns of the meniscus.
- Medial meniscal tears are more commonly longitudinal type, whereas laterally a radial component is more frequent (Klimkiewicz and Shaffer, 2002).

DIAGNOSIS OF MENISCAL INJURY

HISTORY

- Meniscal injury during sport occurs most frequently during noncontact cutting, deceleration, hyperflexion, or landing from a jump.
- Degenerative meniscal injury with aging (>40 years) often occurs after trivial insult. The tear may not be noticed at the time of injury. The mechanical symptoms that follow often trigger the patient to seek attention.
- Mechanical symptoms of popping, catching, locking, or buckling, along with joint line pain are suggestive of meniscal tear. These are nonspecific symptoms, and may be secondary to chondral injury, or patellofemoral chondrosis (Greis et al, 2002*a*).
- Mild synovitis often results from the injury, with swelling present for several days following the event. The synovitis may be recurrent and activity related.

- An audible pop at the time of injury is more characteristic of an ACL tear; however, a meniscus tear is commonly present in this scenario.
- Immediate swelling suggests bleeding, and is frequently not present after isolated meniscus tear; however, may be present with a more peripherally based tear.
- A delayed effusion is more characteristic of meniscus injury, with the production of reactive joint fluid.
- The reporting of loss of motion with a sensation of a mechanical block to extension is suggestive of a displaced meniscus tear (Greis et al, 2002*a*).
- A history of a snapping or popping knee may suggest a discoid variant. Mechanical symptoms present in childhood or adolescence, without a history of trauma, should raise the suspicion of the presence of a discoid meniscus (Rath and Richmond, 2000).
- The complete history should include assessment of the patient's lifestyle, activity level, occupation, and medical history. Younger, more active individuals often require more aggressive management.

PHYSICAL EXAMINATION

- Examination begins with evaluation of gait. A limp is common after meniscus tear, and pain after an acute injury may result in the inability to bear weight.
- Inspection of the knee includes evaluation for an effusion, as well as thigh asymmetry in the setting of a chronic tear.
- Range of motion is assessed in comparison to the opposite extremity. A displaced tear may block the knee from achieving full extension, as well as impair flexion. A mechanical block to motion is termed the *locked knee*.
- Palpation of the joint lines is performed in an effort to elicit tenderness, and may be the best clinical sign of a tear, with 74% sensitivity, and 50% positive predictive value (Greis et al, 2002*a*).
- Pain at terminal flexion or extension may be present, depending on the location of the tear.
- The McMurray test is performed with the patient supine. The hip and knee are flexed, and the foot is alternately internally and externally rotated during application of a circumduction maneuver to the knee. Concurrently, the examiner palpates the posterolateral and posteromedial joint lines.
- Medial meniscal injury is tested by extending the knee with the foot externally rotated. Lateral meniscal injury is assessed with the foot internally rotated.
- A palpable and audible clunk is considered a positive McMurray test. A true positive test is uncommon, even in the presence of a tear, but is nearly 100% specific. The sensitivity of the test is as low as 15% (Greis et al,

2002*a*). More commonly the test elicits pain (Richmond, 1996).
- Cysts at or below the joint line may be palpable, and are highly correlated with meniscal tears, most commonly lateral (Greis et al, 2002*a*).
- No clinical examination finding is consistently predictive of meniscus tear; however, the combination of several positive tests, from the following list is highly predictive of meniscus tear: joint line tenderness, pain on forced flexion, positive McMurray test, and a block to extension.
- Sensitivity of thorough examination reaches 95%, and specificity 72% (Greis et al, 2002*a*).
- Confounding diagnoses include fibrotic plica, fat pad impingement, chondral lesions, and synovitis (Greis et al, 2002*a*).

IMAGING

- Diagnostic studies should begin with plain radiography. Radiographs are assessed for associated skeletal injury, loose bodies, and presence of degenerative changes.
- Radiographs should include a 45° flexed knee PA weight-bearing view for individuals who may have knee arthrosis. Flexion weight-bearing views allow evaluation of the posterior tibiofemoral contact region, which is most frequently involved in early degenerative arthritis. Identification of arthrosis may have significant influence on treatment planning.
- Arthrograms are generally reserved for individuals for whom *magnetic resonance imaging* (MRI) is not possible. This includes individuals with metal implants (pacemaker, aneurysm clips, foreign body, and the like), individuals too large for the MRI equipment, or individuals with severe claustrophobia.
- MRI is the diagnostic modality of choice to evaluate the menisci.
- Accuracy of modern MRI scans in detection of meniscus tears approaches 95% (Greis et al, 2002*a*).
- MRI studies have shown that the meniscal substance is not always homogeneous.
- Abnormal signal has been found in up to 30% of asymptomatic patients without any history of knee injury (Rath and Richmond, 2000).
- Normal anatomic structures adjacent to the meniscus, such as the intermeniscal ligament, and hiatus for the popliteus tendon, can be a source of confusion in interpretation of MRI scans (Greis et al, 2002*a*).
- False positive results occur more frequently than false negative results, which emphasize the need for clinical correlation.
- Routine preoperative MRI scan does not significantly improve diagnostic accuracy over clinical examination

alone (Miller, 1996). Each has accuracy in competitive athletes of approximately 90% (Muellner et al, 1997).
- MRI does provide information regarding the extent of the tear, and identification of occult chondral and osseous injuries.
- Judicious use of MRI is recommended, particularly in patients in whom arthroscopic surgery is anticipated.

MRI INTERPRETATION

- Meniscal signals as shown by MRI have been classified into four grades.
- Grade 0 signal: Uniformly low signal intensity (normal meniscus).
- Grade I signal: Irregular increases in intrameniscal signal.
- Grade II signal: Linear increases in intrameniscal signal, not communicating with the superior or inferior meniscal surface.
- Grade III signal: Abnormal increased signal extends to one meniscal surface.
- Grades I and II have no surgical significance. Grade III signal is visible arthroscopically and represents a meniscus tear.

MENISCUS TEAR PATTERNS

- Meniscus injuries are commonly classified by the description of the pattern of tear.
- Patterns of tear include vertical longitudinal, oblique (flap, parrot-beak), horizontal, radial (transverse), and complex.
- Vertical and oblique patterns constitute approximately 80% of tears (Greis et al, 2002*a*).
- Complex, degenerative tears increase in frequency with age (>40).
- A complete, displaced vertical tear is termed a bucket handle tear, and is the pattern often associated with mechanical block to motion.
- Radial tears disrupt the circumferential fibers of the meniscus, and when they extend to the periphery, result in loss of the load bearing function of the meniscus.

TREATMENT

- Treatment of meniscal injury is influenced by patient factors, as well as the nature of the meniscal pathology. Patient factors include the chronicity of symptoms, tolerance for activity modification following

repair versus resection, tolerance for risk of failure, expectations, age, and underlying condition of the joint (Klimkiewicz and Shaffer, 2002).
- The determinants of successful healing of a torn meniscus include tear location and configuration.
- No more than the peripheral one-third of the meniscus has a vascular supply. Therefore, the central 70–80% demonstrates inferior conditions for healing.
- It is important to classify the location of the tear relative to the blood supply of the meniscus, in order to predict repair potential.
- Tear classification based on location is as follows: red–red tear, located at the meniscal periphery within the vascular zone; red–white, no blood supply from the inner surface of the lesion; and white–white, located in the avascular zone.
- Red–red tears have the greatest potential for healing, and white–white the least (Klimkiewicz and Shaffer, 2002).

NONOPERATIVE MANAGEMENT

- Surgical treatment is recommended for most meniscal tears, except those causing minor symptoms in less active patients.
- If nonoperative management is selected, treatment is directed at minimizing symptoms of pain and swelling.
- A trial of activity modification, rehabilitation, and nonsteroidal anti-inflammatory medications is warranted until symptoms abate. This may be successful; however, symptoms may recur.

OPERATIVE MANAGEMENT

- Arthroscopic treatment of meniscal injuries has become one of the most common orthopedic surgical procedures in the United States (Greis et al, 2002a).
- Operative treatment of meniscus tears is warranted in patients with high physical demands associated with work or sport, as the activity modification required to reduce symptoms often is not acceptable.
- Surgical indications include symptoms that affect activities of daily living, work or sport; failure to respond to nonsurgical management; absence of other causes of knee pain identified by radiographs or other imaging.
- Results of early treatment of peripheral tears (suspected with development of an effusion over the first 48 h) are improved with surgical repair performed within the first 4 months from the time of injury (ideally less than 10 weeks) (Greis et al, 2002b).

- Additional predictors of favorable outcome from repair include peripheral location (within 3 mm of the meniscosynovial junction), patient age less than 30 years, tear length less than 2.5 cm, tear of the lateral meniscus, and simultaneous ACL reconstruction (secondary to intra-articular bleeding and fibrin clot formation) (Greis et al, 2002b; Eggli et al, 1995).
- The goal of meniscal surgery is to maximize meniscal preservation. Tears with the potential to heal should be repaired.
- Tears most likely to heal without treatment include tears less than 10 mm in length, tears with less than 3 mm displacement on arthroscopic probing, partial thickness tears (<50% meniscal depth), and radial tears less than 3 mm in length (Klimkiewicz and Shaffer, 2002).
- Arthroscopic rasping of the tear and synovium, or trephination, of these tears to encourage neovascularization, may encourage healing, and may be successful in as many as 90% of cases (Klimkiewicz and Shaffer, 2002; Greis et al, 2002b).
- Displaced tears that result in a block to motion should be treated expeditiously.

MENISCUS REPAIR

- Repair techniques include open, arthroscopically-assisted, and all arthroscopic repair.
- Traditional techniques for repair utilize suture fixation, passed using a variety of devices that are tied through a posterior counter-incision.
- Meniscus repair implants continue to evolve since their introduction in the mid-1990s. Current generation implants incorporate a suture based repair, and allow for an all arthroscopic technique.
- Criteria for meniscus repair include complete vertical longitudinal tear >10 mm in length, location within the peripheral 10–30% of the meniscus (or within 3–4 mm of the meniscosynovial junction), displaceable more than 3–5 mm on arthroscopic probing, no significant secondary joint degeneration or deformity, and a stable knee (Klimkiewicz and Shaffer, 2002; Greis et al, 2002b).
- Situations not meeting the above criteria must be individualized. It may be appropriate to extend the indications in younger individuals, or in cases where resection would lead to nonfunctional remaining tissue (Klimkiewicz and Shaffer, 2002).
- Suture repairs should be performed with vertical mattress stitches when possible, as these demonstrate superior repair strength compared to the horizontal pattern (Greis et al, 2002b).

PARTIAL MENISCECTOMY

- Meniscal injury leads to partial meniscectomy in the majority of cases, as a result of the anatomy of the tear, underlying degeneration of the substance of the meniscus, or distance from the blood supply (Klimkiewicz and Shaffer, 2002).
- Meniscal tears that do not fall into the category of stable (with possible spontaneous healing), or repairable, should be treated with partial meniscectomy to remove unstable fragments, eliminate mechanical symptoms, and reduce pain and associated swelling (Greis et al, 2002*a*).
- Indications for partial meniscectomy include complete oblique, radial, horizontal, degenerative, or complex tears, and tears located in the white–white zone (Klimkiewicz and Shaffer, 2002).
- The goal during meniscectomy is to remove nonfunctioning tissue, maximize meniscus preservation, and create a stable configuration of the remaining tissue.

OUTCOMES

- As previously outlined, the meniscus serves a chondroprotective function in the knee.
- Precocious arthropathy may result from partial or total meniscectomy. This is thought to be secondary to the increased contact stresses on the articular surfaces.
- Total meniscectomy in previously normal knees results in significant arthrosis in two-thirds of patients by 15 years from surgery (Andersson-Molina, Karlsson, and Rockborn, 2002).
- Better outcome is noted after successful repair compared to resection, with lower incidence of degenerative change after 5 years (Klimkiewicz and Shaffer, 2002).
- More rapid degeneration is noted after lateral meniscectomy compared to medial meniscectomy (Klimkiewicz and Shaffer, 2002; Rodeo, 2001; Jaureguito et al, 1995).
- The factor with the greatest impact on long-term outcome is whether articular damage is present at the time of partial meniscectomy (Greis et al, 2002*b*).
- Other factors that influence risk of future arthritis include amount of resection (more resection, higher risk), type of resection (radial resection destroys the meniscus ability to convert compression forces to hoop stresses), associated instability, overall weight-bearing alignment, body habitus, age, and activity level (Klimkiewicz and Shaffer, 2002).
- Results of partial meniscectomy remain good or excellent in over 90% of patients not demonstrating articular cartilage damage at the time of meniscectomy, and this declines to approximately 60% if

damage is present (Greis et al, 2002*b*). In general, 80–90% of patients have documented good to excellent results within the first 5 years after partial meniscectomy (Klimkiewicz and Shaffer, 2002).
- Functional results do not always correlate with radiographic findings. Up to 50% of patients at 8 years after partial meniscectomy versus 25% in untreated knees will demonstrate radiographic changes (Greis et al, 2002*a*; Klimkiewicz and Shaffer, 2002; Jaureguito et al, 1995).
- Meniscus repair is successful in approximately 80% of cases. Healing rates increase to approximately 95% in the setting of concomitant ACL reconstruction (Greis et al, 2002*b*).

COMPLICATIONS

- Complications specific to meniscus repair include neurovascular injuries.
- The peroneal nerve is at greatest risk with lateral meniscus repair. The popliteal artery, popliteal vein, and tibial nerve are also at risk.
- The saphenous nerve, particularly the infrapatellar branch, is at greatest risk with medial repair.
- Failure of repair resulting in the need for repeat arthroscopy is possible, and the risk increases as indications for repair are extended.
- Meniscus repair done concurrently with ACL reconstruction increases the risk of motion loss; however, the appropriateness of staged repair remains controversial.

MENISCAL SUBSTITUTES

- Substitutes for meniscus tissue injury, or loss, are in development.
- Current replacements include meniscal allograft transplantation and collagen meniscal implants.

MENISCAL ALLOGRAFT TRANSPLANTATION

- Meniscal allograft transplantation has been in human use for over 10 years.
- The allograft tissue is most commonly fresh-frozen or cryopreserved. Fresh allografts have also been used; however, logistical difficulties in the routine use of fresh grafts make them impractical for widespread use (Greis et al, 2002*b*).
- Immune response against the transplant has been shown; however, frank rejection does not appear to occur (Rodeo, 2001).

- The technique of allograft transplantation has proved to be reproducible in terms of healing, and control of postmeniscectomy pain and swelling. The exact indications for allograft transplantation, however, continue to be developed (Rodeo, 2001). When properly indicated, transplant leads to predictable good results in over 90% of patients (Klimkiewicz and Shaffer, 2002).
- Meniscal allograft transplantation may be considered for patients with symptoms referable to a meniscus-deficient tibiofemoral compartment. These symptoms include pain and swelling, more commonly than mechanical symptoms (Klimkiewicz and Shaffer, 2002; Rodeo, 2001).
- It is not possible, at this time, to identify patients that will develop symptomatic arthrosis after meniscectomy, and therefore prophylactic transplantation in the asymptomatic patient after meniscectomy has not been justified (Klimkiewicz and Shaffer, 2002).
- Ideally, an objective marker of early pathologic changes to articular surfaces will be identified to allow identification of appropriate patients for early meniscus replacement. Such markers may be found through advanced imaging techniques, or synovial fluid analysis for cartilage degradation products.
- Transplantation results are poor in cases of advanced joint degeneration, and therefore should only be considered when no more than fibrillation and fissuring of the articular surfaces is present.
- Full-thickness articular cartilage lesions on the flexion weight-bearing zone of the femoral condyle or tibia greater than 10–15 mm in diameter is a contraindication to transplantation (Greis et al, 2002b; Rodeo, 2001).
- Additionally, in order to be a candidate for transplantation, the knee must be stable, without malalignment. An unstable knee must be stabilized, and malalignment requires correction to avoid direct weight bearing through the involved compartment receiving the meniscus transplant (Klimkiewicz and Shaffer, 2002; Rodeo, 2001).

MENISCUS SCAFFOLDS

- Bovine collagen meniscal scaffolds, termed *collagen meniscal implants* (CMI), have been approved for human implantation in Europe, Australia, and Chile. These implants are currently under evaluation in the United States in an ongoing multicenter trial. The scaffold is gradually replaced by meniscus-like tissue as fibrochondrocytes proliferate within the scaffold.

- Preliminary trials have shown that CMI scaffolds demonstrate promise as an alternative to allograft. Patients note subjective improvement in symptoms, with generation of meniscus-like tissue viewed by arthroscopy and histology (Stone et al, 1997).
- Porcine small intestine submucosa, which contains collagen and multiple growth factors, is an alternative scaffold under consideration and currently used in animal trials (Welch et al, 2002).

FUTURE DIRECTIONS

- Future treatments in both meniscus repair and replacement continue to evolve.
- Several growth factors and cytokines are under investigation as potential adjuncts to potentiate healing.
- Meniscal fibrochondrocytes respond with migration and proliferation to growth factors, including *platelet derived growth factor* (PDGF), *hepatocyte growth factor* (HGF), *bone morphogenic protein-2* (BMP-2), *insulin-like growth factor-1* (IGF-1), and *transforming growth factor-beta* (TGF-β) (Bhargava et al, 1999; Ochi et al, 2001).
- Suggested delivery systems for growth factors include impregnated absorbable scaffolds, impregnated fixation devices, or even virus vectors for gene therapy (Martinek et al, 2002).
- Tissue engineering may be the next step in development of a durable meniscal replacement. This technique combines the technology of cell culture, polymer chemistry, and biology to create tissues that are appropriate for tissue replacement or reconstruction. The implant would incorporate fibrochondrocytes that have been multiplied in cell culture, in appropriate shaped polymer scaffolds.

REFERENCES

Andersson-Molina H, Karlsson H, Rockborn P: Arthroscopic partial and total meniscectomy: A long-term follow-up study with matched controls. *Arthroscopy* 18(2):183–189, 2002.

Arnoczky SP, McDevitt CA: The meniscus: Structure, function, repair, and replacement, in *Orthopaedic Basic Science: Biology and Biomechanics of the Musculoskeletal System*, 2nd ed. Rosemont, IL, AAOS, 2000, pp 531–545.

Bhargava MM, Attia ET, Murrell GAC, et al: The effect of cytokines on the proliferation and migration of bovine meniscal cells. *Am J Sports Med* 27(5):636–643, 1999.

Eggli S, Wegmueller H, Kosina J, et al: Long-term results of arthroscopic meniscal repair. *Am J Sports Med* 23:715–720, 1995.

Fairbank TJ: Knee joint changes after meniscectomy. *J Bone Joint Surg [Br]* 30:664–670, 1948.

Greis PE, Bardana DD, Holmstrom MC, et al: Meniscal injury: Part I. Basic science and evaluation. *J Am Acad Ortho Surg* 10(3):168–176, 2002*a*.

Greis PE, Holmstrom MC, Bardana DD, et al: Meniscal injury: Part II. Management. *J Am Acad Orthop Surg* 10(3):177–187, 2002*b*.

Gupte CM, Bull AMJ, Thomas R, et al: A review of the function and biomechanics of the meniscofemoral ligaments. *Arthroscopy* 19(2):161–171, 2003.

Jaureguito JW, Elliot JS, Lietner T, et al: The effects of arthroscopic partial lateral meniscectomy in an otherwise normal knee: A retrospective review of functional, clinical, and radiographic results. *Arthroscopy* 11(1):29–36, 1995.

Klimkiewicz JJ, Shaffer B: Meniscal surgery 2002 Update: Indications and techniques for resection, repair, regeneration, and replacement. *Arthroscopy* 18(9):14–25, 2002.

Levy IM, Torzilli PA, Warren RF: The effect of medial meniscectomy on anterior-posterior motion of the knee. *J Bone Joint Surg [Am]* 64A(6):883–888, 1982.

Levy IM, Torzilli PA, Gould JD, et al: The effect of lateral meniscectomy on motion of the knee. *J Bone Joint Surg [Am]* 71A(3):401–406, 1989.

Lo IKY, Thornton G, Miniaci A, et al: Structure and function of diarthrodial joints, in McGinty JB (ed.): *Operative Arthroscopy*, 3rd ed. Philadelphia, PA, Lippincott Williams and Wilkins, 2003, pp 41–126.

Martinek V, Usas A, Pelinkovic D, et al: Genetic engineering of meniscal allografts. *Tissue Eng* 8:107–117, 2002.

Miller GK: A prospective study comparing the accuracy of the clinical diagnosis of meniscus tear with magnetic resonance imaging and its effect on clinical outcome. *Arthroscopy* 12:406–413, 1996.

Muellner T, Weinstabl R, Schabus R, et al: The diagnosis of meniscal tears in athletes. A comparison of clinical and magnetic resonance imaging investigations. *Am J Sports Med* 25:7–12, 1997.

Ochi M, Uchio Y, Okuda K, et al: Expression of cytokines after meniscal rasping to promote meniscal healing. *Arthroscopy* 17(7):724–731, 2001.

Rath E, Richmond JC: The menisci: Basic science and advances in treatment. *Br J Sports Med* 34:252–257, 2000.

Richmond JC: The knee, in Richmond JC, Shahady EJ (eds.): *Sports Medicine for Primary Care*. Oxford, Blackwell Science, 1996, pp 387–444.

Rodeo SA: Meniscal allografts—where do we stand? *Am J Sports Med* 29(2):246–260, 2001.

Simon SR, Alaranta H, An KN, et al: Kinesiology, in *Orthopaedic Basic Science: Biology and Biomechanics of the Musculoskeletal System*, 2nd ed. Rosemont, IL, AAOS, 2000, pp 730–827.

Stone KR, Steadman JR, Rodkey WG, et al: Regeneration of meniscal cartilage with use of a collagen scaffold. Analysis of preliminary results. *J Bone Joint Surg* 79A:1770–1777, 1997.

Welch JA, Montgomery RD, Lenz SD, et al: Evaluation of small-intestinal submucosa implants for repair of meniscal defects in dogs. *Am J Vet Res* 63:427–431, 2002.

59 KNEE INSTABILITY

Alex J Kline, BA
Mark D Miller, MD

INTRODUCTION

- The bony structure of the knee provides relatively little inherent stability to the joint. In turn, knee stability depends on the intact functioning of the four major knee ligaments as well as the supporting ligamentous structures. Injuries to these structures lead to varying degrees of functional instability in the knee joint.

ANATOMY AND BIOMECHANICS OF KNEE LIGAMENTS

ACL

- The *anterior cruciate ligament* (ACL) originates on the posteromedial aspect of the lateral femoral condyle. From there, it courses anteromedially to insert in a wide, depressed area just anterior to and between the intercondylar eminences of the tibia.
- The ACL is approximately 33-mm long and 11-mm in diameter (Miller, 2000). The blood supply is from the middle geniculate artery. Innervation is via branches of the tibial nerve.
- Often described as having two distinct bundles. The anteromedial bundle is tight in flexion. The posterolateral bundle is tight in extension.
- The primary function of the ACL is to resist anterior translation of the tibia on the femur. Secondary functions include stabilization against excessive varus and valgus stress, stabilizer to hyperextension, proprioception, and the *screw home* mechanism.

PCL

- The *posterior cruciate ligament* (PCL) originates in a comma shaped area on the posterolateral surface of the medial femoral condyle. It runs posterolaterally to insert the tibia in a sulcus approximately 1 cm below the articular surface.
- The PCL is approximately 38-mm long and 13-mm in diameter (Girgis, Marshall, and Al Monajem, 1975). The blood supply is from branches of the middle geniculate and innervation is via branches of the tibial nerve.
- Like the ACL, the PCL is described as having two distinct bundles. The anterolateral bundle is tight in flexion. The posteromedial bundle is tight in extension.

- The primary function of the PCL is to resist posterior translation of the tibia on the femur. Secondary function includes stabilization to varus and valgus stress and a role in the screw home mechanism.
- Accessory meniscofemoral ligaments are variably present and run from the lateral meniscus to the body of the PCL. The anterior meniscofemoral ligament is Humphry's ligament; the posterior meniscofemoral ligament is Wrisberg's ligament.

MCL

- The *medial collateral ligament* (MCL) is composed of superficial (tibial collateral ligament) and deep (medial capsular ligament) fibers. The superficial fibers originate from the posterior aspect of the medial femoral condyle and insert in the proximal tibia approximately 5 cm inferior to the joint line.
- The MCL functions as the primary restraint to valgus stress at the knee.

LCL

- The *lateral collateral ligament* (LCL) consists of a single layer and runs from the lateral femoral epicondyle to the lateral aspect of the head of the fibula. The insertion is proximal and posterior to the insertion of the popliteus tendon.
- The LCL functions primarily to stabilize the knee against varus stress.

MEDIAL AND LATERAL SUPPORTING STRUCTURES

- The lateral and medial supporting structures are best considered in layers.
- Medial Structures
  1. Layer I: Sartorius and fascia
  2. Layer II: Superficial MCL, posterior oblique ligament, semimembranosus
  3. Layer III: Deep MCL, capsule
- Lateral Structures
  1. Layer I: Lateral fascia, iliotibial band, biceps tendon
  2. Layer II: Patellar retinaculum, patellofemoral ligament, LCL
  3. Layer III: Arcuate ligament, fabellofibular ligament, capsule

ACL INJURIES

BASICS

- The ACL is the most commonly injured major ligament of the knee, accounting for nearly 50% of all knee ligament injuries (Hirshman, Daniel, and Miyasaka, 1990). More than 200,000 ACL tears occur in the United States each year (Albright et al, 1999).

Seventy percent of these injuries occur during athletic activities (Hirshman, Daniel, and Miyasaka, 1990).
- Women in competitive sports show an increased predisposition to ACL rupture of two to eight times compared with their male counterparts (Harmon and Ireland, 2000). Theories for increased rates of ACL ruptures in females include increased joint laxity, hormonal influences, intercondylar notch dimensions, and ligament size.
- The most common mechanism of ACL injury is external rotation of the femur on a fixed tibia combined with a valgus load and often is the result of a noncontact pivoting injury. Such twisting or cutting-type injuries commonly occur during skiing, football, and soccer.
- Another common mechanism is hyperextension with internal rotation of the tibia as seen in basketball as the athlete lands while grabbing a rebound. Pure hyperextension can also lead to ACL injury as seen in football injuries. More rarely, hyperflexion injuries can also lead to ACL disruption.
- In approximately 40% of cases, the patient will describe feeling or hearing a pop when the injury occurred (Silbey and Fu, 2001). This is the most reliable factor in the patient history in diagnosing an ACL injury. Most often the patient is unable to continue with athletic activity and a hemarthrosis develops within several hours in 70% of patients (Donaldson, Warren, and Wickiewicz, 1992).

EVALUATION

- As in any orthopedic evaluation, inspection, palpation, and range of motion testing are important in the evaluation of ACL injuries. Ecchymosis and loss of the normal knee contour may be seen and a significant effusion may be present. Examination is most accurate immediately after the injury occurs, before significant pain and swelling are present.
- The Lachman test remains the gold standard for the diagnosis of acute ACL injuries. The patient is placed supine on the examination table with the knee in 20°–30° of flexion and the foot resting on the table. The femur is firmly stabilized with one hand, while the other hand applies an anteriorly directed force on the posterior tibia. The degree of tibial displacement is determined, as is the quality of the endpoint. This test has a sensitivity of 87–98% (Donaldson, Warren, and Wickiewicz, 1992; Jonsson et al, 1982).
- In the Lachman test, laxity is graded as 1+ (0–5-mm displacement), 2+ (5–10-mm displacement), or 3+ (>10-mm displacement) and the endpoint is described as firm or soft.
- The anterior drawer test is less sensitive than the Lachman. The hip is flexed to 45° and the knee is

flexed to 90°. Both thumbs are placed on the joint line, and the tibia is drawn gently forward. The degree of laxity and the quality of the endpoint are evaluated.

- Other evaluations of the acute ACL injured knee include the flexion-rotation-drawer test, the pivot shift test, the MacIntosh test, and the Losee test (Silbey and Fu, 2001).
- Instrumented testing devices strive to minimize interexaminer variability determining the degree of knee laxity. The devices work by tracking motion of the tibial tubercle in relation to the patella, thereby measuring an objective measurement of anterior tibial translation (D'Amato and Bach, 2003). The most commonly cited model is the KT-1000 arthrometer (Medmetric, San Diego, CA) (D'Amato and Bach, 2003).
- The history and physical remains the cornerstone of ACL injury diagnosis. Radiographs can provide important adjunct information in the setting of a torn ACL, especially to include associated injuries. Findings that should be closely evaluated for include avulsion of the tibial spine, Segond fractures, and tibial plateau fractures.
- MRI imaging is now often used to assess the integrity of the ligament and look for associated injury to other structures (menisci, PCL, collateral ligaments). MRI also shows bone contusions in up to 80% of patients (Johnson et al, 1998). It should be stressed that diagnosis of an ACL tear relies most heavily on the history and physical and in the majority of cases the additional cost of the MRI is not warranted.

NATURAL HISTORY

- The menisci are often concomitantly injured with the ACL (Bellabarba, Bush-Joseph, and Bach, Jr, 1997; Fithian, Paxton, and Goltz, 2002). In a review of the literature, Bellabarba et al. reported a 41 to 81% incidence of meniscal tears in acute ACL injuries, and a 58 to 100% incidence in chronic ACL tears 11). With our current knowledge of the fate of the postmeniscectomized knee, it is imperative to identify and repair torn menisci associated with ACL tears when at all possible.
- Chondral injuries are also commonly found in the evaluation of the ACL disrupted knee. Studies show an approximately 20% incidence of chondral injuries in acute ACL tears and 50% or more in chronic ACL patients (Indelicato and Bittar, 1985).
- Development of late degenerative arthritis in the ACL injured knee is controversial. Long-term follow of ACL deficient knees often reveals associated degenerative arthritic changes. These "fairbanks changes" have been correlated with meniscal pathology in some studies (Satku, Kumar, and Ngoi, 1986;

Fowler and Regan, 1987), while others show similar rates of degeneration in ACL deficient knees with or without meniscectomy (Giove et al, 1983; Noyes et al, 1983).

- In addition to the associated injuries listed above, nonoperative treatment also frequently leads to instability with activity. Noyes et al. reported a 65% incidence of giving way during strenuous activity following conservative treatment of ACL tears (Noyes et al, 1983). They also reported that only 19% of nonoperative patients could perform turning or twisting activities. Obviously, many young and athletically active patients will not tolerate such an outcome.

MANAGEMENT

- Decision making concerning the optimal treatment of ACL tears must take into account patient preference, age, activity level, knee instability, and associated injuries. Some older patients who do not engage in strenuous activities may be satisfied with conservative treatments. Other patients will require reconstruction in order to function at an acceptable level.
- Fu et al outlined several indications for ACL reconstruction (Fu and Schulte, 1996): (*1*) Athletically active patients who desire to continue to participate at a high level. (*2*) Patients who present with reparable meniscus tears in addition to the ACL tear. (*3*) Patients with associated grade III tears of other major knee ligaments (PCL, MCL, LCL). (*4*) Patients experiencing instability that is interfering with activities of daily living.
- Several studies have stressed the importance of the timing of ACL surgery. ACL reconstruction surgery too soon after the initial injury is associated with increased incidence of arthofibrosis and decreased range of motion following surgery (Harner et al, 1992). As such, Harner et al recommend waiting 3 to 4 weeks after the acute injury before reconstruction is undertaken (Harner et al, 1992).
- Successful ACL reconstruction relies on grafts that mimic the complex anatomy and biomechanical properties of the native ACL (Miller and Gladstone, 1002). The most commonly used choices today for intra-articular ACL reconstruction are *bone-patellar tendon-bone* (BTB) grafts, quadrupled semitendinosus/gracilis tendon grafts, and quadriceps tendon grafts.
- BTB grafts are generally 8- to 11-mm wide and comprise the central third of the patellar tendon adjacent tibial and patellar bone blocks (Miller and Gladstone, 1002; Fu et al, 1999). This method is popular due to a high initial tensile load and stiffness, and the ability to achieve rigid fixation with the bony ends. Disadvantages are largely due to donor site morbidity.

- Hamstring tendon grafts have received attention because of the potential for lower donor site morbidity (Miller and Gladstone, 1002; Fu et al, 1999). Quadrupling of the grafts allows for increased tensile strength and cross-sectional area. Potential disadvantages of this technique include a longer healing time required for soft tissue to bone fixation.
- The quadriceps tendon graft has been shown to have an adequate tensile load and cross-sectional area for ACL reconstruction (Fu et al, 1999). It serves as an important replacement graft in revision ACL surgeries and in multiple ligament injuries.
- Additionally allograft tissues have been successfully employed in ACL reconstruction. Advantages include decreased operative time, the lack of graft harvest morbidity, and unlimited graft supply. Disadvantages include the potential for disease transmission, delayed graft incorporation, increased cost, and the biomechanical effects of graft sterilization (Miller and Gladstone, 1002; Fu et al, 1999).

PCL INJURIES

BASICS
- Reports of the incidence of PCL injuries vary widely from 3% of all knee ligament injuries in the general population to greater than 38% of such injuries in the emergency room setting (Allen et al, 2002; Clancy et al, 1983; Fanelli and Edson, 1995; Miyasaka and Daniel, 1991). One evaluation of college football players reported chronic PCL injuries in approximately 2% of asymptomatic athletes (Parolie and Bergfeld, 1986).
- Fifty to ninety percent of PCL injuries are associated with injury to other knee structures (Fanelli and Edson, 1995; Clancy, Jr and Sutherland, 1994). Most commonly, the posterolateral structures are involved. In trauma settings up to 95% of PCL injuries have other associated ligamentous injuries to the same knee (Allen et al, 2002).
- The mechanism of injury is most commonly a posteriorly directed force to the anterior of a flexed knee, the so-called *dashboard injury*. In athletics, such injuries can be caused by a fall on a flexed knee with a plantarflexed foot. More rarely, PCL injuries can result from hyperextension or hyperflexion and are often associated with multiple ligament injuries (Allen et al, 2002; St Pierre and Miller, 1999).
- Unlike ACL injuries, the patient with a PCL injury does not usually feel a pop and the athlete may not be able to describe exactly how or when the injury occurred (Shelbourne and Rubinstein, 1994). Patients will often report nonspecific symptoms such as an insecure feeling, a vague aching pain, or difficulty climbing stairs.

EVALUATION
- The posterior drawer test is considered the gold standard of physical examination. The knee is flexed to 90° and the hip to 45°, and the foot is firmly planted on the examination table. Crucial to interpreting this test is recognizing the starting point. There is normally a 10-mm step-off between the medial tibial plateau to the medial femoral condyle with the knee in 90° of flexion. Absence of a normal step-off suggests PCL injury. This test is reported to be 90% sensitive and 99% specific (Pournaras and Symeonides, 1991).
- In the posterior drawer, the degree of laxity can be assessed as follows. Displacement up to 5 mm is grade I, and the tibial condyle remains anterior to the femoral condyle. Five to ten millimeters of displacement is grade II, and the tibia and femur are approximately flush. Greater than 10 mm of displacement is grade III, and the tibia is displaced posterior to the femoral condyle.
- Other techniques include the posterior sag test, prone drawer test, quadriceps active test, dynamic posterior shift test, and the posterior Lachman. Due to the frequent association with posterolateral corner injuries, these structures should also be examined. Such examinations include the reverse pivot shift and External Rotation Thigh Foot Angle tests (Margheritini et al, 2002).
- Stress radiographs should be obtained to evaluate for avulsion fractures involving the PCL, fibular head, or Gerdy's tubercle. In chronic PCL injuries, there may be evidence of medial compartment arthritic changes.
- MRI can also contribute valuable information in the diagnosis of PCL injuries with reported 100% sensitivity in identifying complete PCL disruption (Gross et al, 1992). MRI is also valuable in evaluating for associated injury to other knee structures.

NATURAL HISTORY
- The natural history of the PCL injured knee remains controversial. Some studies show high rates of patient satisfaction, the ability of the patient to return to preinjury athletic participation, and no increased incidence in osteoarthritis following conservative treatment of PCL injuries.
- Other studies indicate that PCL injuries may not be so benign. Multiple studies have demonstrated arthritic changes in the medial compartment and patellofemoral joint with chronic PCL injuries. Other potential deleterious effects include significant limitation in postinjury activities and pain with activity.

MANAGEMENT

- Overall patient selection for operative versus nonoperative treatment is still somewhat ill-defined in part because of the controversy surrounding the natural history of the injury.
- Most avulsion fractures require acute fixation. Injuries with large avulsion fragments can be fixed with reduction and lag screw fixation, while those with small avulsion fragments are better repaired with reduction and suture fixation through small drill holes (St Pierre and Miller, 1999; Meyers, 1975).
- The treatment of midsubstance PCL tears is somewhat more complicated. The severity of injury (grade/amount of posterior translation) and the presence or absence of associated ligament injuries must both be considered. Nonoperative treatment is often advocated for isolated grade I or grade II injuries. Such treatment includes initially splinting the knee in extension, followed by early motion and aggressive quadriceps rehabilitation (St Pierre and Miller, 1999).
- Surgical intervention is indicated for severe grade III PCL injuries, symptomatic chronic PCL tears causing significant pain or instability despite appropriate rehabilitation, and PCL injuries in combination with injuries to the ACL, MCL, or posterolateral structures.
- Traditional single bundle transtibial (anterior-posterior) techniques involve passing a graft through a tibial tunnel and into a femoral tunnel to mimic the native function of the PCL. This technique results in the graft passing over a *killer turn* on the posterior edge of the tibial tunnel and may cause the graft to stretch and loosen with time.
- The double-bundle PCL reconstruction utilizes two femoral tunnels in order to better recreate the functional PCL anatomy of the distinct anterolateral and posteromedial bands. One study indicates that the double-bundle reconstruction using two grafts of a split graft may better reproduce the biomechanical functioning of the native PCL. Again, the killer turn may lead to eventual graft loosening.
- The modified arthroscopic technique developed by Harner et al (Harner, Miller, and Swenson, 1994) places the tendon-bone interface of the graft flush with the intra-articular edge of the tibial bone tunnel thereby effectively reducing the graft bending angle by 50% (Harner, Miller, and Swenson, 1994).
- More recently, tibial inlay reconstruction has been developed (Berg, 1995). This technique utilizes a bone trough at the tibial PCL insertion site rather than the traditional tibial tunnel. The bone block of the graft is directly fixed into the trough, thereby obviating the need to negotiate the killer turn. Studies indicate that this technique results in significantly less posterior laxity and graft degradation as compared

with the traditional transtibial method (Bergfeld et al, 2001).

COLLATERAL LIGAMENT INJURIES

MEDIAL COLLATERAL LIGAMENT

- Most often injured by a direct blow to the lateral side of the knee causing valgus stress. Such a blow may lead to the unhappy triad of ACL, MCL, and medial meniscus tears. Injuries most commonly occur at the femoral insertion of the ligament, and tenderness may be localized to the medial epicondyle.
- Diagnosed by a valgus stress test. This is performed with the knee in 30° of flexion in order to relax the ACL and PCL, making the test more specific for the MCL. At full extension, the MCL, posterior oblique ligament, the medial portion of the posterior capsule, the PCL, and the ACL all contribute to valgus stability (Harmon and Ireland, 2000).
- In chronic tears, radiographs may show calcification at the medial femoral condyle insertion site (the so-called Pellegrini-Stieda sign).
- Most tears are amenable to nonoperative management with a hinged knee brace and range-of-motion exercises. After successful initial rehabilitation, football players may choose to wear a prophylactic brace for the remainder of that season.
- Some Grade III tears associated with associated cruciate ligament injuries or repairable meniscal injuries may require surgery (Indelicato, 1995).

LATERAL COLLATERAL LIGAMENT

- Most commonly injured by direct blow to medial knee causing varus stress. Isolated injuries are quite rare, and as such the knee must be thoroughly evaluated for accompanying injuries.
- Diagnosed by varus stress test. Again, the knee is placed in 30° of flexion so the test is more specific for the LCL. It is also important to assess the function of the peroneal nerve, as it courses around the neck of the fibula and may be injured concomitantly with the LCL. Tests of peroneal nerve function include foot dorsiflexion, foot eversion, and sensation to the lateral lower leg (Silbey and Fu, 2001).
- Isolated LCL injuries are usually treated conservatively.

POSTEROLATERAL CORNER INJURIES

- The primary static stabilizers against abnormal posterolateral movements are the fibular collateral ligament, the popliteus tendon, and the popliteofibular ligament (LaPrade and Wentorf, 2002). Most often, these are injured in combination with either the PCL (most common) or ACL and should be repaired at the time of the cruciate repair. The mechanism of injury is generally a blow to the anteromedial aspect of the knee, hyperextenion, or a varus noncontact injury (LaPrade and Terry, 1997).

- External rotation recurvatum, posterolateral drawer test, reverse pivot shift test, and examination for increased external rotation are all important components of the physical examination. Peroneal nerve function should also be assessed, as 15% of posterolateral corner injuries have concomitant injury to the common peroneal nerve (LaPrade and Terry, 1997). MRI scans may be valuable in assessing what structures are involved in the injury.

- Because of poor results with chronic reconstruction, acute repair is advocated in Grade III posterolateral corner injuries within 1–2 weeks if possible. One of the more popular techniques for repair is the popliteus tendon and popliteofibular ligament reconstruction (Veltri and Warren, 1995).

MULTIPLE LIGAMENT INJURIES

- Knee dislocations leading to multiple ligament injuries are fortunately relatively rare. Oftentimes, knee dislocations lead to tears of both the ACL and PCL as well as supporting ligamentous structures of the knee. Neruovascular injury is often present, and a thorough examination must be performed. Popliteal artery injury occurs in approximately 1/3 of knee dislocations (Cole and Harner, 1999). Early arteriography is advocated to avoid missing potential popliteal artery injuries, as such injuries can lead to ischemia and require eventual amputation.

- Nerve injury is also quite common in knee dislocations. Peroneal nerve injury occurs in between 9 and 49% of knee dislocations (Shields, Mital, and Cave, 1969; Taft and Almekinders, 1994), and tibial nerve damage has also been reported (Welling, Kakkasseril and Cranley, 1981). Additionally, as a result of their traumatic nature, knee dislocations frequently have associated fractures.

- Knee dislocations are described by the relative position of the tibia to the femur. Dislocations can be anterior, posterior, medial, lateral, or a combination of these (rotatory). Anterior dislocations are seen with extreme hyperextension, and posterior dislocations may result from high impact dash-board type injuries (Cole and Harner, 1999). Knee dislocations can spontaneously relocate.

- Immediate surgical management is required for popliteal injuries, open dislocations, irreducible

dislocations, and compartment syndrome. Ligament reconstruction is generally delayed for 1 to 3 weeks (Cole and Harner, 1999).

REFERENCES

Albright JC, Carpenter JE, Graf BK, et al: Knee and leg: Soft tissue trauma, in Beaty JH (ed.): *Orthopaedic Knowledge Update* 6, Rosemont, IL, AAOS, 1999, pp 533–559.

Allen CR, Kaplan LD, Fluhme DJ, et al: Posterior cruciate ligament injuries. *Curr Opin Rheumatol* 14:142–149, 2002.

Bellabarba C, Bush-Joseph CA, Bach BR, Jr: Patterns of meniscal injury in the anterior cruciate deficient knee: A review of the literature. *Am J Orthop* 26:18–23, 1997.

Berg EE: Posterior cruciate ligament tibial inlay reconstruction. *Arthroscopy* 11:69–76, 1995.

Bergfeld JA, McAllister DR, Parker RD, et al: A biomechanical comparison of posterior cruciate ligament reconstruction techniques. *Am J Sports Med* 29:129–136, 2001.

Clancy WG, Shelbourne KD, Zoellner GB, et al: Treatment of knee joint instability secondary to rupture of the posterior cruciate ligament: report of a new procedure. *J Bone Joint Surg Am* 65A:310–322, 1983.

Clancy WG, Jr, Sutherland TB: Combined posterior cruciate ligament injuries. *Clin Sports Med* 13:629–647, 1994.

Cole BJ, Harner CD: The multiple ligament injured knee. *Clin Sports Med* 18:241–262, 1999.

D'Amato MJ, Bach BR: Anterior cruciate ligament reconstruction in the adult, in DeLee JC, Drez D, Miller MD (eds.): *DeLee & Drez's Orthopaedic Sports Medicine: Principles and Practice*. Philadelphia, PA, Saunders, 2003, pp 2012–2067.

Donaldson WF, Warren RF, Wickiewicz T: A comparison of acute anterior cruciate ligament examinations. *Am J Sports Med* 10:100–102, 1992.

Fanelli GC, Edson CJ: Posterior cruciate ligament injuries in trauma patients: Part II. *Arthroscopy* 11:526–529, 1995.

Fithian DC, Paxton LW, Goltz DH: Fate of the anterior cruciate ligament-injured knee. *Ortho Clin of North Am* 33:621–636, 2002.

Fowler PJ, Regan WD: The patient with symptomatic chronic anterior cruciate ligament insufficiency. Results of minimal arthroscopic surgery and rehabilitation. *Am J Sports Med* 15:321–325, 1987.

Fu FH, Bennett CG, Lattermann C, et al: Current trends in anterior cruciate ligament reconstruction. Part 1: Biology and biomechanics of reconstruction. *Am J Sports Med* 27:821–830, 1999.

Fu FH, Schulte KR: Anterior cruciate ligament surgery 1996: State of the art? *Clin Orthop* 325:19–24, 1996.

Giove TP, Miller SJ, Kent BE, et al: Non-operative treatment of the torn anterior cruciate ligament. *J Bone Joint Surg Am* 65:184–192, 1983.

Girgis FG, Marshall JL, Al Monajem ARS: The cruciate ligaments of the knee joint: Anatomical, functional, and experimental analysis. *Clin Orthop* 106:216–231, 1975.

Gross ML, Grover JS, Bassett LW, et al: Magnetic resonance imagine of the posterior cruciate ligament: Clinical use to improve diagnostic accuracy. *Am J Sports Med* 20:732–737, 1992.

Harmon KG, Ireland ML: Gender differences in noncontact anterior cruciate ligament injuries. *Clin Sports Med* 19:287–302, 2000.

Harner CD, Miller MD, Swenson TM: New technique for posterior cruciate ligament reconstruction using fresh-frozen achilles tendon allograft. Presented at the 61st Annual Meeting of the American Academy of Orthopedic Surgeons, New Orleans, February 24, 1994.

Harner CD, Irrgang JJ, Paul J, et al: Loss of motion after anterior cruciate ligament reconstruction. *Am J Sports Med* 20:499–506, 1992.

Hirshman HP, Daniel DM, Miyasaka K: The fate of unoperated knee ligament injuries, in Daniel DM, Akeson WH, O'Connor JJ (eds.): *Knee Ligaments: Structure, Function, Injury, and Repair.* New York, NY, Raven Press, 481–503, 1990.

Indelicato PA: Medial collateral ligament injuries. *J Am Acad Orthop Surg* 3:9–14, 1995.

Indelicato PA, Bittar ES: A perspective of lesions associated with ACL insufficiency of the knee. A review of 100 cases. *Clin Orthop* 198:77–80, 1985.

Jonsson T, Althoff B, Peterson L, et al: Clinical diagnosis of rupture of the anterior cruciate ligament. *Am J Sports Med* 10:100–102, 1982.

Johnson DL, Urban WP, Caborn DM, et al: Articular cartilage changes seen with magnetic resonance imaging-detected bone bruises associated with acute anterior cruciate ligament rupture. *Am J Sports Med* 26:409–414, 1998.

LaPrade RF, Terry GC: Injuries to the posterolateral aspect of the knee: Associateion of injuries with clinical instability. *Am J Sports Med* 25:433–438, 1997.

LaPrade RF, Wentorf F: Diagnosis and treatment of posterolateral knee injuries. *Clin Orthop* 402:110–121, 2002.

Margheritini F, Rihn J, Mausahl V, et al: Posterior cruciate ligament injuries in the athlete: An anatomical, biomechanical and clinical review. *Sports Med* 32:393–408, 2002.

Meyers MH: Isolated avulsion of the tibial attachment of the posterior cruciate ligament of the knee. *J Bone Joint Surg* 57A:669–672, 1975.

Miller MD: Sports medicine, in Miller MD (ed.): *Review of Orthopaedics.* Philadelphia, PA, Saunders, 2000, pp 195–240.

Miller SL, Gladstone JN: Graft selection in anterior cruciate ligament reconstruction. *Ortho Clin North Am* 33:678–683, 1002.

Miyasaka KC, Daniel DM: The incidence of knee ligament injuries in the general population. *Am J Knee Surg* 4:3–8, 1991.

Noyes FR, Mooar PA, Matthews DS, et al: The symptomatic anterior cruciate-deficient knee. Part I: The long-term functional disability in athletically active individuals. *J Bone Joint Surg Am* 65:154–162, 1983.

Parolie JM, Bergfeld JA: Long term results of nonoperative treatment of isolated posterior cruciate ligament injuries in the athlete. *Am J Sports Med* 14:35–38, 1986.

Pournaras J, Symeonides PT: The results of surgical repair of acute tears of the posterior cruciate ligament. *Clin Orthop* 267:103–107, 1991.

Satku K, Kumar VP, Ngoi SS: Anterior cruciate ligament injuries. To counsel or to operate? *J Bone Joint Surg Br* 68:458–461, 1986.

Shelbourne KD, Rubinstein RA: Methodist Sports medicine center's experience with acute and chronic isolated posterior cruciate ligament injuries. *Clin Sports Med* 13:531–543, 1994.

Shields L, Mital M, Cave E: Complete dislocation of the knee: Experience at the Massachusetts General hospital. *J Trauma* 9:192–215, 1969.

Silbey MB, Fu FH: Knee injuries, in Fu FH, Stone DA (eds.): *Sports Injuries: Mechanisms, Prevention, Treatment.* Philadelphia, PA, Lippincott Williams & Wilkins, 2001, pp 1102–1134.

St Pierre P, Miller MD: Posterior cruciate ligament injuries. *Clin Sports Med* 18:199–221, 1999.

Taft T, Almekinders L: The dislocated knee, in Fu F, Harner C, Vince K (eds.): *Knee Surgery.* Baltimore, MD, Williams & Wilkins, 1994, pp 837–858.

Veltri DM, Warren RF: Posteolateral instability of the knee. *Instr Course Lect* 44:441–453, 1995.

Welling R, Kakkasseril J, Cranley J: Complete dislocations of the knee with popliteal vascular injury. *J Trauma* 21:450–453, 1981.

60 THE PATELLOFEMORAL JOINT

Robert J Nicoletta, MD
Anthony A Schepsis, MD

ANATOMY

- The patella is the largest sesamoid bone in the body. Its blood supply arises mainly from the peripatellar plexus. The patella articulates with the femoral sulcus. It is asymmetrically oval in shape with the apex distal. It is enveloped by fibers of the quadriceps tendon and blends with the patellar tendon distally. The patella serves as a fulcrum for the quadriceps muscles. The main biomechanical function of the patella is to increase the moment arm of the quadriceps mechanism.

- The patellar surface is divided into two large facets—medial and lateral, which are separated by a central ridge. The facets are covered by the thickest hyaline cartilage in the body that may measure up to 6.5 mm. The superior three-fourths of patella are articular and the inferior one-fourth is nonarticular. The contact area between the patella and femur varies with knee position. At 10° to 20° of knee flexion the distal pole of the patella contacts the femoral trochlea. As flexion increases, the contact of the patella moves proximally and medially with the most extensive contact being made at approximately 45°. Contact stresses on the patellofemoral joint are higher than any other major weight bearing joint in the body. The contact area and load across the joint increases with knee flexion. Compressive forces on the patella can range from 3.3 times body weight with stair climbing up to 7.6 times body weight with squatting.

- The patellar medial facet varies anatomically. It may be divided into a medial facet proper and a small odd facet. The odd facet may develop as a response to functional loads and does not contact the medial femoral condyle except in extreme flexion.

- Several ossification centers contribute to the patella. Failure of fusion can lead to bipartite patella that can be classified into three types: type I—inferior; type II—lateral; and type III—superolateral (most common). Bipartite patella is most often discovered accidentally during radiographic examination of the knee for another disorder.

- The medial retinaculum is composed of the medial patellofemoral ligament and the medial patellotibial ligament. The *medial patellofemoral ligament* (MPFL) originates from the adductor tubercle and inserts on the medial border of the patella. This ligament plays a major role in preventing lateral displacement of the patella. The lateral retinaculum is composed of a superficial and deep layer and runs from lateral margin of the patella and patellar tendon to the anterior aspect of the iliotibial band.

- The patellar tendon varies in length (average 4.6 cm). It connects the apex of the patella to the tibial tuberosity and is slightly wider proximally than distally.

PATELLAR PAIN

- The single most common cause of knee pain involves pathology related to the patella. Patellar pain or discomfort may be the result of direct trauma, repetitive direct pressure, constant repetitive movements with the knee in a flexed position, malalignment, or a combination of these factors.

- Symptoms of patellar pain that begin during relatively normal activities/sports should alert the physician that the knee was not normal in the first place. If the knee swells significantly within the first 12 to 24 h after traumatic knee injury, this signifies that there is blood or a hemarthrosis within the joint. The most common cause of an acute hemarthrosis after a sports related knee injury is a tear of the anterior cruciate ligament with the second most common cause being a traumatic patellar dislocation/subluxation with bleeding

as a result of either soft tissue tearing, osteochondral fracture or both.

PHYSICAL EXAMINATION

- The physical examination should begin with general inspection for skin abrasions, contusions, or lacerations.

- It is important to document the overall alignment of the leg while the patient is standing, seated, and supine. With the patient supine, patellar alignment and Q angle (angle between *anterior superior iliac spine* (ASIS), patella, and tibial tubercle) are measured. A Q angle of less than 15° is generally considered normal. The Q angle should be assessed with the knee extended and also with the knee flexed 90°. An angle greater than 8° with this method is indicative of an abnormally lateralized patellar vector. If the patella is subluxed, the Q angle reverts to within normal range. Along with Q angle determination, the amount of varus/valgus should be noted. Thigh circumference should be measured at a consistent level above the knee to assess for quadriceps atrophy. Observe patellofemoral tracking with the patient seated over the edge of the table while slowly flexing and extending the knee from 0 to 90°. Observe for high or lateral patellar positioning (grasshopper eyes), small patella, patella alta (the patella faces the ceiling rather than straight ahead), *vastus medialis oblique* (VMO) dysplasia, excessive hit anteversion. Also the examiner should observe for signs of J tracking (the patella deviates laterally in terminal extension).

- Palpate for crepitation, suggesting possible chondral injury, noting the degree of knee flexion that crepitus is present to delineate between proximal and distal lesions. Patellofemoral crepitus is best elicited by having the patient standing and then squatting down with the examiners hands over the patella noting at what arc of motion the crepitus occurs. Retropatellar crepitus that is painful and occurs in either early flexion or terminal extension indicates disease on the distal part of the patella. A painful arc with crepitus in greater degrees of flexion indicates disease on the more proximal portion of the patella. One finger palpation is important to localize tenderness whether it is in the retinaculum or the medial and lateral patellar facets. These are best palpated by placing one finger under the respective facet and pushing the patella over to that side with the other hand. The quadriceps tendon and patellar tendon are also best palpated in a resting position with the knee extended. Point tenderness at the inferior pole of the patella at the attachment of the patellar tendon is typically consistent with

patellar tendonitis or *jumper's knee*. The tenderness is more pronounced with the patellar tendon relaxed with the knee in the extended position. Usually this area is less tender with the knee in the flexed position.
• Lateral displacement may cause apprehension in pts with patellar instability. When assessing for instability, measure patellar mobility (patellar glide). This is based on the maximum amount of passive displacement of the patella (using quadrant system with the patella divided into four vertical quadrants) both medially and laterally with the knee at 30° flexion. This test evaluates the integrity and tightness of the medial and lateral restraints. The passive patellar tilt test determines the tension of the lateral restraints. With the knee fully extended, the patella is manually elevated. A passive tilt of less than 0° (neutral or below the horizontal plane), may imply lateral retinacular tightness and a diagnosis of *excessive lateral pressure syndrome* (ELPS).

RADIOGRAPHS

• The standard patellar radiograph is the merchant view or sunrise view. It is generally performed with the patient supine with the knee flexed 45° to evaluate for articular cartilage loss, tilt, and subluxation. The Laurin view (20° sunrise view) may be more sensitive for delineating subluxation or tilt. A *computed tomography* (CT) scan from 10–60° of knee flexion may be useful to evaluate for tilt, subluxation.

CHONDROMALACIA PATELLA

• Predisposing extrinsic anatomic factors leading to patellofemoral pathology include femoral anteversion, external tibial torsion, foot pronation, and extreme genu varum/valgum. Nonoperative management is the mainstay of treatment of most patellofemoral disorders. Chrondromalacia refers to some type of disruption in the articular cartilage of the the patella that is either painful or nonpainful. Proposed etiologies of chondromalacia include trauma, malalignment, biomechanical, and metabolic. Most patients with symptomatic chondromalacia present with an insidious onset and complain of a dull ache around the anterior knee, pain with loaded flexion activities, particularly descending stairs or a prolonged seated position (theatre sign). Nonoperative management of chondromalacia patella includes rest, flexibility exercises especially of the hamstrings, quadriceps strengthening, and anti-inflammatory medication. Return to play is dictated by symptoms.

SYNOVIAL PLICA

• A synovial plica is a redundant fold in the synovial lining of the knee. This is a normal finding but may become symptomatic when it becomes inflamed or fibrotic. A symptomatic plica is most commonly located on the medial side with a localized tender thickening along the medial border of the patella or condyle on palpation (knee at 45° of flexion). An audible snap with flexion may sometimes be elicited with a plica. Nonoperative management of a synovial plica includes relative rest, flexibility exercises especially of the hamstrings, quadriceps strengthening, and anti-inflammatory medication. If the synovial plica is significantly scarred or fibrotic and cannot be rehabilitated, arthroscopic excision is indicated.

EXCESSIVE LATERAL PRESSURE SYNDROME

• *Excessive lateral pressure syndrome* (ELPS), or lateral facet syndrome, represents a loss of equilibrium of the patella in the trochlea associated with tilt. This results in increased pressure on the lateral patellar facet. This is secondary to a tight lateral retinaculum. The patient with ELPS usually has a spontaneous or posttraumatic onset with patellofemoral arthralgia (dull aching in the center of the knee) and occasionally swelling and giving way may be present. Radiographs or CT of patients with ELPS will usually show lateral patellar tilt on the axial views.

PATELLAR MALALIGNMENT AND INSTABILITY

• Patellar malalignment and instability are two separate issues:
 1. Malalignment indicates maltracking of the patella based on physical examination and imaging studies such as X-rays or CT.
 2. Instability is a functional symptom with the patella transiently displacing (usually lateral) either partially (subluxation) or completely (dislocation). Initial treatment for instability is nonoperative. Surgical correction is indicated when there is failure of nonoperative management or evidence of progressive articular cartilage damage as a result of the instability. Patellar realignment for recurrent instability is categorized as either proximal realignment (tightening, repairing, or reconstructing the medial soft tissue patellar restraints) or distal realignment (transposing the tibial tubercle

medially or anteromedially to correct tubercle malalignment, as documented by an abnormal Q angle). Moving the tibial tubercle medially (distal realignment) cannot be performed before skeletal maturity. Medial patellar instability is uncommon. It occurs most commonly following previous overly restrained lateral procedures.

FRACTURES

• Patellar fractures are most commonly transverse in orientation and are seen best on a lateral X-ray. Vertical fractures are rare and best seen on the sunrise view. Fracture types include undisplaced, transverse, lower or upper pole, comminuted, and vertical. Undisplaced fractures are treated nonoperatively with 6 weeks of bracing/casting in extension followed by progressive range of motion exercises. Displaced fractures are those with at least 3 mm of cortical disruption or 2 mm of articular step off on radiographs. These are treated with *open reduction internal fixation* (ORIF). Fractures that occur with patellar dislocation most commonly involve the lateral condyle or medial patellar facet. With a traumatic avulsion of the VMO in a previous normal knee, surgical repair and early motion is advocated.

BIBLIOGRAPHY

Bentley George, Dowd George: Current concepts of etiology and treatment of chondromalacia patellae. *Clin Orthop* 217–224, 176.

Dye SF, Boll DA: Radionuclide imaging of the patellofemoral joint in young adults with anterior knee pain. *Orthop Clin North Am* 17:249–262, 1986.

Fulkerson JP: Anteromedialization of the tibial tuberosity for patellofemoral malalignment. *Clin Orthop* 176–181, 177.

Fulkerson J, Hungerford D: Disorders of the patellofemoral joint. Baltimore, MD, Williams and Wilkins, 1990.

Fulkerson J, Schutzer S, Ramsby G et al: Computerized tomography of the patellofemoral joint before and after lateral release or realignment. *Arthroscopy* 3:19–24, 1987.

Fulkerson JP, Shea, KP: Current concepts review. Disorders of patellofemoral alignment. *J Bone Joint Surg:* vol. 72–A, No. 9, October 1990, pp 1424–1429.

Gambardella RA: Technical pitfalls of patellofemoral surgery. *Clin Sports Med* 18:897–903, 1999.

Griffiths GP, Selesnick FH: Operative treatment and arthroscopic rindings in chronic patellar tendonitis. *Arthroscopy* 14:836–839, 1998.

Henry, J: Conservative treatment of patellofemoral subluxation. *Clin Sports Med* 8:261–278, 1989.

Huberti HH, Hayes WC: Contact pressures in chrondromalacia patellae and the effects of capsular reconstructive procedures. *J Orthop Res* 6:499–508, 1988.

Hughston JC: Subluxation of the patella. *J Bone Joint Surg* 50–A:1003–1026, July 1968.

Hungerford DS, Lennox DW: Rehabilitation of the knee in disorders of the patellofemoral joint. Relevant biomechanics. *Orthop Clin North Am* 14:397–402, 1983.

Insall J: Chondromalacia patella—patellar malalignment syndrome. *Orthop Clin North Am* 10:117–127, 1979.

Laurin CA, Levesque HP, Dussault, Ret al: The abnormal lateral patellofemoral angle. A diagnostic roentgenographic sign of recurrent patellar subluxation. *J Bone Joint Surg* 60–A:55–60, Jan. 1978.

Merchant A: Classification of patellofemoral disorders. *Arthroscopy* 4:235–240, 1988.

Merchant AC, Mercer RL, Jacobsen RHet al: Roentgenographic analysis of patellofemoral congruence. *J Bone Joint Surg* 56–A:1391–1396, Oct. 1974.

Miller M, Brinker M: *Review of Orthopaedics*, 3rd ed. Philadelphia, PA, Saunders, 2000.

Radin EL: A rational approach to the treatment of patellofemoral pain. *Clin Orthop* 144:107–109, 1979.

Wiles Philip, Andrews PS, Devas MB: Chondromalacia of the patella. *J Bone Joint Surg* 38–B(1):95–113, 1956.

61 SOFT TISSUE KNEE INJURIES (TENDON AND BURSAE)

John J Klimkiewicz, MD

BIOMECHANICS OF TENDON RUPTURES

$$\text{Extensor mechanism force ratio} = \frac{\text{Patellar tendon force}}{\text{Quadriceps tendon force}}$$

• Position of knee flexion of the knee directly affects this ratio. At knee flexion angles <45°, this ratio is >1, while at those a knee flexion angles >45° this ratio is <1 (Huberti et al, 1984).

• At greater than 45°, the patellar tendon has a mechanical advantage and is less susceptible to injury through tensile failure, while at positions less than 45° the quadriceps tendon has a mechanical advantage and is less vulnerable to injury.

• Tendon strain in response to tensile load is up to three times greater at the insertion sites than at the tendon midsubstance. Additionally, collagen fiber stiffness is less at the insertion sites. These biomechanical properties contribute to tendon rupture commonly occurring at their insertion sites rather than at their midsubstance (Zernicke, Garhammer, and Jobe, 1997; Woo et al, 1988).

- Failure usually occurs during rapid eccentric muscular contraction when markedly higher forces can be generated as compared to concentric muscular contraction (Garrett, Jr, 1988).
- Several metabolic diseases or direct steroid injection can predispose to tendon rupture. These conditions include hyperparathryroidism, *calcium pyrophosphate deposition disease* (CPPD), diabetes mellitus, chronic renal disease, gout, systemic lupus erythematosus, and rheumatoid arthritis (Woo et al, 1988; Ford and DeBender, 1979).
- Fluoroquinone antibiotic and isoretinoin treatment have been associated with pathologic tendon alteration and increased incidence of tendon rupture (Williams et al, 2000; Scuderi et al, 1993).

PATELLAR TENDON RUPTURES

- The patellar tendon receives its blood supply from the vessels within the infrapatellar fat pad and retinacular structures (Arnoczky, 1985; Scapinelli, 1968).
- The origin and insertion of the patellar tendon are relatively avascular.
- Ruptures of the patella tendon most typically occur in patients less than 40 years of age and are frequently associated with sporting activities including football, basketball, and soccer (Matava, 1996).
- Ruptures are most common through the tendon–bone junction at the distal pole of the patella.
- Histologic examination of rupture tendon often demonstrates an area of degeneration thought to predispose these patients to injury.
- Previous surgery including total knee arthroplasty, anterior cruciate ligament reconstruction using autograft patellar tendon, and tibial intramedullary nailing have been associated with postoperative patellar tendon ruptures (Crossett et al, 2002; Bonamo, Krinick, and Sporn, 1984; Keating, Orfaly, and O'Brien, 1997).

CLINICAL PRESENTATION

- At time of injury a pop is often heard with an acute onset of pain and swelling. Patient usually unable to actively extend knee or maintain it in an extended position against gravity. Chronic cases present with an extensor lag (Matava, 1996).
- A palpable defect is commonly present just below the distal pole of the patella.

- Concomittant anterior cruciate ligament injuries are not uncommon and should be clinically ruled out.
- Plain radiographs often demonstrate a patella alta in comparison to the opposite knee using the Insall-Salvati Index (Greater than 1.2) (Aglietti, Buzzi, and Insall, 2001).

- Insall - Salvati Index $= \dfrac{\text{Length of patellar tendon}}{\text{Length of patella}}$

    $\times(\text{Normal value } 0.8-1.2)$

- An osseous fragment is present at times at the distal pole of the patella when an avulsion is part of the injury.
- *Magnetic resonance imaging* (MRI) is useful in cases where partial injury is suspected.

TREATMENT

- Partial tendon injuries can be treated conservatively by cylinder cast or brace with the leg placed in full extension for 4–6 weeks followed by progressive range of motion and strengthening.
- Complete ruptures should be directly repaired on an acute basis through transosseous drill holes through the patella. Once secured the knee should have at least 90° of flexion to avoid overconstraint. Primary repairs are often augmented with wire, mersilene tape, suture, or autologous hamstring tendon or iliotibial band (Larson and Lund, 1986).
- Chronic ruptures can involve proximal patellar migration and can often require quadriceps mobilization or V-Y advancement in order to restore patellar height.
- Semitendinosus/gracilis augmentation is recommended in the chronic scenario. Achilles tendon or patellar tendon allograft has often been found useful to replace/reinforce the reconstruction in chronic situations (Hyman, Rodep, and Wickiewicz, 2003).

COMPLICATIONS

- Following surgery include knee stiffness and weakness. Rerupture is rare. Restoration of normal patellofemoral tracking and height at the time of surgery is essential to achieve optimal results. Residual weakness of extensor mechanism is more common in delayed repairs.

QUADRICEPS TENDON RUPTURES

- The quadriceps tendon is a coalescence of tendinous portions of the rectus femoris, vastus lateralis, vastus intermedius, and vastus medialis muscle.

- The quadriceps tendon receives its vascular supply from an anastomatic network including the lateral circumflex femoral artery, descending geniculate artery, and medial/lateral geniculate arteries (Peterson, Stein, and Tillman, 1999).
- There is an avascular region of the deep part of the quadriceps tendon measuring 1.5×3.0 cm.
- Ruptures of the quadriceps tendon most typically occur in patients over 40 years of age and are three times more frequent than patella tendon ruptures. Unilateral injuries are up to 20 times more frequent than bilateral injury (Ilan et al, 2003).
- The site of rupture usually occurs through a degenerative area within the tendon and seldom occurs in younger individuals. Systemic disease can lead to tendon degeneration and predispose to infrequent bilateral tendon ruptures (Lauerman, Smith, and Kenmore, 1987).

CLINICAL PRESENTATION

- Pain is often present before rupture. At time of injury a pop is often heard with an acute onset of pain and swelling.
- In cases of partial injury or complete injuries that do not extend to include the retinacular tissue, the patient may be able to extend and resist gravity with an associated extensor lag but in complete injuries this is not possible.
- A palpable defect at the site of rupture is usually felt just superior to the proximal pole of the patella.
- Plain radiographs often demonstrate patellar baja, an avulsion of the superior pole of the patella, spurring of the superior patellar region, or calcification within the quadriceps tendon. Insall-Salvati ratio less than 0.8 (Aglietti, Buzzi, and Insall, 2001).
- Magnetic resonance imaging is useful adjunct study as it can demonstrate partial ruptures or preexisting disease within the quadriceps tendon.

TREATMENT

- Partial tears are often responsive to conservative treatment when the patient presents primarily with pain and has little loss of strength, retaining the ability to actively extend the knee against gravity.
- Conservative treatment consists of a long leg cylinder cast in full extension for 4–6 weeks, with progressive range of motion and strengthening thereafter for partial injuries.
- Complete ruptures respond best to immediate surgical repair in a direct end-to-end fashion after tendon

debridement of necrotic tissue or with transosseous tunnels through the patella (Rasul and Fischer, 1993).
- Chronic rupture involving more significant tendon retraction often require quadriceps tendon advancement through a tendon Z-plasty or V-Y advancement technique. Interpositional autograft/allograft tendon has been utilized with success in this scenario (Scuderi, 1958).
- Success of repair is direct related to the length of time between injury and the time of surgery, with more chronic repairs producing less favorable outcomes. Age is also a factor with better results in younger patients (Konrath et al, 1998).
- Most common complications following surgery or conservative treatment include decreased quadriceps strength/function with an associated extensor lag and lack of knee flexion.

GASTROCNEMIUS RUPTURE

- Often referred to as *tennis leg*.
- Traumatic injury to middle aged athlete presenting as sudden pain in posterior proximal calf region. Significant pain, swelling, and ecchymosis usually occur with 24 h.
- Involves tearing of the medial head of the gastrocnemius muscle typically at its musculotendinous junction (Miller, 1977).
- Mechanism of injury combines ankle dorsiflexion in combination with knee hyperextension.

DIFFERENTIAL DIAGNOSES

- Differential diagnoses involve plantaris rupture, thrombophlebitis, and an acute compartment syndrome (Severence and Bassett, 1982).
- *Magnetic resonance imaging* (MRI) remains the imaging modality of choice. Ultrasound can be employed to rule out thrombophlebitis.
- Can be associated with an acute compartment syndrome secondary to swelling.

TREATMENT

- Treatment of isolated ruptures of the medial gastrocnemius involves compressive wrapping, activity modification including crutches if necessary, ankle range of motion, ice, and anti-inflammatory medications (Gecha and Torg, 1988).

PATELLAR TENDINITIS

- Caused by activities involving repeated extension of the knee.
- Termed *jumper's knee*, as it's most common in sporting activities such as basketball, volleyball, and soccer. Seen most commonly in younger individuals from their adolescent years to 40 years of age (Feretti et al, 1985).
- Predisposing factors include abnormal patellofemoral tracking, patellar alta, chondromalacia, Osgood-Schlatter disease, and leg length discrepancy.
- Can be confused with Sindig-Larsen-Johansson disease that is a traction apophysitis of the distal pole of the patella that presents with similar complaints in a younger age group.
- Involves the most proximal part of the patellar tendon and its attachment to the distal pole of the patella. This area of tendon is thought to impinge on the adjacent patella during knee flexion causing injury to the tendon (King et al, 1990).
- The affected area of tendon resembles tendonosis in the form of tendon degeneration and not inflammation. Histologically, this tissue is chacterized as undergoing *angiofibroblastic hyperplasia* with fibroblast proliferation, new blood vessel formation, chondromucoid deposition, and collagen fragmentation (Kannus and Jozsa, 1991).

CLINICAL PRESENTATION

- Pain to palpation in the area of tendon involvement just distal its insertion on the inferior pole of the patella.
- Pain is increased with activity requiring knee extension against resistance.
- Tendon may acquire bogginess; however, there is no associated joint effusion.
- Blanzina et al have classified this condition based on the patients' symptoms: (*1*) Pain only after activity. (*2*) Pain is present before activity, and then disappears, only to return near the end of activity with muscular fatigue. (*3*) Pain is constant with both rest and activity. (*4*) Patellar tendon rupture (Blanzina et al, 1973).

RADIOGRAPHIC EVALUATION

- Mainly a clinical diagnosis, but plain X-rays while usually normal, can, at times, demonstrate an osteopenia at the distal pole of the patella, a traction osteophyte in the area of involvement, and calcification of the tendon.

- MRI is the study of choice in the chronic setting as it can clearly identify the area of tendon involvement. This area usually involves the posterior aspect of the tendon in its proximal third (Johnson, Wakely, and Watt, 1996).

TREATMENT

- Conservative treatment is usually successful and includes rest, ice, and anti-inflammatory medication. Therapeutic modalities including ultrasound, ionophoresis, and phonophoresis are helpful in pain relief (Martens et al, 1982; Panni, Tartarone, and Maffulli, 2000).
- Once the pain has subsided, physiotherapy in the form of quadriceps strengthening and hamstring stretching are begun with gradual return to activity.
- An elastic knee sleeve or counterforce brace have also proved beneficial.
- More chronic cases with pathology demonstrable on MRI scan require surgical debridement and excision of the diseased tendon and adjacent bone through either an open or arthroscopic approach (Griffiths and Selesnick, 1998; Romeo and Larson, 1999; Coleman et al, 2000).

QUADRICEPS TENDINITIS

- Not as common as patellar tendonitis but has similar risk factors.
- Repetive microtrauma through overuse can lead to localized degeneration of the quadriceps tendon at its insertion into the superior pole of the patella.
- Chronic symptoms in this area appear to be a risk factor for future tendon ruptue.

CLINICAL PRESENTATION

- Pain with exertion and tenderness over affected area of quadriceps insertion. This most commonly is the lateral aspect of the tendon.
- Radiographs often demonstrate calcification of the tendon at its insertion to the patella or a traction osteophyte at the osseous margin.

TREATMENT

- Treatment is similar to that of patellar tendonitis. Results of conservative treatment are excellent, although more chronic cases can require open surgical debridement (James, 1995).

POPLITEUS TENDINITIS

- Popliteus tendon travels from its origin on the lateral femoral condyle posterolaterally through the popliteal hiatus to insert on the posterior aspect of the proximal tibia (Mann and Hagy, 1977).
- Injuries to this area are a cause of posterolateral knee pain and can occur both acutely (i.e., *anterior cruciate ligament* (ACL) rupture or posterolateral corner injuries) or more chronically as an overuse phenomenon. Chronic injuries most often occur with excessive downhill running or walking (i.e., backpacking) (Nauer and Aalberg, 1985; Mayfield, 1977).

CLINICAL PRESENTATION

- Pain to palpation posterolaterally over the popliteus tendon. This is best appreciated clinically by placing the leg in a figure-of-four position and palpating at the origin of the popliteus just anterior to the lateral femoral epicondyle.
- Differential diagnosis includes iliotibial band syndrome, lateral meniscal tear, and biceps femoris tendonitis.

TREATMENT

- Includes rest and activity modification in the form of eliminating downhill activity. Anti-inflammatory medication as well as physiotherapeutic modalities are also helpful (Mayfield, 1977).

ILIOTIBIAL BAND SYNDROME

- Most common cause of lateral sided knee pain in long distance runners. Also seen in cyclists, weightlifters, football, soccer, and tennis. Often precipitated by downhill running (Orava, 1978).
- Caused by excessive friction between iliotibial band and lateral epicondyle. Knee flexion angle of 30° maximizes friction between these two structures casing an ensuing bursitis.
- Anatomic factors predisposing to this condition include genu varum, tibial varum, varus hindfoot, and compensatory foot hyperpronation.

CLINICAL PRESENTATION

- Lateral sided knee pain that usually is present after initial warm-up that often causes cessation of activity. Pain not present at rest.

- Point of maximal tenderness is approximately 3 cm proximal to lateral joint line over lateral epicondylar region.
- *Ober's* and *Noble's test* are positive and can confirm diagnosis:
- Ober's test: Patient is placed in lateral decubitus position with the affected extremity upwards. The unaffected knee and hip are flexed. The involved knee is flexed and hip hyperextended and abducted. Tightness in the iliotibial tract will prevent the affected extremity from adducting below the horizontal created by the patient's torso (Renee, 1975).
- Noble's test: Patient is in supine position with the knee flexed 90°. Pain is elicited in lateral epicondylar region when the patient's knee is extended between 30° and 40°.
- Radiographs are negative in this condition. MRI can confirm more chronic cases unresponsive to conservative treatment.

TREATMENT

- Conservative treatment focusing on iliotibial tract, hamstring, and hip external rotator stretching combined with strengthening of the hip abductors is usually successful when combined with activity modification and anti-inflammatory treatment. Foot orthotics can also be a useful adjunct in conservative treatment.
- Surgical excision of the posterior aspect of the iliotibial tract overlying the lateral epicondyle at 30°–40° of knee flexion is effective in chronic cases not responding to conservative treatment (Martens, Libbrect, and Burssens, 1989).

PREPATELLAR BURSITIS

- Prepatellar bursa is a potential space of synovial tissue that functions to decrease the friction between the overlying subcutaneous tissue and patella.
- A bursitis can result from an acute injury, infection, systemic disease (i.e., gout), or from chronic activity or overuse (Dawn, 1977).
- Commonly seen in the sport of wrestling (Mysnyk et al, 1986).

CLINICAL PRESENTATION

- Patients typically present with swelling superficial to the patella. Knee range of motion may be limited at the extremes of flexion pending the size of the collection but is painless. There is no associated effusion. Crepitation and thickening of the tissue involving the bursal tissue are often present in more chronic cases.

- Warmth, erythema, and pain to palpation may signify a septic process, but aspiration is necessary to confirm this as not all infected bursae are clinically demonstrable.
- Most common infecting organisms include staphylococcous aureus and streptococcal species.
- On synovial fluid analysis, greater than 75% polymorphonuclear cell differential is most accurate in confirming a septic process. Total white count and glucose levels are less predictable (Ho and Tice, 1979).
- Radiographs are usually negative aside from radiolucency in the area of the bursitis. In cases involving gouty deposits, calcific stippling can be seen.

TREATMENT

- Treatment for aseptic bursitis in this region is activity modification, compressive wrapping, and anti-inflammatory medications. In more chronic situations aspiration in combination with immobilization in extension can be useful.
- Septic or more chronic aseptic processes are best treated with surgical excision via open or arthroscopic techniques. Cases of septic bursitis should be treated with postoperative antibiotics sensitive to the infecting organism (Kaalund, 1998).

PES ANSERINE BURSITIS

- Pes anserine bursa is the synovial tissue overlying the attachment of sartorius, gracilis, and semitendinosis tendons.
- Patients present with pain over this bursal region with often some swelling in this region.
- Differential diagnoses include, medial collateral ligament injury, medial meniscal tear, medial compartmental arthritis, saphenous neuritis, and stress fracture or avascular necrosis of the medial tibial plateau (Larsson and Baum, 1985).

TREATMENT

- Treatment comprises activity modification, anti-inflammatory medications, hamstring stretching, and physiotherapy modalities. Recalcitrant cases often respond to a corticosteroid injection.

SYNOVIAL PLICAE SYNDROME

- Plicae are defined as synovial folds of tissue within the knee. They are described as suprapatellar, infrapatellar, medial, or lateral based on their position within the knee (Dandy, 1990).
- Ninety percent of cadavers studied on anatomic dissection have the presence of at least one of the synovial plicae described.
- Not all plicae are symptomatic. Differential diagnoses include patellofemoral syndrome and meniscal/chondral pathology. Medial plicae are most commonly associated with symptoms. Its presence noted at the time of arthroscopy in all patients ranges from 19 to 70% (Pipkin, 1971; Joyce and Harty, 1984).
- Patients often describe pain over the affected plicae in combination with intermittent snapping or giving way.
- Clinically, this snapping can often be elicited with manipulation of the plicae at varying degrees of flexion between 45° and 60°.
- Radiographic studies including X-rays and MRI are usually negative. The latter is often obtained to rule out other intra-articular pathology.

TREATMENT

- Treatment is usually conservative with *nonsteroidal anti-inflammatory drugs* (NSAIDs) and activity modification. Steroid injections have proven to be effective in more unresponsive cases.
- Arthroscopic resection is limited to those not responding to conservative treatment and has mixed results. Associated chondral injuries or concurrent patellofemoral maltracking have been implicated to athroscopic failures which have been reported to be as high as 30% (Dupont, 1997).

REFERENCES

Aglietti P, Buzzi R, Insall J: Disorders of the patellofemoral joint, in Insall J(ed.): *Surgery of the knee,* 3rd ed. New York, NY, Churchill Livingstone, 930–931, 2001.

Arnoczky SP: Blood supply to the anterior cruciate ligament and supporting structures. *Orthop Clin North Am* 16:15–28, 1985.

Blanzina ME, Kerlan RJ, Jobe FW, et al: Jumper's knee. *Orthop Clin North Am* 4:665–678, 1973.

Bonamo JJ, Krinick RM, Sporn AA: Rupture of the patellar ligament after use of its central third for anterior cruciate ligament reconstruction. A report of two cases. *J Bone Joint Surg* 66–A:1294–1297, 1984.

Coleman BD, Khan KM, Kiss ZS, et al: Open and arthroscopic patellar tenotomy for chronic patellar tendinopathy. *Am J Sports Med* 28(2):183–190, 2000.

Crossett LS, Sinha RK, Sechriest RC, et al: Reconstruction of a ruptured patellar tendon with achilles tendon allograft after total knee arthroplasty. *J Bone Joint Surg* 84–A:1354–1361, 2002.

Dandy DJ: Anatomy of the medial suprapatellar plicae and medial synovial shelf. *Arthrosopy* 6:79–85, 1990.

Dawn B: Prepatellar bursitis: A unique presentation in tophaceous gout in a normourecemic patient. *J Rheumatol* 24:976–978, 1997.

Dupont J: Synovial plicae of the knee. Controversies and review. *Clin Sports Med* 16:87–121, 1997.

Feretti A, Puddu G, Mariani PP, et al: The natural history of jumper's knee. Patellar or quadriceps tendonitis. *Int Orthop* 8:239–242, 1985.

Ford LT, DeBender J: Tendon rupture after local steroid injection. *South Med J* 72:827–830, 1979.

Garrett WE, Jr: Injuries to muscle-tendon unit. *Instr Course Lect* 37:275–282, 1988.

Gecha S, Torg J: Knee injuries in tennis. *Clin Sports Med* 7:435–452, 1988.

Griffiths GP, Selesnick FH: Operative treatment and arthroscopic findings in chronic patellar tendonitis. *Arthroscopy* 14:836–839, 1998.

Ho G, Tice AC: Comparison of nonseptic and septic bursitis. *Arch Int Med* 139:1269–1272, 1979.

Huberti HH, Hayes WC, Stone JL, et al: Force ratios in the quadriceps tendon and ligamentum patellae. *J Orthop Res* 2:49–54, 1984.

Hyman J, Rodep SA, Wickiewicz T: Patellofemoral tendinopathy, in Drez D, DeLee J, Miller M (eds.): *Orthopaedic Sports Medicine: Principles and Practice* 2nd ed. Philadelphia, PA, Saunders, 2003, pp1849–1854.

Ilan DI, Tejwani N, Keschner M, et al: Quadriceps tendon rupture. *J Am Acad Orthop Surg* 11(3):192–200, 2003.

James SL: Running injuries to the knee. *J Am Acad Orthop Surg* 3(6):309–318, 1995.

Johnson DP, Wakely CJ, Watt I: Magnetic Resonance imaging of patellar tendonitis. *J Bone Joint Surg* 78–B:452–457, 1996.

Joyce JJ, Harty M: Surgery of the synovial fold, in Cassells W (ed.): *Arthroscopy: Diagnosis in Surgical Practice.* Philadelphia, PA, Lea & Febiger, 1984, pp 201–209.

Kaalund S: Endoscopic resection of septic prepatellar bursae. *Arthroscopy* 14:757–758,1998.

Kannus P, Jozsa L: Histopathologic changes preceding spontaneous rupture of a tendon. A controlled study of 891 patients. *J Bone Joint Surg* 73–A:1507–1525, 1991.

Keating JF, Orfaly R, O'Brien PJ: Knee pain after tibial nailing. *J Orthop Trauma* 11:10–13, 1997.

King JB , Perry DJ, Mourad K, et al: Lesions of the patellar ligament. *J Bone Joint Surg* 72–B:46–48, 1990.

Konrath GA, Chen D, Lock T, et al: Outcomes following repairs of quadriceps tendon ruptures. *J Orthop Trauma* 12:273–279, 1998.

Larson E, Lund PN: Ruptures of the extensor mechanism of the knee joint. Clinical results and patellofemoral articulation. *Clin Orthop* 213:150–153, 1986.

Larsson LG, Baum J: The syndrome of anserine bursitis. An overlooked diagnosis. *Arthritis Rheum* 28:1062–1065, 1985.

Lauerman WC, Smith BG, Kenmore PI: Spontaneous bilateral rupture of the extensor mechanism of the knee in two patients on chronic ambulatory peritoneal dialysis. *Orthopedics* 10:589–591, 1987.

Mann RA, Hagy JL: The politeus muscle. *J Bone Joint Surg* 59-A:924–927, 1977.

Martens M, Libbrect P, Burssens A: Surgical treatment of iliotibial band friction syndrome. *Am J Sports Med* 17:651–654, 1989.

Martens M, Wouters P, Burssens A, et al: Patellar tendonitis: Pathology and results of treatment. *ACTA Orthop Scand* 53:445–450, 1982.

Matava MJ: Patella tendon ruptures. *J Am Acad Orthop Surg* 4:287–296, 1996.

Mayfield GW: Popliteus tendon tenosynovitis. *Am J Sports Med* 5:31–36, 1977.

Miller W: Rupture of the musculotendinous juncture of the medial head of the gastrocnemius muscle. *Am J Sports Med* 5:191–193, 1977.

Mysnyk MC, Wroble RR, Foster BT, et al: Prepatellar bursitis in wrestlers. *Am J Sports Med* 14:46–54, 1986,

Nauer L, Aalberg JR: Avulsion of the popliteus tendon. *Am J Sports Med* 13:423–424, 1985.

Orava S: Iliotibial friction syndrome in athletes. *Br J Sports Med* 12(2): 69–73, 1978.

Panni AS, Tartarone M, Maffulli N: Patellar tendinopathy in athletes: Outcome of non-operative and operative management. *Am J Sports Med* 28(3):392–397, 2000.

Peterson W, Stein V, Tillman B: Blood supply of the quadriceps tendon. *Unfallchirurg (Ger)* 102:543–547, 1999.

Pipkin G: Knee Injuries: The role of the suprapatellar plica and suprapatella bursae in simulating internal derangement. *Clin Orthop* 74:161–176, 1971.

Rasul AT, Fischer DA: Primary repair of quadriceps tendon ruptures: Results of treatment. *Clin Orthop* 289:205–207, 1993.

Renee JW: The iliotibial band friction syndrome. *J Bone Joint Surg* 57-A:1110–1115, 1975.

Romeo AA, Larson RV: Arthroscopic treatment of infra patellar tendonosis. *Arthroscopy* 15:341–345, 1999.

Scapinelli R: Studies on the vasculature of the human knee joint. *Acta Anat* 70:305–331, 1968.

Scuderi C: Rupture of the quadriceps tendon: Study of twenty tendon ruptures. *Am J Surg* 95:626, 1958.

Scuderi AJ, Datz FL, Valdiva S, et al: Enesthopathy of the patellar tendon insertion associated with isoretinoin therapy. *J Nucl Med* 34:455–457, 1993.

Severence H, Bassett FH: Rupture of the plantaris—Does it exist? *J Bone Joint Surg* 64–A:1387–1388, 1982.

Williams RJ, Brooks DD, Wickiwicz TL, et al: The effect of ciprofloxacin on tendon paratenon, and capsular fibroblast metabolism. *Am J Sports Med* 28:364–369, 2000.

Woo S, Maynard J, Butler D, et al: Ligament, tendon and joint capsule insertions into bone, in Woo S, Buckwalter JJA (eds.): *Injury and Repair of the Musculoskeletal Soft Tissues.* American Academy of Orthopedic Surgeons, Park Ridge, IL, 1988, pp 133–166.

Zernicke RF, Garhammer J, Jobe FW: Human patellar tendon rupture. *J Bone Joint Surg* 59–A:179–183, 1977.

62 ANKLE INSTABILITY

Todd R Hockenbury, MD

DEFINITION OF ANKLE SPRAIN

- An ankle sprain is a tear of the ligaments supporting the ankle joint.
- Ankle sprains are common. They constitute 25% of all sports-related injuries (Mack, 1982).
- Ankle sprains make up 21–53% of basketball injuries and 17–29% of all soccer injuries (Ekstrand and Tropp, 1990; Garrick and Requa, 1988).

ANATOMY AND PATHOPHYSIOLOGY

ANATOMY

- The ankle, or talocrural, joint comprises the talus, tibial plafond, medial malleolus, and lateral malleolus. The distal tibia and lateral malleolus form a mortise, in which the talus sits.
- The talus is wider anteriorly than posterior, thus resulting in a tighter fit and more stable articulation between the talus and mortise during ankle dorsiflexion.
- Ankle joint stability depends on joint congruency and the supporting ligamentous structures.
- The lateral ankle ligaments are the *anterior talofibular ligament* (ATFL), *calcaneofibular ligament* (CFL), and *posterior talofibular ligament* (PTFL). The medial ankle ligaments are the deep and superficial portions of the deltoid ligament.
- The relative strengths soft the ankle ligaments from weakest to strongest are ATFL, CFL, PTFL, and deltoid (Attarian et al, 1985).
- The syndesmotic ligaments connect and stabilize the distal fibula to the distal tibia. The syndesmotic ligaments are the anterior tibiofibular ligament, posterior tibiofibular ligament, transverse tibiofibular ligament, interosseous ligament, and interosseous membrane.
- The subtalar (talocalcaneal) joint lies inferior to the ankle joint and is responsible for hind foot inversion and eversion. Up to 50% of clinical ankle inversion occurs at the subtalar joint (Stephens and Sammarco, 1992).

JOINT MECHANICS

- The ankle is a hinge joint that permits flexion, extension, and rotation. The talus externally rotates with ankle dorsiflexion, and internally rotates during plantar flexion (Sammarco and Hockenbury, 2001).
- The distal fibula externally rotates during ankle dorsiflexion and moves distally during weight bearing, thus deepening and stabilizing the ankle mortise (Wang et al, 1996).
- The ankle mortise widens with ankle dorsiflexion and with weight bearing.
- The ATFL and CFL act synergistically to resist ankle inversion forces. The ATFL resists ankle inversion in plantar flexion and the CFL resists ankle inversion during ankle dorsiflexion.
- The CFL spans both the lateral ankle joint and lateral subtalar joint, thus contributing to both ankle and subtalar joint stability (Stephens and Sammarco, 1992).
- The PTFL limits posterior talar displacement and external rotation (Sarrafian, 1993).
- The deltoid ligament resists ankle eversion, external rotation, and planter flexion. In cases of distal fibular fracture and mortise instability, it restrains lateral talar translation (Harper, 1987).

INJURY MECHANISMS

- The most commonly sprained ankle ligament is the ATFL, followed by the CFL. An isolated CFL tear is rare. A CFL tear is almost always preceded by a tear of the ATFL.
- Lateral ankle sprains occur as a result of landing on a plantar flexed and inverted foot. These injuries occur while running on uneven terrain, stepping in a hole, stepping on another athlete's foot during play, or landing from a jump in an unbalanced position.
- A syndesmotic ankle sprain or *high ankle sprain* occurs as a result of forced external rotation of the foot or during internal rotation of the tibia on a fixed planted foot. A common mechanism is a direct blow to the back of the ankle while the patient is lying prone with the foot externally rotated (Wuest, 1997).
- Isolated deltoid ligament sprains are rare and are usually accompanied by a lateral malleolar fracture and/or syndesmotic injury. The deltoid ligament is injured through a mechanism or external rotation or eversion.

LIGAMENT PATHOPHYSIOLOGY

- Ligamentous injuries undergo a series of phases during the healing process: hemorrhage and inflammation, fibroblastic proliferation, collagen protein formation, and collagen maturation (Akeson et al, 1984; Chvapil, 1967).

- Early mobilization of joints following ligamentous injury actually stimulates collagen bundle orientation and promotes healing, although full ligamentous strength is not reestablished for several months (Noyes et al, 1974; Tipton et al, 1970; Vailas et al, 1981).
- Early treatment focuses on limiting soft tissue effusion, which speeds the healing process by lessening the amount of extracellular fluid and hematoma to be reabsorbed (Hettinga, 1985; Safran et al, 1999a; Thorndike, 1962).

PHYSICAL EXAMINATION

- Lateral ankle swelling and ecchymosis are present and are proportional to the degree of ligament damage.
- Careful one finger palpation is essential to define areas of tenderness and avoid misdiagnosis of associated fractures or tendon ruptures.
- Common fractures that mimic ankle sprains are fractures of the lateral malleolus and medial malleolus, fifth metatarsal base, anterior process of the calcaneus, lateral process of the talus, posterior talar process, talar dome, and navicular.
- Commonly missed tendon injuries are Achilles ruptures, peroneal tendon tears, peroneal tendon subluxation/dislocation, posterior tibial tendon injuries, anterior tibial tendon tears, and flexor hallucis longus tendon ruptures.
- A careful neurologic examination is essential to rule out loss of sensation or motor weakness, as peroneal nerve and tibial nerve injuries are sometimes seen with severe lateral ankle sprains (Nitz, Dobner, and Kersey, 1994).

DIAGNOSTIC TESTS

ANTERIOR DRAWER TEST

- Tests the integrity of the ATFL.
- Performed by stabilizing the anterior tibia just above the ankle with one hand while grasping the posterior heel with the other hand and applying an anteriorly directed force, therefore attempting to translate the talus anteriorly.
- The test should be performed on a relaxed leg with the knee bent and the ankle held in slight plantar flexion.
- Normal anterior talar translation is less than 5 mm. The contralateral asymptomatic ankle should also be tested as a baseline.

INVERSION STRESS TEST OR TALAR TILT TEST

- Tests the integrity of the ATFL and CFL.
- Performed by grasping the heel and inverting the ankle. A clunk may be heard or palpated in unstable ankles, as the medial talar dome impacts the distal tibial medial articular surface, indicating injury to one or both ligaments.
- This test should be performed with the ankle in both dorsiflexion (to test the CFL) and plantar flexion (to test the ATFL).

SUCTION SIGN

- Tests the integrity of the ATFL.
- During performance of the anterior drawer test, an unstable ankle will produce a dimple in the anterolateral ankle as the talus reaches its full anterior excursion. The dimple is formed by negative pressure within the ankle joint (Hockenbury and Sammarco, 2001).

SQUEEZE TEST

- Tests the integrity of the syndesmotic ligaments.
- The squeeze test is performed by placing the fingers over the proximal half of the fibula and thumb around the tibia and squeezing the two bones together. Pain in the distal ankle may indicate a syndesmotic injury (Hopkinson et al, 1990; Ryan et al, 1989).

EXTERNAL ROTATION STRESS TEST

- Tests the integrity of the syndesmotic ligaments.
- The external rotation stress test is performed on the seated patient by externally rotating the foot while stabilizing the tibia with the other hand. Medial ankle pain or lateral talar motion indicates a syndesmotic injury may be present.
- Confirmatory anteroposterior and lateral external rotation stress radiographs will document widening of the syndesmosis and lateral talar subluxation (Edwards, Jr, and DeLee, 1984; Xenos et al, 1995).

IMAGING

OTTAWA ANKLE RULES

- Every sprained ankle does not require screening radiographs.

- Anteroposterior, lateral, and oblique radiographs should be obtained if any of the below criteria are present:
  1. Lateral or medial malleolar bone tenderness is present
  2. Patient unable to bear weight for four steps both immediately post injury and in the emergency department.
- The Ottawa ankle rules do *not* apply in the following settings:
  1. Age less than 18 years
  2. Multiple painful injuries
  3. Pregnancy
  4. Diminished sensation caused by neurologic deficit
- These criteria have been found to be 100% sensitive for detecting fracture while decreasing the incidence of unneeded radiographs (Stiell et al, 1993).

RADIOGRAPHS

- If radiographs are warranted, they should be examined closely for the following fractures that mimic ankle sprains:
  1. Medial or lateral malleolus
  2. Talar dome
  3. Posterior malleolus (posterior distal tibia)
  4. Posterior talar process
  5. Lateral talar process
  6. Anterior calcaneal process
  7. *Flake fracture* off the posterior distal fibular rim, indicating a tear of the superior peroneal retinaculum and peroneal tendon dislocation
  8. Navicular fracture
- Radiographs should also be examined for radiographic evidence of syndesmotic injury:
  1. Widening of the medial clear space of more than 5 mm between the medial talar facet and medial malleolus, produced by lateral talar subluxation, is indicative of a tear of the deltoid ligament and probable syndesmotic ligament instability.
  2. Widening of the tibiofibular clear space of greater than 5 mm or a tibiofibular overlap of less than 10 mm may also indicate syndesmotic injury.

STRESS RADIOGRAPHS

- Not required to make a diagnosis of an acute ankle sprain.
- Used primarily to document mechanical instability as a cause of chronic lateral ankle instability symptoms.
- Can be performed with or without the injection of local anesthetic into the lateral ankle. An injection of 5 cc. of 1% xylocaine into the anterolateral ankle may yield a more reliable test as a result of patient comfort.
- Talar tilt test
  1. The talar tilt test is performed by taking an *anteroposterior* (AP) or mortise view of the ankle while performing an inversion stress on the slightly plantar-flexed ankle.
  2. The talar tilt angle is obtained by measuring the angle subtended by a line parallel to the distal tibial articular surface and a line drawn along the superior articular surface of the talus.
  3. Most authors agree that a difference of 5°–15° in talar tilt between the injured and uninjured side is diagnostic of mechanical ankle instability (Safran et al, 1999b).
- Anterior drawer test
  1. Anterior drawer stress radiographs are performed by taking a lateral radiograph of the ankle while attempting to translate the talus anteriorly within the mortise, as in the clinical anterior drawer test.
  2. The anterior drawer is measured as the shortest distance between a point on the posterior aspect of the distal tibial articular surface and a point on the posterior aspect of the talar dome.
  3. An anterior drawer difference of greater than 3mm between injured and uninjured ankles is thought to be diagnostic of ATFL laxity (Anderson and Lecocq, 1954).
- Stress radiographs for syndesmotic instability
  1. A mortise stress radiograph of the ankle syndesmosis can be obtained by placing an external rotation force on the ankle while stabilizing the proximal tibia with the knee flexed 90°.
  2. Abnormal widening of the mortise and lateral talar shift indicates distal syndesmotic instability.

MRI

- *Magnetic resonance imaging* (MRI) not is needed for diagnosis in the acute setting unless occult fractures or tendon injury is suspected.
- MRI is most useful in diagnosing causes of the chronically sprained ankle and MRI can diagnose talar dome injuries, peroneal tendon tears, bone bruises, or other occult fractures.

CT SCAN

- No needed in the acute setting unless an occult fracture is suspected.
- More valuable than MRI in delineating bone or joint pathology, e.g., talar dome fractures, lateral talar process fractures, tarsal coalition, subtalar arthritis, and loose bodies.

TABLE 62-1 **West Point Ankle Sprain Grading System**

	STAGE 1	STAGE 2	STAGE 3
Edema/ecchymosis	Localized/slight	Localized/moderate	Diffuse/significant
Weight bearing ability	Full or partial without significant pain	Difficult without crutches	Impossible
Ligament pathology	Ligament stretch	Partial tear	Complete tear
Instability testing	None	None or slight	definite
Time to return to sporting activities	11 days	2–6 weeks	4–26 weeks

GRADING

- Grading of ankle sprains helps to guide treatment, rehabilitation, and prognosis. The grade is based on the number of ligaments injured, degree of ligament tearing (partial vs. complete tear), and amount of swelling and ecchymosis.
- *The west point* ankle grading system is a useful tool for grading ankle sprains (Gerber et al, 1998) (see Table 62-1).

INITIAL TREATMENT

P.R.I.C.E., PROTECTION, REST, ICE, COMPRESSION, ELEVATION (SAFRAN ET AL, 1999A)

- **Protection:** Accomplished with the use of taping, a lace up splint, a thermoplastic ankle stirrup splint, a functional walking orthosis, or a short leg cast. Early protected range of motion in a flexible or semirigid orthosis is superior to rigid cast immobilization in terms of patient satisfaction, return of motion and strength and earlier return to function (Klein, Hoher, and Tiling, 1993; Regis et al, 1995). Protected weight-bearing in an orthosis is allowed with weight bearing to tolerance as soon as possible following injury. Crutches are used until pain free weight bearing is achieved.
- **Rest:** Interruption of training in running or jumping sports is essential in limiting swelling and preventing early reinjury. Length of time to return to sports depends on injury grade (see Fig. 62-1).
- **Ice:** Cryotherapy is the application of cold to the ankle in the form of ice bags, a cold whirlpool or a commercially available compressive cuff filled with circulating coolant. Early use of cryotherapy has been shown to enable patients to return to full activity more quickly (Hocutt et al, 1982).
- **Compression:** Compression can be applied to the ankle by means of an elastic bandage, felt doughnut, neoprene or elastic orthosis, or pneumatic device.

- **Elevation:** This initial treatment along attempts to limit the amount of hematoma and extracellular fluid accumulation edema around the ankle in order to speed ligamentous healing.

REHABILITATION—FIVE PHASES (SAFRAN ET AL, 1999B)

- **Acute/P.R.I.C.E.:** Goal is to limit effusion, reduce pain, and protect from further injury.
- **Subacute:** Focus is on eliminating pain, increasing pain-free range of motion, continued protection against reinjury with bracing, limiting loss of strength with isometric exercises, and continued modalities to decrease pain and effusion.
- **Rehabilitative:** Emphasizes regaining full pain free motion with joint mobilization and stretching, increasing strength with isotonic and isokinetic exercises, and propioceptive training.
- **Functional:** Focuses on sports specific exercises with a goal to return the patient to sports participation.
- **Prophylactic:** Seeks to prevent recurrence of injury through preventative strengthening, functional propioceptive drills, and prophylactic support as needed.

TREATMENT OF SYNDESMOTIC LIGAMENT INJURY—HIGH ANKLE SPRAIN

- P.R.I.C.E.
- If the mortise is not widened or fractured, protection is in the form of a short leg cast or brace for 4 weeks, followed by physical therapy.
- In the presence of diastasis between the distal fibula and tibia on X-ray, operative stabilization of the syndesmotic is required with a syndesmotic screw placed through the distal fibula and tibia parallel to the ankle joint.
- The patient should be warned that these injuries result in longer periods of disability than do injuries to the lateral collateral ligaments. In one study, only 44% of 16 patients had an acceptable outcome at 6 months (Gerber et al, 1998).

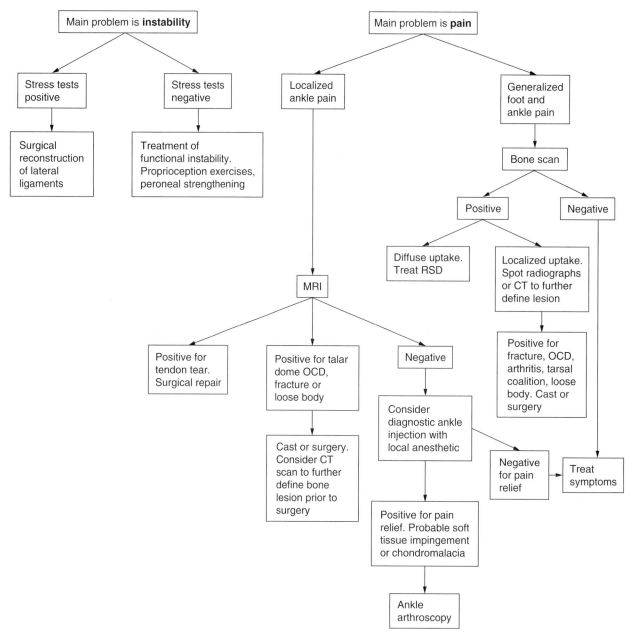

FIG. 62-1 Chronic ankle pain algorithm.

• Heterotopic ossification of the distal syndesmosis has been reported in up to 25% of patients, although no correlation to ossification with functional outcome has been found (Taylor, Englehardt, and Basset, 1992).

NONSURGICAL TREATMENT RESULTS

• Primary ligamentous repair has not been supported by studies comparing early surgery to functional treatment of ankle sprains (Sommer and Arza, 1989; Weise, Rupf,

and Weinelt, 1988; Zwipp et al, 1989). Satisfactory healing of lateral ankle ligaments with the use of a functional ankle brace has been documented by MRI (De Simoni et al, 1996).

• A prospective study of 146 patients with grade 3 ankle sprains who were randomized into operative and nonoperative groups found that the group treated with an ankle orthosis returned to work faster. No difference in joint laxity was found on stress radiographs 2 years post injury (Povacz et al, 1998).

CHRONIC ANKLE PAIN AND INSTABILITY

PAIN VERSUS INSTABILITY

- For residual symptoms following an ankle sprain, initial work-up should center on whether the patient's chief complaint is pain or instability. This determination dictates further work-up on the different sides of the diagnostic algorithm (see algorithm).

CHRONIC ANKLE PAIN

- In a retrospective study of 457 patients treated with immobilization or bracing, 72.6% reported residual symptoms at 6–18 months (Braun, 1999). A study of 96 ankle sprains in *west point* cadets found residual symptoms in 40% of ankles at 6 months post injury (Gerber et al, 1998).
- Common causes of chronic ankle pain are occult fractures, tendon tears, or ankle soft tissue impingement.
- A bone scan (technetium-labeled nuclear medicine study) is an excellent screening test to rule-out occult fractures and to guide further treatment. If the bone scan reveals increased uptake in a discrete area, then a spot radiograph or CT scan is useful in further identifying the exact location of fracture.
- Occult or associated injuries to the tendons of the foot and ankle should also be considered. The physical examination is crucial in testing for tendon integrity, strength, or tendon sheath swelling. MRI is the most useful examination to identify and confirm tendon injuries.
- Injury to the lateral ankle ligaments may produce scarring of the ATFL and joint capsule leading to the formation of *meniscoid tissue* in the anterolateral ankle. This inflamed tissue is pinched between the talus, fibula, and tibia, leading to a condition called anterolateral impingement (Wolin et al, 1950).
- The distal fascicle of the anteroinferior tibiofibular ligament may abrade the anterolateral surface of the talus during ankle dorsiflexion during abnormal anterior translation of the talus (Bassett et al, 1990).
- An anomalous or accessory peroneal tendon may also cause chronic posterolateral ankle pain (Trono et al, 1999). Its presence is confirmed by MRI.

CHRONIC ANKLE INSTABILITY

- If the primary problem is ankle instability, the patient will experience feelings of giving way of the ankle on uneven ground, inability to play cutting or jumping sports, loss of confidence in ankle support, reliance on braces, and give a history of multiple ankle sprains.
- The ankle should be evaluated with stress radiographs. If the stress radiographs are positive for mechanical lateral ligamentous laxity, then surgery is indicated to reconstruct the deficient ligaments.
- If stress radiographs disprove mechanical laxity of the lateral ankle ligaments, then the patient may have functional ankle instability rather than true mechanical ankle instability. Functional instability is the result of deficient neuromuscular control of the ankle, impaired proprioception, and peroneal weakness (Freeman, Dean, and Hanham, 1965; Gauffin, Tropp, and Odenrick, 1988). Treatment in this case should be directed toward restoring peroneal tendon strength, restoring ankle motion, and improving ankle proprioception with physical therapy.
- Other causes for ankle instability not demonstrated by stress radiographs include rotational instability of the talus, subtalar instability, distal syndesmotic (tibiofibular) instability, and hindfoot varus malalignment (Hintermann, 1999).

SURGICAL TREATMENT

INDICATIONS FOR SURGERY

- Multiple episodes of mechanical instability, i.e., difficulty walking on uneven ground, inability to play cutting sports, and lack of confidence in ankle stability
- Demonstration of mechanical instability on stress radiographs
- Failure of a full course of physical therapy emphasizing peroneal strengthening and proprioceptive training
- Failure of a course of bracing

SURGICAL PROCEDURES

- Most procedures are designed to tighten or reconstruct the ATFL and CFL.
- Ankle reconstructive procedures are described either as anatomic or nonanatomic procedures. Anatomic reconstructions attempt to tighten lateral ligaments or transfer tendons into the exact anatomic locations of the ATFL and CFL. Nonanatomic reconstructions use tendon transfers to act as a tenodesis on the lateral side of the ankle, although they do not attempt to place the transferred tendons to the exact anatomic origins of the ATFL or CFL. Most surgeons agree that anatomic reconstructions are preferable.
- The Brostrom procedure is an anatomic reconstruction in which the ATFL and CFL are divided and

imbricated (Brostrom, 1966). Some authors advance the shortened ligaments into the distal fibula. This procedure is sometimes modified by advancing the extensor retinaculum proximally (the Gould modification) to further tighten the lateral aspects of the ankle and subtalar joints (Gould, Seligson, and Gassman, 1980).

- Tendon transfers most commonly utilize one half of the peroneus brevis tendon, which is divided proximally about 15 cm proximal to its insertion in the base of the fifth metatarsal. The transferred peroneus brevis tendon is then passed through holes in the talar neck, distal fibula, and lateral calcaneus in order to reconstruct the lateral ligamentous structures. In lieu of drill holes, the transferred tendon may be sutured directly to bone using suture anchors. A detailed discussion of all these procedures is beyond the scope of this chapter (Sammarco and DiRaimondo, 1988; Sammarco and Idusuyi, 1999; Snook, Chrisman, and Wilson, 1985).

POSTOPERATIVE CARE

- Following lateral ankle ligamentous reconstructive procedures, most postoperative regimens immobilize the ankle in a cast for 4 weeks followed by an orthosis for 4 additional weeks.
- Physical therapy is instituted at 6–8 weeks post surgery with an emphasis on peroneal strengthening and propioceptive training.
- Return to sports occurs at about 3 months postoperative.

REFERENCES

Akeson WH, Woo SLY, Amiel D, et al: The chemical basis for tissue repair, in Hunter LH and Funk FJ (eds.): *Rehabilitation of the Injured Knee*, St. Louis, MO, Mosby, 1984, p 93.

Anderson KJ, Lecocq JF: Operative treatment of injury to the fibular collateral ligaments of the ankle. *J Bone Joint Surg* 36A:825, 1954.

Attarian DE, McCracken HJ, Devito, DP, et al: Biomechanical characteristics of human ankle ligaments. *Foot Ankle* 6:54, 1985.

Bassett FH, Gates III HS, Billys JB, et al: Talar impingement by the anteroinferior tibiofibular ligament. *J Bone Joint Surg* 72A(1):55, 1990.

Braun BL: Effects of ankle sprain in a general clinic population 6 to 18 months after medical evaluation. *Arch Fam Med* 8(2):143, 1999.

Brostrom L: Sprained ankles VI: Surgical treatment of "chronic" ligament ruptures. *Acta Chir Scand* 132(5):551, 1966.

Chvapil, M. *Physiology of Connective Tissue*. London, Butterworths, 1967.

De Simoni C, Wetz HH, Zanetti M, et al: Clinical examination and magnetic resonance imaging in the assessment of ankle sprains treated with an orthosis. *Foot Ankle Int* 17(3):177, 1996.

Edwards GS, Jr, DeLee JC: Ankle diastasis without fracture. *Foot Ankle* 4(6):305, 1984.

Ekstrand J, Tropp H: The incidence of ankle sprains in soccer. *Foot Ankle* 11(1):41, 1990.

Freeman MAR, Dean MRE, Hanham IWF: The etiology and prevention of functional instability of the foot. *J Bone Joint Surg* 47B(4):678, 1965.

Garrick JG, Requa RK: The epidemiology of foot and ankle injuries in sports. *Clin Sports Med* 7(1):29,1988.

Gauffin H, Tropp H, Odenrick P: Effect of ankle disk training on postural control in patients with functional instability of the ankle. *Int J Sports Med* 9(2):141, 1988.

Gerber JP, Williams GN, Scoville CR, et al: Persistent disability associated with ankle sprains: A prospective examination of an athletic population. *Foot Ankle Int* 19(10):653, 1998.

Gould N, Seligson D, Gassman J: Early and late repair of lateral ligaments of the ankle. *Foot Ankle* 1(2): 84, 1980.

Harper M: Deltoid ligament: An experimental evaluation of function. *Foot Ankle* 8:19, 1987.

Hettinga DL: Inflammatory response of synovial joint structures, in Gould JA, Daivies GJ (eds.): *Orthopaedic and Sports Physical Therapy*. St. Louis, MO, Mosby, 1985, p 87.

Hintermann B: Biomechanics of the unstable ankle joint and clinical implications. *Med Sci Sports Exc* 31(7) (Suppl):S459, 1999.

Hockenbury RT, Sammarco GJ: Evaluation and treatment of ankle sprains. Clinical recommendations for a positive outcome. *Phys Sports Med* 29(2):57, 2001.

Hocutt JE, Jaffee R, Rylander R, et al: Cryotherapy in ankle sprains. *Am J Sports Med* 10(5):316, 1982.

Hopkinson WJ, St. Pierre P, Ryan JB, et al: Syndesmosis sprains of the ankle. *Foot Ankle* 10(6):325, 1990.

Klein J, Hoher J, Tiling T: Comparative study of therapies for fibular ligament rupture of the lateral ankle joint in competitive basketball players. *Foot Ankle Int* 14(6):320, 1993.

Mack RP: Ankle injuries in athletes. *Clin Sports Med* 1(1):71, 1982.

Nitz AJ, Dobner JJ, Kersey DK: Nerve injury and Grade II and III ankle sprains. *Am J Sports Med* 13(3):177, 1994.

Noyes FR, Torvik PJ, Hyde WB, et al: Biomechanics of ligament failure: Part II. An analysis of immobilization, exercise, and reconditioning effects in primates. *J Bone Joint Surg* 56A(7): 1406, 1974.

Povacz P, Unger F, Miller K, et al: A randomized, prospective study of operative and non-operative treatment of injuries of the fibular collateral ligaments of the ankle. *J Bone Joint Surg* 80A(3):345, 1998.

Regis D, Montanari M, Magnon B, et al: Dynamic orthopedic brace in the treatment of ankle sprains. *Foot Ankle Int* 16(7):422, 1995.

Ryan JB, Hopkinson WJ, Wheeler JH, et al: Office management of the acute ankle sprain. *Clin Sports Med* 8(3):477, 1989.

Safran MR, Benedetti RS, Bartolozzi AR, III, et al: Lateral ankle sprains: A comprehensive review. Part 1: Etiology, pathoanatomy, histopathogenesis, and diagnosis. *Med Sci Sports Exerc* 31(7)(Suppl.):S429, 1999*a*.

Safran MR, Zachazewski JE, Benedetti, RS, et al: Lateral ankle sprains: A comprehensive review. Part 2: Treatment and rehabilitation with an emphasis on the athlete. *Med Sci Sports Exerc* 31(7)(Suppl.):S438, 1999*b*.

Sammarco GJ, DiRaimondo CV: Surgical treatment of lateral ankle instability syndrome. *Am J Sports Med* 16(5):501, 1988.

Sammarco GJ, Hockenbury RT: Biomechanics of the Foot and Ankle, in Nordin M, Frankel VH (eds.): *Basic Biomechanics of the Musculoskeletal System*, 3rd ed. Baltimore, MD, Lippincott Williams & Wilkins, 2001, p 242.

Sammarco GJ, Idusuyi O: Reconstruction of the lateral ankle ligaments using a split peroneus brevis tendon graft. *Foot Ankle Int* 20(2):97, 1999.

Sarrafian SK: *Anatomy of the Foot and Ankle*. Philadelphia, PA, Lippincott Williams & Wilkins 1993.

Snook GA, Chrisman D, Wilson TC: Long-term results of the Chrisman-Snook operation for reconstruction of the lateral ligaments of the ankle. *J Bone Joint Surg* 67A(1):1, 1985.

Sommer HM, Arza D: Functional treatment of recent ruptures of the fibular ligament of the ankle. *Internat Orthop* 13(2):157, 1989.

Stephens MM, Sammarco GJ: The stabilizing role of the lateral ligament complex around the ankle and subtalar joints. *Foot Ankle* 13:130, 1992.

Stiell, IG, McKnight RD, Greenberg GH, et al: Decision rules for the use of radiography in acute ankle injuries: refinement and prospective validation. *JAMA* 269(9):1127, 1993.

Taylor DC, Englehardt DL, Basset FH, III: Syndesmosis sprains of the ankle: The influence of heterotopic ossification. *Am J Sports Med* 20(2):146, 1992.

Thorndike A. *Athletic Injuries: Prevention, Diagnosis, and Treatment*. Philadelphia, PA, Lea & Febinger, 1962.

Tipton CM, James SL, Mergner W, et al: Influence of exercise in strength of medial collateral ligaments in dogs. *Am J Physiol* 218(3):894, 1970.

Trono M, Tueche S, Quintart C, et al: Peroneus quartus muscle: a case report and review of the literature. *Foot Ankle Int* 20(10):659, 1999.

Vailas AC, Tipton CM, Mathes RD, et al: Physical activity and its influence on the repair process of medial collateral ligaments. *Connect Tissue Res* 9(1):25, 1981.

Wang QW, Whittle M, Cunningham J, et al: Fibula and its ligaments in load transmission and ankle joint stability. *Clin Orthop* 330: 261, 1996.

Weise K, Rupf G, Weinelt J: Die laterale Bandverletzung des OSG beim Sport. *Aktuel Traumatol* 18(Suppl.)l1:54, 1988.

Wolin I, Glassman F, Sideman S, et al: Internal derangement of the talofibular component of the ankle. *Surg Gynechol* 91:193, 1950.

Wuest, TK: Injuries to the distal lower extremity syndesmosis. *J Am Acad Orthop Surg* 5:172, 1997.

Xenos JS, Hopkinson WJ, Mulligan ME, et al: The tibiofibular syndesmosis: Evaluation of the ligamentous structures, methods of fixation, and radiographic assessment. *J Bone Joint Surg* 77A (6):847, 1995.

Zwipp H, Hoffmann R, Wippermann B, et al: Fibulare Bandruptur am oberen Sprunggelenk. *Orthopaedie* 18(4):336, 1989.

63 SURGICAL CONSIDERATIONS IN THE LEG

Gregory G Dammann, MD
Keith S Albertson, MD

INTRODUCTION

- As the number of recreational athletes involved in running and jumping sports has increased, so has the number of patients presenting with exertional lower leg pain. Three diagnoses in the differential diagnosis of exertional leg pain that may require surgical intervention are: exertional compartment syndrome, tibial stress fracture, and posterior tibial tendonitis.

EXERTIONAL COMPARTMENT SYNDROME

- Exertional compartment syndrome is activity related pain caused by an increased intermuscular pressure within an anatomic compartment. In the leg there are four compartments that contain muscle, blood vessel, and nerves. The compartments are enclosed by fascia, which if tight or thickened will not allow the muscle to expand during activity and thus cause compression of all the components of the compartment. The pain of exertional compartment syndrome is most likely caused by ischemia due to decreased blood flow in muscle arterioles.
- Knowledge of the anatomy of the lower leg is vital to the diagnosis of exertional compartment syndrome.
  - The anterior compartment contains the extensor hallucis longus, extensor digitorum longus, peroneus tertius, and tibialis anterior as well as the deep peroneal nerve.
  - The lateral compartment contains the peroneus longus and brevis as well as the superficial peroneal nerve.
  - The superficial posterior compartment contains the gastrocnemius and soleus muscles and the sural nerve.
  - The deep posterior compartment contains the flexor hallucis longus, flexor digitorum longus, and posterior tibialis muscle as well as the posterior tibial nerve.

- There are important aspects of the patient's history that can guide one to consider the diagnosis of exertional compartment syndrome.
  - The patient is usually asymptomatic upon initiating exercise. The pain will begin at a predictable time during the workout.
  - The pain is described as aching or cramping associated with feelings of swelling, fullness, or tightness.
  - Dysesthesias often accompany the pain along the nerve within the affected compartment.
  - Patients may also complain of altered running style. For example, a runner may state that the foot seems to be slapping the ground when the pain comes on.
- Physical examination
  - The physical examination at rest is often normal. In advanced cases, there may be tenderness to deep palpation along the affected compartment.
  - There may be a palpable fascial defect with hernia within the affected compartment.
  - Examination immediately after exercise usually reveals a firm, tender compartment with increased pain on passive stretch.
  - Fascial defects with resultant herniations are more identifiable after exercise.
  - There may be altered sensation in the distribution of the nerve that traverses the affected compartment.
- Compartment pressure testing
  - The most useful diagnostic test in the evaluation for exertional compartment syndrome.
  - Several techniques have been described for measuring compartment pressures: these include needle manometry, wick catheter, and slit catheter. Our preferred method of measuring compartment pressure is with a battery-operated, hand-held, digital, fluid pressure monitor. The Stryker Intracompartmental Pressure Monitor (Stryker Corporation, Kalamazoo, MI) is a convenient and easy to use measuring device for use in clinical setting.
    1. The equipment needed for pressure measurement includes the stryker pressure monitor and a disposable packet designed for use with it (sterile 18 gauge needle, diaphragm chamber, syringe filled with 3 cc of normal saline). Betadine solution, alcohol pads, gauze, a 25–27 gauge needle and syringe for local anesthesia, 1% xylocaine without epinephrine and bupivicaine 0.5% for anesthesia.
    2. The first step is to identify the compartment and sterilize the overlying skin.
    3. The next step is to anesthetize the skin by injecting 1–3 mL of 1% lidocaine without epinephrine subcutaneously being sure to avoid penetration of the fascial compartment.
    4. The third step in the process involves preparing the monitor unit for insertion and measurement. Connect the disposable syringe and the sterile needle to the diaphragm transducer. Turn the unit on and press the syringe until a drop of saline is expressed from the needle tip. Press the "zero" button to clear the unit; however, it is important to zero at the same angle at which the needle will enter the skin.
    5. The measurement should be done by inserting the needle at 90° to the anesthetized skin, through the fascia and into the appropriate compartment. Inject a small amount of saline to ensure a solid fluid column. Wait a few seconds for the reading to equilibrate, record the reading, and remove the needle.
    6. Cover the needle site with a bandage. Instruct the patient on postprocedure complications: infection, neurologic injury, and vascular injury.
    7. To approach the anterior compartment, palpate the tibialis anterior just lateral to the anterior tibial border at the level of the mid-third of the tibia.
    8. To approach the lateral compartment, palpate the muscle bellies of the peroneus longus and brevis at the midpoint between the head of the fibula and lateral malleolus.
    9. To approach the superficial posterior compartment, palpate the muscle bellies of the gastrocnemius and soleus. This is a medial approach just posterior to the medial border of the tibia.
    10. To approach the deep posterior compartment, use the same approach as for the superficial posterior compartment. This compartment can be measured after completing the superficial posterior compartment then advancing the needle until a second "pop" is felt when the fascia is penetrated.
- Compartment pressures should be taken before exercise, 1 min after exercise, and if necessary, 5 min after exercise.
- Compartments can be measured based on history; for example if the history is suggestive on anterior compartment then only that compartment may be measured; however, if the symptoms are vague it may be necessary to measure all four compartments.
- One or more of the following pressure criteria must be met in addition to a history and physical that is consistent with the diagnosis of exertional compartment syndrome. Preexercise pressure >15 mm-Hg, 1 min postexercise pressure >30 mm-Hg, or 5 min postexercise pressure > 20 mm-Hg.

- Indications for surgery
  - Appropriate history for chronic exertional compartment syndrome
  - One minute postexercise compartment pressure greater than 30 mm-Hg
  - The presence of a fascial defect
- Surgical procedures
  - Fasciotomy divides the fascia longitudinally over the entire length of the involved fascia.
  - One or two incision technique may be used.
    1. Risks/benefits of a single incision technique.
       a. Benefit is a smaller skin wound.
       b. Disadvantage is that it is more difficult to ensure the compartment is completely released.
    2. Risks/benefits of a two incision technique
       a. Benefit is that it allows good visualization of the most proximal and distal portions of the compartment to ensure complete compartmental release.
       b. Disadvantage is that there is more scarring.
- Postoperative care
  - A compressive dressing is applied.
  - Crutches are used for comfort for a few days but the patient begins active and passive motion immediately. Patients may begin walking once the wound is healed and light jogging may begin at 2 weeks but no running for 6 weeks. Complete recovery usually takes 3 months (Chang and Harris, 1996).
- Complications
  - Most complications are due to neurovascular injury. A transected sensory nerve is likely to result in permanent numbness and possibly a painful neuroma.
  - Symptoms may return if the compartment is not fully released or is allowed to scar secondary to immobilization.

TIBIAL STRESS FRACTURE

- Stress fractures of the tibia may occur on either the compression or tension side of the cortex.
  - Fractures of the proximal or distal third of the tibia are more likely to occur in compression. These fractures are frequently seen in undertrained or *forced* athletes, such as new military recruits.
  - Midshaft tibial stress fractures occur on the tension side of the bone and usually affect the well conditioned athlete involved in running and jumping sports.
  - Although the vast majority of stress fractures will heal with nonoperative treatment, surgery can be considered for selected individuals.
- Surgical evaluation

- History
  1. Patients usually report a rapid increase in intensity or duration of their workouts 1–2 months prior to the onset of symptoms.
  2. Patients will report dull, achy pain over the shin that began after strenuous exercise. Pain gradually worsens and occurs with nonathletic activities or even at rest.
  3. Initially the pain may be relieved with rest, ice, *nonsteroidal anti-inflammatory drugs* (NSAIDs) but will return as soon as activity resumes.
- Physical examination
  - The hallmark of a stress fracture is localized point tenderness directly over the bone.
  - Occasionally there is palpable bony bump or fullness representing periosteal new bone formation.
  - A tuning fork placed on the bone distant from the suspected fracture site will elicit pain at the fracture site.
- Imaging
  - Plain radiographs should be included as part of the initial evaluation of leg pain in athletes.
    1. X-ray findings include cortical thickening, narrowing of the intermedullary canal, or evidence of periostitis. A complete fracture line may be visualized but this is usually not the case. A linear, unicortical, radiolucency in the anterior tibia represents the dreaded black line of a tension side stress fracture (Green, Rogers, and Lipscomb, 1985).
  - A bone scan is the most sensitive test for stress fracture but has poor specificity (Mubarak and Owne, 1977). A triple phase bone scan may improve specificity. Medial tibial stress syndrome, periostitis, and contusion can all cause increased uptake, but the uptake in these conditions is more diffuse; whereas that of stress fracture is more focal.
  - MRI scan is both specific and sensitive for stress fracture; however, cost is a detractor against routine use.
- Nonoperative treatment
  - Compression side stress fractures
    1. Limiting impact loading is usually sufficient in these fractures. Crutches can be used until the limp resolves. Patient needs to abstain from running or jumping for 8–12 weeks. Nonimpact conditioning activities such as water running, cycling, and elliptical trainer can be used as long as they do not cause pain.
       a. A splint or pneumatic brace may be used for comfort.
       b. A cast may be used but only for a short duration of time to limit atrophy and stiffness.

- Tension sided stress fractures(mid shaft anterior)
    1. These require more aggressive treatment because of the predisposition to nonunion. Immobilization in a nonweightbearing cast for 3–6 months is the standard treatment. If no evidence of healing at 3–6 months, an electrical stimulator may have some benefit.
- Return to play
    1. Patients may return to athletic activity when they have no pain with unprotected daily activity, there is no bony tenderness, and the radiographs show evidence of healing (Green, Rogers, and Lipscomb, 1985).
    2. When patients can walk without pain, they may jog. When they can jog without pain, they may run. When they can run or jump without pain, they may compete.
- Indications for surgery
    1. Surgery should be reserved for patients with anterior tibial stress fractures who fail to heal after 6 months of nonoperative treatment.
    2. Surgery should also be considered for the high-level athlete who is unwilling or unable to comply with a prolonged period of inactivity.
- Surgical procedures
    1. Cortical drilling: In an attempt to stimulate the reparative process, multiple transverse 2–3 mm drill holes are made a few centimeters proximal and distal to the fracture. Cortical drilling is frequently combined with bone grafting.
    2. Bone grafting: Autogenous cancellous bone is harvested from the ipsilateral iliac crest and packed into the fracture gap and around the sides of the fracture site. Healing time may be 5 months from surgery (Wang et al, 1997).
    3. Intramedullary nailing: A reamed nail is recommended to provide a larger contact area and increased stiffness to resist tension across the fracture area better than an unreamed nail.
        a. A short leg splint may provide initial postoperative comfort but this is exchanged for a hinged *walking boot* orthosis as soon as possible.
        b. Knee and ankle motion exercises are begun immediately.
        c. Crutches are used for comfort only and discontinued when weight bearing is well tolerated.
        d. Conditioning with biking, swimming, or water walking can begin within a few weeks.
        e. Impact loading and running may begin as early as 6 weeks with full fracture healing usually taking 6 months.

POSTERIOR TIBIAL TENDON INJURY

- Injury to the posterior tibial tendon may occur from an acute traumatic event, which may signify tendon disruption, or as part of chronic overuse syndrome, which could signify posterior tibial tendonosis.
- Surgical evaluation
    - History: Patients report pain along the medial aspect of the leg posterior to the medial malleolus. The onset of pain is usually gradual with increases in such activities as walking, running, or jumping.
- Physical examination
    - There may be loss of the longitudinal arch and a planovalgus deformity, as evidenced by the too many toes sign. When observing the patient from behind, the affected side will reveal more toes lateral to the heel than the unaffected side.
    - With an attempted single leg heel raise, there is loss of foot supination and heel inversion.
    - There is tenderness to palpation over the course of the tendon.
    - Pain and weakness are present with resisted inversion.
- Imaging
    - The X-ray evaluation should include standing anteroposterior and lateral views.
        1. *Anteroposterior* (AP) view: look for medial talar displacement in relation to the navicular bone.
        2. Lateral view: look for decreased height of the longitudinal arch (Trevino and Baumhauer, 1992).
    - *Magnetic resonance imaging* (MRI) is the test of choice to evaluate the posterior tibial tendon for signs of tenosynovitis versus tendonosis (Trevino and Baumhauer, 1992).
- Nonoperative care
    - Initial management should be nonsurgical.
    - Options for resting the tendon vary from activity modification to immobilization with the use of a short leg walking boot or short leg walking cast.
    - Orthotics should be used to support the arch and relieve stress on the tendon.
    - Corticosteroid injections are not recommended because of the risk of tendon rupture.
- Surgical management
    - Surgery should be considered in those who do not respond to nonsurgical management after 6–12 weeks or those with loss of the arch (Mann, 1993).
    - Surgical options include synovectomy for inflamed synovium and more extensive procedures such as flexor digitorum longus transfer for significant tendon dysfunction.

- Postoperative management
  1. Synovectomy: Immobilization for 10 days to allow wound healing, followed by 3 weeks in a short leg walking cast. After the cast is removed, range of motion exercises and weight bearing are begun as tolerated.
  2. Flexor digitorum longus transfer: Plantar splint for 10 days followed by short leg nonwalking cast for 4 weeks. Then the patient is progressed to short leg walking cast for another 4 weeks. After the casting period, physical therapy is begun with range of motion exercises followed by strengthening exercises for 3–4 months.
- Complications: The complications include infection, *deep venous thrombosis* (DVT), wound dehiscence, and adhesions. One third of patient undergoing tendon transfer will fail to have their arch corrected (Mann, 1993).

REFERENCES

Chang PS, Harris RM: Intramedullary nailing for chronic tibial stress fractures. *Am J Sports Med* 1996:24,688.

Green NE, Rogers RA, Lipscomb AB: Nonunion of stress fractures of the tibia. *Am J Sports Med* 1985:13, 171.

Mann RA: Flatfoot in adults, in Mann RA, Coughlin MJ (eds.), *Surgery of the Foot and Ankle*, 6th ed, St. Louis, Mosby, 1993:757.

Mubarak SJ, Owne CA: Double incision fasciotomy of the lower leg for decompression in compartment syndromes. *J Bone Joint Surg Am* 1977:59A, 184.

Trevino S, Baumhauer JF: Tendon injuries of the foot and ankle. *Clin Sports Med* 1992:11,727.

Wang CL, Wang TG, Hsu TC, et al: Ultrasonographic examination of the posterior tibial tendon. *Foot Ankle Int* 1997: 18,34.

BIBLIOGRAPHY

Albertson KS, Dammann GG: The Leg, in O'Connor FG, Wilder RP (eds.): *The Textbook of Running Medicine,* McGraw-Hill. 2001.

Andrish JT: The Leg, in DeLee JC, Drez D (eds.): *Orthopaedic Sports Medicine: Principles and Practice*, Philadelphia, PA, Saunders, 1994, p 1603.

Davey JR, Fowler PJ, Rorabeck CH: The tibialis posterior muscle compartment: An unrecognized cause of exertional compartment syndrome. *Am J Sports Med* 12:391, 1984.

Detmer DE, Sharpe K, Sufit RL, et al: Chronic compartment syndrome: Diagnosis, management and outcomes. *Am J Sports Med* 13:162–170, 1985.

Giladi M, Milgrom C, Simkin A, et al: Stress fractures: Identifiable risk factors. *Am J Sports Med* 19:647, 1991.

Jones DC, James SL: Overuse injuries of the lower extremity: Shin splints, iliotibial band syndrome, and exertional compartment syndromes. *Clin Sports Med* 6:273, 1987.

Ota Y, Senda M, Hashizume H, et al: Chronic compartment syndrome of the lower leg: A new diagnostic method using near-infrared spectroscopy and a new technique of endoscopic fasciotomy. *Arthroscopy* 15:439, 1999.

Quinn MR, Mendicino SS: Surgical treatment of posterior tibial tendon dysfunction. *Clin Podiatr Med Surg* 8:543, 1991.

Rorabeck CH: The diagnosis and management of chronic compartment syndromes. *Instr Course Lect* 38:466, 1989.

Takebayashi S, Takazawa H, Sasaki R, et al: Chronic exertional compartment syndrome in lower legs: Localization and follow-up with thallium-201 SPECT imaging. *J Nucl Med* 38:972, 1997.

64 TIBIAL AND ANKLE FRACTURES

Edward S Ashman, MD
Brian E Abell, BS, MS IV

TIBIAL FRACTURES

INTRODUCTION

- Fractures of the tibia and fibula are the most common long bone fractures with over 500,000 occurring annually. Tibial shaft fractures are more common in male athletes, particularly soccer players, with an average age of 31 years (Court-Brown and McBirnie, 1995). Many, but not all of these fractures are high energy and are related to motor vehicle accidents or falls.
- The tibia is the most frequent site of stress fractures in the athletic population (Koval and Zuckerman, 2002).
- Surgical emergencies related to tibial shaft fractures include compartment syndrome, open fracture, and neurovascular compromise.
- Common to all tibial fractures is a concern for soft tissue injury. For this reason it is extremely important to therapeutically ice, elevate, and immobilize the injured limb at initial examination.

PHYSICAL EXAMINATION

- The physician must always evaluate and document the neurovascular status of the patient with a suspected

TABLE 64-1 Compartments of the Lower Leg

COMPARTMENT	NERVES	MUSCLES	PAIN WITH MOVEMENT ON PHYSICAL EXAMINATION
Anterior	Deep peroneal	Tibialis anterior Extensor hallucis longus Extensor digitorum	Plantarflexion of the foot Flexion or extension of toes
Deep posterior	Tibial	Tibialis posterior Flexor hallucis longus Flexor digitorum	Extension of toes
Lateral	Superficial peroneal Deep peroneal	Peroneus longus Peroneus brevis	Inversion of the foot
Superfical posterior	Sural	Gastrocnemius Soleus	Dorsiflexion of the foot

tibial fracture. It is most important to evaluate and document the dorsalis pedis and posterior tibial pulses as well as the function of the peroneal nerve.

- The physician must also rule out compartment syndrome in a patient with a fractured tibia. Common sensitive predictors of compartment syndrome are pain with passive stretch of the musculotendinous unit that travels through the respective compartment or sensory loss in the distribution of nerves that traverse the compartment. Further discussion of compartment syndrome can be found in Chapter 56. Table 64-1 outlines the various compartments of the lower leg.
- The joints above and below all tibia fractures must be thoroughly examined. Therefore, a careful clinical and radiologic evaluation and assessment of the ipsilateral knee and ankle is mandatory. The physician should evaluate the range of motion and the integrity of the ligamentous complex at both joints respectively. Studies have shown that there is an increased incidence of ligamentous injury to the knee with fractures of the tibial shaft (Templeman and Marder, 1989).

RADIOGRAPHIC EXAMINATION

- The physician evaluating a tibial fracture must include anterior-posterior and lateral radiographic views of the tibia and three-view radiographs of the ipsilateral knee and ankle.
- *Computed tomography* (CT) may aid in determining the precise location, depth, and articular involvement of tibial plateau and plafond fractures; however, these are not a part of the initial radiological evaluation for fractures of the tibial shaft. Magnetic resonance imaging may be used to investigate stress fractures, but a bone scan is the radiographic study of choice (Daffner and Pavlov, 1992).

- When describing fractures of the tibia, the reporting physician should include the following: open versus closed, proximal versus middle versus distal 1/3, comminution with number of fragments, transverse/spiral/oblique, angulation, shortening or overlap, and displacement.

TIBIAL SHAFT FRACTURES

- Fractures of the tibial shaft are due to varying amounts of energy. High energy fractures more commonly present with a higher likelihood of compartment syndrome, higher likelihood of being open, and tend to be more comminuted with soft tissue damage. Tscherne and Gotzen first described and classified the soft tissue injury associated with these fractures (Tscherne and Gotzen, 1984) (see Table 64-2).
- Treatment options for tibial shaft fractures vary widely and depend upon the degree of comminution, displacement of fragments, and location of fracture. Treatment options range from closed reduction with long leg casting to open reduction with internal fixation or intramedullary nailing. External fixation may be appropriate in cases of open fracture, high energy trauma, and soft tissue injury or infection. Studies have suggested that operative intramedullary nailing is more successful

TABLE 64-2 Soft Tissue Injury Associated with Fractures

GRADE	INJURY
0	Minimal soft tissue damage; indirect violence; simple fracture pattern
1	Superficial abrasion or contusion from internal pressure, mild to moderate fracture configuration
2	Deep, contaminated abrasion with associated contusion; impending compartment syndrome
3	Extensive skin contusion or crush injury; associated muscle injury; major vascular injury; severely comminuted fracture pattern

than cast immobilization in closed tibial fractures even in cases demonstrating significant displacement of fracture fragments (Hooper, Keddell, and Penny, 1991).

- Acceptable postreduction parameters of a tibial shaft fracture are commonly less than 5° of varus or valgus angulation, less than 10° of anterior-posterior angulation, less than 10° of rotational deformity, and less than 1 cm of shortening. Many authors have demonstrated, however, that clinical and radiographic outcomes are often unaffected by various amounts of anterior, posterior, varus, or valgus angulation (Court-Brown, 2001). Compressive forces are necessary for adequate healing as it has been shown that 5 mm of distraction may delay healing up to 1 year (Koval and Zuckerman, 2002).

TIBIAL PLATEAU FRACTURES

- Tibial plateau fractures comprise less than 1% of all fractures and approximately 8% of fractures in elderly patients. In 70 to 80% of the cases, fractures of the tibial plateau occur on its lateral margins (Koval and Zuckerman, 2002).
- Tibial plateau fractures often occur after violent varus or valgus stress coupled with axial loading. For this reason, there are often associated ligamentous or cartilage injuries.
- Tibial plateau fractures are classified according to the Schatzker classification system. Schatzker classified tibial plateau fractures relative to their location and associated articular depression (Merchant and Dietz, 1989) (Table 64-3).
- Tibial plateau fractures can be managed successfully both operatively and nonoperatively. Nonoperative treatment is favored in patients that demonstrate nondisplaced or minimally displaced fractures radiographically and who do not demonstrate ligamentous laxity by physical examination. Nonoperative treatment is also favored in patients with multiple comorbidities or advanced osteoporosis.
- Indications for operative treatment are displaced fractures of the tibial plateau that demonstrate a varying degree of depression, compartment syndrome or neurovascular compromise, instability, or laxity of the knee.

TABLE 64-3   Schatzker's Classification of Tibial Plateau Fractures

TYPE	FRACTURE DESCRIPTION
1	Lateral plateau, split fracture, no associated articular depression
2	Lateral plateau, split fracture with associated articular depression
3	Lateral plateau, moderate articular depression
4	Medial plateau
5	Bicondylar plateau
6	Plateau fracture with metaphyseal-diaphyseal dissociation

All open fractures must also be treated operatively. Research does not support operative intervention in a patient that is neurovascularly intact and demonstrates mild radiographic evidence of articular depression. Jensen et al found no association between the degree of fracture displacement and clinical outcome (Schatzker, McBroom, and Bruce, 1979). Additionally Lucht and Pligaard demonstrated that the majority of patients with up to 10 mm of articular depression had acceptable, functional results at 7 years follow-up (Jensen et al, 1990).

TIBIAL PLAFOND FRACTURES

- Tibial plafond fractures comprise 7 to 10% of all tibial fractures. Fractures of the plafond usually occur following falls from heights with significant axial compression, shear forces at the distal tibial articulation, or a combination of both (Lucht and Pligaard, 1971).
- Patients with plafond fractures are often reluctant to ambulate, with variable gross deformities of the distal tibia or ankle mortise. Patients often present with a great deal of pain and edema.
- Anterior-posterior, lateral, mortise, and 45° oblique views of the ankle are necessary. An occasional CT is required for better understanding of complex fracture patterns and intra-articular involvement.
- Nonoperative therapy is only indicated for nondisplaced fractures or plafond fractures in severely debilitated patients. Operative treatment is ideally aimed at anatomic reduction, but often requires temporary external fixation to relieve articular surface pressure until swelling and inflammation around the joint resolve. There is a high incidence of soft tissue complications if swelling is not controlled at the time of surgery. For this reason, it is particularly important to control associated swelling and edema with ice, elevation, and immobilization.
- Successful anatomic reduction and congruity does not appear to affect patient outcome and rehabilitative success. DeCoster et al demonstrated that the mechanics and energy of the initial insult to the plafond predicted patient outcome measures more reliably than anatomic reduction (DeCoster et al, 1999).

ANKLE FRACTURES

INTRODUCTION

- The true incidence of ankle fractures in the general population is unknown, as it changes with increased participation in athletics and trends in fashion footwear. There is also a great deal of interobserver reliability when it comes to classifying these fractures.

- A great deal of research has been conducted to determine the incidence of age related fractures particularly in the elderly population. Barrett et al analyzed medicare data in 1999 and found that ankle fractures were the fourth most common fracture in the elderly population (65–90 years of age). The study also demonstrated that elderly Blacks were less likely than Whites to fracture the ankle (Barrett et al, 1999).

PHYSICAL EXAMINATION

- The examination of the ankle should begin with a thorough visual inspection noting abnormal swelling, redness, or deformities. The physician should also palpate the ankle to determine the extent of any swelling, identify any abnormal bony prominences or incongruities, determine specific areas of point tenderness or extreme pain, and evaluate the neurovascular status of the patient.
- The neurovascular examination should include an assessment of the dorsalis pedis and posterior tibial pulses. Additionally, the physician should evaluate the capillary refill, light touch, and two-point discrimination distal to the ankle.
- Gross deformity of the ankle is a likely indicator of dislocation, which should be reduced and splinted prior to radiographic examination or further evaluation.
- The physician will then evaluate the range of motion of the ankle. The normal range of ankle motion is 30° of dorsiflexion and 45° of plantarflexion. The range of motion necessary for ankle functionality or ambulation is 10° of dorsiflexion and 20° of plantarflexion (Koval and Zuckerman, 2002).
- It is important to evaluate the stability of the ankle when suspecting a fracture. The squeeze test is performed to rule out disruption of the tibiofibular syndesmosis. The squeeze test is performed by squeezing the leg, approximating the tibia and fibula, at or slightly above the level of the belly of the gastrocnemius. An indicator of syndesmotic disruption is pain at the distal tibiofibular articulation when the squeeze test is performed (Hopkinson et al, 1990). The physician should also perform an anterior-drawer to evaluate the laxity of the complex ligamentous support network of the ankle. Pain with dorsiflexion and external rotation should also be noted as this may represent posterior bony injury or tendinous disruption.

RADIOGRAPHIC EXAMINATION

- The *Ottawa ankle rules* are a valuable guideline in determining the need for radiographic examination in a patient suspected to have an ankle fracture. Radiographic examination is required if the patient is unable to bear weight, if the patient has pain with palpation within 6 cm proximal or distal to the talar articulation, or if the patient has bony tenderness at the posterior edge or tip of either malleoli (Stiell et al, 1993).
- The ankle is best examined radiographically with an anterior-posterior, lateral, and mortise view. Three view radiographs demonstrate greater reliability when compared to various combinations of two view radiographs (Brandser et al). Abnormal radiographic findings are greater than 2 mm of talar tilt (difference in lateral and medial joint spaces in anterior-posterior view), misalignment of the talar dome under the tibia in anterior-posterior or lateral views, and a demonstrated tibiofibular overlap of less than 10 mm in the anterior-posterior view or the mortise view (Marsh and Saltzman, 2001). Stress radiographs may be valuable, but are difficult to standardize. Though normative data is not adequately reported in the literature, the Telos stress device is being used to standardize the amount of stress about the ankle during routine radiographic stress examinations.
- *Magnetic resonance imaging* (MRI) is best suited for the examination of the integrity of the ankle ligaments, and a bone scan is often helpful to rule out osteochondral lesions in patients with chronic ankle injuries.

CLASSIFICATION

- There are three primary classification systems used to define ankle fractures. The Danis-Weber classification is based solely upon the fibula and the location of the fracture in relation to the ankle mortise (Danis, 1949). The Lauge-Hansen classification describes the ankle fracture according to foot position and movement of the foot in relation to the leg (supination-adduction, supination-external rotation, pronation-abduction, pronation-eversion, pronation-dorsiflexion). The most common mechanism of ankle fracture is of the supination-external rotation variety (Lauge-Hansen, 1950). Lastly, the A-O classification is based on the level of the fibula fracture, medial malleolar involvement, and syndesmotic disruption (Orthopedic Trauma Association, 1996). A summary of the aforementioned classifications can be found in Table 64-4.

TREATMENT

- The goal of treatment of ankle fractures is to restore the anatomic congruity of the ankle joint, promote pain free restoration of range of motion, and to restore and maintain fibular length.

TABLE 64-4 Classification Systems of Ankle Fractures

FRACTURE CLASSIFICATION	TYPE	LOCATION OF FRACTURE	ASSOCIATED INJURIES
Danis-Weber	A	Below ankle mortise and tibiofibular articulation	Syndesmosis likely intact
	B	At level of mortise and tibiofibular articulation	Syndesmosis likely intact
	C	Above level of mortise and tibiofibular articulation	Likely disruption of syndesmosis with positive squeeze test
Lauge-Hansen	Supination-adduction	Transverse fracture of lateral malleolus	Stage 1: Tear of lateral ligaments Stage 2: Fracture of medial malleolus
	Supination-external rotation	Avulsion fracture of lateral malleolus	Stage 1: Rupture of anterior tib-fib ligament Stage 2: Spiral or oblique fracture of lateral malleolus Stage 3: Posterior tibial fracture Stage 4: Fracture of medial malleolus or torn deltoid ligament
	Pronation-abduction	Medial malleolus	Stage 1: Torn deltoid ligament Stage 2: Syndesmotic disruption and posterior tibial fracture Stage 3: Oblique fracture of fibula above mortise
	Pronation-external rotation	Medial malleolus	Stage 1: Torn deltoid ligament Stage 2: Syndesmotic disruption Stage 3: Spiral fracture of fibula above mortise Stage 4: Posterior tibial fracture
AO	A	Fibula at or below plafond	Intact or possible avulsions medial and posterior
	B	Fibula at plafond extending proximally	Tib-fib ligaments torn; possible avulsions medially and posteriorly
	C	Fibula above plafond	Syndesmosis always torn; deltoid ligament torn

- Nondisplaced, stable ankle fractures and stable, reduced ankle fractures can be managed nonoperatively with great success. Once swelling is reduced, long leg casting is indicated with transition to short leg cast or fracture bracing after 4 to 6 weeks (Marsh and Saltzman, 2001). Diabetics are a special subgroup of patients that may need more time in the long leg cast before adequate bone growth is evident and are less likely candidates for operative intervention. Recent studies suggest that diabetics have higher postoperative complication rates when compared to nondiabetics. Blotter et al reported a 43% complication rate in diabetics as compared to a 15% complication rate in nondiabetics (Blotter et al, 1999). Diabetics also demonstrate a higher postoperative infection rate after ankle surgery as reported by Flynn et al in 2000 (Flynn, Rodriguez-del, and Piza, 2000).
- Displaced, unstable, open, or unreducible ankle fractures must be treated operatively with reduction and internal or external fixation. Studies have been unable, however, to demonstrate that the accuracy of ankle fracture reduction determines better long term outcome or reduces the amount of intra-articular contact stresses (Vrahas, Fu, and Veenis, 1994).
- Open fractures require emergent orthopedic consult and it is very likely that they will be taken to the operating room immediately. Studies have shown that most open ankle fractures are associated with wounds less than 1 cm long and that infection rates after operative treatment of these fractures is comparable to infection rates seen in the treatment of closed fractures. Chapman and Mahoney demonstrated in their series of open ankle fractures in which immediate fixation was achieved, that the rate of infection in open fracture wounds less than 1 cm was 2% and the rate of infection in open fracture wounds with extensive soft tissue damage and wounds greater than 1 cm was 29% (Chapman and Mahoney, 1976).
- The most important aspects of ankle fracture management are to immediately reduce dislocated ankles prior to radiographic study, clean and dress open wounds in a proper sterile fashion, document and evaluate neurovascular status, and apply a posterior splint with a U-shaped component at the ankle when transporting the patient or preparing them for further work-up by an orthopedic surgeon.

REFERENCES

Barrett JA, Baron JA, Karagas MR, et al: Fracture risk in the U.S. Medicare population. *J Clin Epidemiol* 52:243–249, 1999.

Blotter RH, Connolly E, Wasan A, et al: Acute complications in the operative treatment of isolated ankle fractures in patients with diabetes mellitus. *Foot Ankle Int* 20:687–694, 1999.

Brandser EA, Berbaum KS, Dorfman DD, et al: Contribution of individual projections alone and in combination for radiographic detection of ankle fractures. *AJR Am J Roentgenol* 174(6):1691–7, 2000.

Chapman MW, Mahoney M: The place of immediate internal fixation in the management of open fracture. *Abbott Soc Bull* 8:85, 1976.

Court-Brown CM: Fractures of the tibia and fibula, in Rockwood CA, Green DB, Bucholz RW, et al (eds): *Fractures in Adults*, 5th ed. Philadelphia, PA, Lippincott Williams & Wilkins, 1939–2000, 2001.

Court-Brown CM, McBirnie J: The epidemiology of tibial fractures. *J Bone Joint Surg* 77B:417–421, 1995.

Daffner RH, Pavlov H: Stress fractures: Current concepts. *Am J Radiol* 159:245–252, 1992.

Danis R: Les fractures malleolaires, in Danis R (ed.): *Theories et pratique de l'osteosynthese.* 1949, p 133–165.

DeCoster TA, Willis MC, Marsh JL, et al: Rank order analysis of tibial plafond fractures: Does injury or reduction predict outcome? *Foot Ankle Int* 20:44–49, 1999.

Flynn JM, Rodriguez-del Rio F, Piza PA: Closed ankle fractures in the diabetic patient. *Foot Ankle Int* 21:311–319, 2000.

Hooper GJ, Keddell RG, Penny ID: Conservative management or closed nailing of tibial shaft fractures. *J Bone Joint Surg Br* 73:83–85, 1991.

Hopkinson WJ, St Pierre P, Ryan JB, et al: Syndesmosis sprains of the ankle. *Foot Ankle* 10:325–330, 1990.

Jensen DB, Rude C, Duus B, et al: Tibial plateau fractures: a comparison of conservative and surgical treatment. *J Bone Joint Surg Br* 72:49–56, 1990.

Koval KJ, Zuckerman JD: *Handbook of Fractures.* New York, NY, Baltimore, MD, Lippincott Williams & Wilkins, 2002.

Lauge-Hansen N: Fractures of the ankle: Combined experiemental-surgical and experimental roentgenologic investigations. *Arch Surg* 60:957–985, 1950.

Lucht U, Pligaard S: Fractures of the tibial condyles. *Acta Orthop Scand* 42:366–376, 1971.

Marsh JL, Saltzman C: Ankle fractures, in Rockwood CA, Green DB, Bucholz RW, et al (eds.): *Fractures in Adults*, 5th ed. Philadelphia, PA, Lippincott Williams & Wilkins, 2001, pp 2001–2089.

Merchant TC, Dietz FR: Long term follow-up after fracture of the tibial and fibular shafts. *J Bone Joint Surg Am* 71:599–605, 1989.

Orthopedic Trauma Association: Fracture and dislocation compendium. *J Orthop Trauma* 10:1–55, 1996.

Schatzker J, McBroom R, Bruce D: Tibial plateau fractures: The Toronto experience 1968–1975. *Clin Orthop* 138:94–104, 1979.

Stiell IG, Greenberg GH, McKnight RD, et al: Decision rules for the use of radiography in acute ankle injuries: Refinement and prospective validation. *JAMA* 269:1127–1132, 1993.

Templeman DC, Marder RA: Injuries of the knee associated with fractures of the tibial shaft. *J Bone Joint Surg* 71A:1392–1395, 1989.

Tscherne H, Gotzen L (eds.): *Fractures With Soft Tissue Injuries.* New York, NY, Springer-Verlag, 1984.

Vrahas M, Fu F, Veenis B: Intrarticular contact stresses with simulated ankle malunions. *J Orthop Trauma* 8:159–166, 1994.

65 FOOT INJURIES

Mark D Porter
Joseph J Zubak
Winston J Warme

HINDFOOT/MIDFOOT

BONY

CALCANEAL STRESS FRACTURE

• Stress fractures of the calcaneus are relatively rare, but may be a cause of heel pain in athletes or military recruits who place significant stress on their heels (Pester and Smith, 1992).

• Calcaneal stress fractures usually present as progressive diffuse pain over the entire heel, not localized only to the plantar heel. The physical examination is characterized by tenderness with simultaneous medial and lateral compression of the calcaneus, and there may be mild swelling or erythema. Radiographs may be normal, or a sclerotic vertical band may appear 3 to 4 weeks after the onset of symptoms.

• Technetium bone scan may be necessary particularly for detection of early cases.

• Activity modification is the mainstay of treatment. Weightbearing is as tolerated with crutches. Anti-inflammatories and shock-absorbing heel inserts may be beneficial (Pfeffer, 2001).

NAVICULAR STRESS FRACTURE

• Stress fractures of the navicular are being recognized with increasing frequency in active persons. Diagnosis is often delayed, and outcome often suffers because of lack familiarity with the condition.

• Navicular stress fractures typically present in a running athlete with gradually increasing pain in the dorsal midfoot with radiation of pain down the medial arch. Initial plain films are often normal. It may be necessary to obtain a three-phase bone scan, which is positive early and localizes the lesion well. After a positive bone scan, a computed tomographic scan should be obtained to provide anatomic detail and guide therapy.

- Fractures that are nondisplaced and without comminution respond well to six weeks of nonweightbearing cast immobilization. Displacement, comminution, and delayed or nonunion fractures are indications for surgical open reduction internal fixation (Quirk, 1995; Eric, Coris, and John, 2003).

CALCANEAL ANTERIOR PROCESS FRACTURE

- Fracture of the anterior process of the calcaneus is a common injury that is often misdiagnosed. It has been referred to as "the ankle sprain that does not heal" (Trnka, Zettl, and Ritschl, 1998).
- Patients typically present following a twisting injury with immediate pain on the outer aspect of the mid portion of the foot and discomfort on weightbearing. If the diagnosis is missed initially they may present with prolonged disability and local pain at the calcaneocuboid joint.
- The mechanism can be avulsion of the bifurcate ligament with plantar flexion inversion or direct compression with dorsiflexion eversion.
- Physical examination is notable for swelling at the anterior lateral midfoot and tenderness to palpation at the anterior lateral process of the calcaneus. Standard *anteroposteior* (AP), lateral and oblique films should be obtained. The oblique projection is the most helpful.
- For acute nondisplaced fractures the patient can be treated with a short-leg cast and no weightbearing for 6–8 weeks. Displaced fractures may require open reduction and internal fixation or excision of the fragment and repair of the bifurcate ligament. Neglected injuries may lead to arthrosis of the calcaneocuboid joint (Roesen and Kanat, 1993).

SUBTALAR DISLOCATION

- Subtalar dislocation is most often a result of high-energy trauma, such as motor vehicle accidents; however, it can be a result of sports injuries as well. Eighty percent of dislocations are medial, 20% are lateral. Ten percent are open, and about half have associated fractures. Subsequent osteonecrosis of the talus occurs in about 5–10% of cases (Freund, 1989).
- Closed reduction is performed by flexing the knee and forefoot, applying gentle traction, accentuating and reversing the deformity while applying gentle pressure over the talar head. Reduction may be blocked by longitudinally directed structures, the posterior tibial tendon in the case of lateral dislocations, extensor tendons in medial dislocation. After reduction, treatment is with a short-leg cast for 4 weeks. In the case of open dislocations operative repair followed by prolonged immobilization is required (Bohay and Manoli, 1990).

SUBTALAR INSTABILITY

- Subtalar instability may contribute to lateral ankle instability or may be its own entity. Instability can be produced after lateral ankle sprain or subtalar dislocation by injury to the cervical ligament, lateral talocalcaneal ligament, intraosseous ligament and calcaneofibular ligament (Hertel et al, 1999).
- Patients present with symptoms of lateral ankle instability. Isolated or comorbid subtalar instability can be difficult to identify. Stress radiographs taken in AP subtalar neutral, AP supination stress, lateral Broden, and supination stress Broden can be helpful.
- May require anatomic reconstruction of the involved lateral ankle ligaments (Karlsson and Eriksson, 1997).

POSTERIOR TALAR PROCESS FRACTURE

- Avulsion fracture of the medial tubercle of the posterior process of the talus occurs after forceful dorsiflexion-pronation of the ankle. Generally presents as pain in the posterior medial ankle. The patient may also have tenderness to palpation over the posterior talar beak or pain with plantar flexion.
- Acute fractures that are nondisplaced can be treated by immobilization in a short leg cast. Displaced fractures may require open reduction and internal fixation. Missed fractures do poorly and patients complain of persistent posteromedial ankle pain.
- However, delayed operative excision of missed fractures yields good results (Kim, Berkowitz, and Pressman, 2003; Judd and Kim, 2002).

LATERAL TALAR PROCESS FRACTURE

- Lateral talar process fractures are another frequently underdiagnosed foot injury. Delay in diagnosis can lead to persistent pain and severe degeneration of the subtalar joint. Patients complains of lateral ankle discomfort and increased pain with activity particularly inversion and eversion of the ankle. The usual mechanism is inversion and dorsiflexion with axial load but they can also be caused by eversion load (snowboarder's fracture).
- Examination is characterized by swelling and tenderness over the lateral talar process and pain with forced inversion and eversion. Lateral process fractures are easily missed on routine X-rays. Radiographs taken at 30° plantar flexion and 45° internal rotation may reveal the fracture, but *computed tomography* (CT) is best.
- Nondisplaced fractures can be treated with immobilization in cast or boot. Displaced or intra-articular fractures may be treated surgically by excision of fragment or open reduction and internal fixation (Judd and Kim, 2002; Boon et al, 2001; Cantrell and Tarquinio, 1998).

PAINFUL OS TRIGONUM

- The os trigonum is an ossicle present in 7 to 11% of the population as a continuation of the posterior talar process.
- The painful os trigonum syndrome is one cause of posteromedial ankle pain. This syndrome is most prevalent in athletes who perform frequent or forceful plantar flexion. The condition may be misdiagnosed as other conditions such as Achilles' tendonitis (Martin, 2000).
- Presentation is with pain in the posterior medial ankle. There may be tenderness to palpation over the os or pain with dorsiflexion/plantarflexion, or movement of the great toe. The lateral X-ray may reveal the presence of the os trigonum.
- Initial treatment is conservative with nonsteroidals and activity modification. Surgical excision may be required with failure of nonoperative management (Blake, Lallas, and Ferguson, 1989).

TARSAL COALITION

- Tarsal coalition is fibrous (syndesmosis), cartilaginous (synchondrosis), or osseous (synostosis) bridging of two or more tarsal bones.
- It often presents in older children or adolescents as ankle instability and pain, or painful flat foot and decreased subtalar motion. Pain localized to midtarsal area, exacerbated by standing or athletic activity. Bilaterality is common (as high as 50%). Incidence is less than 1%.
- The etiology is unclear. There may be a congenital form that is autosomal dominant with variable penetrance. Failure of mesenchymal segmentation has been proposed as cause (Pachuda, Lasday, and Jay, 1990).
- In early childhood the union is fibrous and mobile and is thought to become symptomatic as union becomes cartilaginous or osseus.
- Radiographic evaluation should include AP, lateral, and oblique views of the foot. Coalition between the talus and navicular can be seen on the lateral. Coalition between the calcaneus and navicular, and the cuboid and navicular can be seen on the oblique films. Consider axial view of the calcaneus or CT if routine views fail to show abnormality.
- Talonavicular coalition is frequently mild, may present as early as 2–3 years old and respond to treatment with a plastizote shoe insert. Calcaneonavicular coalition commonly presents inpatients between 8–12 years of age. Surgical excision of the coalition may be indicated in patients with a cartilaginous bridge and no degenerative changes in the talonavicular region.
- Talocalcaneal coalition frequently presents during adolescence. It may occur in the anterior, middle, or posterior facet. Treatment with immobilization in a short leg cast may relieve symptoms. Surgical treatment may consist of resection of the coalition or triple arthrodesis (Pachuda, Lasday, and Jay, 1990; Kulik, Jr, and Clanton, 1996; Varner and Michelson, 2000).

TARSOMETATARSAL FRACTURE-DISLOCATIONS (LISFRANC INJURIES)

- Injuries to the tarsometarsal joint are called *Lisfranc injuries* after a French surgeon in the Napoleonic era. Injuries to the tarsometatarsal joint are typically associated with high-energy trauma, but may also occur with lower energy mechanisms in athletics.
- The base of the metatarsals and adjacent tarsals are wedge-shaped, forming a "roman arch" to support the transverse arch of the foot. The second metatarsal base dovetails with adjacent tarsals and metatarsals to form highly stable articulation. The third through fourth metatarsals are connected at their bases by transverse, oblique, and interosseous ligaments. The second metatarsal is connected to the medial cuneiform by the strong Lisfranc ligament.
- Forced plantar flexion may injure the weaker dorsal ligaments. Direct blows to the dorsum of the foot or rotational injuries may also injure the tarsometatarsal joint (Solan et al, 2001).
- Lisfranc injuries may be purely ligamentous without apparent fracture. Consequently they are often missed. Swelling and tenderness in the midfoot without obvious fracture should raise suspicion. Significant soft tissue injury may be associated with tarsometatarsal injuries and may be associated with compartment syndrome. Instability of the tarsometatarsal joints can be determined by palpating the joint while grasping the metatarsal heads and applying a dorsally-directed force, although this may not be tolerated in the acute setting.
- While markedly displaced fracture-dislocations are obvious, some dislocations may spontaneously reduce and non-weightbearing radiographs may appear benign. Three radiographic findings suggest subtle tarsometatarsal injury. The first is disruption of continuity of a line drawn from the medial base of the second metatarsal to the medial side of the middle cuneiform on the AP and oblique views. The second is widening between the first and second rays. Third, the medial side of the base of the fourth metatarsal should line up with medial side of the cuboid on the oblique view. Weightbearing radiographs, if tolerated, provide excellent stress views.
- Successful outcome is predicated upon anatomic reduction. Injuries to the Lisfranc joint are treated by open or closed reduction and stabilization with screws or percutaneous wires, followed by a period

of nonweightbearing immobilization (Arntz, Veith, and Hansen, Jr, 1988; Myerson, 1989; Kuo et al, 2000).

SOFT TISSUE

COMPRESSION NEUROPATHY (JOGGER'S FOOT)

- Entrapment of the medial plantar nerve distal to the tarsal tunnel can cause a neuropathy known as *jogger's foot*. The medial plantar nerve courses plantarward after it exits the tarsal tunnel where it may be compressed by osteophytes from the talonavicular joint or a fibrotic master knot of Henry.
- Patient's complain of pain or numbness of the medial sole of the foot and medial toes.
- Conservative treatment consists of rest, nonsteroidal anti-inflammatories, or soft orthoses. Patients with a planovalgus foot may benefit from a University of California Biomechanics Laboratory (UCBL) orthosis. Injection of corticosteroid with local anesthetic can be diagnostic as well as therapeutic. Surgical release of the medial plantar nerve may be indicated with failure of nonoperative management (DiGiovanni and Gould, 1998).

TARSAL TUNNEL SYNDROME

- Tarsal tunnel syndrome is the most common compression neuropathy of the foot and ankle. Etiology is entrapment neuropathy of the posterior tibial nerve in the tarsal tunnel or one of its terminal branches after leaving the tarsal tunnel. Tarsal tunnel syndrome may be posttraumatic, as result of a space-occupying lesion, accessory muscle, or idiopathic (Schon, 1994).
- The tarsal tunnel is a fibro-osseous tunnel. The osseous boundaries are the medial surface of the talus, the medial surface of the os calcis, the sustentaculum tali, and inferomedial navicular. The fibrous portion of the canal consists of the flexor retinaculum as the roof and the abductor hallucis with its investing fascia.
- Patients complain of burning, tingling, or numbness on plantar aspect of foot and may have night pain, or discomfort with even light bedcovers.
- The physical examination is characterized by a positive Tinel's sign at the tarsal tunnel or reproduction of symptoms with compression for 60 s.
- Other causes of peripheral neuropathy should be considered such as diabetes, hypothyroidism, and alcoholism. Radiographs are obtained to rule out extrinsic bony abnormality. Electrodiagnostic studies are helpful in differentiating from peripheral neuropathy or lumbosacral radiculopathy.
- Conservative treatment consists of avoidance of aggravating activities, control of generalized edema,

if present, with medications or compressive stockings as indicated. Arch supports or medial heel wedges may helpful. Nonsteroidals or injection of corticosteroid into the tarsal tunnel may benefit patients with tenosynovitis. Surgical management consists of complete release of the tibial nerve and all its branches, and has been shown to result in improved outcome measures after failure of conservative management (Lau and Daniels, 1999).

PLANTAR HEEL PAIN

- Plantar heel pain is a common complaint among athletes and military recruits. There are several etiologies for chronic plantar heel pain.
- Plantar fasciitis
  1. Plantar Fasciitis is probably the most common cause of plantar heel pain. Repetitive or acute trauma leads to microtears at the calcaneal insertion of the plantar fascia. The patient typically presents with pain localized to the plantar medial heel. The pain is often worse with the first few steps in the morning or after rest, also with jumping or pushing off.
  2. Radiographs may show a plantar heel spur in 50% of patients with plantar fasciitis and 15% of asymptomatic patients. Bone scan can help differentiate plantar fasciitis from calcanael stress fracture.
  3. Primary treatment of plantar fasciitis is nonoperative, conisisting of Achilles stretching and activity modification. Hand massage, ice massage, or anti-inflammatories may also be helpful. Cushioned heel cups are often prescribed. Injection of corticosteroids with local anesthetic may be considered after failure of other methods. Repeated steroid injection may cause atrophy of the heel fat pad and should be avoided.
  4. Ninety-five percent of patients with plantar fasciitis will have resolution of their symptoms within 12–18 months. For the 5% of patients who fail conservative treatment, surgical release of the plantar fascia may be considered. Although surgery generally results in improvement in symptoms patients should be counseled that recovery can be prolonged, and that exercises to maintain Achilles length must be continued (Pfeffer, 2003).
- Acute *posterior fourchette* (PF) tear
  1. A variation of insertional plantar fasciitis is acute tear of the plantar fascia. Patients present with acute pain or swelling of the plantar foot. A defect in the plantar fascia may be palpable, and loss of arch height may be noted with complete rupture.
  2. Treatment varies with symptoms, ranging from weightbearing as tolerated to nonweightbearing

and cast immobilzation. Physical therapy is begun once the patient can comfortably bear weight (usually about 4–6 weeks). An arch support may be helpful with persistent discomfort associated with loss of arch height.

- Fat pad insufficiency
  1. Fat pad insufficiency is often seen in older athletes or in patients after multiple corticosteroid injections to the heel. Other causes of heel pain should be excluded prior to making the diagnosis of fat pad atrophy. Treatment consists of a viscoelastic heel cup and well-cushioned shoes (Baxter, Thigpen, and Pfeffer, 1989; Karr, 1994).

POSTERIOR HEEL PAIN

- There are several causes of posterior heel pain. In addition to the entities below, inflammatory conditions such as gout, psoriasis, and Reiter's disease must be considered.
  1. Insertional Achilles tendinitis is common in jumping athletes, but may also be precipitated by a direct blow or poorly fitting shoes. On physical examination there is tenderness to palpation directly over the insertion of the Achilles and pain with resisted plantar flexion. Treatment is conservative with *nonsteroidal anti-inflammatory drugs* (NSAIDs), Achilles stretching, and activity modification. Felt or silipose pads placed over the posterior heel may also be beneficial.
  2. Retrocalcaneal bursitis can also present as posterior heel pain and direct tenderness to palpation of the posterior heel. The bursa is a synovial-lined bursa between the posterior calcaneus and the Achilles tendon. Treatment is conservative as for insertional Achilles tendinitis. Rarely, excision of the bursa may be necessary.
  3. Haglund's deformity is an abnormal prominence of the posterosuperior portion of the calcaneus that can be associated with retrocalcaneal bursitis. Initial treatment is conservative as for retrocalcaneal bursitis, but surgical excision of the prominence may be required (Stephens, 1994).

SPRING LIGAMENT RUPTURE

- Rupture of the plantar calcaneonavicular ligament is usually seen to fail secondary to rupture of the posterior tibial tendon in the setting of acquired flatfoot. Rarely, however, acute rupture of the spring ligament can also be a primary cause of painful acquired flatfoot.
- Presentation is similar to that of posterior tibial tendon dysfunction with a progressive painful planovalgus foot. There may be a history of eversion injury. The patient may have difficulty or be unable to perform a single toe raise; however, the tibialis posterior will have full strength on testing. Radiographs may reveal loss of longitudinal arch height.
- Treatment with surgical reconstruction of the spring ligament complex has been reported to be successful (Borton and Saxby, 1997).

FOREFOOT

BONY

METATARSAL STRESS FRACTURE

- Stress fractures account for nearly 5% of all sports injuries. Stress fractures of the metatarsals rank second after the distal tibia in frequency. Among the metatarsal fractures, fracture of the diaphysis of the fifth is most common; however, stress fractures of the fifth must be distinguished from acute traumatic fractures.
- Generally presents with pain of insidious onset, although may present after acute trauma. Patients often relate a history of increased intensity of activity, or changes in footwear or activity surface. Ninety percent of metatarsal stress fractures involve the second, third, or fourth metatarsal.
- Presentation of stress fractures of the metatarsals can be similar to *metatarsophalangeal joint* (MTPJ) synovitis or interdigital neuritis. The pain can be reproduced by pushing the metatarsal upward from below, and is generally more proximal than the pain from MTP synovitis. Diagnosis is confirmed by radiographs. If stress fracture is still suspected and routine radiographs are normal, technetium bone scan may be performed.
- Rest and a stiff wooden-soled shoe are usually sufficient treatment. Occasionally, a short-leg walking cast or walking boot may be required. Symptoms typically resolve in about 4 weeks and activity is resumed gradually (Myerson, Haddad, and Weinfeld, 1997).

FRACTURES OF THE PROXIMAL FIFTH METATARSAL

- There are at least three distinct fracture patterns in the proximal fifth metatarsal, each with its own mechanism of injury, treatment options, and prognosis.
  1. The most common fractures of the proximal fifth metatarsal are avulsion fractures of the tuberosity. The mechanism of injury is thought to be avulsion of the lateral band of the plantar aponeurosis. These fractures are generally extra-articular and rarely displaced. Treatment usually consists of weight-bearing as tolerated in a walking cast or hard-soled shoe until pain subsides. If the fracture is markedly displaced open reduction and internal fixation may be indicated.

2. Fractures just distal to the tuberosity, at the metaphyseal–diaphyseal junction bear the eponym *Jones' fracture.* They are caused by forceful adduction of a plantar-flexed ankle. These fractures demonstrate higher rates of nonunion than tuberosity fractures. Nonoperative treatment consists of nonweightbearing in a short leg cast for 6–8 weeks. If more rapid return to activity is desired for high-level or recreational athletes, operative treatment with an intramedullary screw may be advised. Nonunions or delayed unions are also treated with intramedullary fixation and bone graft.

3. The third fracture pattern of the proximal fifth metatarsal is the diaphyseal stress fracture. Criteria for stress fracture are a history of prodromal symptoms at the lateral aspect of the foot, radiographic evidence of stress phenomena in the bone, and no history of treatment for fracture of the fifth metatarsal. Initial treatment of acute diaphyseal stress fractures of the fifth metatarsal consists of nonweightbearing ambulation in a short leg cast for 6–8 weeks. Stress fractures that go on to become delayed unions or nonunions may require operative intervention (Rosenberg and Sferra, 2000).

HALLUX RIGIDUS

• Hallux rigidus a common disorder, seen in about 1 in 45 individuals over the age of 50. It is characterized by limitation of motion of the first metatarsophalangeal joint, particularly in dorsiflexion. Hallux rigidus has been attributed to many causes, including trauma, inflammatory or metabolic conditions, and congenital disorders.

• Patients present complaining of limitation of motion and pain at the metatarsophalangeal joint with ambulation or athletic activity. A palpable exostosis may be present at the dorsal MTPJ and the patient may have symptoms from footwear impinging on the exostosis or *cheil.*

• Standing AP, lateral, and oblique views reveal narrowing of the joint space and a dorsal osteophyte.

• Initial treatment is nonoperative, consisting of NSAIDs, activity modification to avoid high impact activity. A steel or fiberglass shank in the sole of the shoe can relieve symptoms by limiting dorsiflexion. Rocker bottom shoes and custom insoles may have similar effect. Failure of nonoperative treatment is an indication for surgery. Surgical treatment can consist of cheilectomy, arthrodesis, or Keller arthroplasty (Fleming, 2000).

SESAMOIDS

• Injuries of the sesamoids can cause significant pain and disability for athletes.

1. Stress fracture of sesamoids is associated with insidious pain and may progress to osteonecrosis.

2. The condition must be differentiated radiographically from bipartite sesamoid. Bone scan can be helpful if there is doubt.

3. Initial treatment is with a short leg walking cast. Excision of the sesamoid may be indicated with failure of closed treatment (Biedert and Hintemann, 2003).

• Sesamoiditis

1. Inflammation of the sesamoid complex includes tendinitis of the flexor hallucis longus, synovitis, and chondromalacia of the sesamoids.

2. Presents as insidious onset pain localized to the ball of the foot. Physical examination reveals tenderness to palpation of the sesamoids. Routine radiographs are normal.

3. Metatarsal bars or sesamoid cut-outs can provide relief by shifting weight proximally, off the sesamoids. If necessary, rest can be enforced with the use of a short-leg walking cast. Anti-inflammatories are a useful adjunct. Recalcitrant cases may benefit from a single intra-articular injection of corticosteroid, followed by cast immobilization for 2–4 weeks. Failure of conservative treatment warrants consideration of sesamoidectomy.

• Acute fracture

1. Acute fracture of the sesamoid can occur by compression as in direct blow or a fall from a height, or in tension with violent dorsiflexion of the first metatarsophalangeal joint. Presents with history of identifiable trauma to the region, swelling, ecchymosis, and tenderness to palpation at the plantar MTP joint.

2. In addition to standard AP, oblique, and lateral radiographs, an axial view of the sesamoids should be obtained. Acute fractures can be distinguished from other conditions, such as bipartite sesamoids or osteonecrosis by their radiographic appearance. Acute fractures demonstrate sharp, irregular edges in contrast to the smooth, sclerotic edges of the bipartite sesamoid. Osteonecrosis of the sesamoid is characterized by fragmentation into multiple pieces, often with evidence of remodeling or new bone formation.

3. Treatment for nondisplaced fractures is similar to treatment of sesamoiditis, ranging from hard-soled shoe or metatarsal bar to a short leg walking cast. Treatment of displaced fractures or nondisplaced fractures that fail closed treatment is surgical excision (Grace, 2000).

1ST METATARSALPHALANGEAL JOINT DISLOCATION

• Traumatic dislocations of the first metatarsophalangeal joint are relatively rare, and represent the extreme end of the turf toe continuum. The mechanism is almost always forceful hyperextension. Patients present with a clear history of trauma and painful limitation of motion. Local swelling may obscure obvious deformity. Radiographs reveal the proximal phalanx dislocated dorsally over the metatarsal head.

- The sesamoids may be seen in their normal relationship to each other, indicating that the hallux has dislocated over the metatarsal head and neck with the sesamoids still attached at its base (type I dislocation). This configuration is generally irreducible by closed means.
- Wide separation of the sesamoids indicates rupture of the intersesamoid ligament (type IIA). Fractures of the sesamoids may also be seen (type IIB). Types IIA and IIB are usually reducible by closed manipulation, which should be followed by 3–6 weeks in a short leg walking cast (Jahss, 1980).

SOFT TISSUE

HALLUX VALGUS

- Hallux valgus or bunion deformity is common in the general population and occurs in athletes as well. Hallux valgus in athletes demands different considerations and treatment than in the general population. Hallux valgus occurs with lateral deviation of the great toe and progressive subluxation of the first metatarsophalangeal joint. The medial eminence of the first metatarsophalangeal joint becomes prominent. The overlying soft tissue becomes irritated, swollen, and inflamed creating the bunion (from the Greek for turnip).
- Several intrinsic and extrinsic factors may contribute to hallux valgus. The most important extrinsic factor is constricting footwear. Shoes with heels and a narrow toe box have been associated with bunions. Athletic activities that increase the lateral stress on the first MTP joint can be another extrinsic cause. Intrinsic factors include a pronated foot, contracted heel cord, hypermobility of the first metatarsocuneiform joint, and metatarsus primus varus. Injury to the first metatarsophalangeal joint, such as turf toe or first MTP dislocation may weaken the joint capsule and collateral ligament predisposing to hallux valgus.
- Patients typically present complaining of pain over the medial eminence and irritation with shoe wear. The skin and bursa over the medial eminence may be irritated.
- The patient's feet should be examined sitting and standing. Standing may accentuate the deformity. Range of motion at the first MTP should be noted, as well as any hypermobiltiy at the metatarsocuneiform joint. The foot is examined for pes planus and pronation.

- Radiographic evaluation consists of AP, lateral, and sesamoid views with the patient standing. The angle formed by the proximal phalynx and first metatarsal, or hallux valgus angle is measured. A normal hallux valgus angle is less than 15°. An angle between 15° and 20° is considered mild hallux valgus. Moderate deformity is characterized by a hallux valgus angle between 20° and 40°, with an angle greater than 40° being severe deformity. Other radiographic angles measured include the intermetatarsal angle between the shafts of the first and second metatarsal and the distal metatarsal articular angle, a measurement of joint congruity.
- Initial treatment is conservative. Modification of shoe wear is paramount. Irritation of the medial eminence may be relieved with a wider toe box, shoe stretching, or pads around the bunion. Patients with pes planus may benefit from an orthosis. Contracture of the Achilles if present should be treated appropriately. Persistent pain after exhausting nonoperative treatment options is an indication for surgery. Surgery can result in postoperative restriction of MTP motion, which should be considered by athletes requiring a great range of MTP motion, such as dancers and sprinters (Baxter, 1994; Coughlin, 1997).

METATARSALGIA

- Metatarsalgia is a descriptive term for pain beneath the metarsal heads that may have a number of etiologies including stress fracture, synovitis, Freiberg's infarction, or neuroma. Forefoot pain has been associated with tightness of the gastrocnemius-soleus complex. Patients presenting with forefoot or midfoot symptoms have less dorsiflexion on average than asymptomatic controls (Digiovani et al, 2002).
- Lesser MTPJ synovitis
  - Synovitis of the metatarsophalangeal joint most commonly affects the second metatarsal. It occurs most frequently in middle-aged athletes.
  - Symptoms typically include pain in the forefoot exacerbated by running, walking, or forced dorsiflexion of the MTP joint. On examination there may be swelling dorsally and there is tenderness to palpation of the MTP joint. Radiographs might reveal joint space widening, or joint degeneration. It must be differentiated from other conditions with similar appearance, such as Freiberg's infarction, metatarsal stress fracture, degenerative joint disease. The natural history is one of progression and attrition of the capsule, plantar plate and collateral ligaments leading to subluxation or dislocation of the joints.
  - Treatment is initially conservative, including activity modification, shock absorbing insoles, NSAIDs. Surgical management may be necessary with failure

of conservative treatment and development of deformity (Mizel and Yodlowski, 1995).

- Interdigital neuroma
  - Interdigital neuroma or Morton's neuroma is a common cause of forefoot pain. Classically presents as neurogenic pain in the ball of the foot between the third and fourth toes, less commonly in the other interspaces. It is thought to be caused by irritation of the interdigital nerve as it passes beneath the deep transverse metatarsal ligament. It occurs in all populations, but is most frequently reported in runners and dancers.
  - Palpation of the interspace while compressing the forefoot by pressing on the first and fifth metatarsal heads may reproduce the pain. Radiographs are obtained to rule out other sources of pathology such as metatarsal stress fracture or metatarsaophalgeal joint abnormality.
  - The first stage of treatment is modification of shoe wear, avoiding heels and shoes with narrow toe-boxes that may cause compression of the nerve. Injection of corticosteroid with local anesthetic may give lasting or permanent relief. Failure of conservative treatment is an indication for operative management. Excision of the neuroma has demonstrated good pain relief in 80% of patients (Kay and Bennett, 2003).
- Freiberg's infarction
  - Freiberg's infarction is an osteochondrosis of the metatarsal head. Although it may be an asymptomatic finding on radiographs, it generally involves some pain and limitation of motion. It is more common in women, typically in their late teens and early twenties. Involvement of the second metatarsal head is by far the most common.
  - Patients complain of forefoot pain exacerbated by activity. There is tenderness to palpation about the metatarsal head, with or without edema. Although radiographs may be normal early in the disease process, they typically show subchondral collapse and progressive flattening of the metatarsal head.
  - The goal of treatment is to minimize deformity. Most authors recommend a short leg cast and no weightbearing followed by a gradual return to activity. Several surgical procedures have been proposed to address failure of conservative management. They range from joint debridement to metatarsal osteotomy or excision of the metatarsal head (Katcherian, 1994).

TURF TOE

- Injury to the first metatarsophalangeal joint has ranked third in collegiate athletes after knee and ankle injuries. Forced hyperextension is the most common mechanism, although *metacarpal-phalangeal* (MP) sprain can also be seen with varus or valgus stresses, as well as forced flexion.
- Turf toe is classified into three grades. In grade I the plantar tissues remain intact, symptoms are minimal. There may be minor swelling but no ecchymosis. Grade II injuries represent a partial tear of the capsule. Symptoms are pain, swelling, ecchymosis, restricted motion. The patient will be unable to perform at his usual level of sport. Grade III injuries are complete capsuloligamentous tears. There may have been an occult MP dislocation that spontaneously reduced. In addition to pain, swelling, and ecchymosis, the patient will have difficulty with normal ambulation. Radiographs may reveal sesamoid fracture, diastasis, or periarticular fracture.
- Differential diagnosis includes MP dislocation, acute fracture, stress fracture, osteochondral lesion, and flexor tendinitis. Stability of the MP joint should be assessed. With grade II and III sprains radiographs should be obtained.
- Treatment is generally conservative, consisting of rest, ice, elevation, and possibly anti-inflammatories. Buddy taping or rigid orthoses to limit MP motion may also help. Operative treatment may be indicated in patients with symptoms refractory to conservative management. Surgery may also be indicated for osteochondral fracture, unstable MPJ, or proximal migration of the sesamoids. Turf toe injuries may predispose toward osteoarthritis of the first MTPJ and hallux rigidus (Fleming, 2000; Clanton and Ford, 1994).

REFERENCES

Arntz CT, Veith RG, Hansen ST, Jr: Fractures and fracture-dislocations of the tarsometatarsal joint. *J Bone Joint Surg Am* 70(2):173–181, 1988.

Baxter DE: Treatment of bunion deformity. *Athlete Orthop Clinics* 25:1, 161–175, 1994.

Baxter DE, Thigpen M, Pfeffer GB: Chronic heel pain treatment rationale. *Orthop Clin* 20(4), 1989.

Biedert R, Hintemann B: Stress fractures of the medial great toe and sesamoids. *Foot Ankle Int* 24(2):137–141, 2003.

Blake RL, Lallas PJ, Ferguson H: The os trigonum syndrome. A literature review. *J Foot Surg* 28(4):312–318, 1989.

Bohay DR, Manoli A: 2nd subtalar joint dislocations. *Instr Course Lect* 39:157–159, 1990.

Boon AJ, Smith J, Zobitz ME, et al: Snowboarder's talus fracture. Mechanism of injury. *Am J Sports Med* 29(3):333–382, 2001.

Borton DC, Saxby TS: Tear of the plantar calcaneonavicular (spring) ligament causing flatfoot. *J Bone Joint Surg (Br)* 79-B:4, 641–643, 1997.

Cantrell MW, Tarquinio TA: Fracture of the lateral process of the talus. *Am J Sports Med* 26(2):271–277, 1998.

Clanton TO, Ford JJ: Turf toe injury. *Clin Sports Med* 13(4):731–741, 1994.

Coughlin MJ: Hallux valgus. *Instr Course Lect* 46:357–391, 1997.

DiGiovanni BF, Gould JS: Tarsal tunnel syndrome and related entities. *Foot Ankle Clin* 3:3, 1998.

Digiovani et al: Isolated gastrocnemius tightness. *J Bone Joint Surg* 84-A:962–970, 2002.

Eric E. Coris; John A: Lombardo Tarsal navicular stress fractures. (Radiologic Decision-Making) *Am Fam Phys* 67:85, 2003.

Fleming LL: Turf toe injuries and related conditions, in William F Garrett, Kevin P Speer, Donald T Kirkendall (eds.): *Principles and Practice of Orthopedic Sports Medicine.* Philadelphia, PA, Lippincott Williams, and Wilkins, 2000, pp 965–967.

Freund KG: Subtalar dislocations: A review of the literature. *J Foot Surg* 28(5):429–436, 1989.

Grace DL: Sesamoid problems. *Foot Ankle Clin* 5(3):609–627, 2000.

Hertel J, Denegar CR, Monroe MM, et al: Talocrural and subtalar instability. *Med Sci Sport Exerc* 31(11):1501–1581, 1999.

Jahss MH: Traumatic dislocations of the first metatarsophalngeal joint. *Foot Ankle* 1(1):15–21, 1980.

Judd DB, Kim DH: Foot fractures frequently misdiagnosed as ankle sprains. *Am Fam Phys* 66(5):785–794, 2002.

Karlsson, Eriksson: Subtalar instability. *Sports Med* 24(5):337–346, 1997.

Karr SD: Subcalcaneal heel pain. *Orthop Clinics* 25:1, 161–175, 1994.

Katcherian DA: Treatment of Freiberg's disease. *Orthop Clincs* 25:1, 41–49, 1994.

Kay D, Bennett GL: *Foot Ankle Clin* 8(1):49–59, 2003.

Kim DH, Berkowitz MJ, Pressman DN: Avulsion fractures of the medial tubercle of the posterior process of the talus. *Foot Ankle Int* 24(2):172–175, 2003.

Kulik SA, Jr, Clanton TO: Tarsal coalition. *Foot Ankle Int* 17(5):286–296, 1996.

Kuo RS, Tejwani NC, Digiovanni CW, et al: Outcome after open reduction and internal fixation of Lisfranc joint injuries. *J Bone Joint Surg Am* 82-A(11):1609–1618, 2000.

Lau JTC, Daniels TR: Tarsal tunnel syndrome. *Foot and Ankle Int* 19(11):770–777, 1999.

Martin BF: Posterior triangle pain: The os trigonum. *Foot Ankle Int* 21(8):669–672, 2000.

Mizel MS, Yodlowski ML: Disorders of the lesser metatarsophalngeal joints. *JAAOS* 3(3):166–173, 1995.

Myerson M: The diagnosis and treatment of injuries to the Lisfranc joint complex. *Orthop Clin North Am* 20(4):655–664, 1989.

Myerson MS, Haddad SL, Weinfeld SB: Metatarsal stress fractures clincs. *Sports Med* 16(2):319–339, 1997.

Pachuda NM, Lasday SD, Jay RM: Tarsal coalition: Etiology, diagnosis, and treatment. *J Foot Surg* 29(5):474–488, 1990.

Pester S, Smith PC: Stress fractures in the lower extremities of soldiers in basic training. *Orthop Rev* 21(3):297–303, 1992.

Pfeffer GB: Plantar heel pain. *Instr Course Lect* 50:521–531, 2001.

Pfeffer GB: Plantar heel pain. *Am Fam Phys* 67(1):85–90, 2003.

Quirk R: Stress fractures of the navicular. *Orthop Clin North Am* 26(3):423–432, 1995.

Roesen HM, Kanat IO: Anterior process fracture of the calcaneus, *J Foot Ankle Surg* 32(4):424–429, 1993.

Rosenberg GA, Sferra JJ: Treatment strategies for acute fractures and nonunions of the proximal fifth metatarsal. *JAAOS* 8(5), 2000.

Schon LC: Nerve entrapment, neuropathy and nerve dysfunction in athletes. *Orthop Clinics* 25(1):47–59, 1994.

Solan MC, Moorman CT, 3rd, Miyamoto RG, et al: Ligamentous restraints of the second tarsometatarsal joint: A biomechanical evaluation. *Foot Ankle Int* 22(8):637–641, 2001.

Stephens MM Haglund's: Deformity and retrocalcaneal bursistis. *Orthop Clincs* 25:1, 41–49, 1994.

Trnka HJ, Zettl R, Ritschl P: Fracture of the anterior superior process of the calcaneus: An often misdiagnose fracture. *Arch Orthop Trauma Surg* 117(4–5):300–302, 1998.

Varner KE, Michelson JD: Tarsal coalition in adults. *Foot Ankle Int* 21(8):669–672, 2000.

66 LOWER EXTREMITY STRESS FRACTURE

Michael Fredericson

INCIDENCE

- Stress fractures have been shown to account for 0.7–20% of all injuries presented to sports medicine clinics (Bergman and Fredericson, 1999). A recent prospective study specifically involving US college athletes found that track and field athletes had the highest incidence of stress fractures compared with athletes in other sports, such as football, basketball, soccer, and rowing (Johnson, Weiss, and Wheeler, 1994).
- The site of stress fractures varies from sport to sport. For example, among track athletes stress fractures of the navicular, tibia, and metatarsal are the most common while in distance runners it is the tibia and fibula, and in dancers the metatarsals.

ETIOLOGY

- A stress fracture may be best described as accelerated bone remodeling in response to repetitive submaximal stresses. Histological studies of stress fractures have shown that repetitive response to stress leads to osteoclastic activity that surpasses the rate of osteoblastic new bone formation, resulting in temporary weakening of bone (Fredericson, Bergman, and Matheson, 1997).

- Whether stress fractures occur due to the increased load after fatigue of supporting structures or are due to contractile muscular forces acting across and on the bone is debated; in principle, both factors contribute (Daffner and Pavlov, 1992).

RISK FACTORS

- Most studies of stress injuries mention some alteration in the training program as the most significant factor in the production of injury. It has been well documented that there is an increased injury rate with increasing distance beyond approximately 32 km per week (Macera, 1992).
- Also important is any rapid change in the training program, whether a sudden increase in mileage, pace, volume, or some other factor that has been inserted into the program without adequte time for physiologic adaptation to accommodate the new forces. Hard or cambered training surfaces are also important precursors to lower extremity overuse injuries (Fredericson et al, 1995).
- Two independent anatomic variables were identified as major risk factors for stress fracture: a narrow transverse diameter of the tibial diaphysis and retroversion (increased external rotation) of the hip. Female runners with stress fractures were found to have smaller calf circumference measurements. Statistics suggest that women are at 1.5 to 3.5 times greater risk for sustaining stress fractures than men (Johnson, Weiss, and Wheeler, 1994).

HISTORY

- The typical history of a stress fracture is that of localized pain that is not present at the start but occurs after or toward the end of physical activity. This pattern is opposite to that of many soft tissue injuries that have pain first in the morning and with day to day activities but reduced pain during physical activity.
- The site of development of stress fractures varies from sport to sport. Among track athletes, stress fractures of the navicular, tibia, and metatarsal are the most common; whereas in distance runners they can also be seen in areas such as the femur or sacrum, although stress fractures can involve any bone of the lower extremity (Brunkner et al, 1996).

- A careful history often reveals some change in the training regimen during the preceeding 2 to 6 weeks and it is critical the physician ask detailed questions to identify training errors as a cause.

PHYSICAL EXAMINATION

- The physical examination typically reveals local tenderness and swelling over the involved bone. Other tests for the clinical detection of stress fracture such as the hop test (femoral shaft) and fulcrum test and spinal extension test (pars interarticularis) are helpful but not as reliable as direct palpation (Johnson, Weiss, and Wheeler, 1994).
- As with the history, risk factors that can be detected on physical examination should be evaluated. True leg length discrepancies, femoral neck anteversion, varus or valgus alignment at the knee, tibial torsion, muscle weakness, excessive Q angle, and excessive subtalar pronation or a pes cavus style foot should be noted (Matheson et al, 1987).

IMAGING

- In approximately two-thirds of symptomatic patients, the radiographs are initially negative, and of these only half ever develop positive radiographic findings (Daffner and Pavlov, 1992).
- The most common sign in early stress fracture is a region of focal periosteal bone formation. The "gray cortex" sign (a cortical area of decreased density) may also be seen, and is an early sign of stress fracture (Mulligan, 1995).
- Radionuclide scanning is a more sensitive but less specific method for imaging bony stress injuries. Radionuclide technetium-99 diphosphonate triple-phase scanning can provide the diagnosis as early as 2 to 8 days after the onset of symptoms (Fredericson et al, 1995).
- *Magnetic resonance imaging* (MRI) with fat suppression technique has shown promise in grading the progressive stages of stress fracture severity. A four-stage grading system has been developed: A grade-1 injury simply shows periosteal edema on the fat-suppressed images. Grade-2, abnormal increased signal intensity is seen on fat-suppressed T2-weighted images, and in grade-3 injuries decreased signal intensity is seen on T1-weighted images. In grade-4 injuries an actual fracture line is present and is typically visualized on both T1 and T2-weighted images (Fredericson et al, 1995).
- MRI offers the advantages of multiplanar capability, high sensitivity for pathology, ability to precisely

define the location and extent of bony injury, lack of exposure to ionizing radiation and significantly less imaging time than a triple phase bone scan (Fredericson et al, 1995).

GENERAL PRINCIPLE OF TREATMENT

- Less critical or not-at-risk fractures can be treated with a two-phase protocol. Phase one includes pain control with ice massage and physical therapy modalities.
- Weight bearing is allowed for normal activities within the tolerance of pain. Running is discontinued. A modified activity program such as pool running, rowing, or cycling is designed to maintain strength and fitness but to reduce impact loading to the skeleton.
- Phase two, graduated return to sport, generally begins one week following the resolution of focal bony tenderness. The athlete can return to running, starting at a slow pace for 10–15 min running only every other day for the first two weeks. Then, over a 3- to 6-week period, a gradual increase in distance and frequency is permitted (Fredericson, Bergman, and Matheson, 1997).
- Functional foot orthoses are capable of either reducing abnormal pronation in those patients with a markedly everted rearfoot or providing better shock absorption in athletes with a rigid, inverted rearfoot.
- If there is a positive history of late onset menarche or irregular menses or amenorrhea, then consideration should be given to obtaining a bone mineral density test and endocrine work-up.
- A recent study showed that women with stress fractures in trochanteric bone often have osteopenia (Marx et al, 2001)
- In general, treatment of higher risk stress fractures mandates immediate diagnosis, nonweightbearing, and occasionally internal fixation.

SPECIFIC SITES OF STRESS FRACTURE

PELVIS

SACRUM
- Stress fracture in the sacrum are most common in women distance runners with low bone density, but can be seen in those with normal bone mineralization. These stress fractures tend to involve the anteroinferior aspect of the sacral wing unilaterally (Fredericson, Salamancha, and Beaulieu, 2003).
- MRI is recommended for diagnosis, with intermediate signal intensity on T1-weighted images and high

signal intensity on T2-weighted images (Fredericson, Salamancha, and Beaulieu, 2003).

PUBIC RAMI
- More commonly, a bony stress reaction may develop in runners at the symphysis pubis (osteitis pubis) or at the inferior pubic ramus adjacent to the symphysis and are believed related to overuse of the adductor muscles for pelvic stabilization.
- Treatment for the above pelvic stress fractures requires a period of rest and temporary use of crutches if there is any pain during ambulation. Symptoms usually resolve within several weeks and return to full activity can be safely advised at between 8 and 10 weeks, depending on the severity of injury.

ISCHIUM
- An ischial ramus stress reaction is not considered a true stress fracture, as it is seen in association with proximal hamstring tendinitis or hamstring bursitis, secondary to chronic traction of the muscle origin (Bergman and Fredericson, 1999; Fredericson, Bergman, and Matheson, 1997).

FEMUR

FEMORAL NECK
- Stress fractures of the femoral neck are high risk fractures and should be considered in any athlete, especially a distance runner, who presents with hip, thigh, or groin pain. Pain and symptoms are worse with weightbearing, and there is often reduced range of movement in the hip, particularly internal rotation (Lombardo and Benson, 1982; Keen and Lash, 1992).
- Early detection of femoral neck stress fractures is crucial, as continued stress may lead to a displaced fracture, with associated risk of avascular necrosis and irreversible damages to the joint (Lombardo and Benson, 1982; Keen and Lash, 1992; Volpin et al, 1990).
- Compression fractures are more common in younger athletic patients and are located at the cortex of the lower medial margin of the femoral neck. The early radiographic appearance of these fractures is subtle endosteal lysis or sclerosis along the inferior cortex of the femoral neck, followed by progressive sclerosis and appearance of a fracture line.
- If the radiographic findings are subtle or absent, MRI can be used to detect marrow edema and the presence or absence of a low signal intensity line that indicates a fracture.
- If a stress reaction without a fracture line is detected, treatment is conservative, with a 2- to 3-month period of progressive weight bearing followed by a gradual

return to athletics (Volpin et al, 1990). If a fracture is present, orthopaedic consultation is usually indicated.

FEMORAL DIAPHYSIS

- The femoral diaphysis are relatively common but often misdiagnosed as muscle or tendon injuries. In a study of college athletes, an incidence of 20.6% femoral diaphysis stress fractures was found (Johnson, Weiss, and Wheeler, 1994; Lombardo and Benson, 1982; Hershman, Lombardo, and Bergfeld, 1990).
- MRI shows typically periosteal as well as bone marrow edema involving the medial aspect of the proximal femur at the junction of the proximal and middle thirds of the femoral disphysis (Bergman and Fredericson, 1999; Hershman, Lombardo, and Bergfeld, 1990).
- Physical examination may reveal local tenderness, with normal hip range of motion. Hopping on the affected side will typically reproduce pain in the involved bone. The fulcrum test can be helpful in localizing the anatomic site of involvement (Johnson, Weiss, and Wheeler, 1994).

PATELLA

- Stress fracture of the patella is a rare injury that occurs in jumping sports. It may have an insidious or acute onset (Fredericson, Bergman, and Matheson, 1997).
- The clinical findings are localized tenderness over the patella. Most patellar stress fractures are of the transverse type. These may be confused radiographically with bipartite patella; however, a patella fracture line tends to be more oblique than the bipartite patella.

TIBIA

POSTERIOR-MEDIAL

- The many athletes, particularly runners, with stress fracture of the tibia present with gradual onset of pain along the medial border of tibia aggravated by exercise. Pain may occur with walking, at rest or even at night (Fredericson et al, 1995).
- It is often difficult to clinically distinguish the more severe tibial stress reaction or fracture from the more common medial tibial stress or shin splint syndrome (tibial periostitis). A recent study concluded that the periostitis (seen as periosteal edema on MRI) may be the initial injury on a spectrum that if allowed to progress may evolve into a more serious bone injury (Fredericson et al, 1995; Mubarak et al, 1982).
- The physical examination findings such as localized tibial tenderness and pain with direct or indirect (at a distance from the site of tenderness) percussion over

the involved bone help distinguish that from more common medial tibial stress syndrome (shin splint) (Fredericson et al, 1995).
- The pain is occasionally aggravated by testing muscle strength actively, particularly in those muscles that have origins on the posterior medial border including the soleus (best tested by repetitive toe raises), posterior tibialis, and flexor digitorum longus.
- It is also important to evaluate the runner's lower extremity alignment as well as mechanical gait, such as excessive foot pronation, hindfoot and forefoot varus increasing stress to the tibia during running. Thus, many athletes benefit from a foot orthosis to help control pronation (Bergman and Fredericson, 1999; Fredericson et al, 1995).
- A temporary cessation of running is essential to allow for bony remodeling and repair. This can range from a few days to three weeks for a minor injury to 12 weeks for a severe injury with frank cortical fracture. If there is pain with daily activities a pneumatic tibial brace can be used for immobilizing distal and midtibial injuries (Fredericson et al, 1995).

ANTERIOR-MID-TIBIA

- A typical stress fracture of the anterior cortex of the midtibia occur almost exclusively in athletes performing jumping and leaping activities. These fractures occur on the tension side of bone and are thus prone to delayed union, nonunion, or even complete fracture (Orava and Hulkko, 1984).
- The cortical transverse lesion is known as the dreaded black line for its propensity to nonunion or even progression to a complete fracture that may displace (Orava and Hulkko, 1984).
- These patients require treatment in a nonweightbearing braces for 6 to 8 weeks. Surgical excision and bone grafting or placement of an intramedullary rod is indicated after 3 to 6 months of failed closed management.

TIBIAL PLATEAU

- Stress reaction and fractures occur less frequently in the medial tibial plateau than in the tibial diaphysis. Furthermore, medial tibial plateau stress injuries are often misdiagnosed as per anserinus tendinitis or bursitis (Harolds, 1981).
- If radiographs are positive at presentation, they typically show a linear transverse region of sclerosis 2- to 3-mm wide in the medial plateau close to the level of the epiphyseal scar.
- An MRI examination may demonstrate bone marrow edema of the medial tibial plateau before radiographic sings appear, with periosteal edema present and sometimes presence of a fracture line (Bergman and Fredericson, 1999).

FIBULAR

- Fibular stress fractures are relatively common in runners, with the majority occurring in the distal third of the fibular, just proximal to the tibiofibular ligament attachment (Blair and Manley, 1980).
- These athletes are often found to have a cavus-type foot. The subcutaneous location of the fibula makes it easy to recreate symptoms with direct palpation over the involved bone.
- Radiographs may not be diagnostic, whereas *magnetic resonance* (MR) examination shows focal bone marrow edema and sometimes a well-defined vertical fracture line (Blair and Manley, 1980).
- Fibular stress fractures are noncritical injuries and a return to running program can usually resume after 6 weeks (Bergman and Fredericson, 1999).

Medial Malleolus

- The repetitive stress of running and jumping can create a vertical stress fracture starting at the junction of the medial malleolus and the tibial plafond and continuing proximally and slightly medially.
- Shelbourne et al in 1988 proposed that athletes with radiographic signs of a medial malleolar fracture, especially a displaced fracture, who desire early return to full participation should be treated by open reduction and internal fixation (Shelbourne et al, 1988).
- Stress reactions without frank cortical fracture can be treated with temporary immobilization. Unlimited ambulation in a brace is permitted and a gradual return to running is allowed as symptoms resolve.

Calcaneus

- Calcaneal stress fractures present as heel pain with localized tenderness over the bone, usually in the body of the calcaneus posterior to the talus.
- Pain elicited by squeezing the calcaneus from both sides simultaneously can usually differentiate this condition from retrocalcaneal bursitis, Achilles tendinitis and plantar nerve entrapment (Fredericson, Bergman, and Matheson, 1997).
- Radiographs generally become positive within the first month after pain presentation and show callus formation perpendicular to the trabecular axis of the calcaneus (Bergman and Fredericson, 1999).
- Calcaneal stress fracture is a noncritical stress fracture with rapid healing and return to activity is usually possible by 4 to 6 weeks.

NAVICULAR BONES

- A history of vague, activity-related midfoot pain with associated tenderness over the dorsal border of the navicular near the talonavicular joint (Khan et al, 1994).
- Plain x-ray is rarely helpful in the detection of navicular stress fracture, particularly with an incomplete fracture. Investigation usually requires bone scan or MRI. Computed tomography (CT) is often needed to detect early separation of bone fragments or more clearly define the degree of fracture (Bergman and Fredericson, 1999).
- The most common site of stress fracture within the navicular is the central third, which is an area of relative avascularity. Significant disability can result with delayed diagnosis or inadequate treatment.
- Treatment of an uncomplicated partial stress fracture or nondisplaced complete stress fracture of this bone should include at least 6 weeks of nonweightbearing cast immobilization until the navicular is no longer tender. This is followed by a further 6-week program of rehabilitation (Fredericson, Bergman, and Matheson, 1997).
- Non-union navicular fractures are best treated with screw fixation ± bone grafting.

TALUS, CUBOID, CENEIFORM

- Stress fractures of the talus, cuboid, and cuneiform bones are uncommon. In general, joint involvement, displacement, and nonunion do not occur (Khan, Brukne, and Bradshaw, 1993).
- Treatment can be the same as that for other noncritical stress fracture (Khan, Brukne, and Bradshaw, 1993).
- Stress fractures of the body of the talus, however, can extend into the subtalar joint, which places them into the critical-at-risk category and requires 4 to 6 weeks of cast immobilization and occasionally open reduction and internal fixation (Fredericson, Bergman, and Matheson, 1997; Khan, Brukne, and Bradshaw, 1993).

METATARSALS

- Stress fractures of the metatarsal bones were first described in military recruits as a *march fracture*. The fracture typically occurs in the neck or distal shaft, with the second and third metatarsal most commonly affected (Matheson et al, 1987).
- These are noncritical stress fractures and cross-training can begin as soon as painful ambulation subsides.

- The stress fracture at the base of the second metatarsal is known as the *dancer's fracture*. Pain is noted to be greatest when in the full *en pointe* position. During this maneuver the foot is maximally plantarflexed and weight is borne on the plantar aspect and tip of the first and second distal phalanges (Micheli, Sohn, and Soloman, 1985).
- The dance's fracture should be recognized early and treated with at least 4 weeks of nonweightbearing immobilization (Micheli, Sohn, and Soloman, 1985).
- Stress fractures of the proximal fifth metatarsal diaphysis that occur approximately 1.5 cm distal to the tuberosity are known as the *Jones fracture*. It is important to differentiate this fracture from the acute avulsion fracture of the tuberosity of the 5th metatarsal. The avulsion injury is noncritical and is treated with relative rest then gradual progression. The Jones fracture is notorious for poor healing and requires prolonged weightbearing (6–12 weeks) and often requires screw fixation (Oloff and Schulhofer, 1996).

SESMOIDS

- Sesmoid stress fracture can be particularly disabling and can result in delayed union or nonunion. Passive distal push of the sesmoid, direct tenderness, and sesmoid area pain with stretch of the flexor hallucis suggest the diagnosis.
- Radiographic changes may be difficult to detect sesmoid stress fracture, but occasionally axial views or magnification views can assist in diagnosis. Separation of the sesmoid fragments and irregular edges suggest a stress fracture rather than a bipartite sesmoid. Since a bone scan is nonspecific, CT scan or MRI is often indicated to confirm the diagnosis (Bergman and Fredericson, 1999).
- Rest from the offending activity is clearly advised. Treatment involves casting in a nonweightbearing short leg cast with specific prevention of dorsiflexion for 6 weeks (Oloff and Schulhofer, 1996).

REFERENCES

Bergman AG, Fredericson M: MR imaging of stress reactions, muscle injuries, and other overuse injuries in runners. *MRI Clinics North Am* 7:151–174, 1999.

Blair WF, Manley SR: Stress fracture of the proximal fibula. *Am J Sports Med* 8:212–213, 1980.

Brunkner PD, Bradshaw C, Khan et al: Stress fractures, a review of 180 cases. *Clin J Sport Med* 6(2):85–89, 1996.

Daffner RH, Pavlov H: Stress fracture: Current concepts. *AJR* 159:245–252, 1992.

Fredericson M, Bergman AG, Matheson GO: Stress fractures in athletes. *Orthopaedics* 26(11):961–971, 1997.

Fredericson M, Bergman AG, Hoffman KL, et al: Tibial stress reaction in runners: Correlation of clinical symptoms and scintigraphy with a new magnetic resonance grading system. *Am J Sports Med* 23:472–481, 1995.

Fredericson M, Salamancha L, Beaulieu C: Sacral stress fractures: Tracking down nonspecific pain in distance runners. *Phys Sportsmed* 31(2):31–42, 2003.

Harolds JA: Fatigue fractures of the medial tibial plateau. *Southern Med J* 74:578–581, 1981.

Hershman EB, Lombardo J, Bergfeld TA: Femoral shaft stress fracture in athletes. *Clin Sports Med* 9:111–119, 1990.

Johnson AW, Weiss CB, Wheeler DL: Stress fractures of the femoral shaft in athletes more common than expected: A new clinical test. *Am J Sports Med* 22:248–256, 1994.

Keen JS, Lash EG: Negative bone scan in a femoral neck stress fracture: A case report. *Am J Sports Med* 20:234–236, 1992.

Khan KM, Brukner PD, Bradshaw C: Stress fracture of the medial cuneiform bone in a runner. *Clin Sports Med* 3:262–264, 1993.

Khan KM, Brukner PD, Kearney C, et al: Tarsal navicular stress fracture in athletes. *Sport Med* 17(1):65–76, 1994.

Lombardo, SJ, Benson DW: Stress fractures of the femur in runners. *Am J Sports Med* 10:219–227, 1982.

Macera CA: Lower extremity injuries in runners: advances in prediction. *Sports Med* 13(1):50–57, 1992.

Marx RG, Saint-Phard D, Callahan LR, et al: Stress fracture sites related to underlying bone health in athletic females. *Clin J Sport Med* 11(2):73–76, Apr. 2001.

Matheson GO, Clement DB, Mckenzie DC et al: Stress fracture in athletes: A study of 320 cases. *Am J Sports Med* 15:46–58, 1987.

Micheli LJ, Sohn RS, Soloman R: Stress fractures of the second metatarsal involving Lisfranc's joint in ballet dancer: A new overuse injury of the foot. *J Bone Joint Surg* 67A:1372–1375, 1985.

Mubarak SJ, Guld RN, Lee YF, et al: The medial tibial stress syndrome. A cause of shin splints. *Am J Sports Med* 10:201–205, 1982.

Mulligan EM: The gray cortex: An early sign of stress fracture. *Skeletal Radiol* 24:201–203, 1995.

Oloff LM, Schulhofer SD: Sesmoid complex disorders. *Clin Podiatr Med Surg* 13(3):497–513, 1996.

Orava S, Hulkko A: Stress fracture of the mid-tibial shaft. *Acta Orthop Scand* 55:35–37, 1984.

Shelbourne K, Fisher D, Rettig A, et al: Stress fractures of the medial malleolus. *Am J Sports Med* 16(1):60–63, 1988.

Volpin G, Hoerer D, Groisman G, et al: Stress fractures of the femoral neck following strenuous activity. *J Orthop Trauma* 4:394–398, 1990.

67 NERVE ENTRAPMENTS OF THE LOWER EXTREMITY

Robert P Wilder, MD, FACSM
Jay Smith, MD
Diane Dahm, MD

INTRODUCTION

- Neurological conditions currently account for 10 to 15% of all exercise-inducted leg pain among runners (Smith and Dahm, 2001; McCluskey and Webb, 1999; Massey and Pleet, 1978).
- Among runners, most nerve entrapments occur at or below the knee. In order of decreasing frequency, common nerves affected include the interdigital nerve (interdigital or Morton's neuroma), the *first branch of the lateral plantar nerve* (FB-LPN), *medial plantar nerve* (MPN), *tibial nerve* (TN), *peroneal nerve deep and superficial portions* (DPN and SPN), *sural nerve* (SN), and saphenous nerve (Smith and Dahm, 2001; Schon and Baxter, 1990).
- Nerve entrapment produces neuropathic pain, described as a diffuse, aching, burning discomfort, often accompanied by tingling and cramping. Numbness is less common. Neuropathic pain classically occurs in the nerve distribution distal to the injury site (Smith and Dahm, 2001).
- However, symptoms may affect only a portion of the distal nerve, and may also radiate proximally (called the Valleix phenomenon) (Lau and Daniels, 1999). Symptoms usually occur during and shortly after running, although some syndromes include components of rest and nighttime pain (e.g., tarsal tunnel syndrome).
- Examination findings include tenderness over the affected site and a positive percussion sign (Schon, 1994; Baxter, 1993). The percussion sign, or Tinel's sign, involves percussion along the length of the nerve. Neuropathic pain reproduction with palpation or percussion suggests the possible level of the lesion (Downey and Barrett, 1999; Henderson, 1948).
- Motor or sensory deficits may be subtle requiring focused examination.
- *Double crush* injuries, in which a proximal nerve injury renders the distal portion of the nerve more susceptible to insult, have been reported in the lower limb (Upton and McComas, 1973; Sammarco, Chalk, and Feibel, 1993).
- The majority of entrapment neuropathies are diagnosed clinically, with supportive imaging and

electrodiagnostic (EDX) testing. EDX testing is only occasionally positive, but is useful to exclude alternative neurological conditions (Park and Del Toro, 1998).

COMMON NERVE ENTRAPMENT SYNDROMES

INTERDIGITAL NEUROMA (MORTON'S NEUROMA)

DEFINITION
- Interdigital neuromas commonly affect the third web space, but may rarely affect the second or fourth web spaces.

ANATOMY, PATHOPHYSIOLOGY, AND RISK FACTORS
- At the level of the matatarsal heads, the interdigital nerve passes under (superficial) to the intermetatarsal ligament. During push off, forceful toe dorsiflexion may compress and stretch the nerve beneath the inter-metatarsal ligament (Baxter, 1993). A tumorous mass may develop just distal to the intermetatarsal ligament.
- Risk factors include prolonged walking or running (especially during push-off), squatting, use of high-heeled shoes, or the demi-pointe in ballet (Smith and Dahm, 2001).
- Hyperpronation dorsiflexes the third metatarsal relative to the fourth, exposing the nerve to injury (Schon and Baxter, 1990). Hallux valgus or a hypermobile first ray may lead to callus formation, increasing intermetatarsal pressures. *Metatarsophalangeal joint* (MTJ) synovitis may cause local edema and interdigital nerve compression (Schon, 1994). Soft soled shoes or a heel lift may cause symptoms due to increased toe dorsiflexion.

SYMPTOMS AND SIGNS
- Neuropathic pain between the third and fourth toes, increased with running, walking, toe dorsiflexion, and squatting. Burning/cramping is common, as is night pain.
- Tenderness in the intermetatarsal space. Provocative testing includes squeezing the metatarsals together during palpation (metatarsal squeeze test) with distal radiating neuropathic pain. A click (Mulder's click) may result as the *neuroma* subluxes from between the metatarsals (Schon and Baxter, 1990). A web space sensory deficit is occasionally seen, but no motor deficit is expected to occur along the purely sensory nerve.

DIFFERENTIAL DIAGNOSIS AND EVALUATION

- Differential diagnosis includes proximal and systemic neurological conditions; stress fractures; MTP synovitis, instability or arthritis; and flexor-extensor tenosynovitis (Smith and Dahm, 2001).

TREATMENT

- Activity modification, *nonsteroidal anti-inflammatory drugs* (NSAIDs), physical therapy, biomechanical intervention to reduce toe dorsiflexion, control hyperpronation, and maintain greater metatarsal separation (i.e., a well-padded supportive sole, wide shoe, metatarsal bar or pad, Achilles tendon flexibility, and corticosteroid injections) (McCluskey and Webb, 1999). Surgery is indicated upon failure of conservative care.

TIBIAL NERVE: TARSAL TUNNEL SYNDROME

DEFINITION

- A constellation of processes affecting the TN or it branches at the level of the ankle, producing neuropathic pain along the posteromedial ankle, medial foot, or plantar foot (Smith and Dahm, 2001; Lau and Daniels, 1999).

ANATOMY, PATHOPHYSIOLOGY, AND RISK FACTORS

- The TN originates from the L4-S3 spinal segments and is the larger terminal branch of the sciatic nerve (McCluskey and Webb, 1999). The TN supplies muscular innervation in the posterior thigh and leg, and a cutaneous contribution to the SN, prior to becoming superficial medial to the Achilles tendon and entering the tarsal tunnel posterior to the medial malleolus.
- The tarsal tunnel is a fibro-osseous space formed by the flexor retinaculum, medial calcaneus, posterior talus, distal tibia, and medial malleolus; and extends from the distal tibia to the navicular bone.
- Over 90% of the time, the TN will divide into the MPN and LPN within the tarsal tunnel, typically at the medial malleolar-calcaneal line (Lau and Daniels, 1999). Within 1 to 2 cm below/distal to the medial malleolar-calcaneal line, the MPN and LPN enter separate fibro-osseous canals at the origin of the *abductor hallucis muscle* (AHM) (Schon and Baxter, 1990; Park and Del, 1998).
- *Tarsal tunnel syndrome* TTS can involve the TN, MPN, LPN, and at times the *medial calcaneal nerve* (MCN).
- Risk factors include repetitive trauma and hyperpronation. Compression from stiff orthoses or space-occupying lesions such as an os trigonum, tenosynovitis, tumor, or ganglion is less common.

SYMPTOMS AND SIGNS

- Cramping, burning, and tingling at the medial ankle, medial and/or plantar foot. Diffuse foot pain has been reported. The medial heel is usually spared due to the proximal origin of the MCN. Symptoms increase with activity.
- Examination includes inspection for malalignment, deformity, and muscular atrophy causing or resulting from TTS, such as forefoot pronation, claw toe, talipes calcaneus, or calcaneovalgus. Nerve palpation and percussion testing is completed over the TN and all its terminal branches (Dumitru, 1995). Provocation maneuvers include sustained passive eversion or great toe dorsiflexion to stretch affected nerves, and postexercise examination.
- In severe cases, weakness of toe plantarflexion manifests by reduced push-off on the affected side (McCluskey and Webb, 1999).

DIFFERENTIAL DIAGNOSIS AND EVALUATION

- Differential diagnosis includes polyneuropathy; proximal neuropathy (including *double crush* injuries from radiculopathy or sciatic neuropathy); deep posterior compartment syndrome; popliteal artery entrapment; vascular claudication; venous disease; tenosynovitis or ganglia; plantar fasciitis; tibiotalar or subtalar synovitis, instability or arthritis (Sammarco, Chalk, and Feibel, 1993; Turnipseed and Pozniak, 1992). Examination will help differentiate proximal TN injuries. Tibial nerve injury just distal to the SN contribution will spare lateral calcaneal and foot sensation and gastrocnemius-soleus function. Injury distal to the midportion of the leg will affect plantar sensation and result in claw toe deformity due to imbalance between the affected foot intrinsic and unaffected *flexor digitorum longus* (FDL) and *extensor digitorum brevis* (EDB) muscles (McCluskey and Webb, 1999).
- TTS is primarily a clinical diagnosis. In acute TTS or in failed nonoperative management, MRI is recommended to determine the presence of synovitis or a space-occupying lesion (Frey and Kerr, 1993). EDX studies assist in excluding alternative neurological disorders. They may be positive in up to 90% of patients with well-established TTS, but do not correlate with surgical findings or clinical outcome (Galardi et al, 1994).

TREATMENT

- Activity modification, NSAIDs, neuromodulatory medications (tricyclic and antiseizure medications), physical therapy, and biomechanical interventions. Physical therapy includes (*1*) strengthening the foot intrinsic and medial arch supporting muscles,

(2) Achilles stretching in subtalar neutral, (3) lower limb kinetic chain rehabilitation, and (4) proprioceptive enriched rehabilitation in cases of ankle or subtalar instability (Lau and Daniels, 1999).

- Biomechanical management includes pronation control. If symptoms are reproduced by dorsiflexion, temporal use of a heel lift (in combination with appropriate stretching) may be useful.
- Treatment should address contributing underlying systemic conditions. A steroid injection at the entrapment site may help, provided that the PT tendon is avoided (Lau and Daniels, 1999).
- Surgery may be indicated when nonoperative treatment fails (Lau and Daniels, 1999).

FIRST BRANCH OF THE LATERAL PLANTAR NERVE

DEFINITION
- Isolated LPN entrapments are relatively rare. More commonly, entrapment specifically affects the FB-LPN, sometimes called Baxter's nerve, the *nerve to the abductor digiti quinti muscle* (NADQ), or the *inferior calcaneal nerve* (ICN). FB-LPN entrapment is reported to be the most common *neurological* cause of heel pain (Smith and Dahm, 2001; Baxter and Pfeffer, 1992).

ANATOMY, PATHOPHYSIOLOGY, AND RISK FACTORS
- After penetrating the *abductor hallucis muscle* (AHM) and its fascia, the FB-LPN courses inferiorly, passing between the deep, taut fascia of the AHM medially and the medial, caudal margin of the medial head of the quadratus plantae muscle laterally (Baxter and Pfeffer, 1992). The nerve then abruptly turns laterally, coursing toward the lateral foot between the flexor digitorum brevis and quadratus plantae muscles. The FB-LPN ramifies into three terminal branches supplying the flexor digitorum brevis, the medial calcaneal periosteum, and abductor digiti quinti. The branch to the calcaneal periosteum often supplies branches to the long plantar ligament as well as an inconsistent branch to the quadratus plantae muscle (Schon and Baxter, 1990). There is no cutaneous innervation.
- The actual site of FB-LPN entrapment most commonly occurs at the site of direction change from an inferior to lateral course deep to the AHM (Baxter and Pfeffer, 1992).
- Risk factors include chronic plantar fasciitis and a calcaneal spur.

SYMPTOMS AND SIGNS
- Medial heel pain; no sensory or reflex deficits.

DIFFERENTIAL DIAGNOSIS
- Differential diagnosis includes the following:
  - Plantar fasciitis and fat pad disorder. Sensory losses on the medial heel suggest a disorder affecting the MCN, L4 radiculopathy, plexopathy, or diffuse neurological disease.
  - MRI and EDX testing are not accurate enough to confirm or refute the clinical diagnosis of FB-LPN entrapment, but may assist in differential diagnosis.

TREATMENT
- Nonoperative measures follow treatment principles used for plantar fasciitis. Physical therapy should focus on muscle rebalancing about the ankle-foot and the entire lower limb kinetic chain. Neuromodulatory medication and local corticosteroid injections may be useful.
- Most authors advocate at least 6 to 12 months of nonoperative care prior to considering surgery.
- Decompression includes the deep fascia of the AHM and a portion of the contiguous medal plantar fascia.

MEDIAL PLANTAR NERVE: JOGGER'S FOOT

DEFINITION
- Local entrapment of the MPN results in a syndrome of neuropathic pain radiating along the medial heel and longitudinal arch (Smith and Dahm, 2001).

ANATOMY, PATHOPHYSIOLOGY, AND RISK FACTORS
- After the MPN and LPN exit the tarsal tunnel, each nerve enters a fibro-osseous canal bounded superiorly by the calcaneonovicular or spring ligament and inferiorly by the attachment of the AHM to the navicular bone. The MPN then enters the sole of the foot, passes superficial to the traversing FDL tendon at the master knot of Henry, and continues distally along the *flexor hallucis longus* (FHL) tendon to divide into terminal medial and lateral branches at the level of the base of the first metatarsal. These branches ramify and terminate as three common plantar digital nerves within the medial three web spaces. The MPN is a mixed sensorimotor nerve providing sensation to the medial sole and plantar aspect of the first, second, third, and medial fourth toes, as well as motor innervation to the abductor hallucis, flexor hallucis brevis, flexor digitorum brevis, and first lumbrical muscles.
- MPN entrapment typically occurs at the AHM fibro-osseous canal or master knot of Henry (Baxter, 1993).
- Risk factors include AHM hypertrophy, a valgus running style, functional hyperpronation (e.g., calcaneovalgus, hallux rigids), and high-arched orthoses

(Baxter, 1993). A history of prior ankle injuries with instability is common.

SYMPTOMS AND SIGNS

- Neuropathic medial heel pain radiating along the medial arch toward the plantar aspect of the first and second toes.
- Tenderness at the superior aspect of the AHM at the navicular tuberosity, with distally radiating pain or tingling. Provocative testing includes forceful passive heel eversion, standing on the balls of the feet, or percussion over the nerve. Sensory loss, weakness, or atrophy is rarely reported. The athlete should be examined for ankle instabilities, malalignments, hallux rigidus, AHM hypertrophy, and a valgus running style.

DIFFERENTIAL DIAGNOSIS AND EVALUATION

- Differential diagnosis parallels that of TTS, with the exception of additional local pathological processes.
- Resisted great toe plantarflexion or passive toe dorsiflexion will induce pain with flexor tendonitis, but not typically with nerve entrapment (McCluskey and Webb, 1999). Hindfoot and midfoot synovitis, arthritis, and stress fractures should be considered.
- Evaluation is similar to that for TTS.

TREATMENT

- Treatment principles are parallel to those for TTS. Rigid orthoses should be modified, replaced, or removed to avoid MPN compression. Functional hyperpronation may be addressed.
- Therapeutic injection should avoid direct nerve contact. Surgical release has been successful in refractory cases and is generally a distal extension of the surgery performed for TTS.

COMMON PERONEAL NERVE (CPN)

DEFINITION

- *Common peroneal nerve* (CPN) entrapment typically occurs at the fibular head, proximal to the bifurcation into the SPN and DPN, and produces dorsiflexion weakness and possibly neuropathic pain extending over the anterolateral leg and foot dorsum (Smith and Dahm, 2001).

ANATOMY, PATHOPHYSIOLOGY, AND RISK FACTORS

- The CPN consists of sensory and motor fibers from the L4-S2 segments and is the smaller terminal branch of the sciatic nerve. The CPN separates from the sciatic nerve just above the knee, where it supplies innervation to the short head of the biceps femoris (the only thigh muscle innervated by the peroneal nerve) and divides into the SPN, DPN, and *lateral sural cutaneaous nerve* (LSCN) at the level of the fibular head. The SPN innervates leg lateral compartment muscles, and then emerges from the lateral compartment by penetrating the crural fascia 10.5 to 12.5 cm proximal to the tip of the lateral malleolus. It supplies sensation to the anterolateral leg, and then divides into its terminal medial and intermediate cutaneous branches about 6 cm above the lateral malleolus. These branches enter the foot dorsum superficial to the inferior extensor retinaculum and supply sensation to the foot dorsum, including the medial aspect of the first toe, and the adjacent sides of the third and fourth, and fourth and fifth toes. The DPN traverses the leg anterior compartment, innervating all the muscles including the peroneus tertius, divides into medial and lateral branches 1 to 2 cm proximal to the ankle, and enters the foot deep to the inferior extensor retinaculum. Its medial branch supplies sensation to the first web space, and its lateral branch innervates the EDB as well as local joints. Up to 20% of individuals may have accessory innervation of the EDB from the SPN (McCluskey and Webb, 1999).
- The CPN is vulnerable to compression at the fibular head. Reported etiologies of SPN injury include external compression (knee crossing, bed rest, casts, orthoses), aneurysms, tumors, (e.g., neurofibroma), tibiofibular joint ganglion, fibular head dislocation, Baker's cyst, generalized ligamentous laxity, genu varum, genu recurvatum, and compartment syndrome (Moller and Kadin, 1987; Di Risio, Lazaro, and Popp, 1994; Nagel et al, 1994). Repetitive combined plantarflexion and inversion while running downhill or on uneven surfaces may also produce stretching of the CPN at the fibular head.

SYMPTOMS AND SIGNS

- The DPN is often more severely affected than the SPN. The athlete may report neuropathic symptoms extending into the dorsal foot and toe web spaces. The most common complaint is dorsiflexion weakness.
- The athlete may complain of foot drop, steppage gait, recurrent ankle sprains, and/or an otherwise funny sound when running.

DIFFERENTIAL DIAGNOSIS AND EVALUATION

- Differential diagnosis includes compartment syndrome, sciatic neuropathy, lumbosacral plexopathy and L5 radiculopathy.
- EDX studies may be extremely helpful for localization, prognostication, and differential diagnosis; however, EDX abnormalities may only occur postexercise (Leach, Purnell, and Saito, 1987).

TREATMENT

- Neuromodulatory medications and *transcutaneous electrical nerve stimulation* (TENS), biomechanical interventions to reduce neural tension, dorsiflexion support, and change in running style to avoid excessive varus/recurvatum knee moments. If recovery is prolonged, MRI evaluation may be indicated (Leach, Purnell, and Saito, 1987).

SUPERFICIAL PERONEAL NERVE

DEFINITION

- SPN entrapment typically occurs as the nerve penetrates the crural fascia above the ankle.

ANATOMY, PATHOPHYSIOLOGY, AND RISK FACTORS

- SPN injury at the site of emergence from the lateral compartment may result from sharp fascial edges, chronic ankle sprains (25% of athletes have a history of trauma), muscular herniation, direct contusive trauma, fibular fracture, edema, varicose veins, wearing tight ski boots or roller blades, biomechanical factors (see CPN entrapment, above), and space-occupying lesions such as nerve sheath tumors, lipomas, and ganglia.
- Up to 10% of affected individuals may have chronic lateral compartment syndrome.
- Tight footwear may externally compress the SPN or either of its two terminal branches.

SYMPTOMS AND SIGNS

- Diffuse ache over the dorsolateral foot and less commonly numbness or tingling over the same areas (Schon and Baxter, 1990).
- Examination may reveal percussion tenderness, a fascial defect (60% of patients), or muscular herniation at the exit site approximately 10–13 cm above the ankle. Provocative testing before and after exercise is the most useful clinical indicator of SPN entrapment and includes (*1*) pressure over the exit site during resisted ankle dorsiflexion-eversion, (*2*) pressure over the same area during passive plantarflexion combined with inversion, and (*3*) percussion over the SPN course while passive plantarflexion and inversion are maintained.
- Sensation and EDB bulk may be diminished but are not common findings (Schon and Baxter, 1990).

DIFFERENTIAL DIAGNOSIS AND EVALUATION

- Differential diagnosis resembles that for CPN entrapment. MRI can detect most mass lesions.

TREATMENT

- Treatment parallels that for CPN entrapment, but may also include corticosteroid injection at the site of emergence from the lateral compartment, ankle instability rehabilitation, myofascial release, and use of lateral wedges to decrease nerve stretch.

DEEP PERONEAL NERVE: ANTERIOR TARSAL TUNNEL SYNDROME

DEFINITION

- DPN entrapment is also called *anterior tarsal tunnel syndrome* (ATTS).
- DPN compression occurs in the vicinity of the extensor retinaculum.

ANATOMY, PATHOPHYSIOLOGY, AND RISK FACTORS

- In the anterior leg compartment, the *extensor hallucis longus* (EHL) muscle courses in a medial, oblique direction. The DPN traverses deep to the EHL to course between the EHL and *extensor digitorum longus* (EDL) at the level of the inferior aspect of the superior extensor retinaculum, approximately 3 to 5 cm above the ankle joint. At the level of the oblique superior band of the inferior extensor retinaculum, about 1 cm above the ankle joint, the DPN forms its terminal lateral and medial branches. The lateral branch innervates the EDB muscle. The medial branch courses distally with the dorsalis pedis artery, passing deep to the oblique inferior medial band of the inferior extensor retinaculum, where it may be entrapped by processes affecting the talonavicular joint (Schon and Baxter, 1990).
- Risk factors include trauma, shoe contact pressure (boot top neuropathy, wearing a key under the tongue of the shoe), osteophytic compression, edema, and synovitis or ganglia (Smith and Dahm, 2001).

SYMPTOMS AND SIGNS

- Deep, aching, dorsal midfoot pain and neuropathic symptoms extending into the first web space.
- Percussion along the course of the DPN starting at the fibular head may localize the entrapment.
- Symptom provocation may occur with either plantarflexion or dorsiflexion.

DIFFERENTIAL DIAGNOSIS AND EVALUATION

- Differential diagnosis parallels that for CPN and SPN entrapments, but also includes anterior compartment syndrome.
- EDX can assist in differential diagnosis and localization (e.g., involvement of the EDB or CPN). Compartment pressures and MRI may be useful.

TREATMENT

- Footwear changes to avoid direct pressure, neuromodulatory and anti-inflammatory medication, TENS, ankle stability rehabilitation, and steroid injections.
- Surgery is performed via a dorsomedial approach, and involves partial sectioning of the extensor retinaculum and osteophyte removal.

MISCELLANEOUS NERVE ENTRAPMENT SYNDROMES

MEDIAL CALCANEAL NERVE

- The MCN usually arises from the TN, but may arise from the LPN or at the MPN–LPN bifurcation (Smith and Dahm, 2001).
- The MCN pierces the flexor retinaculum to provide cutaneous innervation to the posterior, medial, and plantar surfaces of the heel, providing no motor innervation.
- Entrapment usually occurs as the MCN pierces the flexor retinaculum. Excessive pronation may be contributory. Direct compression from external sources such as footwear.
- Neuropathic pain is limited to the medial heel and there is no motor or reflex deficit. Symptoms increase with activity. The most useful clinical sign is percussion tenderness and paresthesias when palpating the MCN as it pierces the retinaculum posterior to the TN. Examination will less commonly reveal proximal readiation, or a lamp cord sign (a hypersensitive, tender thickening of the MCN along its oblique-posterior course) (Cohen, 1974).
- Differential diagnosis resembles that for TTS, but medial heel involvement suggests MCN entrapment.
- EDX studies assist in the differential diagnosis, but are rarely useful in making the diagnosis.
- Treatment includes pronation control, corticosteroid injections, and cut-out pads and footwear alterations to reduce direct pressure on the MCN as necessary. The lamp cord sign is often a poor prognostic factor, and surgery is often recommended to remove the pseudoneuroma, often with excellent outcome.

SURAL NEUROPATHY

- The SN is formed by branches of the TN and CPN in the posterior calf, proximal to the lateral malleolus. Two centimeters proximal to the malleolus, the SN provides a sensory branch to the lateral heel, then courses subcutaneously inferior to the peroneal tendons to the base of the fifth metatarsal, where it ramifies into distal sensory branches.

- Etiologies include recurrent ankle sprains, calcaneal or fifth metatarsal fractures, Achilles tendinopathy, space-occupying lesions such as ganglia, direct contusion, footwear-induced pressure, or iatrogenic (post-biopsy neuroma). Symptoms consist of achy, posterolateral calf pain, with neuropathic pain in the SN distribution.
- Examination should include percussion testing along the nerve and provocative testing by passive dorsiflexion and inversion.
- Treatment emphasizes reduction of pressure from footwear, Achilles stretching, neuropathic pain treatment, and ankle stability rehabilitation. Surgery consists of exploration and decompression.

SAPHENOUS NERVE

- The saphenous nerve is the largest cutaneous branch of the femoral nerve. This purely sensory nerve arises from the femoral nerve in the femoral triangle and courses with the femoral artery to the medial knee, where its infrapatellar branch supplies cutaneous sensation to the medial knee. It then courses inferiorly with the saphenous vein to supply cutaneous sensation to the medial calf to the level of the ankle. At the ankle, a branch passes anterior to the medial malleolus to innervate the medial foot. The saphenous nerve is most vulnerable at the medial knee, where it pierces the fascia and emerges from the distal subsartorial canal (Hunter's adductor canal) (Smith and Dahm, 2001).
- Etiologies include entrapment at the adductor canal, pes anserine bursitis, contusion, and postsurgical (knee) iatrogenic injury. The athlete will typically report neuropathic pain and numbness in the area of the medial knee and/or calf, depending on whether there is isolated infrapatellar branch or complete saphenous nerve involvement. There should be no motor deficits.
- Examination includes percussion testing along the nerve starting at the adductor canal, and a search for underlying etiologies. Differential diagnosis includes all proximal femoral nerve, plexus, and root lesions, as well as musculoskeletal disorders about the knee.
- Diagnosis and treatment principles resemble those for SN entrapment, but focus upon different anatomical areas. Surgical release may be necessary.

OBTURATOR NERVE

- *Obturator nerve* (ON) entrapment has received increased attention as a potential source of groin pain in athletes (McCroy and Bell, 1999).

- ON arises from the L2–L4 spinal segments, and exits the pelvis via a fibro-osseous tunnel (obturator canal), in which it divides into terminal anterior and posterior branches. These branches provide the predominant motor innervation to the thigh adductor group and sensory innervation to the distal half to two thirds of the medial thigh. ON entrapments most commonly occur at the exit of the obturator canal (McCroy and Bell, 1999; Bradshaw et al, 1997). The athlete will typically complain of activity-related groin pain of a deep, burning, achy quality.
- EDX studies may reveal fibrillation potentials in the adductor muscles in some cases, but is not uniformly helpful (Bradshaw et al, 1997; Williams and Trzil, 1991). Local anesthetic and corticosteroid injections may assist in making the diagnosis. Surgical treatment may become necessary.

LATERAL FEMORAL CUTANEOUS NERVE: MERALGIA PARESTHETICA

- *Lateral femoral cutaneous nerve* (LFCN) injury has been reported in runners. The LFCN arises from the L2-L3 spinal segments, and typically exits the pelvis via a small tunnel formed by a split in the lateral ilioinguinal ligament at its insertion into the *anterior superior iliac spine* (ASIS) (McCroy and Bell, 1999). Just distal to the tunnel, the LFCN will split into two terminal branches supplying cutaneous innervation to the anterolateral thigh. There is no motor innervation. LFCN injury usually occurs at the level of the ilioninguinal ligament.
- Specific etiologies include rapid weight change, compression from tight clothing or belts, and systematic disease affecting nerves such as thyroid disease and diabetes.
- Burning, aching discomfort over the anterolateral thigh.
- Sensory deficit occurs in the cutaneous distribution. Differential diagnosis includes focal musculoskeletal pathologies, lesions affecting the lumbosacral plexus L2-L3 nerve roots, and systemic disease such as hypothyroidism and diabetes. Local anesthetic and corticosteroid injections may not only be diagnostic, but therapeutic. Treatment involves removal of inciting factors, treatment of neuropathic pain, observation, and injections. Up to 90% of cases resolve with nonoperative management (Williams and Trzil, 1991). Surgical release is sometimes necessary.

MEDIAL HALLUCAL NERVE ENTRAPMENT

- The medial hallucal nerve is a distal terminal branch of the MPN providing sensation to the medial aspect of the great toe. This nerve may rarely be entrapped as it exits the distal end of the AHM, producing medial first MTJ pain.
- Etiologies include pressure from hallux valgus, prominent tibial sesamoid disorders, MTJ disorders, and polyneuropathy.
- Diagnosis is clinical based on symptoms, percussion tenderness or a percussion sign over the nerve.
- Treatment includes removal of inciting factors, and treatment of neuropathic pain as previously described.

REFERENCES

Baxter D: Functional nerve disorders in the athlete's foot, ankle and leg. *Instr Course Lect* 42:185, 1993.

Baxter D, Pfeffer G: Treatment of chronic heel pain by surgical release of the first branch of the lateral plantar nerve. *Clin Orthop* 279:229–236, 1992.

Bradshaw C, McCrory P, Bell S, et al: Obturator nerve entrapment: A cause of groin pain in athletes. *Am J Sports Med* 25:402, 1997.

Cohen S: Another consideration in the diagnosis of heel pain: Neuroma of the medial calcaneal nerve. *J Foot Ankle Surg* 13:128, 1974.

Di Risio D, Lazaro R, Popp A: Nerve entrapment and calfatrophy caused by a Baker's cyst: Case report. *Neurosurgery* 35:333, 1994.

Downey M, Barrett J: Peripheral nerve surgery of the foot and ankle: A review of current principles. *Clin Podiatr Med Surg* 16:175, 1999.

Dumitru D: *Electrodiagnostic Medicine.* Philadelphia, PA, Hanley & Belfus, 1995.

Frey C, Kerr R: Magnetic resonance imaging and the evaluation of tarsal tunnel syndrome. *Foot Ankle* 14:153, 1993.

Galardi G, Amadio S, Marderna L, et al.: Electrophysiologic studies in tarsal tunnel syndrome: Diagnostic reliability of motor distal latency, mixed nerve and sensory nerve conduction studies. *Am J Phys Med* 73:193, 1994.

Henderson W: Clinical assessment of peripheral nerve injuries: Tinel's test. *Lancet* 2:801, 1948.

Lau K, Daniels T: Tarsal tunnel syndrome: A review of the literature. *Foot Ankle Int* 20:201, 1999.

Leach R, Purnell M, Saito A: Peroneal nerve entrapment in runners. *Am J Sports Med* 17:287, 1987.

Massey E, Pleet A: Neuropathy in joggers. *Am J Sports Med* 6:209, 1978.

McCluskey L, Webb: Compression and entrapment neuropathies of the lower extremity. *Clin Podiatr Med Surg* 16:96, 1999.

McCroy P, Bell S: Nerve entrapment syndromes as a cause of pain in the hip, groin, and buttock. *Sports Med* 27:261, 1999.

Moller B, Kadin S: Entrapment of the common peroneal nerve. *Am J Sports Med* 15:90, 1987.

Nagel A, Greenebaum E, Singson R, et al: Foot drop in a long-distance runner. An unusual presentation of neurofibromatosis. *Orthop Rev* 23:526, 1994.

Park T, Del Toro D: Electrodiagnostic evaluation of the foot. *Phys Med Rehabil Clin North Am* 9:871, 1998.

Sammarco G, Chalk D, Feibel J: Tarsal tunnel syndrome and additional nerve lesions in the same limb. *Foot ankle* 14:71, 1993.

Schon L: Nerve entrapment neuropathy, and nerve dysfunction in the athlete. *Orthop Clin North Am* 25:47, 1994.

Schon L, Baxter D: Neuropathies of the foot and ankle in athletes. *Clin Sports Med* 9:489, 1990.

Smith J, Dahm D: Nerve entrapments, in O'Connor F, Wilder R (eds.): *The Textbook of Running Medicine.* New York, NY, McGraw-Hill, 2001.

Turnipseed W, Pozniak M: Popliteal entrapment as a result of neurovascular compression by the soleus and plantaris muscles. *J Vasc Surg* 15:285, 1992.

Upton A, McComas A: The double crush in nerve entrapment syndromes. *Lancet* 2:359, 1973.

Williams P, Trzil K: Management of meralgia parestherica. *J Neurosurg* 74:76, 1991.

68 PHYSICAL MODALITIES IN SPORTS MEDICINE

Alan P Alfano, MD

INTRODUCTION

- The physical modalities use physical forces to speed healing and return an athlete to as full a level of function as possible.
- These agents should not be used in isolation: they are more effective when used as a part of a comprehensive treatment approach including medical and/or surgical intervention as well as exercise and education.

THERAPEUTIC HEAT

- Energy transfer by physical modalities typically occurs by one of three processes: *conduction, convection,* or *conversion.*
- **Conduction:** Heat energy is transferred by contact from the object of highest energy to the object of lowest energy.
- **Convection:** The process of heat energy transfer between a solid object and a moving gas or liquid.
- **Conversion:** The process of energy transfer that involves converting one form of energy to a different form. Use of high frequency sound waves or electromagnetic waves to heat tissue will be discussed.
- Heating modalities are divided into *superficial* and *deep*.

PHYSIOLOGY OF SUPERFICIAL HEAT
- Predominant mode of heating is conduction; however, some superficial applications utilize convection or conversion.

- Superficial heat effects include vasodilitation, pain relief, reduction of muscle tone and spasiticity, increase cellular metabolic activity, decrease joint stiffness, increase soft tissue extensibility, promote hyperemia. Elevation of tissue temperature does not generally exceed 40°C and is usually short lived.
- Causes superficial vasodilitation preferentially.
- May be associated with consensual vasodilitation of areas distant to the area being heated. For example, the contralateral limb.
- Changes of 13 to 15°C in the finger joint may change joint viscosity by about 20% (Wright, 1961).

GENERAL INDICATIONS

- Pain
- Muscle spasm
- Contracture
- Tension myalgia
- Hematoma resolution
- Bursitis
- Tenosynoitis
- Fibromylagia
- Superficial thrombophlebitis
- Acceleration of metabolic process

GENERAL CONTRAINDICATIONS AND PRECAUTIONS

- Acute inflammation, trauma, or hemorrhage
- Bleeding dyscrasia
- Ischemia
- Insensitivity
- Atrophic skin
- Scar tissue
- Inability to communicate

- Poor thermal regulation (systemic applications)
- Malignancy
- Edema

SUPERFICIAL HEAT APPLICATION METHODS

HOT PACKS (HYDROCOLLATOR)

- Transfer of heat energy by conduction
- **Application:** Silicate gel in a canvas cover
- When not in use these packs are kept in thermostatically controlled water baths at 70 to 80°C.
- Used in terry cloth insulating covers or used with towels placed between the pack and the patient for periods of 20 to 30 min.
- **Advantages:** Low cost, easy use, long life, and patient acceptance
- **Disadvantages:** Difficult to apply to curved surfaces
- **Safety:** One should never lie on top on the pack, as it is more likely to cause burns. Towels should be applied between the skin and hydrocollator pack.

HEAT LAMPS

- Heat primarily by the conversion of radiant energy to heat, i.e., the direct application of photons to living tissue leading to heat production.
- **Application:** Simple to use but require some attention to avoid injuries or burn.
- In practice, therapeutic temperatures are usually obtained when the heat sources are about 50 cm from the skin.
- The intensity of heating of point heat sources, such as incandescent bulbs, drops off in accordance with the inverse squared ($1/r^2$) law, the heating effectiveness of linear sources, such as some quartz lamps, may follow a more slowly decreasing $1/r$ relationship.
- **Safety:** These agents produce erythema (known as *erythema ab igne* and *erythema calor*).
- Chronic use may produce a permanent brownish discoloration.

HYDROTHERAPY

- Heat transfer is primarily by convection
  - Uses a fluid medium (usually H_2O) to apply heat and cold.
  - Immersion of large portion of the body in water at neutral temperatures between 36.5 and 40°C for 20 min.

- Water temperatures are limited to about 39°C if a significant fraction of the body is immersed.
- Hydrotherapy medium may be stationary or in motion.

SPECIFIC MODES
- Whirlpool baths and hubbard tanks
  - Tanks range in size/construction from small portable units to treat a portion of a limb to fixed Hubbard tanks for the entire body.
  - Hydrotherapy is expensive in terms of labor and resources.

ADVANTAGES/SPECIFIC USES
- **Wounds and burns:** Hydrotherapy may lessen pain and speed healing of open wounds (Burke et al, 1998; Juve Meeker, 1998).
- Used for wounds and treatments when gentle mechanical debridement, heat, and solvent actions are desired.
- For larger wounds, a 0.9% NaCl solution, improves comfort and lessens the risks of hemolysis and electrolyte imbalance.
- **Musculoskeletal/pain applications:** Hydrotherapy is often used as an adjunct to joint mobilization after cast removal or prolonged mobilization.
- Sitz baths (small warm water bath) for perineal and anal pain
- Used to treat musculoskeletal pain, spasms, and tension myalgia.
- In clinical institutions where disinfecting procedures are followed and areas of stagnant water are avoided, infection appears to be rare.

DISADVANTAGES
- Should not be used with edematous limbs.
- Treatment systems and infection control are time consuming.

CONTRAST BATHS

APPLICATION
- Contrast baths consist of two baths: a warm bath at 38–44°C and a cool reservoir at about 10–18°C.
- Treatment begins by soaking the involved limb in the warm reservoir for about 10 min and then progressing to about four cycles of 1- to 4-min cold and 4- to 6-min warm soaks (Woodmansey, Collins, and Ernst, 1938).

ADVANTAGES/DISADVANTAGES
- Most commonly used to produce reflex hyperemia and desensitization in patients with complex regional pain syndrome I.
- Athletes may find the cold baths uncomfortable.

SPA THERAPY (BALNEOTHERAPY)

- Little research has addressed these issues for athletes.
- In addition, a comparison of the effects of spa therapy, underwater traction, and water jets on low-back pain found no specific benefits attributable to balneotherapy (Konrad et al, 1992).

FLUIDOTHERAPY

APPLICATION

- **Heats by convection:** Fine particles fluidized by turbulent, high-velocity hot air, frequently used in hand therapy.
- Despite wide-spread use, benefits of this high-temperature, remain poorly established (Alcorn et al, 1984; Borrell et al, 1980).
- May be used for analgesia or desensitization.

PARAFFIN BATHS

APPLICATION

- **Heats primarily by conduction:** Liquid mixture of paraffin wax and mineral oil.
- Helpful in the treatment of scars and hand contractures. Temperatures (52 to 54°C) are higher than those of hydrotherapy (<40 to 45°C) but are well tolerated due to the low heat capacity of the paraffin-mineral oil mixture and a lack of convection.
- **Treatment:** Dipping, immersion, occasionally brushed onto the area of treatment
- **Safety:** Burns are the main safety concern with paraffin treatment.
- **Visual inspection is important:** Paraffin bath should have a thin film of white paraffin on its surface or an edging around the reservoir.

DIATHERMY (DEEP HEATING)

- The following differences set diathermy apart form superficial heating:
  a. Produces higher temperatures
  b. Heats tissue faster and heat dissipates more slowly
  c. Predominantly utilizes sound waves or electromagnetic energy

DEEP HEATING MODALITIES

ULTRASOUND

- *Ultrasound* is defined as sound waves at a frequency above the threshold of human hearing (frequencies higher than 20 kHz).

HEATS BY CONVERSION

- Ultrasound uses sound waves to heat tissues. A wide range of frequencies are potentially useful, but in the United States most machines operate between 0.8 and 1 MHz.
- Use piezoelectric transducers to convert electrical energy into sound.

PHYSIOLOGY

- The most vigorous and deeply penetrating heating agent can elevate intramuscular temperatures of by about 3.5 to 4.0°C (Draper et al, 1998).
- Penetration, is not uniform and depends markedly on tissue properties: Ultrasound beam will selectively heat tissue with high water content.
- The ability of ultrasound to heat tissue by the conversion of sound energy into heat is its best-understood capability.
- Nonthermal processes such as *cavitation, shock waves, streaming,* and *mechanical deformation* have been identified.
- Cavitation occurs when small gaseous bubbles are formed in the presence of a high-intensity ultrasound beam and either oscillate stably or grow rapidly in size and collapse (Flint and Suslick, 1991).
- No irreversible harmful effects of cavitation have been demonstrated in animal tissue (Frizzell and Dunn, 1990).
- Streaming is described as movements in water-rich tissues and standing waves. Streaming may damage tissue or possibly speed healing.
- Typical intensity for application is 0.8–1.5 W/cm^2
- Low-intensity ultrasound (15 to 400 mW/cm^2) may also stimulate cell proliferation, protein synthesis, and cytokine production. Although these findings are limited to the laboratory, they furnish some support for the clinical interest in low-intensity ultrasound in wound healing.

ULTRASOUND INDICATIONS

- Tendonitis and bursitis
- Muscle pain and overuse
- Contractures
- Inflammation and trauma
- Scars and keloids
- The evidence is mixed. In most cases, ultrasound comparisons have been done against placebo controls, therefore the relative effectiveness of this agent over that of other conventional approaches is unknown.
- **Fractures:** Low-intensity ultrasound (e.g., 30 mW/cm^2) accelerates bone healing and is approved by the Food and Drug Administration (FDA) for the treatment of some fractures (Hadjiargyrou et al, 1998).

ULTRASOUND PRECAUTIONS

- Ultrasound is typically avoided in the acute stages of an injury due to concerns that it may aggravate bleeding, tissue damage, and swelling.
- The subacute situation may be different, as many feel that ultrasound may speed healing and the resolution of symptoms in the later stages of injury.

PHONOPHORESIS

- Ultrasound may be used to deliver medication into tissues. The active substance is mixed into a coupling medium, and ultrasound is used to drive (phonophores) the material through the skin.
- Phonophoresis with corticosteroids is frequently used in sports medicine.
- Clinical studies are conflicting.
- A comparison of phonophoresis of 0.05% fluocinonide with ultrasound alone. At 1.5 W/cm² both treatments were found beneficial, but indistinguishable in their effects on superficial musculoskeletal conditions (Klaiman et al, 1998).
- Another study did not find lidocaine and corticosteroid phonophoresis more effective than the same treatment with an inert coupling agent (Moll, 1977).

CONTRAINDICATIONS

- Fluid-filled areas (i.e., eye and the pregnant uterus)
- Growth plates, immature or inflamed joints (Dussick et al, 1958; Weinberger et al, 1988; 1989)
- Acute hemorrhages, ischemic tissue, tumors, laminectomy sites, infections, and implanted devices such as pacemakers and pumps
- **Caution:** Relatively contraindicated near metal plates or cemented artificial joints, as the effects of localized heating (Brunner et al, 1958; Gersten, 1958; Skoubo-Kristensen and Sommer, 1982) or mechanical forces on prosthetic-cement interfaces is not well known.

SHORTWAVE DIATHERMY

HEATS BY CONVERSION

- *Shortwave diathermy* (SWD) uses *electromagnetic* (EM) energy to interact with tissue and produce heat.
- Both thermal and nonthermal effects are possible.
- Tissue warming is produced by two processes:
  1. Resistive heating
  2. Degradation of molecular oscillatory motions that EM waves induce when they interact with tissue.
- SWD is the dominant EM diathermy in sports medicine, albeit relatively rarely used in comparison the other heating modalities.
- Most devices operate at 27.12 MHz. The U.S. Federal Communications Commission also approves frequencies of 13.56 and 40.68 MHz for use.

MECHANISM

- An SWD machine is a signal generator that uses either inductive or capacitive electrodes to deliver energy to the body.
- Inductive electrodes act as an antenna, and the body absorbs energy from an EM field produced by the short-wave machine.
- With capacitive electrodes, the portion of the body being treated is placed in series between the electrodes and serves as the dielectric (resistance) between two plates of a capacitor.
- Inductive applicators induce currents that preferentially flow in water-rich tissues such as muscles that are highly conductive.
- Capacitive applicators, on the other hand, heat poorly conductive substances, such as fat preferentially (Kantor, 1981).
- SWD can increase subcutaneous fat temperatures by 15°C and intramuscular temperatures at depths of 4 to 5 cm by 4 to 6°C (Lehmann, DeLateur, and Stonebridge, 1969; Draper et al, 1999).

TECHNIQUE

- Two common inductive applicators are typically utilized (pads or drums).
- Pad applicators are moderately flexible mats that contain a coil.
- Drum applicators are characterized by fixed coils and hinges.

INDICATIONS

- Heating in tissues that are either too deep or too extensive to be treated by other modalities, e.g., the low back, the knee.

PRECAUTIONS AND CONTRAINDICATIONS/SAFETY

- Jewelry is removed.
- Treatment is performed on nonconductive tables.
- Contraindications include metal implants or electrical devices (e.g., joints, pacemakers, pumps, and metallic intrauterine devices), contact lenses, and the menstruating or pregnant uterus.
- Treating the immature skeleton is generally not recommended and has not been well studied.

LOW-POWER AND PULSED ELECTROMAGNETIC FIELD

HEATS BY CONVERSION

- Nonthermal effects can be obtained and tissue heating avoided altogether by using low-power fields delivered in either continuous or pulsed modes.
- Research offers little to support the specificity or certainty of benefits.

THERAPEUTIC COLD

- The cooling agents are often used for their analgesic, metabolic, and perfusion-limiting effects.
- Cooling therapies are restricted to conductive and convective means.

GENERAL INDICATIONS

- Acute musculoskeletal trauma
- Pain
- Muscle spasm
- Spasticity
- Reduction of metabolic activity

GENERAL CONTRAINDICATION AND PRECAUTIONS

- Ischemia
- Insensitivity
- Cold intolerance
- Raynaud's phenomenon and disease
- Severe cold pressor responses
- Cold allergy

PHYSIOLOGY OF CRYOTHERAPY

- Superficial cold produces analgesia (Hartviksen, 1962), reduces metabolic activity, slows and may block nerve conduction (Denys, 1991), decreases muscle tone and spasticity (Knight, 1985; Knutsson and Mattsson, 1969; Miglietta, 1973), and increases gastrointestinal motility (Bisgard and Nye, 1940).
- Ice is the most common cryotherapy agent.
- Skin temperatures initially fall rapidly following the application of ice and then decreased more slowly toward an equilibrium value of 12 to 13°C.
- Long periods have a more pronounced effect. Ice cooling for 20 to 180 min can lower relatively superficial intramuscular temperatures by 6 to 16°C (Denys, 1991; Dussick et al, 1958; Knight, 1985; Lehmann and de Lateur, 1982).
  a. In one study, knee intra-articular temperatures decreased by 6°C after being packed in ice for 3 h. Likewise, blood flow decreased by 20 and 30% in bone and soft tissue, respectively, after 25 min (Oosterveld and Rasker, 1994).
  b. Reduces conduction velocity.
  c. Inhibits the release of histamine.
  d. Slows chemical reactions.
  e. Relative hyperemia after cold application stimulates tissue repair and healing.
- **Technique:** Ice packs, compression wraps are most common.
- Sessions typically last 20 to 30 min.
- Ice massage is a vigorous approach suitable for limited portions of the body. A piece of ice is rubbed over the painful area for 7 to 10 min.
- Iced whirlpools cool large areas vigorously.
- Vapocoolant and liquid nitrogen sprays produce large (as much as 20°C), rapid drops in skin temperature and are used at times to produces superficial analgesia as well as in *spray and stretch* treatments (Oosterveld and Rasker, 1994; Travell, 1952).
- Chemical ice packs are also common.

TRAUMA INDICATIONS
- Cooling applied soon after trauma may decrease edema, lessen metabolic activity, reduce blood flow, lower compartmental pressures, diminish tissue damage, and accelerate healing (Ho et al, 1995; Basur, Shephard, and Mouzas, 1976; Moore and Cardea, 1977; Schaubel, 1946; Bert et al, 1991; Hirase, 1993).
- *Rest, ice, compression, and elevation* (RICE) are the mainstay of treatment
- Cyclic ice application is often recommended (e.g., 20 min on, 10 min off; or 30 min on, 2 h off) for 6 to 24 h (Hartviksen, 1962; Knight, 1985; Sloan, Hain, and Pownall, 1989; Hocutt et al, 1982).
- Opinions regarding usefulness of cryotherapy for injuries more that 24 to 48 h old are divergent.

PRECAUTIONS AND CONTRAINDICATIONS
- When sensation is compromised, circulation is impaired, or tissues are compressed (Barlas, Homan, and Thode, Jr, 1996).
- Rare but possible problems include pressor responses aggravating cardiovascular disease, Raynaud's phenomenon, cold hypersensitivity, urticaria, and cold allergy/cryoprecipitation.

ELECTROTHERAPY

GENERAL INDICATIONS
- Today, high-intensity electrical stimulation is used to strengthen muscles and to move paralyzed limbs.
- Less-intense stimulation produces analgesia and delivers medications percutaneously.
- Stimulation at still lower intensities has gained FDA approval for fracture healing.
- Soft-tissue wounds, osteoporosis, and musculoskeletal pain represent additional potentially important, but still investigational, applications.

SPECIFIC APPLICATIONS

TRANSCUTANEOUS ELECTRICAL NERVE STIMULATORS

- It is clear that *transcutaneous electrical nerve stimulators* (TENS) stimulation produces localized analgesia, and research suggests that stimulation at 110 Hz (as well as HWT at 2 and 60 Hz) results in a hypoalgesia that persists for up to 5 minutes after stimulation is stopped (McDowell et al, 1999)
- Dorsal horn cell activity is reduced following stimulation (Garrison and Foreman, 1996).
- High frequency, low intensity TENS (barely or not perceptible, 10 to 100+ Hz) may work more according to the gate theory than higher intensity low frequency (1 to 4 Hz) stimulation, which may be more dependent on endorphins.
- Electrodes are usually placed over the painful region, but other locations are common.
- TENS units are expensive (often as much as $800) and annoying to put on. Benefits may appear to wane with time; purchase is not warranted unless its improvements persist for several months.

TENS INDICATIONS
- Pain reduction

PRECAUTIONS AND CONTRAINDICATIONS
- Skin irritation and contact dermatitis?
- Cardiac pacemakers may be relatively resistant to TENS signals, but there is at least one report that an intracardiac defibrillator was triggered by a TENS unit (Curwin, Coyne, and Winters, 1999).
- The pregnant uterus should not be treated.

FUNCTIONAL ELECTRIC STIMULATION

MUSCLE STIMULATION
- In summary, electrical muscle stimulation is more effective in maintaining muscle mass after an injury than it is in reversing atrophy once it is established (Baldi et al, 1998).

IONTOPHORESIS
- Iontophoresis uses electrical fields to force charged or polarized substances into tissue (Chantraine, Ludy, and Berger, 1986; O'Malley and Oester, 1955; Hill, Baker, and Jansen, 1981).
- Iontophoretic devices consist basically of a direct-current (possibly pulsed) power source and two electrodes. A dilute solution of the active substance (which must exist in an ionized or polar form) is placed under the electrode of the same polarity, and the device is turned on.

- Medication is not always required as the electric current alone may have therapeutic benefits.
- Despite generalization to materials other than analgesics and rather widespread use, including use in tendonitis, bursitis, and sprains, research support is limited.
- Nonsteroidal anti-inflammatory iontophoresis of lateral epicondylitis may be helpful (Demirtas and Oner, 1998).
- Direct comparison of iontophoresis with oral medication, transdermal patches, or alternative physical therapy approaches is rare.
- **Safety:** Allergies to the materials (pads, electrodes, and medication) used are always possible, and the passage of electrical current into the skin can cause erythema, rashes, and, if the current intensity is high, pain (Berliner, 1997).
- **Wound healing:** Low-frequency microcurrent (e.g., 10 to 200 Hz, <10 mA/cm^2) electric currents and fields designed to accelerate wound healing by neutralizing injury currents or reducing free radical concentrations have gained some notice (Barron, Jacobson, and Tidd, 1985).

INTERFERENTIAL AND KILOHERTZ FREQUENCY CURRENTS
- Skin impedance falls as frequency increases. As a result, stimuli that are painful at the low <70-Hz frequencies of TENS and many muscle simulators are well tolerated at a few thousand hertz.
- There are at least two ways to take advantage of this fact. One of these arranges two sets of electrodes so that two sine waves in the low-kilohertz range differing by 20 to 100 Hz cross. The waves thus interfere with each other and produce beneath the skin barrier a *difference* frequency comparable to that of TENS units and muscle stimulators.
- **Safety:** no conclusive and consistent evidence that EM field exposure causes a significant increase in the risk of cancer, neurobehavioral, or reproductive dysfunction (Kaiser, 1996; 1998).

COMPLEMENTARY AND ALTERNATIVE THERAPIES

- Athletes as well as the general population are intrigued by the potential use of complementary and alternative medicine.

LOW-INTENSITY LASER THERAPY
- Low-power lasers are widely used to treat musculoskeletal injuries, speed healing, and lessen pain.
- Unfortunately, demonstration of clinical benefits has been difficult, and these devices have yet to gain FDA approval for clinical use (Basford, 1995).

Static Magnetic Fields (Magnetic Devices)

• Magnetic discs, pads, bandages, and blankets are promoted in sports, veterinary, and general circulation magazines as a cure for a variety of musculoskeletal injuries.

• Various magnetic products have been studied with field strengths generally in the 300–3,950 Gauss(Gs) range (Vallbona, Hazelwood, and Jurida, 1997; Alfano et al, 2001).

• Results are generally mixed. In one study efficacy has been demonstrated in patients with painful diabetic neuropathy (Weintraub et al, 2003); another study comparing magnet pad versus control groups suffering from fibromyalgia showed statistical significance for pain relief, but no clear functional improvement in the magnet user group (Alfano et al, 2001).

• Observed physiologic effects have included increased nerve excitability (Hong, 1987) and circulatory stimulation (Ohkubo and Xu, 1997).

Acupuncture

• Treatment consists of utilizing acupuncture needles to pierce the skin to differing depths at designated acupuncture points to bring about pain relief or physiologic change.

• Needles are commonly stimulated by hand, electricity, or heat.

• Research is not available regarding treatment of athletic injuries; however, in 1997 the NIH sponsored a consensus panel, which concluded: "promising results have emerged, for example, showing efficacy of acupuncture in adult post-operative and chemotherapy associated nausea and vomiting and in post-operative dental pain. There are other situations such as addiction, stroke rehabilitation, headache, menstrual cramps, tennis elbow, fibromyalgia, myofascial pain, osteoarthritis, low back pain, carpal tunnel syndrome, and asthma, in which acupuncture may be useful..." (NIH, 1997).

REFERENCES

Alcorn R, Bowser B, Henley EJ, et al: Fluidotherapy and exercise in the management of sickle cell anemia. A clinical report. *Phys Ther* 64:1520, 1984.

Alfano AP, Taylor AG, Dunkl PR, et al: Static magnetic fields for the treatment of fibromyalgia: A randomized controlled trial. *J Altern Complement Med* 7(1):53–64, 2001.

Baldi JC, Jackson RD, Moraille R, et al: Muscle atrophy is prevented in patients with acute spinal cord injury using functional electrical stimulation. *Spinal Cord* 36:463, 1998.

Barlas D, Homan CS, Thode JC, Jr: In vivo tissue temperature comparison of cryotherapy with and without external compression. *Ann Emerg Med* 28:436, 1996.

Barron JJ, Jacobson WE, Tidd G: Treatment of decubitus ulcers. A new approach. *Minn Med* 68:103, 1985.

Basford JR: Low intensity laser therapy: Still not an established clinical tool. *Lasers Surg Med* 16;331, 1995.

Basur RL, Shephard E, Mouzas GL: A cooling method in the treatment of ankle sprains. *Practitioner* 216:708, 1976.

Berliner MN: Reduced skin hyperemia during tap water iontophoresis after intake of acetylsalicylic acid. *Am J Phys Med Rehabil* 76:482, 1997.

Bert JM, Stark JG, Maschka K, et al: The effect of cold therapy on morbidity subsequent to arthroscopic lateral retinacular release. *Orthop Rev* 20:755, 1991.

Bisgard JD, Nye D: The influence of hot and cold application upon gastric and intestinal motor activity. *Surg Gynecol Obstet* 71:172, 1940.

Borrell RM, Parker R, Henley EJ, et al: Comparison of in vivo temperatures produced by hydrotherapy, paraffin wax treatment, and fluidotherapy. *Phys Ther* 60:1273, 1980.

Brunner GD, Lehmann JF, McMillan JA, et al: Can ultrasound be used in the presence of surgical metal implants: An experimental approach. *Phys Ther* 38:823, 1958.

Burke DT, Ho CC, Saucier MA, et al: Effects of hydrotherapy on pressure ulcer healing. *Am J Phys Med Rehabil* 77:394, 1998.

Chantraine A, Ludy JP, Berger D: Is cortisone iontophoresis possible? *Arch Phys Med Rehabil* 67:38, 1986.

Curwin JH, Coyne RF, Winters SL: Inappropriate defibrillator (ICD) shocks caused by transcutaneous electronic nerve stimulation (TENS) units [letter, comment]. *Pacing Clin Electrophysiol* 22:692, 1999.

Demirtas RN, Oner C: The treatment of lateral epicondylitis by iontophoresis of sodium salicylate and sodium diclofenac. *Clin Rehabil* 12;23, 1998.

Denys EH: AAEM Minimonograph 14: The influence of temperature in clinical neurophysiology. *Muscle Nerve* 14:795, 1991.

Draper DO, Harris ST, Schulthies S, et al: Hot-pack and 1-MHz ultrasound treatments have an additive effect on muscle temperature increase. *J Athl Train* 33:2, 1998.

Draper DO, Knight K, Fujiwara T, et al: Temperature change in human muscle during and after pulsed shortwave diathermy. *J Orthop Sports Phys Ther* 29:13, 1999.

Dussick DT, Fritch DJ, Kyraizidan M, et al: Measurement of articular tissues with ultrasound. *Am J Phys Med* 37:160, 1958.

Flint EB, Suslick KS: The temperature of cavitation. *Science* 253:1397, 1991.

Frizzell LA, Dunn F: Biophysics of ultrasound, in Lehman J (ed.): *Therapeutic Heat and Cold,* 4th ed. Baltimore, MD, Williams and Wilkins, 1990, pp 404–405.

Garrison DW, Foreman RD: Effects of transcutaneous electrical nerve stimulation (TENS) on spontaneous and noxiously evoked dorsal horn cell activity in cats with transected spinal cords. *Neurosci Lett* 216:125, 1996.

Gersten JW: Effects of metallic objects on temperature rises produced in tissue by ultrasound. *Am J Phys Med* 37:75, 1958.

Hadjiargyrou M, McLeod K, Ryaby JP, et al: Enhancement of fracture healing by low intensity ultrasound. *Clin Orthop* S216:29, 1998.

Hartviksen K: Ice therapy in spasticity. *Acta Neurol Scand* 38;79, 1962.

Hill AC, Baker GF, Jansen GT: mechanism of action of iontophoresis in the treatment of palmar hyperhidrosis. *Cutis* 28:69, 1981.

Hirase Y: Postoperative cooling enhances composite graft survival in nasal-alar and fingertip reconstruction. *Br J Plast Surg* 46:707, 1993.

Ho SS, Illgen RL, Meyer RW, et al: Comparison of various icing times in decreasing bone metabolism and blood flow in the know. *Am J Sports Med* 23:74, 1995.

Hocutt JE, Jr, Jaffe R, Rylander CR, et al: Cryotherapy in ankle sprains. *Am J Sports Med* 10;316, 1982.

Hong CZ: Static magnetic field influence on human nerve function. *Arch Phys Med Rehabil* 68(3):162–164, Mar. 1987.

Juve Meeker B: Whirlpool therapy on postoperative pain and surgical wound healing: An exploration. *Patient Educ Couns* 33:39, 1998.

Kaiser J: Panel finds EMFs pose no threat [news] [see comments] [published erratum appears in *Science* 275:741, 1997]. *Science* 274:910, 1996.

Kaiser J: NIH panel revives EMF-cancer link [news]. *Science* 281:21, 1998.

Kantor G: Evaluation and survey of microwave and radiofrequency applicators. *J Microw Power* 16:135, 1981.

Klaiman MD, Shrader JA, Danoff JV, et al: Phonophoresis verses ultrasound in the treatment of common musculoskeletal conditions. *Med Sci Sports Exerc* 30:1349, 1998.

Knight K: *Cryotherapy: Theory, Technique and Physiology*, 1st ed. Chattanooga, TN, Chattanooga, 1985, p 83.

Knight KL: *Cryotherapy: Theory, Technique and Physiology*, 1st ed. Chattanooga, TN Chattanooga, 1985, p 15.

Knutsson E, Mattsson E: Effects of local cooling on monosynaptic reflexes in man. *Scand J Rehabil Med* 1:126, 1969.

Konrad K, Tatrai T, Hunka A, et al: Controlled trial of balneotherapy in treatment of low back pain. *Ann Rheum Dis* 51:820, 1992.

Lehmann JF, de Lateur BJ: Diathermy and superficial heat and cold therapy, in Kottke FJ, Stilllwell GK, Lehmann JF (eds.): *Krusen's Handbook of Physical Medicine and Rehabilitation*, 3rd ed. Philadelphia, PA, Saunders, 1982, p 275.

Lehmann JF, DeLateur BJ, Stonebridge JB: Selective muscle heating by shortwave diathermy with a helical coil. *Arch Phys Med Rehabil* 50:117, 1969.

McDowell BC, McCormack K, Walsh DM, et al: Comparative analgesic effects of H-wave therapy and transcutaneous electrical nerve stimulation on pain threshold in humans. *Arch Phys Med Rehabil* 80:1001, 1999.

Miglietta O: Action of cold on spasticity. *Am J Phys Med* 52:198, 1973.

Moll MJ: A new approach to pain: Lidocaine and decadron with ultrasound. *USAF Med Service Dig* 30:8, 1977.

Moore CD, Cardea JA: Vascular changes in leg trauma. *South Med J* 70:1285, 1977.

NIH: *Consensus statement on acupuncture.* 15(5):2, Nov. 1997.

O'Malley EP, Oester YT: Influence of some physical chemical factors on iontophoresis using radioisotopes. *Arch Phys Med Rehabil* 36:310, 1955.

Ohkubo C, Xu S: Acute effects of static magnetic fields on cutaneous circulation in rabbits. *In Vivo* 11:221–225, 1997.

Oosterveld FG, Rasker JJ: Effects of local heat and cold treatment on surface and articular temperature of arthritic knees. *Arthritis Rheum* 37:1578, 1994.

Schaubel HJ: The local use of ice after orthopedic procedures. *Am J Surg* 72:711, 1946.

Skoubo-Kristensen E, Sommer J: Ultrasound influence on internal fixation with a rigid plate in dogs. *Arch Phys Med Rehabil* 63:371, 1982.

Sloan JP, Hain R, Pownall R: Clinical benefits of early cold therapy in accident and emergency following ankle sprain. *Arch Emerg Med* 6:1, 1989.

Travell J: Ethyl chloride spray for painful muscle spasm. *Arch Phys Med Rehabil* 33:291, 1952.

Vallbona C, Hazelwood CF, Jurida G: Response of pain to static magnetic fields in postpolio patients: A double blind pilot study. [Comment] *Arch Phys Med Rehabil* 78(11):1200–1203, Nov. 1997.

Weinberger A, Fadilah R, Lev A, et al: Deep heat in the treatment of inflammatory joint disease. *Med Hypotheses* 25:231, 1988.

Weinberger A, Fadilah R, Lev A, et al: Treatment of articular effusions with local deep microwave hyperthermia. *Clin Rheumatol* 8:461, 1989.

Weintraub MI, Wolfe GI, Barohn RA, et al: Static magnetic field theapy for symptomatic diabetic neuropathy: A randomized, double-blind, placebo-controlled trial. *Arch Phys Med Rehabil.* 84(5):736–746, May. 2003.

Woodmansey A, Collins DH, Ernst MM: Vascular reactions to the contrast bath in health and in rheumatoid arthritis. *Lancet* 2:1350, 1938.

Wright V: Quantitative and qualitative analysis of joint stiffness in normal subjects and in patients with connective tissue disease. *Ann Rheum Dis* 20:36, 1961.

69 CORE STRENGTHENING

Joel Press, MD

OVERVIEW

- Core rehabilitation allows the multisegmented spinal column to maintain its center of gravity through multiple ranges of motion, counteracting gravity, and applied forces to decrease torsion and shear on the spinal structures (ligaments, disk, nerve).
- Definition of core
  1. The core is the lumbopelvic hip complex.
  2. The core is where the center of gravity is located and where all movement begins (Clark, Fater, and Reuteman, 2000).

3. An efficient core allows for maintenance of the normal length–tension relationship of functional agonists and antagonists, which allows for the maintenance of normal force–couple relationships in the lumbopelvic hip complex (Clark, Fater, and Reuteman, 2000).

- Why are they important?
1. When a limb is moved, reactive forces are imposed on the spine acting in parallel and opposing those forces producing the movement (Bouisset and Zattara, 1987).
2. The spine is particularly prone to the effect of these reactive forces due to its multisegmental nature and the requirement for muscle contractions to provide stability of the spine (Panjabi, 1992).
3. Without muscular support and contraction, buckling of the spine occurs with compressive forces of as little as 2 kg (Morris, Lucas, and Bresler, 1961).
4. Significant microtrauma of the lumbar spine will occur with rotation of as little as 2° (Gracovetsky, Farfan, and Helleur, 1985).
5. The musculature of the spine has been shown repeatedly to be most important in maintaining spinal stability under various conditions (Gardner-Morse, Stokes, and Lauble, 1995; Solomonow et al, 1998).
6. Function of core muscles: oppose the movements of limbs, hold spine together, and decrease lumbar shearing
7. Muscle dysfunction in low back pain is a problem with motor control in the deep muscles related to segmental joint stabilization (Richardson et al, 1999).
8. Back pain can occur as a consequence of deficits in control of the spinal segment when abnormally large segmental motions cause abnormal deformation of ligaments and pain-sensitive structures (Panjabi, 1992).
   a. Loss of joint stiffness
   b. Increase in mobility and abnormal spinal motion
   c. Changes in the ratios of segmental rotations and translations

WHAT ARE CORE MUSCLES? ANATOMY/ BIOMECHANICS OF THE "CORE"

- Local paravertebral-multifidi
1. Stabilizing role: Protecting articular structures, disks, and ligaments from excessive bending, strains, and injury
2. Multisegmental column is unstable and will buckle under compression at individual joints unless locally stabilized.

3. Short muscles provide local support for longer muscles to work (Bergmark, 1989).
4. Neutral zone control: Little resistance by passive spinal restraints (ligaments).
   a. Sensitive region for stabilization of joints (Panjabi, 1992)
   b. Multifidi contribute to control of the neutral zone (Panjabi, 1991; Steffen, Nolte, and Pingel, 1994; Wilke et al, 1995)
   c. Contribute more than 2/3 of stiffness increase at L4–L5 (Wilke et al, 1995).

- Polysegmental: Erector spinae
1. Important for posture: Contract intermittently during the swaying movements that take place from an upright position.
2. Contraction of the erector spinae extend the trunk, a movement controlled largely by opposing activity of the rectus abdominus.
3. In slow trunk flexion movements, the erector spinae lowers the trunk into flexion (eccentrically contract) against the action of gravity during slow movements (Oddsson, 1990).
4. Role: Balance external loads and minimize forces on the spine (Bergmark, 1989).
5. Only a very small increase in activation of the multifidi and abdominal muscles required to stiffen the spinal segments—5% *maximal voluntary contraction* (MVC) for ADLs and 10% MVC for rigorous activity (Cholewicki, Juluru, and McGill, 1999).
6. Endurance of muscles to maintain stability margin of safety, not absolute strength is most important (McGill and Norman, 1987).

- Abdominals: *transversus abdominus* (TrA), internal, external obliques, and rectus abdominus
1. Contraction of abdominals (esp TrA) the pelvic floor and diaphragm correlate closely with increased abdominal pressure in a variety of postural tasks (Cresswell, Oddsson, and Thorstensson, 1994; Hodges et al, 1997).
2. TrA: Critical in stabilization of lumbar spine (Cresswell, Oddsson, and Thorstensson, 1994).
3. Contracting TrA increased intra-abdominal pressure and tensions thoracolumbar fascia.
4. Helps create rigid cylinder enhancing stiffness of lumbar spine (McGill and Norman, 1987).
5. Rectus abdominus and oblique abdominals are activated in direction-specific patterns with respect to limb movements, thus providing postural support *before* limb movements (Aruin and Latash, 1995; Hodges and Richardson, 1997).
6. Contraction increasing intra-abdominal pressure occurs *before* initiation of large segment movement of the upper limbs (Hodges et al, 1997).

- Quadratus lumborum
  1. Fibers cross link the vertebrae.
  2. From transverse process to rib cage to iliac crests can buttress shearing of spine in all planes.
  3. Active during flexion, extension, and lateral bending—not just a frontal plane muscle
- Diaphragm
  1. In order to minimize the displacement of the abdominal contents within the abdomen and pelvis, it is necessary to elevate the intra-abdominal pressure by simultaneously contracting the diaphragm, the pelvic floor, and the abdominal muscles (Cholewicki, Juluru, and McGill, 1999; Daggfeldt and Thorstensson, 1997).
  2. Diaphragm increases intra-abdominal pressure, segmental unloading of the spine, and increased trunk stability as a consequence.
- Pelvic floor
  1. Coactivation of the TrA and pelvic floor muscles studies support idea of muscle synergy between TrA, abdominals, multifidi, and pelvic floor (Sapsford et al, 2001).
- Lower extremity muscles—gluteus maximus, hamstrings
  1. Hip and pelvic muscles: Base of support for lumbar spine and upper limbs
  2. Thoracolumbar fascia
     a. Covers the deep muscles of the back and trunk (including multifidi)
     b. Connects the lower limbs to the upper via the latissimus dorsi
     c. Internal obliques, TrA, latissimus dorsi, gluteus max
     d. Enhances stiffness of the lumbar spine
  3. Multifidi blend with superior medial aspect of G_{max}
  4. Multifidi attach to sacrotuberous ligaments and mechanically linked to G_{max}

HOW DO WE STRENGTHEN CORE MUSCLES?

- Principles: Eccentric loading prior to concentric contraction
- Combines stretching
- Strengthening
- Balance: Control *center of gravity* (COG) as it moves through various planes of motion shift the COG through various planes.
- Goals of core strengthening exercise:
  1. Improve multifidus activity and endurance.
  2. Restore the control of deep abdominal muscles.
  3. Restore coordination and position sense.
  4. Restore mobility, especially in rotational and lateral flexion directions.

  5. Restore normal gluteal muscle activity and lumbopelvic rhythm.
  6. Train motor and postural control and balance.
  7. Make exercises functional.

THE PRACTICAL STUFF

- Turn on the light.
  1. Abdominal bracing: May require cueing and instruction.
     a. Need core stability for global mobility.
  2. Reeducation of stabilization muscles—pelvic clocks.
     a. Learn how to turn on pelvic and hip muscles.
- Get the engines going.
  1. Abdominal bracing in supine>prone, side lying>quadriped
  2. Progress to kneeling>sitting>standing
- Make it functional and fun to do
  1. Start in pain free ranges
  2. Multiple planes of motions
     a. Frontal plane core
     b. Sagittal plane core
     c. Transverse plane core
  3. Dynamic challenges—easy to hard
  4. Include balance/proprioception
  5. Need to make it subconscious

REFERENCES

Aruin AS, Latash ML: Directional specificity of postural muscles in a feed-forward postural reaction during fast voluntary arm movements. *Exp Brain Res* 103:323–332, 1995.

Bergmark A: Stability of the lumbar spine: a study in mechanical engineering. *Acta Orthop Scand Suppl* 230:1–54, 1989.

Bouisset S, Zattara M: Biomechanical study of the programming and anticipatory postural adjustments associated with voluntary movement. *J Biomech* 20:735–742, 1987.

Cholewicki J, Juluru K, McGill SM: Intra-abdominal pressure for stabilizing the lumbar spine. *J Biomech* 32:13–17, 1999.

Clark MA, Fater D, Reuteman P: Core (trunk) stabilization and its importance for closed kinetic chain rehabilitation. *Orthop Phys Ther Clin North Am* 9:2, 119–132, June 2000.

Cresswell AG, Oddsson L, Thorstensson A: The influence of sudden perturbations on trunk muscle activity and intraabdominal pressure while standing. *Exp Brain Res* 98:336–341, 1994.

Daggfeldt K, Thorstensson A: The role of intra-abdominal pressure in spinal unloading. *Spine* 30:1149–1155, 1997.

Gardner-Morse M, Stokes IAF, Lauble JP: Role of the muscles in lumbar spine stability in maximum extension efforts. *J Orthop Res* 13:802–808, 1995.

Gracovetsky S, Farfan H, Helleur C: The abdominal mechanism. *Spine* 10:317–324, 1985.

Hodges PW, Richardson CA: Feedforward contraction of transverses abdominus is not influenced by the direction of the arm movement. *Exp Brain Res* 114:362–370, 1997.

Hodges PW, Butler JE et al: Contraction of the human diaphragm during rapid postural adjustments. *J Physiol* 505:539–548, 1997.

McGill SM, Norman RW: Reassessment of the role of intra-abdominal pressure in spinal compression. *Ergonomics* 30:1565–1588, 1987.

Morris JM, Lucas DM, Bresler B: Role of the trunk in the stability of the spine. *J Bone Joint Surg (Am)* 43:327–351, 1961.

Oddsson L: Control of voluntary trunk movements in man: mechanisms for postural equilibrium in standing. *Acta Physiol Scan Suppl* 140:595, 1990.

Panjabi MM: The stabilizing system of the spine. Part 1. Function, dysfunction, adaptation, and enhancement. *J Spinal Disord* 5:383–389, 1991.

Panjabi MM: The stabilizing system of the spine. Part II. Neutral zone and stability hypothesis. *J Spinal Disord* 5:390–397, 1992.

Richardson C, Jull G, Hodges P, et al: *Therapeutic Exercise for Spinal Segmental Stabilization in Low Back Pain*. Edinburgh, Churchill Livingstone, 1999.

Sapsford RR, Hodges PW, Richardson CA e et al: Co-activation of the abdominal and pelvic floor muscles during voluntary exercise. Neurourol Urodyn 20:31–42, 2001.

Solomonow M, Zhou BH et al: The ligamento-muscular stabilizing system of the spine. *Spine* 23:2552–2562, 1998.

Steffen R, Nolte P, Pingel TH: Importance of back muscles in rehabilitation of postoperative lumber instability; a biomechanical analysis. *Rehabil (Stutt)* 33;164–170, 1994.

Wilke HJ, Steffen W, Claes LE et al: Stability increase of the lumbar spine with different muscle groups. A biomechanical in vitro study. *Spine* 20:192–198, 1995.

Luoto S, Taimela S, Hurri H et al: Mechanisms explaining the association between low back trouble and deficits in information processing. A controlled follow-up study. *Spine* 21:2621–2627.

Luoto S, Aalto H, Taimela S et al: One-footed and externally disturbed two-footed postural control in chronic low back pain patients and healthy controls. A controlled study with follow up. *Spine* 23:2081–2090, 1998.

Luoto S, Taimela S, Hurri H et al: Mechanisms explaining the association between low back touble and deficits in information processing. A controlled study with follow up. *Spine* 24(3):255–261, 1999.

Panjabi MM: Lumbar spine instability: a biomechanical challenge. *Curr Orthop* 8:100–105, 1994.

Taimela S, Harkapaa K: Strength, mobility, their changes and pain reduction during active functional restoration for chronic low back disorders. *J Spinal Disord* 9:306–312, 1996.

Taimela S, Kankaanpaa M, Luoto S: The effect of lumbar fatigue on the ability to sense a change in lumbar position. A controlled study. *Spine* 249(3):1322–1327, 1999.

BIBLIOGRAPHY

Arokoski JP, Kankaanpaa M, Valta T et al: Back and hip extensor muscle function during therapeutic exercises. *Arch Phys Med Rehabil* 80(7):842–850, 1999.

Hides JA, Richardson CA, Jull GA: Multifidus muscle recovery is not automatic after resolution of acute, first-episode low back pain. *Spine* 21(23):2763–2769, 1996.

Hodges P, Richardson C: Insufficient muscular stabilization of the lumbar spine associated with low back pain: a motor control evaluation of transversus abdominis. *Spine* 21:2640–2650, 1996.

Hodges PW, Richardson CA: Delayed postural contraction of transversus abdominus in low back pain associated with movement of the lumber spine. *J spinal Disord* 11(1):46–56, 1998.

Leinonen V, Kankaanpaa M, Airaksinen O et al: Back and hip extensor activities during trunk flexion/extension; effects of low back pain and rehabilitation. *Arch Phys med Rehabil* 81(1):32–37, 2000.

70 MEDICATIONS AND ERGOGENICS
Scott B Flinn, MD

OVERVIEW

- Many athletes self medicate without medical supervision using both traditional medications and ergogenic aids. Commonly used medications include anti-inflammatory medications used to limit pain and inflammation and presumably speed healing from injury. In overuse injuries, both oral medications and corticosteroid injections are used. Additionally, ergogenic aids are used in an attempt to develop optimal performance as well as to prevent and heal injuries.

MEDICATIONS

NONSTEROIDAL ANTI-INFLAMMATORY DRUGS

- *Nonsteroidal anti-inflammatory drugs* (NSAIDs) are commonly used to treat both acute and chronic injuries.
- Over 50 million people in the United States take daily prescription NSAIDs, with over 100 million Americans using prescription NSAIDs during a year (Simon and Smith, 1998).

MECHANISM OF ACTION

- The major pharmacologic effect of NSAIDs is to inhibit the enzyme *cyclooxygenase* (COX), thus decreasing prostaglandin production. The decreased prostaglandins produce decreased inflammation and promote analgesia in the injured tissue. There are at least two forms of the COX enzyme, COX-1 and COX-2.
- COX-1 is important in the production of prostaglandins involved in the homeostasis of various tissues including renal parenchyma, gastric mucosa, and platelets.
- COX-2 produces prostaglandins involved in pain and inflammation. Most NSAIDs inhibit both COX-1 and COX-2 at various levels, with newer agents (e.g., celecoxib) developed to be more COX-2 selective. Theoretically, this enhances the desired effects while limiting the side effects.
- NSAIDs also have physiologic effects on tissue presumably caused by prostaglandin inhibition. The effects include inhibiting articular cartilage synthesis of glycosaminoglycans, decreasing neutrophil adherence to endothelial cells (although neutrophil metabolic activity does not seem to be affected), and probably inhibiting colorectal tumorigenesis. They are among the few agents known to be chemopreventive (Stanley and Weaver, 1998).

USE IN ACUTE INJURIES

- Studies have been conducted looking at the efficacy of NSAIDs in treating acute injuries, with some studies showing no clinical benefit (Stanley and Weaver, 1998) including studies on exercise induced quadriceps injury and acute hamstring injuries (Yamamoto, 2003; Bourgeois et al, 1999).
- Other studies have shown a benefit: a meta-analysis reviewing 84 articles on ankle soft tissue injuries concluded that early use of NSAIDs relieved pain and shortened the time to recovery. Subjects had less pain, were able to return to training more rapidly, and had better exercise endurance compared to subjects treated with placebo, and had a decrease in the perception of soreness and improved muscular performance after injury (Ogilvie-Harris and Gilbart, 1995).
- Overall, judicious use of NSAIDs for pain control in the acute phase of an injury probably speeds return to sport while not delaying healing.

USE IN CHRONIC INJURIES

- Histopathologic studies of tendons involved in chronic overuse injuries have shown an absence of inflammatory cells, but rather show disorganized fibroblastic or myofibroblastic cells and prominent capillary cell proliferation, often with discontinuity of these cells. This suggests that chronic tendon injuries should be called tendonosis, referring to a degenerative process, instead of tendonitis since inflammation is not a major factor. Although NSAIDs are commonly used in these injuries to treat the chronic inflammation, judicious short-term use of NSAIDs to control pain may still be warranted (Almekinders and Temple, 1998). Treatment for chronic tendon injuries should be directed at correcting the underlying biomechanical cause and properly rehabilitating the injury.

SIDE EFFECTS AND COMPLICATIONS

- Side effects of NSAIDs have a significant impact. It is estimated that over 100,000 hospitalizations occur each year due to NSAID toxicity.
- The most common side effect is dyspepsia, occurring in about 15%.
- The most common serious side effect is *gastrointestinal* (GI) ulceration, which occurs in 2–4% of patients taking the medicine for a year.
- The following risk factors place a patient in a high risk category: past history of upper GI bleeding, past history of ulcer, concurrent anticoagulant use (including aspirin), concurrent corticosteroid use, age over 50, and use of multiple or high-dose NSAIDs.
- The annual incidence of serious NSAID-induced GI complications (i.e., perforation, obstruction, and bleeding) is approximately 0.5% in patients without risk factors.
- GI bleeds are more common in elderly patients with history of ulcers, there is a four- to sixfold relative risk of a fatal GI bleed.
- Coadministration of aspirin and celecoxib produces the same risk of serious NSAID-associated GI complications as coadministration of aspirin and conventional NSAIDs. Therefore if aspirin must be coadministered with NSAIDs (e.g., for prophylaxis against coronary artery disease), less expensive conventional NSAIDs should be used (Schoenfeld, 2001).
- Chronic NSAID use has also been associated with the development of liver injury, chronic renal disease, and rarely in acute renal failure.
- In 10–15% of all asthmatics, NSAIDs have also been associated with *nonimmunoglobulin E* (non IgE) mediated asthma and has been termed *aspirin-induced asthma* (AIA).
- Sometimes, platelet function may be impaired, resulting in prolonged bleeding times.
- There may be an increased risk of thromboembolic events including Myocardial Infarction, especially in those taking COX-2 inhibitors. Patients who are at risk for such an event should be treated with low-dose aspirin whether they are treated with COX-2-specific

inhibitors or nonselective NSAIDs (Mukherjee, 2001).

STRATEGIES TO LIMIT SIDE EFFECTS
- Limit amount and duration.
- Use alternative medication (e.g., acetominophen).
- Use alternative modality for pain control (e.g., ice, electrical stimulation).
- Since GI ulceration is the most common serious side effect, most strategies have focused on reducing this complication.
  - H_2 blockers are largely ineffective except for perhaps duodenal ulcers.
  - The role of sucralafate is not well defined.
  - In a small study performed in Hong Kong, coadministration of *proton pump inhibitors* (PPIs) with conventional NSAIDs reduced recurrent NSAID-associated upper GI bleeding (Schoenfeld, 2001).
  - Although there is no data currently to support coadministration of PPIs with COX-2-selective NSAIDs, it should be considered for patients with multiple risk factors for serious NSAID-associated GI disorders (Schoenfeld, 2001).
  - Misoprostol, a PGE1 analog, has been shown to decrease ulcers and serious GI complication rates up to 40%. It is cost effective in high risk groups, those over 75 with previous ulcer disease, but is not very cost effective in the typically younger otherwise healthy athlete (Maetzel, Ferraz, and Bombadier, 1998).
- Use of COX-2 inhibitors.
  - a. When choosing a COX-2 NSAID to reduce serious NSAID-associated GI complications, stronger evidence indicates that rofecoxib reduces serious NSAID-associated GI complications compared with conventional NSAIDs (Schoenfeld, 2001).
  - b. However, patients receiving celecoxib do not show a statistically significant reduction in serious NSAID-associated GI complications compared with patients receiving ibuprofen or diclofenac unless aspirin use was eliminated (Schoenfeld, 2001).
  - c. It is not known how other NSAID effects (such as that on kidneys, brain and platelets) will be modified by the use of COX-2 inhibitors, and what new toxicities will be experienced until the postmarketing reporting and long-term follow-up studies are performed.
- Use topical preparations of NSAIDs.
  - Topical NSAIDs have serum drug levels of only about 10% of oral medication while showing equivalent tissue concentrations.
  - A meta-analysis of 86 trials using up to 2 weeks of treatment concluded that topical nonsteroidals are effective in relieving pain in both acute and chronic

conditions and have a low incidence of local side effects with systemic side effects no different than placebo (Moore et al, 1998).

CORTICOSTEROIDS

MECHANISM OF ACTION
- Corticosteroids are a class of medications acting on a number of body systems including inflammation. Glucocorticoids downregulate the expression of inflammatory genes in cells, thus decreasing inflammatory cytokines, enzymes, and adhesion molecules, while upregulating the production of anti-inflammatory proteins such as interleukin-1 receptor antagonist and interleukin-10.

RATIONALE FOR USE
- Can be given via various routes including orally, by injection, or transdermally through the use of creams—iontophoresis or phonophoresis.
- Although commonly used for a variety of acute and chronic injuries, most of the literature evaluating steroids for treating sports medicine injuries is retrospective in nature, case series, or anecdotal.
  - Acute injuries.
    - a. The literature has no prospective studies that evaluate the effectiveness of steroids in treating acute injuries. Anecdotally, some clinicians use short courses of oral steroids from 3–5 days on acute injuries including radicular back pain, but this has not been evaluated prospectively. Because of the potential side effects from steroid use, treatment with corticosteroids for acute injuries in the sports setting should be of short duration and left up to the individual clinician to develop any treatment protocol until better information becomes available.
  - Chronic overuse injuries
    - a. Although many chronic tendon injuries seem to be a tendonosis of a degenerative nature and do not involve classic chronic inflammatory cells, clinicians frequently use corticosteroids for these conditions, which often provide the patient with temporary pain control (Almekinders and Temple, 1998).
    - b. The effectiveness of steroids in chronic injuries has not been well investigated by prospective trials.
    - c. Overall, the literature suggests that if steroids are used to treat chronic sports injuries, they should be considered a pain control method.

SIDE EFFECTS AND COMPLICATIONS
- Steroid injection has a low complication rate of 1–2%.
  - Hypopigmentation and fat pad atrophy are the most common long term ill effects.

- Steroid injection directly into a tendon weakens it while injection of the paratenon does not appear to have that effect.
- Long-term therapy or extremely high dosages of steroids may cause avascular necrosis, adrenal suppression, GI ulcer, diabetes, cataracts, and hypertension.

STRATEGIES TO LIMIT SIDE EFFECTS

- Limit usage, usual practice limit is 2–3 times per year for joint injections.
- Treat the underlying cause.
- Direct injection into tendon should probably be avoided although injection into paratenon appears safe.

ERGOGENIC AIDS

DEFINITION

- Ergogenic aids are defined as items designed to increase work or improve performance above that of regular training and diet. Ergogenic aids are usually classified into five groups: mechanical aids such as running shoes, psychologic aids, physiologic aids such as fluids and blood, pharmacologic aids that generally are thought of as requiring a prescription, and nutritional aids.

HISTORY

- In 1994, Congress passed the Dietary Health and Supplement Health Education Act (DHSEA) which substantially changed the regulation and marketing of dietary supplements (Glade, 1997). Essentially, substances can be sold without U.S. Food and Drug Administration (FDA) approval as long as the products are labeled and sold as dietary supplements and the label makes no claim as a drug. These supplements are not held to the same quality control standards as FDA approved drugs; the content and purity of these products is not regulated and may contain too much of the product to none at all (Butterfield, 1996). Furthermore, these substances do not require evaluation for safety or efficacy.
- Despite all this, ergogenic aids are commonly used, sometimes with cataclysmic consequences.

EVALUATING ERGOGENIC AIDS

- Evaluation of ergogenic aids are often difficult to perform. Additionally, the scientific literature usually differs significantly from the advertising on many products (Butterfield, 1996).

- There is no burden of proof on the manufacturer to prove efficacy or product content like there is for drugs (Glade, 1997).
- Products may contain lower amounts of the product than that listed on the label, with some products having zero amount of the supposedly ergogenic substance and while others may be contaminated by the previous drug manufactured in the equipment (Schardt, 1998).
- Furthermore, the placebo effect can have a huge impact on the perceived benefits derived by the user.

EFFICACY OF ERGOGENIC AIDS

- Ergogenic aids can affect various aspects of physical fitness to improve performance. Six components of fitness that may be affected include aerobic fitness, anaerobic fitness, strength, body composition, psychologic factors, and healing of injuries.
- Aerobic metabolism uses oxygen while anaerobic metabolism does not.
- Aerobic fitness is the ability to produce work using aerobic metabolism, generally lasting longer than 1 min and often lasting for hours and is important especially to distance runners. It comprises two parts, maximal aerobic power and aerobic capacity.
- Anaerobic fitness is important in activities generally lasting less than 1 min and are fueled primarily through anaerobic metabolism.
- Maximum strength, usually measured by the one repetition maximum, refers to the amount of power that can be generated in a brief burst fueled by anaerobic metabolism.
- Body composition can effect performance by increasing lean muscle mass to produce more muscles to do the work and by decreasing body fat to decrease the weight that has to be carried through space to the finish line.
- Psychologic factors may affect performance through various mind-body mechanisms including decreased perceptions of fatigue and pain.
- Enhancing the healing of injuries and soreness promotes a more rapid return to training and maintenance of fitness.

SAFETY CONSIDERATIONS

- Ergogenic aids can have side effects like any other substance.
  - Heart attacks, seizures, strokes, coma, and death have been attributed to the use of ergogenic products (Butterfield, 1996).

• Injectable products carry the risk of disease transmission if needles are shared.

ETHICAL AND LEGAL CONSIDERATIONS

• Winning simply through training and ability should be the athletic ideal; it is often not the reality. Athletes are constantly caught in the dilemma of trying to keep up with what their competitors may be trying to do. Many athletes will try these products even though the product has not been shown to work, has serious side effects, or is banned by the sports governing body ruling over the sport in which the athlete is competing.
• In an attempt to keep the playing field level, various amateur and professional organizations have instituted drug policies. These policies are targeted toward substances that may be dangerous, illegal, and/or give an unfair competitive advantage. For example, the use of anabolic steroids had become so widespread by the 1964 Olympics that drug testing began at the 1968 Olympic Games in Mexico City, with the National Collegiate Athletic Association (NCAA) following in 1986.
• The American College of Sports Medicine (ACSM) and other organizations have taken a position on anabolic steroids stating that they are unethical, have dangerous side effects, and their use should be deplored (American College of Sports Medicine, 1987).
• The Anabolic Steroids Control Act of 1990 made anabolic steroids a Schedule III controlled substance.
• Anabolic steroids are not the only substances banned by sports governing bodies such as the International Olympic Committee (IOC) and NCAA. The IOC developed their list in 1967.
• Because of many doping scandals, the U.S. Antidoping Agency (USADA) was formed in 2000 as an independent antidoping organization for Olympic sports in the United States. The list of banned substances for the IOC can be viewed on their website at http://www.usantidoping.org and there is a telephone hotline to answer any questions at 800-233-0393 (U.S. Antidoping Agency, 2003).
• The NCAA has their list at http://www.ncaa.org/sports_sciences/drugtesting/banned_list.html (National Collegiate Athletic Association, 2003).
• Because the lists are continually changing, physicians caring for athletes in these or other organizations should always consult prior to writing a prescription or suggesting over the counter remedies.
• Testing is done using analyzing urine samples through a number of methods, with most confirmatory tests done using gas chromatography/mass spectrometry. In the future, blood or hair samples may be used to detect banned substances.

SPECIFIC ERGOGENIC AIDS

• Specific ergogenic aids will be reviewed here regarding their efficacy, safety, and use in Olympic and NCAA competition. Table 70-1 gives an overview of many ergogenic aids, their effects on the six fitness components and their safety.

TABLE 70-1 Ergogenic Aids, Their Effect on Fitness Components, and Dangerous Side Effects

PRODUCT	AEROBIC	ANAEROBIC	STRENGTH	BODY.COMP	PSYCH	HEALING	DANGER
Amphetamines	+	+	+	+	+	—	+
Anabolic steroids	—	—	+	+	+	?	+
Antioxidants	—	—	—	—	—	?	—
Bicarbonate	—	+	—	—	+	—	—
Blood doping	+	—	—	—	—	—	+
Caffeine	+	+	—	—	?	—	—
Caffeine+ ephedrine	+	—	—	+	?	—	—
Carbohydrate	+					?	
Clenbuterol			?	?	?		
CoQ10						?	
DHEA			?	?			
Ephedrine	+			+	?		+
Ginseng						?	
Glucosamine and chondroitin						?	
Glycerol							rare
Growth hormone				+			?
Hydration	+						
Vitamins							

AMPHETAMINES; DEXEDRINE; RELATED STIMULANTS

EFFICACY

- Amphetamine and dextroamphetamine are stimulants, which are sometimes used to treat obesity and attention deficit/hyperactivity disorder.
  - Acutely, probably improves strength, muscular power (endurance), and time to exhaustion, possibly due to the masking of fatigue (Smith and Beecher, 1959); however, there was no improvement in aerobic power (VO_{2max}) nor running speed.
  - Has been shown to maintain vigilance, reaction time, and cognitive function during sleep deprivation (Chandler and Blair, 1980).
  - Amphetamines also act as appetite suppressants.

SAFETY

- The side effects often depend on dose and can include death from cardiovascular complications including myocardial infarctions and arrhythmias, cerebrovascular accidents, and heat stroke (Smith and Beecher, 1959; Chandler and Blair, 1980).
- Other problems include hypertension, restlessness, vomiting, arrhythmias, and seizures.
- Amphetamine and dextroamphetamine are Class CII medications and are considered potentially addicting, with particular dependency risk with chronic use.

LEGAL

- Amphetamines are banned both by the IOC and NCAA (U.S. Antidoping Agency, 2003; National Collegiate Athletic Association, 2003).

ANABOLIC/ANDROGENIC STEROIDS AND ANDROSTENEDIONE

EFFICACY

- Anabolic steroids have both anabolic (tissue building) and androgenic effects.
- Anabolic steroids have been shown to increase lean muscle mass and strength when used with an adequate diet and with progressive weight training. The effects seem even more pronounced in athletes who use supraphysiologic doses (American College of Sports Medicine, 1987).
- There appears to be no effect on aerobic power, aerobic capacity, or athleticism.

TABLE 70-2 Indications and Contraindications for Anabolic Steroids

INDICATIONS	CONTRAINDICATIONS
Primary hypogonadism	Known or suspected prostate cancer
Hypogonadotropic hypogonadism	Breast cancer in females with high Ca^{2+}
Hereditary angioedema	Breast cancer in males
Antithrombin III deficiency	Nephritis
Anemia from renal disease	Pregnancy or nursing
Catabolic disease such as AIDS	
Delayed onset puberty	

- Enhancement of aggression may also occur.
- Androstenedione is one of the few ergogenic aids, which is converted into testosterone when ingested.

SAFETY

- Anabolic steroids are a class III drug. Legal indications to prescribe and common contraindications to steroids are listed in Table 70-2.
- Anabolic steroids have a long list of reported side effects, some of which may have been exaggerated in the literature.
- An increase in *low-density lipoprotein* (LDL) and decrease in *high-density lipoprotein* (HDL) on average of 50% in both male and female users, combined with hypertension have been shown with no direct link yet to increased cardiovascular mortality is a leading concern (American College of Sports Medicine, 1987; Blue and Lombardo, 1999).
- Adverse effects have been noted in the liver including jaundice, benign tumors, and, rarely, peliosis hepatis (blood filled cysts in the liver) that has caused a few fatalities when the cysts ruptured. Causation of malignant liver tumors has not been proven (Blue and Lombardo, 1999).
- Other side effects include acne, female masculinization (alopecia, hirsutism, clitoromegaly, deepening of the voice), and enhancement of aggression. Side effects of androstenedione are likely to be similar to anabolic steroids.

LONG-TERM SIDE EFFECTS HAVE BEEN HARDER TO ESTABLISH

LEGAL

- Steroids are a Class III controlled substance.
- Banned by IOC and NCAA (American College of Sports Medicine, 1987; U.S. Antidoping Agency, 2003).

- Users attempt to avoid detection by tapering in advance of announced tests, staying within the 6:1 testosterone to epitestosterone level, or using masking agents like diuretics. Recent development of a hair test may change the way testing is done in the future.
- Androstenedione, although banned, currently is not frequently specifically tested (Blue and Lombardo, 1999).

BICARBONATE

EFFICACY

- Thought to act ergogenically by helping to buffer lactic acid during high intensity exercise or through some action of the sodium ion on intravascular volume (Williams, 1995).
- Appears to be effective in reducing acidosis of the muscle cell and blood, decreasing the perception of fatigue, and improving performance and delaying time to exhaustion in high intensity events, and improve performance in highly trained runners in 400, 800, and 1500 m (Williams, 1995).

SAFETY

- Appears safe at doses needed to produce ergogenic effects (Williams, 1995). Excessive doses could lead to alkalosis.
- Major side effect at ergogenic doses is GI distress and diarrhea, which may cause runners to not show the ergogenic effect.

LEGAL

- Bicarbonate is currently not a banned substance.

BLOOD DOPING AND RECOMBINANT ERYTHROPOIETIN

EFFICACY

- Blood doping refers to the process of artificially increasing *red blood cell* (RBC) mass to improve exercise performance. Increasing RBC mass can be accomplished through infusion of RBCs or through the use of the *recombinant erythropoietin* (rEPO) of human hormone stimulating RBC production (Sawka et al, 1996).
- By increasing the RBC mass, oxygen carrying capacity is increased with resultant increase in both maximal aerobic power and aerobic capacity. The increased VO_{2max} and time to exhaustion cause improvements in race performance especially in distance runners (Sawka et al, 1996; Ekblom, 1996).
- Blood doping also seems to help performance in the heat, especially in acclimatized individuals (Sawka et al, 1996).

SAFETY

- Although rare, the major risk from blood transfusions is transfusion reactions. Other complications include infection from the blood or procedure.
- Hyperviscosity can occur with hemoglobin levels over 55%, which may increase the risk of thrombosis causing strokes or myocardial infarction in athletes using rEPO or blood transfusions. It has been postulated that numerous deaths among cyclists have been as a result of rEPO induced hyperviscosity causing vascular sludging and myocardial artery occlusion (Sawka et al, 1996; Eichner, 1992).
- Blood pressure may also be increased by rEPO and is contraindicated in uncontrolled hypertension (Ekblom, 1996).

LEGAL

- Banned by the IOC and NCAA (American College of Sports Medicine, 1987; U.S. Antidoping Agency, 2003).
- Blood transfusions can be detected if homologous blood is used, but autologous blood and rEPO are harder to detect (Sawka et al, 1996). Improved testing including direct measuring of erythropoietin isoforms can be done, but since rEPO currently can only be detected for a few days after administration but has effects that last for weeks, reliable testing is difficult.

CAFFEINE

EFFICACY

- Caffeine enhances performance during both prolonged activity and shorter intense activity, and has been hypothesized to work for runners by increasing free fatty acid production (which would spare muscle glycogen), elevating *adenosine 3',5'-monophosphate* (cAMP) levels in cells, altering the movement of calcium by the sarcoplasmic reticulum, increasing levels of catecholamines, increasing neuromuscular transmissions, and decreasing perceived effort and fatigue (Applegate, 1999).

• The effectiveness of caffeine may not be as great in habitual users or in hot humid environments.

SAFETY

• In normal doses (5–8 mg/kg) caffeine appears safe and produces a few side effects such as diarrhea, insomnia, restlessness, and anxiety.
• Caffeine does not appear to increase risk for heatstroke or compromise cardiovascular activity in endurance performance (Pasman et al, 1995).
• Very high doses, over 10 mg/kg, may cause seizures and overdosing may lead to death.

LEGAL

• Caffeine, although ergogenic at 5–10 mg/kg, is not completely banned by the IOC and NCAA. Habitual users may consume their usual caffeine in small amounts. Ingestion of around 7 mg/kg, roughly two cups of coffee, produce urinary levels close to the limit of 12 mcg/mL for the IOC. The NCAA levels are slightly more liberal at 15 mcg/mL (American College of Sports Medicine, 1987; U.S. Antidoping Agency, 2003).

CLENBUTEROL AND BETA AGONISTS

EFFICACY

• Clenbuterol and other beta 2 agonists like salmeterol and albuterol are used widely as bronchodilators for the treatment of many types of asthma including exercise induced asthma.
• There are no human studies to support athlete's use of clenbuterol for their potential anabolic effects, either as an anabolic steroid substitute or to prevent some of the muscle loss after cessation of anabolic steroids. Animal studies have shown that clenbuterol in high doses increases lean body mass and decreases adipose tissue (Prather et al, 1995).
• However, a study on a relative drug, salbutamol, showed increased quadriceps and hamstring strength, while another showed that 6 weeks of oral albuterol may augment strength gains in isokinetic strength training of the knee (Martineau et al, 1992; Caruso et al, 1995).
• These studies taken together imply that there may be an ergogenic effect of prolonged oral beta 2 agonists on strength, but no ergogenic effect of short term administration of inhaled medicines. Confirmatory studies on humans remain to be done regarding their potential anabolic effects.

SAFETY

• Side effects of beta 2 agonists are common and include tachycardia, tremor, palpitations, anxiety, headache, anorexia, and insomnia. Serious side effects include dysrhythmias, cardiac muscle hypertrophy, myocardial infarction, or stroke (Prather et al, 1995).

LEGAL

• Because of its potential ergogenic effect clenbuterol in all its forms and all oral beta 2 agonists are banned by the IOC and NCAA (American College of Sports Medicine, 1987; U.S. Antidoping Agency, 2003).
• Advances in testing may eventually enable detection of these drugs through hair analysis.
• Clenbuterol is not FDA approved.
• It is interesting to note there was an increase in the percentage of U.S. Olympic athletes with exercise induced asthma from 10% in the 1984 Summer Olympics to over 20% in the 1996 Summer Olympics, thus greatly increasing the number of athletes who can "legally" use these products (Weiler, Layton, and Hunt, 1998).

COENZYME Q10

EFFICACY

• Coenzyme Q10 (CoQ10), also called ubiquinone, is a part of the electron transport system and functions as an antioxidant. Endurance runners sometimes use CoQ10 and other antioxidants.
• In patients with congestive heart failure, CoQ10 improves cardiac function including stroke volume, ejection fraction, cardiac output, and cardiac index (although total work output does not appear to be increased) and may serve a role in postmyocardial infarction patients (Soja and Mortensen, 1997).
• A double blind Finnish study did show an increase in anaerobic and aerobic indices in 25 top level cross country skiers (Snider et al, 1992); however, other studies examining CoQ10 either alone or in combination with other antioxidants have not shown any effect on anaerobic or aerobic performance. More research is required.
• Safety CoQ10 seems safe although there are no long term studies.
• Legal CoQ10 is not on the list of banned substances (American College of Sports Medicine, 1987; U.S. Antidoping Agency, 2003).

DEHYDROEPIANDROSTERONE

EFFICACY

- *Dehydroepiandrosterone* (DHEA) is a hormone secreted by the adrenal gland that is a precursor to both androgens and estrogens.
- Although the FDA banned the manufacture of DHEA as a drug due to insufficient evidence of efficacy and safety, it continues to be available as a nutritional supplement (Sturmi and Diorio, 1998).
- DHEA levels peak at puberty and young adulthood and gradually fade as aging progresses.
- Studies showed that physiologic doses (50 mg/day) and supraphysiologic doses (1600 mg/day) of DHEA increased circulating androgen levels in older women but not in older men (Stricker, 1998).
- DHEA increased androstenedione levels but not testosterone levels and had a small, not statistically significant increase in lean body mass when given at supraphysiologic doses to five young males (Stricker, 1998).
- DHEA did not appear to effect energy or protein metabolism in young males (Welle, Jozefowicz, and Statt, 1990).
- In summary, DHEA does not appear to increase testosterone in young healthy males, and it does not appear to have an ergogenic effect.

SAFETY

- Short-term use of DHEA has been associated with few side effects, but long-term use risks are unknown. There is a theoretical risk of prostate and endometrial cancer as well as gynecomastia. DHEA effects on lipids are unknown (Corrigan, 1999).

LEGAL

- DHEA is currently banned by both the NCAA and IOC and is available only as a nutritional supplement in the United States (American College of Sports Medicine, 1987; U.S. Antidoping Agency, 2003).

EPHEDRINE (MA HUANG) AND RELATED SYMPATHOMIMETICS

EFFICACY

- Ephedrine is a sympathomimetic drug that is the active ingredient in the Chinese herbal medicine *Ma huang*.
- Ephedrine and other sympathomimetics like pseudoephedrine are commonly found in over the counter cold medicines. It acts physiologically to increase heart rate and blood pressure. When used with caffeine, ephedrine has been shown to improve time to exhaustion during exercise tests. When used with caffeine, it also seems to be effective in producing weight loss. Low dose (24 mg) ephedrine did not show an improvement in performance (Sidney and Lefcoe, 1977).
- Pseudoephedrine has not been shown to improve aerobic performance in controlled trials (Swain et al, 1997).
- More research would be needed to find a therapeutic nontoxic dose of ephedrine.

SAFETY

- Higher dose ephedrine has been associated with hemorrhagic stroke.
- Other serious side effects have been reported including nephrolithiasis and, rarely, hepatitis.
- Common side effects include tachycardia, hypertension, anxiety, and arrhythmias.
- Ephedrine has caused fatalities even at recommended over-the-counter doses, prompting the FDA to issue a warning against its consumption in 1996 (U.S. Department of Health and Human Services, 1996). Ephedra's inclusion in over-the-counter products was officially banned by the FDA in 2003.

LEGAL

- Ephedrine and related compounds are banned by the NCAA and IOC (American College of Sports Medicine, 1987; U.S. Antidoping Agency, 2003).

GINSENG

EFFICACY

- Ginseng is a shrub of which there are four varieties whose root is often used as a ergogenic aid. The saponin extracts or glycosides from the root are considered to provide most of the biological activity, but there is a marked lack of quality control and standardization in the amount of saponins available in the products.
- There have been conflicting reports on efficacy, with a few placebo controlled studies showing improvement in maximum aerobic capacity while others did not.
- Recent well designed placebo-controlled, double-blind studies have failed to demonstrate any improvement in

aerobic exercise (Morris et al, 1996; Dowling et al, 1996).

SIDE EFFECTS

• There are few reported side effects with ginseng. Hypertension, anxiety, acne, edema, and diarrhea have been reported with long-term high-dose use.

LEGAL

• Ginseng is not banned by the NCAA or the IOC (American College of Sports Medicine, 1987; U.S. Antidoping Agency, 2003).

GLUCOSAMINE AND CHONDROITIN SULFATE

EFFICACY

• Glucosamine and chondroitin sulfate are substances produced by the body and used in the synthesis of glycosaminoglycans, a significant part of the extracellular matrix of articular cartilage. Studies have shown that supplementation with chondroitin sulfate and glucosamine reduces pain often equal to or above that of NSAIDs in osteoarthritis patients (Deal and Moskowitz, 1999; Morreale et al, 1996)
• Combination products are probably better than using one product alone (Deal and Moskowitz, 1999).

SAFETY

• Short-term studies have not shown any adverse side effects, but there are no long-term studies evaluating safety (Deal and Moskowitz, 1999).

LEGAL

• Glucosamine and Chondroitin sulfate are not banned by the IOC or NCAA (American College of Sports Medicine, 1987; U.S. Antidoping Agency, 2003).

GLYCEROL AND HYPERHYDRATION

EFFICACY

• Theoretically, glycerol can be used to induce a state of hyperhydration that may theoretically aid in distance running in warm environments (Inder et al, 1998).

• In a thermoneutral environment, glycerol hyperhydration did not improve performance in prolonged exercise (Inder et al, 1998); however, when heat stress was added, hyperhydration with and without glycerol significantly prolonged the time to heat exhaustion compared to euhydration (Latzka et al, 1998).

SAFETY

• Glycerol may increase the risk of intraocular and intracerebral dehydration and should not be used in persons with renal disease.

LEGAL

• Glycerol is not banned by the NCAA or IOC (American College of Sports Medicine, 1987; U.S. Antidoping Agency, 2003).

GROWTH HORMONE

EFFICACY

• Growth hormone is secreted by the hypothalamus and is important in the growth and development of normal bones and muscle.
• *Growth hormone* (GH) seems to be intricately related to *insulin-like growth factor I* (IGF-I) and the regulation of insulin.
• GH appears to provide an anabolic effect and increases bone mass and lean body mass while decreasing adipose tissue (Berneis and Keller, 1996).
• Administration of GH in GH deficient individuals has been shown to increase height, decrease body fat, and improve respiratory muscle function, strength, and agility.
• However, in normal individuals, supplementation with GH has never been shown to improve athletic performance (Eichner, 1997).
• Although there are myocardial receptors for GH, administration of *recombinant human growth hormone* (rhGH) did not affect cardiovascular performance as measured by left ventricular ejection fraction, heart rate or blood pressure in seven normal male volunteers (Bisi et al, 1999).
• GH levels can be increased by exercise and the level of release is related directly to exercise intensity, but the duration of the secretion and effects of long-term training are not known (Pritzalff et al, 1999).
• In summary, GH appears to increase lean body mass but does not improve performance.

SAFETY

- The safety of long term administration of GH in non-deficient individuals has not been established. High GH levels causes acromegaly and gigantism.

LEGALITY

- Growth hormone is banned by the IOC and the NCAA but there is currently no way to effectively test for the recombinant form.

VITAMINS AND ANTIOXIDANTS

EFFICACY

- Vitamin and mineral supplementation has been used by athletes for years despite there being no evidence of its effectiveness.
- Vitamin supplementation for 3 months does not seem to affect blood concentrations of the vitamins in athletes who are not vitamin deficient and consumes a well balanced diet (Weight et al, 1988). After 3 to 9 months of multivitamin and mineral supplementation there was no effect seen on exercise performance (Weight, Myburgh, and Noakes, 1988; Singh, Moses, and Deuster, 1992). Unless a nutritional deficiency exists, routine supplementation of vitamins, and minerals is not recommended.
- Antioxidants including vitamin E, vitamin C, beta-carotene (a Vitamin A precursor), and CoQ10 among others. Although animal studies have suggested that muscle injury places oxidative stress on muscles, almost all studies on humans to date have not reported a beneficial effect of antioxidant supplementation on performance. The lone study that did show an effect used N-acetyl-cysteine as the antioxidant and showed an improvement on tibialis anterior contraction force following stimulation to fatigue (Reid et al, 1994). Until more studies show an ergogenic effect, routine supplementation with antioxidants does not appear warranted.

SAFETY

- Supplementation with a multivitamin or antioxidant appears safe; however, in large doses they may become toxic, especially the fat soluble vitamins D, E, A, and K. At high doses, vitamin C and beta-carotene may actually become pro-oxidant.

LEGAL

- Vitamins and antioxidants are not banned by the NCAA or IOC (American College of Sports Medicine, 1987; U.S. Antidoping Agency, 2003).

REFERENCES

Almekinders LC, Temple JD: Etiology, diagnosis, and treatment of tenodonitis: An analysis of the literature. *Med Sci Sports Exerc* 30(8):1183–1190, 1998.

American College of Sports Medicine: The use of anabolic-androgenic steroids in sports. *Med Sci Sports Exerc* 19(5):453–539, 1987.

Applegate E: Effective nutritional ergogenic aids. *Int J Sport Nutr* 9(2):229–239, 1999.

Berneis K, Keller U: Metabolic action of growth hormone: Direct and indirect. *Baillieres Clin Endocrinol Metab* 10(3):337–352, 1996.

Bisi G, Podio V, Valetto MR, et al. Acute cardiovascular and hormonal effects of GH and hexarelin, a synthetic GH releasing peptide, in humans. *J Endocrinol Invest* 22(4):266–272, 1999.

Blue JG, Lombardo JA: Nutritional aspects of exercise. Steroids and steroid-like compounds. *Clin Sports Med* 18(3):667–689, 1999.

Bourgeois J, MacDougall D, MacDonald J, et al: Naproxen does not alter indices of muscle damage in resistance-exercise trained men. *Med Sci Sports Exerc* 31(1):4–9, 1999.

Butterfield G: Ergogenic aids: Evaluating sport nutrition products. *Int J Sport Nutr* 6:191–197, 1996.

Caruso JF, Signorile JF, Perry AC, et al: The effects of albuteol and isokinetic exercise on the quadriceps muscle group. *Med Sci Sports Exerc* 279(11):1471–1476, 1995.

Chandler JV, Blair SN: The effect of amphetamines on selected physiological components related to athletic success. *Med Sci Sports Exerc* 12(1):65–69, 1980.

Corrigan A: Dehydroepiandrosterone and sport. *Med J Aust* 171:206–208, 1999.

Deal CL, Moskowitz RW: Nutraceuticals as therapeutic agents in osteoarthritis. *Rheum Dis Clin North Am* 25(2):379–395, 1999.

Dowling EA, Redondo DR, Branch JD, et al: Effect of Eleutherococcus senticosus on submaximal and maximal exercise. *Med Sci Sports Exerc* 28(4):482–489, 1996.

Eichner ER: Sports anemia, iron supplementation, and blood doping. *Med Sci Sports Exerc* 24(9Supp):S315–S318, 1992.

Eichner ER: Ergogenic aids. *Phys Sportsmed* 25(4):70–83, 1997.

Ekblom B: Blood doping and erythropoietin. *Am J Sports Med* 24(6):S40–S42, 1996.

Glade MJ: The dietary supplement health and education act of 1994-focus on labeling issues. *Nutrition* 13(11/12):999–1001, 1997.

Inder WJ, Swanney MP, Donald RA, et al: The effect of glycero and desmopressin on exercise performance and hydration in triathletes. *Med Sci Sports Exerc* 30(8):1263–1269, 1998.

Latzka WA, Sawka MN, Montain SJ, et al: Hyperhydration: Tolerance and cardiovscular effects during uncompensable exercise-heat stress. *J Appl Physiol* 84(6):1858–1864, 1998.

Maetzel A, Ferraz MB, Bombadier C: The cost-effectiveness of misoprostol in preventing serious gastrointestinal events associated with the use of nonsteroidal antiinflammatory drugs. *Arthritis and Rheum* 41(1):16–25, 1998.

Martineau L, Horan MA, Rothwell NJ, et al: Salbutamol a Beta 2 adrenoceptor agonis increases skeletal muscle strength in young men. *Clin Sci* 83:615–622, 1992.

Moore RA, Tramer MR, Caroll D, et al: Quantitative systematic review of topically applied non-steroidal anti-inflammatory drugs. *Br Med J* 316(7128):333–338, 1998.

Morreale P, Manopulo R, Galati M, et al: Comparison of the anti-inflammatory efficacy of chondroitin sulfate and diclofenac sodium in patients with knee osteoarthritis. *J Rheum* 23(8): 1385–1391, 1996.

Morris AC, Jacobs I, McLellan TM, et al: No ergogenic effect of ginseng ingestion. *Int J Sport Nutr* 6(3):263–271, 1996.

Mukherjee D: Risk of cardiovascular events associated with selective COX-2 inhibitors. *JAMA* 286(8):954–959, 2001.

National Collegiate Athletic Association: *Sports Sciences.* Indianapolis, IN, 2003.

Ogilvie-Harris DJ, Gilbart M: Treatment modalities for soft tissue injuries of the ankle: A critical review. *Clin J Sports Med* 5(3):175–186, 1995.

Pasman WJ, van Baak MA, Jeukendrup AE, et al: The effect of different dosages of caffeine on endurance performance time. *Int J Sports Med* 16(4):225–130, 1995.

Prather ID, Brown DE, North P, et al: Clenbuterol: A substitute for anabolic steroids? *Med Sci Sports Exerc* 27(8):1118–1121, 1995.

Pritzalff CJ, Wideman L, Weltman JY, et al: Impact of acute exercise intensity on pulsatile growth hormone release in men. *J Appl Physiol* 87(2):498–504, 1999.

Reid MB, Stokic DS, Koch SM, et al: N-acetylcysteine inhibits muscle fatigue in humans. *J Clin Invest* 94(6):2468–2474, 1994.

Sawka MN, Joyner MJ, Miles DS, et al: The use of blood doping as an ergogenic aid, ACSM position stand. *Med Sci Sports Exerc* 28(3):i–viii, 1996.

Schardt D: Relieving arthritis, can supplements help? *Nutr Action* Jan/Feb:3–6, 1998.

Schoenfeld P: An evidence-based approach to the gastrointestinal safety profile of COX–2-selective anti-inflammatories. *Gastroenterol Clin North Am* 30(4):1027–1044, viii–ix, 2001.

Sidney KH, Lefcoe NM: The effects of ephedrine on the physiological and psychological responses to submaximal and maximal exercise in man. *Med Sci Sports* 9(2):95–99, 1977.

Simon LS, Smith TJ: NSAID mechanism of action, efficacy, and relative safety. *Managing Arthritis: A Postgraduate Medicine Special Report March*:17–22, 1998.

Singh A, Moses F, Deuster PA: Chronic multivitamin-mineral supplementation does not enhance physical performance. *Med Sci Sports Exerc* 24(6):726–732, 1992.

Smith GM, Beecher HK: Amphetamine sulfate and athletic performance. *J Am Med Assoc* 170:524–557, 1959.

Snider IP, Bazzarre TL, Murdoch SD, et al: Effects of coenzyme athletic performance system as an ergogenic aid on endurance performance to exhaustion. *Int J Sports Nutr* 2(3):272–286, 1992.

Soja AM, Mortensen SA: Treatment of congestive heart failure with coenzyme Q10 illuminated by meta-analysis of clinical trials. *Mol Aspects Med* 18(Supp):S519–S568, 1997.

Stanley KL, Weaver JE: Pharmacologic management of pain and inflammation in athletes. *Clin Sports Med* 17(2):375–392, 1998.

Stricker PR: Sports pharmacology. Other ergogenic aids. *Clin Sports Med* 17(2):283–297, 1998.

Sturmi JE, Diorio DJ: Sports pharmacology. Anabolic agents. *Clin Sports Med* 17(2):261–264, 1998.

Swain RA, Harsha DM, Baenziger J, et al: Do pseudoephedrine or phenylpropanolamine improve maximum oxygen uptake and time to exhaustion? *Clin J Sports Med* 7(3):168–173, 1997.

U.S. Antidoping Agency: USADA Guide to Prohibited Classes of Substances and Prohibited Methods of Doping. www.usantidoping.org.

U.S. Department of Health and Human Services: FDA statement on street drugs containing the botanical ephedrine. April 10, 1996.

Weight LM, Myburgh KH, Noakes TD: Vitamin and mineral supplementation: Effect on running performance of trained athletes. *Am J Clin Nutr* 47(2):192–195, 1988.

Weight LM, Noakes TD, Labadarios D, et al: Vitamin and mineral status of trained athletes including the effects of supplementation. *Am J Clin Nutr* 47(2):186–191, 1988.

Weiler JM, Layton T, Hunt M: Asthma in United States Olympic athletes who participated in the 1996 Summer Games. *J Allergy Clin Immunol* 102(5):722–726, 1998.

Welle S, Jozefowicz R, Statt M: Failure of dehydroepiandrosterone to influence energy and protein metabolism in humans. *J Clin Endocrinol Metab* 71(5):1259–1264, 1990.

Williams MH: Nutrtional ergogenics in athletics. *J Sports Sci* 13:S63–S74, 1995.

Yamamoto DS: Cyclooxygenase-2: From arthritis treatment to new indications for the prevention and treatment of cancer. *Clin J Oncol Nurs* 7(1):21–29, 2003.

71 COMMON INJECTIONS IN SPORTS MEDICINE: GENERAL PRINCIPLES AND SPECIFIC TECHNIQUES

Francis G O'Connor, MD, FACSM

INTRODUCTION

- Injections are a common intervention provided by sports clinicians. Injections can be both diagnostic and therapeutic. If delivered properly and with sound indications, injections can be very rewarding for both the patient and the provider.

- This chapter details the indications, benefits, risks, and technique for administering common injections in sports medicine. These injections, while in most cases simple to administer, should be done only after proper training and appropriate supervision. Most injections are simple to learn (see one, do one, teach one); judgment on their use, however, takes time/effort to acquire.

TABLE 71-1   Classification of Synovial Fluid

CLASSIFICATION	APPEARANCE	WBC	PMNs%	CRYSTALS	CULTURE
Normal	Clear to straw colored	<150	<25	None	Negative
Noninflammatory	Yellow	<3000	<30	None	Negative
Inflammatory	Yellow or cloudy	3000–75,000	>50	None	Negative
Infectious	Yellow or purulent	50,000–200,000	>90	None	Positive
Crystal-induced	Cloudy, turbid	500–200,00	<90	Yes	Negative
Hemorrhagic	Red-brown	50–10,000	<50	No	Negative

SOURCE: O'Connell TX: Interpreting tests from joint aspirates, in Phenninger JL (ed.): *The Clinics Atlas of Office Procedures—Joint Injection Techniques:* vol. 5 (no. 4). December 2002.

INDICATIONS

- Injections/aspirations are indicated for both diagnosis and therapy.
  1. Diagnosis:
     a. Synovial fluid analysis to rule out infection, traumatic, rheumatic, or crystal-induced etiology (see Table 71-1).
     b. To perform a therapeutic trial to differentiate various etiologies
     c. Imaging studies
     d. Synovial biopsy
  2. Therapy:
     a. To remove tense effusions to relieve pain and improve function
     b. To remove blood or pus from a joint
     c. For injection of steroids and other intra-articular therapies
     d. For therapeutic lavage of joints

Risks/Complications (Turner and McKeag, 2002 (see Table 71-2)

- **Infection:** The risk of postinjection infection is extremely rare, on the order of one infection per 20,000 to 50,000 when sterile technique is used.
- **Tendon rupture:** Collagen atrophy and tendon rupture are rare but have been described in the literature. Injections into tendons should be avoided. In addition, injections into the synovial sheath or peritendinous region of major weight-bearing tendons (Achilles, patellar, and plantar fascia) should be done with caution, and the athlete protected from weight-bearing exercise for a period of 2 to 4 weeks.
- **Postinjection flare:** This entity is seen in 2 to 10% of patients. In this setting the patient actually gets worse in the immediate 6–12 h after an injection. The steroid postinjection flare is thought to be secondary to a local reaction to the microcrystalline steroid suspension and is self-limited. The postinjection flare has also been attributed to the preservative that accompanies the anesthetic. The postinjection flare may be treated with ice, activity modification, and a short-course of a *nonsteroidal anti-inflammatory drug* (NSAID). Patients with pain beyond 36 h should be evaluated for a septic joint.

- **Skin atrophy/depigmentation/hyperpigmentation:** When local steroid is applied to close to the surface of the skin, local atrophy as well as depigmentation/ hyperpigmentation can occur. These changes may be irreversible.
- **Hyperglycemia:** In some diabetics there may be short-term difficulties with glycemic control secondary to the local absorption of corticosteroid.
- **Cartilage degeneration:** Limit injections into a weight-bearing joint to no more than three injections per year, as there is some concern about weakening articular cartilage (Turner and McKeag, 2002; Pfenninger, 1994; Genovese, 1998).
- Injection of a steroid/anesthetic agent into a vein or artery.
- **Traumatic injection:** Possible to cause a pneumothorax, damage articular cartilage, local nerves, or soft tissue structures.
- Vasovagal reactions.

TABLE 71-2   Common Adverse Outcomes

COMPLICATION	ESTIMATED INCIDENCE (%)
Postinjection flare	2 to 10
Steroid arthropathy	0.8
Tendon rupture	<1
Facial flushing	<1
Skin atrophy, depigmentation	<1
Iatrogenic infectious arthritis	<0.001 to 0.072
Transient paresis of injected extremity	Rare
Hypersensitivity reaction	Rare
Asymptomatic pericapsular calcification	43
Acceleration of cartilage attrition	Unknown

SOURCE: Gray RG, Gottleib NL: Intra-articular corticosteroids: An updated assessment. *Clin Orthop* 177:253–263, 1983.

CONTRAINDICATIONS

- Cellulitis or broken skin over the needle entry site would increase the risk for infection.
- Anticoagulation or a coagulopathy is a relative contraindication and should be individualized.
- Intra-articular fractures are a contraindication to a corticosteroid injection.
- Septic effusion of a bursa or a periarticular structure.
- Lack of response to prior injections.
- More than three prior injections in the last year to a weight bearing joint.
- Inaccessible joints, e.g., hip, spine, and sacroiliac joint.
- Joint prostheses.

GENERAL PRINCIPLES (White, 2002; Paluska, 2002)

- **Consent:** As there are inherent risks and complications associated with corticosteroid injections, informed consent should be obtained, witnessed, and documented.
- **Equipment:** Most injections are performed using an alcohol, chlorhexidene or povidone-iodine wipe; some authors recommend a sterile scrub before injecting into a large joint. Gloves are another area of controversy; as a rule I teach that sterile gloves are used for a joint and nonsterile gloves for soft tissue structures. Some advocate sterile gloves for all injections, while some authors prefer using the one sterile glove technique. In this technique the physician wears the sterile glove on the noninjecting hand to insure proper positioning after the local prep. Other equipment include the following:
  1. Povidone-iodine wipes or alcohol wipes
  2. Sterile or nonsterile gloves
  3. Sterile drapes: optional
  4. 21 to 27 gauge 1.5-in. needles for injection
  5. 18 to 20 gauge needles for aspirations
  6. 1- to 10-cc syringes for injections
  7. 3- to 50-cc syringes for aspirations
  8. Ethyl chloride surface coolant
  9. 1% lidocaine
  10. 0.5% bupivicaine
  11. 2 × 2 gauze sponges
  12. Band-Aids
  13. Access to equipment to treat severe allergic reactions: oxygen; epinephrine 1:1000; benadryl 25- to 50-mg *intramural* (IM); *advanced cardiac life support* (ACLS) equipment.
- **Anesthesia:** The three main uses of anesthesia include diminishing pain, aiding in diagnosis, and providing a

volume for corticosteroid injections. Although there are many local anesthetics, the two most commonly used are amide compounds, lidocaine, and bupivicaine.
  1. Lidocaine (xylocaine) is available commercially as a 0.5 to 2% concentration. The most commonly utilized is 1%; 2% may be used in small areas where a small volume is required. Time from injection to onset of effect is 1–2 min, with duration of action of approximately 1–2 h. The upper limit of dosing is 10 mL for 2% and 20 mL for 1%; above these levels side effects can be expected.
  2. Bupivicaine (marcaine) is available commercially in 0.25–0.5% concentrations. Time from injection to onset of effect is 5 to 30 min, with duration of action of approximately 8 h. The upper limit of dosing is 30 mL for 0.5% and 60 mL for 0.25%; above these levels side effects can be expected.
  3. Side effects to include anaphylaxis can occur; resuscitation equipment should be available.
  4. An alternative to a local anesthestic injection is topical ethyl chloride. When utilized, however, spray lightly to avoid cold injury and secondary skin changes.
- **Corticosteroids:** Corticosteroids are commonly utilized in musculoskeletal medicine. The corticosteroid treats the local inflammatory response, and not the clinical problem. Steroids have both mineralocorticoid and glucocorticoid effects. The mineralocorticoid effects modify salt and water balance, while the glucocorticoid effect suppresses the inflammatory response. The ideal choice is to use a medication that maximizes the anti-inflammatory effect. Steroids also differ in their solubilities, potencies, and duration of action (see Table 71-3). The duration of the effect is thought to vary inversely with the drug's solubility. Shorter acting agents tend to have a lower incidence of postinjection flare. In general, higher solubility agents (e.g., celestone, dexamethasone, and methylprednisilone) tend to better for soft tissues, while lower solubility agents (e.g., triamcinolone hexacetonide) tend to favor joint injections. Selected dosing is found in Table 71-4.
- **Technique**
  1. Patient: The patient should be in a comfortable position, preferably sitting or lying down. The most important aspect of the patient's position, however, is that the physician injecting is comfortable and can easily identify anatomic landmarks and administer the injection.
  2. Be prepared: Have all your equipment ready so that you can move quickly. Have your combination of steroid and anesthetic already drawn up and ready to go. Remember to use separate needles for drawing up different agents.

TABLE 71-3 Relative Potencies and Solubilities of Corticosteroids

CORTICOSTEROID	RELATIVE ANTI-INFLAMMATORY POTENCY	EQUIVALENT DOSE (mg)	SOLUBILITY	CONCENTRATION (mg/mL)
Short-acting				
Cortisone	0.8	25	NA	25, 50
Hydrocortisone	1	20	0.002	25
Intermediate-acting				
Triamcinolone Hexacetonide	5	4	0.0002	20
Methylprednisilone	5	4	0.001	20, 40, 80
Long-acting				
Dexamethasone Sodium Phosphate	25	0.6	0.01	4, 8
Betamethasone	25	0.6	NA	6

SOURCE: Genovese MC: Joint and soft tissue injection: A useful adjuvant to systemic and local treatment. *Postgrad Med* 103(2):125–134, 1998.

3. Identify structure: Put the skin under traction and identify anatomic landmarks. If needed the skin can be marked with a fingernail, a retracted end of a ballpoint pen, or ink.
4. Aseptic technique: Using nonsterile gloves the area may be cleansed with alcohol, povidone, or betadine. When entering a joint, a sterile prep is recommended.
5. Local anesthesia: The practice of using a preinjection anesthetic varies among practitioners. Some authors will only use local anesthesia when using needles larger than 25 gauge. Prior to a joint prep and injection, I will cleanse only with alcohol swabs and use lidocaine to raise a wheal and numb the tract I am planning to inject. In those cases where I'm not going in a joint, I like to use an assistant to give a quick spray of surface coolant prior to my introduction of the injection needle.
6. Needle insertion: The needle should be an extension of the finger and inserted quickly and preferably perpendicular to the skin. When introducing the agent, aspirate first to insure you are not in the artery or vein. Aspirated contents should be sent for appropriate analysis. The patient should also not be complaining of paresthesias, which would prompt needle repositioning.

TABLE 71-4 Recommended Corticosteroid and Lidocaine Dosages for Injections

SITE OF INJECTION	DOSE OF 1% LIDOCAINE (mL)	DOSE OF TRIAMCINOLONE (mg)	DOSE OF BETAMETHASONE (mg)
DeQuervain's	1–2	40	6
Carpal tunnel	0.5–1	40	6
Trigger finger	1	20	3
Tennis elbow	0.5–1	40	6
Subacromial space	6–8	40	6
Glenohumeral	6–8	40–60	6–9
Acromioclavicular	1–2	40	6
Plantar fascia	1–2	40	6
Anserine bursa	2–3	40	6
Trochanteric bursa	4–5	40–60	6–9
Intraarticular knee	4–6	40–60	6–9
Morton's neuroma	1–2	20–40	3–6
Myofascial	1–2	NA	NA
Iliotibial band	1–2	20–40	3–6
Ankle	2–3	40	6

SOURCE: Stankus SJ: Inflammation and the role of anti-inflammatory medications, in Lillegard WA, Butcher JD, Rucker KS (eds.): *Handbook of Sports Medicine,* 2nd ed. Boston, MA, Butterwoth-Heineman, 1999.

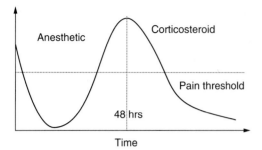

FIG. 71-1 Pain relief and injection therapy.

7. Delivering the steroid: When in a joint the bolus technique can be used; there should be a free flow with no resistance. When injecting near a ligament or tendon some authors recommend a peppering technique. When injecting in a tendon sheath, the ideal injection demonstrates a free low of fluid that fills the sheath. Prior to injection, the patient can be asked to move the affected tendon; if the needle moves this suggests that the clinician is in the tendon and the needle should be backed up.

• **Postprocedure care:** Any afterpain can be relieved with ice or taking a short course of a nonsteroidal anti-inflammatory medication. The patient should be informed that the anti-inflammatory effect of the corticosteroid may not kick-in for 48 to 72 h, and that the anesthetic will quickly wear-off (see Fig. 71-1). It is recommended that strenuous activity be avoided for a period of 10 days to 2 weeks following an injection. Rehabilitative exercise, however, may be commenced within 2 to 3 days.

• **Evidence-based medicine evaluation of steroid injections:** There is currently insufficient quality data to provide a definitive answer on the efficacy of steroid injections. New investigations that are methodologically sound are needed to measure outcomes of steroid injections (McNabb, 2000).

SPECIFIC INJECTIONS (Pfenninger, 1994; Klippel and Dieppe, 1997; Anderson, 1994; Saunders and Cameron, 1997; Safran, 1998)

• **Subacromial space**
  1. Indications: For the relief of pain in subacromial impingement syndrome
  2. Clinical anatomy/Landmarks: Useful landmarks include the *acromioclavicular* (AC) joint, the posterior glenohumeral joint, and the posterolateral corner of the acromion.
  3. Technique: This injection is most easily accomplished with the patient in a seated position. The arm should be in a relaxed position, dependent position; the other arm may be used to provide traction on the shoulder to be injected. The posterior edge of the acromion is palpated, with a recess identified inferior to this edge providing the portal for the injection. The needle is inserted bevel-up in a slightly cephalad angulation, pointed to the AC joint. If bony resistance is felt the needle is most probably in the acromion, and the needle should be redirected inferiorly. Insertion depth is approximately 1 in.
  4. Needle size and dosage: One milliliter of corticosteroid in combination with 6 to 10 mL of long and short acting anesthetics. A 22-gauge long 1½-in. needle is recommended when injecting a large volume.

• **Glenohumeral joint**
  1. Indications: Inflammatory or degenerative arthritis, adhesive capsulitis
  2. Clinical anatomy/Landmarks: Coracoid process, humeral head, and the acromial process of the scapula
  3. Technique: The seated position is most comfortable for this injection. The coracoid process is identified inferomedial to the AC joint, with the anterior glenohumeral joint is inferior to the coracoid and appreciated by internally and externally rotating the shoulder. At the same time the posterior glenohumeral joint can be appreciated. The technique is the same as the subacromial injection; however, the needle is now aimed to the coracoid process. The depth of penetration is approximately 1 in.
  4. Needle size and dosage: A 25-gauge 1½-inch needle is recommended; one mL of corticosteroid can be combined with 5 to 10 mL of anesthetic.

• **Acromioclavicular joint**
  1. Indications: Acromioclavicular degenerative disease
  2. Clinical anatomy/Landmarks: Important landmarks are the clavicle and acromion. The AC joint can be conveniently located by abducting the shoulder.
  3. Technique: The injection is conveniently administered by having the patient in a seated position. The injection is most easily accomplished by coming from above with the needle directed inferiorly. An insertion depth of ⅜ to ½ in. is required. A preinjection radiograph of the angle of the AC joint can be useful.
  4. Needle size and dosage: ½- to 1-in. 25-gauge needle is appropriate; 0.5 mL each of anesthetic and corticosteroid is adequate.

- **Lateral tennis elbow**
  1. Indications: Lateral tennis elbow that fails to improve with conservative therapy
  2. Clinical anatomy/Landmarks: Key landmarks include the radial head, appreciated by pronation and supination of the elbow, and the humeral lateral epicondyle. The most common location of tennis elbow is at the extensor *carpi radialis brevis* origin, which is one fingerbreadth inferior and medial to the lateral epicondyle.
  3. Technique: The injection can be administered in a supine or seated position. If seated, the elbow should be comfortably resting at 90° with the forearm supinated. The area of maximal tenderness is identified, and the needle is inserted at an oblique angle to infiltrate the soft tissues over the extensor aponeurosis. There should be little resistance to the injection; if encountered the needle should be withdrawn until there is little resistance to flow.
  4. Needle size and dosage: A 1-in. 25-gauge needle is recommended; 0.5 mL of corticosteroid should be mixed with 1 to 2 mL of anesthetic.
- **DeQuervain's tenosynovitis**
  1. Indications: This disorder is caused by an inflammation and swelling of the tendons of the abductor pollicis longus and the extensor pollicis brevis at the level of the radial styloid process. Patients who fail to improve with NSAIDs and wrist support may be candidates for an injection.
  2. Clinical anatomy/Landmarks: The anatomic snuffbox is the anatomic landmark. The anterior border is the first dorsal compartment of the wrist (abductor pollicis longus and extensor pollicis brevis) and the posterior border is the extensor pollicis longus tendon.
  3. Technique: This injection can be done in the seated or supine position, with the wrist in a vertical position, resting over a folded towel, with the thumb flexed. The point of maximal tenderness is identified, which is generally over the radial styloid. The needle is inserted bevel-up, directed in an oblique, cephalad angle, nearly parallel to the tendons. If the gap between the two tendons can be appreciated, the needle should be placed in this gap. When the needle is approximately $1/4$ in., an attempt should be made to aspirate, and then gently push the plunger. If there is resistance, the needle should be pulled back, and the process repeated.
  4. Needle size and dosage: 0.5- to 1-in., 25- to 27-gauge needle; 0.5-mL anesthetic and 0.5 mL corticosteroid
- **Carpal tunnel syndrome**
  1. Indications: Carpal tunnel syndrome
  2. Clinical anatomy/Landmarks: Key landmarks include the palmaris longus and flexor carpi radialis tendons, the distal wrist crease and the median nerve. The median nerve lies deep to and between the tendons of the palmaris longus and the flexor carpi radialis at the wrist.
  3. Technique: The injection can be given in the supine position or the seated position. The dorsum of the hand should rest on a folded towel. The needle is inserted just proximal to the distal wrist crease at a 45° angle just ulnar to the palmaris longus and angled toward the index finger. The needle may be felt to pop through the dense transverse carpal ligament. If pain or paresthesias are reported in the palm or fingertips during needle placement, the needle should be withdrawn and reangled prior to reinsertion. Depth of penetration should be approximately $1/2$ in.
  4. Needle size and dosage: A 25- to 27-gauge needle may be used, with 0.5 mL of steroid and a similar dose volume of anesthetic.
- **Trigger finger**
  1. Indications: Trigger finger/stenosing tensosynovitis
  2. Clinical anatomy/Landmarks: The key landmark is the first annular pulley. This condition is secondary to an inflammation and swelling of the flexor tendon of the flexor digitorum superficiales. Repetitive irritation leads to a nodule in this tendon, which becomes obstructed as the nodule passes beneath the pulley, which is proximal to the *metacarpal-phalangeal* (MP) joint.
  3. Technique: The patient may be administered the injection in the seated or supine position. The site for the injection is the distal palmar crease, just proximal to the MP joint. The needle is inserted bevel-up, directed at an oblique angle parallel with the tendon, toward the fingertips. When an increase in resistance is felt, at approximately $1/4$-in. depth, the plunger should be gently pushed. If there is resistance, the needle may be in the tendon, and the needle should be slightly withdrawn, aspirate, and reinjected.
  4. Needle size and dosage: A 25- to 27-gauge needle may be used; a preparation of 0.5 mL corticosteroid with 0.5 mL of anesthetic can be mixed, with half to all of this suspension injected.
- **Trochanteric bursitis**
  1. Indications: Recalcitrant trochanteric bursitis.
  2. Clinical anatomy/Landmarks: The key landmark is the greater trochanteric prominence; most bursitis is posterosuperior to this prominence. This prominence is best appreciated with the patient in a lateral decubitus position.
  3. Technique: The point of maximal tenderness is palpated. The needle should be inserted

perpendicular to the skin; and slowly advanced to the greater trochanter, depth of penetration may vary from $\frac{1}{2}$ to $1\frac{1}{2}$ in. (up to 4–5 in. if there is significant adipose tissue). If paresthesias are appreciated the needle should be withdrawn and reinserted laterally. Once bone is appreciated, the needle should be slightly withdrawn, aspiration performed, and then gentle *peppering* of the bursa is performed.
4. Needle size and dosage: A 21- to 23-gauge needle, $1\frac{1}{2}$-in. long should be used; 1 mL of corticosteroid with 3 to 5 mL of local anesthetic.

• **Knee joint**
1. Indications: Inflammatory or degenerative arthritis
2. Clinical anatomy/Landmarks: Patellar tendon and medial and lateral joint lines
3. Technique: Injections are most easily administered through the lateral joint line recess just lateral to the patellar tendon. This injection can be accomplished in the seated position or in the supine position with the knee flexed to approximately 90°. The portal for injection should be identified as lateral and inferior to the patellar tendon border at the level of the joint line. The needle is directed toward the center of the knee, medially, posteriorly, and slightly cephalad. Depth of insertion is approximately 1 in. One should be careful to insure needle clearance of the fat pad, and avoid injecting the anterior cruciate ligament; there should be a free flow to the injection, with any resistance prompting needle repositioning. An alternative injection technique is to inject the patient in the supine position in the suprapatellar space. This space is most commonly reached by identifying a portal one fingerbreadth superior and one fingerbreadth lateral to the superolateral aspect of the patella.
4. Needle size and dosage: A 22–25-gauge, $1\frac{1}{2}$-in. needle is recommended; 1 mL of corticosteroid should be mixed with 2 to 3 mL of anesthetic.

• **Illiotibial band syndrome**
1. Indications: Recalcitrant illiotibial band friction syndrome
2. Clinical anatomy/Landmarks: The key landmark is the lateral femoral epicondyle, which is the site of repetitive irritation. The bursa lies deep to the illiotibial band just above the lateral condyle of the femur.
3. Technique: The injection may be performed in a seated position or in a lateral decubitus position. The knee should be flexed to 90°, and the maximal point of tenderness identified; the intent is to inject between the epicondyle and the illiotibial band. The skin is entered to the point of maximal tenderness

and angled posteriorly and slightly medially. The needle is inserted to a depth of $\frac{1}{4}$- to $\frac{3}{8}$-in. just above the periosteum. If bone is contacted, withdraw the needle very slightly, aspirate, and then inject. Additionally it is important not to inject the *iliotibial* (IT) band itself; if resistance is felt with injection, withdraw, redirect the needle, aspirate, and inject.
4. Needle size and dosage: A 25- to 27-gauge, 1-in. needle is recommended; 0.5 mL of corticosteroid with 0.5- to 1-mL of anesthetic.

• **Pes anserine bursitis**
1. Indications: Pes anserine bursitis
2. Clinical anatomy/Landmarks: Medial aspect of the proximal tibia, where the sartorious, gracilis, and semitendinosus insert. The Pes is identified by making the patient strongly flex the knee against resistance. The bursa is found as an area of tenderness deep to the insertion.
3. Technique: This injection can be administered in the supine or seated position; I prefer the seated position. The objective of the injection is to slip the needle between the tibia and the pes tendons. The skin should be entered just lateral to the point of maximal tenderness, with the needle angled posteriorly and medially. Depth of insertion is approximately $\frac{1}{4}$ in. If resistance is felt with the injection, withdraw, redirect the needle, aspirate, and inject.
4. Needle size and dosage: A 25-gauge needle, 1-in. long is recommended; 0.5 mL of corticosteroid with 0.5 to 1 mL of anesthetic.

• **Ankle joint**
1. Indications: Diagnostic injection for synovitis; chronic capsulitis. Can be used to treat soft tissue impingement.
2. Clinical anatomy/Landmarks: There is a readily identifiable hollow between the medial malleolus, and the articulation between the tibia and the talus. This area is readily located just medial to the anterior tibial tendon.
3. Technique: The patient may be seated or lying supine with a towel beneath the knee. Distraction of the ankle can be accomplished by an assistant. The skin is entered just medial to the anterior tibial tendon in the anteromedial recess; depth of insertion is approximately $\frac{1}{2}$ to 1 in.
4. Needle size and dosage: A 25-gauge needle, 1- to $1\frac{1}{2}$-in. long may be used; 0.5 mL of corticosteroid may be injected with 3 to 5 mL of anesthetic.

• **Plantar fascia**
1. Indications: Recalcitrant plantar fasciitis
2. Clinical anatomy/Landmarks: Key landmarks include the medial calcaneal tubercle and the

junction between the skin of the sole of foot and the skin of the lower extremity.

3. Technique: This examination is best administered with the patient in the supine position. The needle is inserted medial to lateral toward the point of maximal tenderness, which is generally at the plantar insertion into the medial calcaneal tubercle. Avoid injecting through the plantar fad pad as this may induce fat pad atrophy. If pain is felt radiating across the heel or into the arch, or there is excessive resistance, withdraw, change the angle slightly, and reinsert.

4. Needle size and dosage: A 25- to 27-gauge needle may be used, 1- to $1^{1}/_{2}$-in. long; 1 mL of corticosteroid may be injected with 1 to 2 mL of anesthetic.

• **Morton's neuroma**

1. Indications: Morton's neuroma is thought to be the result of perineural fibrosis of an interdigital nerve.

2. Clinical anatomy/Landmarks: Key are the metatarsal heads.

3. Technique: The point of maximal discomfort should be identified between the metatarsal heads; the neuroma is typically between and slightly plantar to the metatarsal heads. The patient should be placed in the supine position with a pillow under the knee so that the foot can be slightly plantar flexed. The nerve is approached from a dorsal approach, with the needle entering between the metatarsal heads, advanced perpendicular through the transverse tarsal ligament. The depth of insertion is approximately $^{1}/_{2}$-in. A giving way can be felt as the needle passes through the ligament.

4. Needle size and dosage: A 25-gauge 1-in. needle is appropriate; 0.5 mL of corticosteroid with 1 to 2 mL of local anesthetic.

• **Myofascial trigger points**

1. Indications: Diagnosis and treatment of myofascial trigger points

2. Clinical anatomy/Landmarks: Dependent on location of trigger points; knowledge of local anatomy is recommended, as well as knowledge of common trigger point sites and their referral patterns.

3. Technique: Trigger points are often palpable as fusiform firm nodules running parallel to the fibers in a muscle. The nodule should be identified and trapped with the fingers of the nondominant hand. After a sterile prep, the skin is penetrated in a perpendicular fashion with the needle in to the center of the trigger point. Occasionally a local twitch response may be noted, where the muscle twitches as the center of the trigger point is entered.

4. Needle size and dosage: A 25- to 27-gauge needle, 1- to $1^{1}/_{2}$-in. is used; 1 to 5 mL of anesthetic is used for injection.

REFERENCES

Anderson BC: Office orthopedics for primary care. Philadelphia, PA, W.B. Saunders, 1994.

Genovese MC: Joint and soft tissue injection: a useful adjuvant to systemic and local treatment. *Postgraduate Med* 103(2):125–134, 1998.

Klippel JH, Dieppe PA: Practical rheumatology. Baltimore, MD, Mosby, 1997.

McNabb JW: Evidence-based medicine evaluation of steroid injections, in *Joint Injections*. Dallas, TX, AAFP Scientific Assembly Monograph, 2000.

Paluska AS: Indications, contraindications, and overview for aspirating or injecting a joint or related structure, in Phenninger JL (ed.): *The Clinics Atlas of Office Procedures—Joint Injection Techniques:* vol. 5 (no. 4). December 2002.

Pfenninger JL: Joint and soft tissue aspiration and injection, in Pfenninger JL, Fowler GC (eds.): *Procedures for Primary Care Physicians*. St. Louis, MO, Mosby, 1994.

Safran MR: Injections, in Safran MR, McKeag DB, Van Camp SP (eds.): *Manual of Sports Medicine*. Philadelphia, PA, Lippincott-Raven Publishers, 1998.

Saunders S, Cameron G: *Injection Techniques in Orthopedic and Sports Medicine*. Philadelphia, PA, W.B. Saunders, 1997.

Turner JL, McKeag DB: Complications of joint aspirations and injections, in Phenninger JL (ed.): *The Clinics Atlas of Office Procedures—Joint Injection Techniques:* vol. 5 (no. 4). December 2002.

White RD: Supplies and equipment needed for joint injection, in Phenninger JL (ed.): *The Clinics Atlas of Office Procedures—Joint Injection Techniques:* vol. 5 (no. 4): December 2002.

72 FOOTWEAR AND ORTHOTICS

Eric Magrum, PT OCS FAAOMPT
Jay Dicharry, MPT CSCS

ORTHOTICS

INTRODUCTION

• Prescription custom foot orthoses are frequently used as part of a management strategy for the treatment of various lower quarter injuries in the athlete.

• Significant success treating many common lower quarter injuries with orthotic intervention has been shown. James reported 78% of runners were able to return to prior level of running following a knee injury with orthotic management (James, Bates, and

Osternig, 1978). Donatelli reported 96% of patients with knee pain, ankle pain, shin splints, or chondromalacia experienced pain relief and 70% were able to return to prior level of activity (Donatelli et al, 1988). Gross, in a large study, reported 76% of long distance runners had complete recovery or substantial improvement in a variety of lower quarter injuries with orthotic management (Gross, Davlin, and Evanski, 1991). More recently both Nigg (Nigg, Nurse, and Stefanyshyn, 1999) and Nawoczenski (Nawoczenski, Cook, and Saltzman, 1995) agree that at least 70% of runners with lower extremity symptoms will show symptom reduction with orthotic use.

GOALS OF ORTHOTIC MANAGEMENT

- The classic balanced foot orthosis is aimed to allow the subtalar joint to function near and around its neutral position by maintaining the angular anatomical relationships of the forefoot to the rearfoot and the rearfoot to the ground; and control functional pathomechanics in the lower quarter (Foot and Ankle, 2002).
- An orthotic device should alter foot function with the expectation that it will control excessive movement of the foot through the stance phase of gait, through stimulation of the somatosensory system, to promote overall biomechanical efficiency and reduce abnormal tissue stress (Valmassy and Subotnick, 1999; Cornwall and McPoil, 2003).

INDICATIONS

- Numerous clinicians and authors have proposed various indications for the rationale to prescribe custom biomechanical foot orthoses.
  1. Support and correction of rearfoot and forefoot intrinsic deformities (Foot and Ankle, 2002)
  2. Reduce the frequency of lower quarter injuries by altering applied tissue stresses. (James, Bates, and Osternig, 1978; Donatelli et al, 1988; Gross, Davlin, and Evanski, 1991; Gross and Napoli, 1993)
  3. Support or control *range of motion* (ROM) (Nawoczenski, Cook, and Saltzman, 1995; Cornwall and McPoil, 2003; Eng and Pierrynowski, 1993; Nawoczenski, Cook, and Saltzman, 1998; MacLean, 2001; Tillman et al, 2003)
  4. Treatment of postural dysfunction caused by foot abnormalities (Dannanberg and Guiliano, 1999)
  5. Improve sensory feedback and proprioception (Nigg, Nurse, and Stefanyshyn, 1999; Cornwall and McPoil, 2003; Nigg, 2001)
  6. Dissipation of pathologic ground reaction forces, improved shock absorption (Nigg, Nurse, and Stefanyshyn, 1999; MacLean, 2001; Shiba et al, 1995)
  7. Improve neuromuscular responses (Nigg, Nurse, and Stefanyshyn, 1999; MacLean, 2001)
  8. Redistribute plantar weight bearing forces (Cornwall and McPoil, 2003; Landorf and Keenan, 2000; Cornwall and McPoil, 1997; Postema et al, 1998)
  9. Improve lower extremity biomechanics/kinematics:
     a. Decrease amount of pronation, reduce maximal velocity of pronation, reduce time to maximal pronation, and decrease total rearfoot motion. (Cornwall and McPoil, 2003; Razeghi and Batt, 2000; Genova and Gross, 2000)
     b. Significant orthotic effects shown for rotation from heel contact to peak tibial internal rotation, and in the coupling relationship between tibial transverse rotation and calcaneal inversion/eversion. (Nawoczenski, Cook, and Saltzman, 1995; McPoil and Cornwall, 2000)

CLINICAL CONDITIONS

- **Patellofemoral dysfunction:** The successful use of custom foot orthoses as a primary therapeutic intervention for treatment of *patellofemoral pain syndrome* (PFPS) has been well documented in the recent literature. Biomechanical foot orthoses have been shown to be effective as a primary treatment intervention in patients with moderate to severe PFPS allowing faster return to sport. Orthotic management in conjunction with a specific biomechanical exercise program has also been demonstrated to be an effective means of treatment. A significant change in medial patellar glide was shown with a rearfoot medial posted semirigid device. (Donatelli et al, 1988; Gross and Napoli, 1993; Eng and Pierrynowski, 1993; Pitman and Jack, 2000; Way, 1999; Klingman, Liaos, and Hardin, 1997; Powers, Maffucci, and Hampton, 1995; American Physical Rehabilitation Network, 1984; Saxena and Haddad, 1998; Powers, Maffucci, and Hampton, 1995; Benard et al, 2002)
- **Plantar fasciitis:** Semirigid custom orthoses with forefoot medial post and medial longitudinal arch support have been shown to be effective in the management of plantar fasciitis to decrease tissue loading stress, (Benard et al, 2002; Gross, 2001; Sobel, Levitz, and Caselli, 1999; Lynch, Goforth, and Martin, 1998).
- **Posterior tibial tendon dysfunction:** Orthotic management has been described for all four stages based

on progressive deformity and loss of fore/rearfoot flexibility (Benard et al, 2002; Sobel, Levitz, and Caselli, 1999).

- **Lower quarter stress fracture:** Studies using various orthotic devices have been shown to decrease incidence of metatarsal, tibial, and femoral stress fractures with shock absorbing materials as a primary component of the device (Donatelli et al, 1988; Gross, Davlin, and Evanski, 1991; Wayne Decker and Stephen Albert, 2002; Ekenman et al, 2002; Finestone et al, 1999).
- **Medial tibial stress syndrome:** A recent review of the literature concluded there is some evidence for effective prevention of shin splints involving the use of shock-absorbing insoles. Previous reports have demonstrated significant clinical success treating shin splints with various orthotic devices. The American College of Foot and Ankle Orthopedics and Medicine's position statement is that custom foot orthoses can be used to treat the symptoms of shin splints and stabilize the etiology that causes the condition (James, Bates, and Osternig, 1978; Donatelli et al, 1988; Gross, Davlin, and Evanski, 1991; Benard et al, 2002; Thacker et al, 2002).
- **Pes cavus:** Orthotic management of the cavus foot has been described to include an elevated heel, reduced medial arch support, semi-rigid materials, first ray cut-out, and a forefoot valgus wedge. Preliminary data indicate 75% success with this type of device (Benard et al, 2002; Manoli and Graham, 2001).
- **Flexible flat foot:** The symptomatic adult hyperpronated foot has been shown to be effectively treated with various orthotic interventions regarding alleviating pain and deformity (Benard et al, 2002; Sobel, Levitz, and Caselli, 1999; Noll, 2001; Bowman, 1997; Kitaoka et al, 2002).
- **Hallux valgus/Hallux rigidus:** Custom orthoses have been clinically shown to redistribute weight, prevent excessive dorsiflexion forces and improve gait transition with pathology of the great toe (Benard et al, 2002; Churchill and Donley, 1998; Nawoczenski, 1999; Tang et al, 2002).
- **Ankle sprain:** Biomechanical foot orthoses have been shown to be beneficial in improving postural sway, balance, and decreased recurrent inversion ankle injury with jogging following an inversion ankle sprain (Orteza, Vogelbach, and Denegar, 1992; Guskiewicz and Perrin, 1996; Hardoel et al, 2003).
- Low back pain has been shown to be effectively treated with custom fabricated foot orthoses following a comprehensive gait evaluation to address the pathomechanical process to decrease the degree of pain and rate of reoccurrence (Dannanberg and Guiliano, 1999).

TYPES OF ORTHOTICS

- **Accommodative:** A device designed with a primary goal of conforming to the individual's foot allowing plantar-grade floor contact that permits forces to be distributed evenly to the foot (PFA, 1998). An accommodative device allows the foot to compensate and yields to abnormal foot forces. It is primarily prescribed to improve foot function and improve shock absorption for patients who are poor candidates for biomechanical devices secondary to congenital malformations, restrictions of foot or lower quarter motion, neuromuscular dysfunction, insensitive feet, or physiologic old age. Most devices are full length and total contact made of materials such as plastizote, spenco, pelite, sorbathane, *ethyl vinyl acetate* (EVA), and neoprene foam rubber.
- **Biomechanical:** A custom prescription device fabricated specifically to address pathomechanical components of a lower quarter condition by controlling and resisting abnormal compensatory foot forces (Benard et al, 2002). The prescription aspect of the device involves clinical decision making for type of materials to be utilized for rigidity, length of the device (full, metatarsal, or sulcus), degree of correction/posting, and depth of heel seat. Decision making should be based on a comprehensive evaluation of biomechanics and gait.
- **Temporary:** A device fabricated in the clinic primarily for the purpose of assessing the need/benefit for permanent device; unloading tissues for healing; or control hyperpronation. Common materials are aquaplast, or orthopedic felt medial buttress and navicular-sustentaculum tali support (Vicenzino et al, 2000).

SELECTION

- Specific aspects of subjective and objective examination guide clinical decision making for choosing the proper components of a prescription custom fabricated orthoses.
  1. Chief complaint/diagnosis including stage, intensity, severity, and nature of the disorder
  2. Control versus bias of subtalar motion
  3. Mobility of the rearfoot, forefoot, midfoot, first ray: hypermobile → normal → hypomobile
  4. Primary use of the orthoses. Street, sport, or dress shoe to be worn in helps to determine material selection and thickness. Specific sport and competition level also guide choice of components.
  5. Physiologic not chronological age; older patients tolerate semirigid devices better and younger patients tolerate more rigid management.

6. Need for shock absorption to dissipate ground reaction forces.
7. Weight of patient determines durometer (rigidity) of the orthotic.
8. Neurologic or anatomical abnormality helps to determine the need for accommodation with cutouts, pressure distribution modifications, and material selection.

EVALUATION

- Specific components of a lower quarter evaluation are required to develop a treatment plan including custom foot orthotics based on The American College of Foot and Ankle Orthopedics and Medicine (ACFAOM) practice guidelines:
  1. Assessment of ROM, quality of motion and position of the ankle, rearfoot, and rear to forefoot relationship
  2. Testing of specific lower quarter muscle strength
  3. Static stance position
  4. Leg length measurement
  5. Gait analysis
  6. Assessment of position, range, and quality of motion of other lower quarter structures including spine, hip/pelvis, knee complex, 5th ray, 1st ray, 1st *metatarsophalangeal* (MTP), 2–5th MTP joints, and *interphalangeal* (IP) joints (Benard et al, 2002).
- Numerous techniques have been used to capture the foot for fabrication of a custom orthoses (Benard et al, 2002). Plaster casting, preferable when capturing rearfoot to forefoot relationship, is of prime importance for fabrication of a functional device (Laughlin et al, 2002). Weight bearing measures of a loaded foot to determine forefoot posting have been proven reliable and further investigation into clinical application needs to be evaluated for orthotic prescription and fabrication (Cummings and Higbie, 1997). Neutral suspension casting with the foot positioned by holding the sulcus of the 4th and 5th toes obtained in prone or supine is the preferred method for a functional prescription foot orthoses (Benard et al, 2002).
  1. **Plaster cast:** The goal is to capture the relationship of the forefoot to rear foot and reproduce the ideal position of the foot in midstance just prior to heel off.
  2. **Compressive foam box:** Partial weightbearing technique most appropriate for accommodative devices—with the benefits of simplicity of use/clean up; but typically provides an inconsistent representation of forefoot relationship (Benard et al, 2002; Langer, 1996).
  3. **Computer imaging/scanning:** Another technique to capture the contour and shape of the foot for orthotic fabrication where the device is milled from image or a positive model of the foot is created. The benefits of an imaging system are exactness of forefoot to rearfoot relationship for posting, created in partial or nonweightbearing and simplicity of use—with the drawback of expense (Benard et al, 2002).

REQUIREMENTS

- Requirements for successful orthotic intervention are based on patient/condition specific goals developed following a comprehensive subjective and objective evaluation as stated previously. The device must have certain components to increase treatment success and compliance.
  1. Conform precisely to all contours of foot especially heel, calcaneal, and forefoot inclinations
  2. Rigid enough to maintain shape, contour, and angular relationships
  3. Control abnormal motion, allow normal motion, and provide proper sequencing/timing of motion
  4. Improve muscle function
  5. Able to withstand stress and wear
  6. Comfortable to assure compliance
  7. Adjustable
  8. Minimum length ends at least proximal to metatarsal heads
  9. Narrow enough to fit in shoes and allow 1st and 5th rays function

DEVICE ASSESSMENT/USE

- Once the custom orthosis has been fabricated, evaluation of the patient wearing the device must be completed based on goals of management from the initial biomechanical and gait evaluation.
  1. Subjective response
  2. Treadmill/track for 10–20 min
  3. Areas of irritation
  4. Gait changes/corrections
  5. Static correction of calcaneal position
  6. Develop a progressive wear schedule: Typically 1 h first day; gradually increase use 60 min/day; athletic use following tolerance of 4–6 h general use
  7. Proper shoes to work with device are extremely important to maximize the benefits of the device. Some of those basic shoewear components are a stable heel counter, removable insert, and deeper heel cup.

MODIFICATIONS

- Modifications to the device can be made based on specific goals for management of the lower quarter pathology, from the biomechanical evaluation and assessment of the patient using the device.
  1. Metatarsal head cut-out to accommodate a rigid plantar flexed 1st ray
  2. Heel cushioning for increased shock absorption in a rigid cavus foot
  3. Metatarsal pads to redistribute weight from 2–4th metatarsal heads to 1st and 5th with metatarsalgia or Morton's neuroma
  4. Morton's extension to redistribute weight from 2nd to 1st metatarsal
  5. Rigid forefoot extension to limit mobility of great toe with *degenerative joint disease* (DJD) or turf toe
  6. Toe crests can be added to prevent the toes from sliding back over the insole of the shoe and prevent clawing.

CONTROVERSIES/CONCLUSIONS/ FURTHER RESEARCH

- In a review of the literature Pratt judged 40 orthotic related articles using Sackett's "levels of evidence" criterion for scientific merit, and concluded that the literature is rather weak with only one achieving a level of 2 and none achieving a level 1 qualification (Pratt, 2000).
- There are several different classification systems of evaluating foot type that have shown poor inter-rater reliability and measurement accuracy questioning the practical usefulness and validity (Razeghi and Batt, 2000; Finestone et al, 1999; Payne and Chuter, 2001; Ball and Afheldt, 2002*a*).
- There is significant debate whether functional kinematics and pathomechanics of the foot can be based principally on morphology. Mechanisms causing lower quarter injuries are poorly understood with very few adequate randomized controlled studies relating specific foot type or pathomechanics with injury incidence (Razeghi and Batt, 2000; Payne and Chuter, 2001; Ball and Afheldt, 2002*a*).
- Recent research has debated the assumptions that the rearfoot achieves subtalar joint neutral position near midstance in gait and the functional significance of rearfoot neutral (Cornwall and McPoil, 2003; Razeghi and Batt, 2000; Ball and Afheldt, 2002*a*; 2002*b*).
- Studies have shown that static measurements in a classic biomechanical examination are poor predictors of dynamic foot motion (Cornwall and McPoil, 2003;

Payne and Chuter, 2001; Ball and Afheldt, 2002*b*; Heiderscheit, Hamill, and Tiberio, 2001).
- Research evaluating orthotic effectiveness in gait has substantial inadequacies including—various biomechanical assessment tools for gait analysis; nonstandardized orthotic device or footwear; modifications to shoe counter; motion analysis markers on shoe or skin; differences in calibration of equipment; and anecdotal descriptions of gait changes (Cornwall and McPoil, 2003; Landorf and Keenan, 2000; Payne and Chuter, 2001; Ball and Afheldt, 2002*b*).
- The literature demonstrates a lack of controlled studies consistently with poor methodology including variable orthotic prescription, patient presentation, fabrication of the orthoses, and outcome measurement tools (Landorf and Keenan, 2000; Payne and Chuter, 2001).
- Overall throughout the orthotic literature there is a significant amount of inconclusive or conflicting data (Landorf and Keenan, 2000; Ball and Afheldt, 2002*a*; 2002*b*).
- The review of the literature highlights the fact that the current research can be greatly improved upon with further randomized controlled trials for specific measurable clinical outcomes to more effectively prescribe a custom orthotic device for treatment and prevention of lower quarter injuries in our patients and athletes.
- A recent trend in the research proposes orthotic intervention to influence lower quarter dynamic function by increased afferent feedback from cutaneous receptors in the foot; and minimizing muscle activity with the concept combining biomechanical control and proprioceptive feedback with custom fabricated biomechanical orthotics to reduce tissue stress. As with previous work more randomized controlled research must be completed to justify these hypotheses (Nigg, Nurse, and Stefanyshyn, 1999; Nawoczenski, Cook, and Saltzman, 1995; Nigg, 2001; Razeghi and Batt, 2000).

FOOTWEAR

INTRODUCTION

- The running shoe industry changes rapidly with constant revisions and updates to shoe models. Many new marketing techniques have emerged to influence the consumer into believing that one brand is better than another. Clinicians will have better results recommending types of shoes based on construction and features over specific model designations.

- The basis of injury risk lies within the balance of intrinsic and extrinsic control. Intrinsic factors represent each specific athlete's alignment, stability, flexibility, and imbalances that are unique to him or her. Extrinsic factors include surfaces, weather, training programs, and footwear. The intrinsic and extrinsic factors are dependent variables of each other. To assess proper footwear selection, the athlete's intrinsic factors must be assessed to determine the best functional outcome (O'Connor and Wilder, 2001).
- Incorrect footwear choices can exacerbate or cause lower extremity dysfunction, while ideal footwear can help in prevention or even speed healing caused by decreased tissue stress on impaired structures (Stacoff, Kalin, and Stussi, 1991; Nigg et al, 2003; Wakeling, Pascual, and Nigg, 2002; Roberts and Gordon, 2001; Hennig and Milani, 2001; Barnes and Smith, 1994).
- Different shoe constructions in the same runner result in significant differences in peak pressures distribution measured both in and outside the shoe (Sharkey et al, 1995).
- The goal of any shoe/foot interface is to provide cushioning and increase functional stability about the foot's tri-planar motions of pronation and supination throughout the stance phase of gait and provide proper support for the propulsion phase of the gait cycle (Barnes and Smith, 1994).

SHOE CONSTRUCTION AND ANATOMY

- **Upper:** Functional unit is the heel counter. This is a plastic molding that wraps around the heel to control pronation at heal strike. Achilles tab cut-out in the rear of the shoe is made to decrease friction on the Achilles complex. The upper is usually made of highly breathable fabric to minimize heat build up. This may be reinforced by Gore-Tex or similar fabric for water resistance.
- **Lacing:** Round laces slide through holes in the upper more easily than flat laces and reduce pressure points in the dorsum of the foot. Various lacing techniques are available to minimize pressure or increase stability and tension on the foot.
- **Midsole:** Functional part of the shoe. The midsole is usually made up of a mixture of EVA and polyurethane. EVA has the advantage of being light in weight and available in multiple densities so that the manufacturer can manipulate the amount of support for a given shoe type. Polyurethane is heavier, but is longer lasting. Most shoes use a combination of the two to achieve the

desired balance between weight and cushioning. Most shoe companies have developed a trademark insert such as Air, Gel, Grid, Hydroflow, Torsion, Rollerbar, and Adeprene. The goal of these is to increase cushioning, dissipate stress forces, and increase durability, while keeping weight low. Most companies have reinforced areas around the inserts to increase stability where needed.

- **Lastings:** The lasting sits on top of the midsole and is glued or stitched depending on the control requirements. The following are types of lastings: Board-favors motion control. Slip or California-favors cushion and flexibility. Combination-board last rearfoot, and slip last in the forefoot.
- **Insole or Sockliner:** Usually a thin layer of cushion material, mostly to smooth the surface of the foot. The insole does not provide any functional stability to the shoe and usually breaks down in its cushioning properties with 1–2 weeks. This should be removable for replacement with over-the-counter insert or custom orthoses.
- **Outsole:** Most current shoe models are a mixture of carbon rubber for firm support and durability, and softer blown rubber for increased cushioning. Some manufactures utilize a flare in the heel. This can help to increase stability in the rear foot but can also increase the torque moving torsionally through the foot and increase pronation.
- **Last or shape:** This is different from the lasting and is not a separate component of the shoe, but the design element on which the shoe is built. A curved last will encourage pronation, a straight last will provide additional stability, and a semicurved will provide elements of both. (see Table 72-1)

ANATOMICAL DETERMINANTS

- The selection of footwear for the athlete needs to be based on a comprehensive foot and lower quarter assessment to recommend the proper balance of control versus cushion (Frey, 1997).

TABLE 72-1 Three Major Running Shoe Categories

SHOCK ABSORBTION	STABILITY	MOTION CONTROL
Slip or California lasting	Combination lasting	Board lasting
Soft midsole	Medium density midsole	Firm midsole
Curve last	Semi curved last	Straight last
Blown rubber	Mix (blown and carbon rubber)	Carbon rubber

- Foot structure plays a significant role in the quantity of force transmitted to bone and soft tissues (Barnes and Smith, 1994).
- The rigid arch of a cavus foot, while stable, passes on a significant amount of stress up the kinetic chain (Barnes and Smith, 1994). This foot should be shod with a slip lasting, curved shaped last with a soft midsole and no or lateral posting (Foot and Ankle, 2002*b*; Running Course, 2002).
- The flexible or planus foot dissipates considerable vertical force loads inside the foot structure, but needs additional stability control from the shoe to perform (Barnes and Smith, 1994). This foot type would benefit from increased medial support with a firm heel counter, multidensity midsole, and medial heel stabilizer. As the medial posting extends upward toward the toes, the amount of forefoot control increases as well. This foot should be in a straight last (shape) shoe with a board lasting (Foot and Ankle, 2002*b*; Running Course, 2002).
- The athlete's foot type should guide your recommendation toward the ideal last configuration with the goal of increasing shock absorption of the cavus (high) hypomobile arch, increasing stability of the planus (low) arch, or promoting the mechanics of the neutral foot.
- A basic foot assessment is a good starting point. The *wet foot* test has the athlete wet the foot and place it on an absorbent surface to observe the high or low arch alignment of the foot. This test is easily replicated and is a good starting point for foot wear selection; however, several literature references advocate dynamic assessment observing both walking and running gait since a significant proportion of runners do not observe a normal heel–toe gait, but a forefoot contact (O'Connor and Wilder, 2001; Stacoff, Kalin, and Stussi, 1991; Roniger, 2002). It is therefore a good idea to assess the athlete's biomechanics, flexibility, and running pattern when making recommendations.

THE FIVE SHOE TYPES (Foot and Ankle, 2002)

- **Motion control:** Board lasting, dense midsole, straight last, rear and forefoot postings for overpronators and heavy runners
- **Stability:** Combination last, semicurved shape, dense midsole, usually only rear foot posting, usually forefoot cushion, mild pronators, and light runners
- **Cushion:** Slip lasting, soft midsole, curved shape last, cushion in the heel and forefoot, mostly for supinators
- **Trail:** Usually a stability shoe for increased support on uneven surface, carbon rubber for additional durability

- **Racing flats:** Light thin midsole with little to no posting. Not designed for extended mileage due to limited support.

WHAT TO LOOK FOR WHEN BUYING SHOES

- Foot type
- Weight: Heavier runners need increased support and stability
- Type of running: Marathon versus speed work
- Running surfaces/Trails vs. road: Harder surfaces require increased cushion
- Previous pathology and wear patterns
- Heel counter must be perpendicular to supporting surface.
- Try on shoes in early evening as a result of foot swelling during the day.
- Ensure 1/2 in between longest toe and the shoe toe box adequate width (most shoes are a size D).
- Too tight of a shoe can lead to neuroma formation, too short of a toe box can cause black toenail.
- If using orthotics for stability purposes, use board or combination lasting to avoid the orthotic pronating through the shoe.
- Check for toe box for free flex across the metarsal heads.
- Arch cookies are not an effective substitute for a poor fit or performance adaptation since the arch should be not a weight bearing part of the foot.
- Durability: Expect 300–500 mi or 3–6 months out of a pair of shoes prior to midsole break down. Midsoles lose 40% of their cushioning ability after 400–500 mi (Reinschmidt and Nigg, 2000). Breakdown is variable based on weight, shoe type, and foot biomechanics. Look to purchase new shoes when the midsole has shown signs of compression, outer sole has sign of wear, or injury rate increases.

SPECIAL CONSIDERATIONS

- The least amount of pronation occurs while barefoot; however, the greatest amount of torsional loading of the foot also occurs barefoot (Stacoff, Kalin, and Stussi, 1991).
- Midsole characteristics are the primary determinant of the rate of loading imposed during initial ground contact (McCaw, Heil, and Hamill, 2000). Midsole stiffness has a marked effect on proprioception illustrating that peripheral sensory information is a variable in performance (Kurz and Stergiou, 2003).
- Too much or poorly designed cushioning can lead to instability as a result of excess cushioning from the

midsole and less proprioceptive feedback for stability (Barnes and Smith, 1994).

- Shoes with a softer durometer midsole allowed significantly increased pronation and total rear foot movement when compared to medium or hard midsoles (Clarke, Fredrick, and Hamill, 1983).

- With shoe changes, muscle-firing patterns occurred uniquely in a subject specific manner due to anatomical variation in connective tissue density. This demonstrates that shoe construction can be picked for a specific runner to affect treatment and prevention of lower quarter injuries, decrease fatigue, and increase performance (Hennig and Milani, 1995).

- Functional stability of the foot requires effective muscle contraction, coordination, and firing patterns. Fatigued muscle firing patterns cause increased peak strain on the lower extremity, thus leading to injury. This is important since both patellofemoral pain syndrome and osteoarthritis have been linked to abnormal muscle firing patterns (Arrol et al, 1997; Hurley, 1999; Kannus and Nittymaki, 1994; Slemenda et al, 1997).

- Benefits of proper footwear positioning have improved biomechanical disposition toward illiotibial band syndrome and tibial stress syndrome (Barnes and Smith, 1994).

- Despite claims, no manufacturer has successfully achieved energy return in footwear testing. Shoemakers have made functional gains in minimizing energy lost through lightweight alterations in materials (Stefanyshyn and Nigg, 2000).

- Proper footwear has been shown to increase internal stability and decrease onset time to achieve stabilization in the low back via postural changes (Ogon et al, 2001).

- Increases in ankle stability caused by structural support and high collars have not been supported; however, a firm midsole will provide benefits in tactile sensitivity and proprioception, which increase foot position awareness and decrease time to initiation of intrinsic muscles (Barrett, 1993; Robbins and Waked, 1998).

CONCLUSION

- Shoe trends have progressively evolved for today's athletes. While today's research does illustrate benefits in proper shoe construction and use, the shoe changes are often met with compensatory gait patterns (Nigg et al, 2003; Wakeling, Pascual, and Nigg, 2002; Kurz and Stergiou, 2003). These biomechanical changes make it difficult to discern if the benefits are attributed to footwear changes (proprioceptive changes vs. force vector changes). New improved force measuring

devices will increase our accuracy of force vector relationships. These breakthroughs will enable us to increase the specificity of footwear to maximize outcomes and decreases chronic stress levels on the body.

REFERENCES

American Physical Rehabilitation Network: When the feet hit the ground everything changes. Course notes, 1984.

Arrol BE, Ellis-Peleger A, Edwards A, et al: Patellofemoral pain syndrome. A critical review of the clinical trials on non-operative therapy. *Am J Sports Med* 25:207–212, 1997.

Ball K, Afheldt M: Evolution of foot orthotics—Part 1: Coherent theory or coherent practice? *J Manipulative Physiol Ther* 25:116–124, 2002a.

Ball K, Afheldt M: Evolution of foot orthotics—Part 2: Research reshapes long-standing theory. *J Manipulative Physiol Ther* 25:125–134, 2002b.

Barnes RA, Smith PD: The role of footwear in minimizing lower limb injury. *J Sport Sci* 12(4):341–353, 1994.

Barrett JR: High versus low-top shoes for the prevention of ankle sprains in basketball players. A prospective randomized study. *Am J Sports Med* 21(4):582–585, 1993.

Benard M, Goldsmith H, Gurnick K, et al: *Prescription Custom Foot Orthoses Practice Guidelines*. The American College of Foot and Ankle Orthopedics and Medicine, Ellicott, MD, Nov 2002, pp 1–32.

Bowman G: New concepts in orthotic management of the adult hyperpronated foot: Preliminary findings. *J Prosthet Orthot* 9(2):77, 1997.

Churchill R, Donley B: Managing injuries of the Great Toe. *Phys Sports Med* 26(8):280–295, 1998.

Clarke TE, Fredrick EC, Hamill CL: The effects of shoe design parameters on rearfoot control in running. *Med Sci Sports* 15(5):376–381, 1983.

Cornwall M, McPoil T: Effect of foot orthotics on the initiation of plantar surface loading. *The Foot* 7:148–152, 1997.

Cornwall M, McPoil T: *The Foot and Ankle: Current Concepts in Mechanics, Examination, and Orthotic Intervention*. PT 2003: Annual Conference & Exposition of the American Physical Therapy Association. Course Notes. Washington, DC, June 18–22, 2003.

Cummings GS, Higbie EJ: A weight bearing method for determining forefoot posting for orthotic fabrication. *Physiother Res Int* 2(1):42–50, 1997.

Dannanberg H, Guiliano M: Chronic low-back pain and its response to custom-made foot orthoses. *J Amer Pod Med Assoc* 89(3):109–117, 1999.

Donatelli R, Hurlbert C, Conway D, et al: Biomechanical foot orthotics: A retrospective study. *J Orthop Sports Phys Ther* 10:205–212, 1988.

Ekenman I, Milgrom C, Finestone A, et al: The role of biomechanical shoe orthoses in tibial stress fracture prevention. *Am J Sports Med* 30(6):866–870, 2002.

Eng J, Pierrynowski M: Evaluation of soft foot orthotics in the treatment of patellofemoral pain syndrome. *Phys Ther* 73(2):62–70, 1993.

Finestone A, Giladi M, Elad H, et al: Prevention of stress fractures using custom biomechanical shoe orthoses. *Clin Orthop* 360:182–190, 1999.

Foot and Ankle Update: *HEALTHSOUTH Educational Program.* Course notes, 2002.

Frey C: Footwear and stress structures. *Clin Sports Med* 16(2): 249–256, 1997.

Genova J, Gross M: Effect of foot orthotics on calcaneal eversion during standing and treadmill walking for subjects with abnormal pronation. *J Orthop Sports Phys Ther* 30(11):664–675, 2000.

Gross M: Orthoses: Semi rigid orthoses position feet for plantar fasciitis relief. *J Biomech* 802(2):53–60, 2001.

Gross M, Davlin L, Evanski P: Effectiveness of orthotic shoe inserts in the long distance runner. *Am J Sports Med* 19:409–412, 1991.

Gross M, Napoli R: Treatment of lower extremity injuries with orthotic shoe inserts. *Sports Med* 15:66–70, 1993.

Guskiewicz K, Perrin D: Effects of orthotics on postural sway following inversion ankle sprain. *J Orthop Sports Phys Ther* 23:326–331, 1996.

Hardoel H, Rowe B, Quinn K, et al: Intervention for preventing ankle ligament injuries (Cochrane Review). *The Cochrane Library*, Issue 2, 2003.

Heiderscheit B, Hamill J, Tiberio D: A Biomechanical perspective: Do foot orthoses work? *Br J Sports Med* 35(1):4–5, 2001.

Hennig EM, Milani TL: In shoe pressure distribution for running in various types of footwear. *J Appl Biomech* 11:299–310, 1995.

Hennig EM, Milani TL: Pressure distribution measures for evaluation of running shoe properties. *Sportverletz Sportschaden* 14(3):90–7, 2001.

Hurley MV: The role of muscle weakness in pathogenesis of osteoarthritis. *Osteoarthritis* 25:283–298, 1999.

James S, Bates B, Osternig L: Injuries to runners. *Am J Sports Med* 6:40–50, 1978.

Kannus P, Nittymaki S: Which factors predict outcome in the non-operative treatment of patellofemoral pain syndrome? A prospective follow-up study. *Med Sci Sports Exerc* 26:289–296, 1994.

Kitaoka H, Zong-Ping L, Kura H, et al: Effect of foot orthoses on 3-dimensional kinematics of flatfoot: A cadaveric study. *Arch Phys Med Rehabil* 83:876–879, 2002.

Klingman R, Liaos S, Hardin K: The effect of subtalar joint posting on patellar glide position in subjects with excessive rear foot pronation. *J Ortho Sports Phys Ther* 25(3):185–191, 1997.

Kurz MJ, Stergiou N: The spanning set indicates that variability during the stance period of running is affected by footwear. *Gait Posture* 17(2):132–135, 2003.

Landorf K, Keenan A: Efficacy of foot orthoses. What does the literature tell us? *J Am Podiatr Med Assoc* 90(3):149–158, 2000.

Langer S: Custom orthoses: Correct use of foam box casting. *J Biomech* 9:41–44,1996.

Laughlin C, McClay Davis I, et al: A comparison of four methods of obtaining a negative impression of the foot. *J Am Podiatr Med Assoc* 92(5):261–268, 2002.

Lynch D, Goforth W, Martin J: Conservative treatment of plantarfasciitis: A prospective study. *J Am Pod Med Assoc* 88:375, 1998.

MacLean C: Custom foot orthoses for running. *Clin Pod Med Surg* 18(2):217–224, 2001.

Manoli A, Graham B: Cavus foot diagnosis determines treatment. *J Biomech* (1)1–12, 2001.

McCaw ST, Heil ME, Hamill J: Effect of comments about shoe construction on impact forces during walking. *Med Sci Sports Exerc* 32(7):1258–1264, 2000.

McPoil T, Cornwall M: The effect of foot orthoses on transverse tibial rotation during walking. *J Am Podiatr Med Assoc* 90:2–11, 2000.

Nawoczenski D: Nonoperative and operative intervention for hallux rigidus. *J Orthop Sports Phys Ther* 29(12):727–735, 1999.

Nawoczenski D, Cook T, Saltzman C: The effect of foot orthotics on three-dimensional kinematics of the leg and rear foot during running. *J Orthop Sports Phys Ther* 21:317–327, 1995.

Nawoczenski D, Cook T, Saltzman C: The effect of foot structure on the three-dimensional kinematic coupling behavior of the leg and rear foot. *Phys Ther* 78(4):404–416, 1998.

Nigg B: The role of impact force and foot pronation: A new paradigm. *Clin J Sports Med* 11:2–9, 2001.

Nigg B, Nurse M, Stefanyshyn C: Shoe inserts and orthotics for sport and physical activities. *Med Sci Sports Exerc* 31(Suppl): S421–S428, 1999.

Nigg BM, Stefanyshyn D, Cole G et al: The effect of material characteristics of shoe soles on muscle activation and energy aspects during running. *J Biomech* 36(4):569–575, 2003.

Noll K: The use of orthotic devices in adult acquired flatfoot deformity. *Foot Ankle Clin* 6(1):25–36, 2001.

O'Connor F, Wilder R: *Textbook of Running Medicine.* New York, McGraw-Hill, 2001.

Ogon M, Aleksiev AR, Spratt K et al: Footwear affects the behavior of the low back muscles when jogging. *Int J Sports Med* 22(6):414–419, 2001.

Orteza L, Vogelbach W, Denegar C: The effect of molded orthotics on balance and pain while jogging following inversion ankle sprain. *J Athl Train* 27:80–84, 1992.

Payne C, Chuter V: The clash between theory and science on the kinematic effectiveness of foot orthoses. *Clin Podiatr Med Surg* 18(4):705–713, 2001.

PFA: Introduction to pedorthics. Columbia, MD, Pedorthic Footwear Association, 1998.

Pitman D, Jack D: A clinical investigation to determine the effectiveness of biomechanical foot orthoses as initial treatment for patellofemoral pain syndrome. *J Orthot Prosthet* 12(4):110–120, 2000.

Postema K, Burm P, Zande M, et al: Primary metatarsalgia: The influence of a custom molded insole and a rockerbar on plantar pressure. *Prosthet Orthot Int* 22:35–44, 1998.

Powers C, Maffucci R, Hampton S: Rear foot posture in subjects with patellofemoral pain. *J Orthop Sports Phys Ther* 22(4): 155–160, 1995.

Pratt D: A critical review of the literature on foot orthoses. *J Am Podiatr Med Assoc* 90(7):339–341, 2000.

Razeghi M, Batt M: Biomechanical analysis of the effect of orthotic shoe inserts—A review of the literature. *Sports Med* 29(6):425–438, 2000.

Reinschmidt C, Nigg BM: Current issues in the design of running and court shoes. *Sportverletz Sportschaden* 14(3):71–81, 2000.

Robbins S, Waked E: Factors associated with ankle injuries. Preventative measures. *Sports Med* 26(1):63–72, 1998.

Roberts ME, Gordon CE: Orthopedic footwear. Custom-made and commercially manufactured footwear. *Foot Ankle Clin* 6(2):243–247, 2001.

Roniger LR: Shoe science: Stepping up to market challenges. *J Biomech* (4) 23–30, 2002.

Running Course: *HEALTHSOUTH Educational Program.* Course notes, 2002.

Saxena A, Haddad J: The effect of foot orthoses on patellofemoral pain syndrome. *Lower Extremity* 5(2):95–102, 1998.

Sharkey NA, Ferris L, Smith, et al: Strain and loading of the second metatarsal during heel lift. *J Bone Joint Surg* 77A:1050–1057, 1995.

Shiba N, Kitaoka T, Calahan T, et al: Shock-absorbing effect of shoe insert materials commonly used in management of lower extremity disorders. *Clin Ortop Rel Res* 310:130–136, 1995.

Slemenda C, et al: Quadriceps weakness and osteoarthritis of the knee. *Ann Intern Med* 127:97–104, 1997.

Sobel E, Levitz S, Caselli M: Orthoses in the treatment of rear foot problems. *J Am Podiatr Med Assoc* 89(5):220–233, 1999.

Stacoff A, Kalin X., Stussi E: The effects of shoes on torsion and rearfoot motion in running. *Med Sci Sports Exerc* 23(4):482–490, 1991.

Stefanyshyn DJ, Nigg BM: Energy aspects associated with sports shoes. *Sportverletz Sportschaden* 14(3):82–89, 2000.

Tang S, Chen C, Pan J, et al: The effects of a new foot-toe orthosis in treating painful hallux valgus. *Arch Phys Med Rehabil* 83:1792–1795, 2002.

Thacker S, Gilchrist J, Stroup D, et al: The prevention of shin splints in sports: A systematic review of literature. *Med Sci Sports Exerc* 34(1):32–40, 2002.

Tillman M, Chiumento A, Trimble M, et al: Tibiofemoral rotation in landing: The influence of medially and laterally posted orthotics. *Phys Ther Sport* 4(1):34–39, 2003.

Valmassy R, Subotnick S: Orthoses, in Subotnick S (ed.): *Sports Medicine of the Lower Extremity*, 2nd ed. Philadelphia, PA: Churchill Livingston, 1999.

Vicenzino B, Griffiths S, Griffiths L, et al: Effect of antipronation tape and temporary orthotic on vertical navicular height before and after exercise. *J Orthop Sports Phys Ther* 30(6):333–339, 2000.

Wakeling JM, Pascual SA, Nigg BM: Altering muscle activity in the lower extremities by running with different shoes. *Med Sci Sports Exerc* 34(9):1529–1532, 2002.

Way M: Effects of thermoplastic foot orthosis on patellofemoral pain in a collegiate athlete. *J Orthop Sports Phys Ther* 29(6):331–338, 1999.

Wayne Decker, Stephen Albert: *Contemporary Pedorthotics.* Seattle, WA, Elton-Wolf, 2002.

73 TAPING AND BRACING

Tom Grossman
Kate Serenelli, MS, ATC, CSCS
Danny Mistry, MD

INTRODUCTION

• Taping and bracing are essential for the treatment and rehabilitation of injuries. Appropriate taping decreases angular velocity, restricts range of motion, and enhances proprioception. Basic principles that should be adhered to include the following:
1. Use "prewrap" to prevent excoriation of skin.
2. Place joint in the immobilized position.
3. Avoid continuous taping.
4. Keep the roll in hand at all times.
5. Smoothe and mold tape with the free hand.
6. Do not tape after the application of a hot or cold modality (AAOS, 1991).

TAPING

SHOULDER TAPING

• **Acromioclavicular tape:** Used for a sprain of the *acromioclavicular* (AC) joint. The tape should be pulled opposite the direction of displacement to move the clavicle back into the correct anatomical position. (Fig. 73-1)

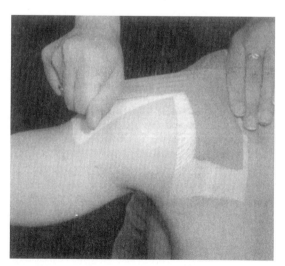

FIG. 73-1 Taping for AC-sprain.

1. Two strips of coverstrip are placed over the AC joint in an anterior to posterior direction. A third strip is placed from the base of the neck to the distal edge of the deltoid.
2. One strip of Leukotape is used to depress the clavicle. The tape is pulled from the anterior to posterior direction.
3. A second strip of Leukotape is used to depress the clavicle from a posterior to anterior direction.
4. A final strip of leukotape is used to depress the clavicle from a proximal to distal direction.

ELBOW TAPING

- Hyperextension: Used for hyperextension injury to the elbow. The Xs should be placed over the injured structure. (Fig. 73-2)
  1. The elbow is covered with prewrap from mid bicep to mid forearm.
  2. Anchor strips are placed at each end of the prewrap.
  3. Two strips are applied creating an X over the joint line (over the cubital fossa).
  4. The finished tape is covered with power flex.

WRIST TAPING

- Wrist hyperextension: Used for hyperextension injury to the wrist. Placing the Xs on the dorsal surface of the hand will also protect the wrist injured from hyperflexion. (Figure 73-3)

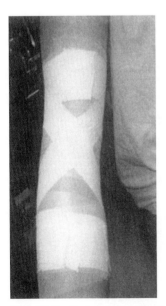

FIG. 73-2 Taping following elbow hyperextension injury.

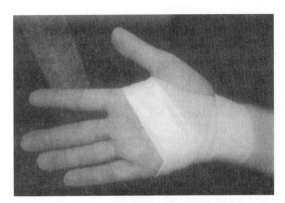

FIG. 73-3 Taping to prevent wrist hyperextension.

1. A strip is begun around the wrist and is continued around the metacarpals distal to the thumb.
2. A strip of elastikon or other stretch tape is used to limit extension. A cut is made in the middle of each end of the strip. The ends are ripped apart and each remaining strip is wrapped around the wrist proximally and the metacarpals distal to the thumb.
3. A strip identical to the first anchor is applied over the elastikon to stabilize the tape.

FINGER TAPING

- **Buddy taping:** Used to immobilize the fingers for sprains or fractures. Strips are placed around adjacent proximal and distal phalanges.
- **Stax splint:** Used to immobilize the *distal interphalangeal* (DIP) joint of the finger in full extension, such as for a mallet finger. The finger is placed in a stax splint with the DIP in full extension. The stax splint is then taped to the finger with a strip of power flex tape (Wang and Johnson, 2001).
- **Checkreins:** To limit abduction. A strip of 1 in. tape is wrapped around the middle phalanx of the injured finger over and around to the adjacent finger. The tape between two fingers (checkrein) is strengthened with a lock strip around the center of the checkrein. Tape is applied around the middle phalanges while allowing enough slack for the strips to touch in the middle.
- **Collateral taping:** Used for ligamentous injury around the proximal interphalangeal joints in order to limit varus, valgus, hyperextension, or hyperflexion. An anchor strip is placed on either side of the *proximal interphalangeal* (PIP). Cross strips (Xs) are then applied across the injured collateral ligament.
- **Thumb spica:** Radial collateral support that protects against an ulnar force. (Fig. 73-4)

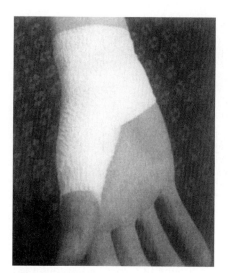

FIG. 73-4 Thumb spica taping.

1. One strip is placed around the wrist. A "figure of eight" is placed around the thumb.
2. A strip of elastikon or other stretch tape is cut in the middle of each end.
3. The ends are ripped apart and each remaining strip is wrapped around the wrist proximally and the thumb distal to the *metacarpophalangeal* (MCP) joint.
4. The tape is covered with figures of eight and around the wrist with stretch tape.

HIP TAPING

• Hip flexor: For hip flexor strain. The patient stands in slight hip flexion. The end of the wrap is placed on the iliac crest and rapped posteriorly around till it meets at the front. This process is then continued around the hip to the opposite iliac crest. The process is repeated with the bandage being overlapped at least by *half-hip*.
• Adductors: For adductor strain the end of the wrap is started at the upper part of the inner thigh, and then wrapped posteriorly around the thigh. The wrap is then drawn across the lower abdominal region and over the crest of the ilium to the opposite side of the body. This process is then continued around the back. The same pattern is repeated and the end of the wrap is secured with $1\frac{1}{2}$ in. adhesive tape.

THIGH TAPING

• Hamstring and quadriceps strain: A bandage is applied in a circular pattern around the thigh or a thigh sleeve is applied over the location of the injury, providing compression and warmth for the injured muscle. A piece of

foam for focal compression such as a pad or piece of felt can be added over the injured area for support and to prevent further injury to the damaged muscle.

KNEE TAPING

• Hyperextension: Used for hyperextension injury, posterior capsule sprain, and hamstring tendon strain. (Fig. 73-5)
    1. With the athlete standing on a heel block to allow slight flexion, anchors are placed around the mid-belly of the quadriceps and the mid-belly of the gastrocnemius. A strip of elastikon or other stretch tape is cut in the middle of each end. The ends are ripped apart and each remaining strip is wrapped around the quadriceps proximally and the gastrocnemius distally.
    2. Second and third strips of elastikon are placed either side of the first strip, overlapping by half.
    3. The underlying tape is closed using stretch tape.
• Knee collateral tape: Can be used for an injury to either collateral ligament.
    1. Two cross strips of coverstrip are applied intersecting the midportion of the collateral ligament.
    2. Leukotape strips are applied over the coverstrip.

LOWER LEG TAPING

• Medial tibial stress syndrome: Used to decrease the symptoms of medial shin pain.
    1. Tape is applied in a rotational pattern, from a medial to lateral direction.
    2. Strips are continued in a proximal direction until the base of the gastrocnemius.

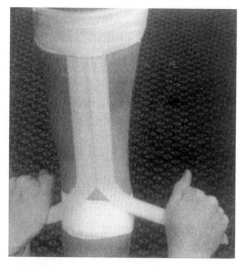

FIG. 73-5 Taping following knee hyperextension injury.

ANKLE TAPING

- **Inversion taping:** Used prophylactically to prevent lateral ankle sprains. (Fig. 73-6)
  1. Anchors are placed around the metatarsals, proximal to the base of the fifth metatarsal and 5 in. proximal to the malleolus, distal to the gastrocnemius muscle belly. A stirrup is placed posterior to the mallelous in a medial to lateral direction, pulling the ankle into dorsiflexion.
  2. The second stirrup is placed directly over the medial mallelous overlapping the first by half. The third is placed anterior to the medial mallelous overlapping the second by half. Each stirrup is followed by a horseshoe placed from posterior to anterior direction.
  3. The heel is then locked for maximum stability. The tape is started high on the instep, pulled along the ankle at an angle and around the heel, under the arch and up to the opposite side until the starting point is reached.
  4. A second heel lock is applied in the same pattern as the first but on the opposite side of the ankle.
  5. A figure of 8 is applied from the bottom of the foot up and around each side of the ankle to form an eight. Then an anchor is applied proximal to the ankle where the first was placed.
- Eversion taping: Same as inversion, but the stirrups are pulled evenly, both medially and laterally.
- Achilles taping: Used to support the Achilles tendon following rehabilitation for Achilles tendonitis.
  1. Anchors are applied approximately 7–9 in. above the malleoli and the other around the foot. These anchors are wrapped around loosely.

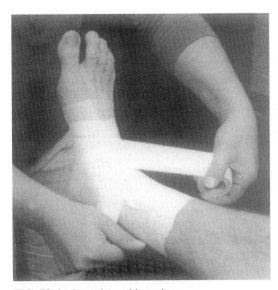

FIG. 73-6 Inversion ankle taping.

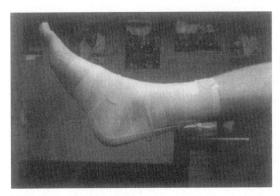

FIG. 73-7 Achilles taping.

  2. A strip of elastic tape is split in the middle of each end. The remaining strips are wrapped around the anchor strips. (Fig. 73-7)
  3. Two additional elastic strips are placed in the same pattern as the first.
  4. However, the strips are started on either side of the ankle and overlapped by half the tape width.
  5. Stretch tape is applied over the tape to close the underlying tape.

FOOT AND TOE TAPING

- Arch tape (low-dye taping): Used for arch support; commonly used for plantar fasciitis (Saxelby et al, 1997).
  1. An anchor strip is placed around the ball of the foot.
  2. A second strip is started on the side of the foot, at the base of the first toe.
  3. The third strip is wrapped around the heel, crossing the arch and returning to the first toe. The fourth strip is placed identical to the third, started on the side of the fifth toe.
  4. This pattern is repeated two to three times over.
  5. Each strip is locked with a piece of tape around the ball of the foot.
  6. Strips are applied to close the underlying arch tape.
  7. The arch tape is covered with stretch tape.
- Toe taping/Buddy taping: Used to immobilize the toes for sprains or fractures. Tape strips are placed around adjacent distal and middle phalanges.

BRACING AND SPLINTING

NASAL FRACTURE

- Nasal shield: Protective shield for nasal fractures—used prophylactically to prevent further injury following nasal bridge fractures.

SHOULDER

- Instability brace: For glenohumeral instability. Brace restricts abduction and external rotation.
- Figure eight brace: For clavicular fractures or training and strengthening the scapular stabilizers.
- Acromioclavicular pad and straps: For AC sprains. The Acromioclavicular joint is protected following sprains of the AC joint with a donut pad held in place by straps wrapped obliquely around the chest and around the upper arm.

ELBOW

- Collateral bracing. Double hinges prevent valgus or varus stress.

WRIST AND THUMB

- Wrist bracing: Wrist brace used to immobilize wrist for wrist sprains.
- Thumb bracing: Thumb with spica brace used to immobilize the thumb and wrist.

BACK

- Back support: Abdominal binder to provide compression and lumbar support.
- Soft cervical collar: Soft cervical collar used to provide support for paraspinal muscle spasm in the absence of vertebral instability.
- Firm cervical collar: Firm cervical collar used to provide support for vertebral instability.

THIGH

- Hamstring and quadriceps sleeve with hip pointer pad to provide protection from repeated contact.

KNEE

- Knee stabilizer: *Anterior cruciate ligament* (ACL) brace for rotational stability.
- Medial and lateral knee stabilizer: Hinge brace for medial and lateral collateral injury. Lateral hinge protects *medial collateral ligament* (MCL); medial hinge protects the *lateral collateral ligament* (LCL). Most commonly used following an injury, these braces have also been widely used prophylactically to prevent injury (especially of the MCL). Current data, however, has not definitively proven that these braces are effective in preventing injury (Martin, 2002).

- Knee patellar strap: Used to provide compression to the patellar tendon in order to relieve symptoms of patellar tendonitis and patellofemoral syndrome.

ANKLE

- Walking boot: Provides immobilization for the ankle foot and toes. It can be either locked to provide no movement or set for different ranges of motion.
- Prophylactic ankle brace: Used either for prophylaxis against ankle sprains or as a substitute to ankle taping.

REFERENCES

American Academy of Orthopedic Surgeons: *Athletic Training and Sports Medicine*, 2nd ed, Parkridge, IL, American Academy of Orthopedic Surgeons, 1991.
Martin TJ: Technical report: knee brace use in the young athlete. *Pediatrics* 108:503–508, 2002.
Saxelby J, Betts R, Bygrave C: Low-dye taping on the foot in the management of plantar fasciitis. The Foot: *Int. J of Clin Foot Science* 7: 205–209, 1997.
Wang QC, Johnson BA: Fingertip Injuries. *Am Family Physician* 63: 1961–1966, 2001.

74 PSYCHOLOGIC CONSIDERATIONS IN EXERCISE AND SPORT
Nicole L Frazer, PhD

INTRODUCTION

- Regarding the psychologic health benefits of physical activity, exercise has been shown to be an effective intervention for depressed and anxious moods (U.S Department of Health and Human Services, 1996). This is an important finding considering that the point prevalence rate for major depression ranges from 5 to 9% for women and from 2 to 3% for men, approximately 3% for generalized anxiety, and between 0.5 and 1.5% for panic disorder (APA, 2000).
1. Noteworthy is a randomized-controlled trial in which older adult men and women, who met Diagnostic and Statistical Manual of Mental Disorders-Fourth Edition (DSM-IV) diagnostic criteria for major depressive disorder, were assigned to 16 weeks of either exercise (30 min of walking

or jogging three times a week) and antidepressant medication (sertraline), or the combination of exercise and medication. Across all three groups, participants had clinically significant improvements in their depression scores at the 16-week follow up. At the 10-month follow-up, those in the only exercise group and the exercise plus antidepressant medication group had a lower rate of relapse and a higher likelihood of being partially or fully recovered than those in the medication alone group (Babyak et al, 2000). An association was also found between exercising on one's own during follow-up and reduced risk of relapse.

2. Studies have also supported a positive impact on affect following exercise (Gauvin, Rejeski, and Norris, 1996; Gauvin, Rejeski, and Reboussin, 2000), and even improvements on some aspects of cognitive function (e.g., scheduling, planning, working memory) (Kramer et al, 1999). For adolescents, an inverse relationship between physical activity and depression has been supported (Sallis, Prochaska, and Taylor, 2000). The aforementioned psychologic health benefits are not exhaustive, but are among those with the most strong and consistent findings (U.S Department of Health and Human Services, 1996).

• More than 360,000 collegiate athletes and almost 6.5 million high school athletes participated in sports during the 1998–1999 school year (Weaver, Marshall, and Miller, 2002). Participating in athletics encourages the development of leadership skills, self-esteem, muscle development, and overall physical health. For children and adolescents, play and sport can enhance physical, psychologic, and social development (Eppright et al, 1997).

• A number of psychologic considerations are relevant in understanding exercise and sport behavior. While not exhaustive, among the most common issues are exercise addiction and overtraining, alcohol use, abuse, and dependence, disordered eating behavior, performance anxiety, recovery from sports injuries, and specialty consultation decision making.

EXERCISE ADDICTION AND OVERTRAINING

• Exercise addiction is the unhealthy reliance on exercise for daily functioning (Barrett, 2003; p 182). More specifically, it comprises dependence, tolerance, and withdrawal factors.

1. An individual who is dependent on exercise has a need to exercise in order to feel good. Exercise is often a primary coping skill in this respect.

2. With tolerance, the individual must continually elevate the level of exercise in order to achieve the same feeling good state.

3. Believed to be a critical component of exercise addiction is the presence of withdrawal symptoms. These symptoms can encompass mood symptoms, such as anxiousness, irritability, depression, and restlessness or even physical symptoms of fatigue 24–36 h after missing a scheduled session of exercise.

• Prevalence rates for exercise addiction are unknown, but it is hypothesized to be a small subset of those who exercise regularly (Barrett, 2003). Additionally, there is no data to suggest that exercise addiction is consistently associated with other addictive behaviors (e.g., alcohol abuse) or psychologic disorders; however, for some individuals, anorexia nervosa and exercise addiction may be comorbid conditions. This has been termed secondary exercise addiction (Barrett, 2003).

• Assessment and treatment for exercise addiction can be difficult as individuals with an exercise addiction do not usually access the healthcare system unless it is for an overuse injury, such as sprains, strains, bursitis, and/or stress fractures secondary to their addictive behavior (Barrett, 2003).

1. To determine the presence of an exercise addiction, the health care provider should explore the patient's motivators for exercise and consequences they experience when they cannot exercise. Any functional impairment associated with maintaining their exercise (e.g., missed work, missed social activities with friends) should also be assessed.

2. Determining the frequency, intensity, and duration of exercise is important. Running is the most commonly associated activity; however, other aerobic activities (e.g., swimming) and team sports (e.g., basketball) also have the potential for exercise addiction (Barrett, 2003).

3. There is no empirically supported treatment for exercise addiction, and treatment can be difficult. The best strategy is to identify and treat the intrapersonal and interpersonal factors for which they are using excessive exercise to cope (Barrett, 2003).

• Overtraining and exercise addiction can be comorbid conditions. Overtraining involves increased training intensity and/or duration without adequate recovery (Sachtleben, 2003). An example would be a runner who trains at increased distances every day without allowing a day of rest or recovery in between sessions. The ultimate result of this behavior is the opposite of what is pursued. That is, a state of staleness or a lack of performance improvement, and possibly even a deterioration in performance may result (Barrett, 2003).

1. Overtraining can be characterized by fatigue, depression, restlessness, and increased resting heart rate to name a few (Sachtleben, 2003).
2. Mood disturbance is one of the key characteristics of the overtraining syndrome, and therefore monitoring of an athlete's mood during increased stress may also be helpful (Sachtleben, 2003). Additionally, athletes who participate in multiple sports and endurance athletes (e.g., marathoners) should be monitored for signs of overtraining due to the nature of their sport behavior (Sachtleben, 2003).

ALCOHOL USE, ABUSE, AND DEPENDENCE

• The most common substance abused by athletes is alcohol (Green and Nattiv, 2003). In a survey of 21,000 college student athletes by the National Collegiate Athletic Association (NCAA) regarding substance abuse habits, 79.5% reported using alcohol in the preceding 12 months. Regarding frequency of alcohol consumption, 69% reported drinking 1–2 times during a typical week. Additionally, 39% reported consuming 3–5 drinks in a sitting, and 30% reported consuming 6–9 drinks in one sitting (NCAA, 1997). Twenty percent also reported that alcohol had a negative effect on their athletic performance.

• The Diagnostic and Statistical Manual of mental Disorders-Fourth Edition-Text Revision (DSM-IV-TR) delineates criteria for whether substance abuse (see Table 74-1) or substance dependence (see Table 74-2)

TABLE 74-1 DSM-IV-TR (2000) Criteria for Substance Abuse

1. A maladaptive pattern of substance use leading to clinically significant impairment or distress, as manifested by one or more of the following, occurring within a 12-month period:
   a. Recurrent substance use resulting in a failure to fulfill major role obligations at work, school, or home (e.g., repeated absences or poor work performance related to substance use; substance-related absences, suspensions, or expulsions from school; neglect of children or household).
   b. Recurrent substance use in situations in which it is physically hazardous (e.g., driving an automobile or operating a machine when impaired by substance use).
   c. Recurrent substance-related legal problems (e.g., arrests for substance-related disorderly conduct).
   d. Continued substance use despite having persistent or recurrent social or interpersonal problems caused by or exacerbated by the effects of the substance (e.g., arguments with spouse about consequences of intoxication, physical fights).
2. The symptoms have never met the criteria for Substance Dependence for this class of substance.

SOURCE: APA: *Diagnostic and Statistical Manual of Mental Disorders*, 4th ed. Text Revision, Washington, DC, American Psychiatric Association, 2000.

TABLE 74-2 DSM-IV-TR (2000) Criteria for Substance Dependence

A maladaptive pattern of substance use, leading to clinically significant impairment or distress, as manifested by three or more of the following, occurring at any time in the same 12-month period:
1. Tolerance, as defined by either of the following:
   a. Need for markedly increased amounts of the substance to achieve intoxication or desired effect.
   b. Markedly diminished effect with continued use of the same amount of the substance.
2. Withdrawal as manifested by either of the following:
   a. The characteristic withdrawal syndrome for the substance (refer to Criteria A and B of the criteria sets for Withdrawal from the specific substances)
   b. The same (or a closely related) substance is taken to relieve or avoid withdrawal.
3. The substance is often taken in larger amounts or over a longer period than was intended.
4. A persistent desire exists to cut down or control substance use along with many unsuccessful attempts to do so.
5. A great deal of time is spent in activities necessary to obtain the substance (e.g., driving long distances), use the substance, or recover from its effects.
6. Important social, occupational, or recreational activities are given up or reduced because of substance use.
7. The substance use is continued despite knowledge of having a persistent or recurrent physical or psychologic problem that is likely to have been caused or exacerbated by the substance (e.g., continued drinking despite recognition that an ulcer was made worse by alcohol consumption).

SOURCE: APA: *Diagnostic and Statistical Manual of Mental Disorders*, 4th ed. Text Revision, Washington, DC, American Psychiatric Association, 2000.

exist. For a diagnosis of alcohol dependence to be made criteria for alcohol withdrawal must be met (see Table 74-3). A helpful screening tool in determining whether the athlete is a recreational drinker or has a more significant problem with alcohol is the CAGE questionnaire (Fleming and Barry, 1992):
1. Have you ever felt you ought to Cut down on your drinking?
2. Have people Annoyed you by criticizing your drinking?
3. Have you ever felt bad or Guilty about your drinking?
4. Have you ever had a drink first thing in the morning to steady your nerves or get rid of a hangover (Eye-opener)?

• One or more positive answers are indicative of hazardous drinking behavior. Two or more positive answers indicate the probability of alcohol abuse and possible dependence. Referral for further assessment and treatment should be made for these individuals.

• The absence of a clinical level of drinking behavior does not diminish the importance of addressing the impact of alcohol use on current sport performance

TABLE 74-3 DSM-IV-TR (2000) Criteria for Alcohol Withdrawal

A. Cessation of (or reduction in) alcohol use that has been heavy and prolonged.
B. Two (or more) of the following, developing within several hours to a few days after Criterion A:
  1. autonomic hyperactivity (e.g., sweating or pulse rate greater than 100)
  2. increased hand tremor
  3. insomnia
  4. nausea or vomiting
  5. transient visual, tactile, or auditory hallucinations or illusions
  6. psychomotor agitation
  7. anxiety
  8. grand mal seizures
C. The symptoms in Criterion B cause clinically significant distress or impairment in social, occupational, or other important areas of functioning.
D. The symptoms are not due to a general medical condition and are not better accounted for by another mental disorder.
Specify if:
  With Perceptual Disturbances

Source: APA: *Diagnostic and Statistical Manual of Mental Disorders*, 4th ed. Text Revision, Washington, DC, American Psychiatric Association, 2000.

(e.g., diminished strength, power, and speed) and the increased potential for risk of injury (Green and Nattiv, 2003).

- According to the NCAA survey, 78% of college athletes reported they began drinking before entering college. Prevention efforts should therefore target student athletes at high school, junior high, and even elementary levels (Green and Nattiv, 2003).
- The use of other drugs by athletes (e.g., anabolic steroids) is of concern and is discussed in greater detail in other chapters. Worth a brief mention here is the use of smokeless tobacco products.
  1. The NCAA 2001 survey reported that 17% of all athletes had used smokeless tobacco. This is a decrease from 28% reported in 1989 (Green and Nattiv, 2003).
  2. According to the 2001 NCAA survey, 41% of baseball players and 29% of football players reported using smokeless tobacco in the past year. The NCAA does ban the use of smokeless tobacco products in NCAA sanctioned events. Minor league baseball has also banned the use of smokeless tobacco products in games, but use is still permitted during games at the major league level (Green and Nattiv, 2003).
  3. Every athlete who uses tobacco products should at least be offered a minimal intervention. An intervention lasting less than 3 min can increase overall tobacco abstinence rates (U.S. Department of Health and Human Services, 2000). Intensive tobacco cessation programs are available to assist individuals in their quit efforts. The more effective

interventions are based on a dose-response relation, with four or more sessions yielding higher abstinence rates (U.S. Department of Health and Human Services, 2000).

DISORDERED EATING BEHAVIOR

- Most athletes experience the same types of mental health problems as that of the general population (Begel and Burton, 2000); however, disordered eating behavior has been identified as being more prevalent amongst athletes and more prevalent in female athletes than male athletes. While there has been variability in prevalence rates reported, a recent study revealed 20% of female and 8% of male athletes met DSM-IV criteria for anorexia nervosa, bulimia nervosa, and eating disorders not otherwise specified compared to 9 and 0.5% for female and male nonathletes (Sundgot-Borgen, Klungland, and Torstveit, 1999).
- The "female athlete triad" was coined by the American College of Sports Medicine in 1992 to describe three interrelated conditions of amenorrhea, osteoporosis, and disordered eating that often occur together in female athletes (Nattiv et al, 1994). This is important given the increase in sports participation by females. For example, in the 1997–1998 school year, 2,570,333 girls participated in high school sports; a significant increase from the 294,015 girls participating in high school sports in the 1971-1972 academic school year (NAGWS, 1999).
- Disordered eating behavior can range from that which meets clinical diagnostic criteria for anorexia nervosa or bulimia nervosa (see Table 74-4) as established in the DSM-IV-TR to subclinical levels of disordered eating behavior, which might include occasional purging, and/or laxative use or diet pill use referred to as "eating disorder not otherwise specified" in the DSM-IV-TR. One subclinical form of anorexia has been referred to by researchers as anorexia athletica (Pugliese et al, 1983; Sundgot-Borgen, 1993).
  1. Symptoms of anorexia nervosa can include compulsive exercising, anxiety at mealtime, a preoccupation with food, calories, and weight, isolation from family and friends and avoiding food related social activities, cutting food into small pieces, extreme sensitivity to cold, sleep disturbances, high consumption of sugar free gum, constipation/bloating, lightheadedness, high intake of caffeine-containing beverages, and amenorrhea (Jacobson, 2003; Wilmore, 1991). Amenorrhea precedes other symptoms of anorexia nervosa in 16% of cases and coincides with the onset of anorexia nervosa in 55% of

TABLE 74-4   DSM-IV-TR (2000) Criteria for Anorexia Nervosa and Bulimia Nervosa

Anorexia Nervosa

1. Refusal to maintain body weight at or above a minimally normal weight for age and height (e.g., weight loss leading to maintenance of body weight less than 85% of that expected: or failure to make expected weight gain during period of growth, leading to body weight less than 85% of that expected).
2. Intense fear of gaining weight or becoming fat, even though underweight.
3. Disturbance in the way one's body weight or shape is experienced, undue influence of body weight or shape on self-evaluation, or denial of the seriousness of the current low body weight.
4. In postmenarcheal females, amenorrhea, i.e., the absence of at least three consecutive menstrual cycles.

   Specify type:
   Restricting type: during the current episode of Anorexia Nervosa, the person has not regularly engaged in binge-eating or purging behavior (i.e., self-induced vomiting or the misuse of laxatives, diuretics, or enemas).
   Binge-Eating/Purging type: during the current episode of Anorexia Nervosa, the person has regularly engaged in binge-eating or purging behavior (i.e., self-induced vomiting or the misuse of laxatives, diuretics, or enemas).

Bulimia Nervosa

1. Recurrent episodes of binge eating. An episode of binge eating is characterized by both of the following:
   a. Eating, in a discrete period of time (e.g., within any 2-hour period), an amount of food that is definitely larger than most people would eat during a similar period of time and under similar circumstances.
   b. A sense of lack of control over eating during the episode (e.g., a feeling that one cannot stop eating or control what or how much one is eating).
2. Recurrent inappropriate compensatory behavior in order to prevent weight gain, such as self-induced vomiting, misuse of laxatives, diuretics, enemas, or other medications; fasting; or excessive exercise.
3. The binge eating and inappropriate compensatory behaviors both occur, on average, at least twice a week for 3 months.
4. Self-evaluation is unduly influenced by body shape and weight.
5. The disturbance does not occur exclusively during episodes of Anorexia Nervosa.

   Specify type:
   Purging type: during the current episode of Bulimia Nervosa, the person has regularly engaged in self-induced vomiting or the misuse of laxatives, diuretics, or enemas.
   Nonpurging type: during the current episode of Bulimia Nervosa, the person has used other inappropriate compensatory behaviors, such as fasting or excessive exercise, but has not regularly engaged in self-induced vomiting or the misuse of laxatives, diuretics, or enemas.

SOURCE: APA: *Diagnostic and Statistical Manual of Mental Disorders*, 4th ed. Text Revision, Washington, DC, American Psychiatric Association, 2000.

cases (Jacobson, 2003). For any athlete presenting with amenorrhea the differential diagnosis should always include anorexia nervosa.
2. Physical signs of anorexia nervosa may include significant weight loss, hyperactivity, distorted body image, rough and/or dry skin, vellous hair on back and extremities, atrophy of breast tissue, bradycardia, hypothermia, low blood pressure/orthostasis, thinning of scalp hair, and carotenemia (Jacobson, 2003).
3. Symptoms of bulimia nervosa can include fatigue, sore throat/chest pain, difficulty swallowing and retaining food, constipation/diarrhea, bloating and abdominal pain, irregular menses, a noticeable weight loss or gain, excessive concern about weight, increasing criticism of one's body/over-concern with personal appearance, secretive behavior, trips to bathroom after meals, weakness, headache, and dizziness (Jacobson, 2003; Wilmore, 1991).
4. Physical signs of bulimia nervosa can include parotid/salivary gland enlargement, puffiness around the face (below cheeks), frequent weight fluctuations, abrasions on the back of the knuckles from inducing vomiting, loss of tooth enamel, and halitosis (Jacobson, 2003).

• There are three main categories of sports where athletes are at greatest risk for developing eating disorders (Sundgot-Borgen, 1993; Jacobson, 2003):
1. Sports emphasizing a lean appearance, such as swimming, diving, synchronized swimming, figure skating, and gymnastics.
2. Sports emphasizing leanness for performance such as track, long distance running, swimming, and cross-country skiing.
3. Sports in which athletes are classified based on weight such as weightlifting, boxing, wrestling, and rowing.

• Early identification and treatment by a multidisciplinary team including a physician, psychotherapist (e.g., psychologist), nutritionist, coaches, and family members has the best prognosis (Jacobson, 2003). Treatment consisting of both individual and group cognitive-behavioral therapy and nutritional counseling has been effective for athletes (Sundgot-Borgen and Sundgot-Schneider, 2001). Continued participation in training and competition must be contingent on adherence with the treatment program.

PERFORMANCE ANXIETY

• Optimal performance comes with a certain level of tension and mental activation (Howe and Ogilvie, 1994; p. 71). For athletes struggling with arousal control, educationally based psychologic interventions have yielded significant improvements in performance. Specifically, Weinberg and Comar (1994) examined 45 studies that used either relaxation-based, cognitive, cognitive-behavioral, or behavioral interventions aimed at improving athletic performance across sports. They found that 38 of 45 studies yielded positive performance outcomes.

- Behavioral strategies for performance enhancement might include the use of visual imagery, diaphragmatic breathing, progressive muscle relaxation, biofeedback, autogenic training, yoga, meditation, and desensitization (Hendrickson, 2003*b*).
  1. Visual imagery can involve imagining a relaxing scene or mental rehearsal of one's performance and a desired course of action.
  2. Diaphragmatic breathing is a simple relaxation technique which involves taking slow, deep inhalations, concentrating on only moving the abdomen, holding each inhalation for a few seconds, and then exhaling.
  3. Desensitization is technique in which the athlete gradually diminishes anxiety associated with certain performance aspects (e.g., free-throws in basketball) or specific anxiety disorders (e.g., social phobia) through gradual exposure, either imaginal or *in vivo*, to the feared or anxiety-eliciting stimuli.
- Cognitive strategies can also help athletes develop a greater sense of arousal control, and more importantly, improve performance. This might include encouraging the athlete to replace any sabotaging negative self-statements (e.g., "I will never make this shot.") with reassuring, realistic self-statements (e.g., "I have made this shot before and will try my best to make it again."). Additionally, goal-setting can be an effective strategy for improving identified areas of performance weakness (Hendrickson, 2003*b*; Robinson, 2001).

INJURY REHABILITATION

- It is estimated that more than 3 million injuries occur each year in the United States to children and adults participating in sports and recreational activities (Bijur et al, 1995; Booth, 1987). The injured athlete may present with a concern about the injury itself, but also with concern over the impact of the injury on present and future performance, and concerns regarding the nature of the rehabilitation process (Robinson, 2001). In fact, Thompson and associates suggest that "Rehabilitation is 75% psychologic and 25% physical" (Thompson, Hershman, and Nicholas, 1990; p 265).
  1. Successful rehabilitation should begin with a comprehensive case-conceptualization using the biopsychosocial model, which then allows target areas for treatment to be effectively identified

TABLE 74-5 Biopsychsocial Factors in Injury Rehabilitation

Physical Factors	Where is the injury? What is the frequency, intensity, and duration of any associated pain? Are there any other current significant medical problems? What is their energy level? How is their sleep? What is their history of sports injuries?
Behavioral Factors	Are they adhering to the rehabilitation program? Do they put forth their best effort at rehabilitation sessions? Are there any substance abuse issues (e.g., alcohol, tobacco, excessive eating)? How have they changed their life since the injury (e.g., have they skipped important responsibilities?)
Cognitive Factors	What is their attitude about the injury, the treatment they have received, and the rehabilitation process? Do they engage in predominantly positive or negative self-statements?
Emotional Factors	Have they recently felt more sad, anxious, upset, and/or irritated than they would have liked? Do they have any fears about returning to their sport? Are they experiencing grief over the loss of their sport or exercise activity?
Relationship Factors	Do they have an adequate social support system? Have coaches and/or teammates been constructive in the rehabilitation process? Have they changed their behavior towards family and friends (e.g., more isolative)? Are they experiencing any relationship difficulties/stressors as a result of the injury?

Source: Robinson CS: Psychology and the injured runner: Recovery enhancing strategies, in O'Connor FG, Wilder RP, Nirschl R (eds.): *Textbook of Running Medicine.* 2001, Chap. 49.

(Robinson, 2001) (see Table 74-5). This will address the three areas of rehabilitation proposed by Steadman (1993) to encompass a complete rehabilitation program. They are physical recovery from the injury itself, specific rehabilitation to the injured area, and psychologic rehabilitation.
  2. Effective treatment must then begin with a thorough understanding of the component parts of the rehabilitation process and a collaborative agreement on specific goals for treatment (Robinson, 2001). Studies have shown that belief in the efficacy of treatment is correlated positively with adherence (Brewer et al, 2003; Duda, Smart, and Tappe, 1989).
- The provider may then choose from among several effective interventions to tailor a rehabilitation program to meet the athlete's needs. This might include the use of imagery and other mental devices, increasing social support, pain management, and/or other cognitive-behavioral techniques such as self-management training (Robinson, 2001).

SPECIALTY CONSULTATION FOR PERFORMANCE ISSUES OR INJURY REHABILITATION CONCERNS

- It is important that physicians be vigilant of symptoms that may warrant referral for more extensive psychologic assessment and treatment (Robinson, 2001). For example, Brewer and associates reported that in a sample of orthopedic patients, 33% percent of injured football players were regarded as depressed (Brewer, Jeffers, and Petitpas, 1994).
- The mnemonic IN SAD CAGES can be utilized as a helpful tool to assess the presence of depressive symptomology (Hendrickson, 2003a):
  1. **In** loss of <u>in</u>terest in pleasurable activities
  2. **S** <u>s</u>uicidal ideation
  3. **A** <u>a</u>ctivity changes (e.g., decreased)
  4. **D** <u>d</u>ysthymia (depressed mood)
  5. **C** <u>c</u>oncentration difficulties
  6. **A** <u>a</u>ppetite changes (increased or decreased)
  7. **G** feelings of <u>g</u>uilt
  8. **E** <u>e</u>nergy changes (usually decreased)
  9. **S** <u>s</u>leep changes (increased or decreased)
- The presence of six or more of these symptoms is indicative of a major depressive disorder.
- Psychologists can assess and treat any clinical significant impairment in mood and/or function that may be involved in the etiology, exacerbation, or maintenance of the patient's current complaints. Psychologic referral may be indicated for refractory cases or when patient present with comorbid mood symptoms (e.g., anxiety, depression, grief) that significantly impact personal, social, and/or occupational functioning (Nideffer, 1983; Miller, Vaughn, and Miller, 1990).

References

APA: *Diagnostic and Statistical Manual of Mental Disorders*, 4th ed. Text Revision, Washington, DC, American Psychiatric Association, 2000.

Babyak M, Blumenthal JA, Herman S, et al: Exercise treatment for major depression: Maintenance of therapeutic benefit at 10 months. *Psychosom Med* 62:633, 2000.

Barrett J.R: Exercise addiction, in Mellion MB, Putakian M, Madden CC (eds.): *Sports Medicine Secrets,* 3rd (ed.): Philadelphia, PA, Hanley & Belfus, 2003, Chap. 32.

Begel D, Burton RW: *Sport Psychiatry: Theory and Practice.* New York, NY, Norton Press, 2000.

Bijur PE, Trumble A, Harel Y et al: Sports and recreation injuries in U.S. children and adolescents. *Arch Pediatr Adolesc Med* 149:1009, 1995.

Booth W: Arthritis institute tackles sports. *Science* 237:846, 1987.

Brewer BW, Cornelius AE, Van Raalte JL et al: Protection motivation theory and adherence to sport injury rehabilitation revisited. *Sport Psychol* 17:95, 2003.

Brewer B, Jeffers K, Petitpas A: Perceptions of psychological interventions in the context of sport injury rehabilitation. *Sports Psychologist* 8:176, 1994.

Duda JL, Smart AE, Tappe MK: Predictors of adherence in rehabilitation of athletic injuries: An application of personal investment theory. *J Sport Exerc Psych* 11:367, 1989.

Eppright TD, Sanfacon JA, Beck NC et al: Sport psychiatry in childhood and adolescence: An overview. *Child Psychiatry Hum Dev* 289:71, 1997.

Fleming MF, Barry KL: *Addictive Disorders.* St. Louis, MO, Mosby, 1992.

Gauvin L, Rejeski WJ, Reboussin BA: Contributions of acute bouts of vigorous physical activity to explaining diurnal variations in feeling states in active middle-aged women. *Health Psychol* 19:365, 2000.

Gauvin, Rejeski, Norris, JL: A naturalistic study of the impact of acute physical activity on feeling states and affect in women. *Health Psychol* 15:391, 1996.

Green GA, Nattiv A: Abuse and addiction: Alcohol and street drugs, in Mellion MB, Putakian M, Madden CC (eds.): *Sports Medicine Secrets,* 3rd ed. Philadelphia, PA, Hanley & Belfus, 2003, Chap. 36.

Hendrickson TP: Psychological problems of the athlete, in Mellion MB, Putakian M, Madden CC (eds.): *Sports Medicine Secrets,* 3rd ed., Philadelphia, PA, Hanley & Belfus 2003a, Chap. 33.

Hendrickson T.P: Psychological techniques to enhance performance, in Mellion MB, Putakian M, Madden CC (eds.): *Sports Medicine Secrets,* 3rd ed. Philadelphia, PA, Hanley & Belfus, 2003b, Chap. 34.

Howe MA, Ogilvie BC: Psychological aspects of sports, in Birrer RB (ed.): *Sports Medicine for the Primary Care Physician,* 2nd ed. Boca Raton, FL, CRC Press, 1994, Chap 9.

Jacobson DL: Eating disorders, in Mellion MB, Putakian M, Madden CC (eds.): *Sports Medicine Secrets,* 3rd ed. Philadelphia, PA, Hanley & Belfus, 2003, Chap. 31.

Kramer A.F., Hahn S., Cohen N.J et al: Ageing, fitness, and neurocognitive function. *Nature* 400:418, 1999.

Miller TW, Vaughn MP, Miller JM: Clinical issues and treatment strategies in stress-oriented athletes. *Sports Med* 9:370, 1990.

NAGWS: National Federation of State High School Athletic Associations, 1999.

NCAA: Study of substance abuse and abuse habits of college athletes. National Collegiate Athletic Association, 1997. (unpublished).

Nattiv A, Agostini R Drinkwater B et al: The female athlete triad: The inter-relatedness of disordered eating, amenorrhea, and osteoporosis. *Clin Sports Med* 13:405, 1994.

Nideffer RM: The injured athlete: Psychological factors in treatment. *Orthop Clin North Am* 14:373, 1983.

Pugliese MT, Liftshitz F, Grad G et al: Fear of obesity: A cause for short stature and delayed puberty. *N Engl J Med* 309:513, 1983.

Robinson CS: Psychology and the injured runner: Recovery enhancing strategies, in O'Connor FG, Wilder RP, Nirschl R (eds.): *Textbook of Running Medicine.* New York, McGraw-Hill, 2001, Chap. 49.

Sachtleben TR: Overtraining, in Mellion MB, Putakian M, Madden CC (eds.): *Sports Medicine Secrets,* 3rd ed. Philadelphia, PA, Hanley & Belfus, 2003, Chap. 35.

Sallis JF, Prochaska JJ, Taylor WC: A review of correlates of physical activity of children and adolescents. *Med Sci Sports Exerc* 32:963, 2000.

Steadman JR: A physician's approach to the psychology of injury, in Heil J (ed.): *Psychology of Sport Injury,* 1993, Chap. 25.

Sundgot-Borgen J: Prevalence of eating disorders in elite female athletes. *Int J Sport Nutr* 3:29, 1993.

Sundgot-Borgen J, Klungland M, Torstveit G: Prevalence of eating disorders in male and female elite athletes. *Med Sci Sports Exerc* 31:5, 1999.

Sundgot-Borgen J, Sundgot-Schneider, H: The long term effect of CBT and nutritional counseling in treating bulimic elite athletes: A randomized controlled study. *Med Sci Sports Exerc* 33:97, 2001.

Thompson TL, Hershman EB, Nicholas JA: Rehabilitation of the injured athlete. *Pediatrician* 17:262, 1990.

U.S. Department of Health and Human Services: Physical activity and health: A report of the Surgeon General. Atlanta, GA, 1996.

U.S. Department of Health and Human Services: Clinical practice guidelines for treating tobacco use and dependence. Rockville, MD, Public Health Service, 2000.

Weaver NL, Marshall SW, Miller MD: Preventing sports injuries: Opportunities for intervention in youth athletes. *Patient Educ Couns* 46:199, 2002.

Weinberg RS, Comar W: The effectiveness of psychological interventions in competitive sport. *Sports Med* 18:406, 1994.

Wilmore JH: Eating and weight disorders in the female athlete. *Int J Sport Nutr* 1:104, 1991.

75 COMPLEMENTARY AND ALTERNATIVE MEDICINE

Anthony I Beutler, MD
Wayne B Jonas, MD

WHAT IS COMPLEMENTARY AND ALTERNATIVE MEDICINE?

- Many different medical systems and medical practices exist in the world today including Traditional Oriental Medicine, Native American Practices, Ayurveda, and Western Biomedicine (to name only a few).
- Western biomedicine is the medicine practiced in American hospitals and taught in American medical schools. Western biomedicine is neither the oldest nor the most widely used medical system in the world today. The World Health Organization estimates that a substantial portion of the world's population receives their medical care outside the Western biomedical system. (Marty, 1997)
- The term "Complementary and Alternative Medicine" or "CAM" is Western biomedicine's term for all medical practices that lie outside its boundaries. CAM's boundaries are imprecise and constantly changing as Western scientific methods are applied to study and establish the efficacy of *outside* medical practices in the treatment of Western biomedical disease states. For instance, is glucosamine supplementation for osteoarthritis pain a Western biomedical therapy or a CAM therapy? (Beutler and Jonas, 2004).

WHO USES COMPLEMENTARY AND ALTERNATIVE MEDICINE?

- Many developing countries rely on CAM practices to provide most of the health care for their citizens.
- Americans spend more than $27 billion each year (most of it unreimbursed by insurance) on CAM practices. Visits to U.S. CAM practitioners rose from 400 million per year in 1990 to 600 million per year in 1996. Forty percent of the U.S. population and 75% of the population of France reported utilizing a CAM practice at least once during the year. (Eisenberg et al, 1998)
- Among Western CAM consumers, 95% use CAM in a complementary fashion or in addition to Western biomedicine. Only 5% use CAM exclusively, or as an alternative to Western biomedicine. (Astin, 1998)
- Studies reveal that CAM users in the United States tend to be more educated, more affluent, more holistic in their view of wellness, and more likely to have chronic pain or a chronic disease than nonusers of CAM (Beutler and Jonas; Eisenberg et al, 1998; Astin, 1998). Past reports indicated that some minorities, such as Blacks, were less likely to use CAM; however, a more recent study specifically designed to assess CAM use among minorities found no difference in CAM use among ethnic groups (Mackenzie et al, 2003). Women consistently use CAM more than men.
- CAM therapies are popular for both major and minor illnesses. Roughly half of patients with *human immunodeficiency virus* (HIV) and half of patients diagnosed with cancer will try CAM therapies to combat their illnesses; however, CAM therapies are less commonly used to treat diseases for which Western biomedicine offers safe, effective treatments. For instance, while 57% of patients with diabetes mellitus type 2 report using CAM treatments, only 20% report trying CAM therapies to treat their diabetes (Yeh et al, 2002).

DO ATHLETES USE COMPLEMENTARY AND ALTERNATIVE MEDICINE?

- No accurate estimate of CAM use among athletes is available (White, 1998); however, anecdotal evidence suggests extremely high rates of CAM use in athletes.

Common sense and common experience suggest that CAM use should be regarded as the rule, not the exception, in athletes.

- Athletes may use CAM therapies to enhance performance, decrease recovery time after workouts, or speed return to play following an injury.
- Examples of CAM treatments commonly used by athletes to enhance performance include caffeine (guarana), creatine, ginkgo biloba, hormone supplements, and ephedra. Examples of CAM treatments typically used for pain control or accelerated return to play include iontophoresis, microcurrent, spinal manipulation, homeopathic arnica, and acupuncture.
- The high pressure and high stakes of athletic competition, together with the exceptionally small margin that separates success from failure, demand that sports medicine physicians exercise great vigilance in protecting the athletes entrusted to their care.

Where Can I Find Good Evidence on CAM Therapies?

- The best type of evidence to use in evaluating a CAM therapy depends on the following:
  1. Risks posed by the therapy
  2. Cost of the therapy
  3. Information preference of the individual patient
  4. Availability of other proven, effective, and safe therapies for the patient's condition
- *Randomized controlled trials* (RCTs) are important for evaluating high risk and/or high cost therapies because RCTs provide essential safety and risk/benefit data; however, RCTs have some important limitations. RCTs are difficult and expensive to sustain for long periods of study. Additionally, the results of an RCT depend greatly on the careful selection of the all-important "control" group (Jonas, Linde, and Walack, 1999).
- Clinical outcomes research is another, less recognized type of research trial that is useful in studying CAM therapies. Outcomes research is more similar to clinical practice than RCTs: It involves a wider range of patients over longer periods of time and allows for variations in care caused by interactions with multiple providers. Outcomes research examines the probability that a therapy will produce a beneficial effect and provides an estimate of how large that effect will be in everyday clinical practice. For long-term, chronic conditions and their therapies, outcomes research often provides the only relevant evidence (Walach, Jonas, and Lewith, 2002).
- Table 75-1 lists a number of sources for obtaining quality evidence on specific CAM therapies and practices.

TABLE 75-1   Internet Resources—Reliable CAM Evidence for Physicians

The Cochrane Library

The library contains a database of systematic reviews featuring RCTs of CAM and conventional therapies, as well as a controlled trials register that provides bibliographic listings of controlled trials and conference proceedings.

Abstracts of the reviews and trials are available free of charge at www.cochrane.org.

Full text copies of all materials are available thru several subscription services including gateway.ovid.com.

PubMed

The most comprehensive and popular medical search engine has new clinical queries filter to assist in limiting your search results. The most comprehensive search is obtained by using the key words "complementary medicine."

Free access at multiple websites including www.pubmed.org

National Center for Complementary and Alternative Medicine

The clinical trials section contains an index of trials by treatment or condition. The index can also be accessed via www.clinicaltrials.gov or thru PubMed.

The NCCAM website is www.nccam.nih.gov.

National Library of Medicine

Powerful search engine allows searches across all government guidelines, plus PubMed. Synonym and related terms search option is very helpful for CAM therapies with multiple common names.

The search engine may be accessed free of charge at hstat.nlm.nih.gov.

Individual guidelines from many government agencies can be found at www.guideline.gov or www.cdc.gov/publications.

Natural Medicines Comprehensive Database

The online database contains comprehensive listings and cross-listings of natural and herbal therapies, including very helpful sections on "all known uses" and "herb-drug interactions." The database also offers an extensive review of the available pharmacologic evidence.

From the publishers of *The Prescriber's Letter*, the database can be accessed via a purchased subscription at www.naturaldatabase.com.

ePocrates Rx Pro

PDA listing of alternative medicines, but does not contain information on nonmedicinal modalities (acupuncture or manipulation). Provides names, common uses, suggested dosages and a multicheck feature that checks the patients medical regimen for drug–drug, herb–herb, and drug–herb interactions.

Alternative medicine content is available only with the purchase of ePocrates Rx Pro, not with the free version of ePocrates Rx. www.epocrates.com.

ABBREVIATION: RCT = randomized controlled trials; CAM = complementary and alternative medicine.

- The patient's individual beliefs and personality can affect the likelihood of therapeutic efficacy. If a patient believes that a specific therapy will alleviate their condition, this prior plausibility has its own therapeutic effect.
- If conventional medicine offers a safe, proven therapy that is acceptable to the patient, any potential CAM therapy must pass equally stringent evidence standards for efficacy and safety before being considered as a viable treatment option.

How do I Advise My Patients About CAM Therapies?

- Ninety-five percent of patients who use CAM therapies also use conventional, Western biomedicine; however, over 60% of these patients do not inform their physicians of their CAM therapy use (Eisenberg et al, 1998). This CAM communication gap results in a wasteful, and potentially dangerous, patient-physician environment.
- Patients who use CAM practices possess character traits that incline them to active participation and partnering in their medical care (Eisenberg, 1997). A physician who refuses to discuss and denies any knowledge of CAM treatments does not alter the patient's need for partnering, but merely forces them to seek association elsewhere—thus widening the already precipitous CAM communication gap.
- Many effective strategies can be used to partner with patients on CAM therapies; however, we recommend the strategy proposed by Jonas. He suggests that depending on the specific patient and the specific treatment, physicians should *protect, permit,* and *promote* CAM therapies (Jonas, 1998).

Protecting From Harm

- Many CAM practices are inherently low risk when performed or prescribed by competent providers; however, herbal remedies and high dose vitamin supplementation (both very popular CAM therapies) can cause serious or fatal consequences (DeSmet, 2002).
- *Natural* does not equal *safe*, contrary to the popular conceived connotation. Herbs and vitamins have real effects, real side effects, and real toxicities. Even without direct toxicity, herb–herb and herb–drug interactions can be severe. Other quality issues, such as contamination, varying potencies, and differing absorption rates abound in the unregulated domain of nutritional supplements (Eisenberg, 1997).
- Biofeedback, meditation, prayer, and acupuncture pose minimal risk for direct toxicity; however, even these safe practices may indirectly result in harm if used in place of more effective treatments. The physician should detail the risks and benefits (both direct and indirect) of all therapeutic options.
- Ephedra (or *Ma Huang*) especially in combination with caffeine (or guaraná), chromium picolinate, and pulsed magnetic field therapy are examples of therapies from which patients should be protected. (See following section on specific CAM treatments.)

Permitting Unproven, Nontoxic Therapies

- Physicians may experience trepidation in allowing patients to engage in unproven practices or therapies.

But if the therapy has no toxicity and is not used in place of a proven-effective treatment, the practice can be safely permitted and may be encouraged.
- The physician's ultimate goal should be to relieve patient suffering. Patients welcome relief—and physicians should do likewise—even should relief come through nonquantifiable means (spiritual effect, placebo effect, prior plausibility). (Moerman and Jonas, 2002)
- Homeopathic arnica, acupuncture, spinal manipulation, ginko biloba supplementation, and many other CAM therapies can be safely permitted when properly administered and appropriately prescribed.

Promoting Proven Treatments

- Physicians should promote safe, effective treatments regardless of their medical system of origin. Western biomedicine has adopted and should continue to incorporate proven techniques and therapies from other systems of medical care (Eisenberg, 1997).
- Glucosamine supplementation is a prime example of a CAM therapy that should be promoted for individuals with knee osteoarthritis.

What's the Current Evidence for or Against Some Popular CAM Treatments?

- Summaries of the evidence for and against a few of the most popular CAM treatments used by athletes and the general population appear below. They are organized into the sections of *Prevent, Permit,* and *Promote.*

Prevent

- Ephedra (*Ma Huang, Herbal Ecstasy, Zhong Mahuang*) (Gilles et al, 1996; Bell et al, 2000; Haller and Benowitz, 2000; Congeni and Miller, 2002)
  1. Primary use: Weight loss or enhanced athletic performance and endurance. Less commonly used for respiratory conditions or asthma.
  2. Evidence: Ephedra can potentiate a small weight loss of 2–5 kg over 6 weeks to 6 months, but only in patients with *body mass index* (BMI) over 30. The weight loss is typically transient and often requires combination the use of other stimulants (i.e., caffeine or guaraná). Multiple studies show no performance enhancing effect unless combined with caffeine/guaraná or used in very high dosages.
  3. Toxicity: High dosages and combination with caffeine known to increase toxicity. High dosages cause dizziness, restlessness, anxiety, palpitations, and hypertension. *Fatal events have been reported.* Capsules have been found to contain many impurities, to include banned substances.
  4. Regulated/Banned: Banned by International Olympic Committee (IOC), likely to be restricted

by Food and Drug Administration (FDA) in near future. Ephedra/caffeine combinations are already banned by FDA. Subsequently sold in combination with guaraná (the herbal and more potent form of caffeine).

5. Conclusion: Ephedra products, especially ephedra/guaraná combinations are banned substances, are not safe, and have been demonstrated to cause considerable harm. As negative publicity builds, Ephedra-free versions of products appear, but there is no evidence that these will be any safer than the original formulations.

• Chromium picolinate (Fox and Sabovic, 1998; McLeod, Gaynes, and Golden, 1999; Speetjens et al, 1999; Beutler and Jonas, 2004).

1. Primary use: Increase lean body mass, improve glycemic control in diabetes.

2. Evidence: While earlier, design-flawed studies suggested some beneficial effects, newer studies show no ergogenic or fat-burning effects. Some studies suggest slight, dose-dependant improvements in diabetes control and lipid profiles.

3. Toxicity: Tremor, along with cognative, sleep, and mood changes have been reported as side effects. Concern exists for potential *deoxyribonucleic acid* (DNA) mutations with long-term exposure to chromium supplementation.

4. Regulated/Banned: No

5. Conclusion: Though inexpensive and minimally toxic with short-term use, real concern exists for DNA mutations with long-term use or high chromium levels. Since the reported benefits are very small and the risk of long-term toxicity potentially great, patients should avoid this supplement.

• *Pulsed electromagnetic field therapy* (PEMF) (Bassett, Payluk, and Pilla, 1974; Aaron, Ciombor, and Jolly, 1989; Hulme et al, 2002)

1 Primary use: Decrease pain and stiffness in osteoarthritis

2. Evidence: The beneficial effect of PEMF therapy in delayed union fractures is well established. Similar magnetic fields have been found to stimulate proteoglycan production *in vitro* chondrocytes; however, despite abundant anecdotal Internet reports, a recent Cochrane review found only three quality articles in the scientific literature. The review found that PEMF produced statistically significant, but clinically insignificant changes in knee *osteoarthritis* (OA) pain and disability. The optimum dosage and frequency of PEMF—as well as acceptable technical standards for the PEMF equipment—remain unknown. The cost of PEMF can exceed $200 per day.

3. Toxicity: Unknown. The effects of pulsed electromagnetic fields on human tissues have not been well-studied.

4. Regulated/Banned: No

5. Conclusion: Patients should be advised that PEMF's small benefits in OA pain and stiffness are outweighed by uncertain side effects, incomplete technical data, and tremendously high cost. Other proven-effective, lower cost treatments for OA exist; and are favored over PEMF therapy.

Permit

• Ginko leaf (Pittler and Ernst, 2000; van Dongen et al, 2000; Oken et al, 1998)

1. Primary use: Combat memory loss and slow progressive dementia. Also used to relieve vascular claudication symptoms.

2. Evidence: Most studies suggest that ginko leaf can slow dementia progression and increase cognitive function in middle-aged adults without subjective memory loss. In some countries, ginko is the standard of care (in place of cholinesterase inhibitors) for Alzheimer's dementia. More limited evidence also suggests that ginko may improve walking distance in vascular claudication.

3. Toxicity: Mild *gastrointestinal* (GI) upset and constipation are the most common side effects reported; however, ginko has anticoagulant properties and lowers the seizure threshold. Ginko has been linked to spontaneous bleeding. It should not be used in patients taking other anticoagulants or in those with a seizure disorder or in combination with other drugs that lower seizure threshold.

4. Regulated/Banned: No

5. Conclusion: In the appropriately selected patients, ginko is a permissible alternative to conventional drug treatments, especially if the patient prefers ginko supplementation.

• St. John's Wort (SJW) (Gaster, 2000; Woelk, 2000; Brenner et al, 2000; Schrader, 2000; Beutler and Jonas, 2004).

1. Primary use: Antidepressant, anxiolytic, anti-insomnia, and adjunct to weight-loss uses are commonly described.

2. Evidence: Most evidence suggests SJW to be effective for mild to moderate depression. SJW may also be effective in obsessive-compulsive disorders. Severe depression is not reliably treated by SJW and higher dosages of SJW increase the risk for severe skin reactions.

3. Toxicity: Insomnia, restlessness, and GI distress are common. Hypericin doses over 5 mg/day increase risk for severe photodermatitis. SJW has fewer side effects than TCA or SSRI antidepressants;

however, the potential for severe herb–herb and drug–herb interactions—including serotonin syndrome—is greater with SJW. SJW can accelerate the metabolism of drugs cleared by the P450 enzyme system and should not be used by those on immunosuppressants or antiviral medications without monitoring.

4. Regulated/Banned: Not banned by athletic regulatory agencies; however, due to the risk of serious drug interactions, the distribution of SJW was recently banned in France. The governments of Japan, the United Kingdom and other European countries are considering similar bans.

5. Conclusion: In monitored patients with mild–moderate depression, SJW therapy is acceptable *if* the patient has a simple, compatible medical regimen and strongly prefers SJW to conventional drug treatment.

• Creatine (Williams, Kreider, and Branch, 1999; Volek et al, 1999; Vandenberghe et al, 1997)

1. Primary use: Decrease workout recovery time; improve muscular strength/athletic performance

2. Evidence: Many studies document increases in repetitive strength tasks of less than 30 s duration. Certain individuals who have low baseline levels of creatine may experience a more pronounced effect.

3. Toxicity: Common side effects include GI upset, diarrhea, and mild muscle cramping. Case reports have attempted to implicate creatine in everything from cardiomyopathy to renal failure to rhabdomyolysis, but these effects are difficult to distinguish from the effects of volume depletion and heat illness. Creatine's ergogenic effects are largely negated by caffeine consumption.

4. Regulated/Banned: Not a banned substance, but the National Collegiate Athletic Association (NCAA) prohibits universities from providing creatine for their athletes.

5. Conclusion: A discussion of risks and benefits is critical to creatine. After thorough discussion with an athlete, creatine use can be permitted in otherwise healthy patients involved in strength-related events. Creatine should not be used in pediatric athletes (unclear safety), athletes with kidney disease, or athletes prone to dehydration (osmotic action of creatine predisposes to dehydration and intensifies subsequent heat illness). For most athletes, creatine has no proven benefit. In fact, the increased body mass (2–4 kg) caused by creatine supplementation may impair performance in endurance events.

• Homeopathy (Arnica) (Ernst and Barnes, 1998; Vickers et al, 1997; Tveiten et al, 1995; Vickers et al, 1998)

1. Primary use: Relief of *delayed onset muscle soreness* (DOMS).

2. Evidence: Homeopathic arnica is more properly viewed as an alternative medical system with many distinct, pharmacologic interventions. No single homeopathic treatment has been conclusively proven to be effective in reducing DOMS. Small trials of diverse remedies offer contradictory conclusions for homeopathy in DOMS. Poor design, differing methodologies, and differing definitions of DOMS predictably plague these trials.

3. Toxicity: No side effects above placebo levels have been reported. Reports of severe allergic reactions appear to be rare. Extreme dilution of homeopathic remedies makes direct toxicity highly unlikely.

4. Regulated/Banned: No. A few states credential homeopathic physicians.

5. Conclusion: The homeopathic system of medicine is complex and has not yet been adequately evaluated; however, its costs and toxicities are low in the hands of trained professionals.

• Acupuncture (Green et al, 2002; Tulder et al, 2002; NIH, 1997; Garvey, Marks, and Wiesel, 1989)

1. Primary use: Relief of low back pain and lateral elbow pain.

2. Evidence: Like homeopathic arnica, acupuncture may be considered as a separate medical system. For lateral elbow pain, a recent Cochrane review found insufficient evidence to make any recommendations. RCTs of acupuncture for low back pain are contradictory and poorly designed. Acupuncture has been proven effective in reducing pain and relief of nausea.

3. Toxicity: Broken needles, pneumothorax and infectious disease transmission are anecdotally reported, but unlikely in the hands of licensed professionals. Pain, fatigue, bleeding, and fainting are the most common side effects.

4. Regulated/Banned: No. Over 30 states license acupuncturists. The FDA has approved acupuncture needles as experimental devices.

5. Conclusion: Given the paucity of evidence, the Cochrane review recommends that effective, proven treatments be considered before acupuncture; however, the costs and risks are sufficiently low that acupuncture use—under the care of a trained professional—can be permitted.

• Chondroitin (Leeb et al, 2000; Leffler et al, 1999; Towheed and Anastassiades, 2000)

1. Primary use: Improving pain and stiffness from OA.

2. Evidence: Several trials suggest (size and design limiting) that chondroitin and ibuprofen are more effective than ibuprofen alone for improving OA

symptoms. Additionally the drugs have different times to onset of action. Ibuprofen reaches maximum efficacy in a matter of days; chondroitin is maximally effective over a few weeks. Chondroitin is typically sold in varying combinations with glucosamine, manganese, and magnesium; however, no data suggests the combination treatment to be more effective than the single agent alone.

3. Toxicity: Mild GI distress is the most common side effect. Combination tablets can exceed safe daily doses of manganese and cause *central nervous system* (CNS) irritability. Chondroitin has a heparinoid structure and may predispose to bleeding if used in with other anticoagulants.

4. Regulated/Banned: No.

5. Conclusion: Though less convincing than glucosamine (see below) some evidence supports chondroitin use in OA. Several studies with 5+ years of follow-up report no adverse events related to chondroitin use. Given the moderately high cost of chondroitin tablets, a 6–8 week trial period is advisable. If no clinical effect is noted during this trial, chondroitin should be discontinued as a result of cost considerations.

• Spinal manipulation (Andersson et al, 1999; Koes et al, 1996; Assendelft et al, 1995)

1. Primary use: Relief of low back pain/stiffness, relief of DOMS, and speeding return to play following low back injury.

2. Evidence: Majority of evidence suggests spinal manipulation to be at least as effective as conventional treatment for low back pain. Nine of ten well-designed RCTs in a recent review concluded that spinal manipulation provided more pain relief than control treatments; however, differences between manipulation techniques make conclusions difficult to generalize. Manipulation may require more physician visits than conventional care, increasing the cost of therapy. Health insurers may reimburse some of this cost.

3. Toxicity: Rare case reports of stoke, paralysis, or spinal chord damage are mostly related to c-spine manipulation and occur at a frequency of one per million of manipulations. No severe complications have been reported from over 15,000 patients enrolled in monitored RCTs.

4. Regulated/Banned: No.

5. Conclusion: Competently performed L-spine manipulation is safe and likely effective for low back pain, although it may be higher cost than other therapies.

• Panax* Ginseng (Allen et al, 1998; Wesnes et al, 2000; Ellis and Reddy, 2002; Yun and Choi, 1998)

1. Primary use: Improve cognitive function, athletic performance, and increase energy.

2. Evidence: Many studies document that *ginseng* supplementation has no ergogenic effects. Similarly, *P. ginseng* has not been shown to improve memory when used alone, but has been demonstrated to have efficacy when combined with ginkgo supplementation in middle-aged individuals.

3. Toxicity: Insomnia, tachycardia and palpitations become more common with high doses. Mastalgia, vaginal bleeding, and amenorrhea are likely related to the estrogenic effects of *ginseng*. Long-term use is not well studied. *Ginseng* will intensify the effects of other common stimulants (caffeine, guaraná, and tea).

4. Regulated/Banned: No.

5. Conclusion: Studies suggest minimal toxicity with short-term use, but long-term use is more difficult to justify since estrogenic risks may outweigh the unclear benefits; however, further studies continue to explore many other possible indications for *ginseng* supplementation.

Promote

• Glucosamine sulfate (Pavelka et al, 2002; Thie, Prasad, and Major, 2001; Foerster, Schmid, and Rovati, 2000; McAlindon et al, 2000)

1. Primary use: Relief of stiffness and pain in OA and *temperomandibular joint dysfunction* (TMJ).

2. Evidence: Multiple trials consistently demonstrate superior efficacy of glucosamine sulfate to placebo. More recent data suggest that glucosamine may provide more pain relief than *nonsteroidal anti-inflammatory drugs* (NSAIDs) after 6 weeks of use. Insufficient data exists to determine if glucosamine slows the rate of OA progression. Knee OA is the most widely studied, but efficacy data also exists for glucosamine in TMJ and OA of the hand and spine.

3. Toxicity: Mild GI distress (comparable to placebo levels) has been reported. Concerns for exacerbations of diabetic control or reactions in patients with shellfish allergy appear to be unfounded.

4. Regulated/Banned: No.

5. Conclusion: Glucosamine is an effective treatment for OA. Glucosamine supplementation should be discontinued if no clinical response occurs after a 6–8 week trial due to its moderate cost.

REFERENCES

Aaron RK, Ciombor DM, Jolly G: Stimulation of experimental endochondral ossification by low-energy pulsing electromagnetic fields. *J Bone Miner Res* 4:227–233, 1989.

Allen JD, McLung J, Nelson AG, et al: Ginseng supplementation does not enhance healthy young adult's peak aerobic exercise performance. *J Am Coll Nutr* 17(5):462–466, 1998.

Andersson, Gunnar GJ, Lucente T et al: A comparison of osteo-pathic spinal manipulation with standard care for patients with low back pain. *NEJM* 341(19):1426–1431, 1999.

Assendelft WJJ, Koes BW, Knipschild PG, et al: The relationship between methodological quality and conclusions in reviews of spinal manipulation. *JAMA* 274(24):1942–1948, 1995.

Astin JA: Why patients use alternative medicine: Results of a national study. *JAMA* 279(19):1548–1553, 1998.

Bassett CA, Payluk RJ, Pilla AA: Augmentation of bone repair by inductively coupled electromagnetic fields. *Science* 184:575–577.

Bell DG, Jacobs I, McLellan TM, et al: Reducing the dose of combined caffeine and ephedrine preserves the ergogenic effect. *Aviat Space Environ* Med 71:415–419, 2000.

Beutler AI, Jonas WB: Complimentary and alternative medicine for the sports medicine physician, in Birrer R, O'Connor F (eds.): *Sports Medicine for the Primary Care Physician*, 3d ed. Boca Raton, FL, CRC Press, 2004.

Brenner R, Azbel V, Madhusoodanan S, et al: Comparison of an extract of Hypericum (LI 160) and sertraline in the treatment of depression: A double-blind, randomized pilot study. *Clin Ther* 22:411–419, 2000.

Congeni J, Miller S: Supplements and drugs used to enhance athletic performance. *Ped Cl North Am* 49:2, 2002.

DeSmet P: Herbal remedies. *N Engl J Med* 347:2046–2056, 2002.

Eisenberg DM: Advising patients who seek alternative medical therapies. *Ann Int Med* 127(1), 1997.

Eisenberg DM, Davis RB, Ettner SL, et al: Trends in alternative medicine use in the United States, 1990–1997: Results of a follow-up national survey. *JAMA* 280(18):1569–1575, 1998.

Ellis JM, Reddy P: Effects of Panax ginseng on quality of life. *Ann Pharmacother* 36:375–379, 2002.

Ernst E, Barnes J: Are homeopathic remedies effective for delayed onset muscle soreness: A systematic review of placebo-controlled trials. *Perfusion* 11:4–8, 1998.

Foerster KK, Schmid K, Rovati LC: Efficacy of glucosamine sulfate in osteoarthritis of the lumbar spine: A placebo-controlled, randomized, double-blind study. Philadelphia, PA, *Am Coll Rheumatol 64th Ann Scientific Mtg,* Oct 29–Nov 2, 2000.

Fox GN, Sabovic Z: Chromium picolinate supplementation for diabetes mellitus. *J Fam Pract* 46(1):83–86, Jan. 1998.

Garvey TA, Marks MR, Wiesel SW: A prospective, randomized double-blind evaluation of trigger-point injection therapy for low-back pain. *Spine* 14:962–964, 1989.

Gaster B: St. John's wort for depression. *Arch Intern Med* 160:152–156, 2000.

Gilles H, Derman WE, Noakes TD, et al: Pseudoephedrine is without ergogenic effects during prolonged exercise. *J Appl Physiol* 81:2611–2617, 1996.

Green S, Buchbinder R, Barnsley L, et al: Acupuncture for lateral elbow pain. *The Cochrane Library:* Vol 4, 2002.

Haller CA, Benowitz NL: Adverse cardiovascular and central nervous system events associated with dietary supplements containing ephedra alkaloids. *N Engl J Med* 343:1833–1838, 2000.

Hulme J, Robinson B, DeBie R, et al: Electromagnetic fields for the treatment of osteoarthritis. *The Cochrane Library:* Vol 4, 2002.

Jonas WB: Alternative medicine—learning from the past, examining the present, advancing to the future. *JAMA* 280:1617, 1998.

Jonas WB, Linde K, Walack H: How to practice evidence-based complementary medicine, in Jonas W, Levin J (eds.): *Essentials of Complementary and Alternative Medicine.* Philadelphia, PA, Lippincott Williams & Wilkins, 1999, pp 72–87.

Koes BW, Assendelf WJJ, Van der Heijde GJ et al: Spinal manipulation for low back pain: An updated systematic review of randomized clinical trials. *Spine* 21(24);2860–2871, 1996.

Leeb BF, Schweitzer H, Montag K, et al: A meta-analysis of chondroitin sulfate in the treatment of osteoarthritis. *J Rheumatol* 27(1):205–211, 2000.

Leffler CT, Philippi AF, Leffler SG, et al: Glucosamine, chondroitin, and manganese ascorbate for degenerative joint disease of the knee or low back: A randomized, double-blind, placebo-controlled pilot study. *Mil Med* 164:85–91, 1999.

Mackenzie ER, Taylor L, Bloom BS, et al: Ethnic minority use of complementary and alternative medicine (CAM): A national probability survey of CAM utilizers. *Altern Ther* 9(4):50–56, 2003.

Marty AT: Fundamentals of complementary and alternative medicine. *Chest* 112(6):16–A, 1997.

McAlindon TE, LaValley MP, Gulin JP, et al: Glucosamine and chondroitin for treatment of osteoarthritis a systematic quality assessment and meta-analysis. *JAMA* 283:1469–1475, 2000.

McLeod MN, Gaynes BN, Golden RN: Chromium potentiation of antidepressant pharmacotherapy for dysthymic disorder in 5 patients. *J Clin Psych* 60(4):237–240, 1999.

Moerman D, Jonas W: Deconstructing the placebo effect and finding the meaning response. *Ann Intern Med* 136:471–476, 2002.

NIH: Acupuncture. NIH Consens Statement Online, 15(5):1–34, Nov 3–5, Dec 30, 1997.

Oken BS, et al: The efficacy of Ginkgo biloba on cognitive function in Alzheimer disease. *Arch Neurol* 55(11):1409–1415, Nov. 1998.

Pavelka K, Gatterova J, Olejarova M, et al: Glucosamine sulfate use and delay of progression of knee osteoarthritis: A 3-year, randomized, placebo-controlled, double-blind study. *Arch Intern Med* 162:2113–2123, 2002.

Pittler MH, Ernst E: Ginkgo biloba extract for the treatment of intermittent claudication: A meta-analysis of randomized trials. *Am J Med* 108:276–281, 2000.

Schrader E: Equivalence of St. John's wort extract (Ze 117) and fluoxetine: A randomized, controlled study in mild-moderate depression. *Int Clin Psychopharmacol* 15:61–68, 2000.

Speetjens JK, Collins RA, Vincent JB, et al: The nutritional supplement chromium(III) tris(picolinate) cleaves DNA. *Chem Res Toxicol* 12(6):483–487, 1999.

Thie NM, Prasad NG, Major PW: Evaluation of glucosamine sulfate compared to ibuprofen for the treatment of temporomandibular joint osteoarthritis: A randomized double blind controlled 3 month clinical trial. *J Rheumatol* 28:1347–1355, 2001.

Towheed TE, Anastassiades TP: Glucosamine and chondriotin for treating symptoms of osteoarthritis. Evidence is widely touted but incomplete. *JAMA* 238(11):1483–1484, 2000.

Tulder MW, van Cherkin DC, Berman B, et al: Acupuncture for low back pain. *The Cochrane Library:* vol. 4, 2002.

Tveiten D, Bruset S, Borchgrevnink CF, et al: Effects of the homeopathic remedy Arnica D 30 on marathon runners: A randomized, double-blind study during the 1995 Oslo Marathon. *Complement Ther Med* 6:71–74, 1998.

van Dongen MC, van Rossum E, Kessels AG, et al: The efficacy of ginkgo for elderly people with dementia and age-associated memory impairment: New results of a randomized clinical trial. *J Am Geriatr Soc* 48(10):1183–1194, 2000.

Vandenberghe K, Goris M, Van Hecke P, et al: Long term creatine intake is beneficial to muscle performance during resistance training. *J Appl Physiol* 83:2055–2063, 1997.

Vickers AJ, Fisher P, Smith C, et al: Homeopathy for delayed onset muscle soreness: a randomized double blind placebo controlled trial. *Br J Sports Med* 31(4):304–307, 1997.

Vickers AJ, Fisher P, Smith C, et al: Homoeopathic Arnica 30× is ineffective for muscle soreness after long-distance running: A randomised, double-blind, placebo-controlled trial. *Clin J Pain* 14:227–231, 1998.

Volek JS, Duncan ND, Mazzetti SA, et al: Performance and muscle fiber adaptations to creatine supplementation and heavy resistance training. *Med Sci Sports Exerc* 1999.

Walach H, Jonas WB, Lewith G: The role of outcomes research in evaluating complementary and alternative medicine, in Lewith G, Jonas W, Walach H (eds.): *Clinical Research in Complementary Therapies*, London, Churchill Livingston, 2002, pp 29–45.

Wesnes KA, Ward T, McGinty A, et al: The memory enhancing effects of a Ginkgo biloba/Panax ginseng combination in healthy middle-aged volunteers. *Psychopharmacology* 152:353–361, 2000.

White J: Alternative sports medicine. *Phys Sports Med* 26(6), 1998.

Williams MH, Kreider RB, Branch JD: Creatine: The power supplement. Champaign, IL, Human Kinetics, 1999.

Woelk H: Comparison of St. John's wort and imipramine for treating depression: Randomized controlled trial. *BMJ* 321:536–539, 2000.

Yeh GY, Eisenberg DM, Davis RB, et al: Use of complimentary and alternative medicine among persons with diabetes mellitus: Results of a national survey. *Am J Public Health* 92(10):1648–1652, 2002.

Yun TK, Choi SY: Non-organ specific cancer prevention of ginseng: A prospective study in Korea. *Int J Epidemiol* 27(3):359–364, 1998.

76 BASEBALL

James R Morales, MD
Dennis A Cardone, DO

OVERVIEW

- America's pastime is one of the most popular sports played today. It has been estimated that more than 19 million children are involved in youth baseball in the United States (Janda et al, 1998).
- Although classified as a "limited contact" sport, the incidence of injury ranges between 2 and 8% of participants per year (Roberts, 2001).
- Serious injuries are associated with blunt chest impact and head and eye trauma. Most injuries involve soft tissue trauma or throwing injuries.

BACKGROUND

- *Biomechanics* of overhand throwing depends on adequate transfer of momentum. This kinetic energy is produced from larger slower muscles and transferred to smaller faster body parts (Newsham et al, 1998).
- *Anatomy* of the shoulder includes the sternoclavicular joint, acromioclavicular joint, glenohumeral joint, and scapulothoracic joint. The glenohumeral joint is a complex joint involving many stabilizers including, the joint capsule, glenoid labrum, glenohumeral ligaments, and the rotator cuff.
- *Anatomy* of the elbow includes the humeroulnar joint, humeroradial joint, and the radioulnar joint. Further components are the medial and lateral collateral ligament complexes. Musculature of the elbow includes

biceps brachii, bracioradialis, brachialis, triceps, aconeus, as well as the supinators and pronators.
- Five phases of throwing: (1) Windup begins with initial movement of pitcher, the deltoid abducts arm, and ends when hands come apart or ball leaves nondominant hand. (2) Early cocking begins when hands come apart, the deltoid abducts arm, infraspinatus and teres minor externally rotate the shoulder, and ends when front leg is extended and strikes ground. (3) Late cocking begins when front foot strikes the ground, glenohumeral joint externally rotates, and ends when shoulder is maximally externally rotated. (4) Acceleration begins with ball moving forward, horizontal adduction and internal rotation of shoulder, and ends when ball is released. (5) Deceleration begins at ball release and ends when motion stops.
- *Deliveries* include overhead, three quarters, and sidearm, each with their own specific risks.

COMMON INJURIES

- *Rotator cuff injuries* vary from mild forms of tendinitis and impingement to complete tears. It is often due to overuse and/or joint instability. Examination findings include positive Neer's sign, positive Hawkin's sign, and pain and weakness with muscle testing. Treatment varies from NSAIDs and physical therapy to surgery, depending on severity.
- *Instability* is often related to a rotator cuff injury and can be due to trauma, poor mechanics and/or overuse. Symptoms include pain with acceleration. Examination findings include positive relocation test, laxity, and weakness with muscle testing. Treatment includes rehabilitation and in some cases surgery.
- *Glenoid labrum injuries* may occur due to trauma, instability, poor mechanics and/or changes in throwing and training. Symptoms include painful clicking,

overhead pain, and pain with acceleration. Examination findings include positive *clunk* test, positive grind test, and positive O'Brien's test. Treatment is surgery if conservative therapies fail.

- *Bennett lesion* is a region of mineralization at the posterior-inferior glenoid rim. This ossification is unique in throwing athletes and often associated with rotator cuff injuries or instability. Symptoms are usually related to secondary shoulder pathology and diagnosis is made with CT scan. Conservative treatment is favored over surgical intervention (De Maeseneer et al, 1998).

- *Osteochondritis dissecans* (OCD) of the humeral capitellum is often due to repetitive valgus stress at radiocapitallar joint. Symptoms include lateral elbow pain associated with throwing and possibly clicking and or locking. Crepitus and limited extension may be found on examination and loose bodies may be seen on plain films. Fractures, avascular necrosis, and accessory centers of ossification have been reported to be associated with OCD (Takahara et al, 1998). Treatment includes rest, ice, NSAIDs and possibly surgery.

- *Ulnar collateral ligament* injury often occurs in throwing athletes from repetitive valgus stress. This stress can cause medial elbow instability and pain. Physical examination findings include decreased extension, and laxity and pain with valgus stressing. Plain films may be negative. Ultrasound and MRI can assist with diagnosis (Sasaki et al, 2002). Treatment includes rest, ice, and NSAIDs. Indications for surgery include chronic instability, failed conservative treatment, or complete 3rd degree tear.

- *Ulnar neuritis* can result from direct trauma, or repetitive overuse. Symptoms include pain at medial elbow, paresthesias throughout arm greatest at 4th and 5th digits. Examination includes pain reproduced with cubital tunnel pressure, positive Tinel's sign, and distal hand weakness. Treatment includes rest, *range of motion* (ROM) exercises, and rarely surgery for failed conservative therapy.

- *Little league elbow* results form repetitive throwing in a skeletally immature athlete, injuring the growth plate. Symptoms include medial elbow pain greatest with throwing. Examination is significant for medial elbow tenderness. Treatment includes rest and throwing modifications.

- *Commotio cordis* is dysrrhythmia or cardiac arrest occurring after a direct blow to the chest. Numerous cases of batters hit by a baseball causing sudden death have heightened awareness and controversy for safer and softer baseball use (Curfman, 1998; Janda et al, 1998). Chest protectors may also be utilized for better prevention (Viano et al, 2000).

- *Head injuries* occur often in baseball due to wild pitches, swinging bats, and hit baseballs often striking fans or spectators. The most common mechanism of injury is direct ball impact to players in the field (Pasrernack, Veenema, and Callahan, 1996).

ASSOCIATED INJURIES

- *Oral cancer* is a concern in many baseball players using chewing tobacco. Education should be directed toward prevention.

- *Abdominal injuries* have been reported from sliding, collisions, falls, and direct impact of the baseball. Common injuries to the abdomen include muscular contusion, rectus sheath hematoma, and spleen and renal damage. Careful evaluation including *computed tomography* (CT) scanning is often necessary to work up abdominal injuries (Riviello and Young, 2000).

- *Aneurysm of mid axillary artery* is rare but has been reported in baseball players and should be considered in the differential diagnosis of a throwing athlete with hand pain and/or paresthesias. This injury can cause embolization to the arm or hand and may be due to the forceful downward displacement of the humeral head or pectoralis minor tendon, damaging the intima in throwing athletes. Treatment is often surgical revascularization (Ishitobi et al, 2001; Todd et al, 1998).

EQUIPMENT

- Baseball equipment includes batting helmets, athletic supporters with cups, cleats, batting gloves, aluminum, or wooden bats, and mouth guards.

- Position specific equipment include mask, chest, throat, and shin protectors for catchers; toe guards for batters and catchers; forearm batting protectors; and gloves or mitts for different fielding positions.

- Recently health care professionals have proposed the implementation of softer baseballs in Little League Baseball to reduce the risk of injury.

REHABILITATION

- Rehabilitation for a baseball player or throwing athlete is often injury specific. Physical therapy should include rehabilitation of the large lower body muscle groups and the smaller muscle groups of the upper extremity. Strengthening often needs to be directed at the rotator cuff and scapular stabilizing muscles.

- The phases of rehabilitation include the acute, recovery, and maintenance phases. The acute phase concentrates on reducing pain and swelling and improving strength. During the recovery phase treatment is focused on pain-free range of motion, strength, and improved stability and function. The maintenance phase of rehabilitation includes increases in power, endurance, strength, and activity specific function.

- *Interval throwing programs* (ITPs) are structured to increase a pitcher's strength and endurance before returning to competitive pitching. ITPs are prescribed after an injury or at the start of preseason training. Programs are designed for players to reach specific goals, often over a period of 3 to 4 weeks. A typical week might comprise 4 days of throwing and 3 days of rest. Throwing days start with warm-ups and stretching and are followed by throwing. Throwing distances are gradually increased throughout the program.

PREVENTION

- Prevention of injuries is directed at proper conditioning, proper mechanics, proper equipment, and avoiding overuse.
- Pitchers throwing more frequent change-ups have a decreased risk of elbow pain compared to pitchers throwing more sinkers (Marshall et al, 2003; Lyman et al, 2001).
- Implementing use of safer equipment including break-away bases, batting helmets with face guards, and lighter mass baseballs in youth play (Janda, 2003).

LITTLE LEAGUE BASEBALL

- For information on Little League Baseball, including policies and rules on such things as restrictions for pitchers, visit their web site at www.littleleague.org.

THE AMERICAN ACADEMY OF PEDIATRICS RECOMMENDATIONS (Washington, 2001)

- Baseball and softball for children 5 through 14 years of age should be acknowledged as relatively safe sports. Catastrophic and chronically disabling injuries are rare; the frequency of injuries does not seem to have increased during the past two decades.
- Preventive measures should be used to protect young baseball pitchers from throwing injuries. These measures include a restriction on the number of pitches thrown in organized and informal settings and instruction in proper training, conditioning and throwing

mechanics. Parents, coaches, and players should be educated about the early warning signs of an overuse injury and encouraged to seek timely and appropriate treatment if evidence of an injury develops.

- Serious and potentially catastrophic baseball injuries can be minimized by the proper use of available safety equipment. This includes the use of approved batting helmets; helmets, masks, and chest and neck protectors for all catchers; and rubber spikes. Protective fencing of dugouts and benches, and the use of break-away bases also are recommended, as is the elimination of the on-deck circle. Protective equipment should always be properly fitted and well maintained. These preventive measures should be used in games and practices and in organized and informal participation.
- Baseball and softball players should be encouraged to wear polycarbonate eye protectors on the batting helmets to reduce the risk of eye injury. These eye protectors should be required for functionally one-eyed athletes (best corrected vision in the worst eye of less than 20/50) and for athletes who have undergone eye surgery or experienced severe eye injuries if the ophthalmologists judge them to be at an increased risk for eye injuries. These athletes also should protect their eyes when fielding by using polycarbonate sports goggles.
- Consideration should be given to using low-impact baseballs and softballs for children 5 to 14 years of age. Particularly, children younger than 10 years should be encouraged to use the lowest impact balls.
- Developmentally appropriate rule modifications, such as avoidance of headfirst sliding, should be implemented for children younger than 10 years.
- Because current data are limited, the routine use of chest protectors is not recommended for baseball players other than catchers.
- Surveillance of baseball and softball injuries should be continued. Studies should continue to determine the effectiveness of low-impact balls for reducing serious impact injuries. Research should be continued to develop other new, improved, and efficacious safety equipment.

REFERENCES

Curfman GD: Fatal impact—concussion of the heart. *N Engl J Med* 338(25):1841–1843, 1998.

De Maeseneer M, Jaovisidha S, Jacobson JA et al: The bennett lesion of the shoulder. *J Comput Assist Tomogr* 22(1):31–34, 1998.

Ishitobi K, Moteki K, Nara S et al: Extra-anatomic bypass graft for management of axillary artery occlusion in pitchers. *J Vasc Surg* 33(4):797–801, 2001.

Janda DH: The prevention of baseball and softball injuries. *Clin Orthop* 1(409):20–28, 2003.

Janda DH, Bir CA, Viano DC et al: Blunt chest impacts: Assessing the relative risk of fatal cardiac injury from various baseballs. *J Trauma* 44(2):298–303, 1998.

Lyman S, Fleisig GS, Waterbor JW et al: Longitudinal study of elbow and shoulder pain in youth baseball pitchers. *Med Sci Sports Exerc* 33(11):1803–1810, 2001.

Marshall SW, Mueller FO, Kirby DP et al: Evaluation of safety and faceguards for protection of injuries in youth baseball. *JAMA* 289(5):568–574, 2003.

Newsham KR, Keith CS, Saunders JE, et al: Isokinetic profile of baseball pitchers' internal/external rotation 180, 300, 450 degrees. *Med Sci Sports Exerc* 30(10):1489 1495, 1998.

Pasrernack JS, Veenema KR, Callahan CM et al: Baseball injuries: A little league survey. *Am Acad Pediatr* 98(3):445–448, 1996.

Riviello RJ, Young JS: Intra-abdominal injury from softball. *Am J Emerg Med* 18(4), 2000.

Roberts DG: A kinder gentler baseball. *Clin Pediatr* 40(4):205–206, 2001.

Sasaki J, Takahara M, Ogino T et al: Ultrasonographic assessment of the ulnar collateral ligament and medial elbow laxity in college baseball. *J Bone Joint Surg* 84–A(4):525–531, 2002.

Takahara M, Shundo M, Kondo M et al: Early detection of osteochondritis dissecans of the capitellum in young baseball players: Report of three cases. *J Bone Joint Surg* 80–A(6): 892–897, 1998.

Todd, GJ, Benvenisty AI, Hershon S et al: Aneurysm of the mid axillary artery in major league baseball pitchers—A report of two cases. *J Vasc Surg* 28(4):702–707, 1998.

Viano DC, Bir CA, Cheney AK et al: Prevention of commotio cordis in baseball: An evaluation of the chest protectors. *J Trauma* 49(6):1023–1028, 2000.

Washington RL : Risk of injury from baseball and softball in children. AAP Recommendations. *Am Acad Pediatr* 107(4), 2001.

77 BASKETBALL

John Turner, MD
Douglas B McKeag, MD, MS

INTRODUCTION

- Basketball has been an organized sport since the 1890s and is considered a limited contact sport. It involves a tremendous amount of running with explosive movements and rapid changes in direction and pace. Extreme stresses on the body during play result in many acute musculoskeletal injuries; while the ability to play year round and at most ages leads to many overuse injuries.

- With the great popularity of basketball most teams at the high school level and beyond have associated physicians who are responsible for injury prevention and medical care; however, care for the athlete falls to the hands of many health care providers since most injuries occur outside of organized play.

- Injury rates in basketball are increasing as popularity rises and the nature of the sport becomes more aggressive.

EPIDEMIOLOGY

- Nearly one million people are involved in basketball injuries each year in the United States. Population based injury rates are 3.9 per 1000 but player injury rates are seen as high as 50% in some European professional leagues (Huget, 1999).

- Studies on high school basketball players have reported injury rates ranging from 15 to 56% (DuRant et al, 1992; Gomez and Farney, 1996; Messina and DeLee, 1999). The largest investigation of high school athletes (12,000 participants) reported injury rates are 28.3% for male and 28.7% for female athletes (Powell, 2000).

- Several studies demonstrate no significant difference in the risk for injury between males and females (Powell, 2000; NCAA, 1998; Kingma, 1998); others have shown that females are more frequently injured (33% vs. 15%). (DuRant et al, 1992)

- College injury rates are 5.7 per 1000 athlete exposures for male and 5.6 for females (NCAA, 1998).

- Between 62 and 64% of injuries in college basketball occur during practice (NCAA, 1998); while 53–58% of high school basketball injuries occur during practice (Powell, 2000).

- Basketball has the highest per capita injury rate for all sports in the age group 14–25 years, ranks second in ages 5–14 years and third in ages 25 years and up (Conn and Gilchrist, 2003).

- A 17.5% of sports related emergency room visits and 13.5% of sports related visits to primary care physicians are basketball related (Cassell and Stathakis, 2003).

- Based on large population based studies, 63.8% of basketball related injuries are cared for in the emergency room.

- Sprains are the most common type of injury in basketball. Sprains account for 32–34% of injuries at the collegiate level (NCAA, 1998) and 47–56% at the high school level. (Messina and DeLee, 1999)

- Following European professional players over two years there were 37 surgeries (8.7%) performed on a total of 423 injuries (Huget, 1999).
- Nonmusculoskeletal problems
- Cumulative data from 3 NBA seasons show 25.9% of reported medical problems were classified as nonathletic related (Steingard, 1993).

INFECTIOUS DISEASE

- Mononucleosis is not specifically seen in basketball more than other sports but must be attentively treated. Resulting splenomegaly and risk of splenic rupture (even in the absence of splenic enlargement) from *epstein barr virus* (EBV) are significant and preclude active participation by an infected individual. Rapid monospot tests can have false negatives in the first 7–10 days so individuals with suspected EBV should be tested for serum antibodies, which are more sensitive in the early course. Since splenic rupture occurs in the first 3–4 weeks after infection, it is recommended to keep players out of activities during this time. Recovery can be prolonged with fatigue that prevents return to play for weeks or months.
- Fungal infections are prevalent in athletes and tinea pedis is the most common dermatophytosis. High top shoes, perspiration, friction, and poor foot care contribute to recurrent problems. Drying feet, changing socks, absorbent powders (without corn starch), and *over-the-counter* (OTC) and prescription antifungals are effective treatment measures. Similar measures should be taken to treat tinea cruris or "jock itch" which is also common in athletes.
- *Upper respiratory infections* (URI) are common in basketball athletes but treatment should vary little from standard measures. Symptomatic treatment including analgesics, decongestants, and antihistamines provide relief for most individuals. These infections are typically viral so antibiotics should be reserved for cases that fail to improve with symptomatic treatment.

CONCUSSION

- Concussion or *mild traumatic brain injury* (MTBI) occurs in basketball from two mechanisms—player-to-player contact or contact with the floor. MTBI results from damage to the brain and functional deficits from rapid, strong compression, shear, or tensile forces to the head.

- Signs and symptoms include loss of consciousness, headache, amnesia, dizziness, nausea, confusion, and visual disturbance. Individuals often have associated subjective complaints including difficulty concentrating, sleep disturbance, emotional lability, behavioral changes, change in smell or taste, poor energy, cognitive decline, and irritability. Recovery is variable and often difficult to assess.
- Mild head injury makes up more than 90% of all MTBI and is difficult to recognize since there is no loss of consciousness but a transient loss of alertness or a brief period of posttraumatic amnesia that may be difficult to recognize (Cantu, 1996).
- The National Athletic Trainers Association injury surveillance program investigated MTBI for three years in high school basketball players from 114 schools. MTBI comprises 4.2% of injuries in males and 5.2% in females. Player collisions are the most likely etiolgy and most of these occur in the open court, not under the basket (Powell, 1999).
- Many concussion guidelines have been published including those by the American College of Sports Medicine, Dr. Robert Cantu, the American Medical Society for Sports Medicine, and the Colorado Medical Society. These guidelines generally utilize neurologic symptoms, sideline memory and functional testing, and loss of consciousness to classify concussion severity.
- Return to play criteria is based on symptom resolution and history of previous concussion. It is often challenging to evaluate concussive symptoms and new evidence suggests cognitive testing should be the main criteria for return to play decisions. Our understanding of concussion, treatment options, and recovery are changing rapidly. Established concussion guidelines are giving way to methods that utilize emerging return to play criteria based on cognitive and neuropsychiatric testing. This allows at risk players, sometimes not clinically symptomatic, to be held while returning recovered players back to competition earlier than previously thought possible.

ASTHMA

- Exercise related bronchospasm is common in all sports. Classic symptoms include shortness of breath with chest tightness, cough, and wheezing. Symptoms typically begin 8–10 min into moderate exercise.
- Pulmonary function tests show a >15% drop in *forced expiratory volume in 1 s* (FEV1), >35% decrease in forced expiratory flow rate, >10% decrease in peak

expiratory flow rate, and an increase in both residual lung volume and total lung capacity (Kobayashi, 2002).

- Diagnosis can be made with history and sideline peak flow testing (screening) or with graded exercise testing with spirometry. Treatment should begin with avoidance of triggers (cold, allergens), cardiovascular training, and proper warm-up. Short acting inhaled beta-agonists relief most symptoms and are readily available for treatment. True underlying chronic asthma with exercise related exacerbation should not be treated with beta-agonist alone as this leads to long-term decline in pulmonary function.

HEAT ILLNESS

- Organized basketball programs typically have access to indoor, climate controlled courts—so heat illness is less of a factor. Most basketball occurs in less organized situations on outdoor courts, which increases the risk of injury. Hydration, monitoring body weight, and attention to early symptoms are required to prevent illness.

CARDIAC

- Basketball involves significant physiologic stress as reflected in findings from professional players. Heart rates average 169 beats per minute and are above 85% predicted maximum for 75% of competitive playing time (McInnes, Jones, and McKenna, 1995).
- Hypertension is seen in basketball even though many players are young. Blood pressure elevation over 140 systolic and 90 diastolic on two separate readings should be investigated. Family history, supplement and medication use, and substance abuse should be considered while investigating other secondary causes.
- Blood pressure should be controlled before allowing exercise. In mild and moderate hypertension, exercise is often part of a treatment plan but in severe hypertension it is contraindicated. When choosing treatment options, medications with negative performance side effects should be limited.
- Sudden cardiac death is extremely rare with estimates ranging from one in 150,000 to one in several million. Preparticipation examination with a focus on history taking is the best method to prevent sudden death. High risk individuals with a family history of premature or sudden death, history of exercise related syncope, or findings of Marfan's syndrome should be identified for further testing.

MUSCULOSKELETAL INJURY TYPES

- **Sprain:** Acute injury to a ligament
  1. Grade 1 (mild): Stretch and microtrauma but no discreet loss of continuity. Examination shows pain with stress testing but no instability.
  2. Grade 2 (moderate): Partial tear of ligament fibers. Examination shows pain with stress testing, partial joint opening but no gross instability. Endpoint usually detected on ligament stress testing.
  3. Grade 3 (severe): Complete rupture of ligament. Examination shows complete joint instability and no endpoint on ligament stress testing.
- **Strain:** Injury to musculotendinous unit from acute trauma. The severity of strains may vary on the basis of the degree of damage to the muscle or tendon fibers.
- **Contusion:** Blunt trauma that causes disruption of underlying soft tissue. This typically involves damage of blood vessels resulting in hemorrhage and visible bruising.
- **Dislocation:** Defined as loss of continuity of a joint. The injury may quickly self-correct, reestablish joint continuity, and never be visualized or remain dislocated. There is a high risk of damage to surrounding soft issues.
- **Fracture:** Disruption of bony tissue that requires immediate attention. Neurovascular compromise and skin integrity must be assessed, as injury to these tissues may change treatment options.

FACIAL AND ORAL INJURIES

- Basketball has no accepted regulations and few players wear face guards for protection against injury. Mouth guards are known to prevent injury but are not generally worn by college or professional players. There is ample contact between players, and most facial injuries result from contact with elbows or fingers from other players. Five to ten percent of basketball injuries involve the face or scalp (Powell, 1989) and an estimated 7500 eye injuries occur annually in the United States (Jones, 1989).
- Most lacerations occur over bony prominences, and fractures must be suspected when significant force is applied and symptoms extend beyond local mild tenderness and ecchymosis.
- Of eye injuries in professional basketball players, eyelid lacerations make up 50%, 28% are periorbital contusions and 12% are corneal abrasions (Zagelbaum et al, 1995).
- Dental injuries are often permanent as teeth do not have much ability to heal. Mouth guards absorb force

and help prevent tooth fracture, jaw injury, and even neck injury. Custom molded guards are inexpensive and preferable to off-the-shelf products.
- Dental literature reports injury rates from 4 to 14%, more occurring in males than females. Most dental trauma occurs to the upper anterior teeth, especially the upper lip and two central incisors. The highest injury rates are in young participants aged 8–15 years (Amy, 1996).
- Mouthguards and protective eyewear have been shown reduce rates of injury (Zagelbaum et al, 1995; Kerr, 1986).

SPINE AND PELVIS

- Back injuries make up more than 5.3% of all basketball injuries (McKay et al, 2001).
- The dynamic nature of basketball including fast changes in direction, repetitive jumping, twisting, rapid starts and stops, high velocity, and overhead arm use produces significant strain on the spine. The vertebral column and intervertebral discs carry 70% of forces and the posterior spine transmits 30%.
- Muscles of the spine and abdominal wall serve as strong stabilizers and create significant motion. Muscular strain resulting in pain and local inflammation is common. Muscular trigger points are another source of pain in athletes and should be treated with stretching, strengthening, direct massage. If this fails to produce results, *nonsteroidal anti-inflammatory drugs* (NSAIDs) can be utilized for general muscle inflammation as well as local treatment with acupuncture or injection with saline, local anesthetics, or corticosteroids.
- Cervical injury from acceleration/deceleration injuries (whiplash) occur in basketball but are less severe than other contact sports. Pain and muscular dysfunction are common but radicular symptoms can be a warning of more significant injury. Treatment includes relative rest, motion and strength exercises, NSAIDs, ice, heat, and modalities. If pain persists consider facet dysfunction or intervertebral disc degeneration.
- Basketball typically involves repetitive extension and hyperextension from rebounding, guarding opponents, and shooting. This can lead to excessive forces on the lumbar spine and injury. Defects of the posterior portions of the vertebra can lead to significant low back pain exacerbated by extension and axial loading.
- Spondylolysis is the presence of a defect in the pars interarticularis from any etiology including congenital defects, chronic stress, or acute fracture. This is the most common source of back pain in people under age

26 (Borenstein and Boden, 1995). Symptoms include low back pain with radiation into buttock and hamstrings from resulting spasm. Pain is worse with standing and back extension and there is an absence of radicular pain. Treatment involves back strengthening with a focus on flexion exercises, avoidance of back extension that produces pain, and analgesia as needed. Radiographs for suspected patients are indicated and may need to be repeated if symptoms persist to detect any instability of the spine.
- Spondylolisthesis is the resulting anterior–posterior subluxation of the one vertebra on another when bilateral defects occur. Slippage greater than 50% may need surgical attention. Otherwise treat patients conservatively with exercise and follow them closely for development of symptoms of nerve root impingement or spinal stenosis. Many athletes can return to basketball after aggressive strengthening and rehabilitation.
- *Sacroiliac* (SI) dysfunction is commonly seen, misdiagnosed, and treated as muscular low back pain and athletes fail to improve significantly. Patients usually cannot find any comfortable position for more than 10–15 min and have pain radiating into the posterior thigh. Pain is worse with motion that involves combined back flexion/extension and trunk rotation. Physical examination with focused attention to palpation of SI joints and functional testing (Faber's test, Gaenslen's test, Gillet's test, Trendelenberg's test) will allow identification and more appropriate treatment.

UPPER EXTREMITY

- There are relatively few upper extremity injuries in basketball due to the nature of the sport. In high school players, 10 to 12% of all basketball injuries occur to the hand and wrist and 2–4% occur to the shoulder. In recreational athletes 39% of all injuries involve the upper extremity.
- The most common upper extremity injuries are sprains and dislocations of the *proximal interphalangeal* (PIP) joints of the finger (Wilson, 1993; Zvijac, 1996).

LOWER EXTREMITY

- Lower extremity injuries account for the majority at every level of competition. Lower extremity injuries account for 51% in recreational players (Kingma, 1998), between 56 and 69% in high school athletes (Gomez and Farney, 1996; Messina and DeLee, 1999; Powell, 2000).

- There is a gender difference with 56–64% of male injuries occurring to the lower extremity and 65–69% in females (Messina and DeLee, 1999; Powell, 2000). This is thought to be due to increase in female knee injury rates compared to males.

KNEE

- Twelve percent of all injuries in male collegiate athletes are knee injuries, while the knee accounts for 19% of injuries in women (Arendt and Dick, 1999).
- Although knee injuries are not the most common type of lower extremity injury they account for most of the lost playing time because the nature of the injuries are more severe (Zvijac, 1996).
- Patellofemoral syndrome is a broad description that characterizes pain and dysfunction of the extensor mechanism of the knee resulting from poor biomechanics (patella tracks laterally) or inflammation that in athletes is usually associated with overuse of the knee. Treatment involves modification of training regimen, ice, NSAIDs, and correction of underlying muscle or bony mal-tracking with quadriceps strengthening. The vastus medialis is responsible for maintaining medial patellar alignment when other forces act to move the patella laterally. If strength training does not correct the problem, taping or functional braces can be helpful.
- Two common causes of anterior shin pain in basketball players are medial tibial stress syndrome (shin splints) and tibial stress fractures. They represent two points on a continuum of muscle overuse leading to periostitis and finally bone degradation. These overuse injuries are characterized with pain on the medial border of the tibia, typically in the lower mid portion. Ice, rest, NSAIDs, correcting foot and ankle biomechanics, and adjusting training regimens will usually improve shin splints.
- Stress fracture symptoms included worsening of typical pain beyond the time of activity and prolonged recovery times from episodes of intense activity or competition. Plain films can show periostitis and stress fractures, but delayed phase bone scans and *magnetic resonance imaging* (MRI) are much more sensitive. Treatment involves an initial period of rest that may include use of removable casts or crutches for pain relief. A very gradual reintroduction of activity with close symptom monitoring will allow for recovery in most cases.
- Patellar tendinitis or Jumpers Knee is common in basketball, found in 40–50% of high level players (Khan, 2003). It results from excessive forces through the extensor mechanism on the anterior knee. Symptoms include anterior knee pain just below the patella that is worse with sitting, squatting, kneeling, or climbing stairs. Point tenderness on the superior pole of the patellar tendon and pain with hyperextension of the knee are seen. An initial phase of symptom reduction with relative rest, ice, and NSAIDs can be followed by strengthening exercises with postactivity ice application. Use of infrapatellar straps or taping is common.
- Osgood-Schlatter disease is an inflammatory apophysitis resulting from excessive pull by the patellar tendon on the tibial tuberosity. It appears in young players typically aged 10 to 15 years during a period of rapid growth combined with intense physical activity. Treatment includes relative rest and analgesia but pain diminishes when growth ceases. Rupture is rare so participation in sports should not be limited.
- *Anterior cruciate ligament* (ACL) injuries account for 10% of male basketball knee injuries while making up 26% of female knee injuries (Sitler et al, 1994). The majority of ACL injuries are noncontact, and involve the player planting and pivoting on the knee.
- ACL injury differences between males and females have been attributed to intrinsic factors such as intercondylar notch size and shape, hormone differences, ACL size, and joint laxity as well as extrinsic factors such as strength, skill, experience, shoewear, and conditioning. There is ongoing debate as to the true mechanism and cause of ACL injuries and differences among the sexes.
- The natural history of ACL tears is early degenerative arthritis to the affected knee. To avoid this, it is generally recommended for athletes to have ACL reconstruction using one of many accepted techniques (patellar autograft, cadaver graft, hamstring autograft, and the like). If patients are not expecting significant continued activity on the knee there are times when rehabilitation and bracing are appropriate.

ANKLE AND FOOT

- Ankle injuries make up 87% of lower extremity injuries and are the most common type seen in basketball (Sitler et al, 1994). Inversion sprains to the anterior talofibular ligament comprise 66% of all ligamentous ankle injuries. Many injuries result from a player landing on another player's foot.
- Ankle taping has been shown to prevent injury (Garrick, 1973) but the concern exists that support from taping declines with time and activity.
- Lace up and semirigid ankle braces also prevent injury and decrease the severity of ligamentous sprain

(Sitler et al, 1994). Players do not like wearing ankle braces but if given a week long break-in period there is no detriment to athletic performance and players feel comfortable (Pienkowski et al, 1995).

- High top shoes are thought to provide added support and have been shown in some studies to reduce ankle injury rates (Garrick, 1973).
- Ottawa ankle rules have a sensitivity of 98% for ankle fractures and should be used. Specificity of the rules varies greatly from 10 to 70% (Bachmann et al, 2003). The rules state that an ankle X-ray is needed if:
  1. There is any pain in the malleolar zone (defined from the tibia and fibula 6 cm above the articulation with the talus, to the bones of the midfoot) and any of these findings:
     a. Bone tenderness at the posterior edge or tip of the lateral malleolus
     b. Bone tenderness at the posterior edge or tip of the medial malleolus
     c. Inability to bear weight both immediately and in the emergency room
  2. A foot X-ray series is required only if there is any pain in midfoot and any of these findings:
     a. Bone tenderness at the base of the 5th metatarsal
     b. Bone tenderness at the navicular
     c. Inability to bear weight both immediately and in the emergency room.
- Ankle sprains should be treated with relative rest, NSAIDS, weight bearing as tolerated, ice, bracing, and physical therapy with a focus on regaining proprioception that helps prevent repetitive injury.
- Navicular stress fractures are the most common stress fractures seen in jumping athletes and present with foot pain that is activity related and may persist to a lesser degree out of activity. Bone scan or MRI is needed for diagnosis as plain films are inadequate. Treatment involves immobilization and nonweight-bearing until the navicular is nontender (Khan, 1994).

REFERENCES

Arendt E, Dick R: Anterior cruciate ligament injury patterns among collegiate men and women. *J Athl Train* 24:86–92, 1999.

Bachmann LM, Koller MT, Steurer J et al: Accuracy of Ottawa ankle rules to exclude fractures of the ankle and mid-foot: A systematic review. *BMJ*, (326):417–423, 2003.

Borenstein DG, Boden SD: *Low Back Pain: Medical Diagnosis & Comprehensive Management.* Philadelphia, PA, WB Saunders, 1995.

Cantu R: Head and neck injuries, in Kibler W (ed.): ACSM's Handbook for the Team Physician. Baltimore, MD, Williams & Wilkins, 1996, pp 188–204.

Cassell EP, Stathakis VZ: Epidemiology of medically treated sport and active recreation injuries in the Latrobe Valley, Victoria, Australia. *Br J Sports Med* 37(5):405–409, 2003.

Conn JM, Gilchrist J: Sports and recreation related injury episodes in the US population, 1997–99. *Inj Prev* 9(2): 117–123, 2003.

DuRant RH, Seymore C, Gaillard G et al: Findings from the preparticipation athletic examination and athletic injuries. *Am J Dis Child* 146:85–91, 1992.

Garrick JG: Role of external support in the prevention of ankle sprains. *Med Sci Sports* 5:200–205, 1973.

Gomez E, Farney WC: Incidence of injury in Texas girls' high school basketball. *Am J Sports Med* 24:684–687, 1996.

Hoffman J: Epidemiology, in McKeag (ed.) *Olympic Handbook of Sports Medicine: Basketball.* Oxford, Blackwell.

Huget J: The pathology of basketball. Report by the Medical Commission of Federation of International Basketball Associations, 1999.

Jones N: Eye injury in sports. *Sports Med* 7(163), 1989.

Kerr I: Mouth-guards for the prevention of injuries in contact sports. *Sports Med* 3(6):415–427, 1986.

Khan KM, Kearney C, Fuller PJ et al: Tarsal navicular stress fracture in athletes. *Sports Med* 17(1):65–76, 1994.

Khan K: Lower extremity considerations, in McKeag (ed.): *Olympic Handbook of Sports Medicine: Basketball.* Oxford, Blackwell, 2003.

Kingma J: Sports members participation in assessment of incidence rate in five sports from records of hospital-based clinical treatment. *Percept Mot Skills* (86):675–686, 1998.

Kobayashi RH: Exercise-induced bronchospasm, anaphylaxis, and urticaria, in Mellion WM, Madden C, Putukian M, Shelton GL (ed.): *The Team Physician's Handbook.* Philadelphia, PA, Hanley & Belfus, 2002, pp 287–293.

McInnes SE, Jones CJ, McKenna MJ: The physiological load imposed on basketball players during competition. *J Sport Sci* 13:387–397, 1995.

McKay GD, Payne WR, Oakes BW et al: A prospective study of injuries in basketball: a total profile and comparison by gender and standard of competition. *J Sci Med Sport* 4(2):196–211, 2001.

Messina DF, DeLee JC: The incidence of injury in Texas high school basketball. *Am J Sports Med* (27):294–299, 1999.

Micheo W: Head and face considerations, in McKeag (ed.): *Olympic Handbook of Sports Medicine: Basketball*: Oxford, Blackwell, 2003.

NCAA: NCAA Injury Surveillance System for All Sports. Overland Park, KA, National Collegiate Athletic Association, 1998.

Pienkowski D, Shapiro R, Caborn DN et al: The effect of ankle stabilizers on athletic performance. *Am J Sports Med* 23: 757–762, 1995.

Powell JW: Sex-related injury patterns among selected high school sports. *Am J Sports Med* (28):385–391, 2000.

Powell JW: Traumatic brain injury in high school athletes. *J Am Med Assoc* 282:958–963, 1999.

Powell, J: Injury toll in prep sports estimated at 1.3 million. *Athl Train* 24:360, 1989.

Sitler M, Wheeler B, McBride J et al: The efficacy of a semirigid ankle stabilizer to reduce acute ankle injuries in basketball. *Am J Sports Med* 22:454–461, 1994.

Steingard S: Special considerations in the medical management of professional basketball players. *Clin Sports Med* 12(2): 239–246, 1993.

Wilson RL: Common hand and wrist injuries in basketball players. *Clin Sports Med* 12:265–291, 1993.

Zagelbaum BM, Hersh PS, et al: The national basketball association eye injury study. *Arch Ophthalmol* 113(6):749–752, 1995.

Zvijac J: Basketball, in Caine CC, Lindner KJ, (eds.): *Epidemiology of Sports Injuries*. Champaign, IL, Human Kinetics, 1996, pp 86–97.

78 BOXING: MEDICAL CONSIDERATIONS

John P Reasoner, MD
Francis G O'Connor, MD

INTRODUCTION

- Acute traumatic brain injuries and permanent and irreversible neurologic dysfunction are the primary medical concerns of boxing and the ringside physician.
- Amateur and professional boxing have unique differences in their approach to providing for the safety of the boxers.
- This chapter discusses the medical considerations required of the ringside physician.

AMATEUR VS. PROFESSIONAL BOXING

- Amateur and professional boxing have many similarities but also many differences (see Table 78-1). An objective assessment of amateur boxing leads to the conclusion that it probably does not involve the same degree of neurologic risk as seen in the professional sport. Shorter competitions, termination of a bout for head blows, and headgear make this understandable.
- Epidemiologic assessments of chronic neurologic sequelae are being surveyed by researchers. The U.S. Olympic Foundation has commissioned the School of Public Health and Hygiene at Johns Hopkins University to design and implement a study to investigate if any excessive medical risks are associated with participation in amateur boxing (U.S. Amateur Boxing, Inc, 2003).

TABLE 78-1   Differences in Amateur and Professional Boxing

	AMATEUR	PROFESSIONAL
1. Governing body	One	Multiple
2. Scoring	All blows equal	Weighted toward knockdown; more subjective
3. Age limit	32 years old	None
4. Competition	3 to 5 rounds of 2 to 3 min each	4 to 12 rounds of 3 min each
5. Referee	Stops contest early	Stops contest late
6. Headgear	Yes	Sparring only
7. Standing 8 count	3 in one round 4 total in bout	Varied
8. Lacerations	Stops contest	Varied
9. Retinal tear	No further competition	Individual decisions
10. Medical suspension	Uniform periods	Varied

MEDICAL RESPONSIBILITIES OF THE RINGSIDE PHYSICIAN (U.S. Amateur Boxing, 2003)

- Prevention and treatment of acute injuries is the primary role of the physician at ringside. This is accomplished through a sound medical plan to cover all aspects of the event—the precompetition phase, the ringside observation, and the postbout examination.

PRECOMPETITION PHASE

- Evaluation of the competition site is mandatory. An area for pre- and postbout assessments should be secure, assessable, and quiet with enough room and light to perform a neurologic examination, treat an injured boxer, and place a cot or stretcher for observation or transportation.
- Identify the nearest emergency room with neurosurgical, ophthalmologic, and dental capabilities. An evacuation route should be mapped out, and the hospital should be notified of the event. Have all emergency numbers available.
- Request to have *emergency medical technician* (EMT) services immediately available. If it is impossible, assure that telephone services are on hand for an emergency call.
- There should be a table large enough to seat ideally three physicians at ringside. It should be situated near a neutral corner with an unobstructed view of the competition.
- A set of steps next to that corner will allow the physician quick and easy access to the ring apron.
- Necessary items for the attending physician are the following:
  1. Stretcher and head board under the ring

2. Oxygen tank with appropriate adaptors and tubing
3. A physician's emergency bag to handle cardiopulmonary resuscitation (i.e., Ambu bag, oral and nasal airways) and to manage an unconscious patient
4. Sterile gauze pads for cuts and epistaxis
5. Disposable examination gloves
6. Otoscope and ophthalmoscope
7. Penlight
8. Blood pressure cuff and stethoscope

- The precompetition physical examination should be coordinated on the day of the scheduled bouts. The objective is to assure that the athlete is fully capable to box—neurologically intact, lacks febrile or contagious conditions, not under the influence of medications, and essentially pain-free.
- The majority of amateur prebout examinations include large numbers of anxious athletes who present without a preparticipation physical examination questionnaire. Nonetheless, the examination can be accomplished in a few minutes.
- Important questions to be answered by the boxer:
  1. When was your last bout?
  2. Do you have any medical problems?
  3. Are you using any medications?
  4. Have you had any recent illness?
  5. Have you ever been knocked out and when?
  6. Do you have a headache or pain anywhere on your body?
- "Yes" to any of these require further investigation for disqualifying factors.
- The following examinations are recommended for the prebout evaluation:
  1. Vital signs
  2. Examination of the eyes for corneal abrasions and hyphema. Check for pupil equality and reactivity. Insure intact visual fields by confrontation to rule out possible retinal detachment. Soft contact lenses may be worn in the ring.
  3. Examination of the ears for tympanic membrane rupture and infection.
  4. Examination of the nose for septal deformities or airway obstruction and of the mouth for loose teeth and oral hardware (i.e., braces and tongue piercing). Piercing hardware must be removed before competition.
  5. Examination of the skin for impetigo or herpetic lesions.
  6. Check heart sounds for murmurs and irregularities.
  7. Examination of the throat and lungs for infection and bronchospasm.
  8. Examination of the central and peripheral nervous systems for focal signs, such as facial or muscular weakness, paresthesia, or ataxia.

TABLE 78-2 Boxing Disqualifying Conditions

Acute illnesses: Acute febrile illnesses
Cardiovascular: Uncontrolled, severe hypertension; evidence of CHF; ectopy (more than 6 per minute)
Respiratory: Acute bronchospasm, evidence of pneumonia or hypoxia; nasal fracture; septal hematoma
Neurologic: Altered mental status, concussion, headache on the day following a match—potential risk for second impact syndrome
Eyes: Visual field defect, hyphema, known or history of retinal detachment, corneal abrasion; uncorrected visual acuity of worse than 20/400 in one or both eyes, or best corrected visual acuity of 20/60 or worse in either eye. Boxers may be permitted soft contacts.
Musculoskeletal: Acute or chronic muscle or joint pain causing significant upper or lower extremity dysfunction that may affect boxer's ability to defend or compete
Internal organs: Enlarged spleen or liver below the costal margin
Skin: Active herpetic lesions; impetigo; open lacerations of the head and neck

SOURCE: U.S. Amateur Boxing: *Ringside Physicians Certification Manual.* Colorado Springs, CO, U.S. Amateur Boxing, 2003.

9. Inspect the hands, upper and lower extremities, as well as the back for any tenderness, swelling, or deformities.
- Contraindications to boxing—a contact sport (see Table 78-2)

RINGSIDE OBSERVATION

- During the bout the physician's role is to study and to observe the individual boxers and the flow of the event. One looks for signs of distress in a boxer during and between rounds. If there is concern, listen and observe to what is being said in the corner by the coaches. The physician can go into a boxer's corner during the rest period if a closer inspection is required. A ringside physician has the right to inspect all first aid equipment intended for use at the event by trainers who are working the corners.
- Generally, the following are the only things allowed in a corner: Vaseline, Adrenalin 1:1000 topical, thrombin, water, ice, gauze pads, towels, sponges, Q-tips, pressure plates for soft tissue swelling and scissors. Artificial skin coverings, liniments, lotions, or any stimulants (such as smelling salts) are not allowed.
- During the action, the boxer's stance and ring movement are key indicators of the skill level and balance. A staggering or running boxer is an indicative of potential trouble. Since effective defense is necessary for safety, its absence mandates cessation of a contest. Early signs of a lapse in defense and of the onset of fatigue are lowered punch counts, lowered arms, and increasing clutches.
- Observation of cumulative trauma is important. Facial swelling, cuts, and epistaxis lead to impaired vision

and mouth-breathing making the boxer susceptible to significant head trauma. This arena is where a referee's level of experience should reflect his or her competence and ability to control the action. The referee may provide this level of safety by closely observing the boxers and their eyes, administering standing "8" counts, and alerting the physicians and corner when there is a concern. If the referee is concerned, then you, as the ringside caretaker, should be alert and ready to render care.

- The physician enters the ring on the referee's request to evaluate a boxer after a stoppage or between rounds. Even without the referee's request, if a serious injury is suspected during competition, the physician should mount the ring apron to suspend or terminate the bout.

- When entering the ring, the physician should do so quickly and confidently carrying gauze pads and a penlight. Remove the boxer's mouthpiece and assure an adequate airway. Though there maybe resistance, a disabled fighter should be made to lie down (if already on the mat) or sit on a stool until fully reactive. When capable walk the fighter to their corner. Establish a baseline neurologic evaluation. Further observation and serial examinations will be necessary by the physician to determine appropriate future care.

- If recovery progresses satisfactorily, the boxer can be released to the care of the coach or responsible family member with instructions on follow-up care and warning signs to notice.

- If the boxer is unconscious or has a period of delayed mental or neurologic recovery, expedite transportation to a hospital using stretcher, supplemental oxygen, and emergency medical services.

- When called to the ringside by a referee to evaluate a boxer, the competition should be stopped if:
  1. Airways are compromised by bleeding or swelling
  2. Significant oral bleeding
  3. Blood draining in the posterior oropharynx caused by epistaxis
  4. Altered mental status
  5. Obvious musculoskeletal dysfunction
  6. Significant facial or lip laceration
  7. Impaired vision caused by swelling, bleeding, or ocular trauma
  8. Possible nasal fracture
  9. Obvious loose or newly missing teeth
  10. A boxer feels he or she cannot continue

POST-BOUT EXAMINATION

- Each contestant must be examined after the bout. For amateurs, a quick evaluation can be performed as they exit the ring. For a more thorough evaluation, the boxer should be taken to the predetermined area away from ringside. For professional bouts, the examination can take place in the individual's locker room.

- Having two to three ringside physicians assure that the contest can continue on schedule when a more thorough postbout examination is necessary. Emergency personnel are a valuable asset in their support of injury care and medical assessments. They should remain on site till they are dismissed by the head physician.

- The brief examination should include observation of the boxer exiting the ring, asking questions to assess their orientation, noticing speech patterns and response, and performing a quick survey of the face, head, mouth, and upper extremities. If there are nonurgent but suspicious findings, have the coach bring the boxer back for a reevaluation after a determined amount of time.

- The criteria for transferring the contestant to the emergency room are as follows:
  1. Lacerations requiring complex repair or extending beyond your level of available care
  2. Altered mental status suggesting a grade 2 concussion or greater
  3. Injuries requiring urgent diagnostic studies such as bloodwork, X-rays, or advanced imaging to determine the level of severity
  4. Injuries requiring splinting or casting

EPIDEMIOLOGY OF INJURIES

- Depending on the study cited, 27 to 93% of boxing injuries involve the head (Caine, Caine, and Linder, 1996; Jordan, 1998). Concussion is the most common neurologic injury while nasal contusion with epistaxis and facial lacerations are the leading nonneurologic injuries. Acute traumatic brain injuries are an unfortunate complication, which include cerebral contusions and intracranial hemorrhage. These are a major concern of the attending physician who must readily recognize their signs and symptoms.

- Musculoskeletal injuries other than the hand and wrist are uncommon in boxers. Based on studies 2 to 46% of injuries occur in the hand and wrist. The second most common is the shoulder. Lower extremity injuries are generally caused by overuse incurred during training (i.e., jogging and jumping rope.).

- Rare injuries such as renal contusion, splenic or hepatic hematomas as well as commotio cordis due to chest impact have been documented in case studies.

REFERENCES

Caine D, Caine C, Linder K: *Epidemiology of Sport Injuries.* Champaign, IL, Human Kinetics, 1996.

Jordan BD: Boxing. in Jordan BJ, Tsairis P, Warren RF (eds.): *Sports Neurology,* 2nd ed. New York, NY, Lippincott-Raven, 1998.

U.S. Amateur Boxing: *Ringside Physicians Certification Manual.* Colorado Springs, CO, U.S. Amateur Boxing, 2003.

79 CREW
Andrew D Perron, MD

OVERVIEW

- Whether on the water or with rowing machines (ergometers), the sport of rowing is rapidly growing at both the recreational and competitive levels. Today, competitive rowing occurs at the Olympic, elite, collegiate, club, and high school levels.
- Virtually all rowing injuries are caused by overuse, and the vast majority of these can be traced to training errors or equipment problems (Karlson, 2000; Hickey, 1997; Edgar, 1995; Redgrave, 1995).

MECHANICS AND EQUIPMENT

- Boats have one, two, four, or eight rowers, who may have either one oar (sweep rowing) or two oars (sculling). Each rower sits in a sliding seat and places his or her feet in a pair of fixed shoes. The oar is held in an outrigger that can be adjusted in multiple ways that can vary the height, position, angle, and load per stroke.
- The rowing stroke begins at the *catch*, where the back and legs are maximally flexed and the arms extended. It is at this point where the oar enters the water. During the *drive* (power) phase of the stroke, the legs are extended, the back opened, and the arms flexed to the chest. At the *finish* the oar is removed from the water and the blade feathered, or turned parallel to the water. Finally, during the *recovery* phase, the body returns to the catch position with legs and back flexed and arms extended.
- Races are usually run over 1000 to 2000 m courses during the *sprint* season of spring and summer. These races are contested with boats side-by-side, and are run at near maximal aerobic capacity, beginning and ending with an anaerobic sprint. A typical sprint race will last 5–8 min. In the fall, *head* races are normally run over a 3 mi course, where the individual boat races against the clock. These competitions are run at a lower intensity than sprint races, with the competitor staying within aerobic capacity, and generally run 15–20 min in duration.

TRAINING

- Rowing, acknowledged as one of the most strenuous sports (Hagerman, 1984), requires high levels of both strength and aerobic capacity. With both a sprint season, and a head season, rowers train nearly year-round. A typical yearly training cycle mandates strength and distance training in the fall, weights and machine training in the winter, and anaerobic work in the spring and summer racing seasons.
- The successful rower usually has a high aerobic capacity, with elite rowers demonstrating VO_{2max} levels of 65 to 70 mL/kg/min (Secher, 1993). The sport favors taller athletes with an extended reach, as they can cover more distance per individual stroke.

COMMON INJURIES

LOW BACK PAIN

- The rowing stroke places a great deal of stress on the low back. It is maximally loaded at the catch, or fully flexed position, which places large forces on both the musculature of the back, and the intervertebral disks (Karlson, 2000; Hickey, 1997; Edgar, 1995). One review on the sport found that back and knee injuries were by far the most common injuries to collegiate rowers (Boland and Hosea, 1991).
- With sweep (one oar) rowing, the back is not only maximally flexed at the catch, but it is also twisted prior to maximal loading in order to extend the athlete's reach. This maximal loading with the back flexed and twisted may result in even more back injury in this patient population (Stallard, 1980), although this has been disputed (Karlson, 2000).
- Back injury syndromes that can be seen include muscular and ligamentous strains, spondylolysis/spondylolysthesis, and lumbar disk herniation (Karlson, 2000; Stallard, 1980; Thomas; George, 2002)
- Specifically for the rower, training errors of distance, technique, or intensity should be addressed. Additionally, a search for mechanical errors should occur,

with modification of equipment as needed to decrease load per stroke, adjust oar/foot height, or even switch side rowed (for sweep rowers) (Karlson, 2000).

OVERUSE KNEE INJURIES

- The rowing stroke maximally loads the knee when it is in the fully flexed position. As a result, patellofemoral pain is a common complaint among rowers. As with patellofemoral problems in other sports, this is more common in women and in those with anatomy that predisposes them to abnormalities in patellar tracking. Tracking problems can be further exacerbated by the position of the shoes fixed in the rowing shell. Their height, spacing, or orientation may be mechanically inappropriate for the rower's anatomy, resulting in increased symptoms (Karlson, 2000).
- Usual treatment of patellofemoral pain, focusing on strengthening of the vastus medialis muscle to improve patellar tracking is recommended. Shoe position should be checked and modified if not appropriate for the athlete.

TENDINITIS (PATELLAR, QUADRICEPS, AND FOREARM)

- Tendinitis can occur in the patellar or quadriceps tendon from repeated flexion/extension with the rowing stroke. Pain is noted over either tendon, worsened by use, and relieved by rest. Usual treatment modalities are employed for relief of symptoms, with a focus on modifying training and equipment errors.
- The rowing stroke predisposes to forearm tendinitis in the dorsal wrist both from tightly gripping the oar during the stroke and from feathering the oar at the finish. Feathering requires rapid extension of the wrist, which further stresses an already strained forearm. Rowers will complain of pain in the dorsal wrist, specifically at the intersection of the first and third dorsal wrist compartments (Karlson, 2000; Edgar, 1995; Fulcher, 1998). Physical examination will reveal pain and swelling at this location, and in more severe cases crepitance may be noted.
- Treatment of forearm tendinitis involves relative rest as well as technique modification. Medical modalities, such as ice, brief immobilization, nonsteroidal anti-inflammatory medications, and on occasion local steroid injection into the affected tendon sheath may all be employed (Fulcher, 1998). Technique modification involves stressing a looser grip on the oar, as well as a grip that places the wrist in as flat a position as possible (Karlson, 2000).

NERVE ENTRAPMENT SYNDROMES

- A number of different nerve entrapment syndromes are seen in rowers. These range from digital nerve compression in individual fingers to carpal tunnel syndrome in the upper extremity and frank sciatica in the lower extremity.
- Digital nerve compression results from a tight grip on the oar with direct pressure on the neurovascular bundle. Equipment and grip modification can alleviate the vast majority of these cases.
- Carpal tunnel syndrome is also frequently the result of an overly tight grip on the oar as well as repeated extension of the wrist at the finish of the stroke. In addition to standard treatment, technique modification, involving a looser grip as well as equipment modification, with shaving the oar handle to give it a smaller diameter may help with these symptoms.
- Sciatica can result from an improperly fitted seat that places pressure on the sciatic nerve. Additionally, there are small holes in the seats of rowing shells designed to fit the ischial tuberosities as the rower moves through the rowing stroke. If the holes are improperly spaced for the individual rower, nerve compression can result with associated numbness. This is especially common if women use seats designed for men that don't accommodate their wider pelvis (Karlson, 2000).

RIB STRESS FRACTURE

- Stress fractures of the ribs have been seen with increasing frequency in rowers (Hickey, 1997; McKenzie, 1989; Brukner and Khan, 1996; Christian and Kanstrup, 1997). This is thought to be secondary to equipment changes that have put more loads on the oar during the stroke (Karlson, 1998). Thought to be caused by the pull of the serratus anterior muscle on the scapula during the rowing stroke, these fractures are seen most frequently in the posteriorlateral region of ribs 5–9 (Karlson, 2000; 1998).
- Rib stress fracture usually presents with slow onset of chest wall pain in the posteriorlateral location. As with other stress fractures, pain is initially only with the inciting activity, but will progress to pain at rest if the overuse continues. Ultimately, a bony callus may be noted at the site of the stress fracture. Diagnosis may be made with a plain film demonstrating callus formation, or a bone scan in questionable cases.
- Treatment for rib stress fracture, as with most other stress fractures, involves rest, frequently for up to 6 weeks to allow complete healing (Karlson, 2000;

Perron, Brady, and Keats, 2001). Prevention with slow progression of load and duration is ideal. Technique modification to unload the oar may also be helpful (Karlson, 2000).

DERMATOLOGIC PROBLEMS

- The skin of the rower is subject to repetitive trauma in the hand, the posterior calf, and the buttock. As a consequence, the rower may have a number of dermatologic complaints referable to these locations.
- The hands of rowers are highly susceptible to blisters, caused by friction with the oar handle. These are considered a badge of honor by experienced rowers, and a right of passage for novices. Rowers rarely wear gloves, as this is felt to interfere with the ability to feel the oar as it passes through the water. Blisters can become secondarily infected, occasionally requiring topical or oral antibiotics in significant cases (Knapik, 1995).
- The buttocks are susceptible to chafing, blisters, callus formation, and abrasions, due to repetitive trauma from the small sliding seat. Blisters can become infected and occasionally require topical or systemic treatment. Changing the seat, use of a foam pad, and judicious use of petroleum jelly can all help to alleviate symptoms.
- *Track bite* is an injury to the skin of the posterior calves. During the rowing stroke, the legs are forcefully extended, and at the finish the posterior lower leg contacts the metal track that the seat slides in. The repetitive trauma of the leg hitting the track can result in skin breakdown, or a track bite. Athletes who hyperextend their knees or row with shoes adjusted into a lower position are particularly at risk for these injuries. These injuries can become superinfected, requiring local or systemic antibiotics. Prevention with padding on the end of the track and/or circumferential leg taping at the point of contact can help to alleviate these injuries.

REFERENCES

Boland AL, Hosea TM: Rowing and sculling and the older athlete. *Clin Sports Med* 10(2):245–256, 1991.

Brukner P, Khan K: Stress fracture of the neck of the seventh and eighth ribs: A case report. *Clin J Sports Med* 6(3):204–206, 1996.

Christian E, Kanstrup IL: Increased risk of stress fractures of the ribs in elite rowers. *Scand J Med Sci Sports* 7(1):49–52, 1997.

Edgar M: Rowing injury: A physiotherapist's perspective. *Sportcare J* 2:32–35, 1995.

Fulcher SM: Upper-extremity tendonitis and overuse syndromes in the athlete. *Clin Sports Med* 17(3):433–448, 1998.

George SZ: Management of the athlete with low back pain. *Clin Sports Med* 21(1):105–120, 2002.

Hagerman FC: Applied physiology of rowing. *Sports Med* 1(4): 303–326, 1984.

Hickey GJ: Injuries to elite rowers over a 10-yr period. *Med Sci Sports Exerc* 19(12):1567–1572, 1997.

Karlson KA: Rib stress fractures in elite rowers: A case series and proposed mechanism. *Am J Sports Med* 26(4):516–519, 1998.

Karlson KA: Rowing injuries. *Phys Sportsmed* 28(4):40–50, 2000.

Knapik JJ: Friction blisters. Pathophysiology, prevention and treatment. *Sports Med* 20(3):136–147, 1995.

McKenzie DC: Stress fracture of the rib in an elite oarsmen. *Int J Sports Med* 10(3):220–222, 1989.

Perron AD, Brady WJ, Keats TA: Principles of stress fracture management. *Postgrad Med* 110(3):115–124, 2001.

Redgrave A: Rowing injuries: An overview. *Sportcare J* 2:28–31, 1995.

Secher NH: Physiological and biomechanical aspects of rowing: Implications for training. *Sports Med* 15(1):24–42, 1993.

Stallard MC: Backache in oarsmen. *Brit J Sports Med* 12(2–3): 105–108, 1980.

Thomas P: Managing rowing backs. *Practitioner* 233(1465): 446–447, 1989.

80 CROSS-COUNTRY SKI INJURIES

Janus D Butcher, MD

INTRODUCTION

BACKGROUND

- Cross-country skiing is one of the three Nordic skiing disciplines along with ski jumping and Nordic combined (skiing and jumping). Most historic references to Nordic skiing discuss its military use. Indeed, the sport of biathlon (skiing and shooting) has it's origin in this historic relationship.
- Cross-country skiing is generally associated with a low injury rate and it is considered to be one of the highest aerobic demand activities. Although generally confined to the northern tier and mountain states, its popularity in the United States continues to grow.
- Cross-country skiing had remained relatively unchanged from its remote beginnings until dramatic innovations in equipment and technique were introduced over the past 20 years. Currently, two very distinct techniques are used, the diagonal stride (classic) and ski-skating (freestyle).

COMPETITION

Elite Level Competition

- The International Ski Federation (FIS) governs international competition. The FIS establishes race rules, schedules, doping control systems, athlete injury surveillance, and most other aspects of World Cup and World Championship racing.
- The specific events held at elite competitions are varied in both distance and technique. Formats include sprint (1 km), sprint relay, middle distance (5 km, 10 km, 15 km), team relay (4 × 5 km, 4 × 10 km), long distance (30 km, 50 km), classic/skate pursuit, and others.
- One unique aspect of elite cross-country skiing is that the athletes frequently compete as both sprinters (1 km) as well as marathon skiers (30 or 50 km) within the same race schedule. Most competitors will train and race in both the classical and skating techniques.

Nonelite Competition

- Marathon distance races are held in nearly all of the countries of Northern, Central, and Eastern Europe as well as Japan, North America, and Australia.
- In the United States a full calendar of local, regional, and national marathon races are scheduled throughout the winter months. The largest of these, the American Birkebeiner is 52 km long with over 7000 participants.
- High school and college cross-country ski teams are common in the Northeast, upper Midwest, and Western states. These competitions include races 5 to 15 km in length with both classic stride and skating formats.

BIOMECHANICS

TECHNIQUE

Diagonal (Classic) Technique

- The diagonal stride technique has been used for centuries and remains a popular style for ski touring and back country skiing.
- In the diagonal stride forward propulsion is accomplished through alternating kick and glide actions of the skis. This requires a full stop of the kick ski to propel the skier forward. Backward slip of the planted ski is limited by the application of high friction kick wax on the cambered portion of the ski surface. The requirement to plant the ski to generate thrust limits the maximum speeds obtainable (Renstrom and Johnson, 1989).
- In the diagonal stride the poles are used primarily for balance but can contribute up to 30% of forward thrust in higher-level skiers (Renstrom and Johnson, 1989). Double poling (planting both poles simultaneously) is utilized as increasing tempo limits the effectiveness of the kick and glide action.

Skating Technique

- Developed in the late 1970s this new technique has rapidly evolved and become the method of choice for most recreational skiers. Skating is the only technique used in both Biathlon and Nordic combined competitions.
- The skating technique generates forward momentum by driving the skis at an angle to the direction of travel in a motion analogous to speed skating. There is no kick phase and thus no stopping of the ski during the cycle. Several different strides (V1 skate, V2 skate, Marathon skate) are utilized depending on terrain and skier tempo.
- Double poling is used in most skating strides to transfer upper body energy to the skiing surface and can provide up to 60% of the forward propulsive force (Smith, 1992).

Biomechanical Comparison of the Techniques

- Skating is much more energy efficient than the diagonal stride technique (Hoffman and Clifford, 1990). In addition, with skating there is no need for a high friction kick wax; so low friction glide waxes can be used along the entire surface of the ski.
- These factors combined with the use of extremely light weight composite construction materials as well as improvements in skiing surface preparation have resulted in a 10–30% increase in average speed since the 1950s (Hoffman and Clifford, 1990; Street, 1992).

INJURY EPIDEMIOLOGY AND PATHOPHYSIOLOGY

OVERALL INCIDENCE

- Historically, the injury rates in cross country skiing are reported between 0.1 and 5.63 injuries per 1000 skiers (Sherry and Asquith, 1987; Boyle, Johnson, and Pope, 1981). The true incidence is difficult to determine as skiing is not generally limited to a confined venue.
- In the limited data available from more controlled circumstances, such as endurance races, the incidence was found to be substantially higher at 10 to 35 per 1000 skiers (Renstrom and Johnson, 1989; Butcher and Brannen, 1998). The majority of these injuries were fatigue related.

CHANGING INJURY PATTERNS

- As the technique and equipment have changed, several equipment-injury relationships have been suggested (Schelkun, 1992; Lawson, Reid, and Wiley, 1992; Lindsay et al, 1993; Bovard, 1994; Dorsen, 1986).
  1. Increased pole length with the skating technique accentuates demands on the shoulder and elbow.

2. Stiffer bindings and rigid boot construction with heel-ski fixation devices in skating equipment may increase the risk of ankle and knee injuries.
- The biomechanics of the new technique are also suggested in the changing injury patterns.
  1. The skating stride places significantly greater demands on the hip adductors and external rotators (Renstrom and Johnson, 1989).
  2. A greater emphasis on upper body strength in the double poling action has been implicated in increasing upper extremity overuse injuries (Dorsen, 1986).

Comparison of Techniques
- Initial reports suggested greater incidence of injury in the skating technique; however this remains unsubstantiated.
- In one recent report of injuries occurring during a long distance event where the skating technique was the dominant style used, the injury rate was found to be higher than reported for similar races in the preskating period (Butcher and Brannen, 1998).

INJURY DISTRIBUTION
- Studies describing the distribution of musculoskeletal injuries in mass participation events demonstrated that lower extremity injuries are somewhat more common than upper extremity injuries (55% vs. 35%) (Sherry and Asquith, 1987).

The Distribution of Injuries
- Sprains/twists 40.4%, fractures 27.4%, contusions 16.4%, lacerations 9.3%, dislocations 5.8%, and other 0.7%
- The most frequently encountered acute orthopedic complaints include thumb ulnar collateral ligament strain, knee medial collateral ligament sprain, and plantar fascia strain.
- The most common overuse injuries include sacroiliitis, 1st *metatarsophalangeal* (MTP) DJD/synovitis, lateral ankle pain, and wrist tendinitis.

MEDICAL PROBLEMS

- Common medical illnesses reported include exhaustion/dehydration, cold injury, *gastrointestinal* (GI) symptoms, photokeratitis, and bronchospasm.

COMMON MEDICAL CONDITIONS

EXERCISE INDUCED ASTHMA
- **Incidence:** *Exercise induced asthma* (EIA) effects up to 35% of winter sports athletes with the highest incidence found in cross-country skiers (Sue-Chu, Larsson,

and Bjermer, 1996; Larsson et al, 1993; Rundell et al, 2000). One study reported 50% of elite cross-country skiers with EIA (Rundell et al, 2000).
- **Pathophysiology:** EIA refers to an inflammatory mediated bronchial response precipitated by exercise. Exercise is a common trigger of symptoms in athletes with classic asthma. There does appear to be a separate population of athletes who exhibit symptoms only with extreme exercise. Etiologic factors are low humidity and temperature of the inspired air and extreme minute volume.
- Typically, the athlete with true exercise induced asthma will develop symptoms only in relatively extreme circumstances. The likelihood of developing symptoms increases with exercise involving a higher minute volume and cold dry conditions.
- **History:** It is common for these athletes to exhibit symptoms intermittently. The usual symptoms include shortness of breath with exercise that is out of proportion to effort, burning chest pain, post exercise cough, and wheezing.
- Other red flags include a history of childhood asthma, frequent upper respiratory illnesses, and a chronic cough.
- **Physical examination:** When symptomatic may demonstrate wheezing otherwise is typically normal.
- **Diagnostic testing:** The majority of testing protocols use running as the exercise challenge with pre- and postexercise pulmonary function test change as the measured variable, and as such have significant limitations when evaluating the cross country skier (see Chapter 23). (Rundell et al, 2000; Eggleston, 1984; Mannix, Manfredi, and Farber, 1999; Garcia de la Rubia et al, 1998; Randolph, Fraser, and Matasavage, 1997; Ogston and Butcher, 2002; Carlsen, Engh, and Mork, 2000; Anderson and Daviskas, 2000; de Bisschop et al, 1999)
- **Treatment:** With classic asthma, the mainstay of therapy is inhaled corticosteroid with inhaled bronchodilator used for symptom management. These athletes should be identified and treated appropriately.
- With EIA, the main goal is prevention of airway irritation and bronchospasm through preexercise administration of medications. Typically a stepped approach is undertaken.

Preventive Medications Include the Following
- Short acting beta agonists (albuterol, pirbuterol), are usually effective and have the advantage of low cost, ease of use, and high compliance.
- Long acting beta agonists (salmeterol)
- Leukotriene inhibitors (montelukast sodium) should be reserved as a second line and should always be used with a beta-agonist as a rescue medication.

• Chromolyn sodium is rarely effective when used alone and tends to be quite expensive in the required dosages.

Moderate to Severe Symptoms
• Athletes who require second-line medications should be further evaluated.
• Addition of a second medication listed above
• Addition of inhaled corticosteroid (budesonide, fluticasone) or beta-agonist/corticosteroid combinations (Advair-Glaxo Wellcome).
  • Inhaled corticosteroid is effective in alleviating the postexercise cough brought on by late phase inflammatory effects of EIA.
• **Doping control:** Care must be taken to ensure compliance with doping control measures in elite level skiers.
• Most asthma medications are restricted and appropriate procedures for documenting their use is required. Recently, the International Olympic Committee (IOC) and FIS have begun requiring documented testing of these athletes prior to the use of asthma medications.
• The USADA hotline is a useful resource for any questions regarding the use of these medications (1-800-223-0393).

COMMON MUSCULOSKELETAL PROBLEMS

SACROILIITIS

• **Pathophysiology:** The *sacroiliac* (SI) joint is a biconcave articulation of the hemipelvis to the sacrum. It has relatively small rotational motion but functions primarily to transmit force from the lower extremity to the spine. Sacroiliac dysfunction is the most common cause of low back pain in the skier.
• Injury can result from direct trauma associated with a fall, but more commonly arises from repetitive loading. Contributing factors in this injury include SI joint hypermobility, excessive shear forces, and relative core strength deficits.
• **Clinical features:** Symptoms stem from inflammation in the SI joint and include local pain at the SI joint that is exacerbated with walking, running, or skiing.
• The athlete will often have associated lateral hip pain and pain at the gluteal prominance. Radicular symptoms are unusual and are associated with piriformis spasm, facet irritation, or concomitant disk disease.
• Examination will typically reveal the following: Tenderness at the SI joint and relative hypomobility on the effected side with a standing knee to chest test
• FABER test (flexion, abduction, and external rotation) will usually elicit symptoms. Neurologic examination is normal.
• **Diagnostic testing:** Radiographs may demonstrate arthrosis or degenerative disease of the lower spine.

• **Treatment:** Pain relief strategies include oral analgesics/anti-inflammatory medications, chiropractic treatment, ice, massage, and stretching.
• Long-term management aims at improving SI function through core stabilization and muscle balance training (Thera-ball program, Pilates, or similar).
• Technique and equipment issues should also be reviewed.

GREATER TROCHANTER BURSITIS
• See detailed description in chapter 57.

RETRO PATELLAR KNEE PAIN (PATELLOFEMORAL DYSFUNCTION)/ILLIOTIBIAL BAND FRICTION SYNDROME
• See detailed descriptions in chapters 60 and 61 respectively.

EXERTIONAL ANTERIOR COMPARTMENT SYNDROME

• **Pathophysiology:** In cross-country skiers, *exertional compartment syndrome* (ECS) typically effects the anterior or lateral compartments representing injury to the tibialis anterior or peroneus brevis muscles respectively.
• ECS is precipitated by exercise induced swelling of the soft tissue in the confined compartment leading to ischemic pain in the effected muscle.
• This is most common in skating technique where the foot is dorsiflexed and everted during ski recovery.
• This injury was very prevalent when the technique was first introduced due to the excessive length of the ski and relatively soft binding used with the classic stride. As equipment has been developed specifically for the skating technique, this has become less common. It is now most commonly seen with the use of combination equipment (designed for both skating and classic technique) and with poorly fitting equipment.
• **Clinical features:** See detailed description of symptoms in chapters 22 and 63.
• **Diagnostic testing:** Pre- and postexercise compartment pressure testing may be helpful although it is difficult to reproduce the specific conditions of skiing in the laboratory (see chapter 22).
• **Treatment:** Includes decreasing compartment inflammation using anti-inflammatory medications and improving function through a balanced stretching and strengthening program.
• Equipment modifications should be made to utilize a skating specific boot-binding-ski system. A stiffer binding and shorter ski may also help.
• In resistant cases a surgical fasciotomy may be necessary (see chapter 63).

PERONEUS TENDON INJURY

• **Pathophysiology:** Injury to the peroneus tendon can occur with an acute inversion dorsiflexion injury or can develop through repetitive overload that leads to tendinitis. With an acute injury, the peroneus tendon can be torn or may be subluxed from the fibular groove with disruption of the overlying retinaculum. Acute injuries occur with both classic and skating techniques, whereas chronic tendinitis is usually seen in the skating technique.

- **Clinical features:** Acute injuries will present with pain, swelling, and bruising along the posterior and inferior fibula. The athlete will often report a pop in association with an appropriate mechanism.
- Following the acute phase, a chronic clicking sensation may be present representing subluxation of the peroneal tendon.
- Peroneal tendinitis will usually present with pain and swelling along the posterior and inferior fibula. Pain will be worse after skiing and will interfere with other activities, such as running and walking.
- Physical examination may demonstrate subluxation of the effected peroneus tendon when compared to the contralateral ankle. Resisted eversion of the foot will reproduce pain.
- **Diagnostic testing:** In most acute injuries, an ankle X-ray is useful to rule out associated fracture.
- In an acute peroneal tear or subluxation, *magnetic resonance imaging* (MRI) evaluation may be helpful to evaluate the extent of injury.
- **Treatment:** Acute strain injuries without a complete tear can be treated with immobilization (either casting or *computer-aided manufacturing* (CAM) walker boot depending on extent of injury). This is typically continued for 4 to 6 weeks.
- Complete tear of the tendon or avulsion of the retinaculum is best managed surgically.
- Tendinitis is managed with temporary immobilization in a CAM walker followed by active rehabilitation incorporating passive stretching and eccentric overload exercise.
- Anti-inflammatory medications may be helpful for pain management. Corticosteroid injection may also address the athlete's discomfort. This is accomplished by injecting a solution of 60 mg of triamcinolone in 2 to 3 cc of 1% lidocaine into the peroneus sheath. An ankle brace or taping may allow the athlete to continue active training during the rehabilitation process.

SKIER'S TOE

- **Pathophysiology:** Skier's toe is a term frequently used to describe pain in the 1st MTP joint.
- This may represent either an acute injury (turf toe or acute sesamoid injury) or chronic problem (hallux rigidus, MTP synovitis, or sesamoiditis).
- In skiers, the chronic form stemming from degenerate joint disease and synovitis is most common and is

associated almost exclusively with the classical technique. The mechanism of injury is repetitive extreme extension of the MTP joint.

- **Clinical features:** Athlete complains of pain, swelling, and limited motion at the great MTP joint.
- Symptoms are exacerbated with classical skiing, running, and other activities involving repetitive forced extension of the toe.
- Physical examination may reveal obvious degenerative changes on inspection of the joint. Tenderness and erythema are common. Pain is exacerbated with passive extension/flexion.
- **Diagnostic testing:** Radiographs will typically demonstrate 1st MTP degenerative disease.
- If a stress fracture or sesamoiditis is suspected a three phase bone scan or limited MRI study may be useful.
- Analysis of joint aspirate may demonstrate uric acid crystals if degeneration is caused by gouty arthritis.
- **Treatment:** Temporary exclusion of the classic technique will help to alleviate symptoms.
- Modifying nonskiing footwear to eliminate flexion with a spring steel insert or rigid orthotic is also beneficial.
- Severe cases may require temporary use of a rocker bottom boot. *Nonsteroidal anti-inflammatory drugs* (NSAIDs) are often helpful.
- In cases with substantial degeneration the athlete may benefit from surgical intervention.

UPPER EXTREMITY

DEQUERVAIN'S TENOSYNOVITIS

- **Pathophysiology:** The repetitive gripping and ulnar/radial deviation motion associated with double poling can lead to tendinitis of the extensor pollicis brevis or abductor pollicis longus. Both tendons occupy the 1st dorsal wrist compartment and are generally both involved.
- Symptoms can be insidious in onset or may arise acutely with a traumatic event. Chronic pain is common if untreated.
- **Clinical features:** Typical symptoms include pain and swelling along the radial aspect of the wrist.
- Pain is precipitated by gripping and rotational motions (removing the lid from a jar or opening a door).
- Examination reveals tenderness along the extensor surface of the thumb, radial wrist, and forearm. Pain is precipitated with resisted thumb abduction or extension. The patient may demonstrate a positive Finklestein's test (see chapter 52).
- **Treatment:** Pain modification via the principles of PRICEMM (protection, rest, ice, elevation, medication, modalities).
- Corticosteroid injection may also be beneficial. Triamcinolone (60 to 80 mg) with 3 cc lidocaine is

injected into the tendon sheath within the 1st dorsal wrist compartment.

- Protective bracing with a thumb spica splint is helpful and may allow the skier to continue to ski while being treated.
- Physical or occupational therapy is often useful to address strength and flexibility issues.
- Surgical treatment (synovectomy) may be necessary in persistent cases.
- Return to skiing when symptom free or if symptom free in appropriate brace.
  1. Several centimeters proximal to the carpus
  2. Symptoms are worse with gripping or twisting motion in wrist.
  3. Examination reveals tenderness and swelling along dorsoradial forearm at the junction of the distal and middle thirds. Pain localized to this area is reproduced with resisted extension of wrist or abduction/extension of the thumb. Crepitance at the intersection is common.
- **Treatment:** Pain management with relative rest, ice, compression, elevation, and physical modalities. Anti-inflammatory medications may be useful for analgesia and swelling.

SKIERS THUMB (ULNAR COLLATERAL LIGAMENT)/ EXTENSOR TENOSYNOVITIS/INTERSECTION SYNDROME
- See detailed descriptions in chapters 52, 53, and 54.

REFERENCES

Anderson SD, Daviskas E: The mechanism of exercise-induced asthma is . . . *J Allergy Clin Immunol* 106(3):453–459, Sep. 2000.

Bovard R: The new ski-skating poles, a role in fracture risk? *Phys Sport Med* 22:41–47, 1994.

Boyle JJ, Johnson RJ, Pope MH: Cross country ski injuries: a prospective study. *Iowa Orthop J* 1:41–48, 1981.

Butcher J, Brannen S: Comparison of injuries in classic and skating Nordic ski techniques. *Clin J Sport Med Apr* 8(2):88–91, 1998.

Carlsen KH, Engh G, Mork M: Exercise-induced bronchoconstriction depends on exercise load. *Respir Med* 94(8):750–755, Aug. 2000.

de Bisschop C, Guenard H, Desnot P, et al: Reduction of exercise-induced asthma in children by short, repeated warm ups. *Br J Sports Med* 33(2):100–104, Apr. 1999.

Dorsen P: Overuse injuries from Nordic ski skating. *Phys Sport Med* 14:34, 1986.

Eggleston PA: Methods of exercise challenge. *J Allergy Clin Immunol* 73(5 Pt 2):666–669, May 1984.

Garcia de la Rubia S, Pajaron-Fernandez MJ, Sanchez-Solis M et al: Exercise-induced asthma in children: A comparative study of free and treadmill running. *Ann Allergy Asthma Immunol* 80(3):232–236, 1998.

Hoffman MD, Clifford PS: Physiological responses to different cross country skiing techniques on level terrain. *Med Sci Sports Excer* 22(6):841–848, 1990.

Larsson K, Ohlsen P, Larsson L et al: High prevalence of asthma in cross country skiers. *BMJ* 307(6915):1326–1329, Nov. 20, 1993.

Lawson SK, Reid DC, Wiley JP: Anterior compartment pressures in cross-country skiers. *Am J Sports Med* 20:750–753, 1992.

Lindsay DM, Meeuwisse WH, Vyse A et al: Lumbosacral dysfunction in elite cross country skiers. *JOSPT* 18(5):580–585, 1993.

Mannix ET, Manfredi F, Farber MO: A comparison of two challenge tests for identifying exercise-induced bronchospasm in figure skaters. *Chest* 115(3):649–653, Mar. 1999.

Ogston J, Butcher J: A sports specific protocol for the diagnosis of exercise induced asthma. *Clin J Sports Med* 12(5):291–295, Sep. 2002.

Randolph S, Fraser B, Matasavage C: The free running athletic screening test as a screening test for exercise induced asthma in high school. *Allergy Asthma Proc* 18(5):311–312, 1997.

Renstrom P, Johnson RJ: Cross country skiing injuries and biomechanics. *Sports Med* 8(6):346–370, 1989.

Rundell KW, Wilber RL, Szmedra L et al: Exercise induced asthma screening of elite athletes: Field versus laboratory exercise challenge. *Med Sci Sports Exerc* 32(2):309–316, 2000.

Schelkun PH: Cross country skiing: Ski skating brings speed and new injuries. *Phys Sports Med* 20(2):168–174, 1992.

Sherry E, Asquith J: Nordic skiing injuries in Australia. *Med J Australia* 146:245–246, 1987.

Smith GA: Biomechanical analysis of cross country skiing techniques. *Med Sci Sports Exerc* 24(9):1015–1022, 1992.

Street GM: Technological advances in cross country ski equipment. *Med Sci Sports Exerc* 24(9):1048–1054, 1992.

Sue-Chu M, Larsson L, Bjermer L: Prevalence of asthma in young cross-country skiers in central Scandinavia: differences between Norway and Sweden. *Respir Med* 90(2):99–105, Feb. 1996.

81 BICYCLING INJURIES
Chad Asplund, MD

INTRODUCTION

- Estimated 100 million riders in 2000 (Mellion, 2001)
- Road cycling
  1. Road racing: Long open road race (40–120 mi)
  2. Criterium: Many laps around a short course
     a. Very popular in America
     b. High potential for crashing
  3. Time trial: Race against the clock with wave start with 1–5 min between riders

- Mountain biking
  1. Downhill: Steep downhill race where focus is on speed. Injuries may occur as safety is sacrificed for speed.
  2. Dual slalom: Two racers compete in downhill ski-style slalom course.
- Touring: Road riding for recreation typically over long distances. Rider may be loaded or nonloaded with panniers/saddlebags.
- Cyclocross: Off-road race in which riders complete a short (1–2 mi) lap multiple times in a set time period. Obstacles are present requiring the rider to mount, dismount, and carry cycle over the course.
- BMX/Trick cycling: Riders compete on ramps with stairs and railings, with multiple aerial stunts. High risk for injury with aerial acrobatics.
  1. Fastest growing segment of U.S. cycling with more than 60,000 riders
  2. Largest portion of child cyclists (Grubb, 2003)

FRAME TYPES

- Standard road: Traditional upright geometry with top tube parallel to ground
- Compact road: Sloping top tube allows rider to fit to a smaller frame, this maximizes stiffness and minimizes weight.
- Mountain/Hybrid: Flatter geometry, heavier bicycle, may have suspension to absorb shock.

FIT

- May be done at a bike shop with Fit Kit or "Size Cycle" (Christiaans and Bremner, 1998).
- Best frame size for a cyclist is as small vertically as possible, with enough length horizontally to allow a stretched out, relaxed upper body. This frame will be lighter and stiffer and handle better. (See Fig. 81-1) (Colorado)

FRAME SIZE

- To ensure proper frame size of bicycle, rider should straddle top of the bicycle wearing riding shoes.
  1. Road bikes:
     a. Standard geometry: 1–2 in. between the crotch and the top tube
     b. Compact geometry: Size determined by top tube length/reach (see below)
  2. Mountain bikes: Determined by reach (see below)
  3. Calculations exist to determine frame size (Colorado):
     a. Inseam height (cm) × 0.67
     b. Mountain bike: Inseam = 10–12 cm

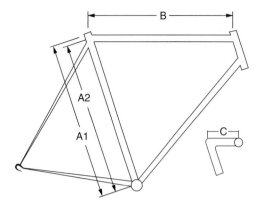

A1 Seat tube length (C–T)
A2 Seat tube length (C–C)
B   Top tube length (C–C)
C   Stem length (C–C)

FIG 81-1 Bike frame dimensions.

SEAT HEIGHT

- Optimal saddle height has been estimated based on maximal power output and caloric expenditure (Burke, 1994).
  1. Calculate height, which will be within a centimeter of 0.883 × inseam length, measured from the center of the bottom bracket to the low point of the top of your saddle. This allows full leg extension, with a slight bend in the leg at the bottom of the pedal stroke.
  2. When seated on bike with pedal at the 6 o'clock position there should be 25–30% flexion in the knee.
  3. Alternatively, the seat may be raised until the hips rock with pedaling, and then lowered until the rocking disappears.

SADDLE POSITION

- Check the position of your forward knee relative to the pedal spindle—for a neutral knee position, you'll be able to drop a plumb line from just below the front of the forward kneecap, and have it bisect the pedal spindle and ball of your foot below. "Keep Over Pedal Spindle (KOPS)" (Burke, 1994)

TOP TUBE LENGTH

- The ideal position varies here more than anywhere else for cyclists, depending on riding style, flexibility, body proportions, and frame geometry, among others. And, your upper body position will evolve with more hours in the saddle.
  1. May be measured by placing your elbow at the fore end of the saddle—your outstretched fingers should touch the handlebars.

HANDLEBAR POSITION

- Most cyclists select a bar that is just as wide as their shoulders, measured as the distance between the shoulder joints. A wider bar opens the chest for better breathing and more leverage, but is less aerodynamic. You'll need to find your own balance between the two.
  1. Handle bar height should always be at or lower than seat height. How low depends on the flexibility and experience of the rider (Mellion, 1991).

CRANK ARM

- Length is based on size and riding style. Shorter crank arms are better for quick acceleration and high cadence. Long crank arms are used for pushing larger gears at lower cadence (Colorado).
  1. To minimize oxygen consumption, crank length is dependent on upper thigh (femur) length: $2.33 \times$ (upper thigh length in cm) $+ 55.8$ (Too, 1990). This roughly translates to the following:
     a. Frame size: <54 cm, 170 mm
     b. 55–61 cm, 172.5 mm
     c. ≥62 cm, 172.5–175 mm

GEARING

EQUIPMENT

- **Chain wheels:** (1) Large chain wheel (usually 53 teeth); (2) Small chain wheel (usually 39 teeth)
- **Cassette:** Clusture of 5–9 gears (cogs) mounted to right of rear wheel

GEAR RATIO

- Number of teeth on chain wheel/Number of teeth on cog
  1. Higher gear ratio requires more strength, endurance and technique, but yields more power
  2. Lower gear ratio allows for more spinning and higher cadence, and without proper technique may yield less power (Mellion, 2001).

CADENCE

- Optimal cadence determined by type of race (TT, climbing, pack riding), strategies, body type, muscle fiber type, training level (Burke, 2002).
  1. High cadences put less strain on trained cycling leg muscles.
  2. Low cadences increase intramuscular pressure, reducing blood flow to the muscles during the power phase of the pedal stroke.
  3. High cadence/low resistance training reduces the incidence of overuse injuries. Cyclists beginning a season, or returning from injury should attempt 500–1000 miles of this type of training.
  4. Cadence is individual, and should be determined on a rider to rider basis.

INJURIES

GENERAL INJURY DATA

- Approximately 1000 deaths; 23,000 hospital admissions; 750,000 emergency room (ER) visits, 1.2 million physician visits per year (Thompson and Rivara, 2001; Hunter, 1998).
- Bicycle crashes are the second leading cause of sports associated serious injury.
- Peak incidence of bicycle related injuries is in the 9–15-year age group.
- Risk factors for injury: Not wearing a helmet, crashes involving motor vehicles, unsafe riding environment, and male sex (Thompson and Rivara, 2001).
- Mountain bikes account for 3.7 of overall injuries, but 51–85% of all mountain bikers sustain injuries each year (Kronisch and Pfeiffer, 2002; Gaulrapp, Weber, and Rosemeyer, 2001).
- BMX bikers are frequently injured doing stunts; 6.3% of all BMX riders sustain injuries in competition (Thompson and Rivara, 2001).

TRAUMATIC INJURIES

UPPER EXTREMITY

- *Fall on outstretched hand* (FOOSH) injuries from falling:
  1. Scaphoid fracture
  2. Distal radius fracture (Colles fracture)
  3. Fractures of the radial head
  4. *Acromioclavicular* (AC) joint separation—usually direct trauma to involved shoulder
     a. Initial treatment is sling, with *range of motion* (ROM) exercises as tolerated.
     b. First and second degree may resume riding as comfort permits.
     c. Third degree may take 4–6 weeks to heal.
     d. Clavicular fracture
     e. If aligned, may return to riding in 48 h.
     f. Nonaligned may return in 4–6 weeks or as pain dictates.

HEAD

- Account for most bicycle related deaths (1000/year)
- Generally preventable with helmets (severity reduced 85–90%) (Thompson and Rivara, 2001; Stephans-Stidham and Mallonee, 2001)

SKIN

- Lacerations
- Abrasions (road rash): Graded as first degree (superficial), second degree (partial thickness), or third degree (full thickness)

- First degree, second degree, and third degree are treated with hydroactive dressings (adaptic) and silvadene or mupuricin ointments
- Larger third degree: Silvadene cream tid or wet to dry dressings
- Tetanus prophylaxis for all abrasions

PELVIC
- Fractures of the superior and inferior rami are the most common pelvic fractures (Baker, 1998).
  1. Stable fractures need pain relief and rest, most heal within 2–3 weeks
  2. Unstable fractures need surgical intervention

VISCERAL
- Mostly caused by handlebars
  1. Abdominal wall—hernia (Holmes, Hall, and Schaller, 2002)
  2. Liver—hematomas (Nehoda et al, 2001)
  3. Spleen—hematoma
  4. Pancreas—hematoma, tears
  5. Bowel—perforation

VASCULAR
- External iliac artery endofibrosis (Abraham, Saumet, and Chevalier, 1997; Morelli and Stone, 2001)
  1. Progressive stenotic intimal thickening of the external iliac artery
  2. Presentation—pain or cramps in buttocks, thighs, or calves; may also present with sensation of the swollen leg with maximal effort or strenuous cycling
  3. Must be seen by physician as soon as possible
  4. Diagnosis
     a. Ultrasound and continuous-wave Doppler of the lower limb
     b. Systolic humeral and posterior tibial arterial pressures with an oscillometer
     c. Arteriorgraphy with femoral Seldinger technique
  5. Treatment
     a. Professional athletes—surgical endarterectomy
     b. Recreational athletes—decrease or switch activity

OVERUSE (FIG. 81-2) (Wilber et al, 1995)

KNEE

Anterior
- Patellar pain syndrome, quadriceps tendinitis, chondromalacia patellae, and patella tendinitits
- **Causes:** Training errors (rapid increase in mileage, high gearing, excessive hills), bicycle fit problems (seat too low or too far forward, malpositioned cleats, crank arm too long), anatomic issues (genu valgus, genu varum, hyperpronation)
- **Treatment:** (1) Review and adjust training plan. (2) Improve bike fit—move seat higher, move saddle posterior; reposition cleats. (3) Correct for lower extremity anatomic abnormalities–consider bicycling orthotics. (4) Rehabilitation and knee strengthening.

Medial
- Irritation of medial patellofemoral ligament, plica, or pes anserine bursitis
- **Causes:** Training errors, cleats with toes pointed out, feet too far apart
- **Treatment:** (1) Review and adjust training plan. (2) Adjust cleats or shorten bottom bracket axle. (3) Possible surgical plica excision or medial patellofemoral ligament release. (4) Rehabilitation and knee strengthening.

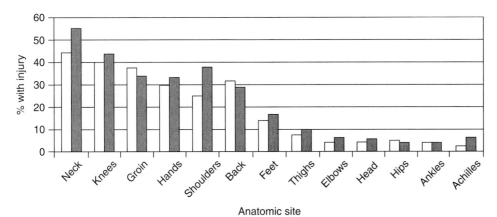

FIG 81-2 Common overuse injuries in Recreational Cyclists. SOURCE: Adapted from Wilber CA, Holland GJ, Madison RE, et al. An epidemiologic analysis of overuse injuries among recreational cyclists. *Int J Sports Med* 1995:16:201–6.

Lateral

- *Iliotibial* (IT) band friction syndrome/tendintitis
- **Causes:** (1) Bicycle-fit problems (improper cleat placement, seat too high or too posterior). (2) Anatomic (hyperpronation, genu varum, tight IT band, leg length discrepancy).
- **Treatment:** (1) Adjust cleats, lower seat, move saddle forward. (2) Consider cycling orthotics. (3) IT band stretching. (4) Rehabilitation and knee strengthening.

Posterior

- Biceps femoris tendinitis, semimembranous tendinitis, posterior capsule strain
- **Causes:** (1) Improper training (too aggressive, too much riding out of saddle. (2) Bicycle fit (saddle too high, too far anterior, cleats improperly set).
- **Treatment:** (1) Review and adjust training plan. (2) Move seat up and/or back, adjust cleats. (3) Rehabilitation and knee strengthening.

SHOULDER

- Weight is borne through shoulder joint
  1. Subacromial bursitis
  2. Rotator cuff tendinitits

NECK

- Common in up to 60% of riders (Mellion, 1994)
  1. Most commonly caused by increased load on the arms and shoulders necessary to support the rider and the hyperextension of the neck in the horizontal riding position.
  2. Bicyclists may develop myofascial trigger points in neck (levator scapula, splenius capitis, trapezius, sternocleidomastoid, infraspinatous, supraspinatous, and rhomboid muscles).
  3. May treat by raising handlebars or shortening the stem extension to reduce the amount of hyperextension of the neck. Strength and flexibility exercises may also be used.

BACK

- The low back muscles are primarily what a cyclist uses for control and generation of power. Chronic fatigue and pain may develop due to position on bike. In older cyclists, may also be a component of degenerative disk changes. Must also consider leg length discrepancy, deconditioning, and other conditions that increase muscle tension (stress, anxiety, depression) (Mellion, 1994).
  1. Management: Strengthening, flexibility, and/or weight loss and posture improvement
  2. On-bike: Change positions, push lower gears, use higher cadence, rise from saddle on climbs.
  3. Review bicycle fit. Move saddle forward—if effective top tube length is too great, extension will exaggerate a lordotic lumbar posture.

HANDS

- Ulnar neuropathy: Ulnar nerve is compressed in Guyon's canal. Pain, numbness, tingling lateral 4th and 5th fingers secondary to compression of the ulnar nerve on the handlebars. May be acute or chronic with sensory changes most often occurring first.
- May be treated with padded gloves, increased handlebar padding, change hand position frequently while riding.
- Carpal tunnel syndrome: Numbness and tingling in thumb, index, middle, and ring fingers caused by median nerve compression.
- Tenosynovitis: Tendons of the extensor pollicis brevis and abductor pollicis longus (De Quervain's). Usually caused in mountain bikers by tight gripping of the handlebars on difficult terrain (Richmond, 1994).

FOOT/ANKLE

- Paresthesias: Numbness and tingling in feet
  1. Cause: Tight shoe straps and increased pressure on pedals
  2. Course: Usually self limited
  3. Management: Loosen straps, ride at higher cadence to reduce pedal pressure
- Metatarsalgia: Pain over metatarsal heads
  1. Cause: Poor foot position, increased pedal pressure. May be caused by pes planus or hyperpronation.
  2. Management: Adjust cleats or consider cycling orthotics.
- Achilles tendonitits
- Plantar fasciitis

HIP

- Trochanteric bursitis: Caused by repetitive sliding of fascia lata over greater trochanter.
- Iliopsoas tendinitis: Pain in medial proximal thigh
  1. Usually because seat is too high.
  2. Lower seat height, evaluate frame size.

GROIN

- Saddle sores: Caused by friction, pressure then infection may be prevented with chamois cream.
- Crotchitis (tinea cruris): More common in women secondary to warmth and wetness.
- Ischial tuberosity tenderness: Eases with continued riding.
- Pudendal neuropathy: Compression of dorsal branch of pudendal nerve between bike seat and pubic symphysis.
  1. May last several minutes to several hours.
  2. May be prevented by adjusting seated position every 5–10 min on the ride or by tilting saddle slightly downward.

ENVIRONMENTAL INJURIES (Baker, 1998; Helzer-Julin, 1994; Bailey, 2000)

• Cyclist may be predisposed to heat and cold injuries and altitude sickness, underscoring the importance of proper clothing, nutrition, hydration, and acclimatization. (Please see chapter 39 for detail.)

EQUIPMENT AND SAFETY

• **Helmet:** Reduce risk of head injuries 74–85% (Thompson and Rivara, 2001; Stephans-Stidham and Mallonee, 2001).
  1. Should be worn snugly in a horizontal position on the head with the straps forming a 'V' around the ears, and held in place with the buckle fastened.
  2. Only 15–25% of children wear helmets correctly (Thompson and Rivara, 2001).
  3. Possible barriers to use of helmets: discomfort, poor fit, cost, underestimation of risk of injury, peer pressure.
  4. Government standards (Mellion, 2001):
     a. Consumer Product Safety Commission (CPSC) mandatory government standard for all helmets made after 1999 incorporates previous volunteer standards from below organizations.
     b. American National Standards Institute (ANSI)—minimum requirement for racing helmets.
     c. Snell Foundation—for children, more stringent than ANSI
• Protective eyewear: Protects from UV radiation, flying objects, and irritants
• Cycling gloves: Cushions hand from road shock, protects hands in falls
• Cycling shorts: Protect inner thigh, groin, and perineum from chafing and pressure trauma.

REFERENCES

Abraham P, Saumet JL, Chevalier JM: External iliac artery end-ofibrosis in athletes. *Sports Med* 24:221–226, 1997.

Bailey DM: Acute mountain sickness: The 'poison of the pass.' *West J Med* 172:399–400, June 2000.

Baker A: *Bicycling Medicine: Cycling Nutrition, Physiology, and Injury Prevention and Treatment for Riders of All Levels.* New York, NY, Fireside, 1998.

Burke ER: Proper fit of the bicycle. *Clin Sports Med* 13(1):1–14, 1994.

Burke ER: Physiology of higher pedaling cadences: Is Lance on to something? *Cycle Sport Journal* Oct 2002, pp 116–118.

Christiaans HH, Bremner A: Comfort on bicycles and the validity of a commercial bicycle fitting system. *Appl Ergon* 29(3):201–211, 1998.

Colorado Cyclist: Bike fit: How to fit your custom bicycle. http://www.coloradocyclist.com/bikefit/, accessed July, 2004.

Gaulrapp H, Weber A, Rosemeyer B: Injuries in mountain biking. *Knee Surg, Sports Trauatol, Arthrosc* 9:48–53, 2001.

Grubb, C: BMX builds racers. *Velonews* 1(1):11, 2003.

Helzer-Julin M: Sun, heat, and cold injuries in cyclists. *Clin Sport Med* 13(1):219–234, 1994.

Holmes JH, Hall A, Schaller RT: Thoracic handlebar hernia: Presentation and management. *J Trauma* 52:165–166, 2002.

Hunter RE: Cycling: Road, velodrome and mountain biking, in Safran MR, McKeag DB, VanCamp SP (eds.): *Manual of Sports Medicine.* Philadelphia, PA, Lippincott-Raven, 1998, pp 551–552.

Kronisch RL, Pfeiffer RP: Mountain biking injuries an update. *Sports Med* 32(8):523–537, 2002.

Mellion MB: Common cycling injuries management and prevention. *Sports Med* 11(1):52–70, 1991.

Mellion MB: Neck and back pain in bicycling. *Clin Sport Med* 13(1):137–164, 1994.

Mellion MB: Bicycling, in Mellion MB (ed.): *Team Physician's Handbook*, 3rd ed. Philadelphia, PA, Hanley & Belfus, 2001, pp 677–695.

Morelli MJ, Stone DA: Bicycling, in Fu FH, Stone DA (eds.): *Sports Injuries: Mechanisms, Prevention, Treatment*, 2nd ed. Philadelphia, PA, Lippincott Williams & Wilkins, 2001, pp 312–319.

Nehoda H, Hochleitner BW, et al: Central liver hematomas caused by mountain-bike crashes. *Injury* 285–287, 2001.

Richmond DR: Handlebar problems in cycling. *Clin Sport Med* 13(1):165–173, 1994.

Stephans-Stidham S, Mallonee S: The prevention of traffic deaths and injuries: The role of physicians. *J Okla State Med Assoc* 94(6):192–193, 2001.

Thompson MJ, Rivara FP: Bicycle-related injuries. *Am Fam Phys* 63:2007–2014, 2017–2018, 2001.

Too, D: Biomechanics of cycling and factors affecting performance. *Sports Med* 10(5):286–302, 1990.

Wilber CA, Holland GJ, Madison RE, et al: An epidemiologic analysis of overuse injuries among recreational cyclists. *Int J Sports Med* 16:201–206, 1995.

82 FIGURE SKATING

Roger J Kruse, MD
Jennifer Burke, MD

INTRODUCTION

SCOPE OF PARTICIPATION

• The U.S. Figure Skating Association (USFSA) is the national governing body for figure skating and includes more than 585 member clubs and over 167,000 members (USFSA Fact Sheet, 2003).

DISCIPLINES

- *Singles Skaters* combine the highest level of athleticism and artistry. These skaters complete multirevolution jumps and spins with rapid footwork sequences, spiral sequences, and connecting moves.
- *Pairs Skaters* skate as a traditional couple, performing not only multirevolution jumps and spins, but also numerous high-risk maneuvers such as throw jumps and overhead lifts.
- *Ice Dancers* skate as a traditional couple, concentrating on speed, body lean, edges, and precise technique. The rules of the sport limit jumps, spins, and lifts, and partner separations.
- *Synchronized Skating* is currently the fastest-growing discipline in figure skating and teams are typically composed of 20 female skaters.

COMPETITION

- In the United States, the competition levels for men and women are preliminary, prejuvenile, juvenile, intermediate, novice, junior, senior, and adult. Participation in each level is generally determined not by age, but by accomplishment of the specific skill tests.
- In competition, singles, pairs, and, synchronized skaters perform two programs, the lengths of which are dictated by level:
  1. The *short program* varies in length with competition level, but not as a function of gender. Senior competitors perform required elements to music that cannot exceed 2 min and 40 s in length.
  2. The *long program* is performed to music that for senior skaters cannot exceed 4 min and 30 s and is generally more difficult.
- Ice dancers perform three programs in competition: one compulsory dance; an original dance that is no longer than 2 min; and a free dance which can be as long as 4 min.

SPORT SCIENCE

ATHLETE ATTRIBUTES

PHYSICAL

- Figure skaters are generally shorter, lighter, and leaner than average (Zeigler et al, 1998). Most figure skaters are right-leg dominant, rotate counter-clockwise and land on their right leg.

PHYSIOLOGY

- Physiologic testing, including VO_{2max}, flexibility, vertical jump, body composition, strength, and power

evaluations, is useful in planning and monitoring training programs (Zeigler et al, 1998). Off-ice training and periodization of training are necessary in order to optimize these elements (Zeigler et al, 1998). While performing a program, a figure skater will reach 90–100% of their maximal heart rate within 30–60 s and then sustain that level of intensity for the duration of the program. Figure skating can be compared to tennis with regard to the necessity of a well-developed anaerobic and aerobic energy system. The effort required for a long program in figure skating can be compared to running a 4-min mi.

NUTRITION

- Skaters, particularly female figure skaters, eat with the goal of achieving or maintaining the lean athletic body type demanded by the sport. Female pair skaters must be lightweight for successful completion of lifts and throw jumps. Female ice dancers are judged on an aesthetically pleasing body line and are typically very thin at higher levels of competition.
- The most common issues encountered are inadequate caloric intake and hydration, as well as inappropriate food choices. More than 1/2 to 2/3 of female figure skaters reported dieting to lose weight (Zeigler et al, 1998). It has been shown that despite relatively low caloric intakes, biochemical measures of overall nutritional status appear to be normal (Zeigler et al, 1998).
- Intake of some micronutrients, including vitamin D and calcium, which affect bone health, is considerably lower than those observed in the general adolescent population (Zeigler et al, 1998; Zeigler, Jonnala-gadda, and Lawrence, 2001).

BONE MASS

- Figure skaters' bone mineral density of the spine and lower extremities has been shown to be significantly higher than in nonskaters, suggesting that intense weight-bearing exercise may protect bone mass, despite inadequate nutritional intake (Slemendra and Johnson, 1993).

PSYCHOLOGY

- More than 85% of the most successful elite skaters are using sports psychology techniques year-round; almost every elite athlete in the United States uses visualization and imagery.
- The abilities to concentrate and refocus are positive predictors of how well athletes will perform. Negative thinking and lack of emotional control are significant issues.
- The relationship of the skater, parent, and coach is a very close one, and the treating physician must communicate with each to optimize treatment compliance

and outcome. Addressing the psychologic impact of an injury is very important to the recovery process.

- As a team sport, team dynamics and team building in synchronized skating are integral to success and must be included in training programs.

EQUIPMENT

BOOTS AND BLADES

- The skating boot is made primarily from leather. A skater's ankles are plantar flexed in the skate due to the height of the boot heel. Some manufacturers make a boot with heat-molded parts in order to customize the fit.
- The design of the skating boot has changed over the past two decades. The boots have become increasingly stiff in response to requests from skaters and coaches to enhance support, slow break down, and accommodate skaters with suboptimal ankle strength and proprioception to improve jump landing success rates.
- Over-the-counter or stock boots and blades are less expensive, less rigid, and can be variable in construction. They are sold as a single unit, with the blade screwed or riveted to the boot. Most elite athletes wear stiff custom-made boots bought separately from the blades.
- New skates and blades can cost well over $1000 and are usually replaced every year. Skaters typically replace boots when the ankle support breaks down. Stock boots are available for half the price of custom-made boots but must be replaced more often.
- Optimal boot fit is necessary to prevent boot-related injuries. The boot should be lightweight (<5% of skater's body weight). It should have a broad forefoot, a well-fitted heel, and a well-padded tongue. New boots should be introduced at the end of the competitive season and never be worn alternately with old boots. There is little room in boots to accommodate orthoses. Additionally, the plantar flexed position in which the boot holds the foot must be accounted for in its orthotic construction.

BIOMECHANICS

JUMPS

- To perform the increasingly difficult triple and quadruple jumps, the athletes are rotating faster, not jumping higher (King DL, Arnold AS, Smith, 1994). Flight times for single, double, and triple jumps are very similar due to nearly identical vertical velocity at takeoffs (King DL, Arnold AS, Smith, 1994).

- An athlete's upper body strength and consequent ability to pull arms against centrifugal forces when initiating jump rotation is correlated positively with the athlete's ability to perform the more difficult jumps.
- Impact forces are greater on landing higher revolution jumps as a result of the decreased time available to dissipate force between the forefoot and rear foot contact with the ice (Lockwood and Gervais, 1997).
- Athletes fail to land multiple revolution jumps or triple-triples because of their inability to attain tight air position efficiently.

SPINS

- Athletes report that spinning requires as much or more energy than jumping. The athlete rotates three to six revolutions per second, creating 200–300 lb of centrifugal force (Nash, 1988). Upper body, lower body, and core strength are all required to keep the arms and legs close to the axis of rotation to counteract the centrifugal force.

TRAINING

GENERAL

- Figure skaters often begin rigorous training as early as 5 years of age, and some are performing jumps requiring two or three revolutions by the age of 8. The more elite athletes can spend up to 45 h a week dedicated to their sport: roughly 15 to 30 h per week on the ice and 5 to 15 h performing off-ice conditioning. Additional time is spent on choreography, music selection, and costume design and fitting.
- Training schedules run virtually year-round with only a small break during the early spring, significantly increasing the risk of overuse injury.

ON-ICE

- A typical on-ice training regimen includes two to three 45-min on-ice sessions throughout the day. Training programs are usually most intense from late spring through summer. During the competitive seasons less time is spent conditioning, and more time is spent perfecting choreography.

OFF-ICE

- Athletes who participate in off-ice programs are stronger, have better-developed aerobic and anaerobic energy systems, jump higher, have more consistent jump landings, have tighter and faster spins, and feel more confident on the ice. Additionally, these athletes may have decreased injury rates for level of participation as well. The number of athletes participating in off-ice training has increased significantly over the past five years.

- Off-ice programs should include core strengthening, plyometrics, and attention to symmetry of limb flexibility and strength, especially hip, ankle, and foot, as well as cardiovascular fitness, including both aerobic and anaerobic fitness. As the athlete spends more time taking part in off-ice conditioning programs, it is important to decrease the time spent on the ice.

MEDICAL ISSUES

MUSCULOSKELETAL ISSUES

GENERAL

- The incidence of injury in figure skating has been calculated to range from 1.37 to 3 per 1000 h of training (Kjaer and Larsson, 1992; Brock and Striowski, 1986). The nature of injuries often varies with the skater's discipline (Smith, 1997).
- The musculoskeletal problems of skaters primarily affect the lower extremity: the knee, foot, and ankles; however, injuries to the hip, pelvis, and spine have increased significantly as program difficulty has increased over the past 10 years. At least half of all injuries are attributed to overuse mechanisms) (Kjaer and Larsson, 1992; Brock and Striowski, 1986) and should be preventable with attention to optimizing flexibility, symmetric strength, and power.

BOOT- AND BLADE-RELATED ISSUES

- The boot and blade are the most important pieces of equipment of the figure skater and are likely contributors to most injuries.
- Boot stiffness, fit, alignment, and weight, as well as blade mount and alignment are issues that can contribute to injury.

LOWER EXTREMITY

Foot

- *Malleolar bursitis* is caused by boot pressure points causing excessive compression and shear forces between malleoli and boots. Both malleoli can be affected. It is generally well tolerated, but can easily become inflamed with minor irritation or boot changes. These types of injuries are treated by operating on the boot, not the skater. Focal stretching/punching out of boot in rub areas, and/or padding placed to distribute compressive forces around the malleoli will typically alleviate the problem. Aspiration and subsequent injection with cortisone and a compressive wrap is tempting, though *infrequently* indicated or beneficial. *Rarely* is surgery required.

- A *pump bump or Haglund's deformity of the calcaneal tuberosity* is caused by a boot heel that is too wide for the skater's heel. This allows the skater's heel to slide up and down within the boot, resulting in callus and bursa inflammation. For nearly all cases, the skate fit should be addressed. It is important that the heel of the boot be sufficiently narrow to prevent up and down motion of the heel. This can be done with padding medial and lateral to the Achilles tendon region, paying special attention not to compress that structure. Small heels lifts may also be helpful to hold the calcaneal tuberosity firmly against the upper part of the skate heel as it curves forward.
- *Tibialis anterior and extensor hallux tendinosis or tenosynovitis* are caused by repetitive dorsiflexion and plantar flexion of the ankle, excessive compression of crossing laces, and abnormal creasing of the boot tongue across the anterior foot. Crepitus over the tendon structure and nodules are not uncommon clinical findings. To prevent anterior compression injuries, the boot tongue should be in a neutral position or slightly medial, especially when the boots are being broken in. If the tongue is properly centralized, anterior tendinitis can still occur, but it can be prevented by padding the boot tongue with closed cell foam or thermoplastic material. A more flexible boot can be preventative.
- *Sinus tarsi pain* is less common and is typically caused by the break-in crease.
- *Achilles tendinosis, partial tears and nodules of the Achilles tendon,* can occur from compression of the tendon with plantar flexion of the foot against the boot, and can also occur during off-ice training with running and jumping. The Achilles tendon is generally protected by the height of the boot heel, though in some cases the posterior portion of the boot can be inappropriately angled forward. Boot modifications may be helpful. Ice dancers often have boots with low cutout areas for the Achilles tendon to improve their line and ability to bend their knees. This modification may be helpful for any skater.
- Other areas that can be irritated include the base of the fifth metatarsal and the tarsal navicular. Metatarsal stress fractures are caused primarily by jumping and the position of the foot in the boot. Corns and calluses on the toes are seen frequently. Typically these are all issues that occur as a result of improper boot fit and can be treated with donut pads, punching out the boot and other modifications to the boot.

Ankle

- Poor ankle proprioception, inversion, and eversion strengths are significant issues among skaters due to the stiffness of the boot and the many hours skaters spent on the ice. Over the past 5 to 10 years, however, attention has been placed on optimizing ankle strength in off-ice programs. In the elite athlete, weakness in the ankle stabilizing structures is much less common.

Lower Leg

- Posterior medial tibial syndrome, peroneal tendinitis, and/or fibular stress syndrome may develop at the level of the top of the boot. These syndromes are typically attributed to weakness of the tibialis posterior and peroneal muscles. They can also be due to relative inflexibility of the gastroc–soleus complex. Continued training with such symptoms can culminate in tibial and/or fibular stress fractures. Treatment and prevention include optimizing flexibility in the gastroc-soleus complex, strengthening of the ankle inverters and averters, evaluation of the boot, and the skater's position within the boot. Orthoses, blade mounting, and padding of the top of the boot may be beneficial.

Knee

- Anterior knee pain is one of the most frequent problems and typically occurs in the "landing leg." The etiologies are multiple and include relative hip weakness, quadriceps weakness, inadequate flexibility of the hip and thigh musculature (Smith, Stroud, and McQueen, 1991), patella shape, and tracking issues. Skaters may also experience patellar compression injuries from falling but rarely experience patellar fracture.
- Infrapatellar and patellar tendinosis are seen in elite skaters and are often very difficult to treat because of the lengthy competitive season. The authors have used prolotherapy with good results.
- Meniscus and ligament injuries are relatively rare in figure skaters, likely due to the lack of fixation of the blade in the ice. Jumps are typically landed as the athlete is skating backward and cocontraction of the quadriceps and hamstring muscles is necessary for control of the landing.

CORE, HIP, AND PELVIS

- Athletes are presenting with an increasing rate of groin, hip flexor, adductor complex, and external and internal oblique injuries. These types of injuries are some of the most common injuries sustained by the most elite athletes. An estimated 25% of national team members from the United States and Canada have been affected by hip flexor injuries in recent years.
- The increase in these types of injuries is attributed to the focus on triple and quadruple revolution. The mechanisms are multifaceted. Skaters perform upwards of 45–60 practice jumps daily. They often have tight hip flexors and asymmetrically strong hip flexors. Additionally, skaters can have relatively weak or asymmetrically strong core musculature and hip stabilizers. Combined, these issues increase the potential for overuse injury.
- Avulsion fractures of the ischium, lesser tuberosity, and crest of the ilium have increasingly been reported in singles and pairs skaters, as well as synchronized skaters. These occur during early phases of growth spurts, and have markedly increased in athletes who perform the more difficult double, triple, and quadruple axel jumps. These injuries are slow to heal and often recur. Proactive evaluation of the athlete for hip strength asymmetry, flexibility, and endurance can be preventive. Additionally, it is important to ensure that an athlete has adequate strength to initiating training for such jumps.

SPINE

- Many skating moves and jump landings require an arched or hyperextended back, placing the posterior elements of the lumbar spine at increased stress and causing potential for lumbar strain, facet pain, posterior iliac crest injury, spondylolysis, and spondylolisthesis. The rigidity of the boot and restricted plantar flexion of the ankle limits adequate knee flexion, therefore the athlete is unable to maintain normal alignment of the spine with jump landings.
- Spondylolysis is often missed by clinicians, and a high level of suspicion is important to diagnose this injury in skaters. A young skater with persistent back pain should be evaluated with X-rays, followed by a *single photon emission computed tomography* (SPECT) bone scan or *computed tomography* (CT) of the area.
- Appropriate therapy includes strengthening of the core musculature to provide control of the trunk and pelvis and to assist in maintaining the alignment of the body during jumps, spins, and lifts, as well as strengthening of the ankle-supporting musculature to permit the use of a more flexible boot, which accommodates greater dorsiflexion during landing.

UPPER EXTREMITIES

- Upper body strength is essential to both jumping and spinning, and pair elements. Many elite skaters have inadequate shoulder stabilizers.
- Synchronized skaters are at increased risk of shoulder and wrist injuries as they often hold onto each other throughout their programs.

MEDICAL CONCERNS

EXERCISE-INDUCED BRONCHOSPASM

- The incidence of *exercise-induced bronchospasm* (EIB) ranges from 33 to 50% in elite skaters in the

United States, with greater prevalence among females and younger skaters (Wilber et al, 1999; Provost-Craig et al).

- Relatively cold air temperatures in combination with questionable air quality from ice resurfacer exhaust fumes, inadequate ventilation systems, and mold in many rinks produces a significant environmental trigger for EIB (Wilber et al, 1999; Provost-Craig et al). Repetitive bouts of extremely vigorous exercise, where HR often reaches 90–100% of predicted maximums during the 1st min of a 4- to 5-min program, also put athletes at increased risk for symptoms of EIB.

- Evaluation for EIB symptoms using self-reported symptoms yields high rates of both false positive and false negative results when correlated with spirometry (Rundell et al, 2001). Ideally, screening for EIB in elite athletes should be carried out using spirometry in a sport-specific environmental setting and under competition level of exertion (Rundell et al, 2000).

- Since spirometry is not easily available at most ice rinks, an athlete can be educated to check their peak flows while at the rink. Peak flows should be obtained before a performance of a long program and at 1 and 5 min after the program is completed. A 10–15% decrease in peak flow can be suggestive of EIB.

- Most skaters respond well to preexercise treatment with an inhaled quick-acting beta agonist, though many elite skaters report a greater improvement in peak flows and symptoms when they use longer-acting beta-agonists because they train intermittently throughout the day at varying intensities. A trial of a long acting beta agonist with an inhaled steroid may be indicated if the athlete's peak flows do not sufficiently improve with single agent therapy.

DISORDERED EATING

- Eating disorders and disordered eating patterns are increasing in frequency among figure skaters. It is unclear what the prevalence is, and whether the risk of eating disorders increases as the skaters climb through the ranks of national and international levels (Ziegler et al, 1998).

MENSTRUAL DYSFUNCTION

- Delayed menarche is not uncommon among female figure skaters. Female figure skaters may have delayed onset of menses by 1 year, and nearly half of menstruating females report irregular or absent cycles (Zeigler et al, 1998). Delays and irregularities are attributed to a high level of training, and inadequate caloric intake with relation to activity level (Williams et al, 1995).

THE FEMALE ATHLETE TRIAD

- As in any sport in which appearance is judged, clinicians must maintain a high level of suspicion for the potential of the continuum of the female athlete triad.

CONCUSSIONS, LACERATIONS, CONTUSIONS

- Skaters involved in pairs skating, ice dancing, and synchronized skating suffer a higher rate of concussions, contusions, and lacerations as compared with single skaters. Frequently, multiple skaters are injured at the same time in synchronized skating.

THE FUTURE

- In summary, at least half of all figure skating injuries are likely preventable due to overuse mechanisms and/or boot and blade issues. New boot design considerations include: flexibility, comfort, support, durability, cushioning of landing impact, ability to plantar and dorsi flex foot to assist with shock absorption from jumping and to assist in power for jump takeoffs, affordability, blade alignment and mounting, weight of boot and blades, and adaptability to orthoses.

- Figure skating is a demanding sport that requires athletes to begin training at a young age and be able to successfully perform jumps of increasing difficulty. Unfortunately, many prepubescent athletes can do a large number of jumps, and while going through puberty, get injured. In order to prevent injuries, studies need to be done incorporating the age as well as the development of the athletes, to determine the exact number of jumps to perform each day. Factors that should be considered include: type of jump, level of mastery, physical issues such as strength and symmetry, hours of on-ice and off-ice training, recovery time between sessions, and time in training cycle.

REFERENCES

Brock RM, Striowski CC: Injuries in elite figure skaters. *Phys Sports Med* 14:111–115, 1986.

King DL, Arnold AS, Smith SL: A kinematic comparison of single, double and triple axels. *J Appl Biomech* 10:51–60, 1994.

Kjaer M, Larsson B: Physiological profile and incidence of injuries among elite figure skaters. *J Sports Sci* 10:29–36, 1992.

Lockwood K, Gervais P: Impact forces upon landing single, double, and triple revolution jumps in figure skaters. *Clin Biomech* (Bristol, Avan) 12(3): S11, Apr. 1997.

Nash HL: U.S. Olympic figure skaters: Honing their performances. *Phys Sports Med* 6:181–185, 1988.

Provost–Craig MA, Arbour KS, Sestili DC, et al: The incidence of exercise–induced bronchospasm in competitive figure skaters. *J Asthma* 33:67–71, 1996.

Rundell KW, Wilber RL, Szmedra L, et al: Exercise-induced bronchospasm screening of elite athletes: field versus laboratory exercise challenge, *Med. Sci. Sports Exerc.* 32:309–316, 2000.

Rundell KW, Im J, Mayers LB, et al: Self-reported symptoms and exercise-induced asthma in the elite athlete. *Med Sci Sports Exerc* 33:209–213, 2001.

Slemendra CW, Johnson CC: High intensity activities in young women: Site specific mass effects among female skaters. *J Bone Miner Res* 20:125–132, 1993.

Smith AD: Skating injuries: A guide to prevention and management. *J Musculoskel Med* 14:10–29, 1997.

Smith AD, Stroud L, McQueen C: Flexibility and anterior knee pain in adolescent elite figure skaters. *J Pediatr Orthop* 11:77–82, 1991.

Wilber RL, Rundell KW, Szmedra L et al: Incidence of exercise-induced bronchospasm in Olympic winter sport athletes. *Med Sci Sports Exerc* 732–737, 1999.

Williams NI, Young JC, McArthur JW et al: Strenuous exercise with caloric restriction: Effect on luteinizing hormone secretion. *Med Sci Sports Exerc* 27:1390–1398, 1995.

Zeigler PJ, Jonnalagadda SS, Lawrence C: Dietary intake of elite figure skating dancers, *Nutr Res* 21:983–992, 2001.

Ziegler P, Hensley S, Roepke JB, et al: Eating attitudes and energy intakes of female skaters. *Med Sci Sports Exerc* 30:583–586, 1998.

Zeigler P, Khoo CS, Sherr B, et al: Body image and dieting behaviors among elite figure skaters. *Int J Eat Disord* 24:421–427, 1998.

2002–2003 USFSA Fact Sheet, U.S. Figure Skating Online – *www.usfsa.org.*

83 FOOTBALL

John M MacKnight, MD

INTRODUCTION

- Sports medicine coverage of American football places unique demands on the sports medicine practitioner. A wide variety of sport-specific conditions and injuries demand that individuals responsible for the care of football teams be well versed in an array of both medical and orthopedic issues. Appropriate planning can minimize the likelihood of athlete injury and help to ensure that athletes are protected and returned to play as quickly as possible.

MUSCULOSKELETAL INJURIES

- Fifty percent of football players at all levels will be injured to some degree in any given season. The majority of these injuries involve the lower extremity with sprains, contusions, and strains being most common. Fractures account for 10% of injuries.

LOWER EXTREMITY INJURIES

MEDIAL COLLATERAL LIGAMENT SPRAIN, KNEE

- The most common knee injury seen in football, resulting from a valgus load to the knee by another player during blocking or tackling.
- Grade-I injuries have stretched but not disrupted the ligament and the knee examination (valgus loading of the knee at 0° and 30° of flexion) reveals no laxity compared to the uninjured side. Grade-II injuries have partial ligament disruption with discernible laxity on valgus testing but preservation of an end point. Grade-III injuries represent full ligament tears with gross laxity and no discernible end point.
- All three grades are generally managed conservatively with icing, *nonsteroidal anti-inflammatory drugs* (NSAIDs), and protective bracing. Even athletes with grade-III injuries may resume sport in protective braces if symptoms allow.
- Many football programs now utilize protective medial stabilizing braces to decrease the incidence of *medial collateral ligament* (MCL) injury, particularly in interior linemen. Although data have not clearly proven their efficacy, they may enhance proprioceptive function and are a reasonable preventative measure for at-risk players.

ANTERIOR CRUCIATE LIGAMENT TEAR

- The most devastating knee injury commonly seen in football. *Anterior cruciate ligament* (ACL) tears generally result from valgus loading of the slightly flexed knee creating significant shear forces on the ACL and subsequent tearing. The majority are noncontact injuries, but the ACL may be torn in a similar contact mechanism to that of the MCL noted above.
- The injury is accompanied by significant pain, immediate swelling, subjective instability of the knee, often an audible "pop" or a sense of tearing inside the knee, and laxity on the Lachman test.
- For competitive athletes, ACL tears will generally require surgical reconstruction. Graft options include patellar tendon, hamstring tendon, or cadaveric grafts. Patellar tendon grafts are generally preferred in athletes but may lead to earlier patellofemoral arthritis than the alternatives. Caution must also be used with

patellar grafting in athletes with prior patellar tendon dysfunction. After 6–9 months of aggressive rehabilitation, functional bracing to protect the reconstructed ACL is generally desirable to aid safe return to full football activities.

THIGH/QUADRICEP CONTUSION

- The most common soft tissue injury in football, resulting from blunt trauma.
- Treatment focuses on limitation of hemorrhage and inflammation while maintaining range of motion and strength. Ice and NSAIDs are appropriate initial interventions. Some practitioners advocate immobilizing the knee in 120° of flexion to limit hemorrhage and hematoma formation.
- Massage and ultrasound should be avoided early in the treatment course to allow for early stabilization of the damaged muscle. Athletes may return to play when they have full range of motion and strength approximating that of the uninjured leg. This injury may lead to myositis ossificans (calcific changes in areas of damaged muscle) in 9–20% of cases if treated inadequately.

TURF TOE

- A sprain of the plantar-capsular ligament complex with associated articular cartilage damage to the metatarsal heads or base of the proximal phalanx.
- The first *metatarsophalangeal* (MTP) joint is the primary area of injury, typically resulting from forced hyperextension of the planted toe on the turf. Athletes experience significant pain, have local swelling, and often limp.
- Artificial turf surfaces and lighter, more flexible shoes have been implicated in a higher incidence of turf toe injuries.
- Management centers on protection of the area with a rigid insert in the shoe to protect against dorsiflexion, donut padding, taping, ice, and NSAIDs. Activity status is as dictated by pain.

HIP POINTER

- Contusion or separation of attached muscle fibers at the superior aspect of the iliac crest as a result of blunt trauma, generally resulting in a significant degree of pain and dysfunction.
- X-rays are generally unnecessary at the time of diagnosis but should be strongly considered for symptoms that are prolonged or increasing.
- Management includes aggressive icing, stretching of the low back and flank muscles, and additional protective padding at the time of return to play.
- Local modalities such as ultrasound or anesthetic/corticosteroid injections may speed the healing response as well.

UPPER EXTREMITY INJURIES

SHOULDER INSTABILITY

- Shoulder instability is a common malady in football athletes as a result of repetitive blows to the shoulder and unusual loading that may arise with blocking and tackling.
- Frank dislocations occur anteriorly in 95% of cases and result from excessive abduction, extension, and external rotational forces.
- Surgery to correct shoulder instability is a frequent consideration as the recurrence rate for subluxations or dislocations is 50%.
- Open stabilization, rather than arthroscopic, is a more predictable means of restoring shoulder stability with excellent maintenance of range of motion and postoperative stability (Pagnani and Dome, 2002).
- Offensive linemen may develop posterior instability from blocking with outstretched arms and repetitively loading the posterior capsule of the glenohumeral joint. Except in extreme cases, aggressive rehabilitation and modification of weightlifting techniques are adequate for management.

JERSEY FINGER

- Forced extension of the actively flexed finger, as in attempting to grasp an opponent for a tackle, may result in avulsion of the flexor digitorum profundus from its insertion on the volar side of the distal phalanx.
- The ring finger is most commonly involved, followed by the middle finger.
- The athlete will feel a pop and the retracted tendon may be palpable proximally in the finger. Examination will demonstrate loss of independent flexion of the distal interphalangeal joint.
- Early surgical repair is the treatment of choice.

SPINAL AND NEUROLOGIC INJURIES

CERVICAL SPINE INJURY

MECHANISM

- Historically, head trauma had been the greatest source of morbidity and mortality in football, generally from subdural hematomas. Better helmet construction decreased such head injuries but fostered technique changes in play, which favored leading with the head and neck for tackling and blocking, so-called "spearing." This dangerous technique led to a marked increase in cervical spine injuries until rule changes were instituted to outlaw spearing in football.
- A review of 1300 cervical spine injuries from the National Football Head and Neck Injury Registry has

documented *axial loading of the cervical spine* as the major mechanism of catastrophic cervical spine injuries (Torg et al, 1990).

• The normal cervical spine is comprised on an arc of vertebral bodies that are able to withstand substantial loading by dissipating forces evenly across each vertebral level; however, when the neck is flexed forward 30°, it becomes a straight segmented column of bones that cannot dissipate force evenly. Axial loading of the neck in this flexposition may then result in excessive forces on the vertebral bodies leading to bony failure, fracture, and cervical spinal cord injury.

CERVICAL CORD NEUROPRAXIA

• Transient reversible deformation of the spinal cord resulting from significant trauma to the neck.
• The etiology of transient quadriplegia.
• Athletes may experience transient *bilateral* (differentiating this entity from a brachial plexus neuropraxia—see below) sensory changes, sensation loss, and variable motor changes including complete paralysis.
• Episodes typically last less than 15 min but may persist up to 2 days.
• A spinal canal: Vertebral body ratio (as determined by lateral radiographs of the cervical spine) of <0.8 has been found reliably in athletes suffering cervical cord neuropraxia (Pavlov et al, 1987). Although this measure has a high sensitivity for cervical cord neuropraxia, it has a low specificity and low positive predictive value and should not be used as a screening tool. In addition, caution must also be used in the interpretation of this ratio in football players because their large vertebral bodies will falsely decrease the ratio in the absence of true cervical spinal stenosis.
• The average rate of recurrence for players who returned to football was 56% (Torg et al, 1997).
• Management of the football player with known cervical spinal stenosis remains controversial as leading authorities in this area have expressed differing opinions with respect to return to play criteria. *Cantu has suggested that cervical spinal stenosis is an absolute contraindication to return to contact sport.* This belief is based on a known predisposition to spinal cord injury in these patients and a higher incidence of permanent neurologic sequelae in this group as compared to those with normal spinal canal volumes (Cantu, 2000; 1997).
• Torg contends that despite its association with transient quadriplegia, cervical spinal stenosis is not reliably associated with catastrophic spinal cord injury and does not mandate exclusion from participation in all cases (Torg and Ramsey-Emrhein, 1997). Torg proposes the following guidelines for participation in this group of athletes:

1. Canal/vertebral body ratio of 0.8 or less in asymptomatic individuals—*no contraindication*
2. Ratio of 0.8 or less with one episode of cervical cord neuropraxia—*relative contraindication*
3. Documented episodes of cervical cord neuropraxia associated with intervertebral disc disease and/or degenerative changes—*relative contraindication*
4. Documented episode of cervical cord neuropraxia associated with *magnetic resonance imaging* (MRI) evidence of cord defect or cord edema—*relative/absolute contraindication*
5. Documented episode of cervical cord neuropraxia associated with ligamentous instability, symptoms of neurologic findings lasting more than 36 h, and/or multiple episodes—*absolute contraindication*

STINGERS/BURNERS

• Brachial plexus neuropraxia resulting from traction or compression of the brachial plexus with violent lateral flexion of the neck.
• The most common nerve injury in football with defensive players most commonly affected.
• Athletes note *unilateral* burning or stinging pain, numbness, or tingling radiating from the supraclavicular area down to the fingers, most commonly in a C5 or C6 distribution. There may be weakness, most commonly of the deltoid, but *no neck pain.* Symptoms typically resolve in minutes. Symptoms that persist suggest more substantial injury to the brachial plexus, including cervical root avulsion, and mandate imaging and appropriate neurologic consultation.
• Athletes may resume competition when they demonstrate full range of motion, full strength, and a normal neurologic examination of the upper extremity.
• Prospective analysis of college football players revealed that a favorable overall spinal canal: vertebral body ratio (>0.9) is associated with a low initial incidence of brachial plexus injury (Castro et al, 1997). Players with multiple such injuries had significantly smaller ratios than those suffering only one event (0.75 vs. 0.87).

SPEAR TACKLER'S SPINE

• Characterized by developmental narrowing of the cervical canal (a canal-vertebral body ratio of <0.8), straightening or reversal of the normal cervical lordosis, and posttraumatic radiographic abnormalities.
• These individuals are at such great risk for permanent spinal cord injury that they should be precluded from participation in tackle football (Torg et al, 1993).

MANAGEMENT OF THE POTENTIAL CERVICAL SPINE INJURY

• Any unconscious athlete or any conscious athlete complaining of neck pain must have the cervical spine immobilized prior to removal from the playing field. This is accomplished by coordinated sports medicine care with a lead care provider at the head and neck to provide traction and stability, particularly if the athlete must be rolled onto their back prior to receiving additional care.

- The helmet should never be removed on the field as the presence of shoulder pads will favor passive hyperextension of the cervical spine and may contribute to further cervical spine or spinal cord injury. The face mask should be removed to allow control of the athlete's airway. Only in an appropriate acute care setting should the helmet and shoulder pads be removed.
- Evaluation includes cervical spine X-rays in several planes and may require *computed tomography* (CT) scanning to rule out fracture in equivocal cases. Football padding has been shown to compromise proper cervical imaging in the hospital setting (Davidson et al, 2001). Consequently, efforts may be undertaken, once in a controlled setting, to remove the helmet and shoulder pads so as not to compromise the quality of cross-table lateral and odontoid view cervical spine X-rays.
- Every potential cervical spine injury must be treated with the same conservative approach and proper technique to prevent unnecessary neurologic compromise.

LUMBAR SPINE INJURY

SPONDYLOLYSIS

- Stress injury to the pars interarticularis in the posterior aspect of the spine as a result of repetitive extension loading. Offensive and defensive linemen are most commonly affected.
- Athletes complain of deep pain in the low back, which is exacerbated by active or passive extension—particularly when standing on one leg. X-rays may reveal a fracture in the pars interarticularis on oblique views or bone scan or MRI may be necessary to make the diagnosis definitively.
- Most athletes respond well to conservative management including rest and rehabilitative activities. Occasionally thoracolumbar bracing may be utilized for additional spinal stability. Most athletes may return in 6–8 weeks if asymptomatic and with objective evidence of fracture healing.

SPONDYLOLISTHESIS

- Displacement of one vertebral body over another as a result of stress injury to the pars interarticularis (a spondylolysis). According to National Football League (NFL) and National Collegiate Athletic Association (NCAA) data (Shaffer, Wiesel, and Lauerman, 1997), approximately 1% of both professional and collegiate football players have a spondylolisthesis.
- The presence of a spondylolisthesis is not a contraindication to playing football but may predispose to pain and associated dysfunction and may also lead to further worsening of the anatomic changes in the spine over time.
- Pathologic forces on both lumbar disks and pars interarticularis have been demonstrated in blocking linemen (Gatt, Jr et al, 1997). The mechanics of repetitive blocking, most notably loaded extension of the lumbar spine, may be responsible for the increased incidence of such injuries in football linemen.

CONCUSSION

GENERAL

- Concussion or *mild traumatic brain injury* (MTBI) is estimated to occur at a rate of 250,000 events per year in football players. Concussion incidence has been found to be highest at the high school (5.6%) and division-III collegiate levels (5.5%) (Guskiewicz et al, 2000), suggesting an association between level of play and risk of injury.
- Mechanisms of injury include a direct blow to the head by an opposing player, whip-like motion of the head and neck in response to a blow delivered to another part of the body, or a blow to the head from hitting the ground. Brain shearing and acceleration/deceleration forces result in a cascade of neurochemical changes including local glucose depletion, edema, and local vascular effects.
- Many athletes either do not realize they have suffered MTBI or fail to report it to their sports medicine staff. Tight ends and defensive linemen are most commonly affected (Delaney et al, 2002), and the majority of concussed football players suffer recurrent concussive injury.

EVALUATION

- Concussed athletes are dazed, disoriented, and may have loss or alteration in consciousness. These manifestations may be mild and transient or prolonged and quite profound. They may complain of dizziness, headache, vision disturbance, and nausea, and they often display changes in personality and behavioral patterns.
- Physical examination is generally within normal limits. In addition to an abbreviated neurologic examination to rule out gross neurologic dysfunction (cranial nerve assessment and gross motor, sensory, and cerebellar testing), sideline neuropsychologic tests should be performed to screen for impairment in general orientation (person, place, time of day, and situation—game, game location, quarter, score, and opponent), short-and long-term memory/recall, and complex processing tasks

such as reciting the months of the year in reverse order. Athletes should always be assessed for the presence of antegrade (since the time of injury) or retrograde (prior to the injury) amnesia.

- Normal testing as above, absence of headache, and return to baseline neurocognitive and emotional states are the key features to the determination of suitability to return to play.

- Previously published concussion guidelines and grading systems (e.g., Cantu, Colorado Medical Society, American Academy of Neurology) have found a poor correlation between the degree of impairment in neuropsychologic testing and the anticipated time to return to play from a concussive injury. For example, loss of consciousness had previously dictated a lengthy period of disqualification. It is now generally accepted that *brief* loss of consciousness (<15 s), in the absence of other classic features of concussion, residual neurologic dysfunction as outlined above, or cervical spine injury does not necessarily preclude return to play even in the same contest. Any athlete suffering a longer period of loss of consciousness should be held from participation and considered for urgent neurosurgical evaluation.

- Emphasis is now being placed on the description of the concussion's characteristics (presence and duration of antegrade or retrograde amnesia, headache, vomiting, vision change, persisting confusion or disorientation, sleep disturbance) as opposed to a specific grade, which had previously dictated a rigid course of management. Concussions are sufficiently heterogeneous that they require flexibility in their diagnosis and management, particularly with respect to return to competitive athletics.

COMPLICATIONS

- The most feared complication of concussion is the "second impact syndrome," a potentially fatal cascade of cerebral hemorrhage and edema resulting from a second concussive blow following incomplete resolution of a first concussive event. Although exceedingly rare, the chance of second impact syndrome should absolutely dictate disqualification until the concussed athlete has completely recovered from their initial injury.

- Neuropsychologic testing has demonstrated the presence of lower cognitive function in collegiate football players with a history of multiple concussions (Collins et al, 1999). Similarly, it is well shown that prior NFL football players have a higher rate of cognitive dysfunction than the general population. In addition, several notable players retired from the NFL as a result of increasing severity and frequency of concussion and a concern about long-term cognitive loss.

- Studies have linked the presence of *apolipoprotein E* (apoE4) genotype and risk for cognitive impairment with head injury. Older professional football players who possessed the apoE4 allele scored lower on cognitive tests than did players without this allele or less experienced players of any genotype (Kutner et al, 2000). The resultant cognitive status of such athletes with repeated head trauma appears to be influenced by this genetic predisposition as well as age and cumulative exposure to contact. Although its utilization as a screening tool is still under study, apoE4 and similar genetic markers may become a practical means of determining an athlete's relative risk for permanent neurocognitive loss in association with head injury in sport.

HEADACHE

- Football-related headache is common with 85% of sampled high school and college football players reporting headache as a result of hitting (Sallis and Jones, 2000). Twenty-one percent reported headache in their previous game; only 19% of those individuals reported the headache to the sports medicine team and only 6% were removed from play.

- Defensive backs (25%), defensive linemen (19%), and offensive linemen (18%) were most likely to have headache related to hitting. Given the high rate of headache and the low rate of serious complications (cerebral hemorrhage, second impact syndrome), the presence of headache, unless persistent or accompanied by other symptoms, does not mandate disqualification from competition.

HEAT ILLNESS

- Heat-related illness in football is common as a result of practice and play in warm weather months and extensive body coverage with heavy padding and helmets, which intrinsically impair heat dissipation.

- Heat illness may manifest as a broad spectrum of conditions including heat cramps, heat syncope, heat exhaustion, and potentially lethal heat stroke.

- Heat cramps, syncope, and exhaustion are characterized by heat-associated physiologic changes that do not result in significant elevations in core body temperature or in central nervous system dysfunction. Heat cramps and syncope may be treated safely with aggressive oral hydration, external cooling measures, electrolyte supplementation, and rest.

- Heat exhaustion is heralded by complaints of dizziness, headache, nausea and vomiting, and generalized weakness and malaise. Core body temperature (measured rectally) is below 104°F, and athletes generally continue to sweat to dissipate heat. Management includes removal from participation, removal of helmet and padding, external cooling measures (cool water immersion, fanning), and *intravenous* (IV) fluids. Resolution of associated symptoms, normal hydration status, and restoration of baseline body weight are necessary prior to resumption of physical activity.

- Heat stroke is defined as core body temperature in excess of 104°F coupled with central nervous system dysfunction characterized by disorientation, confusion, personality change, and even coma. Although the pathophysiology of classic heat stroke includes absence of sweating, athletes with exertional heat stroke may sweat profusely, an important fact to be remembered by care providers.
- Heat stroke is a medical emergency requiring immediate cooling measures such as ice bath immersion and immediate activation of the emergency medical system for rapid transport to a hospital setting where additional aggressive cooling measures may be employed. Consequences of heat stroke may include irreversible brain damage, renal failure, rhabdomyolysis, and death.
- Stimulant supplements such as ephedra and *ma huang* have been implicated in precipitating heat stroke and death in highly competitive athletes. Their detrimental effects are the result of sympathomimetic activity and resultant vasoconstriction during activities which require vasodilation for appropriate heat management.
- *Football players must have free access to water.* Sixteen to twenty ounces of fluid should be consumed 20–30 min prior to activity, and access to water should be ensured throughout the sporting activity. Thirst is a poor measure of hydration status, so athletes must consume fluids regularly during activity regardless of their sense of need to drink. Diet can be utilized to ensure adequate salt and electrolyte replacement, which will aid in overall water balance. Daily weights should be monitored to screen for subclinical dehydration, and participation should be precluded for athletes who are greater than 1–2% below their preexercise baseline weight. Appropriate guidelines for practice duration and attire should be based on *wet bulb globe temperature* (WBGT), which accounts for the heating effects of temperature, humidity, and intensity of sunlight exposure.

SUDDEN CARDIAC DEATH

- Sudden cardiac death in football players is a rare but devastating occurrence. The primary causes of nontraumatic death in athletes include hypertrophic cardiomyopathy, malignant cardiac arrhythmias, heat stroke, asthma, and complications of sickle cell anemia. Screening measures should focus on the identification of such potential conditions or a familial predisposition to them, accepting that such screening methods at present are limited in their yield.

CREATINE

- Creatine is a natural product of muscle metabolism. Its use as a supplement for aiding muscle mass and power development has become widespread, particularly in football athletes. At present, it is generally considered to be safe.
- Studies in collegiate football players have shown that low and high dose creatine supplementation results in significant positive changes in strength, body weight, body composition, lean body mass, and anaerobic muscle endurance and power versus placebo (Wilder et al, 2002; Bemben et al, 2001). There were no differences between the high and low dose creatine groups.
- Creatine use at the high school level is widespread, estimated at up to 50% in the athlete population (McGuine, Sullivan, and Bernhardt, 2001). Use was highest in smaller schools and at higher grade levels. Enhanced recovery following a workout was the most common reason cited for use.

REFERENCES

Bemben MG, Bemben DA, Loftiss DD, et al: Creatine supplementation during resistance training in college football athletes. *Med Sci Sports Exerc* 33(10):1667–1673, 2001.

Cantu RC: Stingers, transient quadraplegia, and cervical spinal stenosis: Return to play criteria. *Med Sci Sports Exerc* 29 (7, Supplement):233–235, 1997.

Cantu, RC: Cervical spinal injuries in the athlete. *Semin Neurol* 20(2):173–178, 2000.

Castro FP, Ricciardi J, Brunet ME, et al: Stingers, the Torg ratio, and the cervical spine. *Am J Sports Med* 25(5):603–608, 1997.

Collins MW, Grindel SH, Lovell MR, et al: Relationship between concussion and neuropsychological performance in college football players. [comment] *JAMA* 282(10):964–970, 1999.

Davidson RM, Burton JH, Snowise M et al: Football protective gear and cervical spine imaging. [comment] *Ann Emerg Med* 38(1):26–30, 2001.

Delaney JS, Lacroix VJ, Leclerc S, et al: Concussions among university football and soccer players. *Clin J Sport Med* 12(6):331–338, 2002.

Gatt CJ, Jr, Hosea TM, Palumbo RC, et al: Impact loading of the lumbar spine during football blocking. *Am J Sports Med* 25(3):317–321, 1997.

Guskiewicz KM, Weaver NL, Padua DA et al: Epidemiology of concussion in collegiate and high school football players. *Am J Sports Med* 28(5):643–650, 2000.

Kutner KC, Erlanger DM, Tsai J et al: Lower cognitive performance of older football players possessing apolipoprotein E epsilon4. *Neurosurgery* 47(3):651–657, discussion 657–658, 2000.

McGuine TA, Sullivan JC, Bernhardt DT: Creatine supplementation in high school football players. *Clin J Sport Med* 11(4):247–253, 2001.

Pagnani MJ, Dome DC: Surgical treatment of traumatic anterior shoulder instability in american football players. *J Bone Joint Surg Am* 84–A(5):711–715, 2002.

Pavlov H, Torg JS, Robie B et al: Cervical spinal stenosis: Determination with vertebral body ratio method. *Radiology* 164(3):771–775, 1987.

Sallis RE, Jones K: Prevalence of headaches in football players. *Med Sci Sports Exerc* 32(11):1820–1824, 2000.

Shaffer B, Wiesel S, Lauerman W: Spondylolisthesis in the elite football player: An epidemiologic study in the NCAA and NFL. *J Spinal Disord* 10(5):365–370, 1997.

Torg JS, Ramsey-Emrhein JA: Suggested management guidelines for participation in collision activities with congenital, developmental, or postinjury lesions involving the cervical spine. *Med Sci Sports Exerc* 29(7, Supplement):256–272, 1997.

Torg JS, Vegso JJ, O'Neill MJ, et al: The epidemiologic, pathologic, biomechanical, and cinematographic analysis of football-induced cervical spine trauma. *Am J Sports Med* 18(1):50–57, 1990.

Torg JS, Sennett B, Pavlov H, et al: Spear tackler's spine. An entity precluding participation in tackle football and collision activities that expose the cervical spine to axial energy inputs. *Am J Sports Med* 21(5):640–649, 1993.

Torg JS, Corcoran TA, Thibault LE, et al: Cervical cord neurapraxia: Classification, pathomechanics, morbidity, and management guidelines. [comment] *J Neurosurg* 87(6):843–850, 1997.

Wilder N, Gilders R, Hagerman F, et al: The effects of a 10-week, periodized, off-season resistance-training program and creatine supplementation among collegiate football players. *J Strength Cond Res* 16(3):343–352, 2002.

84 GOLFING INJURIES

Gregory G Dammann, MD
Jeffrey A Levy, DO

BACKGROUND

- Golf likely was invented in twelfth century in Northern Europe (Mellion, Walsh, and Shelton, 1997).
- First golf course was built in the United States in 1888 (Fu and Stone, 2001). It has significantly grown in popularity during the 1990s with greater than 14,000 golf courses in the United States in 1994 (Metz, 1999).
- The National Sporting Goods Association estimates 18–20 million Americans play golf at least two times per year.

- As a sport, golf is classified as a noncontact, low intensity sport. Only moderate cardiovascular fitness is required.
- Most injuries result from the golf swing, the equipment, or objects, excluding the ball, on the course.

THE GOLF SWING

- The swing comprised of multiple coordinated movements of different parts of the body: the hands, wrists, arms, trunk, and legs.
- There are four phases:
  1. Backswing: Rotation of the trunk, raising the arms, and cocking the wrists while drawing the club head away from the ball. This is often called *coiling*.
  2. Downswing: Movement of the club head toward the ball using the shoulders and uncocking of the wrists. Often called *uncoiling*.
  3. Acceleration and ball strike: The arms and trunk continue to rotate back toward the ball and the wrists are uncocked. The leading wrist also supinates while the trailing wrist pronates. This is the fastest portion of the swing.
  4. Follow through: Momentum of the swing continues with rotation of the shoulders and trunk while raising the arms.

EPIDEMIOLOGY

- The number one site of injury for amateur golfers is the lumbar spine while it is number two for professionals (McCarrol, Rettig, and Shelbourne, 1990; McCarrol and Gioe, 1982). The number one for professionals is the hand/wrist region (McCarrol and Gioe, 1982).
- Twenty-five percent of amateurs are injured due to overuse, 21% from hitting the ground with the club during the swing and 19% are from poor swing mechanics (McCarrol, Rettig, and Shelbourne, 1990).
- Eighty percent of professional injuries occurred secondary to overuse, 12% are from hitting the ground during the swing, and 5% are from twisting the trunk (excessive torque) during the swing (McCarrol and Gioe, 1982).

LOWER BACK INJURIES

- The lumbar spine rotates, sidebends, compresses, flexes, and hyperextends during the golf swings. These movements result in lateral bending, shear, compression, and torsional forces. These forces, especially the shear force, are significantly higher in the amateur versus the professional golfer (Fu and Stonem, 2001).

- The amateur golfer typically has a more varied stance and leans away from the ball at impact and follow through. This results in the "reverse C" position of the lumbar spine at the end of the follow through and increases the torque on the vertebrae (Fu and Stonem, 2001). The professional's swing is smooth and refined from repetition, which results in coordinated muscle firing throughout and an upright stance at the end of follow through (Metz, 1999).

- These increased forces put many golfers at risk for muscle strains, *herniated nucleus pulposus* (HNP), facet arthopathies, and spondylosis/spondylolisthesis.
  1. The lumbosacral strains typically occur during activity and are relieved with rest. There is tenderness over the affected soft tissue area and no radiologic abnormalities.
  2. The HNP and sciatica are almost always associated together. Ninety-five percent of all HNPs occur at L4–L5 or L5–S1 and these nerve roots provide sensory and motor functions to the lower extremity (Fu and Stonem, 2001).
  3. Facet arthropathies and spinal stensois are related as a dysfunction that develops at the posterior facet joints producing a narrowing of the spinal foramen. The pain is often increased with extension and sidebending to the affected side.
  4. Spondylosis (disruption of neural arch) and a resulting spondylolisthesis (anterior displacement of one vertebral body on another) occur from the significant torque produced during the coiling and uncoiling of the lumbar spine. This torque causes fractures at the pars interarticularis, which allows the vertebral body to slide either anteriorly or posteriorly. This displacement can cause impingement of the spinal nerve roots or cord.

- Most injuries can be managed conservatively as greater than 90% recover in 4 weeks after injury (Fu and Stonem, 2001); however, some "red flags" should alert the clinician of underlying pathology: back pain in a patient over 50- or less than 20-year old; a history of cancer; constitutional symptoms of fever, night sweats, weight loss, and the like; bowel and/or bladder dysfunction; and saddle anesthesia. If any of these are positive, a more complete work up with imaging studies would be indicated. If no red flags are present, the patient should be encouraged to perform activities that their pain tolerance allows (active rest), use acetominophen and *nonsteroidal anti-inflammatory drugs* (NSAIDs) as required, perform flexion, and extension strengthening exercises with or without physical therapy and have their golf swing mechanics reviewed on return to play.

SHOULDER INJURIES

- Overuse injuries predominate shoulder injuries in golf (Jobe and Pink, 1996). The leading, nondominant shoulder is typically affected due to its range of motion during the swing. The shoulder goes through internal rotation, adduction, abduction, and then external rotation.

- The acromioclavicular joint or region is the most often injured area followed by impingement and rotator cuff tendinitis, posterior glenohumeral subluxation, rotator cuff tears and glenohumeral arthritis (Mallon and Colosimo, 1995).

- History of the timing of the pain during the swing helps with diagnosis. Anterior leading shoulder pain during the back swing is often a sign of impingement or *acromioclavicular* (AC) joint arthritis.

- Treatment of the degenerative AC joint includes shortening the backswing and weight training with a focus on the rotator cuff muscles. Reviewing the swing mechanics will also be beneficial.

ELBOW INJURIES

- The most common upper extremity injury in the male and female amateur golfer (McCarrol, Rettig, and Shelbourne, 1990). Most elbow injuries occur at impact secondary to the requirement of significant counteracting forearm muscle force to maintain control of the clubface.

- The two most common elbow injuries are medial and lateral epicondylitis. These are most frequently associated with overuse and excessive grip strength (McCarrol, 2001).
  1. Medial Epicondylitis (golfer's elbow)
     a. Overuse injury of medial aspect of elbow involving epicondyle of the humerus, wrist and finger flexor muscles, and pronator muscles.
     b. Right medial epicondylitis in a right handed golfer results from extension of right elbow during impact phase of swing, while right wrist remains dorsiflexed.
  2. Lateral epicondylitis
     a. Overuse injury involving lateral epicondyle of humerus, wrist and finger extensor muscles, and supinator muscles.
     b. Left lateral epicondylitis in a right handed golfer results from forceful contraction of left elbow extensors during impact phase of swing (Metz, 1999).
  3. Three common therapies for these elbow injuries are counterforce bracing, equipment modification, and physical therapy.

a. Counterforce bracing can help provide a reactive force against the contractile muscle and either spread the force over a wider area or decrease the contractile pull on the epicondyle (McCarrol, 2001).

b. Equipment changes such as graphite shafts can help to decrease the force applied to the forearm by decreasing the amount of vibration at impact.

c. Physical therapy can focus on forearm muscle strength, flexibility, and endurance (McCarrol, 2001).

HAND AND WRIST INJURIES

- Tendonopathies are the most common problems seen in the golfer's wrist and are typically secondary to the repetitive movements generated during the golf swing and stress at impact.
- The lead wrist is injured more frequently than the trail wrist because of increased stress with more forceful contact with the ground at impact (McCarrol, Rettig, and Shelbourne, 1990).
- DeQuervain's tenosynovitis involving the first dorsal compartment is a common condition affecting golfers. This results from repeated impact between the club and the ground. The ulnar deviation of the leading wrist at ball impact may stress the tendons in the first dorsal compartment. Poor swing mechanics in which a golfer may prematurely uncock the wrist at the beginning of the downswing rather than during acceleration and ball striking may result in ulnar deviation of the lead wrist too early in the swing. This premature ulnar deviation of the lead wrist can trap the leading thumb between the trailing hand and shaft, which will stress the tendons in the first dorsal compartment (McCarrol, 2001).
- Other tendon groups that may be injured by improper swing mechanics are the extensor carpi ulnaris of the leading arm and flexor carpi radialis and ulnaris of the trailing arm. Hitting a fat shot, which means that the club head strikes the ground too far behind the ball, specifically impacts these tendon groups.
- A traumatic cause of hand and wrist pain in a golfer is a fracture of the hook of the hamate.
  1. They account for 2% of all wrist fractures but 33% of hamate fractures are found in golfers (McCarrol, 2001).
  2. They are the most common fracture in golf.
  3. These occur with the club head striking a rock, tree stump, or too much turf. The butt of the club then impacts into the hypothenar eminence of the lead hand.

4. Carpal tunnel view is the best X-ray view to visualize this fracture. If it is not visible on plain film, then *computed tomography* (CT) scan is the image of choice (Metz, 1999).

- Preventive measures include proper club length with the butt of the club extending slightly beyond the palm of the leading hand rather than dig into the hypothenar eminence.

HIP INJURIES

- The most common hip problem seen in golfers is trochanteric bursitis, which is an inflammatory condition of the bursa overlying the greater trochanter and is usually caused by rotation of the hip during practice, overuse in the frequent golfer, and combined with walking on uneven terrain.
- Treatment involves rest, physical therapy, anti-inflammatory medications, and possibly injection.

KNEE INJURIES

- Knee injuries are not frequently seen in golf; however, when they do occur, they are the result of a valgus stress placed on the trail leg during downward swing and acceleration. The valgus stress combined with knee flexion and rotation can be a cause for meniscal pathology.
- Other knee injuries, such as strains, can be caused by a combination of environmental factors, such as hilly terrain and wet grass causing a player to slip while walking.

SKIN DISORDERS

- Skin cancer is more likely to occur in individuals with fair skin, who sunburn easily and who have increased exposure to *ultraviolet* (UV) light. Golfers spend the majority of their time in sunny locations and often play in the middle of the day when the UV light is most damaging to the skin. Prevention recommendations are that golfers protect their exposed skin with sunscreens and clothing that block these harmful rays.

PSYCHOLOGIC DISORDERS

- The *yips* are an involuntary motor disturbance that affects some golfers. This disorder is described as jerking or spasm of the arms that primarily occurs during putting. It is believed that performance anxiety contributes to the cause of this disorder. No medications have been proven to be of benefit.

REFERENCES

Fu FH, Stone DA: *Sports Injuries*, 2nd ed. Philadelphia, PA, Lippincott Williams & Wilkins, 2001.

Jobe FW, Pink MM: Shoulder pain in golf. *The Clinics of Sports Medicine* 15(1):55–63, 1996.

Mallon WJ, Colosimo AJ: Acromioclavicular joint injury in competitive golfers. *J South Orthop Assoc* 4(4):277–282, 1995.

McCarrol JR: Overuse injuries of the upper extremity in Golf. *Clin Sports Med* 20(3), 2001.

McCarrol JR, Gioe TJ: Professional golfers and the price they pay. *Phys Sports Med* 10(7):64–70, 1982.

McCarrol JR, Rettig AC, Shelbourne KD: Injuries in the amateur golfer. *Phys Sports Med* 18(3):122–126, 1990.

Mellion MB, Walsh WM, Shelton GL: *The Team Physician's Handbook*, 2nd ed. Baltimore, MD, Mosby, 1996.

Metz JP: Managing Golf Injuries. *Phys Sports Med* 27(7), 1999; Philadelphia, PA, Hanley & Belfus, 1997.

85 GYMNASTICS

John P DiFiori, MD
Julie Casper, MD

INTRODUCTION

- Gymnastics is an extremely popular sport in the United States and worldwide. There are an estimated 85,000 competitive gymnasts and an additional three million recreational gymnasts in the United States (USA Gymnastics Online, 2003). Over 1400 participate in National Collegiate Athletic Association (NCAA) gymnastics each year (NCAA Online, 2003).
- Children begin gymnastics training at a very young age. The average age at onset is 5–6 years for girls and 6–7 years for boys (McNitt-Gray, 2001). Most girls reach their highest competitive level by age sixteen (Nattiv and Mandelbaum, 1993).
- Physicians caring for gymnasts must be familiar with the requirements of the sport, common and unique injuries, and potential methods to prevent such injuries.

GYMNASTICS FACTS

- Women and men compete in different individual events. Most gymnasts train for all of the events. Gymnasts acquire new skills for each event via repetition of individual elements and series (groups of elements).
- The competitive levels in women's gymnastics are levels 1–10 and elite, with level 10 and elite being the most advanced. Collegiate gymnasts are typically the equivalent of level 9 or higher. Male gymnasts currently compete in classes 1–7; class 1 is the most advanced. There are also over 150 elite male gymnasts in the United States (USA Gymnastics Online, 2003).
- The *code of points* dictates the degree of difficulty for each skill. There is a specific list of requirements for each level of competition. The *code of points* evolves with the sport and is revised every 4 years, essentially increasing the required levels of difficulty with each revision. The training regimen for gymnastics is rigorous. An advanced or elite level gymnast practices an average of 25–35 h a week throughout the year. Even young, beginning level gymnasts may train 10 h per week or more.
- Special equipment used by gymnasts includes grips with or without wooden dowels for the bars, beam shoes, and wrist supports. Gymnasts may also train using crash mats, foam pits, beam and bar pads, low balance beams, and twisting or spotting belts.

EPIDEMIOLOGY OF INJURY

- Gymnastics has the highest incidence of injury among all women's intercollegiate sports (NCAA Online, 2003). It ranks among the top four men's and women's college sports in total injuries (NCAA, 1997).
- Studies have found that the rate of injury ranges from 5.3 (Pettrone and Ricciardelli, 1987) to 294 (Caine et al, 1989) per 100 participant seasons. This difference has been attributed to variations in the definition of injury, competitive level of subjects, and training hours. The incidence of injury is 0.5 (Lindner and Caine, 1990) to 3.7 (Caine et al, 1989) per 1000 h of exposure. One study found that collegiate gymnasts experienced a new injury in 9% of all exposures (Sands, Shultz, and Newman, 1993).

MECHANISMS OF INJURY

- Both acute and overuse injuries are common in gymnastics. The most common mechanism of acute injury is a missed move, followed by falls from an apparatus and dismounts (Lindner and Caine, 1990). The many hours of training throughout multiple years predispose gymnasts to overuse injuries.

- Injuries increase with the degree of difficulty of gymnastics maneuvers (Pettrone and Ricciardelli, 1987; Caine et al, 1989). Over the time the difficulty of gymnastics skills has continued to increase as equipment and athleticism improve (McAuley, Hudash, and Shields, 1987).
- The equipment itself may predispose to injury due to falls onto the apparatus. In addition, the bar and vault height, springboard placement, and location of mats or spotters are specific for each gymnast. Any unanticipated alteration in these preparations can lead to injury.

INJURY CHARACTERISTICS

- The most common injuries in gymnastics are strains and sprains (Caine et al, 2003).
- Severity of injury has been assessed by calculating the duration of restricted training. While most injuries are minor, resulting in less than a week away from training, 12.5% (Caine et al, 2003) to 25.9% (Caine et al, 1989) result in a time loss of greater than 3 weeks. One study found that the average time until full participation resumed was almost 4.5 weeks per injury (Lindner and Caine, 1990).
- Many gymnasts continue training with pain. Studies have found that as many as 71% of female gymnasts train with an injury (Sands, Shultz, and Newman, 1993). Gymnastics may be unique in that the injured gymnast can alter his or her workout depending on the injury, for example a gymnast with an ankle injury can continue full training on the uneven bars, provided they avoid the dismount.

RISK FACTORS FOR INJURY

- **Level of competition:** Many studies have found that gymnasts at advanced or elite levels suffer more injuries (Caine et al, 1989; Lindner and Caine, 1990; McAuley, Hudash, and Shields, 1987; Caine et al, 2003). This is felt to be due to an increased number of training hours, increased skill difficulty, and less supervision (Caine et al, 1989; 2003). The high prevalence of chronic injuries in this group has been associated with more time spent in the gym (Pettrone and Ricciardelli, 1987).
- **Event:** Multiple studies cite the floor exercise as the most common event for injuries (Pettrone and Ricciardelli, 1987; McAuley, Hudash, and Shields, 1987; Garrick and Requa, 1978). Up to 40% of acute injuries occur during this event (Lindner and Caine, 1990). The fewest injuries occur with the vault. Twisting dismounts and landings are common mechanisms of injury (Pettrone and Ricciardelli, 1987; Caine et al, 1989; Lindner and Caine, 1990).
- **Competition:** Although most injuries occur while training, the incidence when calculated per exposure is higher for competition (Garrick and Requa, 1978). This is especially true among advanced level gymnasts (Caine et al, 2003). The timed warm-up period before a competition seems to be an especially high-risk time for injuries (Caine et al, 2003), perhaps because the gymnasts are in a stressful and hurried situation.
- **Physical characteristics:** Greater body size and body fat percentage have been correlated with higher risk of injury (Caine, 2003b; Steele and White, 1986); however, these studies did not control for such variables as training hours and age (Caine, 2003b).
- **Anatomic location:** Most gymnastics injuries are to the lower extremity (Caine et al, 1989; Dixon and Fricker, 1993).
- **Gender:** Male gymnasts have a higher percentage of upper extremity injuries, while females have relatively lower extremity injuries (Dixon and Fricker, 1993). This variation is likely the result of differences in the events: most men's events such as the parallel bars, high bar, rings, and pommel horse primarily require use of the upper extremities.
- **Age:** Risk of injury may be greater during the adolescent growth spurt (Caine et al, 1989). The rapid change in height alters the moment of inertia for certain skills, requiring gymnasts to make gradual changes in technique. Growth-related changes affecting the articular cartilage and physes may also contribute.
- **Prior injury:** The reinjury rate in gymnastics is high: 32.7% in one year (Caine et al, 1989). As many as one in four injuries is a reinjury (Caine, 2003b). Overuse injuries are especially prone to reinjury, and the lower back is the most common site of recurrent injury (Caine et al, 1989). The high rates of reinjury in gymnasts are felt to be due to premature return to training and inadequate rehabilitation (Caine et al, 1989).

COMMON INJURIES IN GYMNASTICS

- Studies have found that the most common anatomic sites for injury in gymnastics are the ankle, low back, knee, foot, wrist, and elbow (Caine et al, 1989; Lindner and Caine, 1990; Caine et al, 2003; Garrick and Requa, 1978; Caine, 2003*b*; Dixon and Fricker, 1993). The majority of studies have been performed with female gymnasts. The most common injuries will be discussed below.

- **Ankle ligament sprains:** Typically caused by inversion injuries, ankle ligament sprains are the most common acute injuries in gymnastics (Caine et al, 1989; Lindner and Caine, 1990; Dixon and Fricker, 1993). They are usually the result of an incorrect landing or fall. One study found an alarming number of ankle injuries from gymnasts landing with their foot inside a crack in the floor or between mats (Mackie and Taunton, 1994). Evaluation and treatment of gymnasts' ankle injuries are similar to that in other athletes (see Chap. 63).

  1. Gymnasts should initially return to sport with the use of an ankle brace or tape for support. Many gymnasts do not tolerate long-term use of ankle braces since the brace may cause slipping from the apparatus, and it alters their form and appearance. Flesh-colored tape is typically the best-tolerated intervention. There is little information on the use of prophylactic bracing and taping in gymnasts.

- **Low back pain:** Low back pain caused by lumbar strain and sprain injuries is common in gymnasts. It should be managed as with other athletes (see Chap. 42). Repetitive hyperextension, a necessity in gymnastics, predisposes these athletes to chronic injuries of the low back. Strengthening and core stability are especially important in gymnasts. Despite the large number of young gymnasts with back pain, a study comparing former elite gymnasts with age-matched controls concluded that fewer former gymnasts (27%) had subjective back problems than did the controls (38%) (Tsai and Wredmark, 1993).

- **Spondylolysis:** Spondylolysis (or stress fracture of the pars interarticularis) is common in young gymnasts, especially those between the ages of nine and thirteen. It occurs in gymnasts secondary to repetitive flexion and hyperextension of the back: backbends, walkovers, tumbling, and high-impact landings (Goldberg, 1980). The incidence of spondylolysis is higher in gymnasts (11%) than for the general population (5–6%) (Jackson, Wiltse, and Cirincoine, 1976; Fredrickson et al, 1984).

  1. Gymnasts with spondylolysis typically have uni-lateral back pain that localizes to the lumbar area. The pain increases with activity (especially hyperextension) and decreases with rest. Physical examination may find tenderness to palpation at the lower lumbar spine. A single-leg standing hyperextension test (stork test) is sensitive and specific for spondylolysis (Keene, 1983).

  2. Diagnostic testing begins with plain radiographs, which may show the classic pars interarticularis fracture on the oblique view: the "collared scottie dog." *Single photon emission computerized tomography* (SPECT) bone scans are highly sensitive for diagnosing spondylolysis and should be performed to confirm the diagnosis of an active lesion (Moeller and Rifat, 2001). Thin-sliced *computed tomography* (CT) is more specific than bone scan and can also be used to confirm the diagnosis. *Magnetic resonance imaging* (MRI) with thin slices has been reported to be effective in visualizing the pars interarticularis (Udeshi and Reeves, 2000), but more information is needed before the diagnostic role of MRI can be established.

  3. Treatment involves modification of activity (no running, jumping, or gymnastics activities that cause pain) for at least 4 to 6 weeks (Moeller and Rifat, 2001). Physical therapy should target spine stabilization, abdominal muscle strengthening, and hamstring flexibility. The use of bracing is controversial. Some reserve the use of a brace for those patients with no improvement or worsening symptoms during initial therapy. Others may implement bracing if a bone scan demonstrates an active lesion. Decisions regarding bracing should be made on an individual basis (Moeller and Rifat, 2001).

  4. Return to sport depends on progress with activity modification and physical therapy. Many gymnasts can return to a low level of participation after 4 to 6 weeks (Moeller and Rifat, 2001). Activity is then advanced as tolerated. Maintenance exercises should be continued for the remainder of the gymnast's career.

- **Traumatic knee injuries:** Can be severe and disabling (McAuley, Hudash, and Shields, 1987). The typical mechanism is a landing or fall while the gymnast is still completing a twisting rotation. *Anterior cruciate ligament* (ACL), *medial collateral ligament* (MCL), and meniscal injuries are the most common. As a result of the nature of the sport, most gymnasts require surgical reconstruction of an ACL tear in order to continue gymnastics. In young athletes, this procedure is typically delayed until after physeal closure. Gymnasts do not tolerate large knee braces because bulky braces impair the gymnasts' form and appearance. See chapters 57 and 58 for further description of the evaluation and treatment of acute knee injuries.

- **Overuse injuries of the knee:** These injuries result from the repetitive running, jumping, and landing required in gymnastics. Common diagnoses include Osgood-Schlatter disease, patellofemoral disorders, and patellar tendonopathy. Treatment involves relative rest and physical therapy, including strengthening exercises (see Chap. 60 and 61).

- **Sever's disease (calcaneal apophysitis):** This was the most common overuse injury in one survey (Mackie and Taunton, 1994). It occurs in young athletes, typically ages 7–14. The main finding on examination is tenderness at the insertion of the Achilles tendon onto the calcaneus. Sever's disease is a self-limited condition, which resolves when the physis closes. Treatment includes relative rest, ice, heel lifts used on a short-term basis, stretching, and strengthening exercises.
- **Dorsal wrist pain:** Chronic wrist pain affects 46–87% of young gymnasts (DiFiori, Puffer, and Mandelbaum, 1996). Painful dorsiflexion while supporting body weight and dorsal wrist pain, without acute trauma or swelling, characterize gymnast's wrist (McAuley, Hudash, and Shields, 1987). Factors associated with wrist pain include training hours, skill level, and age at initiation of training. It appears to be more common during the adolescent growth spurt. Dorsal wrist pain is associated with radiographic findings of distal radial physeal injury (DiFiori et al, 2002). Cases of premature closure of the distal radial physis have been reported (Albanese et al, 1989).
  1. The mainstay of treatment is reduction of loading to the wrist. Strengthening of the wrist and upper extremity may be helpful. Use of a brace with a hyperextension block may decrease symptoms (Ott, 2002). Premature closure of the distal radial growth plate can result in symptomatic positive ulnar variance (Caine, 2003a). In some skeletally mature gymnasts, an ulnar shortening procedure is required to treat this condition.
- **Elbow dislocations:** Elbow dislocations in gymnasts are typically the result of a *fall on out-stretched hand* (FOOSH) injury (Ott, 2002). As a result, gymnasts are taught never to reach down with their hands when they fall. Elbow joint dislocations require a thorough neurovascular examination, X-rays, and in most cases closed reduction (see Chap. 48).

INJURIES UNIQUE TO GYMNASTICS

- **Clavicular stress fractures:** Clavicular stress fractures are rare but have been described in gymnasts, presumably because of the repetitive forces to which the upper extremity is exposed in activities such as tumbling and vaulting. The injury can be diagnosed with plain radiographs or computed tomography, but an MRI should be done to rule out pathologic causes of the fracture, such as a tumor or cyst. Treatment is conservative. In one report, full training was resumed after eight weeks of upper extremity rest (Fallon and Fricker, 2001).

- **Osteochondritis dissecans of the capitellum:** This is believed to be underrecognized in gymnasts (Ott, 2002). It occurs in young gymnasts with open growth plates, typically ages 10–15, from repeated valgus stress to the elbow. Symptoms include the gradual onset of lateral elbow pain that worsens with activity, inability to fully extend the elbow, and possibly locking or clicking. Management depends on the severity of symptoms and imaging results (see Chap. 49).
- **Forearm fracture:** *Griplock* is an entity unique to gymnastics. Gymnasts wear leather handgrips for bar and ring work. With griplock, the grip accidentally catches on the bar, and while the athlete's momentum carries him or her around the bar, the hand and forearm are kept in a locked position. The result is a serious forearm fracture that may require surgery (Samuelson, Reider, and Weiss, 1996). Griplock is more common in male gymnasts, who use a bar with a smaller circumference, and in gymnasts whose grips are overused and stretched out.
- **Hand blisters/Rips:** Gymnasts frequently train with blisters or *rips* on their hands caused by the friction created between skin and bars. These are difficult to treat and prevent, since usual treatments such as tape or moleskin will not adhere to the hands while practicing. The friction of the bars will usually cause the blister to pop as soon as it arises. These areas should be kept clean to avoid infection. Once an open lesion has dried, the application of a topical antibiotic ointment can be used at night in order to prevent both infection and painful cracking of the lesion.
- **Abdominal wall contusion:** Female gymnasts may develop severe bruising around the lower abdomen and anterior superior iliac spine by doing a beat maneuver on the uneven bars. Gymnasts at the lower competitive levels typically perform this skill, which involves hanging from the high bar and dropping the anterior pelvis and hips onto the low bar. Use of padding may prevent repetitive injury (Weber, 1997). Although painful, the prognosis of this injury is good. Only ice and avoidance are generally required for treatment.
- **Vulvar hematomas:** Vulvar hematomas result from a straddle injury on the balance beam. On most occasions, these falls do not result in significant injury. When a vulvar hematoma develops, incision and drainage can be performed if the hematoma is very large or is expanding (Propst and Thorp, 1998). In minor cases, ice and relative rest are recommended.
- **Heel pad contusions:** Heel pad contusions develop after trauma to the fat pad, usually from a hard landing onto the beam or unpadded floor. If symptoms continue to worsen, radiographs and/or *magnetic resonance imaging* (MRI) should be performed to rule

out a calcaneal stress fracture. Management of heel pad contusions is conservative: ice, rest, anti-inflammatory medications, and a heel cup or donut pad.

OTHER GYMNASTICS-RELATED CONCERNS

CATASTROPHIC INJURY

• Although catastrophic head and neck injuries still occur, the overall number of gymnastics injuries resulting in paralysis or death appears to have declined. In 1976, the trampoline was discontinued as a gymnastics event due to the high number of associated cranial and spinal cord injuries. As a result, the number of head, neck, and spine injuries decreased (Garrick and Requa, 1978).

FEMALE ATHLETE TRIAD

• Although the exact prevalence is unknown, gymnasts are at risk for the female athlete triad of disordered eating, amenorrhea, and osteoporosis (Ott, 2002).
• Eating disorders, ranging from anorexia nervosa and bulimia to less severe forms of disordered eating, are felt to be underdiagnosed.
• The focus on body image may begin at an early age: Girls involved in aesthetic sports such as gymnastics reported higher weight concerns at ages 5–7 than control groups (Davison, Earnest, and Birch, 2002).
• When compared with age-matched controls, gymnasts have a later onset of menarche (Lindholm, Hagenfeldt, and Ringertz, 1994). Menstrual dysfunction occurs more commonly in athletes (3.4–66%) than in the general population (2–5%) (ACSM, 1993); the specific prevalence in gymnasts is unknown. The etiology of menstrual dysfunction in athletes is currently felt to be related to inadequate caloric intake relative to energy expenditure, termed "negative energy balance" (Loucks, Verdum, and Heath, 1998).
• Gymnasts typically have a higher bone mineral density than other athletes, despite the presence of disordered eating and menstrual dysfunction (Robinson et al, 1995). The repetitive impact-loading characteristic of gymnastics training appears to have a salutary effect on bone mineral density, and it seems to offset any negative effects of disordered eating and/or menstrual dysfunction (Robinson et al, 1995).
• Treatment of each component of the female athlete triad involves a multidisciplinary approach: physicians, nutritionists, and psychologists should be involved. Coaches, trainers, parents, and athletes need to be educated regarding the symptoms, signs, and potentially devastating effects of the triad.

PSYCHOLOGIC CONCERNS

• Psychologic stress has been related to increased rates of injury. In one study, injured gymnasts had higher scores for anxiety than healthy gymnasts (Tofler et al, 1996).
• Advanced gymnastics training involves many hours and years of commitment. A gymnast who has created a sense of self-worth primarily on the basis of successes in gymnastics may continue to train long after losing interest in the sport (Tofler et al, 1996). In such cases, gymnasts may create an injury (either imaginary or self-inflicted) in order to discontinue the sport without disappointing family, coaches, or themselves (Tofler et al, 1996).
• Research of gymnasts often finds high rates of nonparticipation (dropouts). Studies have found that from 16.3 to 52.4% of gymnasts may withdraw due to injury (Caine et al, 1989; 2003).

PREVENTION OF INJURY

• Protective equipment may decrease the incidence of injury and should be used when possible. This includes crash mats, pits, low beams, and foam beam and bar covers. Floor mats and pads should be checked often to ensure that there are no cracks that could lead to an ankle injury.
• Some changes aimed at injury prevention in gymnastics have already been made. A safer vault horse was instated at the senior levels in 2001 in order to decrease injuries. Trampoline was discontinued as a fifth event in 1976 as the result of a number of catastrophic injuries. Padded mats are now allowed on the floor exercise at college competitions. Certain high-risk skills, such as the Yurchenko (round-off entry) vault, are restricted to only the most advanced levels.
• As a result of the high rate of recurrent injury, gymnasts should not return to full training until rehabilitation is completed (Caine et al, 1989). Ideally, gymnasts should have a physical therapist or trainer available to guide the return to training. Primary rehabilitation, or prehab, may help to avoid common overuse injuries, such as those to the Achilles tendon or knee (Mackie and Taunton, 1994).
• Injury prevention is of special concern among gymnasts, since young, skeletally immature participants

may incur these injuries. This creates the potential for long-term sequelae. At the present time there is little data regarding the long-term impact of gymnastics injuries. One study evaluated former gymnasts, at an average of 38 months after completing their gymnastics careers, and found that 45% of all injuries were still symptomatic (Wadley and Albright, 1993).

REFERENCES

Albanese SA, Palmer AK, Kerr DR, et al: Wrist pain and distal growth plate closure of the radius in gymnasts. *J Pediatr Orthop* 9:23–28, 1989.

Caine D: Injury and growth, in Sands WA, Caine DJ, Borms J (eds.): *Scientific Aspects of Women's Gymnastics.* Basel, Karger; *Med Sci Sport* 45:46–71, 2003a.

Caine D: Injury Epidemiology, in Sands WA, Caine DJ, Borms J (eds.): *Scientific Aspects of Women's Gymnastics.* Basel, Karger; *Med Sci Sport* 45:72–109, 2003b.

Caine D, Cochrane B, Caine C, et al: An epidemiologic investigation of injuries affecting young competitive female gymnasts. *Am J Sports Med* 17:811–820, 1989.

Caine D, Knutzen K, Howe W, et al: A three-year epidemiological study of injuries affecting young female gymnasts. *Phys Ther Sport* 4:10–23, 2003.

Davison KK, Earnest MB, Birch LL: Participation in aesthetic sports and girls' weight concerns at ages 5 and 7 years. *Int J Eat Disord* 31:312–317, 2002.

DiFiori JP, Puffer JC, Mandelbaum BR et al: Factors associated with wrist pain in the young gymnast. *Am J Sports Med* 24:9–14, 1996.

DiFiori JP, Puffer JC, Aish B, et al: Wrist pain, distal radial physeal injury, and ulnar variance in young gymnasts: Does a relationship exist? *Am J Sports Med* 30:879–885, 2002.

Dixon M, Fricker P: Injuries to elite gymnasts over 10 yr. *Med Sci Sports Exerc* 25:1322–1329, 1993.

Fallon KE, Fricker PA: Stress fracture of the clavicle in a young female gymnast. *Br J Sports Med* 35:448–449, 2001.

Fredrickson BE, Baker D, McHolick WJ, et al: The natural history of spondylolysis and spondylolisthesis. *J Bone Joint Surg Am* 66:699–707, 1984.

Garrick JG, Requa RK: Girls sports injuries in high school athletics. *JAMA* 239:2245–2248, 1978.

Goldberg MJ: Gymnastic injuries. *Orthop Clin North Am* 11:717–726, 1980.

Jackson DW, Wiltse LL, Cirincoine RJ: Spondylolysis in the female gymnast. *Clin Orthop* 117:68–73, 1976.

Keene JS: Low back pain in the athlete: From spondylogenic injury during recreation or competition. *Postgrad Med* 74:209–217, 1983.

Lindholm C, Hagenfeldt K, Ringertz BM: Pubertal development in elite juvenile gymnasts-effects of physical training. *Acta Obtset Gynecol Scand* 73:269–273, 1994.

Lindner KJ, Caine JD: Injury patterns of female competitive club gymnasts. *Can J Sport Sci* 15:254–261, 1990.

Loucks AB, Verdum M, Heath EM: Low energy availability, not stress of exercise, alters LH pulsatility in exercising women. *J Appl Physiol* 84:37–46, 1998.

Mackie SJ, Taunton JE: Injuries in female gymnasts: trends suggest prevention tactics. *Phys Sport Med* 22:40–45, 1994.

McAuley E, Hudash G, Shields K: Injuries in women's gymnastics: The state of the art. *Am J Sports Med* 15:S124–S131, 1987.

McNitt-Gray JL: Gymnastics, in Garrett WE, Lester GE, McGowan J, et al (eds.): *Women's Health in Sports and Exercise.* Rosemont, IL, AAOS, 2001, pp 209–228.

Moeller JL, Rifat SF: Spondylolysis in active adolescents: expediting return to play. *Phys Sports Med* 29:27–32, 2001.

NCAA: NCAA injury surveillance system summary, in Benson M (ed.): *Sports Medicine Handbook,* 9th ed. Overland Park, KA, National Collegiate Athletic Association, 1997, pp 70–79.

Nattiv A, Mandelbaum BR: Injuries and special concerns in female gymnasts. *Phys Sport Med* 21:66–82, 1993.

NCAA Online: At URL: *http://www.ncaa.org/sports_science.* Accessed 5/14/03.

Ott SM: Gymnastics, in Ireland ML, Nattiv A (eds.): *The Female Athlete.* Philadelphia, PA, Saunders, 2002, p 669.

Pettrone FA, Ricciardelli E: Gymnastics injuries: The Virginia experience 1982–1983. *Am J Sports Med* 15:59–62, 1987.

Propst AM, Thorp JM Jr: Traumatic vulvar hematomas: Conservative versus surgical management. *South Med J* 91:144–146, 1998.

Robinson TL, Snow-Carter C, Taafe DR, et al: Gymnasts exhibit higher bone mass than runners despite similar prevalence of amenorrhea and oligomenorrhea. *J Bone Miner Res* 10:26–35, 1995.

Samuelson M, Reider B, Weiss D: Griplock injuries to the forearm in male gymnasts. *Am J Sports Med* 24:15–18, 1996.

Sands WA, Shultz BB, Newman AP: Women's gymnastics injuries: A 5-year study. *Am J Sports Med* 21:271–276, 1993.

Steele VA, White JA: Injury prediction in female gymnasts. *Br J Sports Med* 20:31–33, 1986.

ACSM: The female athlete triad: Disordered eating, amenorrhea, osteoporosis—call to action. *ACSM Sports Med Bull* 28:6, 1993.

Tofler JR, Stryer BK, Micheli LJ, et al: Physical and emotional problems of elite female gymnasts. *N Engl J Med* 335: 281–283, 1996.

Tsai L, Wredmark T: Spinal posture, sagittal mobility, and subjective rating of back problems in former elite gymnasts. *Spine* 18:872–875, 1993.

Udeshi UL, Reeves D: Routine thin slice MRI effectively demonstrates the lumbar pars interarticularis. *Clin Radiol* 55:984, 2000.

USA Gymnastics Online: At URL: *http://www.usa-gymnastics. org/statistics.* Accessed 3/19/03.

Wadley GH, Albright JP: Women's intercollegiate gymnastics. Injury patterns and "permanent" medical disability. *Am J Sports Med* 21:314–320, 1993.

Weber J: Gymnastics, in Mellion MB, Walsh WM, Shelton GL (eds.): *The Team Physician's Handbook,* 2nd ed. Philadelphia, PA, Hanley & Belfus, 1997, p 770.

86 ICE HOCKEY INJURIES

Peter H Seidenberg, MD
Tory Woodard, MD

INTRODUCTION

- Ice hockey is an extremely fast-paced, high-contact game that requires the mastery of many skills (*USA Hockey website*; *Official Rules of Ice Hockey*, 2001; Joyner and Snouse, 2002). Many of these skills (skating, stick handling, body checking, shooting, and goal tending) are unique to the sport (Sim et al, 1988).
- The sport dates back to 1850s, with formal rules first established in Canada in 1881 (*USA Hockey website*; Joyner and Snouse, 2002; Minkoff, Varoltta, and Simonson, 1994; Morgan, 1990).
- In the same time period, equipment specific for ice hockey was developed—hockey ice skates and sticks (*USA Hockey website*).
- It is a National Collegiate Athletic Association (NCAA), international and Olympic sport that made its debut in the Antwerp Olympic Games in 1920 (*USA Hockey website*).
- It is increasing in popularity yearly in the United States. During the 2001–2002 season, there were 525,373 registered players, coaches, and officials in USA Hockey (*USA Hockey website*).
  a. USA Hockey is the governing body for amateur hockey in the United States.
  b. Membership has grown over 176% in the past decade (*USA Hockey website*).
- Women are active participants in all roles in ice hockey.
  a. Females were involved in Canada as early as 1892 (Joyner and Snouse, 2002).
  b. In the 1920s and 1930s, women's leagues were formed in Canada and the United States (Joyner and Snouse, 2002).
  c. After World War II, there was decreased public interest in women's hockey (Joyner and Snouse, 2002).
  d. In the 1960s, women's leagues were restarted in Canada and the United States (Joyner and Snouse, 2002).
  e. The International Ice Hockey Federation coordinated women's world ice hockey tournaments in 1992, 1994, and 1997 (Joyner and Snouse, 2002).
  f. In the 1998 Olympic Games, women's ice hockey first appeared as a medal sport (Joyner and Snouse, 2002).
  g. Today, the NCAA considers female ice hockey an emerging sport (Joyner and Snouse, 2002).
  h. The USA Hockey registrants include 42,292 female players and 1,684 exclusive women's teams (*USA Hockey website*).
  i. Many women are playing on men's teams, even up to the minor league level.
- The physician providing medical care for ice hockey athletes needs to be proficient in treating a wide variety of traumatic and atraumatic problems that range in severity from mild to life-threatening.

EQUIPMENT

- All leagues now require helmets (*Official Rules of Ice Hockey*, 2001), which should fit snugly, and utilize a four-point fit (like football helmets) (Joyner and Snouse, 2002).
  a. The hockey helmet must be able to withstand low mass, high-velocity impacts from the puck and high mass, low-velocity forces from running into the boards (Arheim and Prentice, 1996).
- USA Hockey recommends the use of Hockey Equipment Certification Council (HECC) approved helmets, full face masks, and full mouthpieces for all players during both practices and games (*Official Rules of Ice Hockey*, 2001; Cross and Serenelli, 2003).
- The mouthpiece is to be internal and should cover all the remaining teeth of one jaw. It is required to be colored (not clear) in age 19 and under leagues. A form-fitting mouthpiece is recommended (*Official Rules of Ice Hockey*, 2001).
  a. International play does not require mouthpieces; however, they are still highly encouraged (Joyner and Snouse, 2002).
  b. The purpose of mouthguards is to protect dentition (Labella, Smith, and Sigurdson, 2002).
  c. They may also prevent or decrease the severity of concussion (Arheim and Prentice, 1996; Labella, Smith, and Sigurdson, 2002; Hickey et al, 1967).
- Full facemasks are mandatory for all youth and college leagues (*Official Rules of Ice Hockey*, 2001) and are slowly gaining popularity on the professional level.
- Kevlar throat protectors are required in many leagues and countries (Joyner and Snouse, 2002).
- Gloves, elbow pads, shin pads, shoulder pads, hip pads or padded hockey pants, protective cup, and tendon pads are recommended (*Official Rules of Ice Hockey*, 2001).
  a. There has been a recent trend of wearing hockey gloves with shorter cuffs for the purpose of allowing increased wrist motion (Joyner and Snouse, 2002).

1. This may be at the cost of increased risk of wrist and forearm injury.
   b. Hockey pants have padding to protect from the hips to the top of the knees (*Official Rules of Ice Hockey*, 2001; Joyner and Snouse, 2002).
   c. Shin pads should cover from the top of the knees to the ankles (Joyner and Snouse, 2002).
- All protective equipment except helmets, facemasks, padded hockey gloves, padded hockey pants, and goalie leg pads are worn under the uniform (*Official Rules of Ice Hockey*, 2001).
- Goalkeeper protective equipment (*Official Rules of Ice Hockey*, 2001):
   a. Blocker—worn on stick hand
   b. Trapper glove worn on the nonstick hand. Looks similar to a baseball mitt with protective padding extending up the forearm.
   c. Leg guards up to 12 in. in width on each leg.
   d. Full masks are required. Form-fitting masks are not recommended and are illegal except in adult leagues. Use in adults requires signing a waiver.
   e. Approved HECC helmets are required unless the above formfitting mask includes a back skull plate.
   f. Throat protector
   g. Chest protector
   h. Cup
   i. Goalie skates
- Stick (*Official Rules of Ice Hockey*, 2001):
   a. Made of wood and may have tape covering any part.
   b. The stick length is limited to 63.5 in. and the blade length is limited to 12.5 in. Blade width is limited to 3 in.
   c. The goalkeeper's stick has a wider (up to 3.5 in.) and longer (up to 15.5 in.) blade.
   d. Maximal curve on all sticks is 0.5 in.
- Skates have a protective heel tip (not required for the goalie) (*Official Rules of Ice Hockey*, 2001).
   a. Probably the most important piece of equipment used by the hockey player (Clanton and Wood, 2003).
   b. Speed skates are prohibited (*Official Rules of Ice Hockey*, 2001).
   c. A 10- to 12-in. blade is attached to the base of the boot (*Official Rules of Ice Hockey*, 2001; Joyner and Snouse, 2002).
   d. Many players prefer leather skates that have external plastic shields for ankle support and protection (Green et al, 1976).
   e. Athletes usually prefer ice skates to be snugly fit and may not wear socks so as to improve the feel of the ice (Joyner and Snouse, 2002).
- The puck is made of vulcanized rubber and weighs between 5.5 and 6.0 oz. It is 1-in. thick and 3-in. in diameter (*Official Rules of Ice Hockey*, 2001).
   a. For midget league play, a 4.0-to 4.5-oz puck is recommended (*Official Rules of Ice Hockey*, 2001).
- Equipment that is in poor repair or that has been altered for the purpose of causing harm to other players is prohibited. Use of such equipment results in penalization of the offending player (*Official Rules of Ice Hockey*, 2001).

PHYSIOLOGY OF ICE HOCKEY

- Skating during a game involves repeated accelerations, decelerations, turning, and stopping (Sim et al, 1988; Green et al, 1976).
- The players skate forward, backward, and side to side, often with sudden changes in direction (Sim et al, 1988; Green et al, 1976).
- During competition, players will typically work at >70% of their VO_{2max} with a substantial amount of play at >90% VO_{2max} (Sim et al, 1988; Ferguson, Marcotte, and Montpetit, 1969).
   a. However, with the frequent stoppage of play per shift (on average 2–3) and with 3 to 4 min of rest between shifts, the resulting mean VO_2 consumed per game is 55–66% of maximum (Sim et al, 1988; Ferguson, Marcotte, and Montpetit, 1969).
- Players can lose 4.5 to 6.5 lb via sweat per game (Sim et al, 1988).
- If games are played in consecutive days, glycogen stores are often not replenished (Sim et al, 1988).
- Elite ice hockey players' average 10% body fat (Sim et al, 1988).
- Physiologic differences by position (Sim et al, 1988).
   a. Energy expenditure
      1. Playing time
         i. Goalies have the least number of substitutions and may play an entire game.
         ii. Defensemen have more playing time than forwards and typically have less rest time between shifts.
      2. Goaltending requires quick, short explosive movements interspersed with periods of relative rest.
         i. High reliance on ATP phosphocreatine system.
      3. Forwards and defensemen have a high reliance on both glycolytic and aerobic metabolism.
         i. During games, adult forwards and defensemen skate greater than 4 mi.
         ii. Energy expenditure is one-third aerobic and two-thirds anaerobic.
            a. Postgame lactate increases over eight times the pregame level.

4. Forwards have greater anaerobic activity and typically skate faster than defensemen or goalies.
5. Despite the above differences by position, muscle fiber composition remains equivalent between positions.
  b. Flexibility (Sim et al, 1988)
   1. Goalkeepers are significantly more flexible than forwards or defensemen.
   2. Forwards and defensemen have been found to have equal flexibility.
• Shooting
  a. Properly coordinated acceleration and deceleration of motion of body segments produces maximal velocity (Sim et al, 1988; Alexander, Drake, and Reichenback, 1964).
  b. Motion is concentrated in the lower arm (Sim ct al, 1988; Alexander, Drake, and Reichenback, 1964).
  c. However, maximal velocity is produced through maximal use and full rotation of the trunk (Sim et al, 1988; Alexander, Drake, and Reichenback, 1964; Alexander, Haddow, and Schultz, 1963).
  d. Accuracy of the shot is enhanced via trunk stabilization and restricted use of body segments (Sim et al, 1988; Alexander, Drake, and Reichenback, 1964; Alexander, Haddow, and Schultz, 1963).

EPIDEMIOLOGY OF INJURIES

• Ice hockey is classified as a collision sport by the American Academy of Pediatrics (Anderson, Griesemer, and Johnson, 2000).
• There are many opportunities for injury in this aggressive, fast-paced sport.
  a. Contact/collision with the hard ice surface, unpadded boards, goal posts, equipment from other players (skate blades, sticks), the puck, and the bodies and at times fists of opponents.
   1. In elite hockey, the puck can travel at speeds up to 120 mph, producing impact forces >1250 lb (Sim et al, 1988).
   2. Professional players can skate at speeds up to 30 mph (Sim et al, 1988).
   3. Sliding on the ice after a fall can occur at speeds up to 15 mph (Sim et al, 1988).
  b. Fatigue appears to be a risk factor for injury (Molsa et al, 1997; Stuart, and Smith, 1995; Mair et al, 1996; Smith, and Reischl, 1988).
  c. Equipment that is in poor repair also places the athlete at increased risk for injury; however, even when adequate protection is worn, injury is still possible. Molsa et al. (1997) found that 58% of injuries were on body parts that were covered with protective equipment.

• Overall injury rates
  a. Overall 5.6 injuries per 1000 player-hours (1.5 per 1000 hours in practice, 54 per 1000 hours in games) (Molsa et al, 1997).
  b. Injury is more common in the game setting (76%) than in practice (23%), even though practice represents significantly more time (Molsa et al, 1997). Injuries are thus 25 times more common in game settings (Stuart, and Smith, 1995).
  c. Acute and traumatic injures account for 85%, while overuse injuries represent 15% of all injuries (Tegner, and Lorentzon, 1991).
  d. Approximately 16% of injures are related to rules infractions (Molsa et al, 1997).
  e. During games, Pelletier and colleagues found that 27.1% of injuries occurred during the first period, 35.6% during the second period, and 26.6% during the third period (Pelletier, Montelpare, and Stark, 1993). In contrast, other investigators suggest that 3rd period injuries are roughly equal to 1st and 2nd period injuries combined (Molsa et al, 1997), or are twice as common in the 3rd period (Stuart, and Smith, 1995).
• Age-specific injury rates: Injuries appear to increase with increasing age with a peak in early adulthood (rates are expressed per 1000 player hours of practice time vs. game time) (Stuart, and Smith, 1995).
  a. Youth
   1. Squirt (age 9–10) .... 1.2 versus 0.0
   2. Pee wee (age 11–12) .... 2.2 versus 0.0
   3. Bantam (age 13–14) .... 2.5 versus 10.9
  b. Junior A (age 17–19) .... 3.9 versus 96.1
  c. Intercollegiate (age 18–21) .... 2.3 versus 84.3
  d. Swedish elite (age 19–33) .... 1.4 versus 78.4
• Mechanisms of injuries
  a. Collisions—14 to 65% of all injuries (Sim et al, 1988; Molsa et al, 1997; Stuart, and Smith, 1995; Mair et al, 1996; Smith, and Reischl, 1988; Tegner, and Lorentzon, 1991; Pelletier, Montelpare, and Stark, 1993; Lorentzon et al, 1988; Sane, Ylipaavalniemi, and Leppanen, 1988), with one study showing 29% are caused by unintentional or accidental collisions (Pelletier, Montelpare, and Stark, 1993). Collisions with the boards account for roughly 10% of all injuries (Molsa et al, 1997; Stuart, and Smith, 1995; Mair et al, 1996; Smith, and Reischl, 1988; Tegner, and Lorentzon, 1991; Pelletier, Montelpare, and Stark, 1993; Lorentzon et al, 1988).
  b. Puck—3 to 20% of injuries (Sim et al, 1988; Molsa et al, 1997; Stuart, and Smith, 1995; Mair et al, 1996; Smith, and Reischl, 1988; Tegner, and Lorentzon, 1991; Pelletier, Montelpare, and Stark, 1993; Lorentzon et al, 1988; Sane, Ylipaavalniemi,

and Leppanen, 1988). Puck velocity may reach 120 mph at professional levels (Sim et al, 1988).

c. Stick—8 to 29% of injuries (Molsa et al, 1997; Stuart, and Smith, 1995; Pelletier, Montelpare, and Stark, 1993)

d. Skate—5 to 11% of injuries, often related to lacerations from sharp steel blades (Stuart, and Smith, 1995; Lorentzon et al, 1988)

e. Fighting—3 to 6.5% of injuries (Stuart, and Smith, 1995; Pelletier, Montelpare, and Stark, 1993)

f. Overuse—14.6 % (Tegner and Lorentzon, 1991)

g. Falls—4 to 7% (Molsa et al, 1997; Stuart, and Smith, 1995)

h. Foul play or illegal play—9 to 16% (Molsa et al, 1997)

i. Noncontact injuries—2.2% (Pelletier, Montelpare, and Stark, 1993)

• Type of injury

a. Sprain 31.0% (Pelletier, Montelpare, and Stark, 1993)
1. Average number of days lost from play due to sprains = 13.61

b. Contusion 21.0% (Pelletier, Montelpare, and Stark, 1993)

c. Laceration 13.0% (Pelletier, Montelpare, and Stark, 1993)

d. Strain 11.3% (Pelletier, Montelpare, and Stark, 1993)

e. Fracture 10.2% (Pelletier, Montelpare, and Stark, 1993)
1. Average number of days lost form play due to fractures = 22.22.

f. Concussion 7.5% (Pelletier, Montelpare, and Stark, 1993)

g. General Trauma 5.9% (Pelletier, Montelpare, and Stark, 1993)

• Rate of injury per site (Canadian university athletes) (Pelletier, Montelpare, and Stark, 1993)

a. Head, neck 10.6%

b. Face, eye, ear, jaw, teeth 17.6%

c. Shoulder/clavicle 14.9%

d. Chest, back 4.8%

e. Arm, elbow 3.7%

f. Forearm, wrist, hand 6.9%

g. Hip, groin, abdomen 6.4%

h. Hamstring, thigh 9.0%

i. Knee 18.6%

j. Ankle 3.2%

k. Foot 1.6%

• Injuries related to position on ice

a. Goalkeeper 5.8% (Molsa et al, 1997)

b. Defensemen 31.2% (Molsa et al, 1997)

c. Center 18.5% (Molsa et al, 1997)

d. Wing 36.0% (Molsa et al, 1997)

e. Missing position data 8.5% (Molsa et al, 1997)

f. However, position played has no statistical relationship to days lost from an injury (Ayars, 2000).

INJURIES BY LOCATION

• **Ocular:** Thirty-eight to 47% of sports-related injuries occur in hockey (Pashby, 1988).

a. Most commonly injuries are soft tissue (34%), hyphema (27%), other intraocular injuries (23%), corneal damage (9%), orbital fracture (4%), and ruptured globes (3%) (Pashby, 1988).

b. Pashby (1988) reported that approximately 15% of all eye injured hockey athletes were left with an injury resulting in a legally blind eye (Pashby, 1988).

c. However, 58% of the above would have been preventable with face shields (Pashby, 1988).

• **Concussions:** Management should be as in any other sport.

a. Hockey players sustain head trauma and impact forces from axial loading in a similar mechanism as football players (Cross and Serenelli, 2003).

b. Unlike football, the hockey athlete is also at risk for traumatic brain injury through contact with the hockey puck, which as previously mentioned can reach speeds up to 120 mph (Sim et al, 1988).

c. Concussions account for 7.5% of all hockey injuries (Pelletier, Montelpare, and Stark, 1993).
1. This percentage is likely underestimated, as many injury reporting studies have only looked at injuries that have resulted in time lost from play (Tegner and Lorentzon, 1991; Lorentzon et al, 1988; Lorentzon, Wedren, and Pietila, 1988). Athletes with mild concussions are often only briefly symptomatic and may return to play the same game. As such, many concussions may not have been identified.

d. Benson and associates included mild concussions in their head and neck injury study and found a concussion incidence of 1.53–1.57 per 1000 athlete exposures (Benson et al, 1999).

• **Maxillofacial:** When abrasions and lacerations are excluded, maxillofacial trauma represents 11.5% of hockey injuries (Sane, Ylipaavalniemi, and Leppanen, 1988).

• Blows from the stick represent 54.1% of maxillofacial and dental injuries, while the puck only represents 14.2% of injuries to this same area (Sane, Ylipaavalniemi, and Leppanen, 1988).

• A 69.9% of injuries occur during games with the remainder occurring during practice sessions (Sane, Ylipaavalniemi, and Leppanen, 1988).

- Injury to teeth and alveolar processes represent 84.5% of injuries (Sane, Ylipaavalniemi, and Leppanen, 1988).
  a. Ice hockey accounts for roughly 40% of all sports-related dental injuries (Hayrinen-Immonen et al, 1990).
- Maxillofacial injuries have been drastically reduced since the introduction of mandatory facemasks in many levels of the sport (Sane, Ylipaavalniemi, and Leppanen, 1988).
- 47% of the above reported facial injuries may have been preventable through the use of protective visors (Lorentzon et al, 1988).
- Studies have shown the use of helmets with facemasks significantly reduces (but does not completely eliminate) the incidence of facial lacerations (Benson et al, 1999; LaPrade et al, 1995; Murray and Livingston, 1995).
  a. Number of game induced facial lacerations without facemask = 70 per 1000 player-game hours (Lorentzon et al, 1988; Lorentzon, Wedren, and Pietila, 1988).
  b. Number of game induced facial lacerations with facemask = 14.7–15.1 per 1000 player-game hours (LaPrade et al, 1995).
  c. Number of practice induced facial lacerations without facemask = 21.8 per 1000 player-practice hours (Lorentzon et al, 1988; Lorentzon, Wedren, and Pietila, 1988).
  d. Number of practice induced facial lacerations with facemask = 0.0–0.2 per 1000 player-practice hours (LaPrade et al, 1995).
- Despite facemasks, facial lacerations still occur, and the team physician should be prepared to evaluate and repair these injuries appropriately.
- **Cervical Spine:** The effect of helmet and facemask use on cervical spine injury—the controversy.
  a. After the increased use of helmets with facemasks in ice hockey, there retrospectively appeared to be an increasing incidence of cervical spine injury. Several investigators hypothesize that this is caused as a result of the player wearing a helmet adopting a more aggressive style of play resulting in more cervical injury (Murray and Livingston, 1995; Reynen and Clancy, Jr, 1994). It has been proposed that the protective devices have also altered how officials perceive game situations, leading them to be more lenient in penalization. The net result has been an increase in illegal and injurious behaviors, such as checking from behind (an activity associated with catastrophic cervical spine injury) (Murray and Livingston, 1995).
  b. However, LaPrade and colleagues' prospective study of intercollegiate athletes and facemask use

showed no increase in head and neck injuries (LaPrade et al, 1995).
- Mechanism of injury is axial loading caused by a blow to the head from collision with the boards, other players, the ice, or the goal post (Tator, 1987).
- Many of the reported cervical spine injuries were a result of either illegal play or high-risk aggressive behavior. New rules have been instituted by both the Canadian Amateur Hockey Association and USA Hockey in an attempt to reduce the number of spinal cord injuries. These new rules have moved the action away from the boards and restricted checking; preliminary results appear successful in limiting the incidence of complete spinal cord injuries (Tator, Carson, and Edmonds, 1998).
- **Shoulder:** Clavicle fractures, acromioclavicular joint separations, and glenohumeral subluxation/dislocation are relatively common in ice hockey (Minkoff, Varoltta, and Simonson, 1994; Bahr, Bendiksen, and Engerbretsen, 1995; Thompson, and Scoles, 2000). They usually are a high velocity injury, which is the result of the shoulder be driven into the boards following aggressive body checks.
- **Elbow:** A player who does not wear elbow pads may receive a traumatic olecranon bursitis and/or elbow fracture during collision with the ice or the boards.
- **Wrist, hand:** When hockey players fight (which occurs frequently at higher levels of play), the gloves are typically thrown down, and blows are exchanged using bare hands. The typical street fighter hand injuries can then occur.
- Gamekeeper's thumb (ulnar collateral ligament injury) has been reported (Sim et al, 1988) and is typically due to the player's thumb being hyperabducted when the stick handle is suddenly forced toward the body during a collision with the boards.
- **Wartenberg's syndrome:** In hockey, direct trauma to the superficial radial nerve at the wrist can occur when an opponent strikes the distal forearm with the stick. The athlete will complain of pain and/or parasthesias shooting up the thumb and dorsal wrist in a radial distribution (Nuber, Assenmacher, and Bowen, 1998). Players who use gloves with shorter cuffs (so as to increase wrist mobility) are at increased risk for this injury.
- **Scaphoid fracture:** Mechanism of injury usually is fall on outstretched hand or a dorsiflexed wrist colliding with the boards. The gloves provide some protection against this injury.
- **Chest:** Commotio cordis has been reported in youth ice hockey (Maron et al, 2002). League organizers and physicians should consider having an *automated electric defibrillator* (AED) available at the rink, as there is a 16% survival with rapid defibrillation (Maron et al, 2002).

- **Back:** Back strain and sprain—players skate in a forward flexed position. This combined with the frequent trunk rotation that accompanies shooting and passing can place the player at risk for these injuries.
- Spondylolysis has been reported in ice hockey athletes.
- **Abdomen:** Because of the abrupt and sudden changes in movement (Joyner and Snouse, 2002; Sim et al, 1988), hockey players are at risk for abdominal muscle strain.
- Athletes can sustain traumatic abdominal injury, especially when the handle of the stick is forced into the abdomen during a collision into the boards (which is typically the result of illegal checking).
- **Thigh, groin:** Anterior thigh hematomas may occur as a result of collision with the boards or of blocking a shot puck. These hematomas are at risk for myositis ossificans (Sim et al, 1988) and treatment should be directed at preventing this complication.
  a. If the hematoma is identified immediately after the game, the athlete can be placed in fixed knee flexion for 24 hours in an attempt to tamponade the bleeding thereby decreasing the size of the hematoma.
  b. Old hematomas should not be passively stretched, as this may increase the risk of myositis ossificans.
- Adductor strains are common enough that studies have been performed in an attempt to determine if certain players are at increased risk for this injury and to ascertain what prevention measures can be implemented in an attempt to decrease lost playing time. Hockey players are at risk for this injury as a result of the explosive starts and changes in direction (Joyner and Snouse, 2002).
- Osteitis pubis
- **Knee:** Most common significant lower extremity injury.
  a. Although *anterior cruciate ligament* (ACL) and meniscal injury has been reported, *medial collateral ligament* (MCL) injury is 14 times more common (Molsa et al, 1997).
  b. The ACL appears to be spared because the foot does not lock in position on the ice.
  c. The mechanisms for MCL injury are both contact and noncontact valgus stress to the knee.
- **Ankle:** Ankle sprain—mechanism of injury is dorsiflexion, eversion, and external rotation (Thompson and Scoles, 2000), producing deltoid ligament sprain.
  a. This is in contrast to most other sports where the typical mechanism is plantarflexion, inversion, and internal rotation, producing lateral ligament (especially anterior talofibular ligament) injury.
  b. The mechanism of injury also places the hockey athlete at risk for syndesmotic injury and

Massoneuve fracture (due to transmittal of the force out through the fibula).
  c. Ankle sprains result in 10% of major injuries in ice hockey (defined as absence from sport greater than 28 days) (Molsa et al, 1997).
  d. In an attempt to prevent these debilitating injuries, many hockey players prefer skates that have added external ankle support (Green et al, 1976).
- Boot lace lacerations—the ice skate blade is essentially a 10–12-in. scalpel. The anterior ankle is at risk for laceration of tendons and neurovascular structures because of its proximity to the skates of others. A relatively small laceration can cause damage to these underlying superficial structures (Tator, 1987).
  a. However, most athletes are relatively protected from this injury because of the thickly padded skate tongue over the anterior ankle. Athletes who turn their skate tongue downward (out of personal preference) place themselves at increased risk (Tator, 1987).
- **Foot:** Lace bite (Joyner and Snouse, 2002)—nagging dorsal foot pain and/or parasthesias.
  a. Players often do not wear socks and prefer tight fitting skates as this is thought by athletes to improve performance and speed on the ice. The compression of the laces in such situations can cause extensor tendon and nerve injuries of the dorsum of the foot.
  b. To prevent this injury, the tongue of the boot should remain in a neutral position (Clanton and Wood, 2003).

MEDICAL ILLNESSES

- Indoor ice rinks have ice resurfacing machines called Zambonis that are gas or propane powered. The emissions from the machine coupled with poor ventilation can create increased carbon monoxide levels on the ice.
- Nitrogen dioxide induced lung injury and other indoor air quality syndromes
- Cold induced vasomotor rhinitis
  a. Profuse watery rhinorrhea that typically begins within minutes of skating on the ice. It is thought to be the result of an overly sensitive cholinergic reflex in response to exposure to cold air and changes in humidity (Ayars, 2000; Bousquet et al, 2003).
  b. The athlete has little nasal itching, ocular pruritis, or sneezing, but increased nasal secretions, postnasal drip, sinus headaches, anosmia, and sinusitis are common (Ayars, 2000; Bousquet et al, 2003).
  c. It is a diagnosis of exclusion. Rhinitis caused by infection, allergy, anatomic abnormalities and

eosinophilia should first be ruled out (Ayars, 2000; Bousquet et al, 2003).

d. Many athletes self-medicate with decongestants for this disorder; however, this category of medicines is on the banned substances list for the International Olympic Committee (IOC). There has been some promise in treating this disorder with ipratropium bromide nasal spray, a medication that is not on the prohibited list.

PREVENTION

- Youth hockey programs need to educate players, coaches, and parents of the importance of knowing and following the rules (Anderson, Griesemer, and Johnson, 2000).
- Body checking should not be allowed in youth hockey for children ages 15 and under (Anderson, Griesemer, and Johnson, 2000; Brust et al, 1992).
- Fair-play rules should be used to decrease the incidence of injury in youth hockey. This system gives teams credit for sportsmanship in the final standings of league and tournament play. Teams have points added to their totals for staying under a preestablished limit of penalties per game, while teams that rely on intimidation and foul play have points subtracted. Implementation of this style of play was shown to reduce the number of high school hockey injuries (Roberts et al, 1996).
- Players, coaches, parents, and officials should be educated on the dangers of checking another player from behind (Anderson, Griesemer, and Johnson, 2000).
- The officials and coaches should be encouraged to strictly enforce the rules against illegal body checking.
  a. These forms of checking include boarding, charging, checking from behind, cross checking, elbowing, and roughing.
- Contact with an opposing player made above the shoulder using the fist, forearm, elbow, shoulder, knee or stick must be penalized. If such an act was deliberate, the stiffest sanctions should be used.
- Deliberate attempts to injure other players are illegal and should be heavily penalized.
- Rules against high-sticking should be strictly enforced.
  a. Frequently occurs during a slap shot or when attempting to bat down an airborne puck.
    1. During a slap shot, it is considered high sticking if the stick comes above the level of the waist on the back swing.
      i. Slap shots are illegal in midget play.
    2. Batting a puck down with the stick above the shoulders is also considered high sticking.

- Fighting needs to be discouraged by officials, coaches, players, and players' parents.
- Players should be encouraged or mandated to wear helmets with full coverage facemasks at any level of play for both game and practice situations.
- Ensure adequate ventilation in and monitoring of air quality in indoor ice rinks.
- The medical team providing coverage for ice hockey should have the availability of medical equipment for the stabilization of potentially devastating injury at the ice rink. This should include a spine board, cervical collar, and cardiopulmonary resuscitation equipment (Ghiselli, Schaadt, and McAllister, 2003). The logistics of how to get this equipment to the injured athlete on the ice should be preestablished. The emergency plan should be in place and practiced prior to the beginning of the season so that in the event of a devastating injury, morbidity due to delay in stabilization can be reduced.

REFERENCES

Alexander J, Drake C, Reichenback P: Effect of strength development on speed of shooting in varsity ice hockey players. *Res Q* 35:101–106, 1964.

Alexander J, Haddow J, Schultz G: Comparison of the ice hockey wrist and slap shots for speed and accuracy. *Res Q* 34:259–266, 1963.

Anderson S, Griesemer B, Johnson M: Safety in youth hockey: the effects of body checking. *Pediatrics* 105(3):657–658, 2000.

Arheim D, Prentice W: Protective sports equipment, in *Principles of Athletic Training*. Chicago, Mosby Yearbook, 1996, p 116.

Ayars G: Nonallergic rhinitis. *Immun and Allergy Clin* 20(2):179–192, 2000.

Bahr R, Bendiksen F, Engerbretsen L: Tis the season: Diagnosing and managing ice hockey injuries. *J Musculoskel Med* 12(2):48–56, 1995.

Benson BW, et al: Head and neck injuries among ice hockey players wearing full face shields vs half face shields. *JAMA* 282(24):2328–2332, 1999.

Bousquet J et al: Requirements for medications commonly used in the treatment of allergic rhinitis. European Academy of Allergy and Clinical Immunology (EAACI), Allergic Rhinitis and its Impact on Asthma (ARIA). *Allergy* 58(3):192–197, 2003.

Brust JD et al: Children's ice hockey injuries. *Am J Dis Child* 146(6):741–747, 1992.

Clanton T, Wood R: Etiology of injury to the foot and ankle, in DeLee J, Drez D, and Miller M (eds.): *Delee and Drez's Orthopaedic Sports Medicine* Philadelphia, PA, Saunders, 2003, p. 2265–2267.

Cross KM, Serenelli C: Training and equipment to prevent athletic head and neck injuries. *Clin Sports Med* 22(3):639–667, 2003.

Ferguson R, Marcotte G, Montpetit R: Maximal oxygen uptake test during ice skating. *Med Sci Sports* 1:207–211, 1969.

Ghiselli G, Schaadt G, McAllister DR: On-the-field evaluation of an athlete with a head or neck injury. *Clin Sports Med* 22(3):445–465, 2003.

Green H et al: Time-motion and physiological assessments of ice hockey performance. *J Appl Physiol* 40(2):159–163, 1976.

Hayrinen-Immonen R et al: A six-year follow-up study of sports-related dental injuries in children and adolescents. *Endod Dent Traumatol* 6(5):208–212, 1990.

Hickey JC et al: The relation of mouth protectors to cranial pressure and deformation. *J Am Dent Assoc* 74(4):735–740, 1967.

Joyner D, Snouse S: Skiing, speed skating, ice hockey, in Ireland M and Nattiv A (eds.): *The Female Athlete.* Philadelphia, PA, Saunders: 2002, pp 769–775.

Labella C, Smith B, Sigurdson A: Effect of mouthguards on dental injuries and concussion in college basketball. *Med Sci Sports Exerc* 34(1):41–44, 2002.

LaPrade RF et al: The effect of the mandatory use of face masks on facial lacerations and head and neck injuries in ice hockey. A prospective study. *Am J Sports Med* 23(6):773–735, 1995.

Lorentzon R, Wedren H, Pietila T: Incidence, nature, and causes of ice hockey injuries. A three-year prospective study of a Swedish elite ice hockey team. *Am J Sports Med* 16(4):392–396, 1988.

Lorentzon, R et al: Injuries in international ice hockey. A prospective, comparative study of injury incidence and injury types in international and Swedish elite ice hockey. *Am J Sports Med* 16(4):389–391, 1988.

Mair SD et al: The role of fatigue in susceptibility to acute muscle strain injury. *Am J Sports Med* 24(2):137–143, 1996.

Maron BJ et al: Clinical profile and spectrum of commotio cordis. [comment]. *JAMA* 287(9):1142–1146, 2002.

Minkoff J, Varoltta G, Simonson B: Ice hockey, in Fu F and Stone D (eds.): *Sports Injuries: Mechanisms-Prevention-Treatment.* Baltimore, MD, Williams & Wilkins, 1994, pp 397–444.

Molsa J et al: Ice hockey injuries in Finland. A prospective epidemiologic study. *Am J Sports Med* 25(4):495–499, 1997.

Morgan J: Ice hockey injuries, in Casey M, Forster C, and Hixson E, (eds.): *Winter Sports Medicine.* Philadelphia, PA, FA Davis, 1990, pp 269–274.

Murray TM, Livingston LA: Hockey helmets, face masks, and injurious behavior. *Pediatrics* 95(3):419–421, 1995.

Nuber GW, Assenmacher J, Bowen MK: Neurovascular problems in the forearm, wrist, and hand. *Clin Sports Med* 17(3):585–610, 1998.

Official Rules of Ice Hockey. Chicago, Triumph Books, 2001.

Pashby TJ: Ocular injuries in hockey. *Int Ophthalmol Clin* 28(3):228–231, 1988.

Pelletier RL, Montelpare WJ, Stark RM: Intercollegiate ice hockey injuries. A case for uniform definitions and reports. *Am J Sports Med* 21(1):78–81, 1993.

Reynen PD, Clancy WG, Jr: Cervical spine injury, hockey helmets, and face masks. *Am J Sports Med* 22(2):167–170, 1994.

Roberts WO et al: Fair-play rules and injury reduction in ice hockey. *Arch Pediatr Adolesc Med* 150(2):140–145, 1996.

Sane J, Ylipaavalniemi P, Leppanen H: Maxillofacial and dental ice hockey injuries. *Med Sci Sports Exerc* 20(2):202–207, 1988.

Sim FH et al: Ice hockey injuries. *Am J Sports Med* 16(Suppl 1):S86–S96, 1988.

Smith RW, Reischl SF: Metatarsophalangeal joint synovitis in athletes. *Clin Sports Med* 7(1):75–88, 1988.

Stuart MJ, Smith A: Injuries in junior A ice hockey. A three-year prospective study. *Am J Sports Med* 23(4):458–461, 1995.

Tator CH: Neck injuries in ice hockey: A recent, unsolved problem with many contributing factors. *Clin Sports Med* 6(1):101–114, 1987.

Tator CH, Carson JD, Edmonds VE: Spinal injuries in ice hockey. *Clin Sports Med* 17(1):183–194, 1998.

Tegner Y, Lorentzon R: Ice hockey injuries: Incidence, nature and causes. *Br J Sports Med* 25(2):87–89, 1991.

Thompson G, Scoles P: Bone and joint disorders: sports medicine, in Behrman R, Kliefman R, Jenson H (eds.): *Nelson Textbook of Pediatrics.* Philadelphia, PA, WB Saunders, 2000, p 2111.

USA Hockey website, *www.usahockey.com.*

87 RUGBY INJURIES

Peter H Seidenberg, MD
Rochelle Nolte, MD

INTRODUCTION

- Rugby union is a fast paced contact-collision game with the continuous pace of soccer combined with contact situations similar to those seen in American football.
- It is the fastest growing amateur sport in the United States.
  1. There are greater than 50,000 members in USA Rugby (the governing body for Rugby Union in the United States). (USA Rugby website)
  2. There are 37 local area unions. (USA Rugby website)
  3. The USA national (the Eagles) men's team was established in 1976, and the women's team was established in 1987.
- Rugby is played in over 100 countries worldwide and has a strong tradition in Great Britain, New Zealand, Australia, and South Africa.
  1. Its popularity is second only to soccer in the world (Dexter, 2003).
- World Cup competition occurs every 4 years.
- There are similar sports that are sometimes confused with rugby union such as rugby league and Australian Rules football which will not be discussed in this chapter.

HISTORY

- Rugby is a cross between soccer and football. (Dietzen and Topping, 1999)
- Invented in 1932 when William Webb Ellis picked up the ball and advanced it in a soccer match at Rugby College in England. The only way to stop the runner was to tackle him or her. (Dietzen and Topping, 1999)
- American football evolved from rugby in the late nineteenth century.
- It was an Olympic sport from 1900 to 1924. (USA Rugby website)
  1. The United States won the gold medal in 1920 and 1924.
- After 1924, it was no longer an Olympic sport, and this was followed by decreased popularity in the United States. (USA Rugby website)
- It is currently being considered for reinstatement as an Olympic sport for the 2012 games. (USA Rugby website)

MATCH

- **Goals** (USA Rugby Football Union, 2003)
  1. Where as American football is a game of yardage, rugby union is a game of possession.
  2. The player with possession of the ball is the frontmost player on the attacking team. He or she may advance the ball by running with the ball, kicking it forward, or by passing it backward or laterally to another player on his or her team.
     a. All teammates are behind the ball carrier in support.
     b. Unlike American football, blocking for the ball carrier is not permitted and is penalized as obstruction.
  3. The objective is to maintain control of the ball and touch it down in the try zone (the rugby equivalent of the American football end zone).
     a. Once crossing the try line, the player must touch the ball down on the ground in order to register a try, which is worth 5 points.
     b. The try entitles the scoring team to attempt to kick the ball through the goal posts, which is worth another 2 points.
        i. The kicker takes the ball out of the try zone along a line where the ball was touched down parallel to the touch lines.
  4. An offensive player may also attempt to drop-kick the ball through the goal posts during open play, which is worth 3 points.
  5. The team with the maximum points at the end of the match is the victor.

6. A typical game requires the athlete to cover a distance of 5 to 8 km, running at speeds up to 5–8 m/s (comparable to soccer) (Dexter, 2003).
7. In addition, the rugby player is involved in >1–2 episodes of collision contact per minute (Dexter, 2003).
   a. These equate to approximately 40 tackles and up to 70 rucks and mauls per game.
   b. The forwards sustain an additional 30 scrums and 40 line outs per game.
8. There are few substitutions allowed. The mean duration of high intensity work (sprinting or contact) is 38 s/min with an average workload of 51 min per 80-min match. In comparison, the average American football game has only 10 min of contact or significant exertion per game (Dexter, 2003).

- **Pitch:** The rugby field is called the pitch (USA Rugby Football Union, 2003).
  1. The rectangular field of play (which excludes the goal zones) does not exceed 70 m in width and 100 m in length.
  2. Each try zone is the same width as the remainder of the pitch and is between 10 and 22 m in depth.
  3. The pitch has the following solid lines:
     a. Half-way line or midfield line (half the distance between the try lines)
     b. Ten-meter lines on each side of the half way line
     c. Twenty-meter lines (22 m from the try lines)
     d. Try lines
     e. Dead ball lines (at the deepest portion of the try zone)
     f. Touch lines (side lines)
  4. Dashed lines
     a. Positioned 5 and 15 m parallel to the touch lines.
  5. The goal posts are on the goal line and are in the field of play.
     a. The distance between the posts is 5.6 m in width with a minimum height of 3.4 m.
     b. The crossbar is 3.0 m from the ground.
     c. The posts should be padded (since players can collide with them as they are in the field of play)

- **Rules**
  1. The match is divided into two 40-min halves with a 5–10-min half time (USA Rugby Football Union, 2003).
  2. A player who leaves the match and is substituted may not return to the match.
     a. Exception: A player maybe substituted for a maximum of 15 min for control of bleeding from an injury. After bleeding is controlled, he or she may then return to play. This is commonly referred to as a blood sub.

b. Exception: A referee may permit a substituted tight five player to return to the match to replace an injured player if no eligible player on the team is experienced in these skilled positions.

3. The play clock runs continuously.

4. There is one referee to monitor play. (USA Rugby Football Union, 2003)
   a. Play is stopped only for a penalty, the ball leaving field of play, a score, or a serious injury (in the referee's judgment).
   b. The referee may summon a medical attendant onto to the pitch, or may allow the player to temporarily leave the pitch for medical evaluation.
   c. Even though a medical attendant may be on the pitch evaluating an injured player, the referee may allow play to continue around the injured player.
   d. The medical attendant does not have the power to stop play but does have the ability to determine whether an injured player is allowed to continue to play.

5. Rules have been instituted to decrease the incidence of neck injury in rugby union. The following actions are illegal:
   a. High tackles above the level of the shoulders.
   b. Spearing.
   c. Leaving your feet to make a tackle.
   d. Tackling a player who is in the follow through phase of kicking a ball.
   e. Tackling a player who has jumped in the air to catch a ball.
   f. The tackler must wrap the opposing ball carrier with arms or grasp the player with hands. Tacklers cannot merely hit the opponent with a shoulder or shove him or her.
      i. This rule separates rugby union from other contact-collision sports.
   g. Laws are periodically reviewed and revised by the international rugby board to enhance safety and improve the flow of the game.

• **Positions**

1. There are 15 players on each team with specific positions and responsibilities (USA Rugby Football Union, 2003).

2. Each team ideally has at least 5 to 7 substitutes available.

3. The players numbered 1 through 8 are the forwards and are affectionately referred to as the scrum.
   a. They are generally responsible for gaining and maintaining possession of the ball.

4. Players numbered 9 through 15 are the backs.
   a. They are generally responsible for advancing the ball down the field and defending the open field.

5. Props
   a. Position no. 1—Loose head prop
   b. Position no. 3—Tight head prop
   c. One of three people of the front row, which includes two props on either side of a hooker.
   d. They are responsible for the stability and strength of the front row.
   e. They are generally the stoutest and least aerobically fit on the pitch (Quarrie et al, 1996).

6. Hooker
   a. Position no. 2.
   b. Responsible for hooking (securing the ball with feet) during the scrum
   c. Hooker is in the middle position of the front row of the scrum and is tightly supported by the props on either side, who support the hooker so his or her feet are off the ground. This enables the hooker to hook the ball backward during the scrum.
   d. Hooker is usually slightly shorter and lighter than the props to provide a stable front row platform.

7. Second row/locks
   a. Position nos. 4 and 5.
   b. They are responsible for providing the driving force to the front row of the scrum.
   c. Typically are the jumpers for the line out.
   d. Generally the tallest players on the pitch.
   e. The second and first rows make up the tight five.

8. Flanker/Wing forward
   a. Position nos. 6 and 7.
   b. Together with the eightman make up the loose forwards.
   c. Typically are the first players to leave a scrum.
   d. Generally are the best tacklers and all-around athletes on the team.
   e. Ideal flanker has both size and speed.

9. Eightman
   a. Position no. 8.
   b. Eightman is at the rear end of the scrum and has his or her head between the second row players.
   c. He or she is responsible for providing stability and drive to the scrum.
   d. Generally the tallest loose forward.
   e. He or she needs to be able to reach around the locks hold them securely together.
   f. The eightman is responsible for controlling the ball at the rear of the scrum until the scrumhalf retrieves the ball.

10. Scrumhalf
    a. Position no. 9
    b. Acts as the quarterback of the forwards.
       i. Responsible for offensive and defensive strategy of the forwards during loose play.

ii. Secures the ball from the scrum, rucks, mauls, and tackles.

iii. Is responsible for delivering the ball to the backs for open field play.

c. Scrumhalf is responsible for placing the ball in the tunnel (see scrum below).

d. The scrumhalf is usually smaller and quicker than the other forwards and has a fast and accurate pass.

11. Flyhalf

a. Position no. 10.

b. Acts as the quarterback of the backs and is the first player in the back line.

i. Is responsible for calling back plays.

c. Generally smaller and lighter than other backs with good passing and kicking ability.

12. Centers

a. Position no. 12—inside center

b. Position no. 13—outside center

c. Generally the larger and more physical backs

d. They are often called upon to crash into the competition by intentionally running into defenders to establish a ruck or maul.

13. Wings

a. Position nos. 11 and 14

b. Generally the players who are the quickest and most elusive on the team. They are required to outrun the opposition in open field play.

14. Fullback

a. Position no. 15

b. The last line of defense in rugby

c. Has responsibilities similar to the safety, punter, and punt returner of American football.

d. Essential skills include being able to field a kicked ball, to kick for distance and accuracy, and to be able to consistently tackle in the open field.

• **Formations**

1. Scrum

a. This aspect of the game is tightly controlled by the referee to prevent injury.

b. In preparation for the scrum, each pack assembles under the directions of their individual hooker.

c. After both teams are assembled and stable in the crouched position, the referee will call "Engage!"

i. Engagement is when the two scrums come together forming a tunnel between the front row players.

ii. The referee calling engage is a recent change to enhance safety in the scrum. Previously, the scrums would come together at the end of a cadence called by the hooker of the attacking team.

d. The scrumhalf introduces the ball into the tunnel.

e. The hookers attempt to hook (kick) the ball backward to their own team.

f. After the ball has traveled to the rear of the scrum, the ball can be picked up for advancement.

g. The scrum is used to restart play after the referee has stopped play for minor infringements and at other points in the match.

h. Strategically it is used both offensively and defensively (Milburn, 1993).

i. Offense → base for attacking play

ii. Defense → denying the opponents clean possession

i. The stability of the scrum is determined by the front row's ability to utilize their strength to transmit the force to their opponents (Milburn, 1993).

2. Line out

a. Used to restart play after the ball has gone into touch (out of bounds).

b. There are 2 to 7 forwards from each team arranged in parallel lines that are perpendicular to the touch line.

c. The hooker throws the ball into the tunnel formed by the standing forwards of both teams.

d. Each team has jumpers who will fight for possession of the thrown ball.

e. The jumper is assisted by lifters—two players who grab the jumper above the knees (usually by the shorts) and lift him or her into the air. The lifters also ensure a controlled return to the ground after the jumper has caught the ball. Afterward, a maul (see below) is usually formed.

3. Maul

a. Is formed when the ball carried is stopped by a defender but not taken to the ground.

b. Players from both teams attempt to drive the maul down the field by binding to each other and giving a unified push.

c. Both sides attempt to grab the ball out of the maul to restart open field play.

4. Ruck

a. Is formed when a player is tackled and brought to the ground.

b. The tackled player releases the ball on the ground.

c. The opposing teams come together over the top of the ball in an attempt to drive the other team backward away from the ball.

d. One team must drive the other team completely off the ball before the ball can be picked up.

- **Equipment**
  1. Ball: Appears similar to an oversized, over-inflated, white football.
  2. Boots: The rugby cleats
     a. Typically have removable studs or molded multistudded rubber soles and have cleats similar to soccer. Single toe cleats (as in baseball) are not permitted.
  3. No braces containing metal or hard plastic of any kind (including knee braces) are permitted.
  4. Unlike American football, casts or splints are not permitted to be worn during play.
  5. No jewelry, earrings, hair devices (other than elastic bands), or eye wear (other than contact lenses) are permitted.
  6. Optional equipment
     a. Shoulder pads: Generally a padded pull over top with a maximum thickness of 1/2 in. of foam padding
     b. Mitts: Fingerless gloves
     c. Soft head gear: Scrumcap
     d. Mouth guard
        i. Highly suggested
        ii. Mandatory for high school and below
     e. Shin guards: Thin, 0.5-cm soft padding only—no hard plastic—may be worn under the rugby socks.
     f. Women may wear chest pads—Generally similar to shoulder pads, except padding extends down the front of the chest.

EPIDEMIOLOGY

- Sprains, strains, contusion, abrasions, and lacerations are to be expected in rugby (Dietzen and Topping, 1999).
- A Scottish study found an incidence of injury of 1.45 per 100 player appearances (Dietzen and Topping, 1999).
- Tackling has been sited as the major cause of injury (Dietzen and Topping, 1999).
- The New Zealand Injury and Performance Project found that the location of injuries in this sport is widespread throughout the entire body (Gerrard, Waller, and Bird, 1994). The following are the percent of players that reported an injury at each of the following sites in the previous 12 months.
  1. Head/skull/inner ear—10%
  2. Face/outer ear/eye—19%
  3. Neck—11%
  4. Shoulder/clavicle—21%
  5. Back—17%
  6. Chest and abdomen—4%

  7. Arm/elbow—1%
  8. Wrist/hand/finger—4%
  9. Pelvis/hip/groin—2%
  10. Thumb—18%
  11. Upper leg—19%
  12. Knee—17%
  13. Lower leg—17%
  14. Ankle—24%
  15. Heel/foot/toe—1%
- The same study of total rugby injuries in a year found the following total distribution of injuries (Gerrard, Waller, and Bird, 1994):
  1. Sprains, strains, and other soft tissue injury—74%
  2. Laceration or abrasion—10%
  3. Fracture—7%
  4. Closed head injury—5%
  5. Other—4%
- Injury rates in collegiate and men's club teams range from 13 to 30 per 1000 game hours.
- Injury rates for youth rugby (<18-year old) is generally 8–10 per 1000 game hours (Dexter, 2003; Marshall and Spencer, 2001).
  1. Concussion is the most common head or neck injury with an incidence of 4 per 1000 game hours and is responsible for approximately 25% of all injuries in this age group.
- Women's injury rates occur with less frequency. The ratio of injures of men to women is 4:3.
  1. The exception may be *anterior cruciate ligament* (ACL) injury.
- Australia, New Zealand, South Africa, and the United Kingdom have published papers on the incidence of injuries in rugby for varying age and skill levels. (Quarrie et al, 1996; Chalmers, 1994; Waller et al, 1994; Gerrard, Waller, and Bird, 1994; Quarrie et al, 1995; Bird et al, 1998; Quarrie et al, 2001; Quarrie, Cantu, and Chalmers, 2002; Garraway and Macleod, 1995)
  1. The above cited either facial trauma or sprains and strains are the most common injuries in rugby union.
- In the United States, Wetzler et al published a retrospective study of cervical spine injuries that occurred during the rugby scrum from 1970–1996 (Wetzler et al, 1998).
  1. Total 58% of rugby cervical spine injuries occurred during the scrum (Wetzler et al, 1998).
  2. Total 64% of the above injuries occurred during engagement (Wetzler et al, 1998).
  3. Only 36% of the above occurred when the scrum collapsed (Wetzler et al, 1998).
  4. Hookers accounted for 78% and props were 19% of the injured players. Second row players were the remaining 3% (Wetzler et al, 1998).

- In the United States 47.5% of all rugby cervical spine injuries occurred in hookers versus 18.6% outside of the United States (USA Rugby website; Wetzler et al, 1998).
- Total 57.6% of U.S. catastrophic rugby injuries occur in the scrum in contrast to 41.5% outside of the United States (Dietzen and Topping, 1999; Wetzler et al, 1998).
- It is theorized that the discrepancy may be due to the fact that most rugby players in the United States learn to play the sport at college age or older. This is in contrast to other countries where rugby skills and techniques are learned at a much younger age (Wetzler et al, 1998).
- In the United States, there is not a good database for rugby injuries other than catastrophic.

INJURIES BY POSITION

- The front row is most susceptible to injury during a scrum.
  1. When the ball is put into play during a scrum, the necks of the front row are already in a position of slight flexion.
  2. The two opposing scrums are applying an axial force on the cervical spines that is equivalent to 0.5–1.5 tons (Dietzen and Topping, 1999; Milburn, 1993).
  3. Collapse is often related to the following (Milburn, 1993):
     a. Inappropriately vertical force vectors during engagement
     b. Poor field conditions with poor traction
     c. Inexperience
     d. Fatigue
     e. Playing with injury
     f. Opposing scrum mismatch in terms of size, ability, strength, and experience
- The second row is susceptible to the following injuries:
  1. Neck injury—for the same reasons as the front row but to a lesser extent.
  2. Auricular hematomas, ear avulsions, and head lacerations, as their heads are positioned between the thighs of the front row players.
     a. Often wear scrumcaps or an electrical tape headband to secure their ears to the side of their head.
  3. Susceptible to injuries when they are being lifted during line outs.
- Flanker/Wing forward
  1. Susceptible to injuries in the tackling situation
  2. High incidence of acromioclavicular joint injuries
- Eightman
  1. Susceptible to similar head and facial injuries as the locks because of his or her head position between the locks.

- Scrumhalf
  1. Susceptible to contact injuries while attempting to secure the ball.
- Pack
  1. At risk for contact knee injuries (Dietzen and Topping, 1999).
- Backs
  1. At risk for contact and noncontact knee injuries (Dietzen and Topping, 1999).
  2. Susceptible to injury of the head, neck, and shoulders during tackling (Dietzen and Topping, 1999).
- In rucks, the players on the ground are at risk for abrasions, lacerations, contusions, and orofacial trauma from the cleats of other players.
- In mauls and rucks, players are susceptible to hand and finger injuries from binding to each others' jerseys.
- During tackling, players are at risk for the same injuries as other collision sports.

PREVENTION

- Locks often wear scrumcaps or electrical tape headbands to secure their ears to the side of their head to prevent ear injuries.
- Some players wear shoulder pads to attempt to prevent *acromioclavicular* (AC) joint injuries.
- There are currently no studies to date that show the above measures have prevented injury.
- On the rugby boots, no toe cleats (like baseball cleats) are allowed.
  1. Tackled players are frequently on the ground underneath players from both teams who are attempting to secure the ball with their feet.
- The referee conducts a safety inspection of the pitch and all players prior to the match.
  1. The referee may prohibit a player from participating if unsafe footwear, uniform, illegal equipment, or long fingernails are found.
  2. Medical personnel are encouraged to join the referee for the inspection.
- Since *tight five* players have the highest incidence of cervical spine injury in the United States, they should have extensive practice and instruction prior to competition.
- Depowering the scrum or having uncontested scrums in less experienced play may decrease the risk of cervical spine injury.
- Since fatigue is thought to be a risk factor for injury (Milburn, 1993), all players should maintain a high level of fitness.
- USA Rugby encourages all coaches to complete a series of coaching clinics. These clinics will arm

coaches with techniques to provide proper instruction on some of the more complex skills and techniques of the game.

SIDELINE PREPAREDNESS

- Since the spectrum of injury in rugby union is wide, the physician covering this sport must be well rounded and prepared to handle the variety of acute injuries.
- The nature of the substitution rules of rugby place more pressure on a sideline physician to make a timely decision on fitness to play. Prompt and accurate evaluation is therefore critical. The game continues without a substitution while the physician is evaluating the injured athlete. If another player replaces the injured rugger, he or she cannot return to the match, even if physically capable. Therefore, the coach is anxiously waiting for the physician to tell whether to play one man down till the injured person's return or whether a permanent substitution should be made.
- There is a delicate balance between not prematurely removing an athlete from play versus minimizing the time the team competes one man short while the physician is performing the evaluation.
- Lacerations deserve special mention as the team physician's proficiency in attending to a bleeding wound within the allotted "blood sub" time of 15 min will determine whether an athlete is able to return to play.
- Although rare, catastrophic injury has been reported in rugby union play. An emergency response plan should be preestablished in case of such a situation.

REFERENCES

Bird YN et al: The New Zealand Rugby injury and performance project: V. Epidemiology of a season of rugby injury. *Br J Sports Med* 32:319–325, 1998.
Chalmers, DJ, New Zealand's: Injury prevention research unit: Reducing sport and recreational injury. *Br J Sports Med* 28(4):221–222, 1994.
Dexter WW: Rugby, in Mellion MM, Putukian M, Madden CC (eds.): *Sports Medicine Secrets,* 3rd ed. Philadelphia, PA, Hanley & Belfus, 2003, pp 579–583.
Dietzen CJ, Topping BR, Rugby Football: *Phys Med Rehabil Clin N Am* 10(1):159–175, 1999.
Garraway M, Macleod D: Epidemiology of rugby football injuries. *Lancet North Am Ed* (345):1485–1487, 1995.
Gerrard DF, Waller AE, Bird YN: The New Zealand Rugby injury and performance project: II. Previous injury experience of a rugby-playing cohort. *Br J Sports Med* 28(4):229–233, 1994.
Marshall SW, Spencer RJ: Concussion and rugby: The hidden epidemic. *J Athl Train* 36(3):3334–3338, 2001.
Milburn PD: Biomechanics of Rugby union scrummaging, technical and safety issues. *Sports Med* 16(3):168–179, 1993.
Quarrie KL, Cantu RC, Chalmers DJ: Rugby union injuries to the cervical spine and spinal cord. *Sports Med* 32(10):633–653, 2002.
Quarrie KL et al: The New Zealand rugby injury and performance project: III. Anthropometric and physical performance characteristics of players. *Br J Sports Med* 29(4):263–270, 1995.
Quarrie KL, Handcock P, Toomey MJ et al: The New Zealand rugby injury and performance project. IV. Anthopometric and physical performance comparisons between positional categories of senior A rugby players. *Br J Sports Med* 30:53–56, 1996.
Quarrie KL, et al: The New Zealand rugby injury and performance project: VI. A prospective cohort study of risk factors for injury in rugby union football. *Br J Sports Med* 35:157–166, 2001.
Scher AT: Rugby injuries to the cervical spine and spinal cord: A 10-year review. *Neurol Athl Head Neck Injuries* 17(1):195–206, 1998.
USA Rugby Football Union: *USA Rugby Handbook,* 2002–2003.
USA Rugby website. *History: An American Tradition. www.usarugby.org*
Waller AE, Feehan M, Marshall SW: The New Zealand rugby injury and performance project: I. Design and methodology of a prospective follow-up study. *Br J Sports Med* 28(4):223–228, 1994.
Wetzler MJ, Akpata T, Laughlin W et al: Occurrence of cervical spine injuries during the rugby scrum. *Am J Sports Med* 26:1.(2):177, 1998.

88 RUNNING
Robert Wilder, MD, FACSM

EPIDEMIOLOGY OF RUNNING INJURIES

INTRODUCTION

- There are over 30 million runners of which more than 10 million run on more than 100 days per year.
- One million enter competitive races per year (Epperly, 2001; Van Mechelen, 1992; Jacobs and Berson, 1986).
- Yearly injury incidence rate ranges from 37 to 56% (Epperly, 2001; Van Mechelen, 1992; Jacobs and Berson, 1986; Walter et al, 1989; Lysholm and Wiklander, 1987).
- Injury rate ranges from 2.5 to 5.8 injuries per 1000 h of running (Epperly, 2001; Van Mechelen, 1992;

Lysholm and Wiklander, 1987). The lower rate of 2.5 per 1000 h is seen in long-distance and marathon runners. Sprinters have the highest rate of 5.8 per 1000 h, and middle distance runners are between the two at 5.6 per 1000 h (Lysholm and Wiklander, 1987).

• Despite the relatively high incidence rate of running injuries per runner per year, this incidence rate is still 2 to 6 times lower than in other sports (Epperly, 2001; Van Mechelen, 1992).

COMMON INJURY SITES

• Most running injuries are musculoskeletal overuse syndromes. Seventy to 80% occur from the knee down.
  1. Back   5%
  2. Hip and groin   15%
  3. Knee   40%
  4. Lower leg   20%
  5. Foot and ankle   20%
• Top running injuries (Epperly, 2001; Van Mechelen, 1992)

DIAGNOSIS	PERCENT
Patellofemoral pain syndrome	32.2
Tibial stress syndrome "shin splints"	17.3
Achilles tendinitis	7.2
Stress fractures	7.2
Plantar fasciitis	6.7
Illiotibial band syndrome	6.3
Patellar tendinitis	5.7
Metatarsal stress syndrome	3.3
Adductor strain	3
Hamstring strain	2.6
Posterior tibial tendinitis	2.6
Ankle sprain	2.4
Peroneus tendinitis	1.9
Illiac apophysitis	1.6

• Although there are no age- or gender-related differences, there are differences in injury pattern between sprinters, middle-distance runners, and long-distance runners. Hamstring strains and tendinitis are more commonly seen in sprinters; backache and hip problems are more commonly seen in middle distance runners; and foot problems are more common among long-distance and marathon runners (Lysholm and Wiklander, 1987).

RISK FACTORS FOR RUNNING INJURIES (Epperly, 2001)

• Important risk factors (for which a clear association with injury has been identified)
  1. Training mi per week (risk increases at 20 mi/week; more sharply at 40 mi/week)
  2. Previous running injury (within past 12 months)
  3. Inexperienced runner (running <3 years)
  4. Training intensity (especially with a recent transition)
• Equivocal risk factors (for which evidence demonstrating a clear link with injury is unclear)
  1. Hyper- or hypoflexibility
  2. Stretching exercises
  3. Running shoes
  4. Shoe orthotics
  5. Roadside running
  6. Malalignment problems
• Unrelated risk factors
  1. Age
  2. Gender
  3. Body morphology
  4. Running surface
  5. Cross training
  6. Time of day
  7. Warm-up or cool-down periods

BIOMECHANICS OF RUNNING

THE RUNNING GAIT CYCLE

• During walking, the stance phase occupies 40% of the gait cycle. The stance phase is decreased to approximately 30% while running and 20% while sprinting (Birrer and Buzermanis, 2001).
• Walking differs from running in that walking has two double support periods in stance, whereas running has two periods of double float in swing. Running does not have a period of double support (Birrer and Buzermanis, 2001).

KINEMATICS

• Generally there is an increase in joint range of motion as velocity increases; however, there are no major differences between walking and running kinematics in the coronal and transverse planes. Most kinematic differences occur in the sagittal plane (Birrer and Buzermanis, 2001; Oonpuu, 1990). The body lowers its *center of gravity* (COG) with increased speed by increasing flexion at the hips and knees and by increased dorsiflexion at the ankle (Birrer and Buzermanis, 2001; Mann and Hagy, 1980).
• The hip
  1. The hip demonstrates an overall increase in *range of motion* (ROM) as velocity increases. The most significant motion occurs in the sagittal plane. Most of this increase occurs in flexion, as the

amount of extension actually decreases slightly. Overall ROM was determined to be 43° with maximum flexion and extension—measuring 37 and 6°, respectively, for normal walking. In running, however, overall range of motion was increased to 46° with the hip flexing and never quite returning past neutral into extension (Birrer and Buzermanis, 2001; Oonpuu, 1994).

- The knee
  1. As in the hip, the most significant motion occurs in the sagittal plan. The knee joint demonstrates increased flexion as velocity increases, but extension is, as in the hip, decreased. Maximum flexion in walking reaches 64°, and extension is −8° (8° of flexion). In running, maximum flexion reaches 79°, and extension is −16° (16° of flexion) (Birrer and Buzermanis, 2001; Mann and Hagy, 1980).
- The ankle and foot
  1. Overall ROM at the ankle during walking is estimated to be 30°, with maximum plantar flexion of 18° and maximum dorsiflexion of 12°. Running produces a greater overall ankle ROM of 50° due to increased hip and knee flexion during running (Birrer and Buzermanis, 2001).
  2. At *initial contact,* due to the increased hip and knee flexion the ankle undergoes rapid dorsiflexion during the absorption phase. In running, because the ankle never quite reaches the amount of plantar flexion that it undergoes while walking, the amount of supination in the subtalar joint is limited but the degree of pronation is increased (Birrer and Buzermanis, 2001).
  3. Subtalar motion is determined by muscular activity as well as response to ground reactive forces. Midtarsal joint motion, however, is determined by subtalar position (Birrer and Buzermanis, 2001).
  4. When the calcaneus and the talus are supinated, the axis is such that an increased obliquity is produced across the oblique and longitudinal midtarsal joints. This serves to lock the midtarsal joint functionally, thereby resulting in a decrease in available motion and allowing the foot to become a "rigid lever." This occurs during late terminal stance and preswing. When the calcaneus and talus are pronated, the axis is such that an increased parallelism exists between the oblique and longitudinal midtarsal joints. This results in an increased available motion in these joints, serving to unlock the midtarsal joint and allowing an increased ROM for adaptation to the ground surface as well as absorbing the ground reactive forces, which lets the foot become a "mobile adapter." This occurs during the midstance (Birrer and Buzermanis, 2001).

5. As the foot makes contact with the floor, the pelvis, femur, and tibia begin the process of internal rotation. This internal rotation lasts through loading response and into midstance, resulting in eversion and unlocking of the subtalar joint. This results in subtalar pronation, which allows unlocking of the oblique and longitudinal midtarsal joints, resulting in further pronation. The pelvis, femur, and tibia then begin to rotate externally, which causes inversion and locking of the subtalar joint (Birrer and Buzermanis, 2001).

KINETICS

- Walking produces vertical ground reactive forces equal to 1.3 to 1.5 times body weight (Jacobs and Berson, 1986). During running, these ground reactive forces equal three to four times that of normal body weight (Rodgers, 1988).
- The percentage of muscle activity increases throughout stance phase during running. It is rare to see a muscle group active for more than 50% of the stance phase during walking, but in running, activity is noted for 70 to 80% of the stance phase (Mann).
- During walking, the *gluteus maximus* is active from the end of the swing phase until the foot is flat on the floor. This serves to decelerate the limb and stabilize the hip joint for initial contact. During running, however, it is active from terminal swing through 40% the stance phase. This helps to produce hip extension (Birrer and Buzermanis, 2001).
- The *hip abductors* function during the terminal swing and throughout 50% of the stance phase during walking and running. This serves to stabilize the stance leg pelvis at IC, which prevents excessive sagging of the swing leg (Birrer and Buzermanis, 2001; Inman, 1947).
- The *hip adductors* are active during the last one-third of the stance phase during walking. During running, they are active during the entire stance and swing phases (Birrer and Buzermanis, 2001; Mann).
- The *quadriceps* are active at the end of the swing phase to bring about terminal knee extension and to aid in hip flexion, through a concentric contraction. They also help stabilize the knee joint at initial contact, through an eccentric contraction. In running, they are highly active during the absorption phase of stance to deal with the greater requirements of weight acceptance. They are continually active throughout knee flexion eccentrically to limit the rate at which knee flexion occurs. They are active for 50 to 60% of the running stance phase and for only 25% of the walking stance phase (Birrer and Buzermanis, 2001).

- During walking the *hamstrings* are active at the end of swing phase and into stance phase until the foot is in full contact with the ground. This occurs at about 10% of the walking gait cycle. During running, they are active during the last third of the swing phase during hip and knee extension. Here they are acting concentrically across the hip joint but eccentrically across the knee joint. This action initiates hip extension and resists knee extension simultaneously (Birrer and Buzermanis, 2001).
- During walking, the *anterior tibial muscle* group is active from late stance phase through the swing phase and then for the first 10 to 15% of the next stance phase. This produces dorsiflexion of the ankle during the swing phase through concentric contraction. It also helps to control plantar flexion by initial contact through eccentric contraction, thereby preventing foot slap. During running, they are active from late stance phase, through the swing phase and for the first 50 to 60% of the next stance phase. For their duration of activity they are undergoing concentric contraction. During walking, they decelerate foot plantar flexion at IC; however, during running they appear to accelerate movement of the leg over the fixed foot. In heel strikers, a greater degree of activity is found in the anterior tibial muscle group than in midfoot strikers (Birrer and Buzermanis, 2001).
- Activity of the *posterior leg musculature* begins during terminal swing of gait. During walking, these muscles act to resist forward movement of the tibia over the fixed foot during the stance phase. They are active from 25 to 50% of the stance phase through mostly eccentric contraction. During their last 25% of activity, they undergo concentric contraction to initiate active plantar flexion. During running gait, initial contact is a period of rapid dorsiflexion. Here the triceps undergo eccentric contraction, again to resist this motion. They are active for approximately 60% of the stance phase. Initially they serve to stabilize the ankle joint at initial contact, and then to provide for propulsion (Birrer and Buzermanis, 2001).

COMMON RUNNING INJURIES

PATELLOFEMORAL SYNDROME

- Definition
  1. Pain associated with the articular surface of the patella and femoral condyles.
  2. *Runners knee*—No. 1 presenting complaint to runner's clinics
  3. No. 1 cause lost time in basic training in military recruits

- Diagnosis
  1. Anterior, peripatellar, and subpatellar pain
  2. Increased pain following prolonged sitting (theatre sign) as well as running downhill and walking downstairs.
  3. Apprehension (shrug) sign
  4. Abnormal patella tilt (tilt less than 5° in males and less than 10° in females)
  5. Abnormal patella glide (medial glide less than 2 quadrants, lateral glide in excess of three quadrants)
- Contributing factors
  1. Femoral dysplasia
  2. Patellar facet asymmetry
  3. Malalignments (especially those contributing to excessive pronation)
     a Femoral anteversion
     b. External tibial torsion
     c. Varus ankle, foot
     d. Patella alta, baja
     e. Weak VMO
     f. Tight lateral structures (ITB)
     g. Increased Q angle
- Treatment
  1. Patellofemoral syndrome treatment
     a. Correct biomechanical factors which lead to compensatory subtalar pronation and obligatory internal tibial rotation: genu valgum, tibia vara, hind foot varus, and forefoot pronation
     b. Flexibility: ITB, HS, and gastrocnemius
     c. Manual therapy to stretch tight retinaculum: medial glide and tilt.
     d. Strengthening: Quadriceps, hip abductors and external rotators
        i. Multiangle isometrics
        ii. Short arc terminal extensions (last 30 deg. ROM extension)
        iii. Gluteal strength
        iv. Closed chain strengthening with cocontraction of quads, HS, gastroc soleus
     e. McConnell taping
     f. Bracing (patellar straps and braces)
- Consider with persistent symptoms
  1. *Magnetic resonance imaging* (MRI): Osteochondritis and cartilage injury
  2. Injections: Steroid and synvisc
  3. Surgery: Lateral release if tight retinaculum and realignment

ILIOTIBIAL BAND SYNDROME

- Definition
  1. An overuse tendonopathy of the iliotibial band most commonly as it passes over the lateral femoral condyle
  2. No. 1 cause lateral knee pain in runners

- Diagnosis
  1. Lateral pain and crepitus at lateral femoral condyle (or insertion at Gerdy's tubercle)
  2. Tight ITB on OBER test
  3. Abductor weakness
- Contributing factors
  1. Varus positioning of knee, tibia, and foot
  2. Internal tibial torsion
  3. Excessive supination or pronation
  4. Tightness abductors, adductors, ext rotators, and hip extensors
  5. Abductor weakness
- Treatment
  1. PRICEMM (iontophoresis)
  2. Dual action strap
  3. Foam roller exercise for soft tissue work
  4. Flexibility and strength (hip abductors, adductors, rotators, flexors, and extensors)
- Consider with persistent symptoms
  1. Injection (steroid)
  2. MRI r/o lateral meniscus and other

SHIN SPLINTS

- Definition
  1. Shin splints, or medial tibial stress syndrome, is a clinical entity characterized by diffuse tenderness over the posteromedial aspect of the distal third of the tibia. Shin splints have been reported to account for 12–18% of running injuries (James, Bates, and Ostering, 1978; Briner, Jr, 1988; Gudas, 1980; Pinshaw, Atlas, and Noakes, 1984) and in 4% of all military recruits in basic training (Andrish, Bergfeld, and Walheim, 1974). Women appear more frequently affected than men.
  2. Medial tibial stress syndrome is to be differentiated from stress fractures and exertional compartment syndrome. Although different entities, they may coexist. Plain films are negative (except in cases of previous or coexistent stress fracture). Bone scans will demonstrate characteristic vertical linear increased activity along the tibial periosteum, which differs from the more focal fusiform increased radiotracer uptake exhibited by stress fractures.
  3. Medial tibial stress syndrome is felt by most to represent a periostalgia or tendinopathy along the tibial attachment of the tibialis posterior or soleus muscles. Other proposed etiologies have included posterior compartment syndrome and fascial inflammation. Detmer proposed a classification scheme for medial tibial stress syndrome based on etiology. Type 1 included local stress fractures,

type 2 periostitis/periostalgia, and type 3 due to deep posterior compartment syndrome (Detmer, 1986).
- Diagnosis
  1. Dull ache medial shaft with activity
  2. Tenderness to palpation along shaft
  3. Normal neurovascular examination and X-ray
- Contributing factors
  1. Factors that increase valgus forces and pronation, which then increase eccentric contraction of the soleus and tibialis posterior: femoral anteversion, genu varum, tibia and forefoot varus, and excessive Q angle
  2. Excessive pes planus or cavus
  3. Tarsal coalation
  4. Leg length inequality
  5. Muscle imbalances: Inflexibility of plantar flexors; weakness of dorsiflexors, plantarflexors, and inventors
  6. Extrinsic risk factors include improper shoe wear, a rapid transition in training, inadequate warm-up, running on uneven or hard surfaces, running in cold weather, and low calcium intake.
- Treatment
  1. Flexibility: Gastroc-soleus, tibialis posterior
  2. Strength: Concentric and eccentric including tibialis posterior soleus, tibialis anterior, FH, FDL
  3. Orthotic to control compensatory pronation
  4. Shin sleeve
- Consider with persistent symptoms
  1. Bone scan/MRI r/o stress fx
  2. Compartment testing to r/o compartment syndrome
  3. Consider lumbar radiculopathy

EXERTIONAL COMPARTMENT SYNDROME

- Definition
  1. Chronic exertional compartment syndrome is defined as reversible ischemia secondary to a non-compliant osseofascial compartment that is unresponsive to the expansion of muscle volume that occurs with exercise. Most commonly seen in the lower leg, exertional compartment syndrome in athletes has also been described in the thigh and medial compartment of the foot (Raether and Lutter, 1982; Birnbaum, 1983; Mollica and Duyshart, 2002).
  2. There are four major compartments in the leg. Each is bound by bone and fascia, and each contains a major nerve.
     a. The anterior compartment contains the extensor hallucis longus, extensor digitorum longus, peroneus tertius, and anterior tibialis muscles, as well as the deep peroneal nerve.

b. The lateral compartment contains the peroneus longus and brevis as well as the superficial peroneal nerve.
c. The superficial posterior compartment contains the gastrocnemius and soleus muscles and the sural nerve.
d. The deep posterior compartment contains the flexor hallucis longus, flexor digitorum longus, and posterior tibialis muscles, as well as the posterior tibial nerve. Some authors believe that the posterior tibialis should be considered a separate compartment, since it is surrounded by its own fascia (Albertson and Dammann, 2001).
3. Anterior compartment syndrome is most common (45%), followed by the deep posterior compartment (40%), lateral compartment (10%), and superficial posterior compartments (5%) (Edwards and Myerson, 1996).
- Diagnosis
1. Recurrent exercise-induced leg discomfort that occurs at a well-defined and reproducible point and increases if the training persists. Pain is usually described as a tight, cramplike, or squeezing ache over a specific compartment of the leg. Relief of symptoms only occurs with discontinuation of activity. Examination may or may not demonstrate fascial hernias. In some cases, the classic exertional component is not as evident, and patients complain of pain at rest or with daily activities as well.
2. A neurologic and vascular examination should also be performed with reproduction of the symptoms. Understanding the distribution of nerves and functions of muscles in relation to symptoms can help identify the affected compartment in cases where the pain is not well localized to one specific compartment, or it may help determine which compartments are more severely affected in cases where more than one compartment is involved.
   a. Anterior compartment: Weakness of dorsiflexion or toe extension, paresthesias over the dorsum of the foot, numbness in the first web space, or even transient or persistent foot drop.
   b. Lateral compartment: Sensory changes over the anterolateral aspect of the leg and weakness of ankle eversion. An inversion as well as equinus deformity may also be present.
   c. Superficial posterior compartment: Dorsolateral foot hypoesthesia and plantar flexion weakness
   d. Deep posterior compartment: Paresthesias in the plantar aspect of the foot and weakness of toe flexion and foot inversion.
3. The gold standard diagnostic tool is intracompartment pressure monitoring.

4. One or more of the following pressure criteria must be met in addition to a history and physical examination that is consistent with the diagnosis of *chronic exertional compartment syndrome* (CECS): Preexercise pressure ≥5 mm-Hg, 1-min postexercise pressure ≥30 mm-Hg, or 5-min postexercise pressure ≥20 mm-Hg. Diagnosis may require the *sport specific activity* to induce symptoms and raise intracompartment pressure (Padhiar and King, 1996).
5. Other tools that have been employed in the diagnosis of compartment syndrome include—the triple phase bone scan, MRI, near-infrared spectroscopy, and MIBI perfusion imaging (Wilder).
- Contributing factors
1. Enclosure of compartmental contents in an inelastic fascial sheath, increased volume of the skeletal muscle with exertion due to blood flow and edema, muscle hypertrophy as a response to exercise, and dynamic contraction factors due to the gait cycle.
2. It has also been proposed that myofiber damage as a result of eccentric exercise causes a release of protein bound ions and a subsequent increase in osmotic pressure within the compartment. The increase in osmotic pressure increases capillary relaxation pressure, thus decreasing the blood flow.
3. Rapid increases in muscle size due to fluid retention are also believed to play a role in the development of chronic exertional compartment syndrome in athletes taking the popular supplement creatine (Glorioso and Wilckens, 2001).
- Treatment
1. Conservative measures include relative rest (limiting activity to that level which avoids any more than minimal symptoms), anti-inflammatories, stretching and strengthening of the involved muscles, and orthotics (particularly in cases of excessive pronation).
2. Should symptoms persist despite 6–12 weeks of conservative care, or in cases of extreme pressure elevation, surgical remediation (fasciotomy of the involved compartments with or without fasciectomy) should be undertaken.

ACHILLES TENDONOPATHY

- Definition
1. A spectrum of tissue disorders involving the Achilles tendon and sheath:
   a. Tendinitis
   b. Tendonosis
   c. Peritendonitis
   d. Tear

- Diagnosis
  1. Tenderness at myotendinous junction or insertion
- Contributing Factors
  1. Pronation
  2. Lower extremity varus
  3. Tight heel cord
  4. Weak *dorsiflexors/plantar flexors* (DF/PDF)
- Treatment
  1. Heel lifts
  2. Control pronation
  3. Flexibility (include gastroc and soleus)
  4. Strength (particulary eccentric strength)
  5. Modalities (ionto and cross-friction massage)
- Consider if persistent
  1. Retrocalcaneal bursitis
  2. MRI (evaluate tears)
  3. Immobilization
  4. Lidocaine injections for periotendonitis

PLANTAR FASCIITIS

- Definition
  1. An overload injury including inflammation degeneration, and tearing of the plantar fascia, most commonly at its calcaneal insertion.
- Contributing factors
  1. Tight gastroc soleus, plantar fascia
  2. Rigid rear foot
  3. Over pronation or supination
- Diagnosis
  1. Pain plantar heel worse in a.m. and with activity
  2. Tenderness plantar medial heel
  3. Normal neuro examination
  4. No bony (calcaneal) tenderness
- Treatment
  1. Phase 1:
     a. anti-inflammatories: *Nonsteroidal anti-inflammatory drugs* (NSAIDs) and medrol
     b. Device (CTF brace)
     c. Stretch (gastroc-soleus, plantar fascia, hamstring, ITB)
     d. Strength (foot intrinsics)
  2. Phase 2:
     a. P.T. (phono/ionto, massage)
     b. Continue exercise
     c. Different device (heel cushion)
  3. Phase 3: Night splint
  4. Phase 4,5: Injections (3 max), orthotics
- Consider if persistent
  1. MRI: r/o calcaneal stress injury
  2. EMG/NCS: r/o Medial calcaneal, Plantar neuropathy, and radiculopathy
  3. Surgery if fail conservative care (6 months)

STRESS FRACTURES

- Definition
  1. Failure of bone to adapt adequately to mechanical loads (ground reaction forces and muscle contraction) experienced during physical activity.
  2. Tibial stress fractures predominate in distance runners. Navicular stress fractures predominate in track athletes.
- Diagnosis
  1. Focal tenderness
  2. Recent transition in training
  3. X-ray (often neg., esp. early)
  4. Bone scan (all three phases with increased uptake)
  5. MRI (periosteal and marrow edema $T_2 > T_1$)
- Contributing factors
  1. Rapid transition in training
  2. Osteopenia/Osteoporosis
  3. Menstrual irregularities, in particular amennorrhea >6 months.
  4. Excessive pes cavus (femoral, tibial) or pes planus (metatarsals)
  5. Poor shoe wear
- Treatment
  1. Noncritical: Noncritical stress fractures can be treated with 6–8 weeks of relative rest and include the following: medial tibia, metatarsals 2, 3, 4, and 5 metatarsal avulsion. Athletes may benefit from a short period (i.e., 3 weeks) in a walking boot.
  2. Critical stress fractures require more specific attention due to slower healing and higher rates of nonunion and include the following: femoral neck, anterior tibia, medal malleolus, navicular, and base 5th metatarsal.
     a. Femoral neck
        i. Normal X-ray, no cortical break: Conservative RX, *partial weight-bearing* (PWB) to *weight-bearing as tolerated* (WBAT). Follow clinically and serial MRI 8–12 weeks.
        ii. Cortical break: ortho. Superior (distraction) fractures have a higher incidence of worsening and nonunion than inferior (compression) fractures.
     b. Anterior tibia
        i. Casting versus relative rest up to 6–8 months.
        ii. If no healing: Ortho (transverse drilling, grafting, medullary fixation)
     c. Medial malleolus
        i. Nondisplaced: Boot or aircast 6 weeks
        ii. Displaced or nonunion: Ortho
     d. Navicular
        i. Nonweight bearing 6–8 weeks
        ii. Progressive activity over 6 more weeks

e. Proximal 5th metatarsal
  i. Jones *fracture* (Fx) of proximal diaphysis: Cast, *non weight-bearing* (NWB) 6–10 weeks
  ii. Nonunion: Ortho.

SOME PRACTICAL GUIDELINES FOR CLINICIANS

- Certain injuries require the runner to refrain from running (stress fractures, radiculopathy). With most overuse injuries, however, some level of training may be permitted following the Relative Activity Modification Guidelines (Wilder RP: The Runners Clinics at UVa)
  1. Pain/discomfort should not exceed the mild level (≤3/10 on the 10-point pain scale).
  2. Pain that eases after a warm-up is generally benign, do not run if pain progressively worsens.
  3. Do not run if you are limping or changing your gait mechanics.
- Supplement lost run training with cross-training (aqua running, bike, elliptical).
- Do not increase mileage more rapidly than 10% per week.
- Long run of the week increases no more than 2 mi per week, and should not exceed 30% of one's weekly mileage.
- Change shoes every 350–400 mi.

REFERENCES

Albertson K, Dammann G: The leg, in O'Connor F, Wilder R, (eds.): *The Textbook of Running Medicine*, New York, NY, McGraw-Hill, 2001, pp 647–654.

Andrish JT, Bergfeld JA, Walheim J: *A prospective study on the management of shin splints. J Bone Joint Surg Am* 56(8): 1697–1700, 1974.

Birnbaum J: *Recurrent compartment syndrome in the posterior thigh. Am J Sports Med* 11(1):48–49, 1983.

Birrer R, Buzermanis S, DellaCorte M, et al: Biomechanics of running, in O'Connor F, Wilder R, (eds.): *The Textbook of Running Medicine.* New York, NY, McGraw-Hill, 2001.

Briner WW, Jr: Shinsplints. *Am Fam Physician* 37(2):155–160, 1988.

Detmer DE: Chronic shin splints. Classification and management of medial tibial stress syndrome. *Sports Med* 3(6):436–446, 1986.

Edwards P, Myerson M: Exertional compartment syndrome of the leg: Steps for expedient return to activity. *Phys Sportsmed* 24:1996.

Epperly T, Fields K: Epidemiology of running injuries, in O'Connor F, Wilder R, (eds.): *The Textbook of Running Medicine.* New York, NY, McGraw-Hill, 2001.

Glorioso J, Wilckens H: Exertional leg pain, in O'Conner F, Wilder R (eds.): *The Textbook of Running Medicine.* New York, NY, McGraw-Hill, 2001, pp 181–198.

Gudas CJ: Patterns of lower-extremity injury in 224 runners. *Compr Ther* 6(9):50–59, 1980.

Inman VT: Functional aspects of the abductor muscles of the hip. *J Bone Joint Surg Am* 29:607, 1947.

Jacobs SJ, Berson BL: Injuries to runners: A study of entrants to a 10,000 meter race. *Am J Sports Med* 14(2):151–155, 1986.

James SL, Bates BT Osternig LR: Injuries to runners. *Am J Sports Med* 6(2):40–50, 1978.

Lysholm J, Wiklander J: Injuries in runners. *Am J Sports Med* 15(2):168–171, 1987.

Mann R: Biomechanics of running, in Nicholas J, Hershman E (eds.) *The Lower Extremity and Spine in Sports Medicine,* C.V. Mosby, St. Louis, 1986.

Mann RA, Hagy J: Biomechanics of walking, running, and sprinting. *Am J Sports Med* 8(5):345–350, 1980.

Mollica MB, Duyshart SC: Analysis of pre- and postexercise compartment pressures in the medial compartment of the foot. *Am J Sports Med* 30(2):268–271, 2002.

Oonpuu S: The biomechanics of running: A kinematic and kinetic analysis. *Instr Course Lect* 39:305–318, 1990.

Oonpuu S: The biomechanics of walking and running. *Clin Sports Med* 13(4):843–863, 1994.

Padhiar N, King JB: Exercise induced leg pain-chronic compartment syndrome. Is the increase in intra-compartment pressure exercise specific? *Br J Sports Med* 30(4):360–362, 1996.

Pinshaw R, Atlas V, Noakes TD: The nature and response to therapy of 196 consecutive injuries seen at a runners' clinic. *S Afr Med J* 65(8):291–298, 1984.

Raether PM, Lutter LD: Recurrent compartment syndrome in the posterior thigh. Report of a case. *Am J Sports Med* 10(1): 40–43, 1982.

Rodgers MM: Dynamic biomechanics of the normal foot and ankle during walking and running. *Phys Ther* 68(12):1822–1830, 1988.

Van Mechelen W: Running injuries. A review of the epidemiological literature. *Sports Med* 14(5):320–335, 1992.

Walter SD et al: The Ontario cohort study of running-related injuries. *Arch Intern Med* 149(11):2561–2564, 1989.

Wilder R, Sethi S: Overuse injuries: Tendinopathies, stress fractures, compartment syndrome, and shin splints. *Clin Sports Med* 23:55–81, 2004.

89 SOCCER

Nicholas A Piantanida, MD

INTRODUCTION

- Soccer has a worldwide attraction to at least 40 million people and is the fastest growing sport in America (Hoy et al, 1992; Soccer Industry Counsel of America, 1996).

PHYSICAL DEMANDS OF SOCCER

- The American Academy of Pediatrics classifies Soccer as a contact sport.
- The 26th Bethesda Conference classifies soccer as a low static: high dynamic sport.
- Soccer demands physical strength through the trunk and lower extremity.
- The aerobic challenges of soccer mesh the endurance requirements of a distance runner with the abrupt acceleration demands of a sprinter. The average distance covered by an elite midfield male player is in the 10-km range, with the strikers, and fullbacks and centre-backs covering respectively less. Sprinting comprises 10% of the total distance covered (Reilly and Thomas, 1976).
- Agility and proprioception skills are essential to complete soccer's sport specific tasks to make quick changes in direction and jumps in the air.
- The physiologic demands of soccer require proper nutrition and hydration. The *wet bulb globe temperature* (WBGT) and both exercise duration and the intensity will dictate individual requirements for optimal fluid consumption and frequency. The American College of Sports Medicine recommends activities be halted when WBGTs exceed 82°F (28°C) (Elias, Roberts, and Thorson, 1991).
- Young competitors dehydrated as little as 2% will not only have impairments in performance but have a diminished ability to dissipate heat and are more prone to heat related injury. A 5% drop in body weight during or following a soccer match or practice should sideline that athlete for 24 hours to recuperate fluid losses and to identify an intrinsic etiology such as poor acclimatization, ergogenics, or illness (Elias, Roberts, and Thorson, 1991; Saltin and Costill, 1998) (level of evidence C, expert/concensus opinion).
- It has been demonstrated that carbohydrate ingestion in the fluids before and during soccer activity can delay muscle glycogen depletion (Leatt and Jacobs, 1989) (level of evidence A, randomized controlled trial). In a study by Foster and coworkers, they demonstrated that indoor soccer athletes who drank a glucose polymer enhanced work output and increased time to exhaustion when compared to controls (Foster et al, 1986) (level of evidence A, randomized trial).
- The recommended amount of carbohydrate to maintain glucose levels and spare muscle glycogen is 30 to 60 g/h.

SOCCER INJURY RATES

- The overall injury incidence in soccer is favorable. In comparison with American football, youth athletes playing soccer sustain two to five times fewer injuries (Sullivan et al, 1980).
- Injury rates within the sport of soccer increase with participant age and correlate with the increased intensity of the match. More injuries occur during competitive games than during practice. When a correction is incorporated for exposure rates, senior athletes (age >18) sustain 15 to 30 times as many injuries as youths (Keller, Noyes, and Buncher, 1987).
- Female youths have injury rates over twice as high as male youths. Engstrom and colleagues reported an incidence per 1000 player hours of 12 for girls versus 5 for boys (Engstrom, Johanoson, and Tornkvist, 1991). Schmidt-Olson reported an incidence per 1000 player hours of 17.6 for girls versus 7.4 for boys (Schmidt-Olsen et al, 1991).
- In most studies, ankle sprain is the most common injury type in male and female soccer players (Sullivan et al, 1980; Albert, 1983; Nilsson and Roaas, 1978; National Collegiate Athletic Association, 2000); however, Ekstrand in his study of 256 soccer injuries in senior players found knee injuries in 20% of his athletes and ankle injuries in 17% (Ekstrand and Gillquist, 1983). The difference here possibly reflects self-selection as players who sustained ankle injuries as youth could have left the sport or played with ankle braces as adults. Or, the style of play could follow the finding that 50% of knee injuries are attributed to tackling maneuvers (Nielsen and Yde, 1989) and those players/opponents involved in this high-risk exchange were more commonplace in Ekstrand's study of senior athletes.
- Ankle sprain is implicated as a reinjury 56% of the time (Soderman, 2001).
- Soccer injury rates reported by the National Collegiate Athletic Association (NCAA) use an established injury surveillance system to follow male and female collegiate injuries (Putukian, Mandelbaum, and Brown, 2002).
- Head injuries account for 1.2 to 8% of all injuries, depending on the study. Youth soccer participants suffer more head injuries than adults and this is thought to be attributed to underdeveloped neck muscles to absorb the impact shock, increased ball-weight: head-weight ratio, and, more importantly, improper head ball technique (Keller, Noyes, and Buncher, 1987).
- Injury type follows gender differences. Women soccer players suffer more concussions than men at a ratio 4.3:1 and more *anterior cruciate ligament* (ACL) injuries 1.8:1 (practice) and 5.78:1 (games) (Putukian, Mandelbaum, and Brown, 2002).
- Indoor versus outdoor soccer injury rates are similar in severity and type (Putukian et al, 1996).
- Natural grass versus artificial surface soccer injury rates reflect a higher injury incidence in games played

on grass, where males had six times higher total injuries and female injuries were 4.3 times higher (Soderman, 2001).

SOCCER INJURY CHARACTERISTICS

ANKLE INJURY

- The mechanism of an ankle sprain is often an inversion stress as the talus tilts in plantar flexion to manage tasks such as pivoting, jumping, and hard turns with the ball. In this position the *anterior talofibular ligament* (ATFL) is at maximal tension and most vulnerable to injury. The *calcaneal fibular ligament* (CFL) and posterior talo-fibular ligament follow in order of injury behind the ATFL. The spectrum of severity ranges from a lateral ankle ligament stretch (Grade 1) to partial tear (Grade 2) to complete tear (Grade 3).
- Medial ankle ligament injuries are much more rare due to the dominant strength of the deltoid ligament. Therefore, a medial ankle disruption suggests a high-energy impact and will possibly demonstrate ankle mortise alteration requiring surgical management for fractures and follow a longer recovery period.
- Soccer players are susceptible to high ankle injuries. During collisions or contested balls, the ankle position during impact can be in the talar neutral position, with or without a slight lateral talar tilt. This predisposes the athlete to greater stresses along the calcaneal fibular ligament and the inferior anterior tibial-fibular ligament. Performing a proximal tib-fib "squeeze test" with distal referred pain at the ankle or instability with external foot rotation is suggestive for a high ankle sprain.
- In the ankle with persistent pain and swelling beyond two weeks the differential diagnosis should include talar dome lesions, such as osteochondral fractures or a fracture to the lateral process of the talus. If clinical suspicion is high an MRI should be done.
- The injured soccer player with chronic anterior ankle pain extending on to the midfoot who had an acute axial loading of the fore- and midfoot (kick into the turf) should be evaluated for a bifurcate ligament injury, impingement syndrome (especially for repeat ankle injuries) or Lisfranc fracture. If clinical suspicion dictates and weight bearing X-rays of the ankle/foot are normal then a MRI of the ankle/foot should be done.
- Posterior ankle pain or hind foot pain in a soccer athlete should raise concern in the young athlete (Engstrom, Johanoson, and Tornkvist, 1991; Schmidt-Olsen et al, 1991; Albert, 1983; Nilsson and Roaas, 1978; National Collegiate Athletic Association, 2000; Ekstrand and Gillquist, 1983) for Sever's disease or more commonly retrocalcaneal bursitis with indoor soccer players who have a pattern of repetitive heel trauma against the sideboards. Achilles tendinitis differs from the above two conditions by presenting several centimeters proximally to the tendon insertion into the calcaneus.
- Chronic posterior ankle pain should draw concern for a calcaneal stress fracture as evident by calcaneal squeeze test or an os trigonum fracture. Both can be verified by triple phase nuclear bone scan.

KNEE INJURY

- Soccer players can experience the gamut of overuse and acute knee problems. Youth players are prone to Osgood-Schlatter disease or any other patello-femoral tracking maladies seen in all running sports. Senior soccer players will suffer collateral ligament and meniscal injuries along with the pain of creeping osteoarthritis or patellar chondromalacia.
- With the leg well grounded by the cleats of the soccer shoe, rapid rotational and flexion changes of the trunk or lower leg as in passing the soccer ball may produce sudden rotation of the femur relative to the fixed leg causing meniscal and/or knee ligament injuries. As mentioned earlier, tackling is a high-risk maneuver where knee ligament strain often occurs when a player is tackled with the loaded leg secured to the ground.
- Soccer causes a higher incidence of meniscus injuries, but the extreme morbidity caused by ACL injuries has generated broad investigational research interest.
- Soccer players rupture their ACL through direct contact or noncontact. The latter mechanism is the predominant means for ACL injury in most sports other than skiing; however, Arendt and Dick (Arendt and Dick, 1995) reported that male collegiate soccer players have an equal rate of contact versus noncontact ACL injuries. Female collegiate soccer players follow the usual trend for noncontact ACL injuries but as previously mentioned dominates the males in this injury category.
- The mechanism of noncontact ACL injury follows the common pattern of deceleration coupled with pivoting with internal or external rotation or the awkward landing of a varus or valgus collapsed knee. (Boden et al 2000) studied the mechanism of ACL injury as they investigated 85 athletes with ACL tears. They reported 72% of the ACL tears involved noncontact deceleration occurring at an average knee flexion of 23° at foot strike. (Delfico and Garrett 1998) write that at this angle of knee flexion the maximal anterior tibial translation

occurs coupled with maximal eccentric quadriceps contraction to supply the force in the noncontact rupture of the ACL.

- Contact ACL injuries in male soccer players follow a pattern of collision with a valgus stress to the knee resulting in associated injuries to the menisci, the collateral ligaments, and the articular cartilage.
- In the cases of chondral injuries, extreme stress is placed on the articular cartilage through repetitive abrasive wear of high velocity pivoting and deceleration or the acute disruption of the deep cartilage ultra-structure by large shear forces. Chondral lesions are more often seen on the femoral condyle. Acute X-ray imaging for a swollen knee should include tunnel views to rule out an osteochondral fracture and if present, should be staged by knee MRI and co-managed with an orthopedic surgeon.

LOWER LEG INJURY

- A soccer player's lower leg is vulnerable to abrasions, contusions, and fractures. Shin guards have become the only mandatory protective devices in soccer, but serve primarily to protect the leg from minor soft tissue injuries. (Boden et al) reported in his series of soccer tibial and fibular fractures that 90% occurred in athletes wearing shin guards.
- The more typical scenarios involving lower leg injuries of any severity occur with aggressive slide tackles from behind with injury to the offensive player's fixed leg or when opposing players contest a loose ball in scoring position where a haphazard swinging kick or a lunging foot results in high velocity contact (Boden, 1998).
- With combined tibia and fibula fractures the soccer player is sidelined on average of 40 weeks. Isolated fibula and tibia fractures return to competitive play on average of 18 and 35 weeks, respectively. Both combined tib-fib fractures and isolated tibial fractures have a high incidence of recovery complications (Boden, 1998).
- Overuse injuries to the lower extremity span the broad differential for exertional lower leg pain. These include but are not limited to compartment syndrome, *medial tibial stress syndrome* (MTSS), and stress fractures.
- Anterior tibial compartment syndrome can be insidious with the effort dependent running pain that reduces performance over several months to years. Or in another scenario, an acute compartment syndrome may occur when a player sustains a high velocity kick to the protected or unprotected anterior or lateral lower leg. In both cases, the player may describe

lower leg pain with tingling and/or weakness extending on to the dorsum of the foot. Diagnostic stryker compartment testing and comanagement with an orthopedic surgeon should follow.

- Normal connective tissue and bone adaptation occurs in cyclic progression. Injury patterns for MTSS and stress fractures are multifactorial and are exercise dose dependent where extremes of frequency, intensity, and duration are common contributors.
- Stress fractures and MTSS are diagnostic challenges best differentiated by triple phase bone scan and treated with varying degrees of activity modification.

GROIN INJURY

- The mechanism of groin injury in the soccer athlete is associated with the ball manipulation skills where the leg gets overstretched at the groin while the hip is abducted and externally rotated, sometimes against an opposing force, such as the ground or the opponent. This process of overstretching compromises the adolescent's apophysial pelvic ring or pubic attachments or in the case of the senior player the muscular—tendonous attachments.
- Groin pain can follow a pattern of overuse that starts with adductor muscle tendonopathy. These cases should be distinguished from osteitis pubis and sports hernias, which can present with a similar pain pattern.
- Hip flexor strain to the iliopsoas is common in soccer and is characterized by deep groin pain with an occasional snapping hip sensation or pain extension onto the anterior thigh. Treatment consists of relative rest with stretching of the hip flexors and rotators. An iliopsoas strengthening program should precede the return to competitive play (Morelli and Smith, 2001).
- Groin disruption was named Gilmore's Groin in 1980 following the successful treatment of three professional soccer players who had been sidelined with pain for 3 months. Clinical symptoms include the insidious unilateral pain in the adductor region that progresses with activity and follows a course of post activity aggravation getting out of bed or the car. Examination findings are minimal and variable but may include tenderness and dilation of the internal inguinal ring on scrotal hernia palpation. The features of this condition include torn external oblique aponeurosis, torn conjoined tendon—conjoined tendon tear from the pubic tubercle, dehiscence between conjoined tendon and inguinal ligament, and no palpable hernia. Diagnosis should include stork radiographs to evaluate pelvic stability. Cases that fail the rehabilitative process should go to surgery for repair (Gilmore, 1998).

HEAD INJURY

- Soccer is unique among sports in the role the head functions to purposely assist the player in the sport. One study found that the average soccer player heads the ball up to 10 times per game (Jordan et al, 1996).
- The heading technique is a complex synchronized motion whereby the head strikes forcefully through the ball as the trunk goes into flexion. Maintaining a rigid neck during impact diminishes potential injury from angular head and neck acceleration.
- Speculation exists as to the risk of successive head balls over an extended career of playing soccer. Such subclinical concussions may predispose soccer athletes to brain injury analogous to the *punch drunk* syndrome of chronic progressive traumatic encephalopathy seen in career boxers. In 1995, a limited study by Witol and Webbe captured national attention by implicating the action of heading balls as causing decreased IQ scores (Witol and Webbe, 1995).
- Though this study was never published in a referenced medical journal it generated further research interest to question the validity of heading as a cause for brain injury. In a study by Haglund and Eriksson 1993), they studied *typical headers* soccer players and a control group using neuropyschiatric, radiologic, and *electroencephalogram* (EEG) data and found no differences in the groups. (Jordan et al 1996) analyzed U.S. National Soccer Team players with brain MRI and a head injury questionnaire. This study found no differences in brain anatomy when comparing soccer player MRIs with age matched controlled track athletes, but remarkably the questionnaire identified a new concern for the higher incidence of unrecognized concussions in soccer athletes. (Delaney et al 2002) completed a retrospective study in the Fall 1999 reflecting this same finding that 19.8% of concussed soccer players realized that they had suffered a concussion during the season.
- Therefore, currently with limited research the data suggests that heading the ball is safe; however, many studies are underway and the American Youth Soccer Organization recommends that children under the age of 10 not head the soccer ball.
- Regarding concussions in soccer, they occur many times without acknowledgement from the player. Concussions in soccer are a result of impact with another player, the ground or the goal posts.
- Assessment and management of a head injured soccer athlete should be no different from that of any other athlete. Neuropsychological testing is beneficial if there exists a preevent baseline study for comparison.

Diagnostic studies and return to play criteria are discussed in another section.

EYE INJURY

- The mechanism for eye injuries is usually blunt trauma caused by a kicked ball or the kicking foot. A hyphema is the most common injury type and should be comanaged with an ophthalmologist.

PREVENTION

- Ekstrand et al (Ekstrand and Gillquist, 1983) has demonstrated that in soccer injuries can be reduced by 75% by the implementation of a multilevel approach.
- Training errors need the careful attention of a skilled coaching staff that recognizes that quality is more important than quantity.
- Attention to equipment utilization, including shin guards, and optimal field conditions. WBGT guidelines should direct periods of play or practice and hydration standards.
- Prophylactic ankle taping or bracing in players with clinical instability or history of previous strain.
- Exclusion of players with serious knee instability.
- Educate soccer players on the importance of disciplined play.
- No head balls in children under age 10. Ensure the player learns proper head ball technique.
- Early identification and management of concussions. Preseason standardized neuropsychological testing for patients at risk by history or by position (goalie or forward). Pad goal posts.
- Supervised and progressive rehabilitative process. Return to play decisions following injury should come directly from the team physician and physical therapist. Athletes must demonstrate full range of motion and 90% strength.

REFERENCES

Albert M: Descriptive three-year data study of outdoor professional soccer injuries. *Athl Train* 18:218, 1983.

Arendt E, Dick R: Knee injury patterns among men and women in collegiate basketball and soccer. *AM J Sports Med* 23:694, 1995.

Boden BP: Soccer injuries: Leg injuries and shin guards. *Clin Sport Med* 17:769, 1998.

Boden BP, Dean GS, Feagin JA et al: Mechanisms of anterior cruciate ligament injury. *Orthopaedics* 23(6):573, 2000.

Boden BP, Lohnes JH, Numley JA et al: Tibia and fibula fractures in soccer players. *Arthroscopy* 7:262–266, 1999.

Delaney JS, Lacroix VJ, Leclerc S et al: Concussions among university football and soccer players. *Clin J Sport Med* 12:331, 2002.

Delfico AJ, Garrett WE: Soccer injuries: Mechanisms of injury of the anterior cruciate ligament in soccer players. *Clin Sport Med* 17:779, 1998.

Ekstrand J, Gillquist J: Soccer Injuries and their mechanisms. A prospective study. *Med Sci Sports Exerc* 15:267, 1983.

Elias SR, Roberts WO, Thorson DC: Team sports in hot weather. *Phys Sportsmed* 19(5):67, 1991.

Engstrom B, Johanoson C, Tornkvist H: Soccer injuries among elite female players. *AM J Sports Med* 19:372, 1991.

Foster C, Thompson NN, Dean J et al: Carbohydrate supplementation and performance in soccer players. *Med Sci Sport Exerc* 18:8, 1986.

Gilmore J: Soccer Injuries: Groin pain in the soccer athlete: fact, fiction and treatment. *Clin Sport Med* 17:787, 1998.

Haglund Y, Eriksson E: Does amateur boxing lead to chronic brain damage? *AM J Sports Med* 21:97, 1993.

Hoy K, Lindblad BE, Terkelsen CJ et al: European soccer injuries: A prospective epidemiological and socioeconomic study. *AM J Sports Med* 20:318, 1992.

Jordan SW, Green GA, Galanty HL et al: Acute and chronic brain injury in United States national team soccer players. *AM J Sports Med* 24:205, 1996.

Keller CS, Noyes FR, Buncher CR: The medical aspects of soccer injury epidemiology. *AM J Sports Med* 15:230, 1987.

Leatt PB, Jacobs I: Effect of glucose polymer on glycogen depletion during a soccer match. *Can J Sport Sci* 14(2):112, 1989.

Morelli V, Smith V: Groin injuries in athletes. *Am Fam Physician* 64:1405, 2001.

National Collegiate Athletic Association: *NCAA Injury Surveillance System.* Indianapolis, IND, NCAA, 2000.

Nielsen AB, Yde J: Epidemiology and traumatology of injuries in soccer. *AM J Sports Med* 17:803, 1989.

Nilsson S, Roaas A: Soccer injuries in adolescents. *AM J Sports Med* 6:358, 1978.

Putukian M, Knowles WK, Swere S et al: Injuries in indoor soccer. The Lake Placid dawn to dark soccer tournament. *AM J Sports Med* 24(3):317, 1996.

Putukian M, Mandelbaum BR, Brown DW: Sport specific conditions: Soccer, in Ireland ML, Nattiv A (eds.): *The Female Athlete*, New York, NY, Elsevier Science, 2002, p 711.

Reilly T, Thomas V: An analysis of work-rate in different positional roles in professional football match-play. *J Hum Mov Sci* 2:87, 1976.

Saltin B, Costill DL: Fluid and electrolyte balance during prolonged exercise, in Horton ES, Terjung RL (eds.): *Exercise, Nutrition and Metabolism.* New York, NY, Macmillan, 150–158, 1998.

Schmidt-Olsen S, Jorgensen U, Kaalund S et al: Injuries among young soccer players. *AM J Sports Med* 19:273, 1991.

Soccer Industry Counsel of America: National Soccer Participation Survey. North Palm Beach, FL, American Sports Data, 1996.

Soderman K: The Female Soccer Player: Injury Pattern, Risk Factors, and Intervention. Umea, Sweden, Kerstin Soderman, 2001.

Sullivan JA, Gross RH, Grana WA et al: Evaluation of injuries in youth soccer. *AM J Sports Med* 8:325, 1980.

Witol A, Webbe F: Neuropsychological deficits associated with soccer players. Abstract from proceedings of 1995 American Psychological Association, New York, 1995.

90 SWIMMING

Nancy E Rolnik, MD

EPIDEMIOLOGY

- Swimming is a popular activity with participation from all ages. Young children start competitively swimming around 6 years of age. Masters swimmers include athletes into their 19s and beyond.
- For competitive athletes, swimming is an all-year sport with little rest time. Many swimmers engage in two workouts a day averaging between 8000 to 20,000 yards per day.
- The majority of injuries in swimming are due to overuse with the most frequently injured area being the shoulder. A study of competitive United States swimmers demonstrated that 47% of 13- and 14-year-old swimmers, 66% of 15- to 16-year-old swimmers, and 73% of elite swimmers had history of interfering shoulder pain (McMaster and Troup, 1993).
- Aggressive injury management decreases the swimmer's time out of the water.

STROKE MECHANICS

- Breakdowns in stroke mechanics can lead to injury, so it is important to stress proper swim technique to all swimmers. Returning to basic stroke mechanics can help prevent repetitive injuries.
- Competitive swimming includes four strokes: freestyle, breaststroke, butterfly, and backstroke. The main propulsive forces are generated by the arms and back.
- Regardless of the swimmer's chosen stroke, most training is done freestyle.
- Freestyle stroke phases include a catch, pull, and recovery period. During the out-of-water phase, the

torso rotates as the shoulder exits the water in an abducted and externally rotated position. The elbow should remain above the hand until the hand enters the water fingers first in front and just outside the line of the shoulder. To keep the elbow high, the swimmer must roll the body approximately 45° on the swimmer's long axis. During the underwater phase, the shoulder internally rotates and adducts to propel the body forward. The elbow should point toward the side wall during this phase. The upper trapezius, rhomboids, supraspinatus, and deltoid all function in combination to position the scapula and humerus for hand entry and exit New techniques emphasize an early catch, early exit at the beltline, and a straight through arm pull in lieu of the S-shaped pattern often described (Pink et al, 1991; Schubert, 1990; Johnson, Gauvin, and Fredericson, 2003).

- The flutter kick helps stabilize the swimmer's trunk. This kick starts at the hip and simulates a motion similar to kicking off a loose shoe. The knees should flex only 30–40°. Flexion at the hip is minimal.
- The swimmer must focus on the coordinated motion of both the upper and lower extremity. If the swimmer fails to kick throughout the stroke, the body will lose some of its buoyancy and more drag is created. The upper extremity will then compensate placing more stress at the shoulders.
- Bilateral breathing helps the swimmer develop equal pulling strength in both arms and helps ensure equal body roll on each side (Johnson, Gauvin, and Fredericson, 2003).
- The unique whip kick done in the breaststroke places a valgus stress at the knee. Due to these mechanics, breaststrokers have more knee complaints than swimmers competing in the other strokes.
- When stroke mechanics need correction, the use of an underwater video can help clarify the errors.

UPPER EXTREMITY INJURIES

SWIMMER'S SHOULDER

- Shoulder pain is the most common complaint in competitive swimmers. Nearly 50% of collegiate and master's swimmers report shoulder pain lasting at least 3 weeks (Stocker, Pink, and Jobe, 1995).
- Swimmer's shoulder refers to shoulder tendinopathy or impingement. Typically the swimmer feels maximum pain at the beginning of the pull-through phase. Often the swimmer will swim through this pain for weeks until the pain is present throughout the entire freestyle stroke.

- Fatigue, muscle imbalance, and shoulder laxity contribute to the development of swimmer's shoulder.
- Typical treatment includes ice, rest, anti-inflammatory medication, and occasionally subacromial corticosteroid injection.
- The swimmer should limit the total weekly mileage and swim with various strokes.
- Kickboard workouts can allow the swimmer to maintain fitness while resting the shoulders. The elbow should be flexed to minimize irritation to the shoulder.
- Prevention of future injury includes correcting stroke mechanic problems while strengthening the rotator cuff and scapular stabilizing muscles.
- The serratus anterior, a scapular stabilizer, is one of the most important muscles involved in the freestyle stroke and therapy should be aimed to increase its strength (Pink and Tibone, 2000).
- Swimmers have been shown to have increased shoulder adduction and internal rotation strength, which can lead to an imbalance in the shoulder. The swimmer should focus on creating a balance by strengthening the external rotators (Weldon and Richardson, 2001).

SHOULDER INSTABILITY

- Repetitive shoulder rotation and vigorous flexibility may contribute to stretching of the shoulder capsule leading to possible subluxation.
- Instability can be anterior, posterior, inferior, or a combination. The more unstable the glenohumeral joint, the greater the risk of developing a labral tear—a Hills-Sachs lesion or a Bankart lesion. Radiographs including an axillary view should be obtained. If a labral tear is suspected, an MRI-arthrogram should be ordered.
- The mainstay of treatment is rotator cuff muscle strengthening.
- If instability is persistent despite rehabilitation, surgery to tighten the capsule may be warranted. Warn the swimmer that a more stable shoulder may limit their performance.
- Indication for stretching is limited. If the shoulder capsule is overstretched, the risk for instability and injury is increased (Pink and Tibone, 2000).

ELBOW

- Triceps tendinitis can develop as a result of the full extension necessary in the backstroke.
- The ulnar collateral ligament may be stressed in the recovery phase of the freestyle leading to sprain.
- Treatment with rest, *nonsteroidal anti-inflammatory drugs* (NSAIDs), and ice are appropriate.

LOWER EXTREMITY INJURIES

BREASTSTROKER'S KNEE

- Commonly seen in athletes who do the whip kick in the breaststroke.
- The valgus force created at the knee leads to medial collateral ligament sprain (Rodeo, 1999).
- Often poor kick technique contributes to *medial collateral ligament* (MCL) sprain. The swimmer needs instruction on proper technique for prevention.
- The mainstay of treatment includes rest, ice, and anti-inflammatory medications.

PATELLOFEMORAL PAIN

- The symptoms typical of patellofemoral syndrome also occur in swimmers.
- Treatment includes rest, ice, NSAIDs, and quadriceps strengthening. Swimmers should be encouraged to train using a foam buoy between the thighs in order to rest the knees.
- Some swimmers may benefit from a neoprene patella stabilizing brace, which would substitute for McConnell taping.

FOOT/ANKLE PROBLEMS

- Extensor tendinitis may occur from the flutter kick or dolphin kick.
- Treatment includes rest, ice, and NSAIDs. Rest from the flutter kick is best achieved using a foam buoy.
- A lower extremity stretching program focusing on improved range of motion at the ankle will help in the recovery and prevention.
- Local foot injury can occur if the swimmer kicks the side of the pool or gutter. This usually results in abrasions or contusions but may cause a fracture.
- Proper flip-turn technique will prevent foot injuries.

BACK INJURIES

LOW BACK STRAIN

- The butterfly and breaststroke require hyperextension of the lower back to maintain body position and complete the stroke. The body-roll done by freestyle and backstroke swimmers can also cause strain, especially when the swimmer tires.

- Treatment must include back plus abdominal strengthening and instruction on technique.
- The use of muscle relaxants is controversial.

SPONDYLOLYSIS/SPONDYLOLISTHESIS

- The hyperextension of the back required specifically in the butterfly and breaststroke can predispose a swimmer to the development of a spondylolysis.
- The swimmer will often complain of pain during flip-turns and starts.
- Spondylolysis rarely progresses to spondylolisthesis.
- Rest is the mainstay of treatment. Rarely will the athlete require bracing or surgery.

MEDICAL PROBLEMS COMMON IN SWIMMERS

ASTHMA

- In most of the country, swimmers train in enclosed pools that are both warm and humid. Athletes with asthma often gravitate to this environment because it is less asthmagenic.
- Coaches and trainers need to be aware of the asthmatic swimmer and have appropriate emergency treatment at the pool.
- A study involving the 1998 Winter Olympic games swimmers revealed that 22.4% of swimmers reported either use of asthma medications or diagnosis of asthma or both (Weiler and Edward, 2000).

OTITIS EXTERNA

- Otitis externa, or the more common term *swimmer's ear*, is one of the most common medical problems encountered by daily swimmers. The hours that swimmers spend submerging their ears in pool or open water lead to ear canal maceration and infection.
- Topical treatment is effective. The swimmer should remain out of the pool for 2–3 days.
- Preventive measures include drying the ear with a drying agent such as Vosol otic drops or a homemade mixture of 50% vinegar and 50% alcohol.
- Avoid traumatizing the ear canal with Q-tips.

CONJUNCTIVITIS

- Bacterial conjunctivitis and chemical conjunctivitis present similarly as a red eye. Most bacteria are killed by the pool chlorine so transmission via pool is rare. Goggle wear will help prevent chemical conjunctivitis, which is a self-limiting problem.

SUN DAMAGE

- For those swimmers training in open water, close attention to the skin is important to prevent sun burn.
- Twenty to 30 min prior to swimming, waterproof sunscreen should be liberally applied. There is no consensus on timing of reapplication of sunscreen.

SWIMMER'S XEROSIS

- After hours submersed in the water, the skin becomes dehydrated and pruritic.
- Prevention is the key. Swimmers should apply lotion or body oil to their lightly patted skin after showering. The postswim shower should be short and with warm instead of hot water (Basler et al, 2000).

GREEN HAIR

- Though not harmful, green hair can cause the swimmer undue anxiety.
- Application of 2% hydrogen peroxide to the hair and rinsing this out in 30 min will help remove the discoloration.

REFERENCES

Basler R, Basler G, Palmer S et al: Special skin symptoms seen in swimmers. *J Am Acad Derm* 43(2):299–305, 2000.

Johnson J, Gauvin J, Fredericson M: Swimming biomechanics and injury prevention. *Phys Sportsmed* 31(1):39–56 Jan 2003.

McMaster W, Troup J: A survey of interfering shoulder pain in United States competitive swimmers. *Am J Sports Med* 21(1):67–70, 1993.

Pink M, Tibone J: The painful shoulder in the swimming athlete. *Clin Orthop* 21(2):247–261, 2000.

Pink M, Perry J, Browne A et al: The normal shoulder during freestyle swimming: An electromyographic and cinematographic analysis of twelve muscles. *Am J Sports Med* 19:569–576, 1991.

Rodeo S: Knee pain in competitive swimming. *Clin Sports Med* 18(2):379–387, April 1999.

Schubert, M: *Competitive Swimming: Techniques for Champions*. New York, NY, Winner Circle Books, 1990.

Stocker D, Pink M, Jobe FW: Comparison of shoulder injury in collegiate and master's level swimmers. *Clin J Sport Med* 5(1):4–8, 1995.

Weiler J, Edward R: Asthma in United States Olympic athletes who participated in the 1998 Olympic Winter Games. *Clin Allergy Immunol* 106(2):267–271, August 2000.

Weldon E, Richardson A: Upper extremity overuse injuries in swimming. *Clin Sports Med* 20(3):423–438, July 2001.

91 TENNIS

Robert P Nirschl, MD, MS

EPIDEMIOLOGY

- Tennis injuries are equally divided between the upper and lower body. The most celebrated are tendon overuse of the shoulder and elbow (e.g., rotator cuff tendinosis and tennis elbow).
- Lower extremity problems are typical of other running sports: examples include ankle sprains, leg issues (such as medial gastroc rupture, medial tibial stress syndrome, and Achilles tendinosis), and knee abnormalities such as meniscal cartilage tears and chondromalacia patellae.
- The etiology of the common shoulder and elbow tendonopathies is primarily repetitive overuse and heredity.
- Repetitive overuse in tennis elbow and rotator cuff tendinosis are related to tennis technique and equipment, as well as frequency, duration, and intensity.

PATHOPHYSIOLOGY

- The exact mechanisms of tendon failure are not defined. Mechanical tendon failure is presumed to occur by mechanical collagen disruption, a chemical inflammatory cascade, and vascular distress resulting in tendon degeneration (angiofibroblastic tendinosis).
- The histopathology of angiofibroblastic tendinosis is characterized by nonfunctional vascular and fibroblastic elements, as well as collagen disruption and disorganization. There are no noted inflammatory cells in the histopathology of tendinosis.

CLINICAL FEATURES

- The key symptom in tennis elbow include various stages of pain—pain phases (Nirschl):
  1. Mild pain after exercise activity—resolves within 24 h.
  2. Pain after exercise activity—exceeds 48 h and resolves with warm-up.
  3. Pain with exercise activity that does not alter the exercise.

4. Pain with exercise activity that alters the exercise.
5. Pain caused by heavy activities of daily living.
6. Pain caused by light activities of daily living.
7. Intermittent pain at rest that does not disturb sleep.
8. Constant rest pain (dull aching) and pain that disturbs sleep.

- **Pain location is specific:** In lateral elbow tendinosis, the pain is localized just distal and anteromedial to the lateral epicondyle and along the proximal extensor aspect of the forearm. In medial elbow tendinosis, the pain is focused from the tip of the medial epicondyle and distally 2 to 3 in. down the track of the common flexor origin. In the stroke mechanics of tennis, lateral elbow pain is usually associated with the back hand while medial elbow pain is commonly associated with the forehand and serve.
- Rotator cuff tendinosis also has the pain phase sequence noted for the elbow (see pain phases). Pain is characteristically noted in the anterior shoulder with overhead activities and compression forces such as rolling onto the shoulder during sleep. Full motion is commonly restricted and weakness is common (especially external rotation and abduction). In tennis, shoulder pain is commonly present in the serve, overhead and high backhand follow through.

CLINICAL EXAMINATION

- **Lateral elbow:** The quintessential sign is focused tenderness over the *extensor carpi radialis brevis* (ECRB) just distal and anteromedial to the lateral epicondyle. Pain in the same area is noted with resisted wrist extension or hand shaking. Stability and motion are usually normal.
- **Medial elbow:** The classical sign is tenderness at the tip of the medial epicondyle and distal along the track of the flexor carpi radialis and pronator teres. Provocation pains with resisted wrist flexion and forearm pronation are the norm. A positive Tinel's sign indicative of ulnar nerve sensitivity is often present at the medial epicondylar groove. Motion and stability are usually normal but extension is occasionally restricted. Valgus instability can occur in the uncommon instance of associated medial collateral ligament injury.
- **Shoulder (rotator cuff):** Tenderness is located over the greater tuberosity. If associated *acromioclavicular* (AC) osteoarthritis is present, tenderness will also be noted over the AC joint. Forced forward flexion (impingement sign) elicits pain. Motion may or may not be restricted. Weakness—especially external rotation and abduction—are characteristically present as the specific demands of tennis typically weaken the external rotators and scapular stabilizers. Crepitus with shoulder abduction is often present in

the coracoacromial arch. Instability may be noted but is more likely noted in swimmers and baseball pitchers, rather than tennis players.

DIFFERENTIAL DIAGNOSIS

- **Lateral elbow:** Rarely posterior interosseous nerve entrapment may masquerade as tendinosis. The symptoms are more distal and pain may be elicited with resisted supination. Intra-articular synovitis and lateral plica may occur in combination with tendinosis. Cervical radiculopathy (C7 root) has been known as well to have referred pain at the lateral elbow.

TREATMENT

- The basic treatment of tennis related overuse injuries of the rotator cuff and elbow tendons are improvement of the shoulder and arm and diminution of abusive activity. The biological goals of tissue enhancement are neurovascularization and fibroblastic infiltration with collagen production, thereby altering the devitalized degenerative tendinosis tissue in a positive manner (e.g., cure). The mechanism to accomplish cure is rehabilitative exercise.
- **Pain control:** Pain control may take several forms. It should be noted that pain control does not indicate cure (e.g., neovascularization; fibroblastic proliferation; collagen production; and the restoration of strength, endurance, and flexibility). The concept of pain control is to free the patient from pain inhibition so the curative process of rehabilitative exercise can proceed effectively. The proven approaches to pain control include relative rest and medication (analgesic and anti-inflammatories, both nonsteroidal, and cortisone). Cortisone may be delivered by direct injection, iontophoresis, or orally. The modalities of physical therapy including heat, cold, massage, electrical stimulation, and ultrasound can also be helpful. Recently shockwave therapy has been advanced as a modality of pain control and possibly a cure but evidence is unconvincing at this time. Alternative methods, such as magnets and copper bracelets, have no scientific evidence of effectiveness. Acupuncture has some evidence of temporary pain control but no evidence of biological cure.
- **Rehabilitation:** Resistance exercise is the key component. An effective program includes varying and properly sequenced resistances including isometrics, isotonics, isokinetics, and isoflex (tension cord).
- The cardinal six-exercise arcs for tennis elbow include wrist flexion, wrist extension, pronation, supination, and radial and ulnar deviation. Since the upper arm, shoulder, and upper back are characteristically weak in

tennis, exercises to eliminate these weaknesses must also be addressed.

- Rotator cuff rehabilitation includes all shoulder arcs of motion including abduction, adduction, external, and internal rotation. Scapular stabilizer strengthening is critical and elimination of any abnormal thoracic kyphosis, if possible, is addressed. Full shoulder flexibility is a necessity in this endeavor.
- **Control of force loads:** The basic tenet of overall treatment is a balance between improving the musculoskeletal system (e.g., rehabilitation or surgery) and controlling any injury producing overuse imposed by the sport (in this instance, tennis).
- Tennis stroke mechanics of good quality are essential to controlling any injury producing overuse injuries to the rotator cuff, as well as lateral and medial tennis elbow.
- Integral to quality tennis ground stroke mechanics are to use the lower body often (e.g., running to achieve ideal body position and forward weight transfer at the time of ball impact) and the upper body little (e.g., use wrist and forearm for ball control rather than as a power source).
- Traditional lateral tennis elbow is primarily associated with poor backhand technique (e.g., the power source is the forearm and elbow rather than the shoulder, trunk rotation, and body weight transfer). Conversely, a quality single hand or two-handed backhand stroke minimizes arm use.
- Medial tennis elbow from groundstrokes or the volley is commonly associated with a late forehand stroke. The lower body mechanics include poor weight transfer and body position. In these poor mechanics the wrist must snap (flex) to bring the racquet head in a perpendicular position to the incoming ball. This technique results in overuse of the common flexor origin at the medial elbow. As in lateral elbow, quality mechanics include proper body position as well as trunk and shoulder rotation and a firm, not flexing, wrist at the time of ball impact.
- Medial tennis elbow from serve and overhead may occur from quality stroke mechanics. At the interface of the serve cocking motion and backscratch and as acceleration is initiated the medial elbow is subject to valgus stress. In addition, at ball impact, snapping wrist flexion stresses the common flexors and pronator teres further challenging their origins at the medial epicondyle. Subtle changes in grip position and wrist mechanics often aid medial elbow stress but the gross kinesiology of a quality tennis serve may still be stressful. Medial elbow stresses are exaggerated further in a serve and volley player playing on a slow and watered down clay surface (e.g., a wet heavier tennis ball).

- **Rotator cuff:** The rotator cuff is primarily stressed with the tennis serve and overhead. The basic shoulder position of 90° of abduction and full external rotation at the backscratch followed by racquet head acceleration is a major stressor by increasing tension forces on the rotator cuff. The shoulder, in contradistinction to the elbow is vulnerable with both a quality and inexperienced low quality tennis serve. In addition, the constant stretching of scapular muscle groups in at the deceleration phase of the serve, especially after ball impact, fatigues and weakens the posterior shoulder muscles placing the cuff at further risk secondary to muscle imbalance.
- **Shoulder:** Although the primary pathology is rotator cuff tendinosis, companion issues such as shoulder labral tearing and instability, bursitis, and aggravation of AC osteoarthritis may occur. These tissues are challenged in similar shoulder positions of back scratch and acceleration. The extreme of external rotation at 90° of abduction is most stressful. Quality tennis serve technique, unlike baseball pitching, rapidly progresses to full extension and is therefore somewhat protective. The volume of use in tournament class players often, however, ultimately takes its toll. Inexperienced serve mechanics conversely tends to maintain the more punishing 90° abduction position at ball impact thereby increasing the stresses on the shoulder. This troublesome stroke pattern combined with an age related rotator cuff vulnerability of the older recreational player often incites rotator cuff symptoms.
- **Force load control:** Control of force loads can occur in a variety of ways. Alteration of frequency, intensity, and duration of tennis activity is the initial approach (e.g., relative rest). Tennis instruction, including hitting with a ball machine and against a backboard, increases ball impact per unit of time and is often an inciting factor in the onset of tennis elbow symptoms and is best avoided when the arm is sensitive.
- **Equipment:** Increased force loads have been empirically noted with unduly rigid racquets with tight stringing. In addition, gut strings by anecdotal observation are more forgiving and more protective than synthetic strings. Light racquets (under 10 oz) as well have more limited racquet mass resulting in excess torque forces with off center tennis ball hits. Conversely, ball impacts in the center of percussion, with any racquet (e.g., the sweet spot), are protective.
- **Counter force functional bracing:** For tennis elbow, the counter force concept, introduced by the author in 1972, is to diffuse the concentration of forces from a small to a large area. A wide brace (2 3/4 in. or above) is more protective. Since the forearm is conical in

shape, a curved design is necessary for proper fit and dual tension straps to control tension completely across the entire brace is best.

- **Nonoperative treatment summary:** Tennis, like many other repetitive action sports, alters the musculosketal system in nonhealthful ways. The shoulder and elbow muscle tendon units become fatigued, weakened, imbalanced, and ultimately injured. Rehabilitation exercises to correct these deficiencies are critical to cure. Maintenance exercises that counteract the bodies' maladaptation to tennis mechanics are essential to prevent recurrence.
- The other key component in prevention of the tennis related overuse injuries is to control excessive force overload. These approaches as noted include quality stroke technique, equipment (racquet, strings, and the tennis court surface), the intensity, frequency, and duration of activity and quality counterforce bracing (e.g., curvilinear designs).
- **Treatment surgical:** The goal of nonoperative treatment is to revitalize degenerative tendinosis tissue. If this fails, surgical intervention regarding tennis elbow (medial and lateral) and shoulder tendinosis (including full cuff rupture) can be highly successful. The goal of surgery is to resect the pain producing tendinosis tissue and or repair ruptured tissue.
- The indications for surgery are a failed quality rehabilitation program and an unacceptable quality of life as determined by the patient.
- **Return to tennis stroke mechanics protocol:** After rehabilitation or surgery, the following return to tennis practice schedule protocols are suggested:
  1. Medial tennis elbow practice schedule return guidelines (Table 91-1).

TABLE 91-1   Medial Tennis Elbow Practice Schedule Return Guidelines

TOURNAMENT PLAYER			RECREATIONAL PLAYER*		
DAY	DURATION	TECHNIQUE	DAY	DURATION	TECHNIQUE
1	15 min	B only (2 handed); L (no late strokes)	1	15 min	L only
2	20 min	B (2 handed); L; Few F (2 handed)	2	20 min	L; B
3	30 min	B; L; Few F (not T); F; (no late strokes), (no topspin)	3	35 min	Same as day 2
4	35 min	B; L; BV; F (no T)	4	40 min	L; B; F; BV
5	40 min	B; L; BV; F (no T); Few O (to F court only)	5	45 min	L; B; F; BV; few O
6	45 min	B; L; BV; F; (no T); O (to F court only)	6	1 h	L; B; F; BV; O
7	1 h	Same as day 6	7	1 h	L; B; BV; F; O; few S
8	1 h (a.m.)	B; L; BV; F (no T) FV; (no late strokes ever!)	8	1 h	L; B; F; BV; O; S; F; (No late strokes ever!)
9	1 h	All strokes easy	9		Resume normal practice/play schedule
10	1 h (a.m.) 15 min (p.m.)	Same as day 9 B; L; F			
11	1 h (a.m.) 30 min (p.m.)	B; L; BV; F (not T); O; FV;S; (no T or AT) B; L; BV; F; (no T)			
12	1 h (a.m.) 45 min (p.m.)	B; L; BV; F; O; FV; S; (no T or AT) B; L; BV; F; O			
13	1 h (a.m.) 1 h (p.m.)	Same as day 12 Same as a.m.			
14	1 h (a.m.) 1 h (p.m.)	B; L; BV; F Same as in a.m.			
15		Resume normal practice/play schedule			

Code for Tennis Practice Schedule

F = Forehand	T = Topspin	FV = Forehand volley
AT = American twist	S = Serve	L = Lob
U = Underspin	BL = Backhand lob	B = Backhand
FL = Forehand lob	SL = Slice	O = Overhead
BV = Backhand valley		

Caution

1. Use Medical Count'R-Force® at all times.
2. Hit easily—hit through the ball.
3. Stay in balance.
4. Stay in the hitting zone.
5. No late strokes.
6. Keep eye on ball.
7. Avoid frame shots.
8. Ice sore areas immediately after play.

*Progression for recreational player refers to the actual playing days, not chronological days.

TABLE 91-2   Lateral Tennis Elbow Practice Schedule Return Guidelines

	TOURNAMENT PLAYER			RECREATIONAL PLAYER*	
DAY	DURATION	TECHNIQUE	DAY	DURATION	TECHNIQUE
1	15 min	F only	1	15 min	F only
2	20 min	F; FL; few FV	2	30 min	F; FL; few FV
3	30 min	F; FL; FV; Few O (to F court only)	3	35 min	F; FL; FV; few O
4	35 min	F; FL; FV; O; Few S	4	45 min	F; FL; FV; O
5	40 min	F; FL; FV; O; S (no SL, T, or AT)	5	1 h	F; FL; O; S; Few B (2 handed)
6	45 min	As day 5	6	1 h	F; FV; FL; O; S; BV; (2 handed); B
7	1 h	As day 6	7	1 h	F; FV; L; O; S; B; BV (2 handed); B
8	1 h (a.m.)	F; FL; FV; O; S (no SL or AT); few B (two handed)	8	1 h	F; FV; L; O; S; B
9	1 h	F; FL; FV;O; S (no AT); B (no BV)	9		Resume normal practice/play schedule
10	1 h (a.m.) 15 min (p.m.)	F; FV; L; O; S; (no AT) B; (no U) F; FL; O			
11	1 h (a.m.) 20 min (p.m.)	Same as day 10 Same as day 10			
12	1 h (a.m.) 30 min (p.m.)	Same as day 11 F; FV; L; O			
13	1 h (a.m.) 45 min (p.m.)	F; FV; L; O; S; B; few BV (no U) F; FV; L; O; S			
14	1 h (a.m.) 1 h (p.m.)	F; FV; L; O; S; B; BV Same as in a.m.			
15		Resume normal practice/play schedule			

Code for Tennis Practice Schedule

F = Forehand	T = Topspin	FV = Forehand volley
AT = American twist	S = Serve	L = Lob
U = Underspin	BL = Backhand lob	B = Backhand
FL = Forehand lob	SL = Slice	O = Overhead
BV = Backhand valley		

Caution

1. Use Medical Count'R-Force® at all times.
2. Hit easily—hit through the ball.
3. Stay in balance.
4. Stay in the hitting zone.
5. No late strokes.
6. Keep eye on ball.
7. Two-handed backhand is protective
8. Ice sore areas immediately after play.

* Progression for recreational player refers to the actual playing days, not chronological days.

2. Lateral tennis elbow practice schedule return guidelines (Table 91-2).

BIBLIOGRAPHY

Groppel J, Nirschl RP: A biomechanical and electromyographical analysis of the effects of counter force braces on the tennis player. *Am J Sports Med* 14:42–49, 1986.

Nirschl R: Elbow tendinosis. *Clin Sports Med* 11:851–870, 1992.

Nirschl, R.P: Good tennis is good medicine. *Phys Sports Med* 1:33–41, 1973.

Nirschl RP: Orthopedic concerns for the tennis professional, in Groppel J (ed.): *USPTA Sports Science and Sports Medicine Guide*. Houston, TX, USPTA Publications, 1988, Chap. 3, pp. 19–28.

Nirschl RP, Sobel J: *Arm Care*. Arlington, Virginia, Medical Sports Publishing, 1996.

Nirschl, RP: Prevention and treatment of elbow and shoulder injuries in the tennis player. *Clin Sports Med* 7(2): April 1988.

Sobel J, Nirschl RP: Supplemental exercises for the tennis player, in Groppel J (ed.): *USPTA Sports Science and Sports Medicine Guide*. Chap. 5, p. 49–70.

92   TRIATHLON

Shawn F Kane, MD
Fred Brennan, DO

TRIATHLONS

• A unique multidisciplinary event, including sequential swim, bike, and run legs. The concept was initially developed as an alternative to standard marathon or

10 K training programs. In 1974, members of the San Diego Track Club hosted a first of its kind swim-bike-run event in and around the waters of California's Mission Bay. That three-event race was called a triathlon and still to this day triathlons are one of the most popular worldwide endurance events.

1. John Collins, a veteran of the first Mission Bay Triathlon, was influential in the further development of the sport. He is responsible for combining three endurance events: the Waikiki Rough Water Swim, the Around-Oahu Bike Ride, and the Honolulu Marathon into one of the world's most recognized and demanding competition, The Ironman.
   a. The inaugural race of 1978 was comprised of 12 male competitors, followed by 13 competitors in 1979 including the first female competitor. An article, written by Barry McDermott and published in the May 1979 edition of *Sports Illustrated* increased the race field into the hundreds and brought ABC's Wide World of Sports to the event for its first of an unbroken string of broadcasts.
2. Popularity and continued growth led to the establishment of the International Triathlon Union and the inaugural World Triathlon Championship competition in 1980. Popularity and international recognition resulted in the continued growth of the sport through the 1990s into the new century with the 1994 Goodwill Games, 1995 Pan Am Games, and the 2000 Olympic Games hosting their inaugural triathlon competitions.
   a. 2004 data show there are 200,000–300,000 and 100,000 active triathletes in the United States and Australia respectively (Burns, Keenan, and Redmond, 2003). In 2002, there were 850 sanctioned triathlons in the United States alone.
- Triathlons are a unique sport that encompass all health related variables: cardiorespiratory endurance, body composition, muscular strength, endurance, and flexibility.
- Triathlon governing bodies recognize four standard race types based on distance (Korkia, Tunstall-Pedoe, and Maffulli, 1994).
  1. Sprint (0.75-Km swim, 22-km bike, 5-km run)
  2. Olympic (1.5-Km swim, 40-km bike, 10-km run)
  3. Half-Ironman (1.9-Km swim, 90-Km bike, 21-Km run)
  4. Ironman (3.8-Km swim, 180-Km bike, 42-Km run)

VOCABULARY

- Like all sports, triathlons and triathletes have a unique vocabulary. A few of the more common terms are included here to aid in the understanding of these athletes.

1. Bonking: A reference to when a competitor begins to lose the ability to concentrate, feels disoriented and overly fatigued, and at times is unable to continue on in a race. Bonking occurs when energy intake does not meet energy expenditure and glycogen stores are depleted. The regular intake of carbohydrates during prolonged competitions can prevent this condition from occurring.
2. Transition zone: An area of controlled chaos where athletes change from swimmer to biker and from biker to swimmer, T1 and T2 respectively.
3. Breakaway: When one or more competitors significantly increase their speed in an attempt to create distance between themselves and the rest of the field.
4. Surge: Similar concept to a breakaway in cycling but referring to running.
5. Road rash: Superficial abrasions to the skin usually as the direct result of a bicycle accident.
6. Traumatic tattooing: Skin discoloration resulting from debris that was deeply embedded in the skin following road rash.
7. Brick: A training method or workout used to simulate race conditions. It involves swimming, biking, and/or running all in the same day... one event after another.

INJURY EPIDEMIOLOGY

- Triathletes compete and train in three distinct events, each of which triggers its own set of injuries. Injuries specific to an individual component event of the triathlon will be covered in that specific chapter, here we will try and focus on injuries unique to the triathlete.
- Theoretically, it is possible that triathletes would have fewer overuse injuries compared to other one sport endurance athletes as triathletes spend two-thirds of their time cross-training. The contrary may also be true: triathletes suffer from the cumulative effect of three distinct injury-producing events and are susceptible to more injuries.
  1. Injuries are defined as any musculoskeletal problem that causes a cessation of training for at least one day, a reduction in training mileage, the taking of pain medication, or the seeking of medical aid.
- Research has demonstrated injury rates among triathletes to be anywhere from 37 to 90% annually with roughly 50% of injuries occurring during preseason, 37% occurring during the competition season and the remainder overlapped between seasons.
  1. Overuse injuries are the primary injury for the triathlete and comprise 68 and 78% of the injuries sustained in the preseason and competition season

respectively. Acute injuries caused by trauma make up the difference.

- Injury incidence: A range of 2.5—5.4 injuries per 1000 h of triathlon training and 4.6—17.4 injuries per 1000 h of triathlon competition have been reported. These rates are higher than the reported incidences of 3.9 and 2.5 injuries per 1000 h of training for track and field or marathon running respectively (Burns, Keenan, and Redmond, 2003).
  1. Running causes 65–78%, cycling causes 16–37%, and swimming causes 11–21% of the injuries that triathletes experience (Korkia, Tunstall-Pedoe, and Maffulli, 1994).
     a. Iliotibial band syndrome, patellofemoral pain syndrome, patellar and Achilles tendinitis are common injuries encountered during running.
     b. Aeroneck: Neck pain and stiffness caused by prolonged sitting with the shoulders hunched and the arms tucked tightly in underneath and the neck hyperextended. This is a complaint that many triathletes have after or during the cycling portion of the race.
     c. Patellofemoral pain, quadriceps and calf strains are common cycling injuries (Thompson and Rivara, 2001).
     d. Corneal abrasions: Frequently result from having the goggles kicked off the face at the congested start of the swim phase (Hellemans).
  2. Despite differences in training mileage, duration, and number of workouts per week there has been no reported difference in the injury prevalence, distribution, or severity amongst triathletes who varied in skill from elite to recreational.
  3. Predictors of injury: Is there any one-factor or group of factors that predispose triathletes to an increase rate of injury?
     a. Total weekly training distance, weekly cycling distance, swimming distance, total number of workouts (swimming, cycling, and running) per week but surprisingly not running distance per week are all associated with an increased incidence of running injuries (Williams et al, 1988).
     b. Total amount of time spent running and cycling but not total distance played a role in the incidence of cycling injuries.
     c. The most significant predictor of injury in the preseason is number of years of experience in triathlons, with more experienced triathletes having a higher injury rate (Korkia, Tunstall-Pedoe, and Maffulli, 1994).
     d. The most significant predictor of injury during the season was a history of previous injury and high preseason running mileage.

   e. Training errors, most specifically form and style, have been frequently associated with injuries related to cycling and swimming.
  4. Running is by far the most injury producing aspect of a triathlon. The amount of time and distance covered while conducting cycling and swim training are directly associated with higher rates of running injury, not increased running mileage as one might expect.
     a. It is believed that the extra training put in for the swimming and cycling phases delays muscle recovery enough that the stress for running is magnified and leads to more injuries.

- Specific injury rates
  1. Cardiovascular: Cardiac muscle fatigues and is damaged while performing endurance events similarly to skeletal muscle. Troponin T levels are elevated in 27% of Ironman Triathlon finishers and echocardiograms have demonstrated a 24% reduction in postrace ejection fractions compared to pre-race values. There is no published data concerning the rate of fatal cardiac complications in triathletes. We do know from the marathon literature that it is a very rare, one in 50,000 complications (Mayers and Noakes, 2000).
  2. Gastrointestinal bleeding: About 8 to 30% of marathoners have evidence of intra- or postrace gastrointestinal bleeding. The etiology is believed to be relative intestinal ischemia as a result of blood shunting to exercising muscles.
  3. Abdominal cramping: Associated with competitors who consume a diet high in fiber before the race. It may also be seen with the excess consumption of carbohydrates before or during the race.
  4. Diarrhea (Runners Trots): Abdominal pain and diarrhea associated with prolonged running or biking. This condition is caused by ischemic changes in the bowel as a result of the shunting of blood to exercising muscles. This may occur during or shortly after the completion of the race.
  5. Nausea and vomiting: Eating 30 min before a triathlon is highly associated with vomiting during the swim. A diet high in fat or protein and the consumption of hypertonic beverages results in a high rate of nausea and vomiting amongst competitors.
  6. Hematology: About 30% of triathletes demonstrate microscopic hematuria and 95% have a decrease in haptoglobin after an event. These numbers demonstrate that foot strike hemolysis, renal ischemia, and bladder contusions are frequent occurrences.
  7. Infectious diseases: Fresh water swimming in high-risk areas has resulted in triathletes developing leptospirosis. Lyme disease in endemic areas

may also raise the potential risk to triathletes competing in extreme course triathlons.

8. Sunburn: *Sun protection factor sunscreen of at least 15* (SPF 15), a hat or visor, and UV protective sunglasses are recommended to prevent the burning effects of the sun during training and competition.

TRAINING CONSIDERATIONS

- Triathlons are unique and demanding events that require a dedicated, well-organized training program. Proper training will prepare a competitor for successful completion of the race and minimize the risk of injury while training and while competing.
  1. Training programs need to be customized to meet the competitors' needs—what works for one athlete may not work for another. Recommend that novice competitors check on the abundant resources on the web, in triathlon magazines and from more experienced athletes and develop a program that suits them.
- General triathlon training recommendations
  1. Increase training distance and time by no more than 10% per week.
  2. Incorporate a regular stretching program as part of training.
  3. Insure proper amounts of sleep and appropriate nutrition.
  4. Listen to your body: if you start a workout and feel tired or run-down, reduce the workout to a shorter distance. Pushing yourself and completing the longer workout may do you more harm in the long run.
  5. Swim, bike, and run distances a little further than the race distance—builds confidence that you will be able to complete the race.
  6. Open water swimming is very different from lap swimming in a pool; race day is not the best time to try it for the first time. Training will require some extra personnel as solo open water swimming is not recommended.
  7. Train on the actual race course if it is possible.
  8. Do not train hard the 2 weeks prior to the triathlon; you won't make enough of an improvement to notice but you may hamper your performance.
  9. Get plenty of sleep the night before the race.

BRICK TRAINING

- A combination bike/run workout that is used to help train for probably the toughest part of the race, getting off the bike and onto your feet.
  1. Phrase coined in the late 1980s: Bike – Run – ICK (BRICK) descriptive term for how one's legs feel after the workout.
- Very demanding workouts and should not be routine. The novice triathlete should do only 1–2 before a competition with the more seasoned triathlete doing 3–4 at the most.

NUTRITIONAL CONSIDERATIONS

- Energy expenditure during exercise depends on the duration, frequency, and intensity of the exercise. Energy expenditure and energy intake need to be balanced and appropriate for the specific activity that the athlete is training for or competing in.
  1. Triathlons are incredibly energy expending events, with the average male Ironman competitor requiring 9000 kcal during a race and 3000–6000 kcal during training (DiMarco and Samuels, 2001).
- Triathletes acquire 99% of their energy from the body's endurance or aerobic system. After approximately 2 min of exercise the body switches from anaerobic systems to aerobic systems for energy. ATP-creatine phosphate, glucose, and muscle glycogen provide rapid energy to exercising muscle but are unsustainable over prolonged periods. If carbohydrates are not continued during endurance activities, glycogen stores are depleted in approximately 1 h. The aerobic or endurance system through the utilization of fats via the Krebs cycle and electron transport can produce the large amounts of *adenosine triphosphate* (ATP) required for prolonged activity. More than one energy system may be utilized concurrently. This process is dynamic.
  1. The conversion of energy systems from anaerobic to aerobic is not abrupt and the intensity, duration, frequency, type of activity, and the fitness level of the individual all play a role in determining the conversion point.
  2. Training does not impact the total amount of energy expended during practice or competition but it does change the source of the energy from carbohydrates to fats. A well-trained athlete uses a higher percentage of fat, with long-chain fatty acids being the preferred source, than an untrained person at the same workload.
- The diet of the triathlete should be the same generally well-rounded, balanced diet that is recommended to all adults with some specific changes based on the need of the sport.
  1. The average endurance athlete requires approximately 55 kcal/kg body weight while training. The daily requirements are as follows:

a. About 55–70% (6–10 g/kg body weight or 8–10 kcal/kg body weight) of the diet should be in the form of carbohydrates.

b. About 25–30% of the diet should be from fats.

c. About 12–15% (1–1.5 g/kg body weight) of the diet should be high quality protein (American College of Sports Medicine, 2000).

• Athletes are always looking for something that will give them an advantage over their competitors. There are many ergogenic aids that are available, both legally and illegally, to athletes in an attempt to improve their performance. Carbohydrate loading has been proven to improve performance during endurance events. Caffeine ingestion of 3–5 g/kg also improves endurance performance for many athletes. This dose typically has an ergogenic effect without exceeding those serum levels banned by sport governing bodies (Paluska, 2002).

1. Carbohydrate loading has been a proven method to increase endurance event performance since the late 1960s. This technique has been shown to increase the glycogen stores in the muscles being exercised in events that last longer than 90 min.

2. The older method of depleting glycogen stores, 1 week of exhaustive exercise in conjunction with 3 days of a low carbohydrate (less than 100 g/day) diet prior to 3 days of carbohydrate loading with minimal exercise, is no longer recommended due to significant undesired side effects (irritability, hypoglycemia, stiffness and heaviness of muscles, diarrhea, dehydration, and chest pain in older athletes) (DiMarco and Samuels, 2001).

3. The current recommendations for carbohydrate loading are a diet composed of 60–70% carbohydrates and a decrease in the training regiment during the 3 days prior to competition.

• Athletes need to experiment with an individualized preevent and intraevent fuel source that will help to minimize the risk of glycogen depletion, dehydration and poor performance. Triathletes should never utilize a new hydration–nutrition regimen on race day.

1. High fat and protein containing foods should be avoided in the 3 h prior to competition. About 150–300 g of carbohydrate in any form is recommended. Some competitors recommended 1g/kg of body weight of carbohydrate 1 h before competition. There is no evidence that this will improve performance and is more of an anecdotal recommendation that athletes need to decide for themselves about.

2. About 30–60 g/h of carbohydrate during events that last longer than 1 h has been proven to be beneficial to performance. Glucose and sucrose should be the primary carbohydrates ingested as they provide more energy and have fewer side effects than fructose. Newer studies suggest that a small amount of protein along with carbohydrates may have an even better effect on endurance performance (Convertino et al, 1996).

3. Following postevent rehydration, ingestion of foods high in carbohydrates along with a moderate amount of protein should be consumed to help with the repair and maintenance of muscle tissue.

• Hydration

1. Hydration is the most important factor affecting performance. As little as 2–4% dehydration has been shown to negatively affect performance.

2. Water loss occurs primarily through sweat. Ambient temperature, humidity, exercise intensity, and rate of fluid intake all play a role in the overall hydration status of a competitor. Competitors can lose 2 to 6% of their body weight during a race as a result of sweating. Trained athletes can lose 1–3 L of sweat per hour.

a. Average competitors do not consume enough fluid to negate the fluid lost. Consuming beverages while biking is a little easier and more productive than drinking while running. Elite runners may consume as little as 200 mL of fluid during distance events that last over 2 h.

b. Minimal dehydration leads to impaired heat dissipation due to decreased skin blood flow, decreased plasma volume and can lead to severe hydration that can lead to decreased stroke volume, increased heart rate, and possibly heat stroke.

3. Starting an event hydrated or slightly overhydrated will be beneficial to the competitor, as we know that by the end they will be dehydrated. Competitors need to force hydrate themselves the day prior to the competition and consume 400 to 600 mL up to 2 h prior (Convertino et al, 1996).

4. Ideally an athlete will replace fluids at a rate that equals their loss. A loss of 500 mL of fluid equates to a 1-lb decrease in body weight. This can be an excellent guide to post competition fluid replacement needs (Fieseler, 2001).

5. The frequency and amount of fluid consumed by an endurance athlete is a topic of great interest with recommendations changing as more research on the topic is published. About 150 to 300 mL of water every 15 to 20 min of exercise depending on sweat rate is recommended.

a. Too little or too much hydration each lead to their own set of problems—dehydration and hyponatremia respectively, so consuming the proper amount is paramount to maximizing performance.

b. Current recommendations are for competitors to consume 150 to 300 mL every 15–20 min of exercise. These recommendations can lead to problems for slow competitors who spend a lot of time on the course and as a result can consume large volumes of fluid and possibly develop hyponatremia. On the other hand, elite athletes may consume less than 200 mL of fluid during a standard endurance event (Convertino et al, 1996).

c. Noakes proposes that "back in the pack" competitors be urged to drink *ad libitum* (no more than 400–800 mL/h) instead of the traditional drink as much as possible/force hydration model. In his opinion, this method will maintain competitors' vascular status and minimize their risk for dilutional hyponatremia (Noakes, 2003).

6. Which fluids should be consumed by athletes while training or competing?

a. Competitions lasting less than 1 h—water is the best replacement fluid.

b. Competitions lasting greater than 1 h—a carbohydrate/electrolyte replacement beverage is more appropriate.

1. A 4–8% carbohydrate solution is optimal with 10% carbohydrates being the maximum recommended amount. This will maximize the quick absorption of carbohydrates and minimize potential side effects.

REFERENCES

American College of Sports Medicine: American Dietetic Association and Dietitians of Canada: Joint position statement nutrition and athletic performance. *Med Sci Sports Exerc* 2130–2138, 2000.

Burns J, Keenan AM, Redmond AC: Factors associated with triathlon-related overuse injuries. *J Orhop Sports Phy Ther* 33(4):177–184, 2003.

Convertino VA, Armstrong LE et al: Position stand exercise and fluid replacement. *Med Sci Sports Exerc* 28:I–vii, 1996.

DiMarco NM, Samuels M: Nutritional considerations, in O'Connor FG, Wilder RP (eds.): *Textbook of Running Medicine*, New York, NY, McGraw Hill, 2001, pp 477–489.

Fieseler: The ultramarathoner, in O'Connor FG, Wilder RP (eds.): *Textbook of Running Medicine*, New York, NY, McGraw Hill, 2001, pp 469–477.

Hellemans J: Maximizing Olympic Distance Triathlon Performance—A Sports Medicine Perspective.

Mayers LB, Noakes TD: A guide to treating ironman triathletes at the finish line. *Phys Sportsmed* 28(8), 2000.

Noakes T: Hyponatremia in distance runners: Fluid and sodium balance during exercise. *Curr Sports Med Rep* 1(4):197–207, 2003.

Paluska SA: Caffeine and exercise. *Curr Sports Med Rep* 2(4):213–219, 2002.

Thompson MJ, Rivara FP: Bicycle-related injuries. *Am Fam Phys* 63(10):2007–2014, 2001.

Williams MM, Hawley JA et al: Injuries amongst competitive triathletes. *N Z J Sports Med:* 2–6, 1988.

BIBLIOGRAPHY

Armstrong LE et al: Position stand—heat and cold illnesses during distance running. *Am Coll Sports Med*, 1996.

Bouchama A, Knochel JP: Medical progress: Heat stroke. *N Engl J Med* 346(25):1978–1988, 2002.

Cianca JC, Roberts WO, Horn D: Distance running: Organization of the medical team, in O'Connor FG, Wilder RP (eds.): *Textbook of Running Medicine* New York, NY, McGraw Hill, 2001, pp 489–504.

Collins K, Wagner M et al: Overuse injuries in triathletes. A study of the 1986 Seafair Triathlon. *Am J Sports Med* 17(5):675–680, 1989.

Grange JT: Planning for large events. *Curr Sports Med Rep* 1(3): 156–161.

Korkia PK, Tunstall-Pedoe DS, Maffulli N: An epidemiological investigation of training and injury patterns in British triathletes. *Br J Sports Med* 28(3):191–196, 1994.

Martinez JM, Laird R: Managing triathlon competition. *Curr Sports Med Rep* 2(3):142–146, 2003.

Noakes T: Fluid replacement during marathon running. *Clin J Sports Med* 13(5):309–318, 2003.

93 WEIGHTLIFTING

Joe Hart, MS, ATC
Christopher D Ingersoll, PhD, ATC, FACSM

BASIC MUSCLE PHYSIOLOGY

SKELETAL MUSCLE CONTRACTION

• Several bundles of muscle fibers, called fascicles, comprise a skeletal muscle. A muscle fiber is composed of several myofibrils bundled together. Myofibrils contain a series of sarcomeres arranged end-to-end (Lorenz and Campello, 2001).

• Sarcomeres are the functional and contractile component of skeletal muscle through a dynamic interaction between the proteins actin and myosin.

- According to the sliding filament theory, actin and myosin slide past each other to produce sarcomere shortening. Ca^{2+} is released in the sarcomere in response to an action potential that exposes myosin cross-bridge binding sites on actin. Myosin cross bridges bind to actin and pull actin filaments closer to the center of each sarcomere producing force and stiffness within the skeletal muscle (Lorenz and Campello, 2001).
- Force production by a skeletal muscle can be voluntarily graded; however, the muscle fibers innervated by one motor neuron (i.e., a motor unit) act in an all or none fashion. As more motor units are recruited in a particular skeletal muscle, the muscle produces more force (Lorenz and Campello, 2001).

SKELETAL MUSCLE FIBER TYPES

- There are several different types of muscle fiber based on structure and function. These include Type I, Type IIA, and Type IIB.
- Type I muscle fibers (slow twitch oxidative fibers) have high mitochondria content and a rich blood supply. They are difficult to fatigue but do not provide high amounts of muscle force or tension. Type I fibers act in an aerobic capacity during activity.
- Type IIA muscle fibers (fast twitch oxidative-glycolytic fibers) also have high mitochondria content and are moderately capable of performing aerobic and anaerobic activities.
- Type IIB muscle fibers (fast twitch glycolytic fibers) have sparse mitochondria content and blood supply. They fatigue easily but are capable of producing higher force and tension. Type IIB fibers act in an anaerobic capacity during activity.
- All muscle fibers within a motor unit have the same metabolic characteristics (fiber type); however, skeletal muscles can be composed of different types of muscle fibers based on the metabolic demand of the muscle (Lorenz and Campello, 2001).
- Muscle fiber type composition in human skeletal muscle is genetically determined (Lorenz and Campello, 2001). There is little information regarding muscle fiber type transformations in response to training/exercise.
- Heavy resistance training caused increased type IIA and decreased type IIB fibers, while type I fiber composition in human skeletal muscle was unchanged (Adams et al, 1993).
- Structural and genetic characteristics of muscle fiber types have been modulated with fiber-specific stimulation *in vitro* (Liu et al, 2001); however, it is unknown whether such changes occur in all muscle fiber types or if the transformation will be sustained over time *in vivo*.

- Since muscle fiber composition is genetically determined, athletes may participate in sports or activities that involve muscle contractions that are more natural. Whether a distance runner can train to be a successful power lifter or vice versa is an issue that has not yet been clearly elucidated.

TYPES OF SKELETAL MUSCLE CONTRACTION

- Skeletal muscle can produce joint movements through concentric and eccentric movements. Skeletal muscle contractions produce muscle tension and control body and joint movement.
- Concentric contractions describe a movement that involves shortening of a muscle against a load, whereas eccentric contractions involve controlled lengthening of a muscle against a load.
- Eccentric muscle contractions produce greater muscle force and more myofibrillar disruption than concentric exercise (Gibala et al, 1995).
- Eccentric muscle contractions (often referred to as *negatives* in weightlifting) are more effective in producing strength gains and hypertrophy than concentric contractions (Higbie et al, 1996); however, both eccentric (negative) and concentric (positive) contractions elicit gains in skeletal muscle strength and size (Higbie et al, 1996).
- Isometric muscle contractions produce muscle tension without joint movement. For example, pushing against a wall or contracting the quadriceps muscle while holding the knee motionless at a particular point in the knee range of motion.
- Isotonic muscle contractions produce muscle tension and joint movement against a constant load where rate of movement is variable. For example, a dumbbell curl is a contraction against a constant load that can be voluntarily moved at a self-selected rate. This is the most typical contraction in weightlifting.
- Isokinetic muscle contractions involve a constant rate of joint displacement that is maintained by varying amounts of resistance based on muscle effort. This is uncommon in weightlifting or athletic settings. Isokinetic exercise requires expensive machinery and is usually most applicable in the rehabilitation setting.
- Isotonic and isokinetic muscle movements can be performed through concentric or eccentric muscle contractions.

MUSCLE RESPONSE TO RESISTANCE TRAINING

- Improvements in muscle strength, power, or endurance are best achieved by overloading the muscle(s) being trained.

- The overload principle states that when a muscle is exposed to a stress or load that is greater than what it usually experiences, it will adapt so that it is able to handle the greater load (Lorenz and Campello, 2001; Wathen and Roll, 1994; Kraemer et al, 2002).
- Similarly, the SAID principle (*specific adaptations to imposed demands*) states that a muscle or body tissue will adapt to the specific demands imposed on it. For example, if a muscle is overloaded its fibers will grow in size so it is able to produce enough force to overcome the imposed load (Lorenz and Campello, 2001; Wathen and Roll, 1994).
- Observed strength gains within the first few weeks of a weightlifting program are mostly due to neuromuscular adaptations (Deschenes and Kraemer, 2002). As exercise intensity increases and muscles begin to fatigue, the nervous system recruits larger motor units with higher frequencies of stimulation to provide the force necessary to overcome the imposed resistance (Lorenz and Campello, 2001).
- Early strength gains and increased muscle tension production from training result from a more efficient neural recruitment process as well as more densely packed muscle filaments within the skeletal muscle (Narci et al, 1996).

MUSCLE HYPERTROPHY

- Human muscle hypertrophy occurs when the cross-sectional area of a muscle group increases (Narci et al, 1996; Conroy and Earle, 1994). As a skeletal muscle hypertrophies contractile proteins are synthesized (Deschenes and Kraemer, 2002) and is therefore capable of producing more force.
- Type IIA fibers exhibit the greatest growth while types IIB and I exhibit the least amount of growth in response to resistance training (Deschenes and Kraemer, 2002). Muscle hypertrophy is more common in fast twitch than slow twitch muscles.
- Strength training leads to muscle hypertrophy, increasing muscle mass (Narci et al, 1996).
- Muscle hypertrophy is typically observed with resistance training after 6–7 weeks of strength training (Kraemer et al, 2002; Deschenes and Kraemer, 2002).
- There appears to be a gender difference in the rate at which muscles hypertrophy favoring males (Ivey et al, 2000). Additionally, females lose muscle mass quicker than males when detrained (Ivey et al, 2000).
- Resistance-trained muscles hypertrophy in order to adapt to greater imposed loads (Kraemer, 1994). Hypertrophy of individual muscle fibers contributes to changes in muscle cross sectional area (McCall et al, 1996). Muscle fiber hyperplasia does not appear

to play a role in increased muscle cross sectional area or strength gains in resistance trained men (McCall et al, 1996).

BASIC WEIGHTLIFTING PROGRAMS

- There are several different weightlifting programs that can be customized to an individual or their strength training and athletic goals. An effective program balances muscle overloading with recovery time to facilitate strength gains. Sample weightlifting sets based on the DeLorme and DAPRE methods are presented in Table 93-1.

THE DELORME METHOD

- The DeLorme method is a progressive resistance exercise program based on the overload principle (Deschenes and Kraemer, 2002; Stamford, 1998). This method is based on the 10 *rep max* (RM). First, a weight that the athlete is able to lift 10 times (with the desired muscle group(s)) is determined. A total of three sets of 10 repetitions are performed per session for each muscle at 50, 75, and 100% of the 10 RM. The athlete is encouraged to perform more than 10 repetitions during the third set to serve as an overload to the muscle group being trained. As the athlete's 10 RM increases, so does the resistance in each set respectively (Table 93-1).

DAILY ADJUSTED PROGRESSIVE RESISTANCE EXERCISE

- The *daily adjusted progressive resistance exercise* (DAPRE) method of strength training guides the athlete through four sets of exercise per muscle group or other desired task. DAPRE guidelines provide recommendations for when to increase resistance and how much added resistance is appropriate based on individual performance (Table 93-1). This method is described more thoroughly by Knight (Knight, 1979; 1985).

TABLE 93-1   Weight Lifting Programs

	DELORME	DAPRE
Set 1	50% 10 RM* × 10 reps	50% 6 RM† × 10 reps
Set 2	75% 10 RM × 10 reps	75% 6 RM × 6 reps
Set 3	100% 10 RM × 10 reps	100% 6 RM to failure
Set 4	—	Adjusted‡ weight to failure

*10 rep max = weight with which one can perform 10 consecutive repetitions
†6 rep max = weight with which one can perform 6 consecutive repetitions
‡Adjusted weight: Add 5 lb if >7 reps in third set; subtract 5 lb if <5 reps in third set; no change if 5–7 reps performed in third set

- The first two sets in DAPRE involve 10 reps at 50% and 6 reps at 75% of the athlete's predetermined 6 RM. The 6 RM is termed the "working weight." Repetitions in the third set at 100% of the 6 RM are performed to failure (maximum repetitions). The number of repetitions performed in the third set determines how much resistance to add or drop off for the fourth set. Typically, if five to seven repetitions are performed in the third set, resistance for the fourth set remains the same. If less than five or more than seven repetitions are performed, the resistance in the fourth set is decreased or increased respectively. The *adjusted weight* is used for maximum repetitions in the fourth set. The *working weight* for the next day of resistance training is adjusted based on the number of repetitions achieved in the fourth set similar to the method used to adjust the weight for the fourth set.
- The DAPRE method can be adjusted for each individual based on his or her training goals. Manipulating the amount of weight added to the adjusted weight for the fourth set or the modified working weight for the next day's lift can change the pace of individual programs.

PERIODIZATION

- Periodization involves a gradual decrease in training volume as training intensity increases toward the competitive athletic season (in-season) (Brown, 2001). Periodization has been described previously (Wathen and Roll, 1994; Kraemer et al, 2002; Deschenes and Kraemer, 2002).
- In preparation for athletic competition, periodization begins in the athletic off-season where training volume is high but intensity is low. Initially, strength gains and muscle hypertrophy are the goals of this phase. As training intensity gradually increases through the post-season and into the preseason, training volume decreases. This progression continues through the preseason where sport-specific skill training is maximized to facilitate the transition to competition.

SAMPLE EXERCISES FOR MAJOR MUSCLE GROUPS

- There are several exercises that can be used for each muscle group. The appropriate exercise depends on equipment availability, experience, or preference of the weightlifter, or training goals. Isolated muscle exercises are appropriate for toning and strengthening muscles. Whole-body strength exercises that require coordinated, multiple body segment movements are appropriate to develop power and athletic skill.

UPPER BODY/TRUNK

- Seated military press (deltoid): In the seated position, weighted dumbbells or a bar is lifted above the head and then returned to the anterior shoulders/upper chest.
- Bench press/pec major: While supine on a bench, weighted dumbbells or a bar is lifted off the chest until the arms are fully extended and then slowly back to the chest.
- Bicep curls/biceps brachii: In the seated or standing position, weighted dumbbells or a bar is lifted through the full elbow range of motion from the extended to flexed position, then slowly back to the extended position.
- Triceps extension/triceps brachii: While in the supine position, shoulders flexed to 90° and elbows extended, resistance is lowered by flexing the elbow followed by concentric elbow extension.
- Rows: Trapezuis/rhomboids: In the seated or standing position and shoulders flexed to 90°, arms are drawn back by extending the shoulders and flexing the elbows. Visualize squeezing the back-blades (scapula) together. This exercise can be done with free-weights, resistive bands, or a machine.

LOWER BODY

- Squats/Quadriceps: In the standing position with resistance fixed at the shoulders, the body is lowered by flexing the hips and knees while maintaining upright upper body posture.
- Hamstring curls/Hamstrings: In the prone position, resistance fixed at the distal lower leg is curled toward the hips by flexing the knee. This is usually done with the assistance of a pulley-style machine or can be done in standing with ankle weights.
- Calf raises/triceps surae: In the standing or seated position, the body and added resistance (if desired) is elevated by plantar flexing the ankle joint.

GUIDELINES FOR EXERCISE PRESCRIPTION

TRAINING VOLUME AND INTENSITY

- It is important to consider training volume and intensity of training when designing an effective weightlifting program. The goal of a weightlifting program is to achieve maximal or desired gains while allowing for an appropriate amount of time between sets and between sessions for muscle and body recovery.
- Training volume is determined by multiplying the number of repetitions performed in an exercise session

by the resistance used (Kraemer et al, 2002). Therefore, similar training volumes are achieved when light resistance is used for high repetitions and when heavy resistance is used for low repetitions. In periodized programs, it is appropriate to begin with high training volumes (off-season) and progress to lower volumes at higher intensity (preseason).

- Intensity is analogous to power and is therefore dependent on the amount of resistance as well as the speed of the movement (Wathen, 1994*b*). High training intensities are appropriate in the preseason and can coincide with sport-specific training.
- Overtraining can result in decreases in muscle strength and function. It usually occurs when either training volume or intensity are too great and the body cannot appropriately adapt (Brown, 2001).
- As mentioned earlier in this chapter, muscles will adapt to the specific demands imposed on it. When designing an exercise or weightlifting program it is important to include activities that are specific to the athlete's goals. For example, if an athlete wants to perform movements that require high muscle strength and power, they should train with weights that are closer to their 1 RM and perform fewer repetitions per set (Wathen and Roll, 1994). Likewise, if an athlete wants to perform movements that require endurance, they should use less weight with higher repetitions.
- The athletic year is divided into in-season, post and off-season, and preseason segments. During the postseason and off-season, training should concentrate on recovery from the competitive season and maintain fitness and strength. Strength training can begin in the off-season and gradually progress to power training and sport-specific training during preseason. Strength, endurance, and power maintenance should be performed in-season.

SPECIAL CONSIDERATIONS

- Strength describes the maximum force that can be generated by a muscle, whereas power is the ability of a muscle to generate large forces quickly. Endurance is the ability of a muscle to contract repeatedly and generate forces for long periods of time.
- Training for muscle strength should include training with resistance that is closer to maximum ability with lower repetitions. This type of training is most appropriate in the athletic off-season.
- Training for muscle power involves coordinated movements that encourage speed, accuracy, and fluency. Power training is most appropriate in the athletic preseason and gradually progresses to the competitive season (in-season).
- Strength training in both the anterior and posterior musculature or training both agonist and antagonist muscle

groups is important in an effective strength-training program. It may improve sport or activity specific performance and reduce the risk of injury (Wathen, 1994*a*).
- It is important to incorporate gradual warm-up, cooldown, and flexibility exercises into a strength training regimen to maintain muscle health and fitness, reduce the likelihood of injury or postexercise soreness and to improve athletic and weightlifting performance.
- Supervised and guided strength training programs yield greater strength gains than those who are unsupervised (Mazzetti et al, 2000). Recruiting assistance from exercise physiologists, *certified strength and conditioning specialists* (CSCS), *certified personal trainers* (CPT), or *certified athletic trainers* (ATC) may facilitate strength gains and improve overall outcomes and sport-specific preparedness.
- Finally, athletes are encouraged to participate in weightlifting programs with at least one partner. Weightlifting partners can motivate each other, provide constructive feedback on technique and form and provide spotting for heavy or potentially dangerous lifts. An athlete should never participate in weightlifting alone.

REFERENCES

Adams GR, Hather BM, Baldwin KM et al: Skeletal muscle myosin heavy chain composition and resistance training. *J Appl Physiol* Feb 74(2):911–915, 1993.

Brown LE: Nonlinear versus linear periodization models. *Strength Cond J* 23(1):42–44, 2001.

Conroy BP, Earle RW: Bone, muscle, and connective tissue adaptations to physical activity, in Baechle TR (ed.): *Essentials of Strength Training and Conditioning*. Champaign, IL, Human Kinetics, 1994, pp 435–446.

Deschenes MR, Kraemer WJ: Performance and physiologic adaptations to resistance training. *Am J Phys Med Rehabil* 81(11 Suppl):S3–S16, Nov. 2002.

Gibala MJ, MacDougall JD, Tarnopolsky MA et al: Changes in human skeletal muscle ultrastructure and force production after acute resistance exercise. *J Appl Physiol* 78(2):702–708, Feb. 1995.

Higbie EJ, Cureton KJ, Warren GL et al: Effects of concentric and eccentric training on muscle strength, cross-sectional area, and neural activation. *J Appl Physiol* 81(5):2173–2181, Nov. 1996.

Ivey FM, Roth SM, Ferrell RE et al: Effects of age, gender, and myostatin genotype on the hypertrophic response to heavy resistance strength training. *J Gerontol A Biol Sci Med Sci* 55(11):M641–M648, Nov. 2000.

Knight KL: Knee rehabilitation by the daily adjustable progressive resistive exercise technique. *Am J Sports Med* 7(6):336–337, Nov.–Dec. 1979.

Knight KL: Quadriceps strengthening with the DAPRE technique: case studies with neurological implications. *Med Sci Sports Exerc* 17(6):646–650, Dec. 1985.

Kraemer WJ: General adaptations to resistance and endurance training programs, in Baechle TR (ed.): *Essentials of Strength Training and Conditioning*. Champaign, IL, Human Kinetics, 1994, pp 127–150.

Kraemer WJ, Adams K, Cafarelli E et al: American College of Sports Medicine position stand. Progression models in resistance training for healthy adults. *Med Sci Sports Exerc* 34(2):364–380, Feb. 2002.

Liu Y, Cseresnyes Z, Randall WR et al: Activity-dependent nuclear translocation and intranuclear distribution of NFATc in adult skeletal muscle fibers. *J Cell Biol* 155(1):27–39, Oct. 1, 2001.

Lorenz T, Campello M: Biomechanics of skeletal muscle, in Nordin M, Frankel VH (eds.): *Basic Biomechanics of the Musculoskeletal System,* 3rd ed. Philadelphia, PA, Lippincott Williams & Wilkins, 2001, pp 148–174.

Mazzetti SA, Kraemer WJ, Volek JS et al: The influence of direct supervision of resistance training on strength performance. *Med Sci Sports Exerc* 32(6):1175–1184, June 2000.

McCall GE, Byrnes WC, Dickinson A et al: Muscle fiber hypertrophy, hyperplasia, and capillary density in college men after resistance training. *J Appl Physiol* 81(5):2004–2012, Nov. 1996.

Narci M, Hoppeler H, Kayser B et al: Human quadriceps cross-sectional area, torque and neuralactivation during 6 months strength training. *Acta Physiol Scan* 157(2):175–186,1996.

Stamford B: Weight training basics part 2: A sample program. *Phys Sport Med* 26(3), 1998.

Wathen D: Exercise selection, in Baechle TR (ed.): *Essentials of Strength Training and Conditioning*. Champaign, IL, Human Kinetics, 1994a, pp 416–430.

Wathen D: Load Assignment, in Baechle TR (ed.): *Essentials of Strength Training and Conditioning*. Champaign, IL, Human Kinetics, 1994b, pp 435–446.

Wathen D, Roll F: Training methods and modes, in Baechle TR (ed.): *Essentials of Strength Training and Conditioning*. Champaign, IL, Human Kinetics, 1994, pp 403–415.

94 LACROSSE

CPT Thad Barkdull, MD

INTRODUCTION

• History
  1. Considered to be the oldest sport in North America.
  2. Derived from *baggataway*, a game French observed Native Americans playing in seventeenth century Canada.
  3. Stick, or *lacrosse* used in game comes from appearance similar to bishop's crosier or crosse.
  4. In 1879, Canada formed the National Lacrosse Association (now the Canadian Lacrosse Association).
  5. Eleven U.S. men's college and club teams formed the National Lacrosse Association in 1879.
  6. By 1950, over 200 teams in the United States.
  7. Still the national sport of Canada.
• Demographics (U.S. Lacrosse)
  1. Estimated that 250,000 people played organized lacrosse in 2001.
     a. Over 180,000 men
     b. Over 51,000 women
  2. Nearly 25,000 men in over 400 universities with sanctioned programs.
  3. Over 72,000 men at 1,600 high schools now have varsity programs.
  4. Over 240 universities have sanctioned women's programs for 5,500 women athletes.
  5. There are 160 high school programs for over 15,000 women.
  6. Over 100,000 spectators watched the Division I, II, and III National Championships in 1999.
• The Game (Sherbondy, 2002)
  1. Men's field lacrosse
     a. Ten players per side:
        i. Three attackmen (offense), three defensivemen (defense), three midfielders (both), one goalie (defense).
        ii. Teams may allow a maximum of six players on the offensive half and seven on the defensive half.
     b. The field is 110×60 yards.
     c. Goals are 6-ft square with a 9-ft diameter *crease* around them.
     d. Substitutions may occur during play stoppage or during play (similar to hockey).
     e. Players may pass the ball or run while cradling the ball in their *crosse.*
     f. The object is to score more points than the opponent by putting the ball into the opposition's goal.
     g. Players may hit an opposing player who controls the ball or is within 5 yards of ball.
     h. Players may hit an opponent's stick or gloved hand with their own.
  2. Women's field lacrosse
     a. Twelve players:
        i. One goalie, four attackers, four defenders, three midfielders.
        ii. The field is 120×70 yards.
        iii. No contact between players.
        iv. Restraining Line Rule—only seven offensive and eight defensive players in 30-yard area around goal.
  3. Box lacrosse
     a. Six players per side.
     b. Played in enclosed area.
     c. More contact allowed than field lacrosse.

- Equipment
  1. *Crosse* or stick
     a. Length varies by position.
     b. Made of wood, laminated wood, or synthetic material.
     c. Attackmen and midfielder's sticks must be 40–42-in. long.
     d. Defensivemen's stick must be 52–72-in. long.
     e. The head must be 6.5–10-in. wide, or 10–12-in. for the goalie.
  2. Ball
     a. Made of solid rubber.
     b. 7.75–8 in. in circumference.
     c. 5–5.25 oz.
  3. Personal equipment
     a. Varies by different game and position played.
     b. Required equipment
        i. All players required to wear mouthguards.
        ii. In men's game, helmet with full facemask and padded gloves.
        iii. Women are currently only required to wear mouthguards, though some wear soft helmets (goalies are a notable exception, see below).
     c. Goalies
        i. Both men's and women's games require head, chest, and throat protection.
        ii. The stick has a significantly larger net than other players.
        iii. Athletic cup is optional but highly recommended.
     d. Attackmen
        i. Frequently wear elbow pads, shoulder pads, and rib protectors.
        ii. Sticks tend to be shorter.
     e. Defensivemen
        i. Frequently wear less protective gear in the men's game, often only the required helmet, mouthguard, and gloves.
        ii. Have a much longer stick than other players.
     f. Midfielders
        i. Often wear less protection than attackmen.
        ii. May have longer or shorter stick depending on specialty (defensive midfielders have longer sticks).

INJURY EPIDEMIOLOGY (NCAA INJURY SURVEILLANCE SYSTEM)

- Injury Surveillance System (ISS) was developed by National Collegiate Athletic Association (NCAA) in 1982 to monitor collegiate athlete injury patterns.
- Monitors type of injury, body part injured, severity of injury, field type, field condition, and special equipment worn.

- Data are collected by certified athletic trainers at NCAA-sanctioned schools.
- Reportable injuries must meet specific criteria.
  1. Occurs during practice or contest.
  2. Requires medical attention by athletic trainer or physician.
  3. Causes the student-athlete to miss one or more days of participation beyond the day of injury.
- Data is tabulated as rates per 1000 *athlete exposures* (AE).
- Game data (2002)
  1. Men's
     a. Overall AE: 10.8 (61.8%)—8th out of 16 NCAA sports.
        i. Equates to one injury every six games.
     b. Injuries with 7+ days lost—3.0 (8th)
     c. Injuries requiring surgery—0.9 (8th)
  2. Women's
     a. Overall AE: 8.4 (67.0%)—10th
        i. Equates to one injury every eight games.
     b. Injuries with 7+ days lost—1.7 (13th)
     c. Injuries requiring surgery—0.7 (11th)
- Practice data
  1. Men's
     a. Overall AE: 3.2 (31.2%)—13th
     b. Injuries with 7+ days lost—1.2 (10th)
     c. Injuries requiring surgery—0.2 (10th)
  2. Women's
     a. Overall AE: 3.6 (33.0%)—11th
     b. Injuries with 7+ days lost—1.2 (9th)
     c. Injuries requiring surgery—0.3 (7th)
- Men experienced injury rates more than three times as frequently in game situations than practice.
- Women had more than twice as many injuries in games than practice.
- Severe injuries were more prevalent in men than women during competition, but women experienced a slightly higher proportion of injuries in practice than men, with more severe injury patterns.
- Specific injury patterns (NCAA News, 2002)
  1. Women's (data from 2002 season)
     a. Ankle, lower leg, and knee injuries are most prevalent in practice (43%).
     b. Ankle, knee, and head injuries are most prevalent in game situations (55%).
        i. Sprains, strains, and contusions accounted for the majority of game injuries.
     c. Seventeen percent of injuries were above the neck, with 3% to the eye.
     d. Twenty percent of injuries in games were the result of player–player contact, and 20% from stick–player contact.
  2. Men's
     a. Ankle, knee, and upper leg injuries are most prevalent in practice (47%).

b. Head, upper leg, and knee are most prevalent in game situations (47%).

1. Sprains, strains, and contusions were top three injuries.

c. Player–player contact accounted for 40% of injuries in game situations.

3. Catastrophic injuries (U.S. Consumer Product Safety Commission's National Injury Information, 2001)

a. Data collected from 1982 to 2001.

b. In both high school and college, there have been only four fatalities, four nonfatal (permanent severe functional disability) injuries, and three serious injuries (significant injury without permanent disability) reported as a result of direct competition or practice.

c. Four fatalities have occurred as a result of indirect contact while playing lacrosse (exertional injury or complication of a nonfatal injury).

INJURIES IN LACROSSE

- Noncontact (Matthews, Hinton, and Burke, 2001; Casazza and Rossner, 1999; Bartlett, Cress, and Bull, 1991)

1. Lower extremity

a. Groin, hamstring, and low back strains

i. Associated with twisting motion of the torso.

ii. Common motion during passing, shooting, checking, and scooping ground balls.

iii. Performed at high speeds and with rapid changes in direction.

iv. Cryotherapy and strengthening of affected regional musculature key in return to play and reducing repeat injuries.

b. Knee

i. Similar to other field sports, *anterior cruciate ligament* (ACL) and *medial collateral ligament* (MCL) injuries are not uncommon.

1. Account for fewer than 20% of injuries.

2. MCL more commonly affected than LCL.

3. Because of the MCL's deep attachment to the medial meniscal periphery, meniscal tears should be suspected with higher grade MCL injuries.

4. Typically the result of force on the lateral aspect of knee at full extension, with foot planted.

5. May be the result of a lateral blow, but more often the result of planting and directional change resulting in intolerable stresses on ligaments.

6. Grade I and II may be treated nonsurgically.

7. Cryotherapy, hinged braces, hamstring, and quad strengthening are mainstay of rehabilitation.

8. Recovery may take up to 6 weeks, with hinged brace used in competition for 1–2 months for protection.

ii. Patellofemoral syndrome (PFS)

1. Often seen in female players aged 12 to 15, owing to anatomic stresses.

2. Typically presents as anterior knee pain without any physical findings (i.e., instability or effusion).

3. Risk factors include foot pronation, genu valgus, rotated or tilted patellae, or an increased Q-angle.

4. Strengthening of medial quadriceps (VMO) and hamstrings are mainstay of prevention and treatment.

5. Some significant anatomic abnormalities may require surgical intervention to alleviate symptoms.

c. Ankle

i. Accounts for 16.2% of total injuries in NCAA lacrosse (1994–1996 ISS).

ii. Majority are inversion injuries.

iii. Slight inversion and plantar flexion is the state of least stability, and the point when injury most often occurs.

iv. Ligamentous injuries are most common.

1. *Anterior talofibular ligament* (ATFL), followed by *Calcaneofibular ligament* (CFL), and then *Posterior talofibular ligament* (PTFL).

2. Deltoid ligament injuries are associated with eversion mechanism.

3. Avulsion fractures should be suspected with higher grade ligamentous injuries (grade 2 or higher).

v. Early mobilization for nonfractures is the key to rapid return to healthy play.

1. Consider nonweight bearing exercises (i.e., aqua jogging).

2. Strengthening of evertors, invertors, plantar and dorsiflexors, as well as hip ab- and adductors, and extensors.

3. Final rehabilitation should include dynamic strengthening focusing on proprioception (i.e., slide board, figure 8 running drills).

4. Most sprains will recover in 1 to 3 weeks.

2. Upper extremity

a. Much less common

b. Blocker's exostosis

i. Most often with repetitive stick-to-body contact at deltoid insertion.

ii. Use of appropriate shoulder protection (deltoid cup) important in prevention.

iii. Monitoring for myositis ossificans is important (see Contact.1.c.iv. below).

c. Medial and lateral epicondylitis

i. Usually result of cradling motion in the throwing arm.

ii. Cradling of the ball requires rapid pronation/supination and flexion/extension of the arm.

iii. Stretching of affected muscle groups along with braces to reduce strain at tendinous insertions have proven effective in treating this injury.

3. Others

a. Environmental

i. *Exertional heat illness* (EHI).

1. May occur in both field, usually a spring sport, as well as box lacrosse.

2. Players with more protective equipment (i.e., goalies) at higher risk.

3. Hydration is essential.

4. Monitor players for signs/symptoms of EHI.

5. Provide appropriate water and electrolytes to players during games.

6. Avoid conditions where EHI is more likely.

7. Players showing signs of EHI should be immediately removed from play, equipment removed, and measures taken to decrease body temperature.

b. Abrasions/turf burns

i. More common in box lacrosse or competition on artificial surfaces.

ii. Padding and lubrication with petroleum jelly on at-risk areas may reduce incidence.

iii. Ensure antiseptic cleansing of wound and clean dressings to reduce infection risk.

iv. Prepatellar bursitis is common complication, especially in adolescent athletes.

c. Blisters

i. Occurs in areas of increased friction.

ii. Petroleum jelly, powders, moleskin, nylon socks under thick socks may all help to reduce friction.

iii. Treatment with donut pads to distribute forces away from blister, appropriate cleansing of blister (especially if it has opened).

d. Anterior tibial shin splints

i. Overuse injury.

ii. Associated with fatiguing tibialis anterior that spasms with eccentrically decelerating forefoot.

iii. Irritation of fascia or anterior border of tibia results.

iv. Prevention revolves around proper stretching.

e. Turf Toe

i. Hyperextension of first metatarsal.

ii. Associated with rapid deceleration, commonly on artificial turf.

iii. Inflammatory condition causes chronic pain.

iv. Prevention with proper shoe fit allowing some toe and forefoot movement.

v. Limiting hyperextension by taping is appropriate treatment to allow for return to play.

• Contact

1. Lower extremity

a. Much less common

b. Most often associated with stick-to-body or ball-to-body contact

c. Contusions are common

i. May result from contact with hard rubber ball, which may be propelled at up to 100 mph.

ii. Player controlling the ball is often repeatedly hit in the upper torso and extremities by the defender's stick.

iii. Treated by standard PRICEMM (*protection, rest, ice, compression, elevation, modalities, medication*), may cover area with donut protection to distribute future forces to area around injury.

iv. May be complicated by *myositis ossificans.*

1. Inflammatory bony deposition in muscle from repetitive trauma.

2. Often occurs in vastus lateralis and deltoid insertion of humerus.

3. Areas receiving repeated trauma should be protected with donut and hard plate over area.

2. Upper extremity

a. Olecranon bursitis

i. Often stick-to-body or body-to-ground contact

ii. Many players do not wear elbow pads, and are thus more susceptible to this injury.

iii. Drainage of bursal fluid allows for improvement of symptoms, and may respond to steroid injection into bursal sac; protective gear (i.e., elbow pads) reduces risk of further complication.

b. AC separation

i. Associated with checks into the boards (box lacrosse), stick-to-body contact with a downward blow to the outer aspect of the shoulder and *fall on the outstretched hand* (FOOSH) mechanisms.

ii. AC immobilizers or specific taping systems to hold the distal clavicle in place and allow ligaments to heal in a shortened position.

iii. Reduces later step deformities.

iv. Activity without pain is key to return to play.
c. Scaphoid fracture
  i. Most often from FOOSH injury.
  ii. Immobilization is appropriate treatment.
d. Metacarpal, phalangeal, and interphalangeal joint dislocations
  i. Immediate traction and reduction is ideal.
  ii. Often associated with stick checking or falls where the stick traps the hand/fingers in pathologic manner.
e. Gamekeeper's or skier's thumb
  i. Associated typically with falls in which the thumb is trapped by the stick.
  ii. Hyperextension results in a tear of the ulnar collateral ligament.
  iii. May be complicated by an avulsion fracture from the proximal phalanx (Stener lesion).
f. Forearm fractures
  i. Either from stick-to-body contact during checking or from FOOSH injuries.
  ii. Immobilization is mainstay of treatment.
  iii. Surgical reduction and fixation may be required depending on severity of injury.
g. Shoulder burners (stingers)
  i. Commonly result of stick-to-body contact with a check to the shoulder or a fall onto head or shoulder.
  ii. Downward, forward depression of the shoulder.
  iii. Often present with acute, shooting, shock-like pain in extremity.
  iv. May have some transient motor deficits.
  v. Typically resolves without complication.
• Others
1. Lacerations
  a. Pressure, hemostasis, and suturing if needed
2. Nose bleeds
  a. Hold head forward (player may choke on own blood).
  b. Pressure on lower two-thirds of nostrils.
  c. Packing may aid in tamponading bleed.
3. Concussions
  a. Head injuries account for 3.1% of lacrosse injuries.
  b. Lacrosse helmets are designed to deflect blows from a stick or ball, but are not meant to protect against high-velocity impacts, like being thrust into the boards (box lacrosse), or impact into the ground.
  c. Also common when players are crouched down for scooping ground balls and are struck by another player.
  d. Treatment is based on degree of injury.
    i. Most injury scales refer to amnesia, loss of consciousness, and current mental status as markers of severity.
    ii. When in doubt, withhold player from play till symptom-free and a full assessment can be made.
4. Eye injuries (Waicus, 2002; Webster et al, 1999)
  a. Much more common in women's lacrosse owing to minimal protective gear.
    i. It's felt that appropriate enforcement of the rules for contact will minimize eye and facial injuries.
    ii. Waicus and Webster et al have both argued for mandatory eyewear because of the increased incidence of injury compared to those who wear protective eyewear.
    iii. Others feel that mandatory eyewear will lead to poorer compliance to rules and other head injuries.
  b. Eye protection is available but not required.
  c. May be the result of contact with ball or inadvertent stick contact.
  d. Opponents of mandatory eye protection state that this will encourage more stick-to-body contact, and proper enforcement of current rules are sufficient to protect players.
  e. Traumatic eye injuries should be referred for immediate ophthalmologic examination.
    i. Sunken eyes or extraocular muscle deficiencies may represent periorbital skull fractures.
    ii. Assessment for associated closed head injury may be warranted.
5. Rib fractures and abdominal trauma
  a. Most commonly from stick checking.
  b. Injuries to abdominal organs are uncommon, but should be entertained in cases of significant abdominal pain.
  c. Rib padding may offer some protection.
6. Throat trauma
  a. Usually the result of the ball striking the throat.
  b. Goalies most at risk.
  c. Throat deflectors significantly reduce the incidence of injury.
7. Goalkeeper's thumb (Elkousy et al, 2000)
  a. Fracture of distal or proximal phalanx of thumb.
  b. Typically impact of ball directly on extending thumb as goalie is attempting to save shot on goal.
  c. May require surgical fixation or immobilization.
• May be prevented with rigid covering over distal end of thumb.

REFERENCES

Bartlett B, Cress D, Bull RC: Lacrosse, in Bull RC (ed.): *Handbook of Sports Injuries*. New York, NY, McGraw-Hill, Health Professions Division, 1991, pp 423–451.

Casazza BA, Rossner K: Baseball/lacrosse injuries. *Phys Med Rehabil Clin North Am* 10:141–157, 1999.

Elkousy HA, Janssen H, Ferraro J et al: Lacrosse goalkeeper's thumb. *Am J Sports Med* 28(3):317, 2000.

Matthews LS, Hinton RY, Burke N: Lacrosse, in Fu FH, Stone DA (eds.): *Sports Injuries: Mechanisms, Prevention and Treatment*. Philadelphia, PA, Lippincott Williams & Wilkins, 2001, pp 568–582.

NCAA Injury Surveillance System (ISS), *http://www1.ncaa.org/ membership/ed_outreach/health–safety/iss/index.html.*

NCAA News, *http://www.ncaa.org/news/2002/20020805/awide/ 3916n09.html,* August 5, 2002.

Sherbondy PS: Lacrosse, in Mellion MB, Walsh WM, Madden C, Putukian M, Shelton GL (eds.): *Team Physician's Handbook*, 3rd ed. Philadelphia, PA, Hanley & Belfus, 2002, pp 759–765.

U.S. Consumer Product Safety Commission's National Injury Information Clearinghouse: from *National Center for Catastrophic Sport Injury Research Data Tables,* Nineteenth Annual Report, Fall 1982—Spring 2001; *http://www. unc.edu/ depts/nccsi/AllSport.htm*

U.S. Lacrosse: *http://www.lacrosse.org/*

Waicus KM: Eye injuries in women's lacrosse players. *Clin J Sport Med* 12(1):24–29, 2002.

Webster DA, Bayliss DA, Verel G et al: Head and face injuries in scholastic women's lacrosse with and without eyewear. *Med Sci Sports Exerc* 31(7):938–941, 1999.

95 WRESTLING

Michael G Bowers, DO
Thomas M Howard, MD

INTRODUCTION

- Wrestling is a contact sporting event that matches two competitors against each other physically and mentally. The origins of the sport date back to ancient Greek and Roman Times near 500 B.C.
- There are approximately 400,000 wrestlers of all ages in the United States. As the sport has grown in popularity and participation has increased, it has been noted that there are injuries and conditions that are unique to the sport.

DEFINITION OF TERMS

- **Takedown:** Points given to a wrestler when advantage is gained from a neutral position on feet. This may be achieved by a trip or throw. Dependent on the style of wrestling, higher point values may be given for the more skillful maneuver to achieve the takedown (Kelly and Suby, 2002).
- **Fall:** Also known as a *pin*. Determined by the referee when both shoulders are held to the mat for 1 s. The match is over at this time (Kelly and Suby, 2002).
- **Time advantage:** This is popularly called riding time. Time of control is recorded for both wrestlers and compared. A point is given to the wrestlers if their time is one or more minutes greater than their opponent's (NCAA, 2003).
- **Sparring:** An activity participated in when both of the competitors are in a neutral position on their feet. Usually comprises grappling and blocking in an attempt to achieve a takedown (Kelly and Suby, 2002).
- **Leg wrestling:** Term used to describe the use of legs while on the mat to attempt to control an opponent (Kelly and Suby, 2002).
- **Injury time:** Amount of time allowed to a wrestler to attempt to recover from an illness or injury. The time allotted is a maximum of 90 s throughout the match. Additionally, a competitor may have two time-outs during the match to tend to injuries as long as 90 s of total time is not taken (NCAA, 2003).
- **Blood time:** Time allowed for the evaluation of a bleeding injury. This is different from injury time. The amount of time is at the referee's discretion. Generally blood time has no time limit, but an excessive bleeding injury may be cause for disqualification as determined by the referee and trainer or physician (NCAA, 2003).

WRESTLING STYLES

- **Greco Roman:** A style that was developed and popularized in Europe. Upper body throws are executed with the goal to touch the opponent's shoulders to the mat simultaneously. Points are awarded for skill of throws. At no time are the wrestlers allowed to use their own legs to gain advantage or contact their opponent's legs (Kelly and Suby, 2002).
- **Freestyle:** Used worldwide and in international wrestling meets. A style of wrestling that combines the use of the upper body and legs to execute maneuvers. Points are awarded for exposure of opponent's back to the mat, takedowns, and reversals. Execution

of a more difficult takedown with emphasis on exposure of opponent's back to the mat will increase points awarded. The main objective is to pin the opponent's shoulders to the mat for a 1-s count (Kelly and Suby, 2002).

- **High school/collegiate:** The style of wrestling that is used in the Untied States. Considered similar to freestyle because of the use of upper body and legs. A major difference is that points are awarded for time advantage. Also, a wrestler must ensure the safe return of their opponent to the mat after a throw or a takedown. Emphasis is placed on pinning the opponent (Kelly and Suby, 2002).

INJURY DATA

- Recent NCAA Injury Surveillance System (ISS) data concludes that collegiate wrestling has a relatively high rate of injury at 9.6 per 1000 athlete exposures, second only to spring football (NCAA, 2002–03). Most injuries occur during practice as compared to competition though competition confers a greater risk of injury. The incidence of injury seems to be highest at the beginning of the season as compared to the latter part of the season. Though injuries are common there seemed to be a consensus that most injuries were not serious on the basis of time lost (greater than 7 days) or injuries that required surgery. Comparison of the different weight classes yielded no statistical difference in injury percentages (Jarrett, Orwin, and Dick, 1998).
- The knee is the most commonly injured body part in both practice and competition followed by the shoulder and ankle. The face and neck were the least injured. Sprain was the most common type of injury in practice and competition with fracture being the least common (Jarrett, Orwin, and Dick, 1998).
- During takedowns and sparring is when most injuries occur (Jarrett, Orwin, and Dick, 1998).
- Contact with the opponent as compared to contact with the mat was the most common mechanism of injury (Jarrett, Orwin, and Dick, 1998).

MECHANISM OF INJURIES

- A direct blow from the mat or body contact may result in a laceration or contusion during a takedown or sparring. Potential serious injury may occur after a fall especially if a competitor lands on an opponent after attempting a throw or other types of takedowns (Kelly and Suby, 2002).

- A friction injury may result in lacerations or abrasions. This can occur with continuous body contact or contact with the mat. This may later result in skin infections or bursitis (Kelly and Suby, 2002).
- Sprains and strains may occur after a wrestler uses twisting or leverage maneuvers to gain advantage over an opponent (Kelly and Suby, 2002).
- A competitor may also incur injury to his or her own person while attempting maneuvers (Kelly and Suby, 2002).
- An often overlooked potential mechanism is overuse injuries (Kelly and Suby, 2002).

HEAD INJURIES

- Concussions occur with direct contact with a body part or contact with the mat or floor (Kelly and Suby, 2002). (See chapter 40)
- Lacerations and contusion occur frequently from direct blows from the mat and body parts, such as the head, elbow, and knee. The most common areas are the bony areas around the orbits, zygoma, and scalp. Soft tissues around the mouth and ears are also potential sites. During the match, injury time will be called to evaluate the area. Treatment during the injury time may include using Steri-Strips to provide temporary closure of the wound. Dressing the wound may also be required at this time. The match can continue as deemed by the referee depending on the severity of the injury. After the match, lacerations should be cleaned and dressed properly. Closure of wounds with heavy nylon suture is recommended if necessary (Kelly and Suby, 2002).
- Epistaxis may occur with a direct blow from an opponent or the mat. Blood time will be taken to determine the extent of the injury. Direct pressure and ice may be applied to the nares to reduce the hemorrhage. A pledget or nose plug may be inserted to enable the wrestler to continue the match. Nosebleed QR is a recently developed product that can be inserted into the nose with a swab (Nosebleed). Direct pressure to the involved nostril for 15–30 s is required for the product to work properly. If the hemorrhage continues even after the above treatments are implemented then proper medical attention must be sought.
- Nasal fractures with epistaxis are treated as above. A competitor should be evaluated for nasal bone displacement before return to play. Activity may be resumed when indicated. A protective face mask with proper nasal padding may be used to protect the nose from further injury during competition (Kelly and Suby, 2002).

EAR INJURIES

- Auricular hematomas aka *cauliflower ear* are a common injury for many competitive wrestlers. The advent of wearing properly fitted protective head gear has reduced but not eliminated the incidence of this injury. The pathogenesis of this injury is usually from a direct blow to the soft tissues of the auricle. Fluid collects between the auricular cartilage and the perichondrium disrupting blood flow to the auricular cartilage (Kelly and Suby, 2002).
- Treatment of auricular hematomas requires aspiration or incision and drainage. Without immediate aspiration, new auricular cartilage will form that is tightly encased. This can cause discomfort and eventual disfigurement. Compressive dressings after aspiration are usually applied. These dressings are worn for a period of 3–5 days before reevaluation. Return to play is individualized based on pain and a discussion of risk/benefits of continuing competition with possible fluid reaccumulation (Kelly and Suby, 2002).
  1. One technique described involves suturing the pressure dressing to the auricle with resultant return to play in 24 h with a low incidence of complications (Schuller, Dankle, and Strauss, 1989). This technique involves suturing dental roll on both sides of the pinna with 1.0 nonabsorbable suture.
  2. A second technique involves aspiration followed by a collodion pressure dressing in the antihelix and an Ace wrap to insure uniform pressure in the area of the hematoma. The athlete is then reevaluated in 3–5 days. Earlier return to play is preceded by a careful discussion of risks and benefits.
  3. A dry aspiration represents an organization of the hematoma and the early stages of formation of neo-cartilage consistent with cauliflower ear. Long-term management (otoplasty) is generally deferred until completion of the wrestling season.

NECK INJURIES

- Neck injuries usually occur during takedowns especially throws or when a wrestler is diving for the opponent's legs and the head is the first part of the body that strikes the mat. This may cause injuries, such as strains/sprains, stingers, disk injuries, degenerative joint disease, and even fractures or spinal cord injuries (Kelly and Suby, 2002).
- The etiology of neck injuries is most commonly from hyperextension (Kelly and Suby, 2002).
- A stinger is a neck injury in which the participant has transient burning or shooting pain or paresthesia in an arm directly related to neck or shoulder trauma. This may be from traction on the brachial plexus or from cervical nerve root impingement. Wrestling is second only to football in regards to stinger injuries (Lillegard, Butcher, and Rucker, 1999). (See chapter 65)
- If cervical fracture or spinal cord injury is suspected then prompt medical attention should be sought (Kelly and Suby, 2002).

BACK INJURIES

- Acute back injuries occur most often during takedowns and throws. Mechanisms that may lead to back injury include torsional movements, exertion against resistance, and hyperextension while in the standing position, or hyperflexion while on the mat with an opponent (Kelly and Suby, 2002).
- Chronic or recurrent back pain is not unusual in wrestlers and may include spondylolysis, spondylolisthesis, or sacroiliac dysfunction (Kelly and Suby, 2002).

CHEST INJURIES

- Chest wall injuries may occur in a variety of ways. Strains from torsion, direct blows, compression, and exertion against resistance are the most common mechanisms (Kelly and Suby, 2002).
- These mechanisms may cause rib contusions/fractures, costochondral separations, and abdominal wall strains. Competitors often present with pain on breathing and moving or point tenderness. If a rib fracture is suspected than careful monitoring of the patient must be initiated because of the possibility of a hemothorax or pneumothorax. Prompt medical attention must be sought if this is suspected. Treatment with rest, anti-inflammatory medications, and local steroid injections may be beneficial. Taping or padding of ribs may be instituted after the initial symptoms have been treated (Kelly and Suby, 2002).

SHOULDER INJURIES

- Shoulder injuries comprise approximately 14% of all injuries and rank second to knee injuries. Injuries may include acromioclavicular strain, shoulder dislocation, shoulder subluxation, and sternocalvicular strain. Shoulder instability is not uncommon in wrestlers (Kelly and Suby, 2002).

EXTREMITY INJURIES

- Extremity injuries include injuries to fingers, thumb, hands, and elbows. Injuries to fingers are relatively common. These include finger *proximal interphalangeal* (PIP) dislocations or sprains and subluxation. Sprains may be taped to the adjacent finger to allow use during competition. Dislocations often needed splinted and padded to be functional (Kelly and Suby, 2002).
- Thumb injuries may be much more disabling. Forceful adduction of the thumb during takedowns may damage the ulnar collateral ligament resulting in a *gamekeeper's thumb*. The competitor may not have the grasp strength to be effective against an opponent. Patient will need to be evaluated for possible thumb spica casting and may even need surgery (Kelly and Suby, 2002).
- The elbow may be injured when an outstretched arm contacts the mat in an attempt to break a fall. The elbow at this time will be hyperextended leading to ligamentous injury or even possible dislocation or fracture. Other common injuries include olecranon bursitis from direct trauma (Kelly and Suby, 2002).

KNEE INJURIES

- The most common body part injured. Includes 21% of all total injuries in a recent study. The most common of these injuries are strains/sprains, meniscal/cruciate tears, fractures, subluxation, and bursitis. Collateral ligament injury is the most common type of injury accounting for over 30% of knee injuries. Cruciate ligament injury conversely is much lower (approximately 5%) (Jarrett, Orwin, and Dick, 1998).
- Takedowns and leg wrestling are the most common etiologies of ligament damage (Kelly and Suby, 2002).
- The lead leg used for defense and initiating takedowns is the most vulnerable (Kelly and Suby, 2002).
- Wrestlers tend to have a predilection to injure the lateral meniscus or to have isolated lateral/medial collateral sprains as compared to other sports. Etiologies such as overuse, torsion, hyperextension, and shearing all have additive effects toward injury (Kelly and Suby, 2002).
- Prepatellar bursitis is a common injury because of time spent on the knees while wrestling on the mat or performing takedowns (Kelly and Suby, 2002).

SKIN INFECTIONS

- A problem that is unique to the sport of competitive wrestling is skin infections from various bacteria, viruses, and fungi. Modes of transmission include person to person contact on exposed skin especially abraded skin and contact with poorly disinfected wrestling mats or equipment (Kelly and Suby, 2002). According to recent NCAA ISS reports, skin infections are associated with at least 10% of the time-loss injuries in wrestling (NCAA, 2002–03).
- All participating competitors are subject to entire body examinations including the hair on the scalp and in the pubic areas at weigh-in. If an abraded area or an infectious skin condition cannot be adequately protected the participant can be medically disqualified. Adequately protected is deemed where skin conditions are diagnosed as noninfectious and treated as per guidelines stipulated by a governing body such as the NCAA and are able to be covered with bandage that will withstand the competition (NCAA, 2003).
- Documentation of a competitor's condition will be made available with diagnosis, culture results, and current medical therapy. The decision of the physician or trainer is considered final (NCAA, 2003).
- Bacterial infections of the skin include folliculitis, impetigo, furuncle/carbuncle, cellulitis, and erysipelas. Competitors must not have any new skin lesions for at least 48 h. No moist or draining lesions at time of match. Seventy-two hours of antibiotic therapy must be completed in order to compete (NCAA, 2003).
- Pediculosis- and scabies-infected participants must have been treated with the proper medication and examined before being allowed to participate in any competition (NCAA, 2003).
- Viral infections include herpes gladiatorum, herpes zoster, molluscum contagiosum, and verrucae. Herpes gladiatorum has received much attention because of the high incidence of being contagious and potential for morbidity (Kohl et al, 2002). Wrestlers must be free of systemic illness at the time of competition. Competitors must have been treated for at least 120 h with proper antiviral therapy before and at the time of the event. No new active blisters or lesions may be present 72 h before the medical examination (NCAA, 2003).
  1. Dry lesions must be covered with an impermeable bandage (NCAA, 2003).
  2. Recommended that wrestlers with a history of recurrent herpes gladitorum or labials be on prophylactic therapy after consultation with a team physician (NCAA, 2003).
  3. Herpes zoster infections must have crusted over lesions and the patient cannot be systemically ill before the competition (NCAA, 2003).
  4. Molluscum lesions must be removed by the time of the competition. Localized lesions may be covered with a permeable membrane followed by stretch tape (NCAA, 2003).

5. Verrucae-infected wrestlers are allowed to compete under the following conditions. Lesions on the face must be adequately covered by a mask. Solitary lesions on the face must be removed before the match to allow participation. Verrucae on the hands must be covered (NCAA, 2003).

- Fungal infections such as tinea have also come under scrutiny because of their high mode of transmission. A minimum of 72 h of topical cidal-type antifungal treatment is required for all tinea corporis. Tinea capitis infections must be treated with a minimum of 2 weeks of systemic antifungal therapy. Treated lesions may be examined with a KOH preparation at the discretion of the examining provider. Lesions should be washed with a fungal shampoo followed by an antifungal cream before being covered with a gas-permeable dressing and stretch tape. A competitor will be disqualified if the lesion cannot be covered adequately (NCAA, 2003).
- Teams with recurrent or wide spread infections should thoroughly evaluate procedures for mat maintenance in cleaning and disqualifications of infectious wrestlers.

WEIGHING IN

- Competitors are placed into separate categories based on their body weight called weight classes. These are predetermined in advance by a governing body such as the NCAA. Currently, there are 10 weight classes ranging from 125 lb to heavyweight (183–235 lb) under the NCAA guidelines. High school participants compete in 14 different weight classes ranging from 103–275 lb (NCAA, 2003).
- At the beginning of the season, each wrestler is weighed and a minimum weight for the competitor is established (NCAA, 2003). Nevertheless one study indicated that many wrestlers compete below the minimum weight established (Wroble and Moxley, 1998). Perceived notions such as being stronger at a lighter weight have a major influence on these decisions.
- The minimum wrestling weight is established by a comparison of several different factors. Hydrated body weight is calculated by checking urine specific gravity. If the urine specific gravity is less than 1.020 then the weight is recorded as the hydrated weight. Skin fold measurements of triceps, subscapular areas, and abdomen are measured to calculate the body fat percentage. Fat free body weight is calculated and divided by 0.95. This establishes the *lowest allowable weight—1* (LAW1) which is a measurement of body weight with allowable 5% body fat. This weight is compared to the *lowest allowable weight—2* (LAW2), which is calculated over a set period of time as established by the

NCAA with no more than a 1.5% body weight decrease per week. LAW1 is compared to LAW2 with the higher weight being the set minimal weight. This will be the absolute minimum weight set for the wrestler for the season. A competitor must certify by mid-December in a weight class. At no time after this is a competitor allowed to wrestle at a weight class below the certified weight (NCAA, 2003). The above guidelines encompass the current recommendation of the American College of Sports Medicine that competitors should not compete at a weight in which body fat levels would be less than 5% of their preseason weight (Wroble and Moxley, 1998).

- During the season, wrestlers employ many methods to lose weight to make their respective weight classes. These include vigorous exercise before weigh-in to lose water weight, self imposed dehydration and fasting, and some may even use weight loss pills or diuretics. Acute effects of the above may be loss of strength and stamina, hypovolemia, heat exhaustion or heat stroke, and electrolyte imbalances. Long-term effects of continued rapid weight loss with weight gain may chronically compromise cardiac and renal blood flow. Neuropsychiatric disorders, such as depression, anxiety, bulimia, and anorexia nervosa may become prevalent. Other sequlae may include decreased growth and maturation especially in younger wrestlers (Kelly and Suby, 2002).
- It is important for coaches, trainers, and physicians to properly educate the competitors on the dangers of rapid weight loss. Adequate counseling on nutrition and emphasis on conditioning during the season are paramount. The NCAA attempts to dissuade competitors from the practice of rapid weight loss and gain by decreasing the time between weighing in and the actual match (Kelly and Suby, 2002). By NCAA rules, competitors must weigh in no more than an hour before dual, triangular, and quadrangular matches. In multiteam tournaments wrestlers must be weighed no more than 2 h before the first match (NCAA, 2003).

REFERENCES

Jarrett GJ, Orwin JF, Dick RW: Injuries in collegiate wrestling. *Am J Sports Med* 26: 674–680, 1998.

Kelly TF, Suby JS: Chapter 58: Wrestling, in Mellion MB (ed.): *Team Physician's Handbook*, 3rd ed. Philadelphia, PA, Hanley & Belfus, 2002, pp 614–628.

Kohl TD, Giesen DP, Moyer, Jr, JM, et al: Tinea gladiatorum: Pennsylvania's experience. *Clin Sports Med* 12:165–171, 2002.

Lillegard WA, Butcher JD, Rucker KS: *Handbook of Sports Medicine: A System-Oriented Approach*, 2nd ed. Woburn, MA, Butterworth-Heinemann, 1999, p 69.

NCAA: *Injury Surveillance System for Wrestling*. National Collegiate Athletic Association, 2002–03, pp 1–21.

NCAA: *Wrestling Rules and Interpretations*. National Collegiate Athletic Association, WR 18, WR23–29, WR 71–72, WA 11–14, WA 28–33, 2003.

Nosebleed QR. Biolife. *www.biolife.com*

Schuller DE, Dankle SD, Strauss RH: A technique to treat wrestler's auricular hematoma without interrupting training or competition. *Arch Otolaryngol Head Neck Surg* 115:202–206, 1989.

Wroble RR, Moxley DP: Weight loss patterns and success rates in high school wrestlers. *Med Sci Sports Exerc* 30:625–628, 1998.

96 THE PEDIATRIC ATHLETE

Amanda Weiss Kelly, MD
Terry Adirim, MD

EPIDEMIOLOGY

- Twenty to thirty million children participate in organized athletic programs each year (Radelet et al, 2002).
- About three million pediatric sports injuries occur annually in the United States (Hergenroeder, 1998).
- Twenty-five to thirty percent of these injuries occur during participation in organized sports and 40% in unorganized sports (Hergenroeder, 1998)

FRACTURES IN THE PEDIATRIC ATHLETE

PHYSEAL FRACTURES

- The physis is the weakest structure in the growing skeleton, making it more susceptible to injury than the surrounding muscles, tendons, and ligaments.

SALTER—HARRIS CLASSIFICATION
- The Salter—Harris classification is the most widely used method of describing physeal fractures (Peterson, 1994):
  1. Type I: Through the physis
  2. Type II: Through the physis and metaphysis
  3. Type III: Through the physis and epiphysis
  4. Type IV: Through the metaphysis, across the physis, and through the epiphysis

5. Type V: Crush injury to the physis
6. Type VI: Injury to the periochondrium
- Type I fractures have the best prognosis, with the incidence of growth arrest being rare in these fractures.
- In type II fractures, growth arrest may occur, especially when the fractures occur in certain areas, like the distal femoral physis.
- In type III injuries, growth arrest is rare, but since the joint surface is involved anatomic reduction must be maintained to ensure articular cartilage congruity and prevent future joint degeneration.
- In type IV injuries, there is concern for both growth arrest and articular cartilage congruity.
- Type V injuries are usually diagnosed retrospectively after growth arrest or angular deformity has occurred.
- Finally, in type VI injuries, angular deformities may occur if a bony bridge develops in the perichondrium on one side of the physis.
- Salter-Harris fractures can usually be diagnosed with plain films. But *magnetic resonance imaging* (MRI) and *computed tomography* (CT) are sometimes used to more accurately delineate physeal injuries.

APOPHYSEAL AVULSION INJURIES
- Apophyses are growth plates that add shape and contour, rather than length, to a bone. They are often sites for muscle attachment.
- Apophyseal avulsions typically occur as a result of violent contraction of the attached muscle (Metzmaker and Pappass 1985).
- The pelvis is a common site for avulsion fractures. The *anterior superior iliac spine* (ASIS) can be avulsed by the sartorius muscle with violent extension of the hip, such as when a sprinter takes off from the starting block.
- Violent extension of the hip can also lead to avulsion of the *anterior inferior iliac spine* (AIIS) by the rectus femoris.

- Diagnosis of both injuries can be made with plain radiographs. Treatment is conservative including symptom-limited weight-bearing until pain free, followed by gradual return to activities.
- Recovery from an avulsion injury of the AIIS injury is typically more prolonged than that of an ASIS injury.
- Abrupt contraction of the abdominal muscles, as with a rapid direction change, can lead to avulsion of the iliac crest. Direct trauma can also fracture the iliac crest apophysis. This commonly occurs when an athlete is tackled in football. Plain radiographs may not be as useful for diagnosis in this injury, as displacement may be minimal. MRI or bone scan may be helpful in diagnosing iliac crest avulsion. Treatment is conservative and includes protected weight bearing until the athlete is not in pain followed by progressive return to activity.
- Other sites of avulsion injury in the hip and pelvis include the greater trochanter, lesser trochanter, and ischial tuberosity. Diagnosis and treatment are similar to that mentioned for ASIS and AIIS injuries.
- Tibial tubercle avulsions typically occur while an athlete is jumping, as a result of a violent contraction of the quadriceps. Excessive bleeding and swelling can cause an anterior compartment syndrome, so a careful neurovascular examinaton is essential. Diagnosis can be made with plain radiographs. Long leg cast immobilization with the knee in extension for 3–4 weeks is adequate treatment for nondisplaced fractures. Open reduction with internal fixation is required if there is significant displacement of the fracture fragment.
- Avulsions of the medial epicondyle are common in throwing athletes. The athlete typically reports feeling a snap or pop during the throwing motion. *Anteroposterior* (AP) and lateral elbow radiographs will demonstrate the avulsion. Minimally displaced fractures can be treated with immobilization, while fractures displaced more than 5 mm should receive surgical referral (Wheeless, 2003).
- Vertebral end plate fractures are an avulsion of the ring apophysis of the vertebra. If the avulsion is from the posterior inferior portion of the vertebra, the apophyseal attachment of the associated disc and the apophysis can be displaced into the vertebral canal, causing neurologic symptoms. This injury can be difficult to distinguish from disc herniation. Plain radiographs can show the separated bony fragment, and MRI can demonstrate marrow edema. Treatment is operative removal of the disc and bony fragment.

TORUS FRACTURES

- Torus or buckle fractures are compressive fractures that lead to failure of the bone at the junction of the metaphysis and diaphysis.

- This type of injury only occurs in children, and is possible because of the porous nature of their bones.
- Torus fractures are stable and heal well. They can be treated with splinting or casting for comfort.

GREENSTICK FRACTURES

- Another fracture that only occurs in children, the greenstick fracture refers to an incomplete fracture in the shaft of a long bone. There is disruption of one cortex of the bone and bending on the other. The ability of the pediatric bone to plastically deform allows for the occurrence of this type of fracture.
- Greenstick fractures with minimal angulation can be treated with immobilization.
- Surgical intervention may be required for fractures with significant angulation.

SUPRACONDYLAR FRACTURES

- Supracondylar fractures are very common among 3–11-year-old children.
- Supracondylar factures are the pediatric fractures with the highest risk of complications, particularly neurovascular complications.
- These fractures are usually sustained from a fall on an outstretched hand, but can also occur as a result of direct trauma. A thorough neurovascular examinaton is imperative if a supracondylar fracture is suspected.
- The diagnosis can typically be made with plain AP and lateral radiographs of the elbow.
- Any child with a supracondylar fracture should be referred for evaluation by a pediatric orthopedist, as many require surgical fixation.

OVERUSE INJURIES

- Overuse injuries have become more common in children with the growth of competitive youth sports programs (Difiori, 1999).
- Risk factors for overuse injuries are often divided into intrinsic and extrinsic factors.

INTRINSIC RISKS FOR OVERUSE INJURIES

- Some issues specific to immature skeletons contribute to the risk for overuse injuries in children. For instance, children have growth cartilage in several areas of the skeleton, and it is particularly susceptible to injury from repetitive stress.

- Growth cartilage is found at the articular surface, physes, and apophyses.
- Also, as children experience growth spurts, there are rapid changes in bone length, which can lead to a relative inflexibility of the muscle-tendon units that cross joints. This may predispose the growing athlete to muscular, joint, and physeal injury (Difiori, 1999).
- Abnormalities in alignment may also predispose an athlete to overuse injuries. Pes planus or cavus, over pronation, patellofemoral malalignment, tibial torsion, femoral anteversion and leg length discrepancies may be related to increased risk for overuse injuries in athletes (Difiori, 1999).

EXTRINSIC RISK FACTORS FOR OVERUSE INJURY

- Improper training technique can attribute to the risk for overuse injury.
- Increasing intensity or frequency of training can lead to overuse injury.
- In runners, injury may also result from persistently running the same direction around the track or on the same side of the street.
- Also, parental and coaching pressures to increase the intensity of a child's training can contribute to injuries.
- Improperly fitting or worn out equipment may increase the risk injury. For example, using worn out running shoes or adult sized weight training equipment may predispose the pediatric athlete to overuse injury.

COMMON OVERUSE INJURIES

TRACTION APOPHYSITIS
- A traction apophysitis occurs where a muscle group attaches to a secondary center of ossification.
- It is caused by repetitive stress at these sites that can lead to pain, swelling, and inflammation.
- The diagnosis of an apophysitis can usually be made on physical examinaton. In nonclassic cases, radiographs may help rule out other conditions.
- Osgood-Schlatter disease is an apophysitis of the tibial tubercle. It is associated with inflexibility of the extensor mechanism of the knee. Jumping activities exacerbate Osgood-Schlatter disease, so it is commonly diagnosed in basketball players. Treatment involves relative rest, as well as quadriceps stretching and strengthening.
- Sinding-Larsen-Johansson syndrome is an apophysitis of the inferior pole of the patella, and is similar in cause and treatment to Osgood-Schlatter disease.
- Apophysitis of the medial epicondyle of the elbow is common in throwing athletes. It is often termed "little league elbow."

- Traction on the medial epicondyle occurs as a result of the valgus stress placed on the elbow during the throwing motion.
- Treatment includes relative rest followed by progressive strengthening and gradual return to throwing activities is usually effective as a treatment. Also, the athlete's throwing technique should be evaluated and any errors should be corrected.

OSTEOCHONDRITIS DESSICANS
- *Osteochondritis dessicans* (OCD) is a disorder of growth cartilage where there is a separation of cartilage and subchondral bone from underlying well vascularized bone.
- Common sites for OCD in children include the knee and elbow.
- OCD lesions are usually noted on plain radiographs. MRI can be used to assess the stability of the fragment and viability of subchondral bone.
- In general, younger patients and patients with stable lesions have the best prognosis.
- OCD in the knee is most often found on the medial femoral condyle. Patients usually complain of vague knee pain and intermittent swelling. If the affected fragment has detached from the underlying bone, there may be complaints of locking and catching. If the fragment is stable, a period of rest and a gradual return to activity with physical therapy to improve leg strength may be adequate for treatment. If the articular cartilage is disrupted or a loose body is present, a surgical referral is indicated.
- The capitellum of the elbow is a common site for OCD lesions in throwing athletes and gymnasts. In young patients with stable lesions, treatment includes rest, physical therapy, and instruction in proper throwing technique. If the affected fragment is unstable, surgical referral is indicated.

SHEUERMANN'S DISEASE

- Sheuermann's disease is a common adolescent condition that causes painful dorsal kyphosis, loss of anterior vertebral body height and wedging of the vertebral body (Wheeless, 2003).
- Most patients have tightness of the hamstrings, gluteals and lumbodorsal fascia (Wheeless, 2003).
- The etiology is unclear, but it may be an overuse syndrome.
- Diagnosis can be made with plain radiographs of the thoracic spine, which demonstrate anterior wedging of the vertebral bodies, irregular vertebral end plates, Schmorl's nodes and narrow disc spaces.
- Treatment includes physical therapy for strength and flexibility. Bracing may be used for a period of

9–12 months if kyphosis with Cobb angle >50° is present (Ali, Green, and Patel, 1999).

STRESS FRACTURES

- Stress fractures occur when there is an accumulation of microdamage from repetitive stresses, which outstrips the bone's ability to repair and remodel.
- Stress fractures are most commonly found in the lower extremities, but can also be found in the spine and upper extremity.
- Stress fractures may be diagnosed with plain radiographs, but *single photon emission computed tomography* (SPECT) scan, CT or MRI may be needed.
- Many stress fractures are similar in the adult and pediatric populations, only stress fractures specific to the pediatric population are discussed here.

SPONDYLOLYSIS
- The term spondylolysis refers to a stress fracture of the pars interarticularis of the spine.
- If the fracture is unstable forward displacement of one vertebra on another may result, which is termed *spondylolisthesis*.
- Athletes participating in sports that require repetitive hyperextension, like gymnastics or football, may be at increased risk for spondylolysis.
- Most patients complain of low back pain, which is worse with extension and is relieved by rest.
- Spondylolysis is often be diagnosed with plain radiographs and is best seen on oblique views. It can, however, occur without changes on plain radiographs. In this case SPECT scan can be used to detect the abnormality.
- Treatment includes activity restriction until the patient is asymptomatic, followed by a gradual return to activity. A program of core/lumbar strengthening and flexibility should also be instituted. Some practitioners recommend bracing at diagnosis, others recommend bracing only if the patient continues to have pain, despite adequate rest.
- Prognosis is best in cases where only SPECT scan is positive and there is not yet plain radiographic evidence of disease. In cases where radiographic evidence of spondylolysis is present, the likelihood of healing is lower.
- If spondylolisthesis has occurred, there is no chance for healing.
- Conservative therapy is the most widely recommended treatment for spondylolisthesis.
- The role of surgery is controversial. In cases where neurologic compromise is evident or slipping of the

vertebra progresses, surgical stabilization is recommended (Richardson and Furey, 2000).

PROXIMAL HUMERAL STRESS FRACTURE
- The proximal humeral stress fracture is often referred to as little league shoulder, though it is also seen in other overhead athletes, such as tennis or volleyball players.
- The throwing motion places torsion and distraction forces on the proximal humerus, which when done repetitively can result in proximal humeral stress fracture.
- AP internal and external rotation views of the shoulder with comparison views of the opposite shoulder on radiograph should demonstrate widening of the affected physis.
- Treatment involves cessation of throwing or other overhead activities until the child is asymptomatic, usually about 3 months (Stanitski, DeLee, and Drez, 1994). Then, progressive return to activity is allowed. Throwing mechanics should be evaluated and parents and coaches should be warned not to encourage excessive throwing.

DISTAL RADIUS PHYSEAL STRESS FRACTURES
- Distal radius physeal stress fracture is a Salter-Harris type I stress fracture, which typically occurs in gymnasts.
- It is caused by the unusual amount of weightbearing activities that gymnasts perform with their upper extremities.
- Dorsal wrist pain is the most common symptom.
- The diagnosis may be made with plain radiographs by comparing the affected side to the nonpainful side. Abnormal widening of the physis, beaking of the epiphysis and cystic changes on the metaphyseal side of the bone may be noted on the affected radius; however, MRI may be needed to make the diagnosis if plain radiographs are normal.
- Treatment includes rest until the athlete is asymptomatic, usually 1–3 months. Splinting or casting may be helpful.
- When pain has completely resolved, a gradual return to upper extremity weightbearing is permitted.

ANATOMIC VARIANTS

- Several anatomic variants may predispose the pediatric athlete to pain and injury.

DISCOID LATERAL MENISCUS

- Athletes with discoid lateral meniscus often complain of a snapping sensation with extension of the knee.

- Some discoid menisci are not diagnosed until they are torn, in which case the athlete tends to complain of pain, swelling, and mechanical symptoms.
- Diagnosis can often be made on clinical examinaton.
- MRI can also be used to diagnose meniscal tears and discoid lateral meniscus.
- A torn discoid lateral meniscus requires surgery. If a discoid lateral meniscus is found incidentally, surgery is not indicated.

TARSAL COALITION

- Tarsal coalition is a bony or fibrocartilaginous connection of two or more tarsal bones.
- The most common examples are calcaneonavicular and talocalcaneal coalition. They are often bilateral.
- Symptomatic patients typically complain of vague pain that is insidious in onset. The diagnosis can usually be made on the oblique view of the plain radiograph, but CT scan may be necessary to provide a more detailed view of the anatomy.
- Conservative therapy includes rest, immobilization, shoe inserts, and anti-inflammatory medication.
- In patients who fail conservative therapy, surgical resection of the coalition can be undertaken.

ACCESSORY OSSICLES

- The accessory navicular is an accessory ossicle of the foot into which a portion of the posterior tibialis inserts.
- Athletes involved in sports that stress the posterior tibialis tendon with repetitive changes in direction, like basketball, may develop accessory navicular pain.
- Diagnosis can be made on the lateral or external oblique radiograph of the foot.
- Treatment is typically conservative, with rest, shoe inserts, and, sometimes, immobilization. Excision can be performed if conservative therapy fails.
- The os trigonum is another common accessory ossicle that is found posterior to the talus.
- Sports that involve repetitive plantar flexion, such as ballet, can lead to impingement of the os trigonum between the posterior tibia and calcaneus.
- An os trigonum can usually be seen on lateral radiograph of the ankle.
- Conservative therapy is usually effective. This includes physical therapy for strengthening and flexibility, relative rest, anti-inflammatory medication and, sometimes, immobilization. Excision can be performed if conservative therapy fails.

THE OSTEOCHONDROSES

- The osteochondroses are a group of chronic disorders that involve the epiphyses or apophyses.
- They begin as an avascular necrosis of the epiphyseal center followed by eventual repair and replacement of the ossification center.

PANNER'S DISEASE

- Panner's disease is an osteochondrosis of the capitellum associated with the repetitive trauma from throwing. It involves variations in the normal ossification of the capitellum of the humerus. (Sullivan and Anderson, 2000)
- This condition typically affects children between 5 and 11 years of age.
- The athlete complains of pain with throwing and may have swelling of the elbow.
- Fragmentation of the capitellum is noted on radiograph of the elbow.
- This is a self-limiting disease and can be treated conservatively with activity modification.

LEGG-CALVE-PERTHES DISEASE

- Osteochondrosis of the femoral head is referred to as Legg-Calve-Perthes disease.
- Symptoms include knee or anterior thigh pain and limping after activity.
- AP and frog lateral radiographs of the hip confirm the diagnosis.
- The main goal of treatment is to maintain range of motion and prevent deformity of the femoral head by keeping it contained in the acetabulum.
- Orthopedic referral is indicated.

FREIBERG'S DISEASE

- Freiberg's disease is an osteochondrosis of the metatarsal head.
- It usually affects adolescents.
- Forefoot pain is the typical complaint.
- Flattening of the metatarsal head and fragmentation of the growth plate can be seen on plain radiographs. But, MRI or bone scan may be necessary for diagnosis early in the disease process.
- With early diagnosis, conservative therapy, including relative rest, padding of the affected metatarsal head and orthotics may be successful. With failure of conservative therapy, surgical referral should be made.

SAFETY

HEAT AND COLD ILLNESS

- Children are more susceptible to heat illness than adults.
- Children have a larger body surface area to body mass ratio than adults. This makes children more likely to gain heat from the environment in hot conditions and lose it in cold environments (Sullivan and Anderson, 2000).
- Heat loss in children is even more apparent in water because of the high thermal conductivity of water.
- Compared to adults exercising at a given level, children have increased heat production per kilogram of body mass. This leads to faster increases in body temperature in warm weather, but can be protective when exercise is performed in cold environments (Smolander et al, 1992).
- Another disadvantage for children exercising in warm environments is that the sweating rate in children is lower than in adults. This is particularly important when the temperature of the environment exceeds the skin temperature. In this type of environment, sweat evaporation from the skin is the only means for cooling the body.
- When dehydrated, a child's temperature rises faster than an adult's, increasing the risk for serious heat injury (Sullivan and Anderson, 2000).

HYDRATION

- Children should be well hydrated prior to starting any physical activity (Sullivan and Anderson, 2000).
- During activity, children should be encouraged to drink 120 mL (5 oz) of water every 20 min. Older, heavier children will require 250 mL (9 oz) every 30 min (Sullivan and Anderson, 2000).
- For activities lasting longer than 1 h, a 6% carbohydrate solution with sodium and chloride should be used.
- Beverages should be cold to improve palatability.
- Lightweight clothing should be worn to facilitate sweat evaporation.

SUN EXPOSURE

- Sunscreen with SPF 15 should be applied 20 min prior to sun exposure to reduce the risk for sunburn.
- Sun exposure during childhood has been linked to the development of skin cancer in adulthood.

PROPER EQUIPMENT

- Children should be provided with appropriately sized equipment in good condition for sport participation.
- Padding for football, hockey and soccer is made in children's sizes.
- Weight training equipment can be found in sizes and with weight increments appropriate for children.
- Mouthguards should be worn for all contact sports to prevent dental injury. There is some evidence that mouthguards can prevent head injuries as well.

PRESEASON MEDICAL EVALUATION

- The preparticipation physical examinaton can prevent injury by identifying medical conditions that may be exacerbated by sports participation and musculoskeletal issues that can be addressed and rehabilitated before sports participation.

GROWTH AND DEVELOPMENT

- Some debate exists over whether or not sports participation has an effect on growth.
- Regular physical activity does not appear to have any adverse effects on growth (Sullivan and Anderson, 2000).
- There is some evidence that intense, high-volume training may adversely affect growth.
- It appears that young athletes who experience attenuated growth during training will exhibit catch-up growth when training levels decrease. High intensity exercise, alone, may not account for these effects on growth; inadequate nutritional compensation for a given training volume may also play a role.

STRENGTH TRAINING

- Strength training by children and adolescents when properly supervised is considered safe and efficacious.
- Strength training is often recommended for improvement in sports performance, injury rehabilitation, injury prevention and general health benefits (AAP Committee on Sports Medicine and Fitness, 2001).
- Studies have shown that when properly structured, strength training can increase strength in preadolescents

and adolescents (Falk and Tenenbaum, 1996; Faigenbaum et al, 1996).

- In preadolescents, strength training increases strength, but does not cause muscle hypertrophy (Ramsey et al 1990; Kraemer et al, 1989).
- The 2001 position statement from the American Academy of Pediatrics (AAP) Committee on Sports Medicine and Fitness concludes that there is not enough evidence to assert that strength training programs help prevent sports-related musculoskeletal injuries in preadolescents and adolescents. Nor is there evidence that strength training will decrease the incidence of sports-related injuries.

REFERENCES

AAP Committee on Sports Medicine and Fitness: Strength training by children and adolescents. *Pediatrics* 107(6):1470–1472, 2001.

Ali RM, Green DW, Patel TC: Scheuermann's kyphosis. *Curr Opin Pediatr* 11(1):70–75, Feb, 1999. (Review)

Difiori JP: Stress fracture of the proximal fibula in a young soccer player: A case report and a review of the literature. *Med Sci Sports Exerc* 31(7):925–928, Jul. 1999. (Review)

Faigenbaum AD, Wescott WL, Micheli LJ et al: The effects of strength training and detraining on children. *J Strength Cond* 10:109–114, 1996.

Falk B, Tenenbaum G: The effectiveness of resistance training in children. A meta-analysis. *Sports Med* 3:176–186, 1996.

Hergenroeder AC: Prevention of sports injuries. *Pediatrics* 101(6):1057–1063, June 1998.

Kraemer WJ, Fry AC Frykman PN, Conroy B, et al: Resistance training and youth. *Pediatr Exerc Sci* 1:336–350, 1989.

Metzmaker J, Pappass A: Avulsion fractures of the pelvis. *Am J Sports Med* 13:349, 1985.

Peterson HA: Physeal fractures: Part 3. Classification. *J Pediatr Orthop* 14:439–448, 1994.

Radelet MA, Pephart SM, Rubinstein EN, et al: Survey of the injury rate for children in community sports. *Pediatrics* 110(3):e28, Sep. 2002.

Ramsey JA, Blimkie CJ, Smith K, et al: Strength training effects in prepubescent boys. Issues and controversies. *Med Sci Sports Exerc* 22:605–614, 1990.

Richardson WJ, Furey CG: *Low Back and Lumbar Spine Injuries in Principles and Practice of Orthopaedic Sports Medicine.* Garrett WE, Speer K, Kirkendall DT (eds.). Philadelphia, PA, Lippincott Williams & Wilkins, 2000.

Smolander J, Bar-Or O, Korhonen O, et al: Thermoregulation during rest and exercise in the cold in pre-and early pubescent boys and in young men. *J Appl Physiol* 72:1589–1594, 1992.

Stanitski CL, DeLee JC, Drez D: *Pediatric and Adolescent Sports Medicine.* Philadelphia, PA, Saunders, 1994.

Sullivan JA, Anderson SJ (eds.): *Care of the Young Athlete.* Rosemont, IL, American Academy of Orthopedic Surgeons and American Academy of Pediatrics, 2000.

Wheeless CR: *Wheeless Textbook of Orthopedics,* 2003; http://www.ortho-u.net/o2/157.htm. Accessed 8/4/03.

97 THE GERIATRIC ATHLETE

Cynthia M Williams, DO, MEd

INTRODUCTION

- The population of the United States is aging. In 1900, 4% of the population was 65 years or older. It is now over 13% of the population with projections to be over 20% by 2030 (U.S. Census Internet Release, 2000).
  1. Aging demographics also reveal the "oldest old" those persons age 85 and older are the most rapidly growing group within the population (Federal Interagency Forum on Aging-Related Statistics, 2000).
  2. The aging population is heterogeneous and arbitrary age divisions do not take into account functional abilities, comorbidities, or the presence of other infirmities.
- Physiologic changes associated with aging are important to understand as present day competitive athletes and so called *weekend warriors* approach middle and old age.
- Awareness of the benefits and barriers to maintaining a physically active lifestyle, common injuries and nutritional needs of our aging society is essential to all providers of health care.
- Exercise received an A grading from the USPSTF (U.S. Preventive Services Task Force, 1996/2001). Exercise either in the forms of aerobic training, resistance training, or lifestyle modification has many benefits in older adults, even the oldest-old (Booth et al, 2000).
- A recent American Association of Retired Persons (AARP Research, 2002) survey found 63% of middle aged and older adults knew exercise was critical for maintaining good health and moderate exercise at least three times per week could help them stay fit and healthy; however, 11% of the United States adult population reports regular and vigorous physical activity for 20 min or longer more than twice per week.

1. The long-term effects of a sedentary lifestyle are numerous including functional limitations from chronic disease, obesity, diabetes mellitus, and cardiovascular disease.
2. It has been estimated that 35% of deaths from coronary heart disease, 32% from colon cancer, and 35% from diabetes could be prevented if all Americans exercise.

- Successful aging appears to include a combination of physical, cognitive, and social activities with the most rewards coming from continued physical and mental activity (Pescatello, 2001; Cassel, 2002).
- Even though the prospect of starting an exercise or physical activity program may seem hard or possibly dangerous for many older adults, as a group, they are fairly resilient with respect to cardiovascular endurance and strength even after a period of detraining (Albert et al, 2000; Begum and Katzel, 2000; Sforzo et al, 1995).

BENEFITS OF EXERCISE

- Many factors are associated with older adults participating in regular aerobic exercise as well as being physically inactive (Table 97-1) (Edward, Larson, and Wagner, 1992; Seeman et al, 1995; King et al, 2000).
- Exercise as a form of primary prevention has many benefits even for sedentary older adults (Table 97-2). (DiPietro, 2001; Vita et al, 1998; Miller et al, 2000; Penninx et al, 2001; Speechley and Tinetti, 1991; Gardner, Robertson, and Campbell, 2000; Nowalk et al, 2001; Shephard and Balady, 1999; Hakim et al, 1999; Kasch et al, 1999; Kasch et al, 1999; Hambrecht et al, 1998; Maiorana et al, 2000; Billman, 2002; Pratley et al, 2000; Pescatello and Murphy, 1998; Frontera et al, 1988; Evans, 1995a; 1996; McAuley et al, 2000; Gregg et al, 1998; McMurdo, Mole, and Paterson, 1997; Messier et al, 2000;

TABLE 97-1 Participant and Non-participant Factors Associated with Regular Exercise

POSITIVE FACTORS	NEGATIVE FACTORS
Age	Fear of undue harm from physical activity
Positive health perception	Care-giving responsibilities
Higher levels of education and income	Lack of energy to exercise
Less than two chronic health conditions	Absence of enjoyable scenery
Prior exercise behavior	Infrequent observations of others
Supportive social network.[74–75]	exercising in ones neighborhood.[76]

TABLE 97-2 Benefits of Exercise for Older Adults

Improve and/or maintain muscle strength
Improve and/or maintain endurance and mobility
Retain musculoskeletal integrity
Decreased falls with reduction in overall rate of hip fractures
Prevention of coronary artery disease, hypertension, diabetes mellitus, obesity and osteoporosis
Improved lipid levels including increased HDLc
Improved physical appearance and self-confidence
Improved well-being (less worry, anxiety, and depression)
Enhances regularity of bowels–less constipation

Pescatello, Murphy, and Costanzo, 2000; Pescatello and VanHeest, 2000; Andersen et al, 1999; Miszko and Cress, 2000)

PHYSIOLOGIC CHANGES OF AGING

- Aging is associated with many physiologic changes (Table 97-3).
- The age-associated decrease in muscle mass (sarcopenia) is a direct correlate of the age decrement in strength, which in turn leads to functional impairments and disability (Evans, 2003). Many of the physiologic changes once thought to be part of the aging process are now considered to be more a consequence of disuse and a sedentary lifestyle.
- Aerobic exercise as measured by maximal aerobic capacity (VO_{2max}) declines approximately 1% per decade after the age of 20–25. This decline is seen in both sedentary and competitive older athletes (Mengelkock et al, 1997; Wiswell et al, 2001). It is the best single marker of an individuals cardiovascular fitness.
- In most physiologic systems, the aging process does not result in significant impairment or dysfunction in the absence of pathology; however, stress on physiologic reserves can lead to an inability to complete a task requiring near maximal effort (Fiatarone-Singh, 2002).

TABLE 97-3 Physiologic Changes Associated with Aging

Decreased skeletal muscle mass (sarcopenia)
Decreased basal metabolic rate and energy expenditure (decreased caloric need)
Graying and thinning hair
Decrease in skin and ligamentous and tendon elasticity
Reduction in height (loss of intravertebral disc space height)
Changes in the speed of cognitive processing and retention of new information
Slowing of reaction time
Presbyopia and presbycusis.

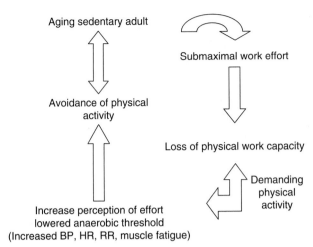

FIG. 97-1 Schema of exercise avoidance.

1. Insidious changes occur over time in sedentary populations leading to a loss of physical capacity and an increased perception of effort at submaximal work (exercise). This leads many adults to avoid exercise, exacerbating age related declines secondary to disuse of biological systems (Figure 97-1).
2. Moderate- to high-intensity activity is a means by which the functional/physiologic losses associated with aging may be altered.

THE AGING MUSCULOSKELETAL SYSTEM (Buckwalter, Heckman, and Petrie, 2003)

• Age-associated musculoskeletal changes play an important role in injuries sustained by the older adults.
  1. Bone mass and strength decrease dramatically with aging. Losses in cortical bone (from increased porosity and endosteal absorption) and cancellous bone (from decreased number of trabeculae) leads to an increasing incidence of vertebral body and long-bone fractures after the age of 50. Women are proportionally more affected than men.
  2. Muscle mass decreases in the size and number of cells resulting in decreased strength.
  3. Articular cartilage undergoes degenerative changes secondary to a decrease in chondrocyte function. Fraying of articular surfaces, decreased tensile stiffness, fatigue resistance, and overall thickness leads to degenerative processes and to the development of osteoarthritis.
  4. Intervertebral discs demonstrate dramatic changes especially in the central region of the disc. The firm fibrous plate develops fissures and cracks that extend centrally with aging leading to disc compression and to the age-related loss of spine height. Changes in proteoglycan, water, and nutrition to the disc lead to disc herniation and changes in disc shape and volume. Stiffness, back and neck pain, loss of mobility, spinal stenosis, and degeneration of the joint facets are common to the aging spinal cord.
  5. Tendons, ligaments, and joint capsules are composed of dense fibrous tissues. Degenerative changes in these tissues lead to low-energy ruptures of the rotator cuff, long head of the biceps, and patellar and Achilles tendons. These tendon and ligamentous ruptures appear to be caused by progressive decline in tensile stiffness and an ultimate load to failure with aging.

FACTORS AFFECTING THE AGING MASTER ATHLETE (Mengelkock et al, 1997; Wiswell et al, 2001; Maharam et al, 1999; Rogers et al, 1990; Pollock et al, 1987; 1997)

• Changes associated with the normal aging process are also found in the master athletes (those older than 40).
• The master athlete continues to maintain muscle mass but it is dependent on strength training and training volume. Table 97-4 outlines changes normally seen with aging and compensatory changes of the master athlete.
• The master athlete is more prone to acute and overuse injuries secondary to slower rates of healing and recovery and lower compliance with rehabilitation.
• The master athlete appears to slow down secondary to a decrease in training intensity, time, and motivation as compared to younger competitive athletes.

COMMON INJURIES IN PHYSICALLY ACTIVE OLDER ADULTS AND ATHLETES (Kannus et al, 1989; Menard and Stanish, 1989; Kallinen and Markku, 1995; Kallinen and Alen, 1994)

• Injuries account for the sixth leading cause of death in older adults, typically from a fall in a frail older individual. Most injuries are related to speed of movement. For women 8 to 21% and in men 9 to 35% of all injuries are related to sports activity (Table 97-5).
• Acute injuries are common in older adults who participate in physical activities that demand a high amount of coordination, balance, and reaction times. These sports include ball games, skiing, and gymnastics.

TABLE 97-4   Physiologic Adaptation of Master Athletes

FUNCTIONAL COMPARTMENT	AGE-RELATED CHANGE	COMPETITIVE MASTER ATHLETE
Muscle	Decreased strength Reduction in muscle area/mass Loss of type 1 (slow-twitch and type 2 (fast twitch muscle fibers)	Maintain type 1 and 2 muscle fibers Mass dependent on strength training Performance dependent on training volume (time and distance)
Cardiovascular	↓ Cardiac output ↓ stroke volume ↓ maximal heart rate (10 beats/min/decade) ↓ aerobic capacity (VO_{2max})	Lower resting heart rate Higher systolic blood pressure Decreased decline in HR_{mas} (4–7 beats/min/decade)
Bone	↓ Bone mineral density	↓ Bone mineral density
Aerobic Capacity (VO_{2max})	≈10% per decade after age 25	≈ 5% per decade after age 25
Performance	Between ages 20–30 near maximal speed and performance	↓ Speed ↓ Strength ↓ Overall performance
Nutrition	↓ Energy requirement (↓ lean body mass; ↓ physical activity)	↑ protein (1.00–1.25 g/kg) Supplement Vitamins D, B_6, B_{12}, E, C, Folate Calcium 1,000–1,500 mg/day Iron 18 mg/day
Water	↓ Thirst mechanism ↑ Output by kidneys	Weigh in before and after workout; replace weight loss with 2 cups of water for each pound lost; Monitor color of urine

Falls, slips, and strains accounted for the majority of these injuries.

- Inflammatory overuse injuries (muscle strain) are common especially to the back and lower extremity.
  1. Strength/power athletes (track and field, sprinters, throwers, power lifters, tennis players) tend to have more injuries of the upper extremities than endurance athletes.
  2. The knee, ankle, and foot account for 39% of all injuries with joint and muscle injuries more common in endurance athletes and muscle and tendon/tendon insertion injuries more common in power/strength athletes.
- There is a higher risk of spontaneous, low energy tears to the rotator cuff, Achilles tendon (peaks in 4th decade), patellar tendon, and medial meniscus. Although not frequently seen, stress fractures of the lower extremity have been found in runners and marchers (Carpintero et al, 1997).

Table 97-5   Common Injuries in Older Athletes

Tendinitis
Patellofemoral Pain Syndrome
Muscle strain
Ligament strain
Plantar fasciitis
Metatarsalgia
Meniscal injuries
Degenerative disc disease
Bursitis
Rotator cuff tear
Subachromial impingement
Achilles tendon tear

- There is no evidence supporting high intensity/high load physical activities promoting degenerative arthritis. Trauma to a joint (hip, knee, ankle) prior surgery, poor alignment, inadequate muscle strength and obesity are more correlated with the development of osteoarthritis. (Buckwalter and Lane, 1997)
- Injuries more commonly occur during competition than during training especially for soccer, football players, and recreational athletes (Murphy, Connolly, and Beynnon, 2003).

DIAGNOSIS AND MANAGEMENT (Epperly; O'Connor et al, 2003)

- Although acute injuries account for a greater number of injuries they are treated as overuse injuries. These injuries may be compounded by osteoarthritis of the knee, hip, wrist, and thumb as well as bursitis of the hip and back and Achilles and rotator cuff tendonitis.
- The diagnosis and management of most injuries involves obtaining a good history and performing an adequate examination. Most elderly athletes do not report injuries immediately, taking a *wait and see* approach. This usually means the acute injury must be treated as if it were chronic (Kallinen and Markku, 1995; Epperly).
- A step-wise approach to management as advocated by O'Connor et al (2003) allows the older adult to go back to full physical activity.

1. Management begins with making a pathoanatomic diagnosis. Examine the entire region in question. In addition any patterns of muscle imbalance and structural malalignment need to be evaluated.
2. Control inflammation to allow injured tissues to repair and heal. This includes a period of rest or activity modification, ice and compression, elevation of effected extremity, and finally strategies to prevent further injury. Medications such as acetominophen or nonsteroidal anti-inflammatory agents may be used to manage pain. Use of steroid is controversial.
3. Promote healing through site-specific rehabilitative exercises and cardiovascular conditioning. This will increase the proliferation of vascular elements and fibroblasts that create collagen deposition and maturation in injured tissue.
4. Begin sport specific rehabilitative exercises when pain free range of motion is achieved and strength and endurance test indicate a return to a preinjury state.
5. Control abuse by educating the older athlete that more is not always better and that overtraining precipitates fatigue, decreases performance, and increases the probability of injury. Emphasis should be placed on a gradual increase in workload and training cycles. Use of bracing and taping can control balance and counter-forces especially during rehabilitation and early resumption of sports activity.

• For older athletes remember that when using any medication "start low and go slow." Using 1/3 to 1/2 the recommended dosing is always a good starting point as is reviewing all other medications for potential drug–drug interactions.
• The older athlete will take longer to heal. Start rehabilitation early and expect the duration of treatment to be twice as long for an athlete of 60 years or more than for a 20-year-old athlete and three times as long for those older than 75.

PROMOTING LIFESTYLE PHYSICAL ACTIVITY IN OLDER ADULTS (Christman and Andersen, 2000; Evans, 1999)

• Encourage all older adults to participate in physical activity. The explanation for promoting this change should include the overall benefits of exercise as well as the potential risks of engaging in exercise, with emphasis on the benefits that the individual will gain. (Table 97-2).
• Obtain a detailed exercise history to include the patient's lifelong pattern of activities and interests;

activity level in the past 2–3 months to determine a current baseline; concerns and perceived barriers regarding exercise including issues regarding perceived lack of time, unsafe environment, cardiovascular risks, and limitations of existing chronic diseases; level of interest and motivation for exercise; and social preferences regarding exercise (Christman and Andersen, 2000).
• The discussion should be documented with a recommendation by the American Heart Association for an informed consent for exercise training to be place in the patient's record (Fletcher et al, 2001). A detailed history of cardiovascular risk factors and disease is a must.
• A physical examination should be performed with emphasis on the following:
1. The cardiopulmonary systems
2. Any limiting conditions including visual or musculoskeletal impairments
3. Evaluate the strength of the quadriceps and ankle. An elderly patient should be able to generate enough force to generate 50% of his or her body weight. Physical therapy is indicated for strengthening if weakness is perceived in these muscle groups.
4. Flexibility of the hips and ankles should be evaluated as well as sensory testing on the plantar surface and dorsum of the feet.
5. The feet, lower legs, knees, thighs, and trunk should be inspected for deformities and joint pain in an attempt to prescribe the right exercise to minimize pain and discomfort.
• The American College of Sports Medicine recommends stress testing for any older adult who intends to begin a vigorous exercise program such as strenuous cycling or running (American College of Sports Medicine, 2000).
1. Conditions that are absolute and relative contraindications to exercise stress testing or embarking on an exercise program should be evaluated (Fletcher et al, 2001).
• Finally an exercise prescription should be written on a prescription pad to strengthen the endorsement for increased physical activity. The prescription should include frequency, intensity, type, and time of exercise (Will, Demko, and George, 1996).
• It is important to start low and go slow especially if the older adult has been relatively sedentary.
1. It is more important to get the older adult doing any physical activity than to prescribe something that is unattainable.
2. The health of older adults may be better served if they perform a little more exercise or activity than the previous week, attempting to incorporate the

activity into their normal daily lives such as walking to a store or gardening.

3. The goal should be for the person to feel pleasantly tired a few hours after the activity with the aim to increase the activity slowly until a desired level of fitness is obtained (Shephard and Balady, 1999).

THE EXERCISE PRESCRIPTION

- The exercise prescription should include both aerobic and resistance exercise.
  1. Aerobic exercise in the form of walking from a more moderate to vigorous pace is very attainable for most if not all community dwelling elders especially if barriers of environment and safety are taken into account.
  2. Aerobic exercise should be performed on most days of the week with the goal of achieving 30 min of moderate to vigorous intensity exercise daily (Christman and Andersen, 2000; Evans, 1999). This can also be achieved by splitting the 30-min goal into two or three sessions.
  3. Discuss "warming up and warming down" as part of the prescription (Seto and Brewster, 1991) as this will prevent musculoskeletal injuries, catecholamine burst, reduce the risk of arrhythmias and fainting, and allow for central venous return.
  4. Resistance training is necessary to counter the muscle atrophy of aging and disuse (Frontera et al, 1988; Evans, 1996; Fiatarrone et al, 1990). Current research indicates that for healthy persons of all ages even those with chronic diseases, a single set of 15 repetitions performed a minimum of 2 days per week can develop and maintain muscle mass, endurance, and strength (Taaffe et al, 1999).
     a. Each work-out session should include 8–10 different exercises that train the major muscle groups, targeting the lower back, abdominals, leg extensors and flexors, chest, biceps, triceps, shoulder, and calf and hip abductors and adductors (Feigenbaum and Pollock, 1999).
     b. To minimize the possibility of orthopedic risk, the exercise should start at a lower intensity level such as 10 repetitions and with low weight and progress slowly over 2–4 weeks.

NUTRITION

- Nutrition has been named a priority for Healthy People 2010 (U.S. Department of Health and Human Services, 2000). An individual's age, chronic diseases, functional impairments, polypharmacy, and age-related physiologic and socioeconomic changes may all act in concert to make an older adult nutritionally at risk.
- Good general nutrition beginning early in life and maintained throughout the life span is important for overall health and is one approach to successful aging. Nutrition has been associated with a reduction in disability and death from heart disease and with its social and nurturing aspects that may lead to increased physical activity, physical functioning, independence, and overall quality of life (Evans, 1995b).
- Guidance on proper nutrition may impact the overall health of the older athlete than actually enhance performance (Rock, 1991).

NUTRITIONAL REQUIREMENTS FOR OLDER ADULTS (Evans, 1995b; Rock, 1991; Morley, 1988; Ausman and Russell, 1999; Casa, 2003)

- Physiologic changes associated with aging can have an impact on the older adult's nutritional requirement (Tables 97-6, 97-7). Nutritional advice for the aging athlete will more likely affect his or her overall health rather than improve performance.
- A multivitamin supplement may be indicated for older individuals consuming 1000 kcal/day or less. Important vitamins and minerals for older individuals include vitamin D and B_{12}, iron (18 mg/day), and calcium 1500 mg/day.
- Dehydration is a particular problem of the elderly and often goes unrecognized.
- Dehydration may be responsible for 7% of hospitalizations in community dwelling elders. Dehydration is usually the result of excessive losses or inadequate intake.
- Among the older athlete, dehydration is common especially if there is poor education on hydration, improper timing of consumption of meals, poor vigilance to hydration state, and in general overall poor physical conditioning.

TABLE 97-6 Nutrition and Physiologic Changes in the Elderly

SYSTEM/PHYSIOLOGIC CHANGE	RESULTANT AFFECT
Taste and smell; progressive loss of taste buds; decreased saliva production	Decreasing food intake secondary to perceived changes in palatability
Decreased metabolic rate secondary to decreased lean muscle mass	Decreasing caloric consumption
Decreased gastrointestinal motility; slower gastric emptying	Early satiety
Decreased ability to concentrate urine	Decreased thirst and dehydration

TABLE 97-7 Nutritional Requirements with Aging

Calorie Requirements:
- < 50 years ol age: 2300 Kcal for 77 kg male and 1900 Kcal for 65 kg female.
- 51–75 years of age: 2070 Kcal for men and 1710 Kcal for women
- >75 years of age 1800 Kcal for men and 1500 Kcal for women

Protein: 0.8 to 1 g/kg/day or about 12–14% of total calories; 1.0–1.5 g protein/day athletes

Dietary carbohydrate: 50 and 100 g/day (55 to 60% of total calories); 60–70% of total calories for endurance athletes.

Fat: 30% or less of calories with 10% saturated and 10–15% monounsaturated and nor more than 10% polyunsaturated (liquids at room temperature).

Dietary cholesterol: 300 mg or less per day

Fiber: 25 g/day.

- The U.S.A. Track and Field Advisory Panel recently made recommendations as to proper hydration during track and field events. These recommendations would probably meet the standards of any sporting event (Casa, 2003).

  1. Thirst should be used as an indicator of dehydration during a sporting event. Since older adults in general have a decreased thirst mechanism, it is incumbent on the health care provider to educate the older athlete about replacing fluids when the sensation of thirst is perceived. Because of the blunting of the thirst mechanism a rule of thumb for fluid replacement is to consume two cups of water before exercise and about 200–400 mL of water for every 20–30 min of activity (Rock, 1991). Fluid replacement with solutions containing 4–10% carbohydrate may enhance performance for older athletes participating in endurance events.

  2. The older athlete needs to understand the effects of overhydration—resulting in exertional hyponatremia (serum Na <130 mmol/L) especially if the individual is also on a low salt diet. The older athlete should be made aware that this condition is more common in sporting events lasting longer than 4 h (marathons), low-intensity endurance events, and by drinking large volumes of water without adequate sodium replacement.

REFERENCES

AARP Research: Exercise, attitudes and behaviors: A survery of midlife and older adults. http://research.aarp.org/health/exercise_1.html. Accessed August 29, 2002.

Albert CM, Mittleman MA, Chae CU et al: Triggering of sudden death from cardiac causes by vigorous exertion. *N Engl J Med* 343:1355–1361, 2000.

American College of Sports Medicine: *ACSM's Guidelines for Exercise Testing and Prescriptions*, 6th ed. Baltimore, MD, Lippincott: Williams & Wilkens, 2000.

Andersen RE, Wassen TA, Bartlett SJ et al: Effects of lifestyle activity vs structured aerobic exercise in obese women: A randomized trail. *JAMA* 281:335–340, 1999.

Ausman LM, Russell RM: Nutrition in the elderly, in Shils ME, Olson JA, Shike M, Ross AC (eds): *Modern Nutrition in Health and Disease*, 9th ed. Baltimore, MD, Lippincott: Williams & Wilkens, 1999, pp 869–881.

Begum S, Katzel LI: Silent ischemia during voluntary detraining and future cardiac events in master athletes. *J Am Geriatr Soc* 48:647–650, 2000.

Billman GE: Aerobic exercise conditioning: A nonpharmacological antiarrhythmic intervention. *J Appl Physiol* 92:446–454, 2002.

Booth FW, Gordon SE, Carlson CJ et al: Waging war on modern chronic diseases: Primary prevention through exercise biology. *J Appl Physiol* 88:774–787, 2000.

Buckwalter JA, Heckman JD, Petrie DP: Aging of the North American population: New challenges for Orthopaedics. *J Bone Joint Surg* 85:748–758, 2003.

Buckwalter JA, Lane NE: Athletics and osteoarthritis. *Am J Sports Med* 25:873–881, 1997.

Carpintero P, Berral FJ, Garcia-Frasquet A et al: Delayed diagnosis of fatigue fractures in the elderly. *Am J Sports Med* 25:659–662, 1997.

Casa DJ: Proper hydration for distance running: Identifying individual fluid needs. http://www.usatf.org. Accessed July 7, 2003.

Cassel CK: Use it or lose it: Activity may be the best treatment for aging. *JAMA* 288:2333–2335, 2002.

Christman C, Andersen RA: Exercise and older patients: guidelines for the clinician. *J Am Geriatr Soc* 48:318–324, 2000.

DiPietro L: Physical activity in aging: Changes in patterns and their relationship to health and function. *J Gerontol [Ser A]* 56A (Special Issue II):13–22, 2001.

Edward K, Larson E, Wagner E: Factors associated with regular aerobic exercise in an elderly population. *J Am Board Fam Pract* 5:467–474, 1992.

Epperly TE: The older athlete, in Birrer RB: *Sports Medicine for the Primary Care Physician*, 2nd ed. Boca Raton, FL: CRC Press, 1994. pp 189–196.

Evans WJ: Effects of exercise on body composition and functional capacity of the elderly. *J Gerontol [Ser A]* 50A:147–150, 1995a.

Evans WJ: Exercise, nutrition, and aging. *Clin Geriatr Med* 11:725–734, 1995b.

Evans WJ: Reversing sarcopenia: How weight training can build strength and vitality. *Geriatrics* 51:46–53, 1996.

Evans WJ: Exercise training guidelines for the elderly. *Med Sci Sports Exerc* 31:12–17, 1999.

Evans WJ: Exercise for successful aging, in Tallis RC, Fillit H M (eds.): *Brocklehurst's Textbook of Geriatric Medicine and Gerontology,* 6th ed. London, Churchhill Livingston 2003, pp 855–861.

Federal Interagency Forum on Aging-Related Statistics: *Older Americans 2000: Key Indicator of Well-being.* Feveral

Interagency Forum on Aging-Related Statistics, Washington, DC: US Government Printing Office. August 2000.

Feigenbaum MS, Pollock ML: Prescription of resistance training for health and disease. *Med Sci Sports Exerc* 31:38–45, 1999.

Fiatarrone MA, Marks EC, Ryan ND et al: High-intensity strength training in nonagerians. *JAMA* 263:3029–3034, 1990.

Fiatarone-Singh MA: Exercise comes of age: Rationale and recommendations for a geriatric exercise prescription. *J Gerontology: Med Sci* 57A:M262–M282, 2002.

Fletcher GF, Balady GJ, Amsterdam EA et al: AHA scientific statement: Exercise standards for testing and training; a statement for healthcare professionals from the American Heart Association. *Circulation* 104:1694–1740, 2001.

Frontera WR, Meredith CN, O'Reilly KP et al: Strength conditioning in older men: Skeletal muscle hypertropy and improved function. *J Appl Physiol* 64:1038–1044, 1988.

Gardner MM, Robertson C, Campbell AJ: Exercise in preventing falls and fall related injuries in older people: A review of randomized controlled trials. *Br J Sports Med* 34:7–17, 2000.

Gregg EW, Cauley JA, Seeley DG et al: Physical activity and osteoporotic fracture risk in older women. The Study of Osteoporotic Fractures Research Group. *Ann Intern Med* 129:81–88, 1998.

Hakim AA, Curb JD, Petrovitch H et al: Effects of walking on coronary heart disease in elderly men: The Honolulu Heart Program. *Circulation* 100:9–13, 1999.

Hambrecht R, Fiehn E, Weigl C et al: Regular physical exercise corrects endothelial dysfunction and improves exercise capacity in patients with chronic heart failure. *Circulation* 98:2709–2715, 1998.

Kallinen M, Alen M: Sports-related injuries in elderly men still active in sports. *Br J Sports Med* 28:52–55, 1994.

Kallinen M, Markku A: Aging, physical activity and sports injuries: An overview of common sports injuries in the elderly. *Sport Med* 20:41–52, 1995.

Kannus P, Niittymaki S, Jarvinen M et al: Sports injuries in elderly athletes: A three-year prospective, controlled study. *Age Aging* 18:263–270, 1989.

Kasch FW, Boyer JL, Schmidt PK et al: Aging of the cardiovascular system during 33 years of aerobic exercise. *Age Aging* 28:531–536, 1999.

King A, Castro C, Wilcox S et al: Personal and environmental factors associated with physical inactivity among different racial-ethnic groups of US middle-aged and older-aged women. *Health Psychol* 19:354–364, 2000.

Maharam LG, Bauman PA, Kalman D et al: Master athletes: Factors affecting performance. *Sports Med* 28:273–285, 1999.

Maiorana A, O'Driscoll G, Cheetham C et al: Combined aerobic and resitance exercise training improves functional capacity and strength in CHF. *J Appl Physiol* 88:1565–1570, 2000.

McAuley E, Blissmer B, Katula J et al: Physical activity, self-esteem, and self-efficacy relationshps in older adults: A randomized controlled trial. *Ann Behav Med* 22:131–139, 2000.

McMurdo ME, Mole PA, Paterson CR: Controlled trial of weight bearing exercise in older women in relation to bone density and falls. *BMJ* 314:569, 1997.

Menard D, Stanish WD: The aging athlete. *Am J Sports Med* 17:187–196, 1989.

Mengelkock LJ, Pollock ML, Limacher MC et al: Effects of age, physical training, and physical fitness on coronary heart disease risk factors in older track athletes at twenty-year follow-up. *J Am Geriatr Soc* 45:1446–1453, 1997.

Messier SP, Royer TD, Craven TE et al: Long-term exercise and its effect on balance in older osteoarthritic adults: Results from the fitness, arthritis, and seniors trial (FAST). *J Am Geriatr Soc* 48:131–138, 2000.

Miller ME, Rejeski J, Reboussin BA et al: Physical activity, functional limitations, and disability in older adults. *J Am Geriatr Soc* 48:1264–1272, 2000.

Miszko TA, Cress ME: A lifetime of fitness: Exercise in the perimenopausal and postmenopausal woman. *Clin Sports Med* 19:215–232, 2000.

Morley JE: Nutrition in the elderly. *Ann Intern Med* 109:890–904, 1988.

Murphy DF, Connolly DA, Beynnon BD: Risk factors for lower extremity injury: A review of the literature. *B J Sports Med* 37:13–29, 2003.

Nowalk MP, Prendergast JM, Bayles CM et al: A randomized trial of exercise programs among older individuals living in two long-term care facilities: The FallsFREE program. *J Am Geriatr Soc* 49:859–865, 2001.

O'Connor FG, Howard TM, Fiesler CM et al: Managing overuse injuries: A systemic approach. http://www.physsportsmed.com/issues/1997/05may/oconnor.htm. Accessed May 2003.

Penninx B, Meissier SP, Rejeski J et al: Physical exercise and the prevention of disability in activities of daily living in older persons with osteoarthritis. *Arch Intern Med* 161:2309–2316, 2001.

Pescatello LS: Exercising for health: The merits of lifestyle physical activity. *West J Med* 174:114–118, 2001.

Pescatello LS, Murphy D: Lower intensity physical activity is advantageous for fat distribution and blood glucose among viscerally obese older adults. *Med Sci Sports Exerc* 9:1408–1413, 1998.

Pescatello LS, Murphy D, Costanzo D: Low-intensity physical activity benefits blood lipids and lipoproteins in older adults living at home. *Age Aging* 29:433–439, 2000.

Pescatello LS, VanHeest JL: Physical activity medicates a healthier body weight in the presence of obesity. *Br J Sports Med* 34:86–93, 2000.

Pollock ML, Foster C, Knapp D et al: Effect of age and training on aerobic capacity and body composition of master athletes. *J Appl Physiol* 62:725–731, 1987.

Pollock ML, Mengelkoch LJ, Graves JE et al: Twenty-year follow-up of aerobic power and body composition of older track athletes. *J Appl Physiol* 82:1508–1516, 1997.

Pratley RE, Hagberg JM, Dengel DR et al: Aerobic exercise training-induces reductions in abdominal fat and glucose stimulated insluin responses in middle-aged and older men. *J Am Geriatr Soc* 48:1055–1061, 2000.

Rock CL: Nutrition of the older athlete. *Clin Sport Med* 10:445–457, 1991. Rogers MA, Hagberg JM, Martin WH et al: Decline in VO$_{2max}$ with aging in master athletes and sedentary men. *J Appl Physiol* 68:2195–2199, 1990.

Seeman TE, Berkman LF, Charpentier PA et al: Behavioral and psychosocial predictors of physical performance: MacArthur studies of successful aging. *J Gerontol Med Sci* 50A:M177–M183, 1995.

Seto JL, Brewster CE: Musculoskeletal conditioning of the older athlete. *Clin Sports Med* 10:401–430, 1991.

Sforzo GA, McManis BG, Black D et al: Resilience to exercise detraining in healthy older adults. *J Am Geriatr Soc* 43:209–215, 1995.

Shephard RJ, Balady GJ: Exercise as cardiovascular therapy. *Circulation* 99:963–972, 1999.

Speechley M, Tinetti M: Falls and injuries in frail and vigorous community elderly persons. *J Am Geriatr Soc* 39:46–52, 1991.

Surveillance for five health risks among older adults, 1993–1997. *MMWR Morb Mortal Wkly Rep* 48(SS08):89–130, 1999.

Taaffe D, Duret C, Wheeler et al: Once-weekly resistance exercise improves muscle strength and neuromuscular performance in older adults. *J Am Geriatr Soc* 47:1208–1214, 1999.

U.S. Census Internet Release: Population projections of the United States by age, sex, race and hispanic origin:1995–2050. Current Population Reports, P25-1130. Release date: Janurary 13, 2000.

U.S. Department of Health and Human Services: Healthy People 2010: Understanding and improving health. Washington, DC, US Department of Health and Human Services, 2000

U.S. Preventive Services Task Force: *Guide to Clinical Preventive Services*, 2nd ed. Updates available online at http://www.ahrq. gov. Baltimore, MD, Williams & Wilkens, 1996/2001.

Vita AJ, Terry RB, Huber HB et al: Aging, health risks and cumulative disability. *N Engl J Med* 338:1035–1041, 1998.

Will PM, Demko TM, George DL: Prescribing exercise for health: A simple framework for primary care. *Am Fam Phys* 53:579–585, 1996.

Wiswell RA, Hawkins SA, Jaque SV et al: Relationship between physiological loss, performance decrement, and age in master athletes. *J Gerontol Med Sci* 56A:M618–M626, 2001.

98 THE FEMALE ATHLETE

Rochelle M Nolte, MD
Catherine M Fieseler, MD

INTRODUCTION

- In 1971, there were fewer than 300,000 girls participating in high school athletics, compared to 3.7 million boys. Title IX was passed in 1972, mandating nondiscrimination in all extracurricular activities and varsity athletics that received federal funding.

In 2000, there were 2.7 million girls involved in high school sports compared to 3.8 million boys (Slater and Stone, 2002).
- Benefits of exercise for girls and women include decreased cholesterol levels and heart disease, decreased incidence of breast, endometrial, gall bladder, and colon cancer, improved self-image, body-image, and sense of well-being, increased confidence and improved social skills and decreased school dropout rates, and decreased rate of unwanted or unplanned pregnancy (Lopiano and Modern, 2000).

ANATOMY AND PHYSIOLOGY

- Prior to puberty, there are no gender differences in testosterone and estradiol concentrations (Strickland and Metzl, 2002).
- Girls start puberty an average of 2 years earlier than boys.
- Peak height velocity for girls ranges from 10.5 to 13 years and for boys, 12.5 to 15 years (Sanborn and Jankowski, 1994).
- Menarche occurs approximately 1 year after peak height velocity.
- Adult height is reached by age 17 to 19 years for girls and by age 20 to 22 for boys.
- Skeletal maturity is completed by age 18 to 19 for girls and age 21 to 22 for boys.
  1. Overall, osseous development correlates better with sexual maturation than does age, height, or weight (Sanborn and Jankowski, 1994).
- VO_{2max} averages around 50 mL/kg/min in prepubescent children, and changes little in boys throughout puberty, but decreases in girls with puberty secondary to a change in body composition and a decreased percentage of lean body mass.
- After puberty, metabolically active muscle averages 40–45% of total body weight in boys, but only 35–38% in girls (Lillegard, 2001).
- Women on average are shorter, weigh less, and have shorter limbs and smaller articular surfaces, narrower shoulders and smaller thoraces, and a wider pelvis in relation to their waist and shoulders than men. Women have less muscle mass per total body weight than equally trained and conditioned men. The average young adult female has approximately 20 to 27% body fat, while the average young adult male has 12 to 18% body fat (Sanborn and Jankowski, 1994; Fieseler, 2001).
- Women have a smaller heart size, smaller stroke volume, and higher heart rate for a given submaximal cardiac output (Mittleman and Zacher, 2000).

EATING DISORDERS AND THE FEMALE ATHLETE TRIAD

- The *female athlete triad* has three components: (1) disordered eating, (2) amenorrhea or oligomenorrhea, and (3) decreased bone mineral density.
- Eating disorders are characterized by disturbances in eating behavior, body image, emotions, and relationships. Tables 98-1 to 98-3 exhibit the diagnostic criteria, whereas Tables 98-4 and 98-5 demonstrate signs, symptoms, and medical complications of eating disorders.
  1. Anorexia nervosa is an extreme version of restrictive eating behavior in which an individual continues to starve and feel fat, even though she (female athlete) is 15% or more below her ideal body weight.
  2. Bulimia nervosa has cycles of recurrent binge-eating with a feeling of loss of control followed by inappropriate compensatory behavior.
  3. *Eating disorders not otherwise specified* (EDNOS) is also included in the DSM-IV and includes patients who have eating disorders but do not meet the exact diagnostic criteria of anorexia nervosa or bulimia nervosa.
  4. Disordered eating includes the entire spectrum of abnormal eating behaviors that may not fit any of the DSM-IV criteria for eating disorders.
- Disordered eating can have devastating effects on psychologic well-being, skeletal health, and other physiologic problems such as dehydration, electrolyte disturbances, thermoregulatory and cardiac disturbances, loss of muscle mass, and decreased performance in addition to other medical complications.
- The disordered eating can lead to an energy deficit that leads to menstrual irregularity and an increased risk of stress fractures and premature osteoporosis.

TABLE 98-1 Diagnostic Criteria for Anorexia Nervosa

A. Refusal to maintain body weight at or above a minimally normal weight for age and height (e.g., weight loss leading to maintenance of body weight less than 85% of that expected; or failure to make expected weight gain during period of growth, leading to body weight less than 85% of that expected).

B. Intense fear of gaining weight or becoming fat, even though underweight.

C. Disturbance in the way in which one's body weight or shape is experienced, undue influence of body weight or shape on self-evaluation, or denial of the seriousness of the current low body weight.

D. In postmenarcheal females, amenorrhea, i.e., the absence of at least three consecutive menstrual cycles. (A woman is considered to have amenorrhea if her periods occur only following hormone, e.g., estrogen, administration.)

  Restricting Type: During the current episode of anorexia nervosa, the person has not regularly engaged in binge-eating or purging behavior (i.e., self-induced vomiting or the misuse of laxatives, diuretics, or enemas)

  Binge-Eating/Purging Type: During the current episode of anorexia nervosa, the person has regularly engaged in binge-eating or purging behavior (i.e., self-induced vomiting or the misuse of laxatives, diuretics, or enemas)

SOURCE: American Psychiatric Association: *Diagnostic and Statistical Manual of Mental Disorders,* 4th ed. 2000.

TABLE 98-2 Diagnostic Criteria for Bulimia Nervosa

A. Recurrent episodes of binge eating. An episode of binge eating is characterized by both of the following:
  a. Eating, in a discrete period of time (e.g., within any 2-h period), an amount of food that is definitely larger than most people would eat during a similar period of time and under similar circumstances.
  b. A sense of lack of control over eating during the episode (e.g., a feeling that one cannot stop eating or control what or how much one is eating)

B. Recurrent inappropriate compensatory behavior to prevent weight gain, such as self-induced vomiting; misuse of laxative, diuretics, enemas, or other medications; fasting; or excessive exercise.

C. The binge eating and inappropriate compensatory behaviors both occur, on average, at least twice a week for 3 months.

D. Self-evaluation is unduly influenced by body shape and weight.

E. The disturbance does not occur exclusively during episodes of anorexia nervosa.

  Purging Type: During the current episode of bulimia nervosa, the person has regularly engaged in self-induced vomiting or the misuse of laxatives, diuretics, or enemas.

  Nonpurging Type: During the current episode of bulimia nervosa, the person has used other inappropriate compensatory behaviors, such as fasting or excessive exercise, but has not regularly engaged in self-induced vomiting or the misuse of laxatives, diuretics, or enemas.

SOURCE: American Psychiatric Association: *Diagnostic and Statistical Manual of Mental Disorders,* 4th ed. 2000.

TABLE 98-3 Eating Disorder Not Otherwise Specified

The *eating disorder not otherwise specified* category is for disorders of eating that do not meet the criteria for any specific eating disorder. Examples include the following:
  1. For females, all the criteria for anorexia nervosa are met except that the individual has regular menses.
  2. All the criteria for anorexia nervosa are met except that, despite significant weight loss, the individual's current weight is in the normal range.
  3. All the criteria for bulimia nervosa are met except that the binge eating and inappropriate compensatory mechanisms occur at a frequency of less than twice a week or for a duration of less than 3 months.
  4. The regular use of inappropriate compensatory behavior by an individual of normal body weight after eating small amounts of food (e.g., self-induced vomiting after the consumption of two cookies).
  5. Repeatedly chewing and spitting out, but not swallowing, large amounts of food.
  6. Binge-eating disorder: Recurrent episodes of binge eating in the absence of the regular use of inappropriate compensatory behaviors characteristic of bulimia nervosa.

SOURCE: American Psychiatric Association: *Diagnostic and Statistical Manual of Mental Disorders,* 4th ed. 2000.

TABLE 98-4   Signs, Symptoms, and Medical Complications of Anorexia Nervosa and Bulimia Nervosa

Orofacial

Perimolysis
Dental caries
Cheilosis
Enlargement of the parotid gland
Submandibular adenopathy

Cardiovascular

Postural and nonpostural hypotension
Acrocyanosis
Electrocardiographic abnormalities: Low voltage, prolonged QT interval, and prominent U waves
Sinus bradycardia
Atrial and ventricular arrhythmias
Left ventricular changes: Decreased mass and cavity size
Mitral-valve prolapse
Cardiomyopathy (caused by ipecac poisoning)

Gastrointestinal

Esophagitis hematemesis (including the Mallory-Weiss syndrome)
Delayed gastric emptying
Decreased intestinal motility
Constipation
Rectal prolapse
Gastric dilatation and rupture
Abnormal results on liver-function tests
Elevated serum amylase level

Endocrine and metabolic

Hypokalemia (including hypokalemic nephropathy)
Hyponatremia, (rarely) hypernatremia
Hypomagnesaemia
Hyperphosphatemia
Hypoglycemia
Hypothermia
Euthyroid sick syndrome
Hypercortisolism, elevated free cortisol level in urine
Low serum estradiol level
Decreased serum testosterone level
Amenorrhea, oligomenorrhea
Delay in puberty
Arrested growth
Osteoporosis
Lipid abnormalities
Obesity

Renal

Renal calculi

Reproductive

Infertility
Insufficient weight gain during pregnancy
Low-birth-weight infants

Integumentary

Dry skin and hair
Hair loss
Lanugo
Yellow skin caused by hypercarotenemia

Neurologic

Peripheral neuropathy
Reversible cortical atrophy
Ventricular enlargement

Hematologic

Anemia
Leukopenia
Neutropenia
Thrombocytopenia

SOURCE: Becker: *N Engl J Med*, 340(14):1092–1098, 1999

TABLE 98-5   Abnormalities That May Indicate an Undisclosed Eating Disorder

Somatic

Arrested growth
Marked change or frequent fluctuation in weight
Inability to gain weight
Fatigue
Constipation or diarrhea
Susceptibility to fractures
Delayed menarche
Hypokalemia, hyperphosphatemia, metabolic acidosis or alkalosis, or high serum amylase levels

Behavioral

Change in eating habits
Difficulty eating in social settings
Reluctance to be weighed
Depression
Social withdrawal
Absence from school or work
Deceptive or secretive behavior
Stealing (e.g., to obtain food)
Substance abuse
Excessive exercise

SOURCE: Becker: *N Engl J Med* 340(14):1092–1098, 1999.

- Risk factors for disordered eating and the female athlete triad include the following:
  1. Chronic dieting
  2. Low self-esteem
  3. Family dysfunction
  4. Physical abuse
  5. Biological factors
  6. Perfectionism
  7. Lack of nutrition knowledge
  8. An emphasis on body weight for performance or appearance
  9. Pressure to lose weight from parents, coaches, judges, and peers
  10. A drive to win at any cost
  11. Self-identity as an athlete only (no identity outside of sports)
  12. A sudden increase in training
  13. Exercising through injury
  14. Overtraining (especially when undernourished)
  15. A traumatic event such as an injury or loss of a coach
  16. Vulnerable times such as an adolescent growth spurt, entering college, retiring from athletics, and postpartum depression
- Any athlete with one of the diagnostic criteria of the female athlete triad should be evaluated for the other two by a thorough history and a physical examination.
  a. Laboratory tests that may be helpful include the following:
     1. *Complete blood count* (CBC)
     2. Electrolytes, calcium, magnesium, phosphorus, *blood urea nitrogen* (BUN), creatinine, cholesterol, albumin, and total protein

3. Urinalysis
4. Pregnancy test
5. Follicle stimulating hormone
6. Estradiol
7. Prolactin
8. Thyroid function tests

b. An electrocardiogram may also be indicated as some patients may develop cardiac rhythm disturbances, including prolongation of the QTc.
- Treatment for disordered eating requires a multidisciplinary team, including a physician, psychologist, and a nutritionist.
  a. Treatment includes the following:
     1. Recognition of the problem
     2. Identification and resolution of psychosocial precipitants
     3. Stabilization of medical and nutritional condition
     4. Reestablishment of healthy patterns of eating
- Medication is not generally helpful in the treatment of anorexia, but fluoxetine, a selective serotonin reuptake inhibitor, has been approved by the U.S. Food and Drug Administration (FDA) for the treatment bulimia. (Hudson et al, 1988).
  a. Desipramine and imipramine have also been used in the treatment of bulimia. (Hay, Bacaltchuk, and Bulimia, 2002)
- Indications for inpatient treatment for a patient with an eating disorder include the following:
  a. Very low body weight (<75% of expected body weight)
  b. >15% loss of initial body weight
  c. Rapid (>10% in 1–2 months) weight loss
  d. Cardiac arrhythmias
  e. Electrolyte imbalances
  f. Suicidal ideation
  g. Temperature <36°C
  h. Pulse <45 bpm
  i. Orthostatic pulse differential >30 bpm
  j. Patient not responding to outpatient treatment (Becker et al, 1999)

AMENORRHEA

- Primary amenorrhea is defined as delayed menarche, or the absence of menses by the age of 16 (Bruckner, Fricker, 1998).
- Athletes who begin intensive training before puberty, especially gymnasts and ballet dancers are at risk of developing primary amenorrhea (Marshall, 1994).
- Evaluation of a patient with amenorrhea should include a thorough history, including pubertal milestones in the patient and other female relatives.

  a. A lack of any pubertal development can indicate hypothalamic, pituitary, or gonadal failure.
  b. An interruption of normal pubertal development can indicate ovarian failure, or pituitary failure, as happens with a pituitary neoplasm.
  c. Normal breast and pubic development in the absence of menstrual periods can indicate an abnormality of the reproductive organs.
- Other history should include a training and dietary history, a thorough history of past medical problems and treatments, medications, including over-the-counter medications such as diuretics, laxatives, or ipecac, and supplements such as ephedra, a thorough family history, and psychologic screening for evidence of increased stress, depression, anxiety, obsessive or compulsive personality traits, or symptoms of an eating disorder.
  a. Athletes who associate more stress with their sport and competition are more likely to be amenorrheic (Marshall, 1994).
- A thorough physical should include vital signs, height, weight, body fat, arm span, Tanner stage, any characteristics of chromosomal anomalies, any traits of androgen excess, fundoscopic examination and visual field confrontation, evaluation for galactorrhea, palpation of the thyroid, and a pelvic examination. Imaging studies may include a *computed tomography* (CT) or *magnetic resonance imaging* (MRI) to rule out a pituitary adenoma if indicated.
- Laboratory testing for amenorrhea is shown in Fig. 98-1. The progestin challenge is done by giving medroxyprogesterone as a 10-mg daily dose for 5–10 days. This testing is appropriate for both primary and secondary amenorrhea.
- Secondary amenorrhea is the absence of menstrual bleeding in a woman who has previously had menstrual cycles (Marshall, 1994).
- One commonly used definition of secondary amenorrhea is "the absence of menstrual cycles for a length of time equal to the total time of the three previous menstrual cycles" (Marshall, 1994). Some other definitions are "the absence of menstrual cycles for 6 months," and the International Olympic Committee definition of "one period or less per year."
- In hypothalamic amenorrhea, the pulsatile *gonadotropin releasing hormone* (GnRH) is abnormal. Rarely, this can be caused by a tumor or trauma or developmental defect. More commonly, it is thought that psychologic and/or physical stress affects neurohormones that regulate GnRH, leading to hypothalamic amenorrhea (Marshall, 1994).
- Exercise-related amenorrhea can be considered a subset of hypothalamic amenorrhea, which also includes amenorrhea related to anorexia nervosa, weight loss, and psychologic stress. It is, however, a

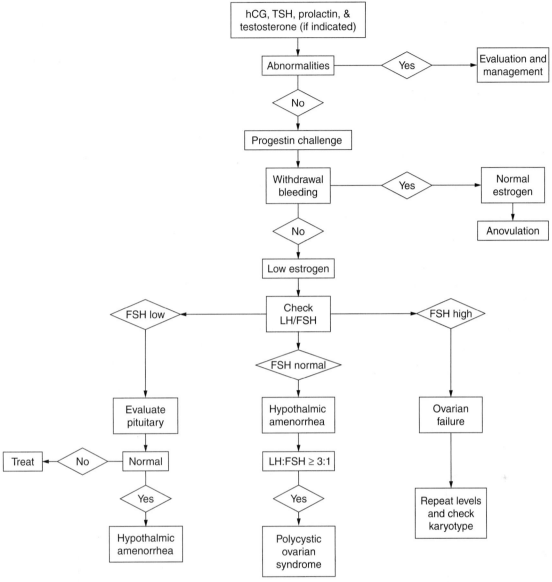

FIG. 98-1 Laboratory Evaluation of Amenorrhea. Source: Adapted from: Fieseler CM. Special considerations for the female runner. *Journal of Back and Musculoskeletal Rehabilitation.* Vol. 6. 1996.

diagnosis of exclusion. Pregnancy is the most common cause of amenorrhea in sexually active women, and must be excluded. Other diagnoses to rule out include *polycystic ovarian syndrome* (PCOS), Asherman's syndrome, and thyroid or pituitary abnormalities.

- If a woman over the age of 30 is presenting with secondary amenorrhea, other etiologies to be considered are premature ovarian failure, endometrial hyperplasia, and carcinoma.
- Exercise-related amenorrhea is thought to be secondary to an energy deficit from an inadequate caloric intake in relationship to energy expenditure. It is thought that girls or women who are having menstrual irregularities secondary to an energy deficit are at risk

of decreased *bone mineral density* (BMD) as well. The primary treatment that is recommended at this time is correcting the energy deficit by increasing caloric intake to the point that there is a spontaneous return of menses. This has been associated with an increase in bone mass as well.

OSTEOPOROSIS

- Osteoporosis is characterized by microarchitectural deterioration of bone tissue leading to enhanced skeletal fragility, low bone mass, and an increased risk for fracture.

a. The World Health Organization has established diagnostic criteria for osteoporosis based on bone density measurements.

b. Osteoporosis is defined as a bone mineral density greater than 2.5 SD below the mean BMD of a young adult woman at her peak bone mass (T-score).

c. Osteopenia is defined as a BMD between 1 and 2.5 SD below the mean.

d. A BMD within 1 SD of the mean is considered normal.

• There is some controversy about whether these criteria are appropriate to use when evaluating adolescents and young women with low bone mass secondary as part of the female athlete triad, as the criteria were established to be used when evaluating post-menopausal women.

• The female athlete triad leads to decreased BMD because bone growth and development is dependent on mechanical, nutritional, and hormonal influences. Women and girls with an energy deficit resulting from decreased caloric intake are at risk of having decreased BMD. Studies have also found a linear relationship between the degree of menstrual dysfunction and vertebral bone density (Vuori and Heinonen, 2000).

• The standard method of diagnosing osteoporosis is by *dual X-ray absorptiometry* (DEXA), which is used to measure bone density at various places, usually the hip, spine, and distal radius. These measurements are used to generate the above mentioned T-score, and an age-matched Z-score.

• It's estimated that 30 million women in the United States have osteoporosis and the estimated direct medical costs for treating osteoporosis are $16 billion annually (National Osteoporosis Foundation, America's Bone Health, 2002).

• The U.S. Preventive Services Task Force recommends BMD screening by DEXA for women over age 65, or over age 60 for women identified as being high risk for developing osteoporosis (US Preventive Services Task Force, Recommendations and Rationale, 2002).

• Nonmodifiable risk factors for osteoporosis (Lane, 2002):
  a. Age
  b. Sex
  c. Race
  d. Family history of osteoporosis
  e. Past history of low-trauma fracture

• Modifiable risk factors for osteoporosis (Lane, 2002).
  a. Low body weight
  b. Low calcium intake
  c. Tobacco use
  d. Excessive alcohol use
  e. Lack of weightbearing exercise

  f. Low muscle mass
  g. Estrogen deficiency (including history of oligomenorrhea, amenorrhea, and delayed menarche)

• Nonpharmacologic measures used in the prevention and treatment of osteoporosis include the following (Becker et al, 1999; Lane, 2002; Cundy et al, 2002; Meier, 1997; Bonjour et al, 1997):
  a. Ensuring adequate caloric intake to meet energy needs, and maintain regular menses if premenopausal
  b. Weightbearing exercise (although it has been shown that weightbearing exercise cannot overcome the bone loss associated with amenorrhea secondary to inadequate caloric intake) (Klibanski et al, 1995; Nattiv, Callahan, and Kelman-Sherstinsky, 2002)
  c. Decreasing tobacco and alcohol use

• Nutritional measures used in the prevention and treatment of osteoporosis include the following:
  a. Calcium intake of 1500 mg daily—divided into three doses containing at least 500 mg of elemental calcium to ensure absorption.
  b. Vitamin D 800 IU daily

• Pharmacologic treatments for pre- and post-menopausal osteoporosis include estrogen, bisphosphonates, *selective estrogen receptor modulators* (SERMs), and calcitonin. These antiresorptive agents are indicated for the prevention and treatment of post-menopausal osteoporosis.

• There are currently no pharmacologic treatments approved by the FDA to treat premenopausal osteoporosis.

• It is thought that the primary problem in the young female athlete is decreased bone formation rather than premature bone loss, so the antiresorptive treatments may not address the problem of adolescent osteopenia/osteoporosis. There is also the concern of possible teratogenic effects if bisphosphonates are used in women of child-bearing age.

• Adequate nutrition and weightbearing exercise during the adolescent years is important for achieving peak bone mass. On average, 92% of the total body BMD is attained by age 18, and 99% is attained by age 26.

• Different sites appear to mature at different ages. Peak bone mass appears to be complete by age 16 in the femoral neck, while the bone mass in the lumbar spine appears to increase into the third decade (Weaver et al, 2001).

• While amenorrhea is associated with osteopenia, using oral contraceptive pills to induce menses has not been shown to increase bone mass in the absence of improved nutrition and calcium intake. In fact, some studies have shown that oral contraceptives may actually cause a further decrease in BMD in adolescent athletes (Weaver et al, 2001).

- In a study of estrogen administration in young women with anorexia nervosa, overall there was no significant difference in bone mass after 1.5 years between the treatment and control groups, although it appeared that the estrogen did help a subgroup of patients who had body weights <70% of ideal body weight; however, a more marked improvement in BMD was obtained with recovery from the eating disorder and gaining weight to ≥85% of ideal body weight and having spontaneous return of normal menstrual function with administration of estrogen (Klibanski et al, 1995).

URINARY INCONTINENCE

- Urinary incontinence is defined by the International Continence Society as the "involuntary loss of urine, which is objectively demonstrable and is a social and hygienic problem." (Elia, 1999)
- *Stress urinary incontinence* (SUI) is the most common type of urinary incontinence, with a prevalence of 10–70% in women between ages 15 and 65. (Bo and Borgen, 2001; Nygaard, 1997; Nygaard, Glowacki, and Saltzman, 1996; Nygaard et al, 1990)
- SUI is the involuntary loss of urine related to increased intra-abdominal pressure with such activities as sneezing, coughing, running, jumping, or heavy lifting.
- Risk factors for SUI include anything that increases intra-abdominal pressure and anything that could weaken the pelvic floor muscles, such as pregnancy and delivery, or decreased estrogen.
- Athletes involved in high-impact activities such as gymnastics (dismount/tumbling) or basketball or volleyball are at risk for SUI during competition or practice (Elia, 1999; Resnick, 1997).
- Management of SUI is directed at correcting the underlying pelvic relaxation. Treatment for mild SUI usually includes pelvic floor strengthening exercises. For women with evidence of vaginal and urethral atrophy secondary to estrogen deficiency, topical or systemic estrogen can be prescribed. For women with severe pelvic relaxation and prolapse, a temporizing measure such as a pessary may be used, but definitive therapy will probably require an invasive treatment such as injection therapy or a surgical repair.

EXERCISE IN PREGNANCY

- Physiologic changes of pregnancy include an increase in blood volume and cardiac output that can have an effect on the maternal response to exercise as early as the first trimester, as these changes happen before uterine and fetal growth (Clapp, 2000).
- Blood volume increases by almost 50% at term.
- The increase in plasma volume occurs before the increase in red cell mass, leading to a dilutional anemia in the second trimester that is partially corrected at term.
- Resting heart rate increases 10 to 15 bpm during pregnancy, and stroke volume and cardiac output also increase (Christian et al, 2002).
- Blood pressure usually falls slightly; reaching a nadir in the second trimester, then slowly rises to prepregnancy levels by term.
- Tidal volume, minute ventilation, and oxygen consumption all increase in pregnancy.
- The usual increases in pulse, cardiac output, blood pressure, and temperature with exercise are slightly blunted in pregnancy.
- Progesterone and relaxin increase pelvic and joint laxity in pregnancy.
- There is no evidence that exercise has a detrimental effect on pregnancy or labor, or fetal well-being (Clapp, 2000).
- Exercise during and after pregnancy has been shown to have a positive psychologic effect (Christian et al, 2002).
- The babies of regularly exercising women appear to tolerate labor well, and have been shown to have a similar head circumference and length, but lower body fat than babies born to nonexercising mothers (Clapp et al, 2002).
- Positive effects of exercise during pregnancy that have been reported include—a tendency to deliver 1 week earlier than nonexercising women, a decreased rate of interventions during labor, including pitocin use and cesarean section, decreased pain perception, and being more than twice as likely to progress from 4 cm to completely dilated in under 4 h, and an average second stage of 36 min versus 60 min in controls (Clapp, 2000; Christian et al, 2002).
- Exertion at altitudes up to 6000 ft appears to be safe, but engaging in physical activities at higher altitudes carries various risks, and women who travel to higher altitudes should be aware of the signs and symptoms of altitude sickness, for which they should cease activity and descend to a lower altitude (Clapp, 2000).
- Scuba diving should be avoided throughout pregnancy as the fetus is at increased risk of decompression sickness secondary to the inability of the fetal pulmonary circulation to filter bubble formation. (American College of Obstetricians and Gynecologists, 2002)
- Absolute contraindications to aerobic exercise during pregnancy:
  a. Hemodynamically significant heart disease
  b. Restrictive lung disease
  c. Incompetent cervix/cerclage

d. Multiple gestation at risk for premature labor
e. Persistent second- or third-trimester bleeding
f. Placenta previa after 26 weeks of gestation
g. Premature labor during the current pregnancy
h. Ruptured membranes
i. Preeclampsia/pregnancy-induced hypertension
• Relative contraindications to aerobic exercise during pregnancy:
a. Severe anemia
b. Unevaluated maternal cardiac arrhythmia
c. Chronic bronchitis
d. Poorly controlled type 1 diabetes
e. Extreme morbid obesity
f. Extreme underweight (*body mass index* or BMI <12)
g. History of extremely sedentary lifestyle
h. Intrauterine growth restriction in current pregnancy
i. Poorly controlled hypertension
j. Orthopedic limitations
k. Poorly controlled seizure disorder
l. Poorly controlled hyperthyroidism
m. Heavy smoker
• Warning signs to terminate exercise while pregnant:
a. Vaginal bleeding
b. Dyspnea prior to exertion
c. Dizziness
d. Headache
e. Chest pain
f. Muscle weakness
g. Calf pain or swelling (need to rule out thrombophlebitis)
h. Preterm labor
i. Decreased fetal movement
j. Amniotic fluid leakage
• There are currently no definitive guidelines for elite or endurance athletes during pregnancy. Elite athletes have to deal with the changing physiology of pregnancy, which may necessitate changing their exercise regimen.
• After the first trimester, the uterus can cause obstruction of venous return in the supine position, so athletes will have to adjust weight-training and floor exercises appropriately.
• Motionless standing also causes a significant decrease in cardiac output and should be avoided as much as possible.
• The increased oxygen consumption of pregnancy will lead to most women experiencing a decline in their exercise tolerance.

REFERENCES

American College of Obstetricians and Gynecologists: Exercise during pregnancy and the postpartum period: ACOG committee opinion no. 267. *Obstet Gynecol* 99(1):171–173, 2002.

Becker AE, Grinspoon SK, Klibanski A et al: Current concepts: Eating disorders. *N Engl J Med* 340(14):1092–1098, 1999.

Bo K, Borgen JS: Prevalence of stress and urge urinary incontinence in elite athletes and controls. *Med Sci Sports Exerc* 33(11):1797–1802, 2001.

Bonjour JP et al: Calcium-enriched foods and bone mass growth in prepubertal girls: A randomized, double-blind, placebo-controlled trial. *J Clin Invest* 99(6):1287–1294, 1997.

Bruckner P Fricker P: Endocrinologic conditions, in Fields KB, Fricker PA (eds.): *Medical Problems in Athletes:* Chap. 28. Oxford, UK: Blackwell Science 1998.

Christian JS, Christian SS, Stamm CA et al: Physiology and Exercise, in Ireland ML, Nattiv A (eds.): *The Female Athlete:* Chap. 20. New York, NY, Elsevier Science 2002.

Clapp JF: Exercise during pregnancy: A clinical update. *Clin Sports Med* 19:2, 2000.

Clapp JF et al: Continuing regular exercise during pregnancy: Effect of exercise volume on fetoplacental growth. *Am J Obstet Gynecol* 186(1):142–147, 2002.

Cundy T et al: Menopausal bone loss in long-term users of depot medroxyprogesterone acetate contraception. *Am J Obstet Gynecol* 186(5):978–983, 2002.

Elia G: Stress urinary incontinence in women. *Phys Sportsmed* 27:1, 1999.

Fieseler CM: The female runner, in O'Connor FG, Wilder RP (eds.): *Textbook of Running Medicine:* Chap. 34. New York, NY, McGraw-Hill, 2001.

Hay P, Bacaltchuk J: *Bulimia Nervosa, Clinical Evidence Concise: Issue 8.* BMJ Publishing Group, 2002, pp 182–183.

Hudson JI et al: Fluvoxamine in the treatment of binge-eating disorder: A multicenter placebo-controlled double-blind trial. *Am J Psych,* 155(12):1756–1762, 1988.

Klibanski A et al: The effects of estrogen administration on trabecular bone loss in young women with anorexia nervosa. *J Clin Endocrinol Metab* 80(3):898–904, 1995.

Lane JM: Osteoporosis in Ireland ML, Nattiv A (eds.): *The Female Athlete:* Chap. 26. New York, NY, Elsevier Science 2002.

Lillegard WA: Special considerations for the pediatric running population, in O'Connor FG, Wilder RP (eds.): *Textbook of Running Medicine:* Chap. 33. New York, NY, McGraw-Hill, 2001.

Lopiano DA: Modern history of women in sports: Twenty-five years of title IX. *Clin Sports Med* 19:2, 2000.

Marshall LA: Clinical evaluation of Amenorrhea in active and athletic women. *Clin Sports Med* 13:2, 1994.

Meier DE: Osteoporosis and other disorders of skeletal aging, in Cassel CK et al (eds.): *Geriatric Medicine:* Chap. 27 3rd ed. New York, NY, Springer-Verlag, 1997.

Mittleman KD, Zacher CM: Factors influencing endurance performance, strength, flexibility and coordination, in Drinkwater BL (ed.): *The Encyclopedia of Sports Medicine: Women in Sport: vol. 8,* Chap. 2. London, Blackwell Science, 2000.

National Osteoporosis Foundation, America's Bone Health: The state of osteoporosis and low bone mass in our nation. www.nof.org. 2002.

Nattiv A, Callahan LR, Kelman-Sherstinsky A: The female athlete triad, in Ireland ML, Nattiv A (eds.): *The Female Athlete:* Chap. 24. New York, NY, Elsevier Science, 2002.

Nygaard IE: Does prolonged high-impact activity contribute to later urinary incontinence? A retrospective cohort study of female olympians. *Obstet Gynecol* 90(5)718–722, 1997.

Nygaard IE, DeLancey JO, Arnsdorf L et al: Exercise and Incontinence. *Obstet Gynecol* 75(5):848–851, 1990.

Nygaard IE, Glowacki C, Saltzman CL: Relationship between foot flexibility and urinary incontinence in nulliparous varsity athletes. *Obstet Gynecol* 87(6):1049–1051, 1996.

Resnick NM: Urinary incontinence, in Cassel CK et al (ed.): *Geriatric Medicine:* Chap. 48, 3rd ed. New York, NY, Springer-Verlag, 1997.

Sanborn CG, Jankowski CM: Physiologic considerations for women in sport. *Clin Sports Med* 13(2):315–327, 1994.

Slater CA, Stone JA: Participation and historical perspective, in Ireland ML, Nattiv A (eds.): *The Female Athlete:* Chap. 2. New York, NY, Elsevier Science, 2002.

Strickland SM Metzl JD: Growth and development, in Ireland ML, Nattiv A (eds.): *The Female Athlete:* Chap. 22. New York, NY, Elsevier Science, 2002.

US Preventive Services Task Force, Recommendations and Rationale: Screening for osteoporosis in postmenopausal women. Agency for Healthcare Research and Quality, 2002.

Vuori I, Heinonen A: Sport and bone, in Drinkwater BL (ed.): *Women in Sport: Volume VIII of the Encyclopaedia of Sports Medicine:* Chap. 19. London, Blackwell Science, 2000.

Weaver CM et al: Impact of exercise on bone health and contraindication of oral contraceptive use in young women. *Med Sci Sports Exerc* 33(6):873–880, 2001.

99 SPECIAL OLYMPICS ATHLETES

Pamela M Williams, MD
Christopher M Prior, DO

SPECIAL OLYMPICS INTERNATIONAL

- Background: Founded in 1968 by Eunice Kennedy Shriver, Special Olympics is an international organization serving more than 1 million persons with mental retardation in over 200 programs more than 150 countries. Eligible athletes are given the opportunity to participate in training and competition that challenges each athlete to their fullest potential, regardless of the athlete's level of ability.
- Mission and goals: The Special Olympics' mission is to provide year round sports training and athletic competition for people with mental retardation. The programs provide opportunities for athletes to develop physical fitness and to experience the camaraderie of sport and the spirit of sportsmanship. The ultimate goal of the program is to use sport as a medium to aid persons with mental retardation in participating as productive and respected members of society.
- Athlete's oath: "Let me win. But if I cannot win, let me be brave in the attempt."
- Eligibility: To be eligible to participate, an individual must be at least eight years of age and:
  - Have been identified by an agency or professional as having mental retardation
  - Have a cognitive delay as determined by standardized measures
  - Have significant learning or vocational problems due to cognitive delays that require or have required specially designed instruction
  - Age restrictions: Children who are at least 6 years old may participate in age-appropriate training programs but may not compete. There is no maximum age limitation for participation.

OFFICIAL SPORTING EVENTS

- Official sports: Special Olympics International (SOI) currently recognizes 26 official sports. These are divided into Summer and Winter games as listed in Table 99-1.
- Demonstration sports: Demonstration sports, officially termed recognized sports, may be incorporated into events as determined by the hosting site in conjunction with SOI and may become official sports when adequate national programs include the event in their national games. Recent examples include kayaking, pitch and putt, and judo.
- Prohibited sports: Prohibited sports are those that have been identified as a result of their unreasonable risk to the health and safety of Special Olympics athletes. Currently prohibited sports include boxing, fencing, shooting, karate, and other martial arts.
- Levels of participation: Special Olympics athletes are divided by sex, age, and ability.

TABLE 99-1   Special Olympics Sports

SUMMER GAMES		WINTER GAMES
Aquatics	Gymnastics	Alpine skiing
Athletics	Powerlifting	Cross country skiing
Badminton	Roller skating	Figure skating
Basketball	Sailing	Floor hockey
Bocce	Softball	Snowboarding
Bowling	Table tennis	Snowshoeing
Cycling	Team handball	Speedskating
Equestrian	Tennis	
Football (Soccer)	Volleyball	
Golf		

PREPARTICIPATION EXAMINATION

- Goals of the preparticipation examination:
  - To identify medical and orthopedic conditions that may affect safe or effective athletic participation.
  - To review the chronic medical status of the Special Olympics athlete and identify need for special assistance or restrictions.
- SOI requirements:
  - Preparticipation questionnaire: The athlete or the athlete's guardian, parent, or caseworker completes a standardized, comprehensive health history every 3 years. The health data documented in the preparticipation questionnaire is listed in Table 99-2.
  - Preparticipation examination (PPE): A physical examination of each athlete is required on entry into the program and a minimum of every 3 years thereafter. A new examination is required whenever an athlete develops a new medical problem.
    1. Examination guidelines: No specific examination requirements have been mandated except for the evaluation of Down syndrome athletes for atlantoaxial instability, if they will be participating in an activity that may involve hyperextension or flexion of the neck or upper spine. The general approach to the PPE should be similar to that applied to athletes without disabilities, as demonstrated in the *Preparticipation Physical Evaluation Monograph*, 2nd edition.
    2. Abnormal examination
       a. Sport-significant abnormalities are identified in up to 40% of PPE on Special Olympic athletes.

TABLE 99-2   Health Data from the Preparticipation Questionnaire

Heart disease/heart defect/hypertension	Chest pain or fainting spells
Seizures or epilepsy	Concussion or serious head injury
Diabetes	Heat stroke/exhaustion
Down syndrome and history of cervical spine imaging	Exercise induced wheezing
Sickle cell disease/trait or any bleeding diathesis	Impaired motor ability and/or use of wheelchair
Serious bone or joint disorders	Hearing impairment and/or use of hearing aid
Emotional, psychiatric, or behavioral problems	Vision impairment and/or use of corrective lenses
Absence of vision/blind in one eye	Dentures or false teeth
Absence of one kidney or testicle	Allergies (medications, food, or insects)
Major surgery or illness	Immunization status, including date of last tetanus
Parent or sibling with premature cardiac disease	Current medications and dosages

- b. Guidelines from the *Preparticipation Physical Evaluation Monograph*, 2nd edition, select American Academy of Pediatrics (AAP) position statements and the 26th Bethesda Conference, along with subspecialty consultation, should be utilized to guide the individual assessment of qualification for participation when a medical condition is identified, which may increase the risk of injury or may be adversely affected by sport.
- Special Olympic athlete profile
  - Gender breakdown: Male = 60%, female = 40%
  - Average age of athletes: 22 years
  - Average number of sports competed in: 1.6 events
  - Prevalence of the most commonly identified health conditions:
    1. No health problems indicated: 50%
    2. Chronic medication use: 25–30%
    3. Vision impairment: 15–27%
    4. Emotional, psychiatric, or behavior problems: 18%
    5. Hearing impairment: 8–10%
    6. Seizure disorder: 8–12 %
- Down syndrome athlete
  - Definition: Down syndrome is the most common human malformation pattern and results from trisomy of chromosome 21. Its incidence is currently estimated at 1 in 600–800 live births. Medical problems are frequent and have a significant impact on sports participation. Orthopedic problems occur because the chromosomal abnormality results in a defect in production of normal collagen. The abnormal collage produced results in generalized ligamentous laxity and decreased muscle tone. Up to 30% of Special Olympics athletes have Down syndrome.
  - Relative risk of injury: 3.2 times greater than other Special Olympics athletes.
  - Atlantoaxial instability
    1. Definition: Atlantoaxial instability (AAI) denotes laxity of the transverse ligament of C1 (atlas) which stabilizes the articulation of the odontoid process of C2 (axis) with C1. As a result of increased mobility, C1 may spontaneously sublux on C2 with resultant compression of the cervical spinal cord.
    2. Incidence: Approximately 15% of children with Down syndrome have radiologic evidence of AAI, which may also occur in patients with rheumatoid arthritis and bone dysplasias.
    3. Cause for concern: AAI can lead to frank atlantoaxial dislocation, a life-threatening condition, manifest as abnormal gait, neck pain, limited neck mobility, head tilt, incoordination,

clumsiness, and changes in bowel and bladder control. Paraplegia, hemiplegia, quadriplegia, and death are rare, but reported, outcomes.
4. SOI policy: Since 1983, Special Olympics has required screening for atlantoaxial instability in athletes with Down syndrome before participation in any high risk sport that places excess stress on the head or the neck.
   a. High risk activities: Butterfly stroke and diving starts in swimming, diving, pentathlon, high jump, squat lifts, equestrian sports, artistic gymnastics, football (soccer), alpine skiing, and any warm-up exercise placing undue stress on the head and neck.
   b. Participation is permitted in these activities if:
      i. An athlete undergoes an examination, including X-rays, by a physician who understands atlantoaxial instability and who determines that the athlete does not have atlantoaxial instability.
      ii. An athlete (or parent/guardian of a minor) with known atlantoaxial instability confirms in writing own decision to participate regardless of risk and two licensed medical physicians certify in writing that they have explained these risks and that, in their judgment, the athlete's condition does not preclude the athlete from participating.
5. Screening controversy: In 1995, the AAP Committee on Sports Medicine and Fitness abandoned its previous recommendation of universal preparticipation radiographic screening of all Down syndrome athletes due to unproven value of radiographs in detecting patients at risk. AAP now recommends careful neurologic evaluation annually of Down syndrome athletes for symptoms and signs consistent with spinal cord injury. Symptoms of AAI include neck pain and stiffness, torticollis, progressive weakness or change in sensation in any extremity, decreasing endurance, loss of bowel or bladder control or a change in bowel habits, increased clumsiness or change in gait pattern. Neurologic signs include sensory deficits, spasticity, hyperreflexia, clonus, extensor-plantar reflex, and other upper motor neuron and posterior column signs.
6. Diagnosis: AAI is screened with lateral radiographs of the cervical spine in flexion, extension, and neutral. The atlantodens interval (ADI), the distance between the odontoid process of the axis and the anterior arch of the atlas, is calculated. The ADI is normally less than 2.5 mm. An ADI greater than 4.5 mm is abnormal.

7. Restrictions: In addition to the guidelines mandated by SOI, any symptomatic athletes regardless of ADI and those with an ADI greater than 6 mm should be restricted from all strenuous activities and evaluated for possible operative stabilization of the cervical spine.
8. Screening intervals: Screening for AAI should be initiated when an individual with Down syndrome starts school, plans to participate in any high-risk activity or if the individual has neurologic symptoms. Although no evidence in the literature currently supports the need for follow-up imaging, many physicians still recommend repeat screening at 3- to 5-year intervals till skeletal maturity is achieved. The presence of neurologic symptoms at any time is a reason for further evaluation and screening radiographs.

INJURY AND ILLNESS PATTERNS

- Incidence of injury and illness
  1. Incidence of illness and injury at state, national, and international competitions has ranged from 2.8 to 13%.
  2. Majority of athletes are seen for acute, minor injuries particularly sprains and strains to the lower extremities.
  3. Seizures account for 7–10% of all encounters.
  4. Athletic injury claims are greatest for athletics, basketball, and softball.
  5. Injury rates are less than those reported for the physically disabled athlete and the able-bodied athlete.
  6. Sport-specific injuries are similar for Special Olympics athletes and able-bodied athletes.
- Summer sports
  - Injuries and illness patterns: Epidemiologic data have been reported for multiple state, national, and international events. The most commonly encountered illnesses and injuries are listed in Table 99-3.

TABLE 99-3 Summer Sport Injuries and Illness

INJURIES	ILLNESSES
Abrasion	Heat-related illness
Strain	Gastrointestinal discomfort
Sprain	Seizure
Contusion	Headache
Laceration	Asthma
Blister	Diabetes management
Nail avulsion	Sunburn
Fracture	Conjunctivitis
	Dermatitis
	Insect bite

TABLE 99-4   Injuries and Illnesses for Team U.S.A. First International Special Olympics Winter Games Austria, 1993

INJURIES	ILLNESSES
Abrasion	Respiratory illness
Strain	Dehydration
Sprain	Behavioral/psychiatric
Contusion	Gastrointestinal illness
Laceration	Dermatologic problem
Blister	Canker sores, gingivitis
Fracture	

- Winter sports
  - Surveillance data: Limited published data is available on injury and illness patterns in Special Olympic Winter Sports. Injuries and illness encountered by Team USA at the First International Special Olympics Winter Games in 1993 in Austria are included in Table 99-4.

EVENT COVERAGE

- General considerations: Coverage of Special Olympics events is a dynamic process that frequently relies heavily on past event experiences. A systematic approach, such as the one outlined in event planning below, ensures success.
- Minimal medical facilities: SOI mandates the following be present for large competitions:
  1. A qualified *emergency medical technician* (EMT) be in attendance or readily available at all times.
  2. A licensed medical professional must be on-site or on immediate call at all times during the competition.
  3. First aid areas must be clearly identified, adequately equipped and staffed by a qualified EMT for the duration of the event.
  4. An ambulance with *advanced cardiac life support* (ACLS) capabilities, including equipment for handling seizures, must be readily available at all times.
- Event planning
  - Crowd size: Estimated event attendance determines the personnel, supplies, and evacuation routes. Each community event is a potential mass casualty event.
  - Environmental concerns: Climate, geography, and time of day of the event need to be considered along with the availability of adequate shelters from sun, rain, and cold. Access to and availability of drinking water and restrooms should be identified. Fluids must be provided for athletes and drinking breaks encouraged minimizing risk of heat-related illnesses. Special Olympics athletes often lack the normal perception of thirst.

- Population: Each Special Olympics athlete population has its own unique composition of ages and illnesses. Preevent screening of the ages and disabilities of the athletes may assist in preparing for unique issues that may arise.
- Injury rates: As discussed above, prior experiences have shown that rates will be similar to other events involving able-bodied athletes.
- Transportation: On-field transportation to transfer athletes to an aid station may include golf carts or stretchers. Ambulances are most commonly used for transport to hospitals. Helicopters have been used at larger events where distance or traffic may have resulted in unacceptable transportation times.
- Evacuation routes: Routes need to be well planned, clear, accessible, and secure.
- Security: The role of security is to assist with locating those with medical needs, to assure appropriate identification of athletes and personnel, and to maintain crowd control and evacuation routes.
- Supplies needed: The items needed are similar to other community sports events. An *automated external defibrillator* (AED) and lorazepam or diazepam are also recommended.
- Site layout: The location and quantity of aid stations required will be determined by the number of participants and by the quality and quantity of geographic sites. The need for a central aid station alone or in conjunction with multiple peripheral venues will be further determined by potential patient loads, ability to transport patients, potential holding capacity, and shelter availability. Site selection should also take into account visibility, accessibility, and proximity to evacuation routes.
- Medical records: Records should be maintained in a central location and be readily transported to the treating provider owing to the complexity of preexisting medical conditions. Athlete's current medications, allergies, and medical conditions may be listed on the back of the identification badge.
- Medical reporting: The use of standard forms assists in tracking supplies used, and incidence and types of injuries including time of day and location.
- Communication: Medical directors must be in contact with event organizers, as well as in contact with each on-site medical station, local medical facilities and EMS. Cellular phones, two-way radios, and pagers are useful tools.
- Local resources: Resources should be solicited from local ambulance services and hospitals. These resources should be advised of the specifics of the event so they can plan and prepare, as well.
- Scope of care: Most care provided at the event will involve general first aid. *Advanced trauma life support*

(ATLS) and ACLS, though rarely needed, should only be provided if resources and trained providers are available. Most situations will involve initial stabilization only with rapid transport of those who require more than basic first aid.

- Personnel: Medical practitioners may include a diverse group of providers ranging from physicians to EMTs. All must work within their level of training and scope of practice.
- Malpractice/liability: Good Samaritan laws will apply in some states. Medical practitioners should discuss coverage with event providers and their individual insurance company to determine the need for additional event coverage.
- Insurance: Most athletes are covered by individual insurance plans. SOI maintains an umbrella insurance plan that covers medical cost of emergency care required at games.
- Pre-event medical briefs
  1. Participant education: Competitors and volunteers should be educated on the available medical services, the identification of providers and the location of aid station locations. Eating a low fat, complex carbohydrate diet to reduce the incidence of abdominal pains is recommended. Further, reminders should be given for athletes to take their chronic medications and consume appropriate fluids.
  2. Medical volunteers: A briefing should occur before the event and prior to each shift. Points to review include—incidence and types of injuries anticipated, scope of care, documentation, schedules, communication, and site layout.

ILLNESS AND INJURY PREVENTION

- Training: Coaching promotes proper technique and appropriate assignment to ability groups. The use of protective equipment is no different than use by able-bodied athletes; however, the use of mouth guards and protective eyewear is often lacking by Special Olympics athletes.
- Safety precautions
  - Sport-specific medical and safety requirements are contained in the Official Special Olympics Sports Rules.
  - Protective eyewear is required for monocular athletes participating in dynamic reactive sorts (such as basketball, volleyball, and softball) and strongly recommended for athletes who wear street glasses and participate in these activities.
  - Protective headgear must be worn by athletes participating in cycling, equestrian, floor hockey,

softball (for batters and base runners), speed skating, and alpine skiing (for giant slalom and downhill events).

- Seizure precautions
  - Well-controlled seizure disorder: Risk for seizure during participation is minimal. Full participation in activities is generally allowed. Athletes are permitted to swim under direct one-on-one visual supervision of a qualified lifeguard who is trained in *cardiopulmonary resuscitation* (CPR) and who is aware of the individual's condition.
  - Poorly controlled seizure disorder: Even when seizures are not completely controlled, sports participation is permitted; however, the following sports should be avoided: swimming, power lifting, and sports involving heights such as gymnastics, diving, or horseback riding.
  - Supervision: Athletes with seizure disorders should be chaperoned at all times, reminded to take chronic medication at events and stay well hydrated.
  - Management of the seizing athlete: Most seizures will be short, self-limited, and followed by a postictal state. With status epilepticus, pharmacologic intervention may be indicated. After protecting the athlete from further injury and stabilizing the airway, antiepileptic benzodiazepines such as lorazepam (initial dose: 0.05–0.1 mg/kg up to 3–4 mg IV) or diazepam (initial dose: 0.2–0.5 mg/kg up to 5–10 mg IV or 0.2–0.3 mg/kg/dose rectal gel) may be administered. The athlete with status epilepticus should be transported immediately for further evaluation and management. In addition, any athlete with new onset seizure needs to be transported and evaluated.
  - Return to play: If a self-limited seizure occurs during an event, the athlete should not participate further that day. If there is no recurrence overnight, the athlete may safely return to competition the next day. Individuals with petit mal (absence) seizures may be considered as exceptions to this rule and may be considered for return to play on the same day.
- Injury surveillance: Ongoing surveillance is a key to identifying sports that may result in injury or factors that may predispose Special Olympics athletes to injury or illness.
- Immunizations: Recommended immunizations include: hepatitis A, hepatitis B, *measles-mumps-rubella* (MMR), tetanus, and influenza. Immunization status should be closely reviewed for those participating in regional, national, and international games.
- Healthy athletes initiative:
  1. Established in 1996 to improve each athlete's ability to train and compete through better fitness and health.

2. On-site event affiliated programs involve dentistry, optometry, audiology, nutrition, podiatry, physical therapy, and health educators.
3. Data on the health status and needs of people with mental retardation is collected, analyzed, and used for planning, programs, and policy development.
4. Current initiatives: Special Smiles, Lions Clubs International Opening Eyes, Healthy Hearing, Health Promotion, and FUN fitness.

BIBLIOGRAPHY

American Academy of Pediatrics, American Academy of Family Physicians, American Orthopedic Society for Sports Medicine, American Medical Society for Sports Medicine, American Osteopathic Society for Sports Medicine: Preparticipation physical evaluation monograph, 2nd ed. New York, NY, McGraw Hill, 1997.

American Academy of Pediatrics, Committee on Sports Medicine and Fitness: Atlantoaxial instability in Down syndrome: Subject review. *Pediatrics* 96:151–154, 1995.

American Academy of Pediatrics, Committee on Sports Medicine and Fitness: Medical conditions affecting sports participation. *Pediatrics* 107:1205–1209, 2001.

Batts KB, Glorioso JE, Williams MS: The medical demands of the special athlete. *Clin J Sport Med* 8:22–25, 1998.

26th Bethesda Conference: Recommendations for determining eligibility for competition in athletes with cardiovascular abnormalities. *J Am Coll Cardiol* 24:845–899, 1995.

Birrer RB: The special Olympics: An injury overview. *Phys Sportsmed* 12:95–97, 1984.

Carek PJ, Dickerson LM, Hawkins A: Special Olympics, special athletes, special needs? *J S C Med Assoc* 98:183–186, 2002.

Fountain NB, May AC: Epilepsy and athletics. *Clin Sports Med* 22:605–616, 2003.

Galena HJ, Epstein CR, Lourie RJ: Connecticut State Special Olympics: Observations and recommendations. *Conn Med* 62:33–37, 1998.

McCormick DP: Medical coverage for Special Olympics games, in *Team Physician's Handbook*, 2nd ed. Philadelphia, PA, Hanley & Belfus, 1997.

McCormick DP, Niebuhr VN, Risser WL: Injury and illness surveillance at local Special Olympic games. *Br J Sports Med* 24:221–224, 1990.

Perlman SP: Special Olympics athletes and the incidence of sports-related injuries. *J Mass Dent Soc* 43:44–46, 1994.

Pizzutillo PD: The cervical spine in the child, in *Delee and Drez's Orthopaedic Sports Medicine*, 2nd ed. Philadelphia, PA, Saunders, 2003.

Robson HE: The Special Olympics games for the mentally handicapped—United Kingdom 1989. *Br J Sports Med* 24:225–230, 1990.

Smith BJ: Treatment of status epilepticus. *Neurol Clin* 19:347–369, 2001.

Smith D: Health care management of adults with Down syndrome. *Am Fam Phys* 64:1031–1040, 2001.

Special Olympics: www.specialolympics.org. Retrieved October 15, 2003.

Zupanc ML: Sports and epilepsy, in *Delee and Drez's Orthopaedic Sports Medicine*, 2nd ed. Philadelphia, PA, Saunders, 2003.

100 THE DISABLED ATHLETE

Paul F Pasquina, MD
Halli Hose, MD
David C Young, MD

INTRODUCTION

• "Athletic competition is inherent to the human spirit" (Bergeron, 1999). This holds true for persons with or without disabilities.
• There are an estimated 43 million disabled people in the United States.
• Approximately 12% of the school-aged population in the United States has a disability.
• There are two to three million recreational and competitive disabled athletes in the United States.
• Of the estimated 43 million disabled, over 60% never participate in any physical or social activity.
• While many opportunities exist for individuals with disabilities, the two most limiting factors for participation in athletics are awareness and access (Wu and Williams, 2001). Healthcare practitioners should make every effort to inform these individuals of the multiple opportunities and encourage their participation.
• Federal Rehabilitation Act—1973
  • Prohibits exclusion of otherwise qualified individuals from participation in federally funded programs.
• The Americans with Disabilities Act of 1990 (ADA)
  • Legal statutes govern whether team physicians can determine participation eligibility.
  • Informed consent—allows athlete greater responsibility in decision making.
  • Extends rights to include private sectors.
  • Requires reasonable accommodations.

HISTORY

• Perhaps the two most well-known competitions that exist for individuals with disabilities are the *Special Olympics* and *Paralympics*. The goal of each is very different. The goal of the Special Olympics is participation and typically involves individuals with mental handicaps. The goal of the Paralympics is winning, involving individuals with various physical disabilities who compete nationally and internationally to determine who the best is.

- In 1924, the first international competition for athletes with physical disabilities, the International Silent Games, was held. The first winter Paralympic games were held in 1976 and were hosted in Ornskoldsvik, Sweden.
- In the United States, the Committee on Sports for the Disabled is a subcommittee of the U.S. Olympic Committee (USOC). It recognizes seven national disabled sports organizations: U.S.A. Deaf Sports Federation, Disabled Sports U.S.A., Dwarf Athletic Association of America, Special Olympics International, U.S. Association for Blind Athletes, U.S. Cerebral Palsy Athletic Association, and Wheelchair Sports U.S.A.

DEFINITIONS/CLASSIFICATIONS

- World Health Organization (WHO)
  - Impairment: Any loss or abnormality of psychologic, physical, or anatomical structure or function.
  - Disability: Any restriction or lack (resulting from an impairment) of an ability to perform an activity in the manner or within the range considered normal for a human being.
  - Handicap: A disadvantage for a given individual, resulting from an impairment or a disability that limits or prevents the fulfillment of a role that is normal (depending on age, sex, and social and culture factors) for that individual.
- National Collegiate Athletic Association (NCAA)
  - A disabled athlete is one who is confined to a wheelchair; deaf, blind, or missing a limb; has one of a pair of organs; or a behavioral, emotional or psychologic disorder that substantially limits a major life activity.
- Classification systems for disabled athletes are more complicated than those for able-bodied athletes. These systems are both sports and impairment specific and are different for each organization. Every effort is made to ensure competition exists between individuals of similar impairments. For example an individual with a transfemoral (above-knee) amputation, would be at a disadvantage racing an individual with a transtibial (below knee) amputation. Team sports, generally involve a point system, where individuals are assigned a point value based on their impairment level. Lower numbers are given to athletes of higher level impairments, and fairness in competition between

teams is achieved by limiting the total amount of points each team may have on the court at anytime. In addition, limitations and regulations are also placed on adaptive equipment, e.g. size and features of wheelchair and prosthetic device.

BENEFITS OF SPORTS AND EXERCISE

- Research has shown that physical fitness and sports participation offer both physical and psychologic health benefits to individuals of all ages, including those with disabilities (Johnson et al, 1998; Weiss and Beck, 1973).
- These benefits include self-image, body awareness, motor development, and mood.
- Athletes with disabilities demonstrate increased exercise endurance, muscle strength, cardiovascular efficiency, and flexibility; improved balance; and better motor skills compared with individuals with disabilities who do not participate in athletics.
- Individuals with amputations who participate in athletics have improved proprioception and increased proficiency in the use of prosthetic devices.
- Disabled athletes have fewer cardiac risk factors, higher *high-density lipoprotein* (HDL) cholesterol, and are less likely to smoke cigarettes than those who are disabled and nonactive.
- Athletes with paraplegia are less likely to be hospitalized, have fewer pressure ulcers, and are less susceptible to infections than nonactive individuals with paraplegia.

PREPARTICIPATION ASSESSMENT

- Preparticipation assessments (PPA) should be performed in a systematic comprehensive fashion similar to that performed for able-bodied athletes.
- Sports medicine practitioners should not be overly focused on the athlete's impairment/disability, and miss common medical issues.
- Careful evaluation of the athlete's wheelchair, prosthetics, orthotics, and assistive/adaptive devices should also be performed prior to competition. This is usually facilitated by consultation with the individual's Orthotist, Prosthetist, or other health care specialists with experience in this area.
- Sports medicine practitioners, who are not familiar with certain impairments, should solicit assistance from practitioners with more experience. This often requires a team approach. For example a physician specializing in sports medicine may have little experience in spinal cord injuries, while a spinal cord injury specialist may have even less experience in sports

medicine. Together, however, they can jointly assess an individual and clear them safely for participation.

- Practitioners should avoid mass screening stations for individuals with disabilities in favor of private office setting visits.
- It is recommended that the PPA be performed by a medical team that is involved in the longitudinal care of the disabled athlete, as knowledge of baseline functioning is essential.
- Individuals with conditions such as osteogenesis imperfecta, arthrogryposis, hemophilia, high cervical lesions, or those missing one of a paired set of organs should avoid contact sports or sports with a high risk of falling.
- The specific elements required in the PPE are determined by the sport, the level of participation, the athletic organization, the clinical indications, and the athlete. The PPE should provide information to guide the athlete, trainer, coach, and team physician toward safe participation, activity limitations, and disability-specific training.
- The objectives of the examination include the following:
  - Identify conditions that may require further medical evaluation before the athlete enters into training, require close supervision during training, and may predispose to injury.
  - Determine the athlete's general health to assess fitness level and performance.
  - Counsel on health-related issues and methods for safe participation.
  - Provide referral for identified conditions that require further evaluation and/or monitoring to physicians familiar with the disability and the management of the identified conditions.
- In addition to the standard components of a history, the elements of the history for an athlete with a disability also should include athletic goals, pre-disability, present level of training, sports participation, over-the-counter (OTC) agents taken, presence of impairments, past family cardiopulmonary history, level of functional independence for mobility and self-care, and needs for adaptive equipment.
- The elements of the disability and sports-specific physical examination are tailored for the individual. Sensory deficits, neurologic deficits, joint stability and *range of motion* (ROM), muscle strength, flexibility, skin integrity, medications, and adaptive equipment needs must be assessed. During the musculoskeletal examination of an athlete who uses a wheelchair, evaluate the stability, flexibility, and strength of the commonly injured sites (e.g., shoulder, hand and wrist, and lower extremities) as well as the trunk.
- Special attention should be made during the PPA for skin breakdown on insensate pressure areas as well as sites that come in contact with orthotics/prosthetics. Also a careful history of heat/cold injuries and changes in neurologic function should be solicited.
- During the musculoskeletal examination of an individual who has had a *lower extremity* (LE) amputation, assess the stability, flexibility, and strength of the trunk, as well as the hip girdle and the unaffected and affected LE with or without the prosthesis.
- For individuals with *upper extremity* (UE) amputations, the stability, flexibility, and strength of the shoulder girdle must be assessed in the unaffected and affected extremity with and without prosthesis, in addition to a trunk and LE evaluation.
- For the athlete with brain injury, stroke, or *multiple sclerosis* (MS), it is prudent to assess the limitations of the unaffected and affected areas based on mobility and sports-specific tasks.
- Cardiovascular and pulmonary examinations can identify conditions that can cause cardiopulmonary collapse or disease progression. Suggested guidelines for cardiovascular screening of the athlete are available from the American Heart Association, American College of Cardiology, and American College of Sports Medicine.
- A PPE is performed upon entry into sports and should be repeated at least every 2–3 years. An interim examination prior to each sport season may be necessary if the athlete's health condition changes.

EPIDEMIOLOGY

- Injury patterns for disabled athletes are similar to those for athletes without disabilities; however, location of injuries appears to be disability and sport dependent. Lower extremity injures are more common in ambulatory athletes (visually impaired, amputee, cerebral palsy), whereas upper extremity injuries are more frequent in athletes who use a wheelchair (Ferrara and Peterson, 2000).
- A 3-year, cross-disability prospective study found the injury rate of disabled athletes to be 9.30/1000 athlete-exposures (Ferrara and Buckley, 1996). An injury rate less than what has been reported in college football (12.0–15.0/1000) and college soccer (9.8/1000), but higher than that reported in men's and women's college basketball (7.0/1000 and 7.3/1000 respectively) (Buckley and Powell, 1982; Buckley, 1982).
- A 6-year longitudinal study on reported injuries from disabled sports organizations, revealed illnesses (29.8%) were the most common, followed by muscular strains (22.1%), tendonitis (9.5%), sprains (5.8%), contusions (5.6%), and abrasions (5.1%). The body part most commonly injured was the thorax/spine

(13.3%), followed by the shoulder (12.8%), the lower leg/ankle and toes (12.0%), and the hip/thigh (7.4%) (Ferrara et al, 2000).

- Injury rates and patterns, as observed at the 1996 Paralympic summer games suggests a decreasing incidence of shoulder injuries, likely as a result of injury prevention strategies (Nyland et al, 2000).
- Wheelchair users are at a significant increased risk of upper extremity entrapment neuropathies, like carpal tunnel syndrome, with a reported prevalence rate of between 50 and 73%; however, it appears that wheelchair athletes have a lower prevalence than nonathletes (Boninger et al, 1996; Brunham and Steadward, 1994).
- With regards to winter sports, studies have shown that disabled athletes have a lower incidence of injuries than able-bodied skiers.

INJURIES AND COMPLICATIONS

MUSCULOSKELETAL

- Musculoskeletal injuries, especially those related to overuse are common in both able- and disabled-bodied athletes. Wheelchair athletes are at particular risk for shoulder, elbow, and wrist injuries given the repetitive use of their upper body as well as their altered body mechanics and posture. Since wheelchair athletes are dependent on wheelchair use during their daily activities, *relative rest* treatment presents a unique challenge in this population. Therefore prevention of these injuries is paramount.
- Shoulder injuries (Curtis and Black, 1999): Wheelchair athletes are at particular risk of rotator cuff injury especially if they participate in throwing, racquet sports, or basketball. Muscle imbalance, particularly involving weakness of the external rotators and scapular retractors (rhomboids, levator) plays a critical role in contributing to subacromial impingement syndromes.
- Elbow injuries: Medial and lateral epicondylitis are common elbow injuries in wheelchair athletes and should be treated similar to able-bodied athletes. Particular attention should be made to ensure proper throwing and racquet/golf swing mechanics to avoid reinjury. Repetitive falls are also frequent in team sports such as wheelchair basketball. Therefore the provider should have a high index of suspicion for fracture, traumatic arthritis, or olecronon bursitis.
- Wrist injuries: DeQervain's tenosynovitis, scapholunate dissociation instability, scaphoid fractures, capal instability, *triangular fibrocartilage complex* (TFCC) tears, and early osteoarthritis exist in both disabled- and able-bodied athletes.

NEUROLOGIC INJURIES (Groah and Lanig, 2000)

- Although wheelchair users have greater incidence of upper extremity entrapment neuropathies, there is no clear evidence that wheelchair athletes are at greater risk than wheelchair nonathletes.
- Carpal tunnel syndrome: Carpal tunnel syndrome (CTS) is the most common nerve injury, occurring in up to 67% of wheelchair users. The syndrome is caused by entrapment of the median nerve at the wrist. Symptoms typically involve numbness and parasthesias to the thumb through ring finger. Physical examination findings may include a positive Tinel sign at the wrist, a positive Phalen's test, and decreased sensation especially to two-point discrimination in the median nerve distribution. In severe cases thenar atrophy may be present. Confirmatory diagnosis is made by *electrodiagnostic testing* (EDX). This is also helpful to rule out other etiologies of parasthesias to include cervical radiculopathy, plexopathy, or diffuse polyneruopathy. Treatment includes decreasing the pressure, swelling, and inflammation within the carpal tunnel through relative rest, wrist splints set in a neutral position, *nonsteroidal anti-inflammatory drugs* (NSAIDs), and often steroid injection. If symptoms persist or worsen, surgical release is indicated.
- Ulnar neuropathy: This is the second most common upper extremity neuropathy and typically occurs at either the wrist (Guyon's canal) or elbow (Cubital tunnel syndrome). Both syndromes may present with small finger parasthesias and decreased sensation in the ulnar nerve distribution as well as weakness of the hand intrinsic muscles. Weakness may be elicited with a positive Froment's sign. Typically, however, with entrapment at Guyon's canal strength to the *abductor digiti minimi* (ADM), *flexor digitorum profundus* (FDP), and *flexor carpi ulnaris* (FCU) are spared as is the sensory distribution of the dorsal ulnar cutaneous nerve. Confirmatory diagnosis is made by EDX. X-rays or even *magnetic resonance imaging* (MRI) of the wrist or elbow may be warranted to rule out possible fracture or mass causing compression on the ulnar nerve. Treatment is similar to that of CTS, although for cubital tunnel syndrome, splinting or padding is applied to the elbow to decrease pressure to the nerve and avoid excessive elbow flexion especially at night while sleeping.
- Radial neuropathy: It occurs rarely in wheelchair users; however, should be considered in athletes who complain of elbow or forearm pain as well as those demonstrating weakness with finger and wrist extension. It should also be considered in individuals with chronic or refractory lateral epicondylitis. Entrapment

of the radial nerve typically occurs as it pierces the supinator muscle (Archade of Frohse).

- Neuroma: Neuroma formation may occur especially in the residual limb of amputees. Symptoms typically include sharp/lancinating pain during direct pressure on the neuroma. This may significantly impact on the athlete's ability to wear the prosthesis both during athletics as well as daily activities. The neuroma can often be visualized by MRI. Treatment should start with providing pressure relief, through prosthetic socket modification. Often a local injection with a combination of anesthetic and steroid is needed. In addition, *tricyclic antidepressants* (TCA) or anti-seizure medications may be helpful at diminishing the pain. Surgical excision is indicated for refractory cases.

SKIN INJURIES

- Wheelchair athletes are at particular risk for traumatic injuries to their hands and fingers from contact with the wheel, spokes, hand brakes, or the wheelchair of an opponent. In addition, chafing may occur to the inner aspect of the arm from contact with the wheel. Protection through the use of gloves or padded sleeves will reduce injuries.
- Multiple skin disorders may arise in the residual limb of an amputee, which are typically related to poor skin care or a poorly fitting prosthesis. Amputee athletes should be educated on the proper care of their limbs and be monitored closely during the initial phase of athletic activity with a new prosthesis.
- Athletes who wear prostheses are at risk for skin breakdown in areas in contact with the prosthesis. Strategies used to decrease risk include a proper prosthetic fit and an adequate suspension system, assessment for a silicone liner, adequate cushioning with socks and padding, and sports-specific biomechanics training with the prosthesis. Avoiding a moist skin environment also helps.
- Pressure sores are always a risk for insensate skin. Wheelchair athletes should perform daily skin checks and practice good pressure relief techniques (lifting off of their seat or weight shifting) throughout the day. Sports chairs may offer better maneuverability and aerodynamics, but often do so at the expense of pressure distribution, therefore wheelchair athletes should be especially cautious when using a new chair or starting a new sport.
- The most common areas at risk for pressure sores in wheelchair athletes include the sacrum and coccyx, ischial tuberosity, posterior knee, foot, and shoulder blade. Strategies used to decrease risk include methods to reduce friction forces (padding) and moist skin environments (moisture-wicking clothing).
- The following classifications (based on depth of involvement) are according to the National Pressure Ulcer Advisory Panel:
  a. Grade 1: Nonblanchable erythema
  b. Grade 2: Partial thickness breakdown through the epidermis
  c. Grade 3: Full thickness breakdown at the dermis into the subcutaneous tissue
  d. Grade 4: Deep tissue breakdown to the fascia, muscle, bone, or joint

MEDICAL ISSUES (Dec, Sparrow, and McKeag, 2000)

THERMOREGULATION (Price and Campbell, 1999; Armstrong et al, 1995)

- Individuals with neurologic impairments, especially spinal cord injuries, have impaired autonomic control of *heat generation* through shivering or *heat dissipation* through sweating, vascular redistribution, and vasodialation. Therefore they are at particular risk for thermal injuries.
- Proper clothing, hydration, and avoidance of activities during extreme temperatures are imperative for injury prevention. Athletes participating in cold whether sports should carefully inspect their digits frequently to avoid frostbite injury given their impaired sensation to recognize early symptoms. Early signs of heat injury may include erratic wheelchair propulsion. Local cooling strategies, such as ice to the axilla, groin, and neck are inadequate to properly reduce an athlete's core body temperature. Therefore cold water immersion is recommended for the treatment of hyperthemia with careful monitoring of core body temperature to avoid overcooling.
- Amputee athletes may experience excessive heat or sweating at the interface of their residual limb with their prosthetic socket. Care must be taken to avoid skin maceration, breakdown, and infection. Frequent socket or liner changing and residual limb care is imperative to avoid injury. Persistent problems may necessitate a change of socket or liner material.

AUTONOMIC DYSREFLEXIA (Pasquina, Houston, and Belandres, 1998)

- Athletes with *spinal cord injuries* (SCI) at or above the T6 level are at risk for autonomic dysreflexia, a condition typically resulting from a noxious stimulus below the level of the SCI injury causing a sympathetic reflex that perpetuates uncontrolled by the central nervous system. This can be a life-threatening condition.

- Common noxious stimuli, which may serve as triggers, include pressure sores, infections, heterotopic ossification (HO), tight clothing, soft tissue injuries, fractures, bladder distension, and constipation.
- Initial symptoms include facial flushing, headache, hypertension, sweating, tachycardia, and bradycardia. If left untreated the condition may lead to seizure or even death.
- Treatment should begin with sitting the patient upright, then finding and eliminating the cause of the noxious stimulus. Sublingual nifedipine, nitropaste, or other fast acting short duration hypotensive agents may be needed if the systolic blood pressure does not respond to initial management.
- Some athletes may try to use this condition to enhance their performance by increasing norepinepherine release and improving oxygen utilization. This is commonly referred to as "boosting" and is dangerous to the athlete's health.

HETEROTOPIC OSSIFICATION

- Individuals with traumatic brain, spinal cord, or burn injuries are at risk for developing HO typically in the soft tissue surrounding large joints or fractures.
- Typical symptoms include pain, warmth, and erythema.
- Diagnosis is made by bone scan early in the disease process and later by plain radiographs. Treatment includes NSAIDs, etidronate, or radiation. Surgical excision should only be considered once ossification has completed.

SPASTICITY

- Spasticity is an increase in resistance of muscle tone from an upper motor neuron injury.
- Spasticity can result in reduced mobility and ability to perform *activities of daily living* (ADL), and may lead to increased risk of pain, skin breakdown, and contractures.
- Multiples medications are currently available to help manage spasticity. They include baclofen, tizanidine, diazepam, dantrolene, clonidine, and botulinum toxin injections. All have side effects and therefore should be screened during the athletes PPA.
- Increases in spasticity may be the first indication of an underlying problem such as bowel or bladder distension, infection, pressure sore, fracture, HO, or other injury.

OSTEOPOROSIS

- Osteoporosis is a common occurrence in neurologically disabled athletes.
- Risk factors for osteoporosis include advanced age, female sex, thin body habitus, White race, immobility, decreased weight-bearing activities, paralysis, alcohol, tobacco, caffeine, and some medications.
- Wheelchair athletes are at increased risk for fracture after a fall. Practitioners should therefore have a lower threshold for obtaining radiographs on disabled athletes.
- Adequate padding is essential for wheelchair athletes, and all athletes should be taught proper fall techniques to prevent injury.
- Calcium and vitamin D supplementation are recommended for prevention. Bisphosphonates can be used when osteoporosis is documented.

DEEP VENOUS THROMBOSIS

- Venous stasis resulting from paralysis increases the risk of *deep venous thrombosis* (DVT). The risk is even greater during a period of hypovolemia or hypoviscosity as seen with blood doping or *erythropoietin* (EPO) use. DVT may lead to thrombophlebitis or pulmonary embolism.
- Symptoms of DVT may include lower extremity swelling, erythema, increased spasticity, or autonomic dysreflexia; however, signs and symptoms may be deceiving therefore the practitioner should always maintain a high index of suspicion. *Pulmonary embolism* (PE) may present as shortness of breath, chest pain, or even fever.
- Diagnosis is made by doppler ultrasound or venogram. Treatment includes anticoagulation medications.

SYNCOPE

- Syncope is the complete loss of consciousness and postural tone. The differential diagnoses include disorders divided into vascular, cardiac, neurologic, and miscellaneous categories.
- The most common etiology of syncope in the athlete is neurocardiogenic syncope (vasovagal or neurally mediated hypotension syncope).
- The differential diagnoses of syncope in athletes who are disabled include neurologic physical disability-related syncope or near-syncopal events, which may result from a number of conditions, including hypovolemia, orthostatic hypotension, seizure, *transient ischemic attacks* (TIAs), or stroke.

- Management involves prevention. Conservative measures such as local mechanical support (supportive pressure gradient stockings and abdominal binders when the patient is in an upright position) can be effective, but sometimes pharmacologic interventions, such as sodium chloride tablets or midodrine, are considered.

SPECIAL POPULATIONS AND SPECIFIC SPORT ADAPTATION

- Adapted sports are designed to depart as little as possible from the original versions. The following is an overview of each sport and its adaptations.
- Archery
  - Adaptive equipment is allowed, including the following:
    1. Trigger releases
    2. Wrist/elbow supports
    3. Standing supports
    4. Bow supports
- Basketball
  - Five players on a regulation court, following the rules of the NCAA. There can be special rules, such as no contact, no dribbling, and lower baskets.
- Bowling
  - Unmodified, except for the use of devices such as bowling sticks and prostheses. Special Olympics regulations allow target bowl (i.e., regulation pins, 2-lb ball, and short and carpeted lanes) and frame bowl (i.e., plastic pins, plastic ball, and short lane).
- Football
  - Rules vary from league to league.
- Hockey
  - Floor hockey is played in a gymnasium with a felt disc, struck with wooden hockey sticks, or fiberglass rods.
  - Sled hockey is played on an ice rink. Pics are used to propel the sleds as well as strike the puck.
- Racquetball
  - Racquetball follows the rules of the American Amateur Racquetball Association. In some divisions, multiple bounces are allowed.
- Skiing
  - Athletes with hemiplegia or amputees can use one ski and two outriggers or two skis and two outriggers. Sit-skis and monoskis are also available for participants with muscular dystrophy, spina bifida, paraplegia, and cerebral palsy.
- Soccer
  - Follows the rules of the U.S. Soccer Federation. The field size (usually 80 × 60 m) and the number of players (generally seven) are flexible, as goal size (for athletes with cerebral palsy).

- Swimming
  - Flotation devices can be used in competition in some divisions.
- Table tennis
  - U.S. Table Tennis Association regulations are used.
  - Often no distinction between disabled and able-bodied competition.
- Tennis
  - Wheelchair tennis is played on a regulation-sized tennis court by USTA rules, except two bounces are allowed.
- Track and field
  - Utilize same rules as able-bodied competitors.

CONTACT INFORMATION

- America's Athletes with Disabilities
  143 California Ave
  Uniondale, NY 11553
- American Wheelchair Bowling Association
  2912 Country Woods Lane
  Palm Harbor, FL 34683–6417
  727–734–0023
- American Wheelchair Table Tennis Association
  23 Parker St
  Port Chester, NY 10573
- Association of Disabled American Golfers
  7700 E Arapahoe Rd, Suite 350
  Englewood, CO 80112
- Disabled Sports – USA
  451 Hungerford Drive, Suite 100A
  Rockville, MD 20850A
  301–217–0960 http://www.dsusa.org
- International Wheelchair Basketball Federation
  1 Meadow Close
  Shavington, Crewe
  Cheshire CW2 5BE England
  011–44–127–066–8789
- International Wheelchair Tennis Federation
  Bank Lane, Roehampton
  London SW15 5XZ, England
  011–44–181–876–6464
- National Wheelchair Basketball Association
  710 Queensbury Loop
  Winter Garden, FL 34787
- National Wheelchair Tennis Association
  940 Calle Ananecer, Suite B
  San Clemente, CA 92672
- Special Olympics and Special Olympics International
  Kennedy Foundation
  1325 G Street, Suite 500
  Washington, DC 20005
- http://www.specialolympics.org

- U.S. Cerebral Palsy Athletic Association
  scpaa@mail.bbsnet.com
  http://www.uscpaa.org
- U.S. Olympic Committee/U.S. Paralympic Committee
  One Olympic Plaza
  Colorado Springs, CO 80909
  719–390–8900
- http://www.olympic.usa.org
- U.S. Tennis Association
  70 West Red Oak Lane
  White Plains, NY 10604
  914–696–7000
  www.usta.org
- Universal Wheelchair Football Association
  University of Cincinnati
  Raymond Walters College
  9555 Plainfield Rd
  Cincinnati, OH 45236–1096
- USA Deaf Sports Federation
  911 Tierra Linda Dr
  Frankfort, KY 40601–4633
  TTY 801–393–7916
- U.S. Association for Blind Athletes
  33 North Institute Street
  Brown Hall, Suite #015
  Colorado Springs, CO 80904
  719–630–0422
- http://www.usaba.org
- U.S. Disabled Ski Team
  PO Box 100
  Park City, UT 84060
  435–649–9090
  www.usaskiteam.org
- U.S. Wheelchair Swimming, Inc.
  c/o Wheelchair Sports, USA
  3595 E Fountain Blvd, Suite L-1
  Colorado Springs, CO 80910
  719–574–1150
- Wheelchair Sports USA
  3595 East Fountain Blvd, Suite L-1
  Colorado Springs, CO 80910
  719–574–1150
- http://www.wsusa.org
- Wheelchair Track and Field-USA
  2351 Parkwood Rd
  Snellville, GA 30039
  http://www.wsusa.org

REFERENCES

Armstrong LE, Maresh CM, Riebe D et al: Local cooling in wheelchair athletes during exercise-heat stress. *Med Sci Sports Exerc* 27(2):211, 1995.

Bergeron JW: Athletes with disabilities. *Phys Med Rehabil Clin N Am* 10(1):213, 1999.
Boninger ML, Robertson RN, Wolff M et al: Upper limb nerve entrapments in elite wheelchair racers. *Am J Phys Med Rehabil* 75:170, 1996.
Brunham RS, Steadward RD: Upper extremity peripheral nerve entrapments among wheelchair athletes: Prevalence, location, and risk factors. *Arch Phys Med Rehabil* 75:519, 1994.
Buckley WE: Five year overview of sport injuries: The NAIRS model. *J Phys Educ Rec Dance* 17:36, 1982.
Buckley WE, Powell JP: NAIRS: An epidemiological overview of the severity of injury in college football. *J Athl Train* 18:279, 1982.
Curtis KA, Black K: Shoulder pain in female wheelchair basketball players. *J Orhop Sports Phys Ther* 29(4):225, 1999.
Dec KL, Sparrow KJ, McKeag DB: The physically-challenged athlete medical issues and assessment. *Sorts Med* 29(4):245, 2000.
Ferrara MS, Buckley WE: Athletes with disabilities injury registry. *Adapt Phsy Act Q* 13:50, 1996.
Ferrara MS, Peterson CL: Injuries to athletes with disabilities: Identifying injury patterns. *Sports Med* 30(2):137, 2000.
Ferrara MS, Palutsis GR, Snouse S et al: A longitudinal study of injuries to athletes with disabilities. *Int J Sports Med* 21:22, 2000.
Groah SL, Lanig IS: Neuromusculoskeletal syndromes in wheelchair athletes. *Semin Neurol* 20(2):201, 2000.
Johnson RJ, McCray JC, Menconi et al: Secondary conditions following spinal cord injury in a population based sample. *Spinal Cord* 36:45, 1998.
Nyland J, Snouse SL, Anderson M et al: Soft tissue injuries to USA paralympians at the 1996 summer games. *Arch Phys Med Rehabil* 81:368, 2000.
Pasquina PF, Houston RM, Belandres PV: Beta blockade in the treatment of autonomic dysreflexia: A case report and review. *Arch Phys Med Rehabil* 79:582, 1998.
Price MJ, Campbell IG: Thermoregulatory and physiological response of wheelchair athletes to prolonged arm crank and wheelchair exercise. *Int J Sports Med* 20(7):457, 1999.
Weiss M, Beck J: Sport as part of therapy and rehabilitation of paraplegics. *Paraplegia* 11:166, 1973.
Wu SK, Williams T: Factors influencing sport participation among athletes with spinal cord injury. *Med Sci Sports Exerc* 33(2):177, 2001.

BIBLIOGRAPHY

Dexter, WW: *Disabled Athlete*. ACSM Team Physician course, San Antonio, TX, May 1999; Burnham R, Newell E, Steadward R: Sports medicine for the physically disabled: The Canadian team experience at the 1988 Seoul Paralympics Games. *Clin J Sports Med* 1(3):193–196, 1991.
Dummer G, Bazylewicz W, Bonnar K et al: Disabled sports. Michigan State University Department of Kinesiology Web site. Available at http://ed-web3.educ.msu.edu/kin/.
Ferrara MS, Davis RW: Injuries to elite wheelchair athletes. *Paraplegia* 28(5):335–341, June 1990.

Ferrara MS, Buckley WE, McCann BC: The injury experience of the competitive athlete with a disability: Prevention implications. *Med Sci Sports Exerc* 24(2):184–188, Feb. 1992.

Harris P: Self-induced autonomic dysreflexia ('boosting') practiced by some tetraplegic athletes to enhance their athletic performance. *Paraplegia* 32(5):289–291, May 1994.

Lai AM, Stanish WD, Stanish HI: The young athlete with physical challenges. *Clin Sports Med* 19(4):793–819, Oct. 2000.

Malanga G, Filart R: Athletes with disabilities. Emedicine article at emedicine@com, May 2002.

Myers A, Sickels T: Preparticipation sports examination. *Adolesc Med* 25(1):225–236, March 1998.

NCAA: *NCAA Sports Medicine Handbook*, 2002–2003.

Patel DP, Gerydanus DE: The pediatric athlete with disabilities. *Pediatr Clin North Am* 49(4), Aug. 2002.

Shepard RJ: Benefits of sport and physical activity for the disabled: Implications for the individual and for society. *Scand J Rehabil Med* 23(2):51–59, 1991.

Taylor D, Williams T: Sports injuries in athletes with disabilities: Wheelchair racing. *Paraplegia* 33:296–299, 1995.

Valliant PM, Bezzubyk I, Daley L: Psychological impact of sport on disabled athletes. *Psychol Rep* 56(3):923–929, June 1985.

Wheeler G, Cumming D, Burnham R: Testosterone, cortisol and catecholamine responses to exercise stress and autonomic dysreflexia in elite quadriplegic athletes. *Paraplegia* 32(5):292–299, May 1994.

101 THE ATHLETE WITH A TOTAL JOINT REPLACEMENT

Jennifer L Reed, MD

BACKGROUND

- Over 594,000 hip and knee replacement operations were performed in the United States in 2000 (American Academy of Orthopedic Surgeons, 2003).
- The prevalence of shoulder arthroplasty in 1998 was 15,266 with 8556 hemiarthroplasties and 6710 total shoulder athroplasties (Mendenhall, 2000).
- Pain remains the primary indication for joint replacement operations; however, disability and reduced function associated with a painful or stiff joint is increasingly seen as an appropriate indication for joint replacement.
- On average, a modern total joint replacement has a >90% chance of surviving 10 to 15 years (Diduch et al, 1997; Knutson et al, 1994).
- Dislocation, periprosthetic fracture, and implant breakage are possible, but uncommon, complications of athletic activity. More salient concerns include implant loosening from periarticular osteolysis and excessive joint bearing surface component wear.

- Athletic activity increases stress on implant fixation, and several studies have suggested that use and activity levels contribute to loosening rates associated with total joint arthroplasty (Schmalzried et al, 2000).
- Active, high-demand patients place arthroplasty implants at increased risk for loosening and wear.
- Patients under 60 years of age are 30% more active on average than patients 60 years of age or older (Zahiri et al, 1998).
- In the Swedish National Hip and Knee Arthroplasty Registers, 10-year revision rates among younger men were 3 to 4 times greater when compared to older patients (Knutson et al, 1994; Malchau, Herberts, and Ahnfelt, 1993).
- Published guidelines concerning activity after total joint arthroplasty discourage high levels of activity (Engh and Ing, 1999).
- Prospective, randomized studies on athletic activity after joint replacement and its effect on implant survivorship are not available (Healy, Iorio, and Lemos, 2001).
- Current recommendations are largely based on the opinions of orthopedic surgeons. Tables 101-1 to 101-3 represent activity recommendations compiled from surveys of the Hip, Knee, and American Shoulder and Elbow Societies conducted in 1999 (Healy, Iorio, and Lemos, 2001).
- A recently published review article by Kuster suggests that recommendations be made according to scientific knowledge including a biomechanical analysis of the joint loads during the sport in question (Kuster, 2002).
- Issues that should be taken into account for each patient and sporting activity include:

WEAR OF TOTAL JOINT REPLACEMENTS
- Up to 500,000 submicron-sized polyethylene particles are released with each step (Schmalzried and Callaghan, 1999). These small particles can activate macrophages that produce factors such as prostaglandins and interleukins thought to explain the progressive osteolysis and subsequent implant loosening.
- Another major long-term problem is polyethylene wear itself. The total volume of wear particles produced strongly depends on the number of steps, the load applied, and the roughness of the joint surfaces (Kuster and Stachowiak, 2002).
- Activity levels can vary tremendously from patient to patient. At least one study has shown that wear is clearly a function of use and not time (Schmalzried et al, 2000).

TABLE 101-1   Activity After Total Hip Arthroplasty—1999 Hip Society Survey

RECOMMENDED/ ALLOWED	ALLOWED WITH EXPERIENCE	NOT RECOMMENDED	NO CONCLUSION
Stationary bicycling	Low-impact aerobics	High-impact aerobics	Jazz dancing
Croquet	Road bicycling	Baseball/softball	Square dancing
Ballroom dancing	Bowling	Basketball	Fencing
Golf	Canoeing	Football	Ice skating
Horseshoes	Hiking	Gymnastics	Roller/inline skating
Shooting	Horseback riding	Handball	Rowing
Shuffleboard	Cross-country skiing	Hockey	Speed walking
Swimming	—	Jogging	Downhill skiing
Doubles tennis	—	Lacrosse	Stationary skiing*
Walking	—	Racquetball	Weight lifting
—	—	Squash	Weight machines
—	—	Rock climbing	—
—	—	Soccer	—
—	—	Singles tennis	—
—	—	Volleyball	—

* NordicTrack, Logan, Utah.

TABLE 101-2   Activity After Total Knee Arthroplasty—1999 Knee Society Survey

RECOMMENDED/ ALLOWED	ALLOWED WITH EXPERIENCE	NOT RECOMMENDED	NO CONCLUSION
Low-impact aerobics	Road bicycling	Racquetball	Fencing
Stationary bicycling	Canoeing	Squash	Roller blade/inline skating
Bowling	Hiking	Rock climbing	Downhill skiing
Golf	Rowing	Soccer	Weight lifting
Dancing	Cross-country skiing	Singles tennis	—
Horseback riding	Stationary skiing*	Volleyball	—
Croquet	Speed walking	Football	—
Walking	Tennis	Gymnastics	—
Swimming	Weight machines	Lacrosse	—
Shooting	Ice skating	Hockey	—
Shuffleboard	—	Basketball	—
Horseshoes	—	Jogging	—
—	—	Handball	—

*NordicTrack.

TABLE 101-3   Activity After Total Shoulder Arthroplasty—1999 American Shoulder and Elbow Society Survey

RECOMMENDED/ ALLOWED	ALLOWED WITH EXPERIENCE	NOT RECOMMENDED	NO CONCLUSION
Cross-country skiing	Golf	Football	High-impact aerobics
Stationary skiing*	Ice skating	Gymnastics	Baseball/softball
Speed walking and jogging	Shooting	Hockey	Fencing
Swimming	Downhill skiing	Rock climbing	Handball
Doubles tennis	—	—	Horseback riding
Low-impact aerobics	—	—	Lacrosse
Bicycling, road and stationary	—	—	Racquetball, squash
Bowling	—	—	Skating, roller/inline
Canoeing	—	—	Rowing
Croquet	—	—	Soccer
Shuffleboard	—	—	Tennis, singles
Horseshoes	—	—	Volleyball
Dancing: ballroom, square, and jazz	—	—	Weight training

*NordicTrack.

JOINT LOAD AND MOMENTS DURING SPORT ACTIVITIES

- Tables 101-4 and 101-5 summarize published data regarding hip and knee joint loads during various daily and athletic activities (Kuster, 2002).
- As a general guide, the following hip and knee joint loads can be assumed. During daily activities, loads of up to 3 to 4 × *body weight* (bw) occur, while during sporting activities loads of 5 to 10 × bw might occur.
- Cycling appears to be the most joint friendly with forces averaging between 1.2 and 1.5 × bw at the hip and knee (less than the forces experienced while walking).
- A key consideration for both walking and jogging: the hip and knee joint loads increase as speed increases. During fast running, the knee joint load can reach 10 × bw or more.
- For activities such as skiing, joint loads can vary significantly depending on style, terrain, and experience. Short turns, large moguls, and inexperience all translate into larger joint loads.

TABLE 101-4 Hip Joint Loads During Different Activities

ACTIVITY	HIP JOINT LOAD (X BW)
Standing on two legs	0.8
Standing on one leg	3.2
Straight leg raise	1.9
Walking at 1 km/h	2.9
Walking at 5 km/h	4.7
Jogging at 5 km/h	5.0
Jogging at 7 km/h	5.4
Stumbling	8.7
Cycling low resistance (40 W)	0.5
Cycling high resistance	1.4
Jogging at 12 km/h	6
Alpine skiing long turns, flat slope	4.5
Alpine skiing long turns, steep slope	6
Alpine skiing short turns, flat slope	5.5–6
Alpine skiing short turns, steep slope	7–8
Alpine skiing small moguls	8–9
Alpine skiing large moguls	10–15
Cross-country skiing classical	4–5
Cross-country skiing skating	4.5
Walking at natural speed	3.2–6.2
Stair ascent	3.4–6
Car entry	5–8
Car exit	4.5–8
Bath entry	4.6–6.6
Stair ascent	5
Stair descent	5.6
Ramp ascent	6.8
Ramp descent	6.5

ABBREVIATION: bw = bodyweight.
SOURCE: Adapted with permission from Kuster, 2002.

TABLE 101-5 Knee Joint Forces During Different Activities

ACTIVITY	KNEE JOINT LOAD (X BW)
Walking at 5.4 km/h	3.4–4
Walking	3.0
Walking at 5 km/h	2.8
Walking at 7 km/h	4.3
Walking	3.5
Cycling at 120 W	1.2
Stair ascent	4.3
Stair ascent	5.0
Stair descent	3.8
Stair descent	6
Ramp ascent	4.5
Ramp descent	4.5
Ramp descent at 5.4 km/h	7–8.5
Squat descent	5.6
Isokinetic knee extension	Up to 9
Jogging at 9 km/h	8–9
Jogging at 12.6 km/h	10.3
Running at 16 km/h	up to 14
Bowling on asphalt alleys	up to 12
Skiing medium steep slope	—
beginner	10
skilled skier	3.5

ABBREVIATION: bw = bodyweight.

RECREATION OR EXERCISE

- It is important to consider whether an activity will be performed for exercise or for recreation.
- In order to maintain cardiovascular fitness, the American College of Sports Medicine recommends aerobic exercise at least three times a week for 30 min or more.
- Joint wear shows a strong correlation to load. Therefore, the most prudent recommendation would be to engage in activities with lower joint loads, such as cycling, swimming, and walking, to maintaining cadiovascular fitness.
- Activities with high joint loads, such as running or tennis, should not be performed as regular endurance activities; however, if patients would like to resume certain high load activities for recreation, such as skiing 1 or 2 weeks a year or hiking on the weekends, this may be acceptable (Kuster, 2002).
- Even when engaging in high load sports recreationally, every effort should be made to reduce the joint forces as much as possible. For example, using ski poles while hiking down hill can reduce the load at the knees by as much as 20% (Schwameder et al, 1999).

EXPERIENCE AND PREOPERATIVE ACTIVITY LEVEL OF PATIENT

- The preoperative activity level is a strong predictor of sporting activities postoperatively.

- Patients who have achieved high levels of skill in athletics have the best chance of safely resuming these activities (Healy, Iorio, and Lemos, 2001).
- Preliminary evidence from Switzerland suggests that individuals not regularly active, out of practice, or inexperienced are at higher risk for sporting accidents (Economic benefits, 2001).
- Joint loads can be significantly increased for beginners compared with experienced individuals.

DIFFERENCES BETWEEN JOINT TYPES (I.E., THA VS. TKA)

- When considering appropriate sporting activities for total *knee* joint replacement patients—one must consider not only joint loads, but also the knee flexion angle of the peak load.
- In many total knee designs, the femoral and tibial components are conforming near extension and nonconforming in flexion (Kuster et al, 2000). Hence, delamination and polyethylene destruction can occur during activities like hiking or running where high joint loads occur between 40° and 60° of knee flexion (Kuster, 2002).
- It is prudent to be more conservative after *total knee arthoplasty* (TKA) than after *total hip arthoplasty* (THA) when considering activities with high joint loads in knee flexion.
- When considering athletic activity for *shoulder* arthroplasty patients, one must differentiate between the dominant and nondominant arm, especially in sports requiring throwing motions (Healy, Iorio, and Lemos, 2001).

SURGICAL FACTORS

- A comprehensive discussion of surgical factors is beyond the scope of this chapter; however, some important factors to consider include: (1) the importance of an anatomically and biomechanically accurate joint reconstruction with a well-designed implant and a properly balanced soft tissue or muscular envelope; (2) the surgical approach (for example, lateral versus posterolateral for THA); (3) fixation (cemented versus uncemented); and (4) component selection materials (ceramic versus polyethylene articular surface).

CONCLUSIONS

- In the absence of prospective randomized controlled trials, physicians have a duty to use the currently available scientific knowledge to educate their patients regarding the risks and benefits of individual athletic activities following joint replacement.

- Patients should not be discouraged from participating in reasonable athletic activity when they prepare and train for the activity, and when they understand the risks.
- Ultimately, whether to engage in a particular sporting activity after total joint replacement is up to each individual patient. Patient must make the final decision.

REFERENCES

American Academy of Orthopedic Surgeons: *Arthroplasty and Total Joint Replacement Procedures*. United States 1991–2000; AAOS on-line Service. http://www.aaos.org/wordhtml/research/stats/arthropl.htm. Accessed April 01, 2003.

Diduch DR, Insall JN, Scott WN et al: Total knee replacement in young, active patients: long-term follow-up and functional outcome. *J Bone Joint Surg Am* 79(4):575–582, 1997.

Economic benefits of the health-enhancing effects of physical activity: First estimates for Switzerland [position statement]. *Sportzmedizin Sportraumatol* 49(3):131–133, 2001.

Engh EA, Ing CA: Activity after replacement of the hip, knee or shoulder. *Orthopedics* (Special Edition) 5:61–65, 1999.

Healy WL, Iorio R, Lemos MJ: Athletic activity after joint replacement. *Am J Sports Med* 29(3):377–388, 2001.

Knutson K, Lewold S, Robertson O et al: The Swedish knee arthroplasty register: A nation-wide study of 30,003 knees 1976–1992. *Acta Orthop Scand* 65(4):375–386, 1994.

Kuster MS: Exercise recommendations after total joint replacement: A review of the current literature and proposal of scientifically based guidelines. *Sports Med* 32(7):433–445, 2002.

Kuster MS, Stachowiak GW: Factors affecting polyethylene wear in total knee replacement. *Orthopedics* 25(2 Suppl.):S235–S242, 2002.

Kuster MS, Horz S, Spalinger E et al: The effects of conformity and load in total knee replacement. *Clin Orthop* 375:302–312, 2000.

Malchau H, Herberts P, Ahnfelt L: Prognosis of total hip replacement in Sweden: Follow-up of 92,675 operations performed 1978–1990. *Acta Orthop Scand* 64(5):497–506, 1993.

Mendenhall S: Editorial. *Orthopedic Network News* 11(January): 7, 2000.

Schmalzried TP, Callaghan JJ: Wear in total hip and knee replacements. *J Bone Joint Surg Am* 81(1):115–136, 1999.

Schmalzried TP, Shepherd EF, Dorey FJ et al: Wear is a function of use, not time. *Clin Orthop* 381:36–46, 2000.

Schwameder H, Roithner R, Muller E et al: Knee joint forces during downhill walking with hiking poles. *J Sports Sci* 17 (12):969–978, 1999.

Zahiri CA, Schmalzried TP, Szuszczewicz ES et al: Assessing activity in joint replacement patients. *J Arthroplasty* 13:890–895, 1998.

102 CANCER AND THE ATHLETE

Brian Whirrett, MD
Kim Harmon, MD

INTRODUCTION

- Cancer in athletes is a topic that has not received much attention from the sports medicine community. With increasing media coverage of elite athletes and their battles with cancer, this topic has become increasingly relevant to physicians and their patients. Athletes such as Lance Armstrong, Andres Galarraga, and Scott Hamilton have brought hope to those battling cancer and have inspired many to return to physical activity and even elite competition.
- Because of increased numbers of participants in physical activity it is more likely that the physician will encounter active people and athletes who also have neoplastic disease.
- The sports medicine physician needs to be aware of the following:
  - Keys to the early diagnosis of cancer in active people
  - Malignancies that present with musculoskeletal symptoms
  - Exercise prescription
  - The effects of exercise on immune function
  - The benefits of exercise in cancer patients
  - The value of exercise for the prevention of cancer

PREPARTICIPATION EXAMINATIONS

- Keep in mind potential red flags suggesting neoplasm.
- A history of night sweats, fatigue, unintentional weight loss, decreasing performance, treatment resistant pain, and recurrent infections suggest the need for further investigation.
- Social history should be reviewed. Tobacco abuse can lead to lung or mouth cancers. Environmental exposure to chemicals or excessive *ultraviolet* (UV) light should prompt a screen for skin or other malignancies. Use of anabolic steroids increases the risk of hepatoma.
- A family history of malignancy is important, particularly in cancers that have a strong genetic link.
- The physical examination should include a skin examination to exclude melanoma or other skin cancers. Adenopathy, particularly if a mass is enlarging, nontender and fixed, suggests lymphoma or metastatic

disease. Excessive ecchymoses can represent leukemia. Conjunctival pallor from anemia can be present with neoplasm that infiltrates the bone marrow, or from occult blood loss in *gastrointestinal* (GI) malignancies. Testicular cancer frequently presents as testicular mass or swelling. The abdomen should be examined for masses and hepatomegaly.

MALIGNANCY MASQUERADING AS MUSCULOSKELETAL PAIN

- There are many medical illnesses that can present as musculoskeletal pain. Cancer is no exception and is the diagnosis that should remain in the differential.
- Warning signs that musculoskeletal pain may represent a malignancy include musculoskeletal pain unrelieved by rest, unrelenting pain, night pain, or pain that does not improve despite appropriate therapy over a 4–6-week period.
- Cancers that commonly present as musculoskeletal pain (Contran):
  - Primary osteosarcoma typically occurs in young persons under the age of 20 with a male predominance. Sixty percent of osteosarcomas arise in the knee and should remain in the differential when examining nontraumatic knee pain. Fifteen percent of osteosarcomas arise in the hip or pelvis and 10% in the shoulder. The presenting complaint of patients is typically pain, swelling, and tenderness.
  - Chondrosarcoma comprises 20% of all malignant bone tumors. It usually presents in the third decade or beyond as an ill-defined pain and mass. The hip, pelvis, femoral diaphysis, ribs, and proximal humerus are the most common sites.
  - Ewing's sarcoma is a neoplasm that afflicts the young. It is rare past second or third decade of life with a 2:1 male predominance. It commonly presents as pain, swelling, and tenderness of the affected part, dilated veins, elevated temperature, and sedimentation rate. It shares many of the same symptoms and signs of osteomyelitis and can be easily confused. X-ray changes may be only a small focus of ill-defined lucency initially, but eventually will progress to a large area of bony lysis. *Onion-skin layering* of bone is the classic appearance on X-ray and is created by subperiosteal new bone formation.
  - Most giant cell tumors occur between 20 and 40 years of age with a slight female predominance. The usual presentation is nonspecific local pain, tenderness, and functional disability. These tumors may grow large enough to produce an externally palpable mass. On X-ray a large, lytic *soap-bubble* lesion is seen.

- Ninety percent of rhabdomyosarcomas occur before the age of 20 and usually present as an enlarging mass.
- Multiple myeloma needs to remain in the differential in anyone presenting with back pain, particularly if they are over 50. It can also present as chest pain. The pain usually does not occur at night. It is induced by movement it is easily confused with mechanical back pain. Diagnosis is made by the presence of Bence-Jones protein in the urine.

EXERCISE PRESCRIPTION

- No specific guidelines exist for exercise prescription in patients with cancer. The approach to starting an exercise regimen should be multidisciplinary, involving physicians, physical therapists, nutritionists, and other local rehabilitation resources. Each program must be designed individually, based on clinical status, complications, and risk factors for exercise.
- Patients undergoing chemotherapy, radiation, and hormone therapy for cancer have very different complications (Table 102-1). Side effects of the agents used in treatment should be understood before a patient is given clearance for exercise.
  - Cancer treatment may cause osteoporosis and bony metastasis may weaken bone leading to a higher risk for pathologic fracture. In patients with osteoporosis, vigorous, open-chained activity should be avoided. Instead, alternatives such as biking, swimming, water aerobics, or stair climber should be considered. Bone-density testing is helpful in guiding

TABLE 102-1   Common Side Effects of Chemotherapy/Radiation

Dehydration
Catabolic state
Electrolyte imbalance
Anemia
Thrombocytopenia
Secondary malignancy
Cardiomyopathy
Arrhythmia
Congestive heart failure
Coronary artery vasospasm
Pulmonary fibrosis
Diarrhea/vomiting
Immunosuppression
Osteoporosis
Radiation necrosis (CNS, GI tract, Respiratory)
Neuropathy

ABBREVIATION: CNS = central nervous system; GI tract = gastrointestinal tract.

exercise choice. Bisphosphonates should be considered in osteoporotic patients.
- Fatigue is a common side effect of both cancer and its treatment. A search for other etiologies such as anemia, secondary malignancy, electrolyte imbalance, dehydration, and improper nutrition (catabolic state) should be undertaken and corrected if possible. Exercise has many positive effects in patients receiving chemotherapy. A low to moderate intensity aerobic exercise regimen can reduce fatigue associated with chemotherapy. Schwartz et al. enrolled 72 newly diagnosed patients with breast cancer and recorded daily levels of fatigue as they followed a moderate intensity exercise regimen. Results showed a significantly reduced fatigue level and improved functional ability over an 8-week exercise program (Schwartz et al, 2001).
- Cardiac complications may be a side effect of some chemotherapeutic agents, particularly the anthracyclines. These put patients at high risk for cardiac arrhythmia, cardiomyopahty, heart failure, and coronary vasospasm. Exercise stress testing may need to be performed prior to any exercise prescription in this subset of patients.

EXERCISE AND IMMUNE FUNCTION

- Macrophages, natural killer cells, and polymorphonuclear neutrophils are the first line of defense against cancer. It is unclear what effects exercise can have on the function of these cells. The "inverted-U" hypothesis suggests there is an optimal level of physical activity that results in enhanced immune function and protection from the development of cancer. The two ends of the "U" represent sedentary people on the one end and those who engage in chronic, intense, and exhaustive exercise on the other end. Both of these groups may have an increased susceptibility to cancer compared to moderately physically active persons (Woods et al, 1999).
- Studies examining the effect of immune function during cancer treatment have mixed results.
  - In a study examining children with acute lymphocytic leukemia, there were nonsignificant decreases in T-cells (Shore and Shepard, 1999).
  - Another study looking at participation in an exercise program after peripheral blood stem cell transplantation found that exercise did not facilitate or delay immune cell recovery (Hayes et al, 2003).
- Three of four studies measuring immune function status in cancer survivors reported significant improvements in immune function status as a result of exercise (Fairey et al, 2002).

BENEFITS OF EXERCISE IN THE CANCER PATIENT

- There are many proven benefits of exercise in the cancer patient. Aerobic exercise can improve quality of life and psychologic health in cancer patients undergoing treatment (Mock et al, 2001; Dimeo et al, 1999) and in cancer survivors (Burnham and Wilcox, 2002; Courneya et al, 2003).
- Exercise has been shown to reduce fatigue in cancer patients and can be prescribed as primary therapy. (Dimeo, Rumberger, and Keul, 1998; Dimeo et al, 1999; Mock et al, 2001; Scwartz et al, 2001)
- Exercise has been well-studied in the patient with prostate cancer.
  - In addition to prostatectomy and radiation therapy, many men are placed on antiandrogen therapy, which can reduce bone density, reduce lean muscle mass, and cause fatigue. Resistance exercise in men undergoing androgen deprivation can reduce fatigue, and improve quality of life and overall muscular fitness (Segal et al, 2003).
  - There is debate about the effect of exercise on *prostate-specific antigen* (PSA) levels (Kratz et al, 2003; Leventhal et al, 1993; Oremek and Seiffert, 1996). A set of guidelines from the U.K. Department of Health recommends that PSA testing not be performed for 48 h after vigorous exercise to avoid confusion or misinterpretation (Weston and Parr, 2003).

EXERCISE FOR PREVENTION OF CANCER

- While treatment of the athlete with cancer may prove to be more challenging, the prevention of cancer should be where physicians are focusing their attention. There are nearly 170 observational epidemiologic studies of physical activity and cancer risk (Friedenreich and Orenstein, 2002). Exercise is frequently used as a modifier of coronary artery disease risk, and the same advice should be applied for the prevention of certain cancer.
- Exercise can be safely advised for most patients given its large benefit and relatively low risk. While exercise can be safely prescribed, not every form of cancer has had a proven preventive benefit from exercise (Byers et al, 2002). There is insufficient data to support exercise as a preventative mechanism in lung, testicular, ovarian, kidney, pancreatic, thyroid, and melanoma. Studies are difficult to interpret because

of confounding variables such as smoking status and lifestyle.

- The American Cancer Society 2001 guidelines (Byers et al, 2002) compiled evidence in support of various risk factors and potential modifiable lifestyle issues in prevention of cancer.
- Colon cancer
  - There was convincing evidence that regular, moderate to vigorous physical activity helped prevent colon cancer. There have been 51 studies conducted with 43 reporting a positive result. The risk reduction averaged 40–50% and up 70% reductions were found with the highest activity levels. The effect did not appear to be compounded by other risk factors for cancer such as dietary intake or body mass index (Friedenreich and Orenstein, 2002; McTeirnan et al, 1998).
  - Exercise may decrease colon cancer rates because of decreased gastrointestinal transit times that decrease mucosal exposure to carcinogens. Exercise may also increase the level of prostaglandin F, which inhibits colonic cell proliferation. It is also hypothesized that bile acids secretion may be lower in physically active persons and confer a protective effect.
- Breast cancer
  - There is also convincing evidence that breast cancer risk can be reduced with regular exercise. Thirty-two of 44 studies have shown positive effects of exercise on cancer prevention. The inconsistent outcomes in breast cancer may be related to differences in the etiology of breast cancer among different subgroups (Friedenreich and Orenstein, 2002; McTeirnan et al, 1998).
  - Physical activity may lower levels of biologically available sex hormones. A decreased lifetime exposure to estrogen may mitigate breast cancer risk. Physical activity affects ovarian estrogen production, increases sex hormone-binding globulin, and may decrease body fat secondarily decreasing fat-produced estrogen.
  - A recent investigation (Dorn et al, 2003) studied physical activity and breast cancer risk in pre- and postmenopausal women. Their results indicate a protective effect on both pre- and postmenopausal women who performed strenuous physical activity. This effect was seen in women who exercised 3.5 h or more per week on average. An even stronger protective effect was noted in those women who reported that level of activity 20 years prior to the investigation. Risk of cancer was reduced by almost 50%.
- Endometrial cancer
  - Nine of 13 studies found a decrease in the risk of endometrial cancer with physical activity. Some

evidence suggests higher intensities confer a greater level of protection (Friedenreich and Orenstein, 2002).

- Many risk factors are similar for both breast and endometrial cancer. Decreased risk of endometrial cancer most likely stems from the same estrogen decreasing effects of exercise on estrogen.
- Prostate cancer
  - The evidence for an association between physical activity and prostate cancer is less convincing than for breast and colon cancer and is classified as probable. Fifteen or 30 studies have found a reduction in physically active men regarding prostate cancer. It may be that activity done at an early age may be more protective than exercise later in life, but most studies have been performed on older men (Friedenreich and Orenstein, 2002).
  - Lower levels of free testosterone occur with exercise-induced increases in sex-hormone binding globulin.
- One way physical activity may prevent cancer is through weight control. There are several biological mechanisms associated with excess weight, particularly abdominal adiposity that could contribute to cancer. Reduced weight and increased physical activity are associated, but each appears to confer an independent benefit in cancer reduction (Friedenreich and Orenstein, 2002).
- Moderate to vigorous activity should be performed at least 45 min most days of the week to achieve maximum preventive effect for colon and breast cancer. According to the American College of Surgeons (ACS) guidelines, moderate activities are defined as a brisk walk. Vigorous activities are those that use larger muscle groups, cause sweating, and increase pulse and respirations (Byers et al, 2002).

REFERENCES

Burnham TR, Wilcox A: Effects of exercise on physiological and psychological variables in cancer survivors. *Med Sci Sports Exerc* 34(12):1863–1867, 2002.

Byers T, Nestle M, McTiernan A et al: American Cancer Society guidelines on nutrition and physical activity for cancer prevention: Reducing the risk of cancer with healthy food choices and physical activity. *CA Cancer J Clin* 52:115, 2002.

Contran: *Robbins Pathologic Basis of Disease*, 6th ed. Philadelphia, PA, Saunders, 1999.

Courneya KS, Mackey JR, Bell GJ et al: Randomized controlled trial of exercise training in postmenopausal breast cancer survivors: Cardiopulmonary and quality of life outcomes. *J Clin Oncol* 21(9):1660–1668, 2003.

Dimeo F, Rumberger BG, Keul J: Aerobic exercise as therapy for cancer fatigue. *Med Sci Sports Exerc* 30(4):475–478, 1998.

Dimeo F, Fetscher S, Lange W et al: Effects of aerobic exercise on the physical performance and incidence of treatment-related complications after high-dose chemotherapy. *Blood* 90():3390–3394, 1997.

Dimeo FC, Stieglitz RD, Novelli-Fischer U et al: Effects of physical activity on the fatigue and psychological status of cancer patients during chemotherapy. *Cancer* 85(10):2273–2277, 1999.

Dorn J, Vena J, Brasure J et al: Lifetime physical activity and breast cancer risk in pre- and postmenopausal women. *Med Sci Sports Exerc* 35(2):278–285, 2003.

Fairey AS, Courneya KS, Field CJ et al: Physical exercise and immune system function in cancer survivors. *Cancer* 94(2):539–551, 2002.

Friedenreich CM, Orenstein MR: Physical activity and cancer prevention: Etiologic evidence and biologic mechanism. *J Nutr* 132:3456S–3464S, 2002.

Hayes SC, Rowbottom D, Davies PS et al: Immunological changes after cancer treatment and participation in an exercise program. *Med Sci Sports Exerc* 35(1):2–9, 2003.

Kratz A, Lewandrowski KB, Siegel AJ et al: Effect of marathon running on total and free serum prostate-specific antigen concentrations. *Arch Pathol Lab Med* 127(3):345–348, 2003.

Leventhal EK, Rozanski TA, Morey AF et al: The effects of exercise and activity on serum prostate specific antigen levels. *J Urol* 150(3):893–894, 1993.

McTiernan A, Ulrich C, Slate S et al: Physical activity and cancer etiology: Associations and mechanisms. *Cancer Causes Control* 9:487–509, 1998.

Mock V, Pickett M, Ropka ME et al: Fatigue and quality of life outcomes of exercise during cancer treatment. *Cancer Pract* 9(3):119–127, 2001.

Oremek GM, Seiffert UB: Physical activity releases prostate-specific antigen from the prostate gland into blood and increases serum PSA concentrations. *Clin Chem* 42(5):691–695, 1996.

Scwartz AL, Mori M, Gao R et al: Exercise reduces daily fatigue in women with breast cancer receiving chemotherapy. *Med Sci Sports Exerc* 33(5):718–723, May 2001.

Segal RJ, Reid RD, Courneya KS et al: Resistance exercise in men receiving androgen deprivation therapy for prostate cancer. *J Clin Oncol* 21(9):1653–1659, 2003.

Shore S, Shepard RJ: Immune responses to exercise in children treated for cancer. *J Sports Med Phys Fitness* 39(3):240–243, 1999.

Weston R, Parr N: New NHS guidelines for PSA testing in primary care. *Lancet* 361:89–90, 2003.

Woods JA, David JM, Smith JA et al: Exercise and cellular innate immune function. *Med Sci Sports Exer* 31(1):57–66, 1999.

103 THE ATHLETE WITH HIV

Robert J Dimeff, MD
Andrew M Blecher

EPIDEMIOLOGY

WORLDWIDE

- According to the *centers for disease control* (CDC), there were 42 million people with *human immunodeficiency virus* (HIV)/*acquired immunodeficiency* (AIDS) through December 2002.
- Last year there were 5 million new cases of HIV/AIDS and 3.1 million AIDS deaths.

THE UNITED STATES

- According to the CDC there were 816,149 HIV/AIDS patients in the United States through December 2001.

IN ATHLETES

- The incidence and prevalence of HIV/AIDS in athletes is unknown, but there are several high profile elite and professional athletes who have acquired HIV including Earvin "Magic" Johnson in 1991 (competed in NBA and 1992 Summer Olympics with HIV), Greg Louganis (competed in 1988 Olympics with HIV), and Tommy Morrison (professional boxing).
- In addition, several professional athletes have died from AIDS, including Jerry Smith (National Football League or NFL), Alan Wiggins (Major League Baseball), Esteban DeJesus (boxing), Tim Richmond (stock car driver), Robert McCall (figure skating), and Arthur Ashe (professional tennis player, Wimbledon, and U.S. Open Champion).
- Fears of the widespread dissemination of HIV throughout professional sports have been fueled by such reports as in 1991 when two Canadian physicians announced a woman who died of AIDS had disclosed that she had sexual intercourse with 30–70 different hockey players in the National Hockey League (NHL) (Johnston, 1994).
- In intercollegiate athletics, a survey of National Collegiate Athletic Association (NCAA) institutions concerning HIV/AIDS policies was conducted almost one decade ago. Eight institutions reported they had known HIV positive athletes in their institutions that

had not been diagnosed with AIDS. These athletes were still participating in sports at three of those institutions. Four institutions reported athletes with AIDS. One of those was still participating in intercollegiate athletics (McGrew et al, 1993).

PATHOPHYSIOLOGY

DEFINITION

- HIV is a human retrovirus, which targets and infects CD4+ T helper cells. It replicates within the CD4 cells and causes cell death.
- AIDS is a chronic illness with an average natural history of >10 years. It is the result of a progressively immunocompromised state due to quantitative and functional defects in CD4+ T helper cells. The decline in CD4 cells results in decreased function of the immune system and the development of opportunistic infections and certain malignancies (Eichner and Calabrese, 1994).

NATURAL HISTORY OF DISEASE

- Following the initial exposure to HIV, the individual may develop an acute and self-limited viral-like syndrome, or seroconversion may occur silently without symptoms.
- Following infection and seroconversion is a period of clinical latency that may last a decade or more. During this time the infected person has normal performance and exercise function.
- As the infection progresses and the immune system becomes compromised, the individual may develop symptoms such as fevers, lymphadenopathy, fatigue, and weight loss.
- An AIDS defining illness occurs as the immune system continues to decline and the infected individual becomes susceptible to opportunistic infections ranging from mild candidiasis to life-threatening *pneumocystis carinii pneumonia* (PCP). Malignancies such as lymphoma may also arise. Muscle wasting also occurs through mechanisms that are not completely understood (Eichner and Calabrese, 1994).

TRANSMISSION

- The virus is found in all body fluids including blood, semen, vaginal and cervical secretions, breast milk, and amniotic fluid. The highest concentration is in the *cerebrospinal fluid* (CSF). It is also found in low concentrations in tears, sputum, saliva, and urine but it is not considered to be highly infectious in these forms unless they are blood tinged. No HIV has been found in sweat (LeBlanc, 1993).

- Primary routes of transmission include intimate sexual contact; parenteral exposure to blood, blood products, or blood containing body fluids; and materno-fetal transmission.
- HIV is not transmissible through casual contact, swimming pools, mosquitoes, saliva, sweat, tears, urine, feces, and inanimate objects (i.e., wrestling mats, toilet seats, and sinks) (Dorman, 2000).

DIAGNOSIS

SCREENING TESTS

- HIV antibodies are low or absent in the first few weeks of infection. They may not be produced until 6 weeks after infection and in some instances may not be detectable until up to 6 months after infection. This is referred to as the "window period." Therefore, antibody testing following possible exposure is recommended at 6 weeks, 3 months, 6 months, and 1 year.
- The most commonly used screening test is the *enzyme-linked immunosorbant assay* (ELISA). This test can identify HIV antibodies in the blood with a sensitivity of up to 99.5% (ELISA tests have also been developed to identify HIV antibodies in saliva or urine). The specificity of the ELISA test, however, is lower and may lead to false positive results. Therefore, a positive ELISA must be confirmed with further testing.
- In standard laboratories, if the ELISA test is positive it is automatically repeated. Two positive ELISA tests are routinely then confirmed by the Western Blot test, which identifies antibodies to proteins of a specific molecular weight. It is only after these confirmatory tests are positive that an HIV antibody test should be reported as being a positive test.

FOLLOW-UP TESTING

- The viral load test is performed via *polymerase chain reaction* (PCR) or *branched DNA* (bDNA) testing and can detect the HIV virus in the blood. Some viral load tests are sensitive enough to detect as few as five or less copies of HIV in the blood.
- Although it can be used for diagnostic purposes in some instances, the viral load test is commonly used in the known HIV positive patient to help assess prognosis and help manage therapy. It is usually suggested

that a baseline measurement be obtained and then the test be rechecked within 2–8 weeks of initiating or changing treatment. It can then be followed every 3–4 months.

- Viral genotype and phenotypic resistance assays can also help guide specific antiretroviral therapy.
- T-cell tests can identify the CD4 count and the CD4:CD8 ratio in the blood. This information can be used to assist with managing treatment and initiating prophylaxis therapy for opportunistic infections.

ATHLETE SPECIFIC CONCERNS

EFFECTS OF HIV ON THE ATHLETE

EXERCISE AND THE IMMUNE RESPONSE IN HEALTHY ATHLETES

- According to the theory of psychoneuroimmunology, any stress may be capable of altering immune function. Exercise is one such stress.
- Immunologic changes with exercise include *white blood cell* (WBC) increases with brisk exercise, which may even occur with heavy exertion of only 30 s. *Polymorphonuclear neutrophils* (PMNs), monocytes, lymphocytes, and natural killer cells also increase. This increase is caused by increased cardiac output; displacement of WBCs from reserve pools in the lung, liver, and spleen; and an increase in epinephrine, which evokes granulocytosis and lymphocytosis. The function of natural killer cells may also increase as a result of the release of cytokines during exercise. This response falls off if a person becomes accustomed to an exercise bout, suggesting that the response is the result of stress and not the inherent effects of exercise itself.
- The lymphocytosis of exercise is brief and after exercise the lymphocyte count will fall within 5 min. A further delayed fall to below baseline occurs over the next hour due to the effects of cortisol, which after exercise is no longer opposed by epinephrine. Counts return to baseline within 24 h.
- Conversely, a leukocytosis and delayed rise in PMNs is mediated by cortisol, which releases PMNs from bone marrow. This returns to baseline in about 24 h. Strenuous exercise may also evoke an acute phase reactant response and activate complement, and release tumor necrosis factor, interferons, interleukins, and other cytokines (Eichner and Calabrese, 1994).
- Chronic exercise can have a negative effect on immune function if there are prolonged periods of intense training. *Natural killer* (NK) cell count and leukocyte function has been shown to decline in swimmers and runners during periods of intense training. Overtraining

is also associated with a possible increase in upper respiratory tract infections (Mackinnon, 2000).

EXERCISE AND THE IMMUNE RESPONSE IN HIV POSITIVE ATHLETES

- There is a definite link between moderate exercise and a strengthened immune response in HIV positive subjects. Increases in CD4 levels caused by aerobic exercise have been shown in asymptomatic patients with HIV. Exercise has also been shown to lower anxiety and tension levels in HIV positive individuals (LaPerriere et al, 1991). Evidence also indicates that even individuals with advanced HIV infection (AIDS-related symptoms or AIDS-defining opportunistic infections) respond to an exercise regimen with increased CD4 counts and an increased CD4:CD8 ratio (Eichner and Calabrese, 1994).
- However, with intense exercise, HIV-infected subjects may have an impaired ability to mobilize neutrophils and natural killer cells. This has been shown in response to 1 h of exercise at 75% VO_{2max} (Ullum et al, 1994).
- Weight training may enhance muscle strength, bulk, and function in HIV+ individuals. It may therefore mitigate AIDS-related muscle wasting (Feller and Flanigan, 1997).
- Nonimmunologic effects of HIV on the athlete include—cardiac effects (a decreased VO_{2max} due to deconditioning, which may be reversible with aerobic training), pulmonary effects (certain infectious diseases like PCP may have restrictive ventilatory effects), hematologic effects (anemia may be a primary manifestation of HIV disease or may be a side effect of antiretroviral therapy and could cause a reduction in maximal oxygen uptake and lower the lactic acidosis threshold impairing physical performance), and muscular effects (some retrovirals may induce mitochondrial myopathies or severe resting lactic acidosis) (Stringer, 2000).
- Exercise recommendations for HIV positive athletes: Moderate exercise may be beneficial both physically and psychologically, but strenuous exercise may be detrimental (Feller and Flanigan, 1997). Additionally, although the exercise demands of high-level and professional athletics may be safe and beneficial, the possible detrimental effects of psychologic stress must be assessed on an individual basis (Eichner and Calabrese, 1994).
- Exercise is safe and beneficial for the HIV-infected person. HIV-infected individuals should begin exercising while healthy, and attempt to maintain their exercise program through the course of their illness. HIV-infected persons can use exercise to help manage their illness and improve their quality of life.

- For healthy, asymptomatic HIV positive individuals, unrestricted exercise is acceptable. Avoidance of overtraining should be emphasized. Stress related to competition should be minimized. Moderate exercise (40–60% VO_{2max}) or heavy aerobic exercise (60–80% VO_{2max}) can be recommended depending on patient preference and motivation. An exercise program prescription should be 1h/day, 3×/week, for 6–12 weeks.
- For individuals with advanced HIV infection with mild to moderate symptoms or lower CD4 counts (<200), competition, restrictive training schedules, and exhaustive exercise should be avoided. Physical activity and moderate exercise training should be encouraged under close supervision.
- Athletes with frank AIDS may remain active on a symptom-related basis but should avoid strenuous exercise and reduce or stop training during acute illness.
- Caveats: A complete physical examination should be undergone to assess the overall health and status of HIV infection before beginning an exercise program. Cardiopulmonary exercise testing with gas exchange measurements (to exclude subtle cardiopulmonary markers of occult infection, anemia, myopathies, and the like) should be performed before determining an exercise prescription, especially in patients with low CD4 counts or high viral loads (Eichner and Calabrese, 1994; Stringer, 2000).

TREATMENT

- Treatment goals should include attempts to—suppress viral replication, suppress evolution of resistant strains, increase CD4 cell counts, prevent disease progression, improve energy levels, decrease weight loss, promote weight gain, and preserve quality of life and prolong survival.
- Antiretroviral medications: Include nucleoside *reverse transcriptase inhibitors* (RTIs), *nonnucleoside reverse transcriptase inhibitors* (NTRIs), and *protease inhibitors* (PIs).
- Recommendations on treatment regimens are constantly changing as a result of finding the correct balance between optimizing the patient's immunologic/virologic outcome versus reducing the toxicity of antiretroviral therapy and the development of drug resistant HIV strains.
- Current recommendations suggest that *highly active antiretroviral therapy* (HAART) should be started when CD4 counts drop to 200 cells/uL or the HIV viral load is >55,000 copies/mL. Earlier treatment may improve immunologic/virologic outcomes, but it increases drug toxicity and the development of resistance. Patients must strive for perfect adherence to

antiretroviral regimens to try and prevent the development of resistance (Armstrong, Calabrese, and Taege, 2002).

- Drug toxicities include myopathy, neuropathy, pancreatitis, cardiomyopathy, bone marrow suppression, nephrotoxicity, lactic acidosis with hepatic steatosis (potentially fatal), osteonecrosis, osteoporosis, hyperglycemia, hyperlipidemia, and lipodystrophy. All these, even in their mildest forms, could have severe effects on an athlete's performance.

- A new class of medications—"fusion inhibitors" (enfuvirtide is the first one on the market)—may prove to be a tremendous advancement in HIV therapy. They prevent HIV from entering immune cells before it has a chance to replicate. They will be especially important for drug-resistant HIV. The current drawbacks to this treatment include subcutaneous administration and a very high cost, which may be prohibitive (Jellin, 2003).

- Immunonutrients and future therapy: Future therapy for HIV will include the development of an HIV vaccine and possibly immune therapy. Another exciting new area of HIV research is the role of immunonutrients, such as glutamine, argenine, and cysteine.

- Glutamine and argenine are amino acids that are required for proper functioning of the immune system. These amino acids are used during exercise and it has been hypothesized that a deficiency in these nutrients can have a detrimental effect on immune function. Therefore, supplementation may be beneficial for immune function.

- Glutamine and argenine supplementation may improve the cytokine profile and have an immunologic benefit in HIV+ patients. One study showed improved weight gain with argenine supplementation; however, if any clinical benefit does exist at all, it requires large doses (greater than 12 g/day). At this time there is insufficient evidence to support supplementation in healthy individuals, but supplementation in those suffering from chronic or acute infections may have some benefit (Field, Johnson, and Pratt, 2000).

- Cysteine supplementation in HIV+ individuals may slow disease progression or prevent muscle wasting. But while some preliminary studies have shown promise, further study is needed before recommendations can be made (Droge and Holm, 1997).

EFFECTS OF HIV ON SPORTS PARTICIPATION

RISK OF TRANSMISSION

- To caregivers: There are currently no reports of transmission of HIV from an athlete to a health care provider on the sidelines or in the training room.

- Determining theoretical risk to the athletic health care provider is based on data on health care professionals exposed to HIV by needlestick. The risk of seroconversion has been reported as ranging from 0.2 to 0.4% in various studies.

- Additionally, there are seven reports of health care workers who have contracted HIV from infected blood splashed onto their mucous membranes or skin. The risk from exposure to mucous membranes or damaged skin is estimated at approximately 0.1%. This is rare because it requires both a portal of entry and prolonged exposure to large amounts of blood (Gerberding, 1995).

- To other athletes: No transmission of HIV during sports has ever been documented; however, two reports of transmission of HIV during bloody fistfights have been verified by the CDC (Feller and Flanigan, 1997).

- In determining theoretical risk, the following should be taken into account: the risk of injury and death during sports is much higher than the risk of contracting HIV; the conditions for a blood-born pathogen to be transmitted during sports include (1) the presence of an infected athlete, (2) a bleeding wound or exudative skin lesion in the infected athlete, (3) a skin lesion or exposed mucous membrane on a susceptible athlete, and (4) sustained contact between the portal of entry on the susceptible athlete and the infective material (Dorman, 2000; Mast et al, 1995).

- The potential risk of HIV transmission during professional football has been estimated at less than 1 per 85 million game contacts (Brown et al, 1995).

- Off of the field situations: Athletes are more at risk of contracting HIV off of the field than on the field.

- Off of the field situations in which athletes may more commonly put themselves at risk for contracting HIV include—sexual contact, use of injectible steroids or other drugs with shared needles or paraphernalia, tattoos, and body piercings.

- One study showed there might be a higher proportion of risky lifestyle behaviors among intercollegiate athletes compared to nonathletes. This included number of sexual partners and episodes of sexually transmitted diseases (Nattiv and Puffer, 1991); however, this may not be the case when female athletes are studied separately from males. A study of the risk of HIV in female intercollegiate athletes (based on sexual activity and *intravenous* (IV) drug use) showed high levels of health risk behaviors; however, female athletes showed fewer risky behaviors than their nonathlete peers (controls were matched for age, education, and ethnic status) (Kokotailo et al, 1998).

- In the realm of the professional athlete, the rate of risky behavior is unknown, but anecdotal evidence suggests that their celebrity status may lead to higher risks (Johnston, 1994).

PREVENTION

- Education for all athletes: Physicians should educate athletes about risky behaviors and to consider HIV testing on a voluntary basis. Education should include discussions on abstinence, safe sex, and use of shared needles or personal items such as razors, clippers, and earrings that may be contaminated with blood.
- Universal precautions: Coaches and athletic trainers should receive training in universal precautions and prevention of HIV transmission. Additionally, Occupational Safety and Health Administration (OSHA) has standards concerning the reduction of occupational exposure to blood-born pathogens, which may be applicable to the athletic training room. To reduce transmission of HIV and other infectious agents, the following universal precautions should be taken:
    1. Athletes with skin wounds and potentially infectious skin lesions should be securely covered with bandages and wraps before competition.
    2. Athletes participating in sports with extensive skin-to-skin contact (i.e., wrestling) should be excluded from matches or practice when skin wounds or lesions are contagious or cannot be securely covered.
    3. Ambu bags and oral airways should be available for use for *cardiopulmonary resuscitation* (CPR).
    4. Athletic trainers and health care personnel should use disposable, preferably sterile, examination gloves when treating athletes who are bleeding. Hands should be washed after gloves removal.
    5. When a sports participant sustains a laceration or wound with substantial bleeding, the injury should be treated promptly. Blood should be washed off thoroughly with soap and water. Emergency care should not be delayed if gloves are not available. A bulky towel may be used to cover the wound until an off-the-field location is reached and gloves can be used for definitive treatment. The athlete should be allowed to return only after the wound has been securely covered or wrapped.
    6. Small amounts of dried blood on uniforms or equipment do not constitute a risk for transmission and do not warrant changing; however, if uniforms or equipment appear wet with blood or if blood has penetrated both sides of the uniform fabric it should be changed at the next stoppage of play.
    7. After each practice or game, any uniforms or equipment soiled with blood should be laundered using standard laundry cycles.
    8. Disposable toweling or absorbent cleaning material should be used to clean environmental surfaces if more than a few drops of blood are present. Clean with soap and water or a germicide registered with the Environmental Protection agency, or a 1/100 dilution of bleach in tap water (one cup bleach to 4 gallons water).
    9. Receptacles should be available for uniforms soiled with bodily fluids. Sharps containers should be used for needles or scalpel blades.
    10. Rules forbidding activities such as biting, scratching, fighting, or other unsportsmanlike behaviors that may lead to bloody contact should be strictly enforced (AAP, 1999; NCAA Guideline 2h, 2000; Dorman, 2000; Mast et al, 1995).
- Recommendations and restrictions for the HIV positive athlete: The most widely used recommendations regarding restriction of the HIV positive athlete from competition come from the American Academy of Pediatrics (AAP) and the NCAA.
- AAP recommendations: Athletes infected with HIV should be allowed to participate in all competitive sports. Physicians should respect the right to confidentiality including not disclosing infection status to participants or to staff of athletic programs. Physicians should counsel the known HIV-infected athlete of the theoretical risk of contaminating others during sports involving blood exposure especially wrestling and boxing. Physicians should strongly encourage the HIV-positive athlete to consider another sport (AAP, 1999).
- A 1993 survey of NCAA institutions concerning HIV/AIDS policies showed that 3% of respondents either restricted or intended to restrict participation of HIV-positive athletes; 15 institutions' policies restricted participation in some form: six barred the HIV-positive athlete from any sport, and nine barred the HIV positive athlete from selected sports including hockey and wrestling (McGrew et al, 1993).
- However, as of the year 2000, NCAA recommendations clearly state that HIV-positive student-athletes should be allowed to participate in intercollegiate athletics based on the individual's health status. The student-athlete should be allowed to play if asymptomatic and there is no evidence of immune function deficiency; however, the intensity of training and stress of competition should be taken into account to prevent the deterioration of the student-athlete's health status (NCAA Guideline 2h, 2000).
- Mandatory testing: The AAP, NCAA, American College of Sports Medicine, Canadian Academy of

Sports Medicine, CDC, International Federation of Sports Medicine, International Olympic Committee, and the World Health Organization all do not recommend mandatory screening of athletes for HIV. Any testing that is performed (mandatory or voluntary) should be accompanied by pre- and posttest counseling, should incorporate confidentiality measures, should address the question of frequency of the testing and should adhere to local and federal law.

- The 1993 survey of NCAA institutions concerning HIV/AIDS policies found that routine HIV testing for athletes occurred in 4% of institutions and only two were mandatory (McGrew et al, 1993).
- To date, none of the four major professional sports leagues in North America have adopted mandatory HIV testing. But, many professional athletes have publicly called for mandatory testing including Wayne Gretsky (NHL) and Kevin Johnson (NBA). In the NFL, the New York Giants and the Philadelphia Eagles tested players and personnel in 1991 and 1992 despite some of the players being unaware of the testing (Johnston, 1994).
- In 1988 the Nevada Boxing Commission mandated HIV testing for all boxers fighting in Nevada and a positive result would disqualify a boxer from fighting. In 1996, after Tommy Morrison tested positive, New York, New Jersey, Washington, Oregon, Arizona, and Puerto Rico joined Nevada in requiring HIV testing for all boxers (Feller and Flanigan, 1997).

LEGAL IMPLICATIONS

- Of testing: In considering whether mandatory HIV testing is ethical and/or legal, we must consider three questions: (1) Does the proposed testing policy serve an ethically acceptable purpose? (2) Is mandatory testing necessary and effective for achieving that purpose? (3) Does mandatory testing violate the individual rights of the athlete?
- Ethically acceptable purpose? The protection of the HIV-infected athlete and the protection of uninfected athletes from transmission are ethical purposes. Using test results for discrimination against HIV-infected athletes is unethical.
- Necessary and effective? Since HIV transmission on the playing field has never been documented and the risk is theoretically low, mandatory testing is not necessary.
- Violation of individual rights? Mandatory testing does violate the individual athlete's right to privacy, but the question for the professional athlete is if this intrusion may be permitted under the agreement to participate in that profession.
- Arguments in favor of permitting violations of the right to privacy cite existing exceptions to HIV testing

without consent including criminal justice settings, life insurance underwriting purposes, defense department and military recruits, immigrants to the United States, State Department foreign service personnel, and the Federal Bureau of Prisons for prison inmates.

- In terms of the professional athlete's right to privacy, a professional team's standard player contract (which is usually determined by the players' collective bargaining agreement) defines the consequences of failure to maintain physical fitness or failure to pass the preseason medical examination to include suspension or termination of a player's contract. Proponents of mandatory testing argue that an athlete's acceptance of a standard player contract negates any invasion of privacy. They argue that an athlete's privacy is no more violated by HIV testing than by other routine medical tests required by team and league policies.
- However, without clear affirmative answers to all three questions, most law theorists conclude that mandatory testing is both unethical and illegal (Johnston, 1994).
- In spite of this, professional boxers are subjected to mandatory testing without proof of the necessity of testing to protect the safety of the infected athlete or other competitors (Feller and Flanigan, 1997).
- The Nevada Boxing Commission's mandatory testing program has yet to be contested in court.
- Of restriction from competition: The Americans with Disabilities Act and the Rehabilitation Act of 1973 do not allow discrimination against people who have contagious diseases who are otherwise qualified to participate. Concern regarding the potentially harmful effects of competition on the immune system of the HIV-positive athlete has not been viewed as legally valid grounds for exclusion from sanctioned athletic events (Johnson, 1992).
- Some courts have ruled that without sufficient medical reason, an HIV-positive athlete cannot be excluded from a sport (School Board of Nassau County, Florida vs. Arline, 480. U.S. 273[1987]).
- However, other courts (Doe vs. Dolton elementary school district number 148, 694 F supp. 440 [1988]) have permitted schools to prohibit HIV-positive students from school-sponsored contact sports because of the perceived risk of transmission and another court upheld the decision to exclude an HIV positive athlete from contact Karate. (Montalov vs. Radcliffe, 167 F. 3d 873 [4th Cir. 1999], cert. Denied, 120 S Ct. 48 1999.)
- Unfortunately, these types of decisions may set precedents leading to personal tragedies such as that of professional boxer Ruben Palacio who in 1993 won the Featherweight World Championship Title after 12 long years in boxing. On the eve of his first title

defense he was subjected to mandatory HIV testing and tested positive. The World Boxing Organization stripped him of his title and refused to allow him to compete (Johnston, 1994).

REFERENCES

Armstrong W, Calabrese L, Taege A: HIV update 2002: Delaying treatment to curb rising resistance. *Clev Clin J Med* 69(12):995–999, Dec. 2002.

Brown LS, Jr, Drotman DP, Chu A et al: Bleeding injuries in professional football: Estimating the risk for HIV transmission. *Ann Intern Med* 122:271–274, 1995.

Dorman JM: Contagious diseases in competitive sport: what are the risks? *J Am Coll Health* 49(3):105–109, Nov. 2000.

Droge W, Holm E: Role of cysteine and glutathione in HIV infection and other diseases associated with muscle wasting and immunologic dysfunction. *FASEB J* 11(13):1077–1089, Nov. 1997.

Eichner ER, Calabrese LH: Immunology and exercise. Physiology, pathophysiology, and implications for HIV infection. *Med Clin North Am* 78(2):377–388, Mar. 1994.

Feller A, Flanigan TP: HIV-infected competitive athletes. What are the risks? What precautions should be taken? *J Gen Intern Med* 12(4):243–246, Apr. 1997.

Field CJ, Johnson I, Pratt VC: Glutamine and argenine: Immunonutrients for improved health. *Med Sci Sports Exerc* 32(7suppl):S377–S388, Jul. 2000.

Gerberding JL: Management of occupational exposures to bloodborne viruses. *NEJM* 332:444–451, 1995.

AAP: Human immunodeficiency virus and other blood-borne viral pathogens in the athletic setting. Committee on Sports Medicine and Fitness, American Academy of Pediatrics. *Pediatrics* 104(6):1400–1403, Dec. 1999.

Johnston JL: Is mandatory HIV testing of professional athletes really the solution? Case Western Reserve University School of Law. *Health Matrix Clevl* 4(1):159–203, Spring 1994.

Johnson RJ: HIV infection in athletes: What are the risks? Who can compete? *Postgrad Med* 92:73–75, 79–80, 1992.

Kokotailo PK, Koscik RE, Henry BC et al: Health risk taking and human immunodeficiency virus risk in collegiate female athletes. *J Am Coll Health* 46(6):263–268, May 1998.

LaPerriere A, Fletcher MA, Antoni MH et al: Aerobic exercise training in an AIDS risk group. *Int J Sports Med* 12(Suppl 1):S53–S57, 1991.

LeBlanc KE: The athlete and HIV. *J La State Med Soc* 145(11):493–495, Nov. 1993.

Mackinnon LT: Chronic exercise training effects on immune function. *Med Sci Sports Exerc* 32(7suppl):S369–S376, Jul. 2000.

Mast EE, Goodman RA, Bond WW et al: Transmission of bloodborne pathogens during sports: Risk and prevention. *Ann Intern Med* 122(4):283–285, Feb. 15, 1995.

McGrew CA, Dick RW, Schniedwind K et al: Survey of NCAA institutions concerning HIV/AIDS policies and universal precautions. *Med Sci Sports Exerc* 25(8):917–921, Aug. 1993.

Nattiv A, Puffer JC: Lifestyles and health risks of collegiate athletes. *J Fam Pract* 33:585–590, 1991.

NCAA Guideline 2h: Blood-borne pathogens and intercollegiate athletics. Overland Park, KS, National Collegiate Athletic Association, August 2000.

Jellin JM (ed.). *Presc Lett* 10(4):23, Apr. 2003.

Stringer WW: Mechanisms of exercise limitation in HIV+ individuals. *Med Sci Sports Exerc* suppl:S412–S421, Apr. 2000.

Ullum H, Palmo J, Halkjaer-Kristensen J et al: The effect of acute exercise on lymphocyte subsets, natural killer cells, proliferative responses, and cytokines in HIV-seropositive persons. *J AIDS* 7:1122–1132, 1994.

RADIOGRAPHIC LINES AND ANGLES IN SPORTS MEDICINE

Peter H Seidenberg, MD

CERVICAL SPINE—LATERAL

RETROPHARYNGEAL SPACE
- Distance from the posterior pharyngeal wall to the anteroinferior aspect of C-2.
- Normal is <7 mm.

RETROTRACHEAL SPACE
- Distance from the posterior wall of the trachea to the anteroinferior aspect of C-6.
- Normal in adults is <22 mm.
- Normal in children is <14 mm.

ANTERIOR VERTEBRAL LINE
- Drawn along the anterior margins of the vertebral bodies.
- Should run smoothly without angulation or disruption.

POSTERIOR VERTEBRAL LINE
- Drawn along the posterior margins of the vertebral bodies.
- Outlines anterior margin of spinal canal.
- Should run smoothly without angulation or disruption.

SPINOLAMINAR LINE
- Drawn along the anterior margins of the bases of the spinous processes at the junction with the lamina.
- Outlines posterior margin of the spinal canal.
- Should run smoothly without angulation or disruption.

POSTERIOR SPINOUS LINE
- Drawn along the tips of the spinous processes from C-2 to C-7.
- Should run smoothly without angulation or disruption.

CLIVUS–ODONTOID LINE
- Drawn from the dorsum sellae along the clivus to the anterior margin of the foramen magnum.
- Should point to the junction of the anterior and middle thirds of the tip of the odontoid process.

TORG RATIO
- Used to check for presence of developmental cervical stenosis.
- Spinal canal to vertebral body ratio.
- Distance spinolaminar line to posterior aspect of vertebral body/diameter of vertebral body
  - Normal >1.0
  - Abnormal <0.8

McRae's LINE
- Diameter of line drawn through foramen magnum opening.
- Normal: Tip of odontoid process of axis should be at or below McRae's line.

CHAMBERLAIN'S LINE
- Posterior edge of foramen magnum to the most posterior aspect of the hard palate.
- Normally odontoid tip 3 mm above Chamberlain's line.
- More than 6.6 mm above this line signifies cranial settling.

McGREGOR'S LINE
- Most posterior aspect of hard palate to the lowest border of the posterior skull.
- Normal: Tip of odontoid process <4.5 mm above line

SPACE AVAILABLE FOR CORD (SAC)
- Also known as spinal canal width.
- Posterior aspect of odontoid process or vertebral body to the nearest posterior structure.
- Normal @ craniocervical junction: 13–14 mm
- Normal below C2: 12 mm
- Significance: Cord compression

ATLANTAL DENS INTERVAL (ADI)
- Distance from anterior border of odontoid to posterior border of atlantal ring.
- Normal: <3 mm (adults); <4 mm (children)
- Significance: Atlantoaxial instability
- ADI 10–12 mm: All ligaments ruptured

THORACIC AND LUMBAR SPINE

COBB ANGLE
- Degree of scoliotic curvature on *anteroposteior* (AP) radiograph.
- Select vertebrae most tilted from horizontal above and below apex of curve.
- Line drawn along superior surface of upper vertebra and along lower surface of lower vertebra.
- Method 1
  - Perpendiculars are drawn to each line.
  - Where perpendiculars intersect: Cobb angle
- Method 2
  - Where lines drawn along superior surface of upper vertebra and along lower surface of lower vertebra intersect.
- Both methods produce equivalent angles.
- Normal = 0°
- Can use same method to measure *kyphosis* and *lordosis* on lateral films.

CENTRAL SACRAL LINE
- Drawn through center of sacrum and perpendicular to line connecting the tops of the iliac crests.
- Patient must be standing and pelvis level.
- Normal: Line passes through each vertebrae up the spine.
- Vertebrae bisected by this line in scoliosis patients are considered stable (surgery).

HARRINGTON STABLE-ZONE LINES
- Parallel lines through lumbrosacral facets
- Normal: All vertebrae fall between these lines.
- Vertebrae within this zone are stable (surgery for rod placement).

SCOTTY DOG
- Used for diagnosis of spondylolysis on oblique views of the lumbar spine.

- The neck of the "Scotty Dog" appears to have a collar on it.
- Signifies fracture of the pars interarticularis.

SACRAL INCLINATION
- Relationship of sacrum to the vertical plane.
- Method of measuring the lumbosacral kyphosis in patients with higher degrees of spondylolisthesis.

SLIP ANGLE
- Angle between intersection of lines drawn along posterior border of S1 and the inferior endplate of L5.
- Method of measuring the lumbosacral kyphosis in patients with higher degrees of spondylolisthesis.
- Used in evaluating and describing L5–S1 spondylolisthesis.
- Normal <0°.
- Greater than 45° has a higher risk of slip progression.

PERCENTAGE SLIP
- Percentage of anterior displacement of the superior vertebra on the lower body.
- Used in evaluating, describing, and grading spondylolisthesis.
- Grade I slip: 0–25% displaced
- Grade II slip: 25–50% displaced
- Grade III slip: 51–75% displaced
- Grade IV slip: 76–100% displaced
- Grade V slip: >100% displaced

SHOULDER, CLAVICLE, PROXIMAL HUMERUS

ACROMIAL TYPE
- Useful in the evaluation of rotator cuff impingement.
- Describes morphology of acromium as viewed on outlet view of plain radiographs or T1 coronal oblique view of *magnetic resonance imaging* (MRI) as depicted above.
- Type 1: Flat
- Type 2: Curved
- Type 3: Hooked

ACROMIOHUMERAL INTERVAL
- AP shoulder with humerus in neutral rotation.
- The minimum distance between inferior surface of the acromion and the articular cortex of the humerus.
- Normal: 7–11 mm
- Greater than 7 mm thought to be at risk for impingement of the rotator cuff tendons and an indicator of a possible rotator cuff tear.

WIDTH OF ACROMIOCLAVICULAR JOINT SPACE
- Normal: 0.3–0.8 mm
- If >0.8 mm, consider the following:

- Acromioclavicular separation
- Osteolysis of the distal clavicle

CORACOCLAVICULAR DISTANCE (CCD)
- Normal: 1.0–1.3 cm
- Greater than 1.3 cm considers Grade II or higher acromioclavicular separation.
  - Grade I: CCD = 1.0–1.3 cm
  - Grade II: CCD = 1.0–1.5 cm
  - Grade III: CCD ≥ 1.5 cm

ANGLE BETWEEN HUMERAL HEAD AND HUMERAL SHAFT
- The angle formed between a line bisecting the shaft of the humerus and a line bisecting the head of the humerus.
  - Normal = 135°
  - An angle ≤90° or >180° signifies a fracture that may require surgical reduction.

DISTAL HUMERUS, ELBOW, AND PROXIMAL FOREARM

BAUMANN'S ANGLE
- AP elbow
- Used to evaluate suspected elbow fractures in skeletally immature patients.
- The angle of the distal lateral humeral condylar physis relative to the metaphysis.
- Normal: 8–20°
- An absolute number degree is not as significant as difference from the contralateral side.

CARRYING ANGLE
- AP elbow
- Longitudinal axis of humerus to forearm.
- Normal: 15° children <4-year-old; 17.8° adults
- No significant difference between males and females.

HUMERAL-LATERAL CONDYLAR ANGLE
- Lateral view of elbow.
- Longitudinal axis of humerus relative to axis of lateral condyle.
- Normal: Symmetric, 40°
- If abnormal, consider supercondylar fracture.

ANTERIOR HUMERAL LINE
- Lateral view of elbow.
- Line down anterior humerus through lateral condyle.
- Normal: Line should pass through middle third of lateral condyle ossification nucleus.
- If abnormal, suspect supracondylar fracture.

ANTERIOR FAT PAD
- Lateral elbow radiograph.
- Normally a thin radiolucent line over the coronoid fossa.

- If displaced anteriorly from the fossa, suspect capsular distention secondary to a fracture causing a hemarthrosis.

POSTERIOR FAT PAD
- Lateral elbow radiograph.
- Over olecranon fossa.
- If seen, considered diagnostic of an intra-articular elbow fracture.
- Only seen with significant hemarthrosis of the joint.

RADIOCAPITELLAR LINE
- Lateral elbow radiograph.
- A line drawn bisecting the long axis of the radius and head of the radius should intersect the capitellum regardless of the degree of elbow flexion or extension.
- If it does not, suspect fracture of proximal radius or distal humerus.

HAND AND WRIST

LATERAL WRIST RADIOGRAPHS

RADIAL AXIS
- Longitudinal axis of radius.
- Runs through the center of the medullary canal at 2 and 5 cm proximal to the radiocarpal joint.

LUNATE AXIS
- Bisector of lunate.
- Runs perpendicular to the tangent of the two distal poles.

CAPITATE AXIS
- Longitudinal axis of capitate.
- Bisects the proximal and distal poles.

GENERAL RULES OF THE RADIAL, LUNATE, AND CAPITATE AXES
- All three should form one line on the lateral wrist view.
- If the lunate is subluxed:
  - Line of axes of radius and capitate will not bisect the lunate.
  - The radial and capitate axes will transect only a small portion or none of the lunate.
- With extension, capitate and lunate should both extend relative to radial axis.
- With flexion, capitate and lunate should both flex relative to radial axis.
- Asynchronous movement with flexion or extension suggests carpal instability.

SCAPHOID AXIS
- Bisector of the scaphoid.
- Bisects proximal and distal poles.

RADIOLUNATE ANGLE
- Long axis of radius to long axis of lunate.
- Normal 0°
- Above 15° flexion: VISI
  - Triquetrolunate dissociation
  - May also occur with scapholunate (less likely than DISI)
- Above 10° extension: DISI
  - Scapholunate dissociation

CAPITOLUNATE ANGLE
- Intersection of capitate and lunate axes
- Normal: 0–30°
- Above 30° Carpal instability

SCAPHOLUNATE ANGLE
- Scaphoid axis to lunate axis
- Normal: 30–60°
- If scaphoid fx and angle >60°: Internal fixation
- Above 80° with dorsiflexion: DISI

DISI
- Dorsal intercalated segment instability.
- Scapholunate angle >60°
- Capitolunate angle >30°
- Significant for ligamentous instability of the carpal bones of the wrist.

VISI
- Volar intercalated segment instability.
- Scapholunate angle <30°
- Capitolunate angle >30°
- Significant for ligamentous instability of the carpal bones of the wrist.

RADIOCARPAL JOINT ANGLE
- The volar tilt of the radiocarpal joint.
- Angle between a line drawn 90° to radial axis and line along distal volar and dorsal tips of radius.
- Normal 1–23°
- Important for reduction of distal radius fxs
- More than 5 mm shortening or >20° dorsal angle: Poor outcome if not surgically managed.

AP WRIST

ULNAR VARIANCE
- Measured in millimeter.
- Normal: 0 mm
- Positive ulnar variance: Articular surface of ulna more distal than articular surface of radius.
- Negative ulnar variance: Articular surface of radius more distal than articular surface of ulna.
- Positive ulnar variance is believed to be a risk factor for *triangular fibrocartilage complex* (TFCC) tear.

RADIAL INCLINATION
- Line from ulnar to lateral side of the distal radius and line perpendicular to axis of radius.
- Normal: 15–30°

SCAPHOLUNATE SPACE
- Normally <2 mm
- Above 2 mm suggests scapholunate dissociation.
- The clenched fist view may be necessary to bring out the widening of the space.
- Compare to the unaffected side.

FINGER

V SIGN OF JOINT INCONGRUITY
- Used when investigating for *proximal interphalangeal* (PIP) joint subluxation.
- Lateral view of the finger.
- Normal: Parallel congruity between the dorsal base of the middle phalanx and the head of the proximal phalanx.
- If the middle phalanx is dorsally subluxed onto the proximal phalanx, the incongruity will result in a "V" between the two articular surfaces.

HIP/PELVIS

ANGLE OF FEMORAL NECK
- Angle formed between a line bisecting the femoral diaphysis and a line bisecting the femoral head.
- Normal: 125–135°
- If <125 or >135°, suspect femoral neck fracture.

ILIOPECTINEAL LINE
- Also known as iliopubic or arcuate line
- Most medial border of pelvic ring.
- Normal: Cortical continuity
- Disruption of cortical continuity: Fracture of anterior column of acetabulum

ILIOISCHIAL LINE
- From most distal juncture of ischium and sacrum to border of ischium and ischial tuberosity to distal juncture of ischium with pubic ramus.
- Defines the medial border of the posterior column of the acetabulum.
- Formed by the posterior portion of the quadrilateral plate of the iliac bone.
- Normal cortical continuity.

- Disruption: Fracture of posterior column of acetabulum.

TEARDROP
- Vertical tear drop shaped line, medial to femoral head.
- Cortical border of quadrangular plate.
- Normal: Teardrop shape
- Disruption: Fracture or penetration through acetabulum into pelvis.
- Femoral head >5–8 mm lateral teardrop: Lateral displacement of femoral head from osteophyte or intra-articular loose body.

PERKIN'S VERTICAL LINE
- Vertical line drawn through upper outer rim of acetabulum.

HILGENREINER'S LINE
- Horizontal line drawn between inferior parts of the ilium.
- The femoral head ossification center should lie in the distal medial quadrant formed by the Hilgenreiner's and Perkin's lines.

SHENTON'S LINE
- Traces the arc of the obturator foramen and the medical femoral neck.
- Disrupted in dislocation of the hip.
- May not appear intact in normal children until age 1.

ACETABULAR INDEX (HILGENREINER'S ANGLE)
- Line drawn along roof of acetabulum; intersecting with Hilgenreiner's line.

AGE	GIRLS	BOYS
Birth	<36°	<30°
6 months	<28°	<25°
1 year	<25°	<24°
7 years	<19°	<18°

- Angles greater than above at risk for progressive dysplasia.

EPIPHYSEAL ANGLE
- Line along proximal femoral epiphysis intersecting with Hilgenreiner's line.
- Normal: <25°
- Developmental coxa vara 40–70°.

WIBERG'S CENTER EDGE ANGLE (CE ANGLE)
- Formed by two lines originating from center of femoral head:

- One perpendicular to a line connecting the centers of the two femoral heads, drawn superiorly into the baseline of the acetabulum.
- One connecting the center of the femoral head with the superior femoral lip.
- Decreased in dysplasia of the acetabulum

AGE (YEARS)	LOWEST NORMAL CE ANGLE VALUE
5–8	19°
9–12	12–25°
13–20	26–30°

KLINE'S LINE
- Line drawn along the superior femoral neck.
- Normal: Symmetrical R and L
- If the line transects less of the femoral physis on one side, suggests slipped capital femoral epiphysis.

KNEE

Q ANGLE
- *Anterior superior iliac spine* (ASIS) to center of patella and tibial spine to center of patella.
- Normal <10–15° male; <15–20° female

INSALL RATIO
- Lateral X-ray with knee flexed 30°.
- Ratio of length of patella to length of patellar tendon.
- Normal = 1:1
- 0.8 or less Patella alta
- 1.2 or more Patella baja

SULCUS ANGLE
- On merchant view.
- Line across lowest part of intracondylar sulcus to highest points on medial and lateral condyles.
- Normal: 126–150°
- Larger angles associated with patellar subluxation/dislocation.

CONGRUENCE ANGLE
- On merchant view.
- Line from apex of sulcus angle to lowest point of patellar articular ridge and a line that bisects the sulcus angle.
- Normal: −6° (male); −10° (female)
- Above 15° abnormal and associated with patellar subluxation/dislocation.

LATERAL PATELLOFEMORAL ANGLE
- On merchant view.
- Line drawn down the lateral surface of the patella and line drawn along the medial and lateral femoral condyles.

- Normal angle opens laterally.
- Parallel or medial opening associated with patellar subluxation/dislocation.

FOOT AND ANKLE

BOHLER'S ANGLE
- Lateral foot or ankle.
- Angle formed by the intersection of a line drawn from posterosuperior margin of the calcaneal tuberosity and a line drawn from the tip of the posterior facet through the superior margin of the anterior process of the calcaneus.
- Used in evaluation of possible calcaneal fractures.
- Normal: 20–40°

GISSANE'S ANGLE
- Lateral foot or ankle.
- Angle of the articulation of the talus and calcaneus.
- Used in evaluation of possible calcaneal fractures with subsequent subtalar instability.
- Normal: 120–145°.

INTERMETATARSAL ANGLE
- AP foot.
- Line drawn through axis of 1st and 2nd metatarsals.
- Normal: <9°
- If >15° and correcting hallux valgus, proximal metatarsal osteotomy may be required.

FIRST METATARSAL ANGLE
- AP foot.
- Line drawn through axis of 1st metatarsal and proximal phalanx.
- Normal: <20°
- Increased in hallux valgus.

AP TALOCALCANEAL ANGLE (KITE'S AP ANGLE)
- AP foot.
- Longitudinal axis of talus and longitudinal axis of calcaneus.
- Normal: 20–40°
- Decreased in clubfoot and hindfoot varus.

ANTERIOR DRAWER STRESS RADIOGRAPH
- Anterior ankle drawer is performed by the examiner.
- Radiograph is taken during *stress* of the anterior drawer.
- Comparison is made with unaffected ankle.

- Measure the shortest distance between the talar dome and the posterior margin of the tibial articular surface.
- Anterior translation >8 mm or 5 mm greater than the unaffected side.

TALAR TILT STRESS RADIOGRAPH
- Talar tilt is performed by the examiner.
- Radiograph is taken during stress of the talar tilt.
- Comparison is made with unaffected ankle.
- Angle is measured between two lines drawn along tibial plafond and talar dome.
- Normal is <15° or a difference of <10° when compared to the normal size.

BIBLIOGRAPHY

Casillas MM: Ligament injuries of the foot and ankle in adult athletes, in DeLee JC, Drez D, Miller MD (eds.): *DeLee and Drez's Orthopaedic Sports Medicine Principles and Practice*, 2nd ed. Philadelphia, PA, Saunders, 2003.

Coughlin MJ: Conditions of the forefoot, in DeLee JC, Drez D, Miller MD (eds.): *DeLee and Drez's Orthopaedic Sports Medicine Principles and Practice*, 2nd ed. Philadelphia, PA, Saunders, 2003.

Eiff MP, Hatch RL, Calmbach WL: *Fracture Management for Primary Care.* Philadelphia, PA, Saunders, 1998.

Greenspan, Adam: *Orthopedic Radiology: A Practical Approach*, 3rd ed. Philadelphia, PA, Lippincott Williams & Wilkens, 2000.

Hak DJ, Gautsch TL: A review of radiographic lines and angles in orthopedics. *Am J Orthop*, Aug 1999.

Herman MJ, Pizzutillo PD: Cervical spine disorders in children. *Orthop Clin North Am* - 30(3):457–466, Jul. 01, 1999.

Keats, TE, Sistrom, C: Atlas of Radiologic Measurement. St. Louis, MO, Mosby, 2001.

Larsen CF, Mathiesen FK, Lindequist S: Measurements of carpal bone angles on lateral wrist radiographs. *J Hand Surg* 16A:888–893, 1991.

Magee, David J: *Orthopedic Physical Assessment*, 3rd ed. Philadelphia, PA, Saunders, 1997.

McAlindon, Robert J: On field evaluation and management of head and neck injured athletes. *Clin Sports Med* 21(1):1–14, Jan 2002.

Simon RR, Koenigsknecht SJ: *Emergency Orthopedics*. East Norwalk, CT, Appleton & Lange, 1987.

Wimberly RL, Lauerman WC: Sponylolisthesis in the Athelte. *Clin Sports Med* 21(1):133–145, Jan. 2002.

INDEX